I T

PHYSICIAN ASSISTANT

A Guide to Clinical Practice

Fifth Edition

Ruth Ballweg, MPA, PA-C, DFAAPA
Associate Professor and Section Chief
MEDEX Northwest
Department of Family Medicine
School of Medicine
University of Washington
Seattle, Washington

Edward M. Sullivan, MS, PA-C
Physician Assistant
J. Kirkland Grant Obstetrics and Gynecology Practice
Sunnyvale, Texas

Darwin Brown, MPH, PA-C, DFAAPA
Assistant Professor
University of Nebraska Medical Center
Physician Assistant Program
Omaha, Nebraska

Daniel T. Vetrosky, PhD, PA-C, DFAAPA
Associate Professor
University of South Alabama
Department of Physician Assistant Studies
Pat Capps Covey College of Allied Health Professions
Mobile, Alabama

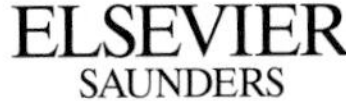

ELSEVIER
SAUNDERS

1600 John F. Kennedy Blvd.
Ste 1800
Philadelphia, PA 19103-2899

PHYSICIAN ASSISTANT: A GUIDE TO CLINCAL PRACTICE ISBN: 978-1-4557-0657-0

Notices

Knowledge and best practice in this field are constantly changing. As new research and experience broaden our understanding, changes in research methods, professional practices, or medical treatment may become necessary.

Practitioners and researchers must always rely on their own experience and knowledge in evaluating and using any information, methods, compounds, or experiments described herein. In using such information or methods they should be mindful of their own safety and the safety of others, including parties for whom they have a professional responsibility.

With respect to any drug or pharmaceutical products identified, readers are advised to check the most current information provided (i) on procedures featured or (ii) by the manufacturer of each product to be administered, to verify the recommended dose or formula, the method and duration of administration, and contraindications. It is the responsibility of practitioners, relying on their own experience and knowledge of their patients, to make diagnoses, to determine dosages and the best treatment for each individual patient, and to take all appropriate safety precautions.

To the fullest extent of the law, neither the Publisher nor the authors, contributors, or editors assume any liability for any injury and/or damage to persons or property as a matter of products liability, negligence or otherwise, or from any use or operation of any methods, products, instructions, or ideas contained in the material herein.

Library of Congress Cataloging-in-Publication Data
Physician assistant : a guide to clinical practice / [edited by] Ruth Ballweg ... [et al.]. —
5th ed.
p. ; cm.
Includes bibliographical references and index.
ISBN 978-1-4557-0657-0 (pbk. : alk. paper)
I. Ballweg, Ruth.
[DNLM: 1. Physician Assistants—United States. 2. Clinical Competence—United States. 3. Delivery of Health Care—methods—United States. 4. Professional Role—United States. W 21.5]
610.7372069—dc23 2012041600

Senior Content Strategist: Kate Dimock
Senior Content Development Strategist: Janice Gaillard
Publishing Services Manager: Patricia Tannian
Senior Project Manager: Claire Kramer
Designer: Steven Stave

Printed in China

Last digit is the print number: 9 8 7 6 5 4 3 2 1

CONTRIBUTORS

Diane D. Abercrombie, PhD, PA-C
Program Director and Chair
Associate Professor
University of South Alabama
Physician Assistant Studies
Mobile, Alabama

Linda G. Allison, MD, MPH
Associate Professor, Pharmacy Science
Belmont College of Pharmacy
Belmont University
Nashville, Tennessee

David P. Asprey, MA, PhD
Professor and Program Director
Physician Assistant Program
College of Medicine
University of Iowa
Iowa City, Iowa

Patrick C. Auth, MS, PhD, PA-C
Department Chair
Hahnemann Physician Assistant Department
Drexel University
Philadelphia, Pennsylvania

Ruth Ballweg, MPA, PA-C, DFAAPA
Associate Professor and Section Chief
MEDEX Northwest
Department of Family Medicine
School of Medicine
University of Washington
Seattle, Washington

J. Dennis Blessing, PhD, PA-C
Associate Dean for South Texas Programs
School of Allied Health Sciences
Professor and Chair
Department of Physician Assistant Studies
The University of Texas Health Sciences Center at San Antonio
San Antonio, Texas

Anthony Brenneman, MPAS, PA-C
Director and Associate Professor
Department of Physician Assistant Studies and Services
Carver College of Medicine
University of Iowa
Iowa City, Iowa

Darwin Brown, MPH, PA-C, DFAAPA
Assistant Professor
University of Nebraska Medical Center
Physician Assistant Program
Omaha, Nebraska

Lawrence Carey, PharmD
Clinical Associate Professor
Department of Pharmacy Practice
Temple University School of Pharmacy
Course Consultant and Lecturer in Phamacotherapy
Physician Assistant Studies Program
Philadelphia University
Philadelphia, Pennsylvania

James L. Cary, MHA, PA-C, DFAAPA
Senior Partner–Cary & Associates, LLC
Panama City, Florida

R. Monty Cary, MEd, PA-C, DFAAPA
Senior Partner–Cary & Associates, LLC
Las Vegas, Nevada

R. Scott Chavez, MPA, PhD, PA, CCHP-A
Vice President
National Commission on Correctional Health Care
Chicago, Illinois

John L. Chitwood, MS, MPAS, MA, PA-C
Colonel (Ret.) U.S. Air Force
San Antonio, Texas

Torry Grantham Cobb, MPH, MHS, DHSc, PA-C
Dartmouth Medical School
Hanover, New Hampshire
Dartmouth-Hitchcock Medical Center
Lebanon, New Hampshire

Roy H. Constantine, MPH, PhD, RPA-C
Assistant Director of Mid-Level Practitioners
St. Francis Hospital–The Heart Center
Roslyn, New York
Professor of Health Sciences
Trident University International
Cypress, California
Lecturer
Physician Assistant Program
Weill Cornell Medical College and Graduate School
New York, New York

Dan Crouse, MPAS, PA-C
Program Director
Division of Physician Assistant Studies
University of Utah
Salt Lake City, Utah

Linda M. Dale, DHEd, PA-C
Associate Professor, Program Director
Physician Assistant Program
Heritage University
Toppenish, Washington

Ann Davis, MS, PA-C
Senior Director of State Advocacy and Outreach
Advocacy and Government Relations
American Academy of Physician Assistants
Alexandria, Virginia

Walter A. Eisenhauer, MEd, MMS
Professor
Physician Assistant Studies
Lock Haven University
Lock Haven, Pennsylvania

Timothy C. Evans, MD, PhD, FACP
Associate Professor of Medicine
Department of Medicine
Senior Medical Director
MEDEX Northwest Physician Assistant Training Program
School of Medicine
University of Washington
Seattle, Washington

Shani D. Fleming, MPH, MS, PA-C
Clinical Coordinator
Physician Assistant Program
Anne Arundel Community College
Arnold, Maryland

F. J. (Gino) Gianola, PA
MEDEX Northwest Physician Assistant Section
Department of Family Medicine
School of Medicine
University of Washington
Seattle, Washington

Anita Duhl Glicken, MSW
President, NCCPA Foundation
Atlanta Georgia
Former Associate Dean of Physician Assistant Studies
School of Medicine
University of Colorado at Denver Anschutz Medical Campus
Aurora, Colorado

Constance Goldgar, MS, PA-C
Associate Program Director and Assistant Professor
Department of Family and Preventive Medicine
University of Utah Physician Assistant Program
Salt Lake City, Utah

J. Kirkland Grant, MD, FACOG
Chairman
Department of Obstetrics and Gynecology
Mesquite Community Hospital
Mesquite, Texas

Jim Hammond, MA, PA-C
Professor and Director
Physician Assistant Program
James Madison University
Harrisonburg, Virginia

Virginia Hass, RN, DNP, PA-C, FNP-C
Associate Program Director
Family Nurse Practitioner/Physician Assistant Program
Department of Family and Community Medicine
University of California, Davis
Sacramento, California

Ky Haverkamp, PA-C
Lecturer
MEDEX Northwest Division of Physician Assistant Studies
School of Medicine
University of Washington
Physician Assistant
Family Practice
Group Health
Seattle, Washington

Lawrence Herman, MPA
Director of Primary Care
Physician Assistant Studies
New York Institute of Technology
Old Westbury, New York

Theresa V. Horvath, MPH, PA-C
Associate Professor and Program Director
Hofstra University Department in Physician Assistant Studies
Hempstead, New York

L. Jill Jones-Hester, PA-C
Physician Assistant
North Texas Infectious Disease Consultants
Dallas, Texas

Kathy A. Kemle, MS, PA-C
Assistant Professor
Family Medicine
School of Medicine
Mercer University
Macon, Georgia

Vasco Deon Kidd, MPH, MS, DHSc, PA-C
University of Texas Health Science Center at San Antonio
San Antonio, Texas

William C. Kohlhepp, DHSc, PA-C
Professor of Physician Assistant Studies and Associate Dean, School of Health Sciences
Quinnipiac University
Hamden, Connecticut

Kristine J. Kucera, MPAS, DHS, PA-C
Adjunct Clinical Professor
Physician Assistant Studies
The University of Texas Southwestern Medical Center
Physician Assistant
Texas Dermatology Associates
Dallas, Texas

David H. Kuhns, MPH, PA-C, CCPA, DFAAPA
Consultant on International Physician Assistant Education
Advisor to the University of Aberdeen (Scotland) Physician Assistant Programme
Advisor to the Royal College of Surgeons in Ireland
Advisor to the European Physician Assistant Cooperative (EuroPAC)
Adjunct Faculty, Arcadia University Assistant Program
Glenside, Pennsylvania

Barbara Coombs Lee, JD, FNP
President
Compassion and Choices
Denver, Colorado

H. James Lurie, MD
Associate Professor Emeritus
MEDEX Northwest Division of Physician Assistant Studies
School of Medicine
University of Washington
Seattle, Washington

H. William Mahaffy, PA-C
Senior Physician Assistant
Hospital Medicine
Evangelical Community Hospital
Lewisburg, Pennsylvania

Steven Meltzer, BA, BHSc, PA-C
Director, Outreach and Eastern Washington Education Programs
MEDEX Northwest Physician Assistant Program
University of Washington
Spokane, Washington

Mindy G. Milton, MPA, PA-C
Faculty Family Nurse Practitioner/Physician Assistant Program
Department of Family and Community Medicine
University of California, Davis
Sacramento, California

Dawn Morton-Rias, EdD, PA-C
Dean and Assistant Professor
College of Health Related Professions
State University of New York Downstate Medical Center
New York, New York

Debra S. Munsell, DHSc, PA-C
Program Director, Physician Assistant Studies
Associate Professor
Interdisciplinary Human Studies
Louisiana State University Health Science Center
New Orleans, Louisiana

Martha Petersen, MPH, PA-C
Associate and Academic Director, Assistant Professor
Physician Assistant Institute
University of Bridgeport
Bridgeport, Connecticut

Maura Polansky, MS, MHPE, PA-C
Program Director, Physician Assistant Education
Physician Assistant
Department of Gastrointestinal Medical Oncology
University of Texas MD Anderson Cancer Center
Houston, Texas

Harry Pomeranz, MS, PA-C
Academic Coordinator
Graduate School of Medical Sciences
Physician Assistant Program
Weill Cornell Medical College
New York, New York

Michael L. Powe, BS
Vice President, Reimbursement and Professional Advocacy
American Academy of Physician Assistants
Alexandria, Virginia

Timothy Quigley, MPH, PA-C, DFAAPA
Director of Student Affairs
MEDEX Northwest Division of Physician Assistant Studies
School of Medicine
University of Washington
Seattle, Washington

Michael Rackover, MS, PA-C
Program Director and Associate Professor
Physician Assistant Program
Philadelphia University
Philadelphia, Pennsylvania

Maryann Ramos, MPH, PA-C
Adjunct Assistant Professor of Health Care Sciences
Physician Assistant Program
School of Medicine and Health Sciences
The George Washington University
Physician Assistant
DiLorenzo Tricare Health Clinic at the Pentagon
Walter Reed Army Medical Center
Washington, District of Columbia

Terry Scott, MPA, PA-C
Program Director
MEDEX Northwest
Department of Family Medicine
Physician Assistant Program
University of Washington
Seattle, Washington

Freddi Segal-Gidan, PhD, PA-C
Assistant Clinical Professor
Neurology and Gerontology
University of Southern California
Keck School of Medicine
Los Angeles, California
Director
Rancho/USC California Alzheimer's Disease Center (CADC)
Rancho Los Amigos National Rehabilitation Center
Downey, California

Albert Simon, DHSc, MEd, PA
Vice Dean
School of Osteopathic Medicine in Arizona
A.T. Still University
Mesa, Arizona

Anna Mae Smith, MPAS, PA-C
Program Director/Associate Professor
Physician Assistant Program
Lock Haven University
Lock Haven, Pennsylvania

Howard Straker, MPH, PA-C
Director of Community Medicine
The George Washington University Physician Assistant Program
School of Medicine and Health Sciences
The George Washington University
Washington, District of Columbia

Ernest L. Stump, MSW, ACSW
Assistant Director/Behavioral Scientist
Altoona Family Physicians Family Medicine
Altoona Regional Health System
Altoona, Pennsylvania

Edward M. Sullivan, MS, PA-C
Physician Assistant
J. Kirkland Grant Obstetrics and Gynecology Practice
Sunnyvale, Texas

Lois C. Thetford, PA-C
Seattle Didactic Faculty
MEDEX Northwest
Department of Family Medicine
School of Medicine
University of Washington
Seattle, Washington

Mary Vacala, ATC, MS, MSPAS, PAC, DFAAPA
Physician Assistant
Orthopedic Sports Medicine
Chatham Orthopaedic Associates
Savannah, Georgia

Stephane VanderMeulen, MPAS, PA-C
Assistant Professor
Physician Assistant Program
University of Nebraska Medical Center
Omaha, Nebraska

Daniel T. Vetrosky, PhD, PA-C, DFAAPA
Associate Professor
University of South Alabama
Department of Physician Assistant Studies
Pat Capps Covey College of Allied Health Professions
Mobile, Alabama

Linda J. Vorvick, MD
Medical Director
MEDEX Northwest Division of Physician Assistant Studies
School of Medicine
University of Washington
Seattle, Washington

Lisa K. Walker, MPAS, PA-C
Master of Physician Assistant Studies
Franklin Pierce University
West Lebanon, New Hampshire

Durward A. Watson, BS
Associate Professor
Interdisciplinary Human Studies
Louisiana State University Health Science Center
New Orleans, Louisiana

Emily WhiteHorse, MA, PA-C
Educational Consultant
West Sacramento, California

Keren H. Wick, PhD
Assistant Professor
Director of Research and Graduate Programs
MEDEX Northwest Physician Assistant Program
School of Medicine
University of Washington
Seattle, Washington

Gwen Yeo, PhD
Director Emerita, Senior Ethnogeriatric Specialist
Stanford Geriatric Education Center
School of Medicine
Stanford University
Stanford, California

FOREWORD

Thirty-one years ago, doctors were in short supply. Nurses were even scarcer. The old model of the doctor, a receptionist, and a laboratory technician was inadequate to meet the needs of our increasingly complex society. Learning time had disappeared from the schedule of the busy doctor. The only solution that the overworked doctor could envisage was more doctors. Only a doctor could do doctors' work. The lengthy educational pathway (college, medical school, internship, residency, and fellowship) must mean that only persons with a doctor's education could carry out a doctor's functions.

I examined in some detail the actual practice of medicine. After sampling the rich diet of medicine, most doctors settled for a small area. If the office was set up to see patients every 10 to 15 minutes and to charge a certain fee, the practice conformed. If the outcome was poor, or if the doctors recognized that the problem was too complex for this pattern of practice, the patient was referred.

Doctors seeing patients at half-hour or 1-hour intervals also developed practice patterns and set fee schedules to conform. The specialists tended to treat diseases and leave the care of patients to others. Again, they cycled in a narrow path.

The average doctors developed efficient patterns of practice. They operated 95% of the time in a habit mode and rarely applied a thinking cap. Because they did everything that involved contact with the patients, time for family, recreation, reading, and furthering their own education disappeared.

Why this intense personalization of medical practice? All doctors starting practices ran scared. They wanted to make their services essential to the well-being of their patients. They wanted the patient to depend on them alone. After a few years in this mode, they brainwashed themselves and actually believed that only they could obtain information from the patient and perform services that involved physical contact with the patient.

During this time I was building a house with my own hands. I could use a wide variety of materials and techniques in my building. I reflected on how inadequate my house would be if I were restricted to only four materials. The doctor restricted to a slim support system could never build a practice adequate to meet the needs of modern medicine. He or she needed more components in the system. The physician assistant (PA) was born!

Nurses, laboratory technicians, and other health professionals were educated in their own schools, which were mostly hospital related. The new practitioner (the PA) was to be selected, educated, and employed by the doctor. The PA—not being geographically bound to the management system of the hospital, the clinic, or the doctor's office—could oscillate between the office, the hospital, the operating room, and the home.

A 2-year curriculum was organized at Duke Medical School with the able assistance of Dr. Harvey Estes, who eventually took the program under the wing of his department of Family and Community Medicine. The object of the 2-year course was to expose the student to the biology of human beings and to learn how doctors rendered services. On graduation, PAs had learned to perform many tasks previously done by licensed doctors only and could serve a useful role in many types of practices. They performed those tasks that they could do as well as their doctor mentors. If the mentor was wise, the PA mastered new areas each year and increased his or her usefulness to the practice.

Setting no ceilings and allowing the PA to grow have made this profession useful and satisfying. Restricting PAs to medical supervision has given them great freedom. Ideally, they do any part of their mentors' practice that they can do as well as their mentors.

The PA profession has certainly established itself and is recognized as a part of the medical system. PAs will be assuming a larger role in the care of hospital patients as physician residency programs decrease in size. As hospital house staff, PAs can improve the quality of care for patients by providing continuity of care.

Because of the close association with the doctor and patient and the PAs' varied duties, PAs have an intimate knowledge of the way of the medical world. They know patients, they are aware of the triumphs and failures of medicine, and they know how doctors think and what they do with information collected about patients. For these reasons, they are in demand by all businesses that touch the medical profession. One of the first five Duke students recently earned a doctoral degree in medical ethics and is working in education. The world is open, and PAs are grasping their share.

We all owe a debt of gratitude to the first five students who were willing to risk 2 years of their lives to enter a new profession when there was little support from doctors, nurses, or government. From the beginning, patients responded favorably, and each PA gained confidence and satisfaction from these interactions. Patients made and saved the profession. We hope that every new PA will acknowledge this debt and continue the excellent work of the original five.

†Eugene A. Stead Jr, MD
Florence McAlister Professor Emeritus of Medicine, Duke University Medical Center, Durham, North Carolina

---

†Deceased.

PREFACE

Welcome to the fifth edition of *Physician Assistant: A Guide to Clinical Practice!* The history and utilization of this publication mirror the expansion of the physician assistant (PA) profession. The first edition, published in 1994, was the first PA textbook to be developed by a major publisher and was at first considered to be a potential risk for the company. Ultimately, it came to seen as a major milestone for our profession. Our first editor, Lisa Biello, attended the national PA conference in New Orleans and immediately saw the potential! She made a strong case to the W.B. Saunders Co. for the development of the book. Quickly, other publishers followed her lead. Now there are multiple PA-specific textbooks and other published resources for use in PA programs by practicing physician assistants.

The first edition was written at a time of rapid growth in the number of PA programs and in the number of enrolled PA students. Intended primarily for PA students, the textbook was also used by administrators, public policy leaders, and employers to better understand the PA role and to create new roles and job opportunities for PAs.

The second edition was expanded and updated to reflect the growth of the PA profession.

The third edition included eight new chapters and a new format. This format included Case Studies, which illustrated the narrative in "real-life" terms; Clinical Applications, which provided questions to stimulate thought, discussion, and further investigation; and a Resources section, which provided an annotated list of books, articles, organizations, and websites for follow-up research. With the third edition, the book became an Elsevier publication with a W.B. Saunders imprint.

The fourth edition had a totally new look and was also the first edition with an electronic platform. Most important, the textbook's content was reorganized to make it more responsive to the new *Physician Assistant Competencies*, which were approved by all four major PA organizations in 2006. (See "Appendix: Competencies for the Physician Assistant Profession.") New sections on professionalism, practice-based learning and improvement, and systems-based practice address specific topics delineated in the competencies. Sections covering materials that had become available in other books (e.g., physical examination and detailed history-taking skills) were omitted. Significant new material was added on the international PA movement, professionalism, patient safety, health disparities, PA roles in internal medicine and hospitalist settings, and issues in caring for patients with disabilities.

The fifth edition again has new content on the electronic health record, population-based practice, the new National Commission on Certification of Physician Assistants specialty recognition process, health care delivery systems, and mass casualty/disaster management.

Many PA programs find the textbook useful for their professional roles course and as a supplement to other core courses. PA students have found the chapters on specific specialties helpful in preparing for clinical rotations. PA graduates thinking about changing jobs and encountering new challenges in credentialing will find a number of relevant examples. All practicing PAs will find the new material useful as they continue their lifelong learning in a rapidly changing health care system. Health care administrators and employers can benefit from an overview of the profession, as well as information specific to PA roles and job descriptions. Policy analysts and health care researchers will find a wealth of information at the micro and macro levels. Developers of the PA concept internationally will find what they need to adapt the PA profession in new settings. Finally, potential PAs can be informed and inspired by the accomplishments of the profession.

Although Dr. Eugene Stead died in 2005, we have decided to continue to use the foreword that he wrote for this book. Encouraged by Dr. Stead and by countless colleagues, students, and patients, we hope that this textbook will continue to serve as a significant resource and inspiration for the PA profession.

Ruth Ballweg, MPA, PA-C, DFAAPA
Edward M. Sullivan, MS, PA-C
Darwin Brown, MPH, PA-C, DFAAPA
Daniel Vetrosky, PhD, PA-C, DFAAPA

ACKNOWLEDGMENTS

As we reach the fifth edition, we want to thank the many individuals—across time—who have made this textbook possible. Much of the success of this textbook has had its roots in physician assistant (PA) educational networks. Not only did we want to create a book that would be a critical resource for PA students and educators, but also we wanted to create new publishing opportunities for many of our colleagues to become contributors. A major strength of the textbook has always been the inclusion of a wide range of faculty members from PA programs from all regions in the United States. We especially want to acknowledge the contribution and leadership of Sherry Stolberg, who served as our coeditor for the first, second, and third editions. When Sherry decided not to continue as an ongoing editor beyond the third edition, we were able to recruit Darwin Brown and Dan Vetrosky as new coeditors. They have brought new energy, new ideas, and new contacts to the fourth and fifth editions, for which we are grateful.

This textbook would not be possible without the support of our colleagues, students, friends, and loved ones who have helped us to continue to move this project ahead. The patience and good humor of our spouses, Cindy Sullivan, Jeanne Brown, Penny Vetrosky, and the late Arnold Rosner, have been critical to this project. Our children, Pirkko Terao, Dayan Ballweg, Chris Sullivan, and Alex, Tim, and Jackson Brown, provided us with their valuable opinions and perspectives.

We gratefully acknowledge our editors over time, including Lisa Biello, Peg Waltner, Shirley Kuhn, Rolla Couchman, John Ingram, Kate Dimock, and our content development specialist, Janice Gaillard. The input from these individuals has resulted in the substantial improvements in this publication over time. Although new authors have joined us for each edition, contributors to prior editions of this book deserve our appreciation for their participation as well: Beth Anderson, Phyllis Barks, Stephen Bartholomew, Susan Blackwell, Dennis Bruneau, Pat Connor, Steven Curley, Lee Daly, Bill Duryea, Bill Finerfrock, Diana Garcia, Ron Garcia, David Gwinn, Nelson Herlihy, Jeff Hummel, Paul Jacques, Debbie Jalbert, Robert W. Jarski, David Jones, Jimmy Keller, Martha Kelly, Timothy King, Gerald Marciano, Ann M. Meehan, Anthony Miller, Venetia Orcutt, Paula Phelps, David Pillow Jr, Nanci Cortright Rice, Karen Sadler-Sparks, John M. Schroeder, Jay Slotkin, Martin L. Smith, Walter Stein, Kimberly Suggs, Peggy Valentine, Mary Em Wallace, John White, Lynda White, John Yerxa, and Sarah Zarbock.

Thanks to the faculty and staff of the MEDEX Northwest PA Program at the University of Washington. Sally Mantz was critical to this publication. She has worked closely with Elsevier content development specialists to edit and reformat incoming chapters and to meet project deadlines. Keren Wick's meticulous technical writing skills—and experience with the content of prior editions—allowed us to provide additional support to some authors. We all feel privileged to have had the opportunity to serve as editors for this important book.

Physician Assistant: A Guide to Clinical Practice has benefited from the feedback of PA educators and students. We hope you will continue to provide us with your opinions and suggestions.

CONTENTS

SECTION I

OVERVIEW

CHAPTER 1

HISTORY OF THE PROFESSION AND CURRENT TRENDS

Ruth Ballweg

CHAPTER CONTENTS

What was to become the physician assistant (PA) profession has many origins. Although it is often thought of as an "American" concept—using former military corpsmen to respond to the access needs in our health care system—the PA has historical antecedents in other countries. Feldshers in Russia and barefoot doctors in China served as models for the creation of the PA profession.

FELDSHERS IN RUSSIA

The *feldsher* concept originated in the European military in the 17th and 18th centuries and was introduced into the Russian military system by Peter the Great. Armies of other countries were ultimately able to secure adequate physician personnel; however, because of a physician shortage, the large numbers of Russian troops relied on feldshers for major portions of their medical care. Feldshers retiring from the military settled in small rural communities, where they continued their contribution to health care access. Feldshers assigned to Russian communities provided much of the health care in remote areas of Alaska during the 1800s.[1] In the late 19th century, formal schools were created for feldsher training, and, by 1913, approximately 30,000 feldshers had been trained to provide medical care.[2]

As the major U.S. researchers reviewing the feldsher concept, Victor Sidel[2] and P. B. Storey[3] described a system in the Soviet Union in which the annual number of new feldshers equaled the annual number of physician graduates. Of those included in the feldsher category, 90% were women, including feldsher midwives.[3] Feldsher training programs, which were located in the same institutions as nursing schools, required 2 years to complete. Outstanding feldsher students were encouraged to take medical school entrance examinations. Roemer[4] found in 1976 that 25% of Soviet physicians were former feldshers.

The use of Soviet feldshers varied from rural to urban settings. Often used as physician substitutes in rural settings, experienced feldshers had full authority to diagnose, prescribe, and institute emergency treatment. A concern that "independent" feldshers might provide "second-class" health care appears to have led to greater supervision of feldshers in rural settings. Storey[3] describes the function of urban feldshers, whose roles were "complementary" rather than "substitutional," as limited to primary care in ambulances and triage settings and not involving polyclinic or hospital tasks. Perry and Breitner[5] compare the urban feldsher role with that of U.S. PAs:

> Working alongside the physician in his daily activities to improve the physician's efficiency and effectiveness (and to relieve him of routine, time-consuming tasks) is not the Russian feldsher's role.

CHINA'S BAREFOOT DOCTORS

In China, the *barefoot doctor* originated in the 1965 Cultural Revolution as a physician substitute. In what became known as the "June 26th Directive," Chairman Mao called for a reorganization of the health care system. In response to Mao's directive, China trained 1.3 million barefoot doctors over the subsequent 10 years.[6]

The barefoot doctors were chosen from rural production brigades and received their initial 2- to 3-month training course in regional hospitals and health centers. Sidel[2] comments that the barefoot doctor is considered by his community, and apparently thinks of himself, as a peasant who performs some medical duties rather than as a health care worker who performs some agricultural duties.

Although they were designed to function independently, barefoot doctors were closely linked to local hospitals for training and medical supervision. Upward mobility was encouraged, in that barefoot doctors were given priority for admission to medical school. In 1978, Dimond[7] found that one third of Chinese medical students were former barefoot doctors.

The use of feldshers and barefoot doctors was significantly greater than that of PAs in the United States. Writing in 1982, Perry and Breitner[5] noted:

> Although physician assistants have received a great deal of publicity and attention in the United States, they currently perform a very minor role in the provision of health services. In contrast, the Russian feldsher and the Chinese barefoot doctor perform a major role in the provision of basic medical services, particularly in rural areas. The "discovery" in the United States that appropriately trained nonphysicians are perfectly capable of diagnosing and treating common medical problems had been previously recognized in both Russia and China.

By 2007, we can no longer say that PAs "perform a very minor role in the provision of health services." In contrast, the numbers of both feldshers and barefoot doctors have declined in their respective countries owing to a lack of governmental support and an increase in the numbers of physicians.

DEVELOPMENTS IN THE UNITED STATES

Beginning in the 1930s, former military corpsmen received on-the-job training from the Federal Prison System to extend the services of prison physicians. In a 4-month program during World War II, the U.S. Coast Guard trained 800 purser mates to provide health care on merchant ships. The program was later discontinued, and, by 1965, fewer than 100 purser mates continued to provide medical services. Both of these programs served as predecessors to those in the federal PA training programs at the Medical Center for Federal Prisoners, Springfield, Missouri, and Staten Island University Hospital, New York.

In 1961, Charles Hudson, MD, proposed the concept at a medical education conference of the American Medical Association (AMA). He recommended that "assistants to doctors" should work as dependent practitioners and should perform such technical tasks as lumbar puncture, suturing, and intubation.

At the same time, a number of physicians in private practice had begun to use informally trained individuals to extend their services. A well-known family physician, Dr. Amos Johnson, publicized the role that he had created for his assistant, Mr. Buddy Treadwell. The website for the Society for the Preservation of Physician Assistant History provides detailed information on Dr. Johnson and tells more about how Mr. Treadwell served as a role model for the design of the PA career.

By 1965, Henry Silver, MD, and Loretta Ford, RN, had created a practitioner-training program for baccalaureate nurses working with impoverished pediatric populations. Although the Colorado program became the foundation for both the nurse practitioner movement and the Child Health Associate PA Program, it was not transferable to other institutions. According to Gifford, this program depended ". . . on a pattern of close cooperation between doctors and nurses not then often found at other schools."[8] In 1965, therefore, practical definition of the PA concept awaited establishment of a training program in local circumstances that could be applied to other institutions.

DEVELOPMENTS AT DUKE UNIVERSITY

In the late 1950s and early 1960s, Eugene Stead, MD, developed a program to extend the capabilities of nurses at Duke University Hospital.[9] This program, which *could* have initiated the nurse practitioner movement, was opposed by the National League of Nursing. The League expressed the concern that such a program would move these new providers from the ranks of nursing and into the "medical model." Simultaneously, Duke University had experience with training several firemen, ex-corpsmen, and other non–college graduates to solve personnel shortages in the clinical services at Duke University Hospital.[9]

The Duke program and other new PA programs arose at a time of national awareness of a health care crisis. Carter and Gifford[10] described the conditions that fostered the PA concept as follows:

1. An increased social consciousness among many Americans that called for the elimination of all types of deprivation in society, especially among the poor, members of minority groups, and women.
2. An increasingly positive value attached to health and health care, which produced greater demand for health services, criticism of the health care delivery system, and constant complaints about rising health care costs.
3. Heightened concern about the supply of physicians, their geographic and specialty maldistribution, and the workloads they carried.
4. Awareness of a variety of physician extender models, including the community nurse midwife in America, the "assistant medical officer" in Africa, and the feldsher in the Soviet Union.
5. The availability of nurses and ex-corpsmen as potential sources of manpower.
6. Local circumstances in numerous hospitals and office-based practice settings that required additional clinical-support professionals.

The first four students—all ex-Navy corpsmen—entered the fledgling Duke program in October 1965. The 2-year training program's philosophy was to provide students with an education and orientation similar to those given the physicians with whom they would work. Although original plans called for the training of two categories of PAs—one for general practice and one for specialized inpatient care—the ultimate decision was made to focus on skills required in assisting family practitioners or internists. The program also emphasized the development of lifelong learning skills to facilitate the ongoing professional growth of these new providers.

CONCEPTS OF EDUCATION AND PRACTICE

The introduction of the PA presented philosophical challenges to established concepts of medical education. E. Harvey Estes, MD,[11] of Duke, described the hierarchical approach of medical education as being "based on the assumption that it was necessary to first learn 'basic sciences,' then normal structure and function, and finally pathophysiology . . . ." The PA clearly defied these previous conventions. Some of the early PAs had no formal collegiate education. They had worked as corpsmen and had learned skills, often under battlefield conditions. Clearly, their skills had been developed, often to a remarkable degree, before the acquisition of any basic science knowledge, or any knowledge of pathologic physiology.

The developing PA profession was also the first to officially share the knowledge base that was formerly the "exclusive property" of physicians:

> Prior to the PA profession, the physician was the sole possessor of information, and neither patient nor other groups could penetrate this wall. The patient generally trusted the medical profession to use the knowledge to his benefit, and other groups were forced to employ another physician to interpret medical data or medical reasoning.
>
> The PA profession was the first to share this knowledge base, but others were to follow—such as the nurse practitioner.[11]

Thirty years later, it is common to see medical textbooks written for PAs, nurse practitioners, and other nonphysician providers. Such publications were relatively new approaches for gaining access to medical knowledge at a time when access to medical textbooks and reference materials was restricted to physicians only. The legal relationship of the PA to the physician was also unique in the health care system. Tied to the license of a specific precepting physician, the PA concept received the strong support of establishment medicine and ultimately achieved significant "independence" through that "dependence." In contrast, nurse practitioners (NPs), who emphasized their capability for "independent practice," incurred the wrath of many physician groups, who believed that NPs needed supervisory relationships with physicians to validate their role.

Finally, the "primary care" or "generalist" nature of PA training, which stressed the acquisition of strong skills in data collection and problem solving, as well as lifelong learning, made the PA extraordinarily adaptable to almost any patient care setting. The dependent status of PA practice provided PAs with ongoing supervision and almost unlimited opportunities to expand skills as needed in specific practice settings. In fact, the adaptability of PAs has had both positive and negative impacts on the PA profession. Although PAs were initially trained to provide health care to the medically underserved, the potential for the use of PAs in specialty medicine became "the good news and the bad news." Sadler and colleagues[12] recognized this concern early on, when they wrote (in 1972):

> The physician's assistant is in considerable danger of being swallowed whole by the whale that is our present entrepreneurial, subspecialty medical practice system. The likely co-option of the newly minted physician's assistant by subspecialty medicine is one of the most serious issues confronting the PA.

A shortage of PAs in the early 1990s appeared to aggravate this situation and confirmed predictions by Sadler and colleagues[12]:

> Until great numbers of physician's assistants are produced, the first to emerge will be in such demand that relatively few are likely to end up in primary care or rural settings where the need is the greatest. The same is true for inner city or poverty areas.

Although most PAs initially chose primary care, increases in specialty positions raised concern about the future direction of the PA profession. The Federal Bureau of Health Professions was so concerned about this trend that at one point, federal training grants for PA programs required that all students complete clinical training assignments in federally designated medically underserved areas.

MILITARY CORPSMEN

The choice to train experienced military corpsmen as the first PAs was a key factor in the success of the concept. As Sadler and colleagues[12] pointed out, "The political appeal of providing a useful civilian health occupation for the returning Vietnam medical corpsman is enormous."

The press and the American public were attracted to the PA concept because it seemed to be one of the few positive "products" of the Vietnam War. Highly skilled, independent duty corpsmen from all branches of the uniformed services were disenfranchised as they attempted to find their place in the U.S. health care system. These corpsmen, whose competence had truly been tested "under fire," provided a willing, motivated, and proven applicant pool of pioneers for the PA profession. Robert Howard, MD,[13] of Duke University, in an AMA publication describing issues of training PAs, noted that not only were there large numbers of corpsmen available but also using former military personnel prevented transfer of workers from other health care careers that were experiencing shortages:

> . . . the existing nursing and allied health professions have manpower shortages parallel to physician shortages and are not the ideal sources from which to select individuals to augment the physician manpower supply. In the face of obvious need, there does exist a relatively large untapped manpower pool, the military corpsmen. Some 32,000 corpsmen are discharged annually who have received valuable training and experience while in the service. If an economically sound, stable, rewarding career were available in the health industry, many of these people would continue to pursue such a course. From this manpower source, it is possible to select mature, career-oriented, experienced people for physician's assistant programs.

The decision to expand these corpsmen's skills as PAs also capitalized on the previous investment of the U.S. military in providing extensive medical training to these men.

Richard Smith, MD, founder of the University of Washington's MEDEX program, described this training:

> The U.S. Department of Defense has developed ways of rapidly training medical personnel to meet its specific needs, which are similar to those of the civilian population. . . . Some of these people, such as Special Forces and Navy "B" Corpsmen, receive 1400 hours of formal medical training, which may include nine weeks of a supervised "clerkship." Army corpsmen of the 91C series may have received up to 1900 hours of this formal training.

Most of these men have had 3 to 20 years of experience, including independent duty on the battlefield, aboard ship, or in other isolated stations. Many have some college background; Special Forces "medics" average a year of college. After at least 2, and up to 20, years in uniform, these men have certain skills and knowledge in the provision of primary care. Once discharged, however, the investment of public funds in medical capabilities and potential care is lost, because they work as detail men, insurance agents, burglar alarm salesmen, or truck drivers. The majority of this vast manpower pool is unavailable to the current medical care delivery system because, up to this point, we have not devised a civilian framework in which their skills can be put to use.[14]

OTHER MODELS

Describing the period of 1965 to 1971 as "Stage One—The Initiation of Physician Assistant Programs," Carter and Gifford[10] have identified 16 programs that pioneered the formal education of PAs and nurse practitioners. Programs based in university medical centers similar to Duke emerged at Bowman Gray, Oklahoma, Yale, Alabama, George Washington, Emory, and Johns Hopkins and used the Duke training model.[8] Primarily using academic medical centers as training facilities, "Duke-model" programs designed their clinical training to coincide with medical student clerkships and emphasized inpatient medical and surgical roles for PAs. A dramatically different training model developed at the University of Washington, pioneered by Richard Smith, MD, a U.S. public health service physician and former Medical Director of the Peace Corps. Assigned to the Pacific Northwest by Surgeon General William Stewart, Smith was directed to develop a PA training program to respond uniquely to the health manpower shortages of the rural Northwest. Garnering the support of the Washington State Medical Association, Smith developed the MEDEX model, which took a strong position on the "deployment" of students and graduates to medically underserved areas.[15] This was accomplished by placing clinical phase students in preceptorships with primary care physicians who agreed to employ them after graduation. The program also emphasized the creation of a "receptive framework" for the new profession and established relationships with legislators, regulators, and third-party payers to facilitate the acceptance and utilization of the new profession. Although the program originally exclusively recruited military corpsmen as trainees, the term *MEDEX* was coined by Smith not as a reference to their former military roles but rather as a contraction of "*Med*icine *Ex*tension."[16] In his view, using MEDEX as a term of address avoided any negative connotations of the word *assistant* and any potential conflict with medicine over the appropriate use of the term *associate*. MEDEX programs were also developed at University of North Dakota School of Medicine, University of Utah College of Medicine, Dartmouth Medical School, Howard University College of Medicine, Charles Drew Postgraduate Medical School, Pennsylvania State University College of Medicine, and Medical University of South Carolina.[15]

In Colorado, Henry Silver, MD, began the Child Health Associate Program in 1969, providing an opportunity for individuals without previous medical experience but with at least 2 years of college to enter the PA profession. Students received a baccalaureate degree at the end of the second year of the 3-year program and were ultimately awarded a master's degree at the end of training. Thus, it became the first PA program to offer a postgraduate degree as an outcome of PA training.

Compared with the pediatric nurse practitioner educated at the same institution, the child health associate, both by greater depth of education and by law, could provide more extensive and independent services to pediatric patients.[10]

Also offering nonmilitary candidates access to the PA profession was the Alderson-Broaddus program in Phillipi, West Virginia. As the result of discussions that had begun as early as 1963, Hu Myers, MD, developed the program, incorporating a campus hospital to provide clinical training for students with no previous medical experience. In the first program designed to give students both a liberal arts education and professional training as PAs, Alderson-Broaddus became the first 4-year college to offer a baccalaureate degree to its students. Subsequently, other PA programs were developed at colleges that were independent of university medical centers. Early programs of this type included those at Northeastern University in Boston and at Mercy College in Detroit.[16]

Specialty training for PAs was first developed at the University of Alabama. Designed to facilitate access to care for underserved populations, the 2-year program focused its entire clinical training component on surgery and the surgical subspecialties. Even more specialized training in urology, orthopedics, and pathology was briefly provided in programs throughout the United States, although it was soon recognized that entry-level PA training needed to offer a broader base of generalist training.

CONTROVERSY ABOUT A NAME

Amid the discussion about the types of training for the new health care professionals was a controversy about the appropriate name for these new providers. Silver of the University of Colorado suggested *syniatrist* (from the Greek *syn*, signifying "along with" or "association," and *iatric*, meaning "relating to medicine or a physician") for those health care personnel performing "physician-like" tasks. He recommended that the term could be used with a prefix designating a medical specialty and a suffix indicating the level of training (aide, assistant, or associate).[17] Because of his background in international health, Smith believed that *assistant* or even *associate* should be avoided as potentially demeaning. His term *MEDEX* for "physician extension" was designed to be used as a term of address, as well as a credential. He even suggested a series of other companion titles, including "Osler" and "Flexner."[14]

In 1970 the American Medical Association (AMA)–sponsored Congress on Health Manpower attempted to end the controversy and endorse appropriate terminology for the emerging profession. The Congress chose *associate* rather than *assistant* because of its belief that *associate* indicated a more collegial relationship between the PA and supervising physicians. *Associate* also eliminated the potential for confusion between PAs and medical assistants. Despite the position of the Congress, the AMA's House of Delegates rejected the term *associate*, holding that it should be applied only to physicians working in collaboration with other physicians. Nevertheless, PA programs, such as those at Yale, Duke, and the University of Oklahoma, began to call their graduates *physician associates*, and the debate about the appropriate title continued. A more subtle concern has been the use of an apostrophe in the PA title. At various times, in various states, PAs have been identified as *physician's assistants*, implying ownership by one physician, and *physicians' assistants*, implying ownership by more than one physician; they are now identified with the current title *physician assistant* without the apostrophe.

The June 1992 edition of the *Journal of the American Academy of Physician Assistants* contains an article by Eugene Stead, MD, reviewing the debate and calling for a reconsideration of the consistent use of the term *physician associate*.[18]

The issue concerning the name resurfaces regularly, usually among students who are less aware of the historical and political context of the title. More recently, however, a name change has the support of more senior PAs who are adamant that the title "*assistant*" is a grossly incorrect description of their work. Although most PAs would agree that *assistant* is a less than optimum title, the greater concern is that the process to change it would be cumbersome, time consuming, and potentially threatening to the PA profession. Every attempt to "open up" a state PA law, with the intent of changing the title, would bring with it the risk that outside forces (e.g., other health professions) could modify the practice law and decrease the PA scope of practice. Similarly, the bureaucratic processes that would be required to change the title in *every* rule and regulation in each state and in every federal agency would be incredibly labor intensive. The overarching concern is that state and national PA organizations would be seen by policymakers as both self-serving and self-centered if such a change were attempted. This has become a particularly contentious issue among PAs since nurse practitioner educators have chosen to move to a "doctorate in nursing practice" by 2015. In 2011, American Academy of Physician Assistants (AAPA) President Robert Wooten sent a letter to all PAs describing a formal process for collecting data regarding PA "opinions" about the "name issue" on the annual AAPA census for review by the AAPA's House of Delegates.

PROGRAM EXPANSION

From 1971 to 1973, 31 new PA programs were established. These startups were directly related to available federal funding. In 1972, Health Manpower Educational Initiatives (U.S. Public Health Service) provided more than $6 million in funding to 40 programs. By 1975, 10 years after the first students entered the Duke program, there were 1282 graduates of PA programs.

From 1974 to 1985, nine additional programs were established. Federal funding was highest in 1978, when $8,686,000 assisted 42 programs. By 1985, the AAPA estimated that 16,000 PAs were practicing in the United States. A total of 76 programs were accredited between 1965 and 1985, but 25 of those programs later closed (Table 1-1). Reasons for closure range from withdrawal of accreditation to competition for funding within the sponsoring institution and adverse pressure on the sponsoring institution from other health care groups.

PA programs entered an expansion phase beginning in the early 1990s when issues of efficiency in medical education, the necessity of team practice, and the search for cost-effective solutions to health care delivery emerged. The AAPA urged the Association of Physician Assistant Programs (APAP) to actively encourage the development of new programs, particularly in states where programs were not available. Beginning in 1990, APAP created processes for new program support, including new program workshops, and ultimately a program consultation service (Program Assistance and Technical Help [PATH]) to promote quality in new and established programs.

TABLE 1-1 **Distribution of Closed Physician Assistant Training Programs by State**

State	Program
Alabama	University of Alabama, Birmingham
Arizona	Maricopa County Hospital Indian HSMC, Phoenix
California	U.S. Navy, San Diego (now Uniformed Services PA Program in San Antonio) Loma Linda University PA Program
Colorado	University of Colorado OB-GYN Associate Program
Florida	Santa Fe Community College PA Program*
Indiana	Indiana University Fort Wayne PA Program
Maryland	Johns Hopkins University Health Associates
Mississippi	University of Mississippi PA Program
Missouri	Stephens College PA Program
North Carolina	Catawba Valley Technical Institute University of North Carolina Surgical Assistant Program
North Dakota	University of North Dakota
New Hampshire	Dartmouth Medical School
New Mexico	USPHS Gallup Indian Medic Program
Ohio	Lake Erie College PA Program Cincinnati Technical College PA Program
Pennsylvania	Pennsylvania State College PA Program Allegheny Community College
South Carolina	Medical University South Carolina
Texas	U.S. Air Force, Sheppard PA Program
Virginia	Naval School Health Sciences
Wisconsin	Marshfield Clinic PA Program

From Oliver DR. Third Annual Report of Physician Assistant Educational Programs in the United States, 1986-1987. Alexandria, VA: Association of Physician Assistant Programs, 1987.

*Transferred to another sponsoring institution (University of Florida, Gainesville).

These services were ultimately disbanded as the rate of new program growth declined.

The PA profession has engaged in an ongoing and lively debate about the development of new PA programs. By 2011, 159 programs were accredited, compared with 56 programs in the early 1980s. The difficulty lies in the impossibility of making accurate predictions about the future health workforce, a problem that applies to all health professions. Expanded roles of PAs in academic medical centers (as resident replacements), in managed care delivery systems, and in enlarging community health center networks have created unpredicted demand for PAs in both primary and specialty roles. The major variable, aside from the consideration of the ideal "mix" of health care providers in future systems, has to do with the *number* of people who will receive health care and the *amount* of health care that will be provided to each person. If, for example, the health reform legislation that was signed into law by President Obama in 2010 is fully implemented on schedule in 2014, the demand for all types of clinicians will rise dramatically. These projections are driving the expansion of current programs and the development of new ones.

Other features of the new program debate include concerns about the locations of new programs (heavily concentrated in the Northeast), the nature of sponsoring institutions (liberal arts colleges unattached to academic health centers or "for-profit" institutions), and the access to academic degrees (community colleges). Current policy studies from a variety of sources (APAP Blue Ribbon Report, the Pew Report on PAs in Managed Care) recommend careful monitoring of the supply of PAs, along with other health care providers. Although neither the AAPA, the APAP, nor the Accreditation Review Committee on Physician Assistants (ARC-PA) can stop the development of new PA programs, the trend is to recommend caution in preventing the overdevelopment of new programs on the basis of careful analysis of employment trends and health care projections.

Unfortunately, much of the concern about the health care workforce has focused primarily on physician supply (see "Physician Supply Literature" in the Resources section) without including PAs and NPs in economic formulas. As a result, American medical and osteopathic schools have been urged to expand their class size and to create new campuses to serve underserved groups. PA programs are concerned about the impact of medical school growth on access to clinical training sites, as well as on the development of PA jobs. Overall, however, it would appear that new models of medical training include increasing emphasis on interdisciplinary teams and greater integration of medical students, residents, and PA students on most patient care services.

Funding for Programs

The success of the Duke program, as well as that of all developing PA programs, was initially tied to external funding. At Duke, Stead was successful in convincing the federal government's National Heart Institute that the new program fell within its granting guidelines. Subsequently, Duke received foundation support from The Josiah Macy, Jr. Foundation, the Carnegie and Rockefeller Foundations, and the Commonwealth Fund.[10]

In 1969, federal interest in the developing profession brought with it demonstration funding from the National Center for Health Services Research and Development. With increasing acceptance of the PA concept and the demonstration that PAs could be trained relatively rapidly and deployed to medically underserved areas, the federal investment increased. In 1972, the Comprehensive Health Manpower Act, under Section 774 of the Public Health Act, authorized support for PA training. The major objectives were education of PAs for the delivery of primary care medical services in ambulatory care settings; deployment of PA graduates to medically underserved areas; and recruitment of larger numbers of residents from medically underserved areas, minority groups, and women to the health professions.

PA funding under the Health Manpower Education Initiatives Awards and Public Health Services Contracts from 1972 to 1976 totaled $32,669,565 for 43 programs. From 1977 to 1991, PA training was funded through Sections 701, 783, and 788 of the Public Health Service Act. Grants during this period totaled $87,927,728 and included strong incentives for primary care training, recruitment of diverse student-bodies, and deployment of students to clinical sites serving the medically underserved. According to Cawley,[19] as of 1992 "This legislation . . . supported the education of at least 17,500, or over 70% of the nation's actively practicing PAs." Unfortunately, this high level of support did not continue and with lesser funding for primary care, programs followed medical schools into specialty practice models. Today the majority of the nation's PAs—and the program's from which they graduated—have unfortunately not been exposed to the primary care values and experiences that characterized and defined the early PA concept.

During the period of program expansion, the focus of federal funding support became much more specific and fewer programs received funding. Tied to the primary care access goals of the Health Resources and Services Administration (HRSA), PA program grants commonly supported less program infrastructure and more specific primary care initiatives and educational innovations. Examples of activities that were eligible for federal support included clinical site expansion in urban and rural underserved settings, recruitment and retention activities, and curriculum development on topics such as managed care and geriatrics.

An important trend was the diversification of funding sources for PA programs. In addition to federal PA training grants, many programs have benefited from clinical site support provided by other federal programs, such as Area Health Education Centers (AHECs) or the National Health Service Corps (NHSC). Also, many programs now receive expanded state funding on the basis of state workforce projections of an expanded need for primary care providers.

Unfortunately, federal Title VII support for all primary care programs (including family medicine, pediatrics, general internal medicine, and primary care dentistry) began to erode in the late 1990s. Federal budget analysts believed that the shrinking number of graduates choosing primary care employment was a signal that federal support was no longer justified. The federal Title VII Advisory Committee on Primary Care Medicine and Dentistry—which includes PA representatives—was formed to study the problem and recommend strategies. Title VII and Title VIII Reauthorization was delayed until the passage of overarching health reform legislation in 2010. The American Association of Medical Colleges (AAMC) described this legislation:

> The Affordable Care Act (P.L. 111-148 and P.L. 111-152) included numerous provisions that reauthorize the health professions education and training programs under Title VII and VIII of the Public Health Service Act for the first time in a decade. The legislation also authorized several new workforce education and training programs under Title VII, including training programs for rural physicians, direct care workers, mental and behavioral health professionals, public health workers, and loan repayment programs for the pediatric and public health workforce, among others.[20]

PA programs immediately benefitted from available funding through traditional 5-year training grants and two one-time only grant programs for (1) educational equipment, including simulation models and teleconferencing hardware and (2) expansion grants to add more training slots for students who were willing to commit themselves to primary care employment. For the first time, PA training grants were expanded from 3 years to 5 years but were limited to $150,000 per grant.

ACCREDITATION

Accreditation of formal PA programs became imperative because the term *physician assistant* was being used to label a wide variety of formally and informally trained health personnel. Leaders of the Duke program—E. Harvey Estes, MD, and Robert

Howard, MD—asked the AMA to determine educational guidelines for PAs. This request was consistent with the AMA's position of leadership in the development of new health careers and its publication of *Guidelines for Development of New Health Occupations.*

The National Academy of Science's Board of Medicine had also become involved in the effort to develop uniform terminology for PAs. It suggested three categories of PAs. Type A was defined as a "generalist" capable of data collection and presentation and having the potential for independent judgment; type B was trained in one clinical specialty; type C was determined to be capable of performing tasks similar to those performed by type A but not capable of independent judgment.

Although these categories have not remained as descriptors of the PA profession, they helped the medical establishment move toward the support of PA program accreditation. Also helpful were surveys conducted by the American Academy of Pediatrics and the American Society of Internal Medicine determining the acceptability of the PA concept to their respective members. With positive responses, these organizations, along with the American Academy of Family Physicians and the American College of Physicians, joined the AMA's Council on Medical Education in the creation of the "educational essentials" for the accreditation of PA training programs. The AMA's House of Delegates approved these essentials in 1971.

Three PAs—William Stanhope, Steven Turnipseed, and Gail Spears—were involved in the creation of these essentials as representatives of the Duke, MEDEX, and Colorado programs, respectively. The AMA appointed L.M. Detmer administrator of the accreditation process. In 1972, accreditation applications were processed, and 20 sites were visited in alphabetical order, 17 of which received accreditation. Ultimately, the accreditation activities were carried out by the Joint Review Committee, which was a part of the AMA's Committee on Allied Health Education and Accreditation (CAHEA). John McCarty became the Administrator of the ARC-PA in 1991 and is the first PA to serve in this role. Later, the Joint Committee was renamed the Accreditation Review Committee (ARC). In 2000, the ARC became an independent entity, apart from the CAHEA, and changed its name to the Accreditation Review Commission. Current members of the ARC include the Association of Physician Assistant Programs, American Academy of Physician Assistants, American Academy of Family Physicians, American Academy of Pediatrics, American College of Physicians, American College of Surgeons, and American Medical Association.

CERTIFICATION

Just as an accreditation process served to assess the quality of PA training programs, a certification process was necessary to ensure the quality of individual program graduates and become the "gold standard" for the new profession. In 1970 the American Registry of Physician's Associates was created by programs from Duke University, Bowman Gray School of Medicine, and the University of Texas, Galveston, to construct the first certification process. The first certification examination, for graduates from eight programs, was administered in 1972. It was recognized, however, that the examination would have greater credibility if the National Board of Medical Examiners administered it. During this same period, the AMA's House of Delegates requested the Council of Health Manpower to become involved in the development of a national certification program for PAs. Specifically, the House of Delegates was concerned that the new professional role should be developed in an orderly fashion, under medical guidance, and should be measured by high standards. The cooperation of the AMA and the National Board of Medical Examiners ultimately resulted in the creation of the National Commission on Certification of Physician Assistants (NCCPA), which brought together representatives of 14 organizations as an independent commission. Federal grants contributed $715,000 toward the construction and validation of the examination.[10]

In 1973, the first NCCPA national board examination was administered at 38 sites to 880 candidates. In 1974, 1303 candidates took the examination; in 1975, there were 1414 candidates. In 1992, 2121 candidates were examined. In 1997, the examination was administered to 3728 candidates. In 2002, 4918 candidates took the Physician Assistant National Certifying Examination (PANCE) (3995 first-time takers). In 2006, 5495 candidates (4522 first-time takers), and, in 2007, an estimated 5836 candidates took the PANCE, of whom 4736 were first-time takers (personal communication from Janet Lathrop, Executive Director, NCCPA, January 2012).

Now administered only to graduates of ARC-PA accredited PA programs, the NCCPA board examination was originally open to three categories of individuals seeking certification:

- Formally trained PAs, who were eligible by virtue of their graduation from a program approved by the Joint Review Committee on Educational Programs for Physician's Assistants.
- Nurse practitioners, who were eligible provided that they had graduated from a family or pediatric nurse practitioner/clinician program of

at least 4 months' duration, affiliated with an accredited medical or nursing school.

- Informally trained PAs, who could sit for the examination provided that they had functioned for 4 of the past 5 years as PAs in a primary care setting. Candidate applications and detailed employment verification by current and former employers provided data for determination of eligibility.[21]

Since 1986, only graduates of formally accredited PA programs have been eligible for the NCCPA examination.

The NCCPA's assignments include not only the annual examination but also technical assistance to state medical boards on issues of certification. The NCCPA website, NCCPA Connect, includes a listing of all currently certified PAs as a resource for employers and state licensing boards.

The NCCPA also administers a recertification process, which includes requirements to complete and register 100 hours of continuing medical education (CME) every 2 years and to sit for recertification examinations every 6 years. The first recertification examination was given in 1981. The move toward recertification was seen as placing PAs in a leadership position among health professionals; both CME and examination were included as quality-assurance mechanisms.

Recertification initially became a focus of controversy among PAs, many of whom were concerned that a primary care examination potentially discriminated against specialty PAs. The supporters of the recertification examination stressed the primary care role of PAs, even in specialty practice. After years of internal controversy within the PA profession, an alternative route for recertification that did not require a proctored examination—Pathway 2— was approved in 1991. Both the certification and recertification examinations were computerized in 1999, allowing greater access and availability for new graduates and practicing PAs. The certification examination is now administered throughout the year in three separate windows of availability. The recertification examination is given twice each year. In 2010 the Pathway 2 option was discontinued to be consistent with a move away from nonproctored examination, as is the case for other health professional groups.

A recent development for the NCCPA is the development of voluntary recognition for specialty training and education. Called Certificates of Added Qualification (CAQ), the process is modeled after similar acknowledgments in Family Medicine. NCCPA's decision to create the CAQ was based on a long process that involved requests from PA specialty groups, a history of inquiries from institutional credentialing and privileging bodies, a series of meetings involving partnerships between specialty PAs and supportive parallel physician organizations, and a long exploration of possible options.

The final decision—to try the CAQ process with five specialties—was sharply criticized by the AAPA, who feared that any specialty process threatens the generalist image. Ultimately, the NCCPA decided that it was better for them to move in this direction rather than have external for-profit organizations create certification processes without PA input. The five specialties chosen were cardiovascular surgery, orthopedics, nephrology, psychiatry, and emergency medicine. Teams composed of representatives of MD and PA specialty organizations worked together to create the CAQ process.

The NCCPA describes the process:

> To qualify for a specialty CAQ, PAs must first satisfy two basic pre-requisites: (1) current PA-C certification and (2) possession of a valid, unrestricted license to practice as a PA in at least one jurisdiction in the United States or its territories, or unrestricted privileges to practice as a PA for a government agency. (Note: If a PA holds licenses in multiple states, all of the licenses must be unrestricted.)
>
> For PAs meeting those basic prerequisites, the CAQ process includes **four core requirements:** (1) Category I specialty CME, (2) one to two years of experience, (3) procedures and patient case experience appropriate for the specialty, and (4) a specialty exam.
>
> The first three core requirements may be completed in any order. Once those are complete, PAs are eligible for the exam.
>
> The cost of this program is just \$350, including a \$100 administrative fee and a \$250 exam registration fee.
>
> The two-hour CAQ exams include 120 multiple-choice questions administered in two blocks of 60 questions with 60 minutes to complete each block.
>
> Once awarded, a CAQ will be valid for a period of ten years (provided that licensure status and PA-C certification are maintained).[22]

The first examinations were administered on September 12, 2011. At the time of this writing, the outcomes have not yet been released.

In 2005, the NCCPA created a separate NCCPA Foundation to promote and support the PA profession through research and educational projects. The Foundation supports the work of the NCCPA for the advancement of certified physician assistants and the benefit of the public. PA Foundation activities have included a PA Ethics Project with the Physician Assistant Education Association, a Best Practice Project focusing on the relationships between PAs and their supervising physicians, and a research grants program.

In 2010 the NCCPA welcomed the Society for the Preservation of Physician Assistant History and was moved into its infrastructure. Originally founded in 2002 as a free-standing organization for educational, research, and literary purposes, the Society's mission is to serve as the preeminent leader in fostering the preservation, study, and presentation of the history of the PA profession by creating and presenting an online virtual repository of historic and current information on the PA profession. The Society's projects include an archive of PA historical items, the extensive website on PA history designed to serve as a resource for PA students, practicing PAs and researchers, as well as the PA History Center housed in the North Carolina Academy's headquarters in Raleigh-Durham, North Carolina. An 11-member board governs the Society and provides leadership for history activities with support from NCCPA staff.

ORGANIZATIONS

AAPA

What was to become the American Academy of Physician Assistants was initiated by students from Duke's second and third classes as the American Association of Physician Assistants. Incorporated in North Carolina in 1968 with E. Harvey Estes, Jr., MD, as its first advisor and William Stanhope serving two terms as the first president (1968-1969 and 1969-1970), the organization's original purposes were to educate the public about PAs, provide education for PAs, and encourage service to patients and the medical community. With initial annual dues of $20, the Academy created a newsletter as the official publication of the AAPA and contacted fellow students at the MEDEX program and at Alderson-Broaddus.

By the end of the second year, national media coverage of emerging PA programs throughout the United States was increasing (Figure 1-1), and the AAPA began to plan for state societies and student chapters. Tax-exempt status was obtained, the office of president-elect was established, and staggered terms of office for board members were approved.

Controversy over types of PA training models offered the first major challenge to the AAPA. Believing that students trained in 2-year programs based on the biomedical model (type A) were the only legitimate PAs, the AAPA initially restricted membership to these graduates. The Council of MEDEX Programs strongly opposed this point of view. Ultimately, discussions between Duke University's Robert Howard, MD, and MEDEX Program's Richard Smith, MD, resulted in an inclusion of graduates of all accredited programs in the definition of *physician assistant*, and thus in the AAPA.

At least three other organizations also positioned themselves to speak for the new profession. These were a proprietary credentialing association, the American Association of Physician Assistants (a group representing U.S. Public Health Service PAs at Staten Island); the National Association of Physician Assistants; and the American College of Physician Assistants, from the Cincinnati Technical College PA Program. AAPA President Paul Moson provided the leadership that "would result in the emergence of the American Academy of Physician Assistants as the single voice of professional PAs" (W. D. Stanhope, C. E. Fasser, unpublished manuscript, 1992).

This unification was critical to the involvement of PAs in the development of educational standards and the accreditation of PA programs. During Carl Fasser's term as AAPA President, the AMA formally recognized the AAPA, and three Academy representatives were formally appointed to the Joint Review Committee.

During the AAPA presidency of Tom Godkins and the APAP presidency of Thomas Piemme, MD, the two organizations sought funding from foundations for the creation of a shared national office. Funding was received from the Robert Wood Johnson Foundation, the van Ameringen Foundation, and the Ittleson Foundation. Because of its 501(c)(3) tax-exempt status, APAP received the funds for the cooperative use of both organizations. "Discussions held at that time between Piemme and Godkins and other organizational representatives agreed that in the future, because of the limited size of APAP . . . funds would later flow back from the AAPA to APAP"[23] (W. D. Stanhope, C. E. Fasser, unpublished manuscript, 1992). Donald Fisher, MD, was hired as executive director of both organizations, and a national office was opened in Washington, D.C. According to Stanhope and Fasser, "a considerable debt is owed to the many PA programs and their staff who supported the early years of AAPA."

AAPA constituent chapters were created during President Roger Whittaker's term in 1976. Modeled after the organizational structure of the American Academy of Family Physicians, the AAPA's constituent chapter structure and the apportionment of seats in the House of Delegates were the culmination of initial discussions held in the formative days of the AAPA. The American Academy of Family Physicians hosted the AAPA's first Constituent Chapters Workshop in Kansas City, and the first AAPA House of Delegates was convened in 1977.

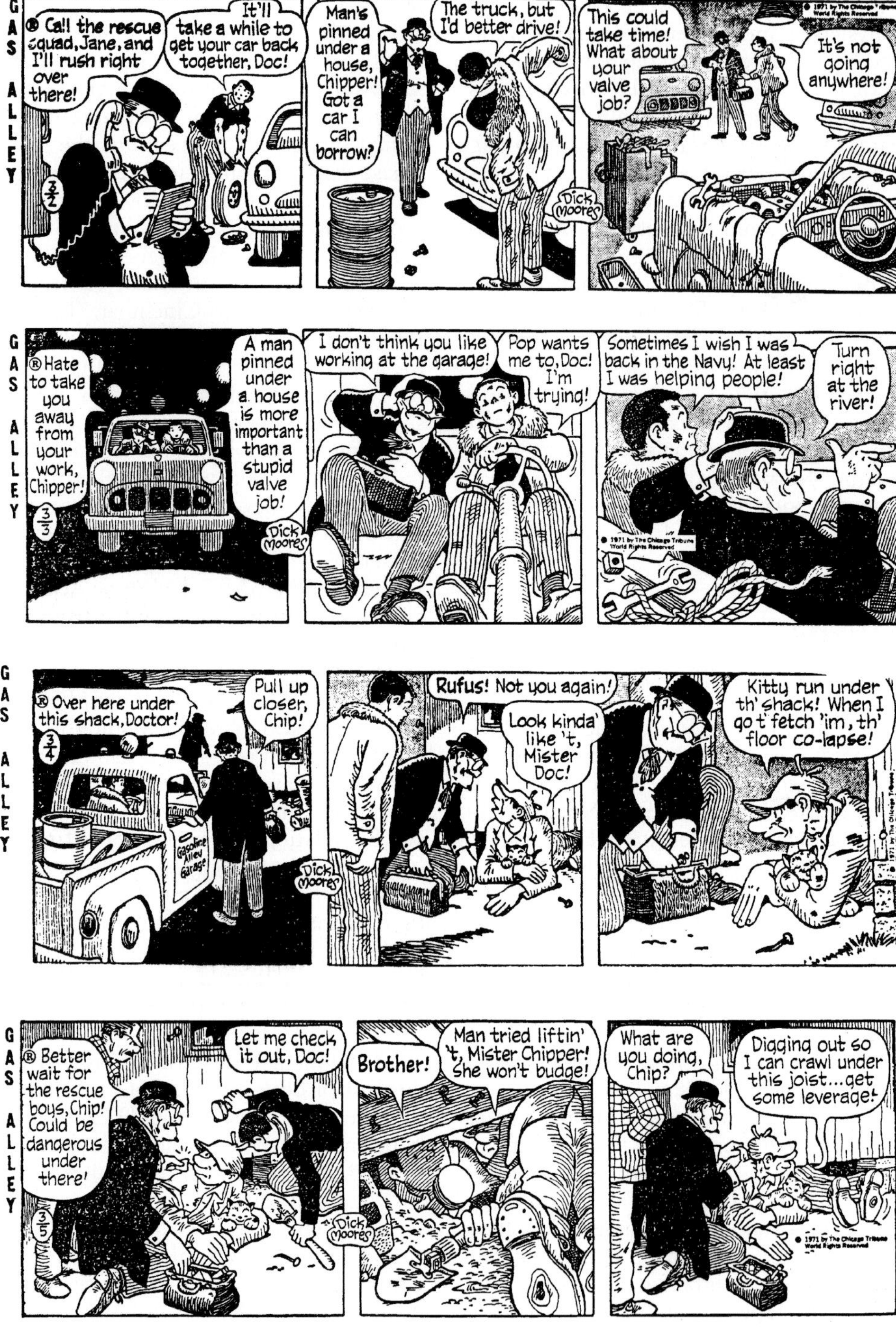
GAS ALLEY
® Call the rescue squad, Jane, and I'll rush right over there!
It'll take a while to get your car back together, Doc!
Man's pinned under a house, Chipper! Got a car I can borrow?
The truck, but I'd better drive!
This could take time! What about your valve job?
It's not going anywhere!
® Hate to take you away from your work, Chipper!
A man pinned under a house is more important than a stupid valve job!
I don't think you like working at the garage!
Pop wants me to, Doc! I'm trying!
Sometimes I wish I was back in the Navy! At least I was helping people!
Turn right at the river!
® Over here under this shack, Doctor!
Pull up closer, Chip!
Gasoline Alley Garage
Rufus! Not you again!
Look kinda' like 't, Mister Doc!
Kitty run under th' shack! When I go t' fetch 'im, th' floor co-lapse!
® Better wait for the rescue boys, Chip! Could be dangerous under there!
Let me check it out, Doc!
Brother!
Man tried liftin' 't, Mister Chipper! She won't budge!
What are you doing, Chip?
Digging out so I can crawl under this joist...get some leverage!
Dick Moores

FIGURE 1-1 ■

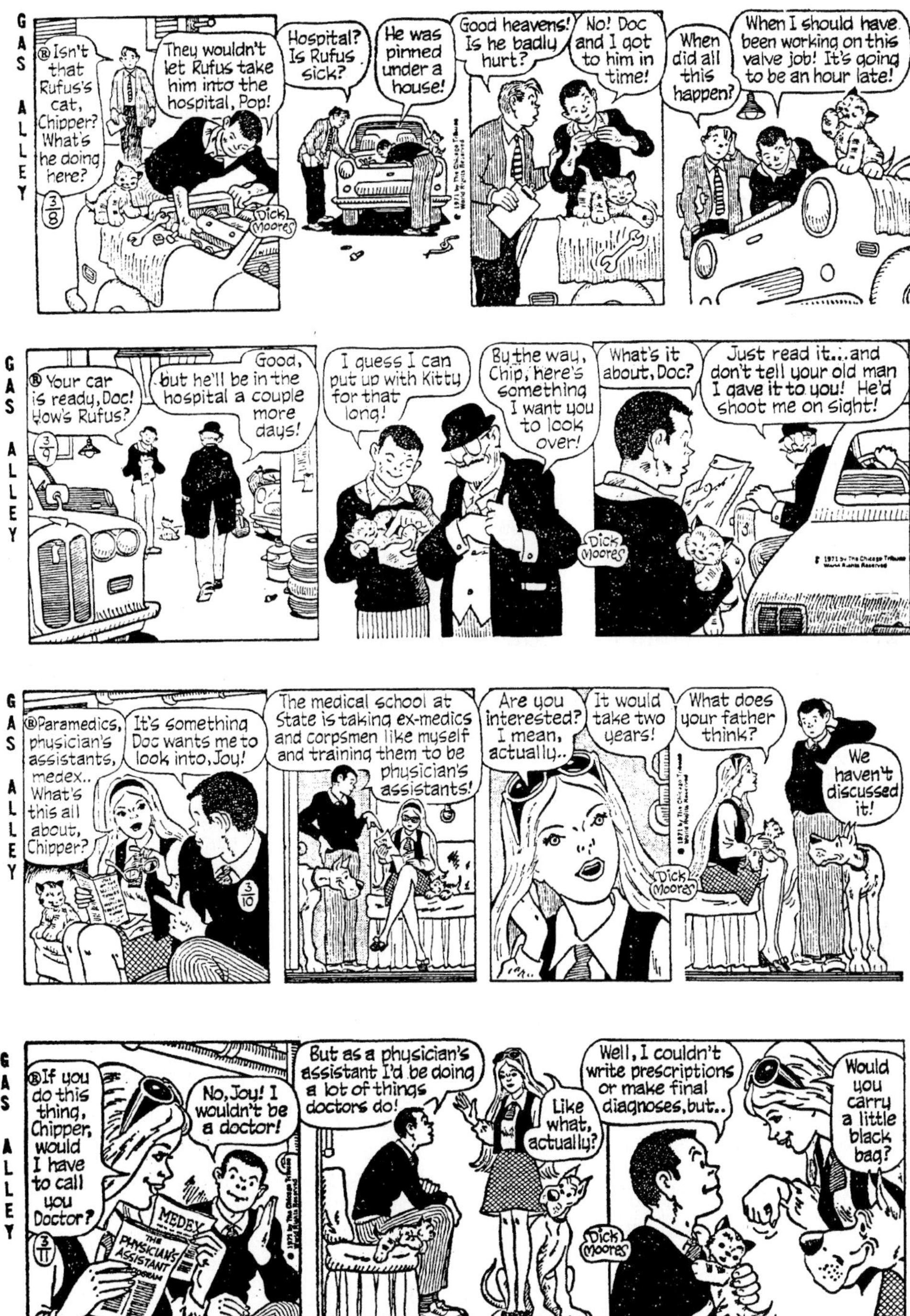
GAS ALLEY
Isn't that Rufus's cat, Chipper? What's he doing here?
They wouldn't let Rufus take him into the hospital, Pop!
Hospital? Is Rufus sick?
He was pinned under a house!
Good heavens! Is he badly hurt?
No! Doc and I got to him in time!
When did all this happen?
When I should have been working on this valve job! It's going to be an hour late!
GAS ALLEY
Your car is ready, Doc! How's Rufus?
Good, but he'll be in the hospital a couple more days!
I guess I can put up with Kitty for that long!
By the way, Chip, here's something I want you to look over!
What's it about, Doc?
Just read it... and don't tell your old man I gave it to you! He'd shoot me on sight!
GAS ALLEY
Paramedics, physician's assistants, medex.. What's this all about, Chipper?
It's something Doc wants me to look into, Joy!
The medical school at State is taking ex-medics and corpsmen like myself and training them to be physician's assistants!
Are you interested? I mean, actually..
It would take two years!
What does your father think?
We haven't discussed it!
GAS ALLEY
If you do this thing, Chipper, would I have to call you Doctor?
No, Joy! I wouldn't be a doctor!
But as a physician's assistant I'd be doing a lot of things doctors do!
Like what, actually?
Well, I couldn't write prescriptions or make final diagnoses, but..
Would you carry a little black bag?
MEDEX
THE PHYSICIAN'S ASSISTANT PROGRAM
Dick Moores

FIGURE 1-1, cont'd For legend see facing page.

Throughout its development, the American Academy of Physician Assistants has been active in the publication of journals for the profession. As the first official journal of the AAPA, *Physician's Associate* was originally designed to encourage research and to report on the developing PA movement. With the consolidation of graduates of all programs into the AAPA, the official academy publication became *The PA Journal, A Journal for New Health Practitioners*. In 1977, *Health Practitioner* became the official magazine of the AAPA, followed by *Physician Assistant* in 1983 and *The Journal of the American Academy of Physician Assistants* in 1988. A new monthly publication, *PA Professional*, has recently been created by the AAPA to feature news, policy issues, and the successes of individual PAs. *Clinician Reviews* and *Physician Assistant*, published by external publishers, also offer medical articles and coverage of professional issues for PAs. In addition to formal publications, the AAPA's website provides the most current information about current practice, policy, and advocacy issues for PAs and their employers.

Governed by a 13-member Board of Directors, including officers of the House of Delegates and a student representative, the Academy includes 10 standing committees and four councils. Specialty groups and formal caucuses bring together academy members with a common concern or interest.[24]

The AAPA's Student Academy is composed of chartered student societies from each PA training program. Each society has one seat in the Assembly of Representatives, which meets at the annual conference and elects officers to direct Student Academy activities.

The Academy also includes a philanthropic arm, the Physician Assistant Foundation, whose mission is to foster knowledge and philanthropy that promotes quality health care. Specifically, the Foundation states that it strives to:

- Award scholarships to deserving PA students across the country to help alleviate the cost of education.
- Provide grants to PAs and PA students who are making a difference in communities across the United States.
- Support PAs who bring high-quality health care to underserved populations internationally.[25]

The annual conference serves as the major political and continuing medical education activity for PAs, with an average annual attendance of 7000 to 9000 participants. A list of past and present AAPA presidents is provided in Table 1-2. A history of conference locations is given in Table 1-3. Table 1-4 lists presidents of the Student Academy (SAAPA) from the AAPA.

TABLE 1-2 **AAPA Presidents**

1968-69	William D. Stanhope, PA
1969-70	William D. Stanhope, PA
1970-71	John J. McQueary, PA
1971-72	Thomas R. Godkins, PA
1972-73	John A. Braun, PA
1973-74	Paul F. Moson, PA
1974-75	C. Emil Fasser, PA-C
1975-76	Thomas R. Godkins, PA
1976-77	Roger G. Whittaker, PA*
1977-78	Dan P. Fox, PA
1978-79	James E. Konopa, PA
1979-80	Ron Rosenberg, PA
1980-81	C. Emil Fasser, PA-C
1981-82	Jarrett M. Wise, RPA
1982-83	Ron I. Fisher, PA
1983-84	Charles G. Huntington, RPA
1984-85	Judith B. Willis, MA, PA
1985-86	Glen E. Combs, PA-C
1986-87	R. Scott Chavez, PA-C
1987-88	Ron L. Nelson, PA-C
1988-89	Marshall R. Sinback, Jr., PA-C
1989-90	Paul Lombardo, RPA-C
1990-91	Bruce C. Fichandler, PA
1991-92	Sherri L. Stuart, PA-C
1992-93	William H. Marquardt, PA-C
1993-94	Ann L. Elderkin, PA
1994-95	Debi A. Gerbert, PA-C
1995-96	Lynn Caton, PA-C
1996-97	Sherrie L. McNeeley, PA-C
1997-98	Libby Coyte, PA-C
1998-99	Ron L. Nelson, PA-C
1999-2000	William C. Kohlhepp, MHA, PA-C
2000-2001	Glen E. Combs, MA, PA-C
2001-2002	Edward Friedmann, PA-C
2002-2003	Ina S. Cushman, PA-C
2003-2004	Pam Moyers Scott, MPAS, PA-C
2004-2005	Julie Theriault, PA-C
2005-2006	Richard C. Rohrs, PA-C
2006-2007	Mary P. Ettari, MPH, PA-C
2007-2008	Gregor F. Bennett, MA, PA-C
2008-2009	Cynthia Lord
2009-2010	Stephen Hanson, MPA, PA-c
2010-2011	Patrick Killeen, MS, PA-C
2011-2012	Robert Wooten, PA-C
2012-2013	James Delaney, PA-C

*Deceased. From American Academy of Physician Assistants, Alexandria, Virginia, 2011.

TABLE 1-3 AAPA National Conference Locations

1973	Sheppard Air Force Base, Texas
1974	New Orleans, Louisiana
1975	St. Louis, Missouri
1976	Atlanta, Georgia
1977	Houston, Texas
1978	Las Vegas, Nevada
1979	Fort Lauderdale, Florida
1980	New Orleans, Louisiana
1981	San Diego, California
1982	Washington, D.C.
1983	St. Louis, Missouri
1984	Denver, Colorado
1985	San Antonio, Texas
1986	Boston, Massachusetts
1987	Cincinnati, Ohio
1988	Los Angeles, California
1989	Washington, D.C.
1990	New Orleans, Louisiana
1991	San Francisco, California
1992	Nashville, Tennessee
1993	Miami Beach, Florida
1994	San Antonio, Texas
1995	Las Vegas, Nevada
1996	New York, New York
1997	Minneapolis, Minnesota
1998	Salt Lake City, Utah
1999	Atlanta, Georgia
2000	Chicago, Illinois
2001	Anaheim, California
2002	Boston, Massachusetts
2003	New Orleans, Louisiana
2004	Las Vegas, Nevada
2005	Orlando, Florida
2006	San Francisco, California
2007	Philadelphia, Pennsylvania
2008	San Antonio, Texas
2009	San Diego, California
2010	Atlanta, Georgia
2011	Las Vegas, Nevada
2012	Toronto, Canada
2013	Washington, D.C.

From American Academy of Physician Assistants, Alexandria, Virginia, 2011.

TABLE 1-4 Student Academy Presidents

1972-1973	J. Jeffrey Heinrich
1973-1974	John McElliott
1974-1975	Robert P. Branc
1975-1976	Tom Driber
1976-1977	John Mahan
1977-1978	Stephen Nunn
1978-1979	William C. Hultman
1979-1980	Arthur H. Leavitt, II
1980-1981	Katherine Carter Stephens
1981-1982	William A. Conner
1982-1983	Michael J. Huckabee
1983-1984	Emily H. Hill
1984-1985	Thomas J. Grothe
1985-1986	Gordon L. Day
1986-1987	Patrick E. Killeen
1987-1988	Keevil W. Helmly
1988-1989	Toni L. Deer
1989-1990	Paul S. Robinson
1990-1991	Jeffrey W. Janikowski
1991-1992	Kathryn L. Kuhlman
1992-1993	Ty W. Klingensmith Flewelling
1993-1994	Beth A. Griffin
1994-1995	Ernest F. Handau
1995-1996	Beth Grivett
1996-1997	James P. McGraw, III
1997-1998	Stacey L. Wolfe
1998-1999	Marilyn E. Olsen
1999-2000	Jennifer M. Huey-Voorhees
2000-2001	Rodney W. Richardson
2001-2002	Abby Jacobson
2002-2003	Andrew Booth
2003-2004	Annmarie McManus
2004-2005	Lindsey Gillispie
2005-2006	Trish Harris-Odimgbe
2006-2007	Gary Jordan
2007-2008	Gary Jordon
2008-2009	Michael T. Simmons
2009-2010	Kate Lenore Callaway
2010-2011	Michael Shepherd
2011-2012	Peggy Diana Walsh
2012-2013	Emilie Suzanne Thornhill

From American Academy of Physician Assistants, Alexandria, Virginia, 2011.

Legislative and leadership activities for the Academy take place at the annual leadership event—now called Capital Connections. Capital Connections—scheduled for March of each year—also provides the opportunity for lobbying of state congressional delegations in Washington, D.C. AAPA regional meetings also provide annual opportunities for leadership development and skill building. Key to the success of the American Academy of Physician Assistants is a dedicated staff at the national office in Alexandria, Virginia. Under an executive vice president who is responsible to the AAPA Board of Directors, four senior vice presidents and seven vice presidents manage Academy activities related to governmental affairs, education, communications, member services, accounting, and administration.

APAP to PAEA

Composed of member programs rather than individuals, the Association of Physician Assistant Programs evolved from the original American Registry of Physician's Associates, which was formed in a collaboration by training programs at Duke University, Bowman Gray School of Medicine, and the University of Texas, Galveston. The Registry was originally created "to determine the competence of Physician's Associates" through the development of a national certifying examination. After these functions were subsequently assumed by the National Board of Medical Examiners, and ultimately the National Commission on Certification of Physician Assistants (NCCPA) in 1972, the Registry became the Association of Physician Assistant Programs (APAP).

Led by Alfred M. Sadler, Jr., MD, as its first president, the Association of Physician Assistant Programs evolved as a network within which member programs could work on "curriculum development, program evaluation, [and] the establishment of continuing education programs"; the APAP was also developed to "serve as a clearing house for information and define the role of the physician assistant."

Like the Association of American Medical Colleges, the Association of Physician Assistant Programs (now the Physician Assistant Education Association, PAEA) represents educational programs, whereas the American Medical Association and the American Academy of Physician Assistants represent individual practitioners.

For many years, the educational offices were located in the AAPA building in Alexandria, Virginia. A change in both the name and the structure of the organization occurred in 2004. APAP became the Physician Assistant Education Association (PAEA), and the organization relocated to separate office space in Alexandria. PAEA, governed by an eight-member Board of Directors, including a student representative, hold its major annual meeting in the late fall, as well as meetings in conjunction with the AAPA annual May meeting. Ten standing committees and two institutes do the work of the organization, as well as special committees and task forces, which are assigned to deal with specific concerns or emerging issues. PAEA is also organized by regional consortia, which meet on individual schedules to consider regional training and professional issues. APAP Presidents are listed in Table 1-5.

PAEA offers an online directory of PA programs as a resource for program applicants. In 2001 the organization began a nationwide centralized electronic application process (CASPA) to streamline PA program application. Although not all programs currently participate in CASPA, the goal is that this service will serve the same function as the American Medical College's Application Service (AMCAS) process used extensively by U.S. medical schools. AMCAS serves as both the medical school admissions gateway and the provider of important data

TABLE 1-5 **PAEA Presidents**

1972-1973	Alfred M. Sadler, Jr., MD
1973-1974	Thomas E. Piemme, MD
1974-1975	Robert Jewett, MD
1975-1976	C. Hilmon Castle, MD
1976-1977	C. Hilmon Castle, MD
1977-1978	Frances L. Horvath, MD
1978-1979	Archie S. Golden, MD
1979-1980	Thomas R. Godkins, PA
1980-1981	David E. Lewis, Med
1981-1982	Regional D. Carter, PhD, PA-C
1982-1983	Stephen C. Gladhart, EdD
1983-1984	Robert H. Curry, MD
1984-1985	Denis R. Oliver, PhD
1985-1986	C. Emil Fasser, PA-C
1986-1987	Jack Liskin, MA, PA-C
1987-1988	Jesse C. Edwards, MS
1988-1989	Suzanne B. Greenberg, MS
1989-1990	Steven R. Shelton, MBA, PA-C
1990-1991	Ruth Ballweg, PA-C
1991-1992	Albert F. Simon, Med, PA-C
1992-1993	Anthony A. Miller, Med, PA-C
1993-1994	Richard R. Rahr, EdD, PA-C
1994-1995	Ronald D. Garcia, PhD
1995-1996	Janet Hammond, MA, PA-C
1996-1997	J. Dennis Blessing, PhD, PA-C
1997-1998	Donald L. Pedersen, PhD, PA-C
1998-1999	Walter A. Stein, MHCA-PA-C
1999-2000	P. Eugene Jones, PhD, PA-C
2000-2001	Gloria Stewart, EdD, PA-C
2001-2002	David Asprey, PhD, PA-C
2002-2003	James F. Cawley, MPH, PA-C
2003-2004	Paul L. Lombardo, MPS, RPA-C
2004-2005	Patrick T. Knott, PhD, PA-C
2005-2006	Dawn Morton-Rias, PD, PA-C
2006-2007	Anita D. Glicken, MSW
2007-2008	Dana L. Sayre-Stanhope, EdD, PA-C
2008-2009	Justine Strand de Oliveira, DrPH, PA-C
2009-2010	Ted Ruback, MS, PA
2010-2011	Kevin Lohenry, PhD, PA-C
2011-2012	Anthony Brenneman, MPAS, PA-C

From Association of Physician Assistant Programs, Alexandria, Virginia, 2011.

regarding the applicant pool and long-term graduate career trajectories.

A major function of PAEA is also the support of PA program faculty. An online newsletter, *PAEA Networker*, provides information on PAEA activities and educational opportunities. PAEA's formal publication, *The Journal of Physician Assistant Education*, offers articles on a range of PA educational issues. PAEA also promotes professional development and scholarly activity through the Faculty Development and Research Institutes.

TRENDS

Although the first PA programs were developed with the primary purpose of training male military corpsmen, the demography of the profession soon changed, largely because the PA profession developed in historical context with both the women's and the civil rights movements. Early articles and promotional materials for PAs described the new provider almost universally as "he." In 1966, Eugene Stead, MD, explained:

> Our intent is to produce career-oriented graduates. Since the long-range goals of most females remove them from continued and full-time employment in the health field, we anticipate that the bulk of the student body will be males. This is not meant to exclude females, for those who can present credentials which would assure the Admissions Committee of proper intent should be considered in the same light as male applicants.[26]

In fact, there were many "career-oriented" women seeking exactly this type of training. By the mid-1970s, the PA profession was quickly evolving—fueled not only by the need for changes in the health care system but also by the attraction to the profession of strong, motivated women seeking a new and open-ended health career. PA program brochures included photographs of both male and female students, and marketing for the PA profession began to focus on the diversity of individuals entering the profession. In 1972, 19.9% of PA students were women; in 1976, 32.8% were women; and by 1981-1982, the distribution of graduates was nearly equal.[27,28] The percentages of women entering U.S. medical schools for the same years were 16.8%, 23.8%, and 30.8%, respectively.[29] By the late 1990s, there was some concern that the PA profession might become a female-dominated profession because women filled more than 60% of the training slots. The move to master's degrees seems to have accelerated the increase in the number of women in PA programs. Researchers have yet to fully explore this phenomenon and its potential impact on the PA profession.

PA programs also immediately focused on recruiting minority candidates for PA training. PA programs to train American Indians and Alaskan Natives were established at Indian Health Service hospitals in Phoenix, Arizona, and Gallup, New Mexico. Programs were also established at Drew University, Howard University, and Harlem Hospital with initiatives to train African Americans for inner-city practice. In addition, federal funding guidelines encouraged other PA programs to emphasize the recruitment and training of minority PAs. Since 1987, 20% of all PA students have been minorities. Nevertheless, the recruitment of minorities into the PA profession is an ongoing issue. In 1977, Ruth Webb of the Drew program challenged "each and every PA to accept the responsibility for seeking out five minority applicants during the coming year. Your minimum goal would be to have at least one of them accepted into your parent program."[30] This challenge is equally appropriate today as an ongoing issue.

NATIONAL HEALTH POLICY REPORTS

Two national reports, one by the Institute of Medicine in 1978 and the other by the Graduate Medical Education National Advisory Committee (GMENAC) in 1981, had a major impact on both PAs and nurse practitioners.

In 1978, the National Academy of Sciences Institute of Medicine (IOM) issued its "Manpower Policy for Primary Health Care." Strongly supporting PAs and NPs, the IOM statements included the following recommendations[31]:

- For the present time, the numbers of PAs and NPs being trained should remain at the current level.
- Training programs for family physicians, PAs, and NPs should continue to receive direct federal, state, and private support.
- Amendments to state licensing laws should authorize, through regulations, PAs and NPs to provide medical services, including prescribing drugs when appropriate and making medical diagnoses. PAs and NPs should be required to perform the range of services they provide as skillfully as physicians, but they should not provide medical services without physician supervision.

Emphasizing the value of primary care, the IOM report stressed that even with the projected increase in the supply of physicians, PAs and NPs have an important role to play in the delivery of primary care.[31]

Charged by the U.S. Secretary of Health, Education and Welfare, a national advisory committee began in 1976 to examine the physician supply issue. The report by GMENAC, published in 1981 and seen as a major turning point in the history of American health care, projected an oversupply of physicians by 1990. Strategies for correcting this oversupply included reducing medical school enrollments, limiting the use of foreign-trained physicians, and reviewing the need to train nonphysician providers. According to Cawley, "Many people who supported PAs during the times of physician shortage viewed an excess of physicians as signaling the discontinuation of federal funding for PA programs and the exit of PAs from the medical scene." Although federal funding was not completely eliminated, it was significantly reduced, from $8,262,968 in 1980 to $4,752,000 in 1982. The reduced funds could assist only 34 programs, rather than the previous 43, and the amounts per program were significantly cut.

In retrospect, there were significant flaws in the assumptions of the GMENAC process. Among the issues that could not be predicted were the impact of HIV, the greater usage of physician services, the shortening of physician workweeks, and the changing lifestyles of physicians. As a result, questions remain about the existence of a physician shortage, and the general understanding is that the United States has a physician maldistribution. As Cawley states, "Any perceived negative impact of the rising physician numbers on the vitality of the PA profession has failed to occur."[32] According to Schafft and Cawley,[32] "The most significant outcome of the study was a gradual awareness that the profession would have to reevaluate its mission and redirect its efforts to validate its existence."

"FUTURES" EVENTS

Two PA symposia in the mid-1980s looked toward the future of health care and the position of PAs in that future. The AAPA sponsored an October 1984 symposium entitled "The Future of Health Care: Challenges and Choices." In the foreword to the Symposium's Executive Summary,[34] 1984 AAPA President Judith Willis described the event and its outcomes:

- In bringing together the symposium panelists, health care practitioners, and policymakers, the American Academy of Physician Assistants hoped to explore concrete problems facing the health care sector in the coming decades—manpower, services, financing technology—as well as provide a forum to focus on the challenge for the future of health care in the United States.
- If there were a consensus from the symposium presentations and workshops, it would be that the future of health care is dependent not so much on biomedical techniques, but rather on how care is delivered and who controls the practice of medicine.

In 1986 the APAP formed an Ad Hoc Futures Committee, which devoted its midyear meeting to the study of the Physician Assistant of the Future and created a vision document recommending directions for PA education. Portions of the vision document read as follows[34]:

- *Professional and Practice Characteristics:* The PA career will include expansion into many different roles: clinical, nonclinical, and combinations of the two. There will be more horizontal and vertical career mobility than at present. PAs will continue to be dependent practitioners in the sense of being supervised by physicians but will have increased performance autonomy. PAs will be part of a multidisciplinary approach to community medical practice. PAs will become more active in anticipating and meeting the health care needs of society.
- *Public Policy Issues:* PAs will respond by mastering the political skills necessary to become more involved in policy decisions affecting health care delivery. Such skills and involvement will be directed toward establishing great uniformity of laws and regulations governing PA practice and facilitating practice reciprocity among states.
- *Entering the Profession:* Applicants and entering PA students will have strong prior academic preparation. . . . More students will enter with bachelor's degrees than now, and some will enter seeking graduate-level education.
- *Education:* Primary care will remain the focus of entry-level education for the PA profession. Baccalaureate degrees will remain the most common credential awarded for entry-level education, but other kinds of credentials will be preserved for some students. Programs will employ as faculty PAs who are trained as teachers, and physicians will continue to be integrally involved in PA education. The number of postgraduate residency programs in clinical specialties will increase. Some postgraduate training will follow a fellowship model, and some will offer a master's degree on completion.

From the vantage point of 2012, the predictions of both the AAPA and the APAP futures projects provided guidance for the further development and evolution of the PA profession. What was not "predicted" was the move toward specialty practice, the extensive development of new programs at the master's degree level, or the passage of health reform legislation finally bringing health care to larger percentages of the U.S. population.

CURRENT ISSUES AND CONTROVERSIES

The development of any new career brings with it controversies and concerns. The late 1960s heralded the creation of the PA and the successful implementation of the pilot projects that would serve as the foundation for subsequent PA training. In the 1970s, enthusiastic new PAs pioneered the role in a variety of settings, practice acts were put in place in most states, and professional organizations were established at national and state levels. The 1980s saw both the continued training of PAs and questions about where PAs fit in the health care system. Although the GMENAC report resulted in a backlash against PAs and nurse practitioners through fewer federal dollars for training, the late 1980s found PAs being used in a wider range of practice settings than had ever been dreamed of by the founders.

During the 1990s, our attention was focused on training and utilization; however, there was new appreciation for the political context of health care in a rapidly changing society. Federal health workforce policy documents were paralleled by similar state documents that acknowledged state-specific issues. Most frequently, these documents called for a maintenance or expansion of the primary care workforce and acknowledgment of the valuable roles that PAs play in any health care system on the basis of their generic primary care training, their adaptability, and their willingness to rapidly respond to the needs of specific health care "niches." In the second decade of the 21st century, we continue to market the profession as one solution to access to care. Competing priorities are now more evident. Medical specialists—many of whom trained alongside PAs—are demanding PAs as part of their practice team. An emphasis on high quality combined with initial moves to population-based care delivery is also creating opportunities for PAs.

Health Workforce and Demand Issues

In a health care system with either a shortage or at least a maldistribution of physicians, determination of the appropriate number of PAs and nurse practitioners involves a controversial calculation. PAs and NPs speak with a louder political voice than in the past, but their relatively small numbers compared with more powerful physician organizations sometimes leave their message muffled by comparison.

Development of managed health care systems and greater attention to accessible, cost-effective, and high-quality care make PAs desirable in many clinical settings. PA training programs find that many new graduates have signed employment contracts before graduation. Other graduates have a difficult time making choices among a variety of job opportunities.

We had all hoped that one outcome of the health reform process would be some "reality-based" workforce projections. Unfortunately, the groups that worked on this issue were limited by the impossibility of such a prediction. (See the previous discussion of this issue in this chapter.) The Council on Graduate Medical Education (COGME), an arm of the Division of Medicine of the Health Resources and Services Administration, convened the Advisory Group on Physician Assistants and the Workforce in 1994.[35] The result was a report, *Physician Assistants in the Health Workforce*, that projected future needs for PAs but fell silent (as do other workforce reports of the time) on the actual numbers of providers needed in the "new" health system. The recommendations of the report included the following:

1. Expand the output of PA educational programs.
2. Increase the level of federal grant support for PA educational programs.
3. Provide increased funding to expand the supply of PA graduates.
4. Retain primary care as the dominant theme of PA education.
5. Provide incentives in Title VII–authorized PA grant programs that encourage sponsoring academic institutions to integrate clinical educational experiences among various health professions.
6. Include incentives in federal grants supporting PA educational programs to reward, maintain, and improve efforts in the recruitment of students and faculty from minority, disadvantaged, and ethnic groups.
7. Provide incentives in federal PA and other grant programs to encourage the recruitment of PA students from rural areas and the use of rural preceptorships that facilitate the return of these graduates to rural practice.
8. Recommend that the Secretary of Health and Human Services develop a plan encouraging PA educational programs to recruit and retrain honorably discharged military personnel, particularly those from underrepresented minority and ethnic groups.
9. Promote health services research that examines clinical effectiveness, patient outcomes,

and resident-substitution ratios when PAs are used in graduate medical education staffing positions.

Although some of these recommendations may have served as the basis for some of the "debates" described earlier, the primary intent of the report was to provide greater clarification about the important role of PAs in meeting the nation's health care needs. A secondary intent was to create a policy document that would prevent some of the backlash against PAs and NPs that had occurred as a result of the GMENAC report.

Primary Care versus Specialization

PAs were created to respond to the primary care access problem in this country. Although changing job patterns reflect, in part, the high demand for a relatively small number of available PAs, many leaders are concerned that the move away from primary care will lead to decreased federal support for PA training and utilization. Other PA leaders actively encourage the move toward specialization as a strategy to enhance what they see to be the visibility and status of the profession. Increasingly this debate is interwoven with the parallel debate about physician deployment and the fact that "PAs go where physicians go." As more new physicians choose specialty practice over primary care, they will need PAs as their colleagues in the specialties. Even in small towns, an MD/PA specialty team may be more cost-effective—and viable—than two physicians.

Federal and state policymakers continue to be concerned about training PAs for the purpose of providing primary care, especially to underserved populations. Government-funded training initiatives not only place increasing importance on training in medically underserved clinics (urban and rural) but also promise to put more pressure on programs to encourage students to seek employment in these settings. These trends have a significant impact on recruitment, selection, and training patterns of PA programs. They also have the effect of putting PA educators in direct conflict with those PA leaders who believe that the future of PAs lies exclusively in the specialties and subspecialties. Over time, some PA programs have chosen to opt out of governmentally funded training opportunities rather than deal with the increasingly restrictive training and reporting requirements that accompany these funds.

In 2006, the specialty debate escalated when an external organization threatened to develop specialty examinations and specialty certification for PAs. Although historically opposed to this type of recognition of specialty practice, the NCCPA responded by announcing to the AAPA House of Delegates that they would explore the process of creating a formal specialty recognition process—one that would not replace the initial certification examination (PANCE) or the recertification examination (PANRE). In June of 2006, NCCPA sponsored a forum of PA specialty organizations and representatives of the AAPA and PAEA. Participants shared the concern that an external body should not have the power to influence the basic principles and structure of the PA profession, although not everyone agreed about what should be done about it. The issue was further complicated by several other issues, including increasing emphasis on "quality initiatives" in health care delivery systems, the demand for more specific documentation of training and experience by hospital credentialing and privileging committees, and the changing demographics—with respect to prior clinical experience—of the pool of new graduates.

Although the AAPA continued to oppose a policy of specialty recognition, the NCCPA moved ahead with an exploration of specialty recognition, which would be voluntary and would not replace the PANCE process. Working with the PA specialty organizations that were seeking this type of recognition, the NCCPA began to design a voluntary process that would recognize both experience and education. The new National Commission on Certification of Physician Assistants (NCCPA) process for Certificate of Added Qualification (see Chapter 5) was first offered to certified PAs in five specialties beginning in 2011.

In the midst of this controversy are many unanswered questions. There is little research about the actual tasks of PAs within specialty practices. Many specialty PAs contend that they are hired by specialists to provide "primary care" to the specialist's patients. If this is the case, a myriad of secondary questions need to be answered about the reimbursement levels for these services, as well as the specialist's ability to supervise services that he or she may not have been trained to provide. Similarly, what role does the "primary care" function of the PA in a specialty practice play in retaining patients in the specialty practice, and is that role appropriate?

Other specialty PAs maintain that they carry out many of the same specialty tasks as their supervising physicians and therefore create significant income streams for the practice. This role of PA specialty practice brings with it the potential need for additional specialty educational opportunities (e.g., residencies, fellowships, online learning materials) and eventually specialty recognition.

A broader view of the "primary care versus specialization" issue is to see both trends as a positive demonstration of the flexibility of PAs to respond to a rapidly changing health care system. The generalist nature of PA training, required by accreditation, allows PAs maximum mobility within the health care system. Unlike physicians, whose relatively early specialization leaves little opportunity for redirection, PAs may move back and forth from primary care to the specialties throughout their careers. Research tracing PA career patterns may help us to better understand the implications of these transitions.

Who Speaks for Us

The growth of the PA profession has also brought with it the expansion of professional organizations, both nationally and at the state level. PA training programs are often seen as the source of information about state or regional issues. State medical boards and the NCCPA also provide information about PA roles and utilization.

There is always an ongoing tension, which is probably not limited to PAs, about who speaks for our profession and the consistency of the messages that are delivered. Lobbying efforts by the AAPA in Washington, D.C., benefit from input from both constituent chapters and individual PAs. Professional staff members cannot be expected to be the exclusive voices of the PA profession. PA programs and state chapters must work together to provide consistent messages. This reality requires the willingness of PAs to be visible and involved not just in health care but in the political process as well.

Degree Issues

In the closing moments of the AAPA Cincinnati Conference in 1987, the House of Delegates passed a resolution supporting a baccalaureate degree as the entry-level credential for PAs. Immediately following that action, the membership of the APAP passed an opposing resolution stating that the AAPA stance was "premature."

The proponents of bachelor's degrees for PAs held that the lack of a degree requirement decreased the credibility of the PA profession and created a barrier to the expansion of PA practice in some states. Opponents of the degree requirement believe that it limits entry to PA training, especially for rural "second career" applicants, who have little access to formal academic prerequisites.

Proponents of degrees further maintained that the requirement of a degree gave PAs upward mobility, particularly within federal and academic systems. Opponents, citing trends away from primary care in other professions associated with advanced degrees, asserted that the focus on degrees was a move away from the primary-care mission of the PA profession.

Central to this issue is the definition of the "gold standard" for PA training and certification. Passing the NCCPA entry-level examination, coupled with graduation from a CAHEA-accredited program, is currently the recognized credential for practice in most states. Proponents of degrees believe that the latter give PAs credibility in addition to that provided by NCCPA certification. Opponents of the degree requirement point out that many other professionals, including physicians, are credentialed by competency-based training and examination rather than by degree.

The 1992 AAPA House of Delegates again considered the degree requirement as part of the required "Sunset Review" of policies. After heated discussion, they tabled the position paper on degrees prepared by the Education Council. In 2000 the AAPA House of Delegates adopted resolutions stating that PA education should be conducted at the graduate level and supporting credentials awarded to students that are reflective of the graduate level of education.[36] A policy paper prepared by the Association of Physician Assistant Programs in the same year acknowledged the increasing numbers of master's degree programs and supported the movement of programs to this degree level, but it also recognized that individual programs must maintain their unique missions of service and access. It was acknowledged that advanced degrees could be a barrier to this mission.

With the development of new PA programs in the 1990s, many new programs were created at the master's level. Soon, other programs began their transition to the master's level. Even programs housed in community colleges began to develop linkages with graduate institutions to create pathways to graduate degrees for their students. Programs remaining at the bachelor's degree level are now relatively few in number, and many of them are in the planning process for a move to advanced degrees.

There is still concern that graduate programs decrease access to PA programs for many candidates, particularly those from diverse backgrounds and rural communities. Regardless of one's opinion on this issue, PA program graduates from programs at all levels must be monitored so that any trends, positive or negative, can be tracked.

Although it may still be too early to determine the impact of master's level training on the PA profession, this transition creates the opportunity for research on the applicant pool and deployment patterns and, ultimately, for assessing the effect of advanced degrees on the profession's track record of improving health care access.

The recent decision by nurse practitioners to create a Doctorate in Nursing Practice as their entry-level degree has raised the question of whether the PA profession plans this same move. Students are encouraged to review the nursing literature on this issue listed in the Resources section at the end of this chapter. Although the nurse practitioner profession's agenda is clearly different from the PA profession's with respect to independent practice, this development raises questions for us about the role of "terminal degrees" in any profession and the impact that the creation of PA degrees at the doctorate level would have on our support from physicians.

International Developments

By the mid-1990s, other countries were becoming interested in the PA profession and individual PAs, and PA programs began working with governments and institutions to transfer the profession overseas. Activities have included the development of international rotations for PA students, the creation of demonstration projects employing U.S. PAs to illustrate the PA concept, and the initiation of PA educational programs. Initially both AAPA and PAEA created infrastructure to support these activities, including sessions at the AAPA and PAEA annual conferences to showcase the profession to visiting international representatives and the creation of networking opportunities for international visitors considering the development of the PA profession in their countries. The NCCPA created a position for a Director of International Relations designed to build and maintain relationships that would support international development of the PA concept and create opportunities to provide technical assistance on the creation of certification processes internationally. Several new international organizations focusing on international PA educational processes and opportunities have arisen. In addition, PA educators are increasingly becoming involved in global health education organizations to bring together all health professions.

An interesting aspect of PA international activities has been the question of whether the expectation is that other countries will simply "adopt" the PA profession as is or whether they will "adapt" it to make it better fit each country's unique circumstances and needs. Tied to this issue is the question of whether the intent is for PAs to be mobile and transferable internationally or whether it is more appropriate for PAs (or whatever name/title is chosen by a specific country) to remain in their home countries to alleviate domestic workforce shortages.

CASE STUDY 1-1

The development of the PA profession internationally creates a number of dilemmas—many of which have already been played out in the United States. However, it is reasonable to expect that other countries may come to different solutions to these issues on the basis of their adaptation of the PA model.

The first issue is the model of training. Countries with medical education systems based on the United Kingdom model admit students into a 6-year medical program after high school. As a result, the master's degree model of PA training is nontransferable because the length of PA training would be equivalent to a medical education.

A second issue is utilization. Some countries think that specialty PAs are a solution to maldistribution with respect to primary care and specialties. Adequate numbers of specialty PAs could eliminate the need for training large numbers of physician specialists and also be a cost-saving strategy for high-volume but low-intensity specialty procedures.

Thirdly, a more culturally appropriate and positive name for the profession might be developed in light of the U.S. experience with a dissatisfying name.

Relationships with Physicians

It is critical that PAs be clear about their relationships with physicians. Because of concern that PAs might be lumped into the excessively generic term, *nonphysician providers*, AAPA President William H. Marquart clarified the AAPA's position on independent practice in a letter to John L. Clowe, MD, president of the American Medical Association, dated May 11, 1993; he wrote, in part:

> Physician assistants do not seek independent practice, direct reimbursement from third-party payers, or federal preemption of state practice acts . . .
>
> All actions affirm positions held by the profession since its inception 25 years ago: that PAs practice with physician supervision and that third-party coverage of PA services should be paid to the PA's employer.
>
> PAs and advance practice nurses are frequently referred to as nonphysician or mid-level providers, and, regrettably, people sometimes fail to draw a distinction between the two professions. We felt it would be appropriate at this time to let you know that PAs maintain a strong belief in the need to work closely with physicians.

M. Roy Schwarz, MD, the AMA's Senior Vice President for Medical Education, responded on May 25, 1993, to the letter as follows:

> I am very pleased to have an official confirmation of your posture concerning independent practice. . . . . Having been involved in the original development of the MEDEX Program at the University of Washington, and having watched the physician assistant movement develop, I could not be more pleased with its evolution and the performance of its people.
>
> You have undoubtedly seen me quoted in newspapers concerning the nursing agenda and their quest for the independent practice of primary care. I never intended [to include], nor have I included physician assistants in those comments. . . . I have clearly indicated in every interview that physician assistants do not have this as their goal, that they are completely satisfied with their present role, and that their relationship with medicine is an excellent one. Your letter reaffirms that conviction, and I appreciate having it. My best to you and your colleagues as you go about serving America's needs.

CASE STUDY 1-2

The history of the PA profession in Washington State illustrates how critical and positive interaction with a state medical association has facilitated the development of PA practice.

1968: The Washington State Medical Association (WSMA) was a partner with the University of Washington School of Medicine in the creation of the MEDEX Northwest physician assistant program. This support was based on the need for health care in rural communities and the premise that the additional support and care provided by MEDEX graduates would result in the retention of rural physicians within the communities.

1971: The Washington State Medical Association sponsored an amendment to the medical practice act allowing physician assistants to practice under the supervision of a practicing physician. This pioneering legislation was sponsored by a physician/legislator, James McDermott, MD, who now serves in the U.S. Congress.

1977: With the endorsement of the WSMA, the Board of Medical Examiners amended its Rules and Regulations to allow PAs to write prescriptions.

1982: Physician assistants were invited to join the Washington State Medical Association. The Washington Academy of Physician Assistants (WAPA) was allowed a voting seat in the WSMA House of Delegates, and WAPA became a participant in the Interspecialty Council.

1986: The Washington State Medical Association House of Delegates passed a resolution to place a PA on the Board of Medical Examiners.

1987: The Washington State Legislature passed legislation to place a PA on the Board of Medical Examiners who would vote on PA matters.

1990: Washington PA status is changed from "registered" to "licensed" by legislative action, with the support of the WSMA. The PA on the Board of Medical Examiners is given full voting privileges.

1991: Again by legislative action, with the support of the WSMA, a PA is added to the Medical Disciplinary Board and is given full voting privileges.

1993: Washington passes "Single Licensure Law" for PAs, thus increasing the flexibility of PA utilization.

Since 1993, WAPA has worked with the WSMA to introduce, support, and pass various pieces of legislation relating to PA scope of practice. The WAPA delegates in the WSMA House of Delegates raise the issue. Subsequent discussion and successful resolutions allow WSMA lobbyists to introduce PA-supportive legislation and to effectively lobby for these bills along with practicing PAs and their supervising physicians. In 2007, for example, three bills were passed by the Washington State Legislature to clarify the authority of PAs to execute and certify forms for the Department of Labor and Industries and to sign and attest to other state-issued documents, including determination of disability parking privileges.

In the mid-90s, WSMA also authorized a WAPA liaison to their Board of Trustees. This position is in addition to a designated PA seat in the WSMA Interspecialty Council, composed of representatives of all WSMA specialty organizations. In addition, WAPA leadership has access to WSMA leadership training opportunities, including an annual leadership retreat.

Interactions with Nurse Practitioners

The changing health care system, as well as common concerns for access and primary care services, encourages alliances between PA and NPs—at academic, clinical, and individual levels. These alliances are facilitated by what is now a clearer definition of similarities and differences between the two groups. Although NPs regard "independent practice" as an essential feature of the professional identity of nursing, PAs continue to believe that "independence through dependence" and strong relationships with physician preceptors are essential features of their profession. NPs have chosen to define themselves by advanced academic degrees as a justification of independent practice and have recently made a decision to move to a Doctorate in Nursing Practice. PAs recognize the NCCPA examination as the gold standard of their profession. The NP applicant pool is almost totally limited to individuals with nursing degrees, whereas PAs have broader entry criteria encompassing both first-career and second-career individuals. Both groups believe that competent nonphysician providers can increase access to care, especially primary care services. Both groups believe that nonphysician providers are part of the cost-effective solution to our health care crisis. Each group can benefit from a better understanding of the other's education/training and practice issues. Ongoing interactions between PAs and NPs, particularly in recognition of their similarities and differences, benefit all of us (Table 1-6).

CONCLUSION

The social change theory, which holds that "it takes society 30 years, more or less, to absorb a new technology into everyday life,"[37] can be applied to PAs. Created during a time of chaos within the health care system, the PA profession is now, more than ever, a solution to access, efficiency, and economic problems in health care. Although consumers are not yet 100% informed about PAs, more and more have been the recipients of PA care. Evolving health care delivery systems—with emphasis on quality and efficiency—require that PAs be part of the provider mix. The range of opportunities for PA employment is limitless in both primary care and the specialties. International applications of the PA movement, including demonstration projects and the creation of educational programs, create opportunities to increase global health care access. Maintaining a flexible, responsive stance will continue to be the most important strategy for the PA profession—domestically and internationally.

TABLE 1-6 **PAs and NPs**

	Nurse Practitioners	Physician Assistants
Students	BSN nurses	Wide range of experienced health care personnel
Gold standard	Degrees	National certifying examination
Model and language	Nursing	Medical
Educators/role models	NPs, nursing educators	Physicians, PAs
Licensure	Board of Nursing	Board of Medicine
Legal	Independent	Dependent
Scope of practice	Specific	Negotiated
Value added	"Caring Approach"	Physician-PA Relationship Medical Education Continuity

CLINICAL APPLICATIONS

1. Research the history of the PA profession in your state. What, if any, was the involvement of the state medical association in the creation of the practice "environment"? Who were the key PAs in the formation of the state academy? If one does not exist, prepare a chronological list of state academy presidents and conference locations.
2. Keep a longitudinal diary of the issues that are your personal, local, state, regional, and national concerns regarding the PA profession. These might include specific licensure or reimbursement issues, or even your personal reflections on the changes occurring across time. Use this diary as a personal history of your PA career. You might want to include your successful application to PA school as the first item in this diary.
3. Review the issues raised in Case Study 1-1. Identify an international setting with a health workforce shortage and consider how you might adapt the PA profession, as you understand it, to the needs of that setting.

KEY POINTS

- The PA concept has its roots in similar roles first created in Russia by Peter the Great (feldshers) and in China (barefoot doctors). In addition, roles such as the Purser's Mate in the U.S. Merchant Marine and informal physician extender roles in the offices of individual physicians paved the way for the American Medical Association* to consider a new role in American medicine.

- Several models of PA training and practice eventually coalesced into the PA that we know today. Duke University focused on an academic medical center role, the MEDEX program trained PAs to work in rural and underserved communities with an emphasis on primary care, the University of Colorado created a pediatric role, Alderson Broadus worked to recruit individuals from small Appalachian communities, and the University of Alabama designed a surgical program. The PA movement is supported by four distinct organizations—each with its own well-defined role: The American Academy of Physician Assistants (AAPA), the Physician Assistant Education Association (PAEA), formerly known as the Association of Physician Assistant Programs (APAP), the National Commission on Certification of Physician Assistants (NCCPA), and the Accreditation Review Commission on Education for Physician Assistants (ARC-PA.)

*Medical schools and physician organizations, such as the AMA, were strong supporters of the PA concept and provided input into accreditation, certification, and the development of regulatory processes.

References

1. Fortuine R. Chills and Fevers: Health and Disease in the Early History of Alaska. Fairbanks: University of Alaska Press; 1992.
2. Sidel VW. Feldshers and feldsherism: the role and training of the feldsher in the USSR. N Engl J Med 1968;278:935.
3. Storey PB. The Soviet feldsher as a physician's assistant. Washington, DC: Geographic Health Studies Program; 1972, US Dept of Health, Education, and Welfare Publication No. (NIH), p. 72–58.
4. Roemer MI. Health Care Systems in World Perspective. Ann Arbor, MI: Health Administration Press; 1975.
5. Perry HB, Breitner B. Physician Assistants: Their Contribution to Health Care. New York: Human Sciences Press; 1982.
6. Basch PF. International Health. New York: Oxford University Press; 1978.
7. Dimond EG. Village health care in China. In: McNeur RW, (ed). Changing Roles and Education of Health Care Personnel Worldwide in View of the Increase in Basic Health Services. Philadelphia: Society for Health and Human Values; 1978.
8. Gifford JF. The development of the physician assistant concept. In: Alternatives in Health Care Delivery: Emerging Roles for Physician Assistants. St Louis: Warren H. Green; 1984.
9. Fisher DW, Horowitz SM. The physician assistant: profile of a new health profession. In: Bliss AA, Cohen ED, (eds). The New Health Professionals: Nurse Practitioners and Physician's Assistants. Germantown, MD: Aspen Systems Corp; 1977.
10. Carter RD, Gifford JF. The emergence of the physician assistant profession. In: Perry HB, Breitner B, (eds). Physician Assistants: Their Contribution to Health Care. New York: Human Sciences Press; 1982.
11. Estes EH. Historical perspectives—how we got here: lessons from the past, applied to the future. In: Physician Assistants: Present and Future Models of Utilization. New York: Praeger; 1986.
12. Sadler AM, Sadler BL, Bliss AA. The Physician's Assistant Today and Tomorrow. New Haven, CT: Yale University; 1972.
13. Howard R. Physician Support Personnel in the 70s: New Concepts. In: Burzek J, (ed). Chicago: American Medical Association; 1971.
14. Smith RA, Vath RE. A strategy for health manpower: reflections on an experience called MEDEX. JAMA 1971;217:1365.
15. Smith RA. MEDEX. JAMA 1970;211:1843.
16. Myers H. The Physician's Assistant. Parson, WV: McClain Printing Company; 1978.
17. Silver HK. The syniatrist. JAMA 1971;217:1368.
18. Stead EA. Debate over PA profession's name rages on. J Am Acad Physician Assist 1992;6:459.
19. Cawley JF. Federal health policy and PAs: two decades of government support have contributed to professional growth. J Am Acad Physician Assist 1992;5:682.
20. Weissman E, Tucker C, (eds). Association of American Medical Colleges, 2011 Annual Report. 2012. p. 5–7.
21. Glazer DL. National Commission on Certification of Physician's Assistants: a precedent in collaboration. In: Bliss AA, Cohen ED, (eds). The New Health Professionals: Nurse Practitioners and Physician's Assistants. Germantown, MD: Aspen Systems Corp; 1977.
22. National Commission on Certification of Physician Assistants. Specialty Certificates of Added Qualifications (CAQs). *http://www.nccpa.net/SpecialtyCAQs.aspx*. Accessed December 5, 2011.
23. Stanhope WD. The roots of the AAPA: the AAPA's first president remembers the milestones and accomplishments of the Academy's first decade. J Am Acad Physician Assist 1993;5:675.
24. American Academy of Physician Assistants. Constitution and bylaws. Membership Directory 1997-1998. Alexandria, VA: American Academy of Physician Assistants; 1997.
25. American Academy of Physician Assistants. *http://www.aapa.org/pa-foundation*. Accessed December 5, 2011.
26. Stead EA. Conserving costly talents: providing physicians' new assistants. JAMA 1966;19:182.
27. Light JA, Crain MJ, Fisher DW. Physician assistant: a profile of the profession, 1976. PAJ 1977;7:111.
28. Selected Findings from the Secondary Analysis. 1981 National Survey of Physician Assistants. Rosslyn, VA: American Academy of Physician Assistants; 1981.
29. American Medical Association. Annual report on medical education in the United States, 1987-88. JAMA 1988;260:8.
30. Webb R. Minorities and the PA movement. Physician Assist 1977;2:14.
31. Stalker TA. IOM report: the recommendations and what they mean. Health Pract Physician Assist 1978;2:25.
32. Schafft GE, Cawley JF. The Physician Assistant in a Changing Health Care Environment. Rockville, MD: Aspen Publishers; 1987.
33. Physician Assistants for the Future. An In-depth Study of PA Education and Practice in the Year 2000. Alexandria, VA: Association of Physician Assistant Programs; 1989.
34. A Symposium: The Future of Health Care: Challenges and Choices, Executive Summary. Alexandria, VA: American Academy of Physician Assistants; 1984.
35. Physician Assistants in the Health Workforce, 1994. Rockville, MD: Bureau of Health Professions, Health Resources and Services Administration; 1994.
36. AAPA House of Delegates. AAPA Policy Manual, H-P-200.2.1 and H-P-200.2.2. Adopted 2000.
37. Cringely RX. Accidental Empires. New York: Harper Collins; 1993.

The resources for this chapter can be found at www.expertconsult.com.

CHAPTER 2

International Development of the Physician Assistant Profession

David H. Kuhns

CHAPTER CONTENTS

The physician assistant (PA) profession was created more than 40 years ago, rooted firmly in the U.S. military medical training model and influenced by "genetic links" from the Chinese barefoot doctors and the Russian feldshers. It is fascinating to now observe how, from these humble sources, the seeds of the PA profession have been dispersed around the world. Perhaps it is the timing, that now, when the need for skilled medical providers continues to grow worldwide, the harsh economic realities reinforce the idea that not everyone can become a doctor, nor can everyone afford to have a doctor treat every ailment. Jane Farmer's evaluation of the Scottish PA pilot considered the international PA movement by saying that "the current wave of international development in deploying and training PAs can . . . be viewed in alternative ways. First, it could be viewed as a "fashion." The PA profession is neatly packaged, emanates from the United States (as many health system fashions do), has some assiduous "product champions," and is promoted in a panacea-like way. Alternatively, PAs can be viewed as *the* profession, designed as uniquely adaptable (i.e., moving from the United States to other parts of the world at this time *expressly because* it can meet the world's current health workforce gaps).[1] This chapter reviews international PAs that are analogs of the American PA model and therefore knowingly excludes many other nonphysician clinicians (NPCs) who contribute substantially to health care delivery around the world. It is important to acknowledge that no slight is intended by this distinction. Rather, it is my attempt to say the role of all NPCs, including PAs, is on a continuum. NPCs can be viewed as either complementing existing health services provided or actually substituting NPC services for those usually done by physicians, especially in the developing countries. This chapter focuses on those models that are complementing existing services.

It is also important to acknowledge that this is intended as an overview of the current state of affairs. It is not intended to be a comprehensive, in-depth report on the PA model worldwide.

The chapter first examines those countries where either, after 10 years of experience, rapid and significant advances are being made or the concept is so nascent that there is little to report. Then, with a case-study approach, the chapter explores some of the common and diverse issues and challenges faced as the PA model evolves.

THE NETHERLANDS

In the 11 years since the first PA students started in 2001 at the University of Applied Sciences in Utrecht, the Dutch PA profession has grown to a population of more than 800. There are also 140 students annually across Utrecht and four other training programs: HAN University of Applied Sciences in Arnhem/Nijmegen, Holland University of Applied Sciences in Amsterdam, Hanze University of Applied Sciences in Groningen, and Rotterdam University. The 30-month national curriculum differs from other traditional international PA models in the integration of their didactic and clinical education. While students are learning the core knowledge and skills required for all PAs, each student simultaneously receives additional clinical expertise in a designated medical specialty by actually working in that area each week. As a result, the PA student has both didactic and clinical days interspersed throughout the duration of their training. Because they are actually working in the clinical area, they are also paid for that work. The education is at the graduate level, and all students must have extensive clinical experience before entry. Fully qualified PAs are known as master physician assistants. Dutch PAs are working across all areas of medicine and, because of their unique approach to their training, are found in subspecialty areas in greater numbers than PAs elsewhere.

Under the leadership from the Netherlands Association of Physician Assistants (NAPA), the Dutch PA profession is making significant advances, the most substantial coming in early 2012 with the inclusion of prescriptive practice and the authorization for PAs to perform technical procedures (i.e., endoscopy and cardioversion), which had previously been limited to doctors. NAPA has become the model for successful implementation of the PA role that other countries can emulate.

NAPA is also at the forefront of efforts to standardize the PA role across the European Union (EU). NAPA leads on the development of the European Physician Assistant Cooperative (EuroPAC), which has the objectives of protecting the title of PA and enabling "professional portability," whereby any European-trained and qualified PA would be granted reciprocity within the other countries of the EU.[2]

INDIA

The Indian Physician Assistant profession, with a focus on training surgical PAs, started in 1992 under the auspices of the Madras Medical Mission, guided by Dr. K. M. Cherian, a renowned cardiac surgeon (G. Sundar, e-mail, October 10, 2011). Today, 20 years later, there are more than 500 qualified PAs and seven PA programs, either university based or hospital based. At the time of their qualification, Indian PAs are, on average, between ages 22 and 24 years and are evenly split by gender.

Like the American experience, there are different academic credentials associated with Indian PA training. Programs range in length from 2 to 4 years. They also vary from baccalaureate, to postgraduate diploma (as per the U.K. approach), to a master's level degree. Regardless of the degree offered, Indian PA programs follow an American-style PA curriculum, but they have adapted it to fit the specific needs of their medical system. As a result, there are apparently no PAs working in primary care. Instead, most are working in cardiology, cardiac surgery, general inpatient medicine, or neurology.[3]

GERMANY

With three 3-year baccalaureate programs in science PA in Germany in 2012, there are students in the pipeline but no graduates yet. The programs are Duale Hochschule Baden-Württemberg in Karlsruhe, the Steinbeis-Hochschule in Berlin, and the Mathias Hochschule in Rheine. Because it is still so early in the evolution of the German PA, there is no formal registration for or recognition of the PA. However, it is anticipated that graduate PAs will work under the delegatory capacity allowed under current German law.[4]

SAUDI ARABIA

The first PA program in the Middle East, offered by the Medical Services Directorate of Ministry of Defense and Aviation in The Kingdom of Saudi Arabia, was launched in September 2010 at the Prince Sultan Military College of Health Professions in Dharhan, Saudi Arabia. A team of experienced American PA educators follows a traditional American-style PA model curriculum, with a 28-month postgraduate curriculum. The program, a collaborative effort with the Prince Sultan Military College of Health Sciences and the George Washington University Medical Faculty Associates in the Department of Emergency Medicine, trains 40 PAs per year, with their eventual deployment across all divisions of the Saudi military. This is expected to be the first of several PA programs for the country. The first class will graduate in February 2013 (A. Keim, personal correspondence, January 2012).[5]

Of particular interest is that Saudi PAs will in fact be known as *APs*, as in *assistant physicians*, because of an issue with how the original physician assistant title is translated into Arabic.

AFGHANISTAN

Afghanistan, with a history of more than 30 years of armed conflict and with the resulting extensive disruption of the national medical infrastructure, is one of the most underresourced health systems in the world. With only 2.1 physicians per 10,000 population, compared with a regional average of 11 physicians per 10,000 population,[6] the need to quickly increase the overall size of the health workforce is essential.

As part of the effort to address some of these inequities, the NATO Training Mission in Afghanistan developed a PA course, which was launched in October 2010. The primary goals of this program are to both increase the overall numbers of clinicians and to improve the skill levels of the clinicians in the Afghan National Army.

The Afghan PA program, located at the National Military Hospital Compound in Kabul, offers a 12-month didactic curriculum, derived from existing U.S. and Canadian military medical courses and then augmented with a month-long pharmacology course. In addition, there is a 16-week clinical phase, offering experience in "sick call" and emergency medicine/trauma. A Tactical Combat Care Course will complete the training, with the expectation that PAs will be ready to face the challenges of providing medical care in a war zone.[7]

It is expected that they will eventually graduate 65 qualified PAs per cohort. Of particular note is that the program has both male and female students. Although female PAs will not be part of active combat units, they will work in district military hospitals.

According to Canadian Forces PA, Master Warrant Officer Kelly Humphreys, who serves as PA Adviser to the Armed Forces Academy of Medical Sciences (AFMAS), "the AFMAS PA program could address many of their health care shortfalls in the urban areas, as well as out in the more remote locations" (K. Humphreys, e-mail, November 19, 2011).

(Plans are under way for expansion of the PA model into the civilian medical system in Afghanistan as well.)

SOUTH AFRICA

The Physician Assistant equivalents in South Africa are called *clinical associates* (CAs), a concept first considered by the National Health Council in 2002. CAs were formally introduced by their Health Ministry in 2008 as a means to address chronic health workforce shortages, especially in rural and otherwise underserved areas of the country. The "brain drain" of the medical workforce of South Africa had resulted in a loss of almost 40% of their doctors through emigration in the past 15 years.

The Twinning Project, funded by the U.S. government through both the President's Emergency Plan for AIDS Relief (PEPFAR) and the Centers for Disease Control/South Africa and administered through the American International Health Alliance, was launched in 2010 and "twinned" South African Clinical Associate schools with American PA programs.[8] As a result, Walter Sisulu University (in the Eastern Cape Province) is twinned with the University of Colorado, the University of Pretoria with Arcadia University, and the University of Witwatersrand (in Johannesburg) with Emory University. These initiatives allow for the exchange of the expertise of long-standing American PA programs with the newly developed South African institutions. In addition, there are faculty and student exchanges.

All CA programs follow a 3-year curriculum, which is competency based and delivered in a variety of formats. This leads to a bachelor of clinical medical practice degree. Qualified CAs are registered with the Health Professions Council of South Africa. The first cohorts of CAs graduated in January 2011 and are now working in district hospitals. (Perhaps it is because the South African government is driving the CA project that it has faced fewer challenges than other international PA projects.)

CASE STUDIES

Canada

As of January 2012 there were about 370 Canadian certified physician assistants (CCPAs), who trained through either a Canadian or an American program. The first three civilian university-level PA training programs started in 2008, joining with the longer established Canadian Forces PA program; combined they produce 80 new graduates per year. The Canadian PA model was developed first in the military as an advanced medical technician called a *medical assistant* during the Korean War; the training transitioned to the present PA concept in 1984.[9]

In the civilian health care sector PAs are already regulated professionals in some provinces, whereas in other provinces so-called demonstration projects, meant to show PA effectiveness, are under development. Meanwhile, the PA role in the civilian sector is expanding, especially as new initiatives are under way to enhance existing medical services and to decrease wait times.

The Canadian PA is a health care clinician academically and nationally qualified to provide medical services to patients in a wide range of settings and in a variety of roles. All PAs work in collaboration with a physician; the scope of practice is determined by observations, comfort levels, and in the negotiated role required of the physician practice and PA qualification. The scope of practice is summarized as those duties authorized by a physician that the physician is qualified to perform and is comfortable delegating. A PA can collect a history, order appropriate diagnostics, reach a differential diagnosis, and prescribe appropriate treatment.[10]

Each province has its own medical act that further delineates the degree of delegation and supervisory requirements. For example, Manitoba first introduced PAs in 1999, under the title of CA. In 2009, those regulations were amended to permit practice under the title of PA. Also in 2009, the College of Physicians and Surgeons of New Brunswick amended the New Brunswick Medical Act (1981) to include PAs. Alberta is the only Canadian Province with a voluntary PA (nonregulated) registry that is held by the College of Physicians and Surgeons of Alberta. Efforts are currently under way to regulate PAs in Ontario, where they currently practice under the supervision of a physician and are only able to perform controlled acts under delegation.

The highest concentration of PAs (50%) in Canada is found in Ontario. What had started as the first emergency medicine projects in 2007 has since expanded to include various demonstration projects in family medicine and community health teams, medical and surgical specialties, and long-term care facilities.[11] New Brunswick has introduced PAs into emergency departments. Alberta has several pilot projects introducing PAs into occupational industrial medicine.

In 2003, the Canadian Medical Association (CMA) Board of Directors approved an application from the Canadian Association of Physician Assistants (CAPA) to include PAs within the CMA accreditation process (CMA Acceditation Report). The CMA first accredited the PA program delivered by the Canadian Forces Medical Services School in 2004. As part of the professional recognition requirements, CAPA structured the Physician Assistants Certification Council of Canada (PACCC) to establish an independent national certification examination and registry. The first national examination was held in 2005. In 2009, CAPA refined their *National Competency Profile and PA Scope of Practice*. The national competency profile (NCP) defines the core competencies that a generalist PA should possess on graduation and is the accepted standard in Canada.[12]

The PA profession, still in the early stages, has a solid foundation and is expected to continue to grow throughout the Canadian health care system (Fig. 2-1, Table 2-1).

Australia

Despite a high standard of living and a health care system rated as one of the best in the world, Australia struggles with a relative shortage of doctors, particularly in rural, indigenous, and public health sectors. To put this into context, first consider the demographics of the "Land Down Under": it has a population of approximately 22.5 million people living on a surface area not much smaller than the United States. Six states and two territories are united into the Commonwealth of Australia. The majority of the population dwells in five southeastern (capital) cities and the

Numbers of Enrolled and Graduated Students Reported by the Canadian PA Education Programs

Academic Institution/Length of Training	Program Inception	No. Graduating Classes (No. Students Graduated per Year)	Total Graduates as of January 2012
University of Manitoba/26 months	August 2008	2010 (10), 2011 (13)	23
McMaster University/24 months	September 2008	2010 (21), 2011 (24)	45
Canadian Forces Health Services Training Centre/24 months	September 2002	2004 (24), 2005 (22), 2006 (21), 2007 (14), 2008 (20), 2009 (23), 2010 (22), 2011 (19),	163
The Consortium of PA Education (University of Toronto, Northern Ontario School of Medicine, and Michener Institute of Applied Health)/24 months	January 2010	Course of Study completed in January 2012; inaugural graduation: June 2012	17

From Jones I. President's Report 2011 Canadian Association of Physician Assistants, Oct 29, 2011.

surrounding metropolitan areas. Eighty-five percent of the population occupies just 1% to 2% of the landmass. The remaining 15% of people live in regional cities or rural and remote environments. There are vast areas of outback or "the bush," with low population density, minimal infrastructure, and poor access to goods and services including health care.[13]

Australia's Department of Health and Aging, charged with setting national health policy, established Medicare as a comprehensive health care system that facilitates access by all eligible Australian residents to either free or low-cost medical and public hospital care; supplemental insurance coverage also allows for utilization of private health services.[13]

Like many developed nations, Australia relies heavily on international medical graduates (IMGs), with 43% of doctors currently working being foreign born.[13] Rural health care is especially dependent on IMGs, who represent more than 40% of all rural general practitioners (GPs).[14]

The PA prototype, having been under study since 1999, is especially viewed as being able to address those sectors that are especially strained: rural and remote settings, indigenous communities, the military, and urban public health facilities.[4] Despite this, proponents have made minimal progress, due in large part to federal and state politics, as well as a complicated, insular health care bureaucracy. Opposition from the Australian Medical Association (AMA), the Queensland Nurses Union (QNU), and the Australian Medical Student Association (AMSA) has also slowed momentum. Some of their concerns are understandable and often bear a noteworthy similarity to criticisms voiced early in the development of the PA profession in the United States. However, the AMA bases its fears on the potential for compromised quality of care and possible threats to patient safety, as well as increased competition for already oversubscribed clinical training resources by medical schools.[15]

In response to increasing demand and the worsening shortage of doctors, the subsequent expansion of the number of medical schools already places additional strain on existing clinical training sites and supervisors. A high attrition rate of doctors from the baby boomer generation, coupled with a declining number of entrants into general practice and an unwillingness of young doctors to adopt the lifestyles of their predecessors or practice outside major metropolitan areas, will continue to aggravate ongoing health care manpower inadequacies, in particular rural and remote general practice.[16]

It has not been all doom and gloom for the PA concept in Australia but more a case of two steps forward, one step back. Two independently evaluated pilot studies completed in South Australia and Queensland in 2010 found the PA model had no negative impact on junior doctor training opportunities and actually augmented the medical education experience in some cases.[17]

Under the direction of American PA educator Karen Mulitalo, the University of Queensland (UQ) rolled out the first PA program in mid-2009. The initial students were pioneers, committing to the challenging curriculum without governing policy or regulations in place at any level. Regrettably, just before graduating the inaugural class in June

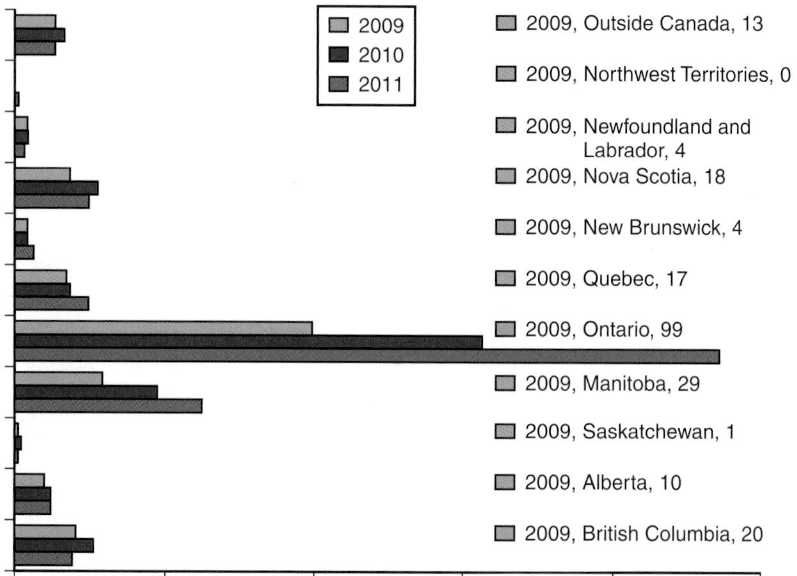

FIGURE 2-1 Province of clinical practice and number of physician assistants. (From Jones I. President's Report 2011 Canadian Association of Physician Assistants, Oct 29, 2011.)

2011, UQ opted to close the PA Program, effective immediately following graduation of the second class in June 2012. Mostly blamed on financial shortfalls, but undoubtedly influenced by political opposition, the decision was disappointing but not totally unexpected. Preserving some measure of hope for the program, the Head of School, Medicine, stated that, "if commitment to the development of a physician assistant workforce arises, the University will give serious consideration to reactivating the program."

Confident that the PA concept remains viable, James Cook University (JCU) School of Medicine & Dentistry (SMD) in Townsville, Queensland, launched a PA program in January 2012. Like UQ, this endeavor is also under the auspices of two American PA educators. The 3-year *course*, as it is called, has a focus on providing PAs to rural, remote, tropical, and indigenous locations. In contrast to the classic self-contained U.S. PA program the course is fully integrated into the SMD, sharing staff and resources. In turn, both PA educators carry responsibilities for portions of the medical student curriculum. The PA curriculum is delivered in a blended format, combining six intensive (2-week) campus residential blocks over the first 24 months interspersed with distance-based learning. The third year will consist of clinical training. The course is designed for mature health care professionals with extensive clinical experience; the average age of the first cohort ($n = 20$) is 41. Academic leaders at James Cook have further demonstrated support of PA competency by employing a third American PA to work exclusively with medical students.

With its emphasis on rural and remote health, tropical medicine, and the health of indigenous Australians, James Cook University is recognized internationally for its involvement in socially responsible medical education. It is thus particularly well suited to house a PA curriculum that has a mission of bettering health care for underserved populations. Several other institutions including Edith Cowan University in Perth, Western Australia, and the University of Adelaide in South Australia continue to monitor the situation and consider a possible launch of PA courses in the future.

In addition to the completion of the pilots and the presence of two educational courses, there have been other positive events. Even though PAs are not yet formally recognized, employment is occurring at a grassroots level, with PAs currently employed in aboriginal health, refugee health, hospital-based surgical service, and orthopedics. At this early phase of the PA profession, they still lack access to Medicare billing and are not yet able to prescribe.

TABLE 2-1 Timeline of Canadian Physician Assistant Development

Year	Event
1984	The Canadian Forces expands the capability of the medical assistant, paving the way for the development of the physician assistant model.
1990	The idea of the physician assistant (PA) was further promoted in a time of limited resources within the military structure.
1992	Canadian Forces adopts the term PA for senior med tech.
1998	Strategic Planning in the Department of National Defence *Project Rx2000* recognizes that the role of the military PA needs to be standardized for integration into the civilian health care environment.
1999	Manitoba Medical Act designates clinical assistants including PAs as certified clinical assistants
1999	Canadian Academy of Physician Assistants is chartered.
2003	The Canadian Medical Association recognizes the PA as a "health care professional."
2003	First formally recognized civilian PA begins work in Manitoba.
2004	Canadian Forces Health Services Training Centre (CFHSTC) is granted accreditation of its PA program by the Canadian Medical Association Conjoint Accreditation Process.
2005	CFHSTC inaugurates its first class (16) as an accredited education institution.
2006	*HealthForceOntario (HFO)* project is implemented. Among its many goals is the staffing of emergency departments and clinics with PAs and IMGs working as PAs.
2008	University of Manitoba inaugurates its first class of 12 PA students.
2008	McMaster University inaugurates its first class of 23 PA students.
2009	CAPA (now Canadian *Association* of Physician Assistants) becomes incorporated by *Industry Canada.*
2010	*Consortium for PA Education* (the University of Toronto, the Michener Institute for Applied Health Sciences, and the Northern Ontario School of Medicine) begins its class of 22 students.
2010	Alberta becomes the fourth province to recognize PAs.
2010	University of Manitoba and McMaster University graduate first civilian classes.
2011	Application for regulation in Ontario submitted to the Ontario government.

The most favorable development has been that the Australian College of Rural and Remote Medicine, the first major medical association to officially support PAs in their policy statement of October 2011, urged the continued advancement of the delegated practice model and utilization of PAs. In 2012 PA proponents remain hopeful that upcoming national recommendations for addressing health workforce shortages will advocate strongly for PAs.[18]

United Kingdom

The first PAs to work in the United Kingdom were two expatriate Americans who in 2003 were recruited for primary care posts. They worked in the Black Country, so-called from its days as an industrial hub but now an economically distressed and medically underserved area of England's West Midlands; this area encompasses Birmingham, the United Kingdom's second largest metropolitan area.

Initial efforts by the British at "growing their own" PAs started in 2002 with pilot training programs for what was called health care practitioners (HCPs) at St. George's University of London and Kingston University. The HCP model then evolved into the medical care practitioner (MCP). The first U.K. PA program was started at the University of Wolverhampton in 2004. The first substantive PA programs, as defined by class size, were launched in 2007 when the University of Birmingham and University of Wolverhampton each started with cohorts of 15 or more, and St. George's in London relaunched with a similar sized cohort in 2009. These programs follow a national curriculum and are taught at the postgraduate diploma (PgDip) level.[19]

A setback to the British PA movement was the closure of the PA program at the University of Birmingham in 2011, the consequence of loss of the original champions within the university hierarchy and opposition from certain quarters within the local National Health Service. The University of Wolverhampton's program was suspended at the same time, but, as of January 2012, it is anticipated that it will resume within the year. Meanwhile, the St. George's program in London has doubled its entry cohort, and a new program was launched in October 2011 at the University of Aberdeen, Scotland. As a result, there is no expected decrease of overall PA student numbers across the United Kingdom.

U.K.-trained PAs were originally expected to work in primary care, which at the time was anticipating a significant shortage of workers in underserved areas. Accordingly, the Competency and Curriculum Framework developed by the Department of Health was focused on primary care. However, implementation of the European Working Time Directive significantly limited work hours for doctors in training to less than 48 hours per week. As a result, the demand has grown for PAs to work in hospital and specialty practices, while fewer are working in general practice (outpatient medicine). Revisions to the CCF are presently under way to reflect the shift to a broader approach, including hospital-based practice.[20] Despite a decade of PAs working in the National Health Service, there is still no official recognition or registration of PAs by the British government. The professional organization for British PAs, U.K. Association of Physician Assistants (ukapa.co.uk), has developed an interim measure, a "managed voluntary register" as a means of identifying the PA workforce; it provides the necessary continuing education British PAs need to maintain their qualification. Until officially recognized, British PAs face the hardship of not having prescriptive practice, thus limiting their overall effectiveness. Despite these challenges, demand for PAs continues to increase. As of January 2012, there are about 150 PAs in the United Kingdom, including about 20 Americans and at least 1 Canadian.

There is an initial qualifying examination, akin to the Physician Assistant National Certifying Exam (PANCE) in the United States. The British version is a two-part process, a 200-question multiple-choice examination and 16-station Objective Structured Clinical Examination (OSCE). Of significance is that the 90% of the written examination is derived from a subset of the National Commission on Certification of Physician Assistants (NCCPA) question bank, which has then been edited, reviewed, and validated by both British PAs working clinically and PA academics. Minor changes were made to language and laboratory values in order to make the questions appropriate to the British medical system. Inclusion of these American questions recognizes that there is a core of medical knowledge that is shared by all PAs, in any country. It is for that reason that Australia is developing a similar examination model using the NCCPA test bank.

WHERE NEXT?

Many other countries, including New Zealand, Japan, Singapore, China, Belgium, France, Spain, Ireland, Switzerland, and Bulgaria, have expressed varying degrees of interest and enthusiasm in the PA model. The coming years will likely continue the further development of the PA role as nations look for ways to address the growing demands on their medical delivery system and explore options to achieve a cost-effective and efficient health care system.

KEY POINTS

- The PA profession is in various states of development in numerous countries in the world. Important issues in their utilization include structures for education, certification, and regulation.
- Case studies of PAs in Canada, Australia, and the United Kingdom provide examples of the profession in three early stages of development. The U.S. experience has provided role models and guidance for each of these developments through the "export" of U.S. PAs and U.S. PA educators who have assisted in the adaptation of the concept to the needs of the specific countries.
- In addition to the development of PA educational programs, the successful implementation of the PA concept in other countries includes issues of funding, deployment, and regulation, which all need careful consideration.

ACKNOWLEDGMENTS

A debt of gratitude is owed to the following contributors to this document:
Ruth Ballweg, MPA, PA-C, Associate Professor and Section Chief MEDEX Northwest PA Section, University of Washington, Seattle, Washington
Michael Dryer, PA-C, DrPH, Chair Department of Medical Science and Community Health, Arcadia University, Glenside, PA
Allen Forde, PA-C, MPAS, Senior Lecturer, James Cook University School of Medicine & Dentistry, Townesville, Australia
Anita Duhl Glicken, MSW, Associate Dean for Physician Assistant Studies, University of Colorado School of Medicine, Director, CHA/PA Program, Denver, Colorado
K.D. Humphreys, CD, CCPA, Master Warrant Officer, Canadian Forces, PA Advisor, National Military Hospital, Kabul, Afghanistan
Ian W Jones, MPAS, PA-C, CCPA, Program Director University of Manitoba Physician Assistant Education Program, Past President, Canadian Association of Physician Assistants

References

1. Farmer J, Curry M, West C, et al. Evaluation of Physician Assistants to NHS Scotland 2009, *http://www.abdn.ac.uk/crh/uploads/files/PA%20Final%20report%20Jan%2009%20version%205.pdf*; Accessed December 2011.
2. Merkle F, Ritsema T, Bauer S, et al. The physician assistant: shifting the Paradigm of European medical practice? HSR Proceedings in Intensive Care and Cardiovascular Anesthesia 2011;3(4): 255.
3. Indian Association of Physician Assistants website. *http://www.iapaonline.org*; Accessed December 10, 2011.
4. Duale Hochschule Baden-Württemberg Karlsruhe/Baden-Württemberg Cooperative State University Karlsruhe. *http://www.dhbw-karlsruhe.de/allgemein/newssingle/article/studiengang- physician-assistantarztassistent-organisiert-tagung/64/*; Accessed October 12, 2012.
5. Kuhns D, Tozier W, Hearn D. Physician Assistants and Military Medical Services (Poster) for the Annual Conference of the American Academy of Physician Assistants, Las Vegas, June 1-4, 2011.
6. World Health Organization. *http://www.who.int/gho/countries/afg.pdf*; Accessed November 20, 2011.
7. NATO Training Mission—Afghanistan. *http://ntm-a.com/wordpress2/archives/2175*; Accessed November 20, 2011.
8. Clinical Associates website. *http://www.twinningagainstaids.org/documents/CABoolketFinal_lowres.pdf*; Accessed January 4, 2012.
9. Hooker R, MacDonald K, Patterson R. Physician Assistants in the Canadian Forces. Mil Med 2003;168(11):948.
10. Canadian Association of Physician Assistants. Scope of Practice and National Competency Profile. Ottawa: Canadian Association of Physician Assistants, 2009.
11. Mikhael N, Ozon P, Rhule C. Defining the Physician Assistant Role in Ontario. Toronto: HealthForce Ontario, 2007.
12. Jones IW, Hooker RS. Physician assistants in Canada: update on health policy initiatives. Can Fam Physician 2011;57:e83.
13. Australia. Federal Court. Australian Government, Department of Foreign Affairs and Trade. *http://www.dfat.gov.au/facts/healthcare.html*.
14. Gorman DF, Brooks PM. On solutions to the shortage of doctors in Australia and New Zealand. Med J Aust 2009;190(3):152.
15. Forde A, O'Connor T. Augmenting the rural health workforce with physician assistants. Tenth National Rural Health Conference paper, 2009.
16. Forde A, et al. Should Australian Universities Be Producing Physician Assistants? Informational paper distributed to the Medical Deans of Australia and New Zealand Annual Conference. Alice Springs: Flinders University, 2009.
17. Evaluation of the Queensland Physician`s Assistant Pilot—Final Report. *www.health.qld.gov.au/publications/pa_eval_final.pdf*; Accessed October 12, 2012.
18. Position Statement on Physician Assistants. Australian College of Rural and Remote Medicine, October 2011.
19. UK Association of Physician Assistants website. *www.ukapa.co.uk*; Accessed October 12, 2012.
20. Merkle F, Ritsema T, Bauer S, et al. The physician assistant: shifting the Paradigm of European medical practice? HSR Proceedings in Intensive Care and Cardiovascular Anesthesia 2011;3(4):255.

CHAPTER 3

EDUCATION

Dawn Morton-Rias • Jim Hammond

CHAPTER CONTENTS

In this chapter, some of the characteristics of physician assistant (PA) education and contributions made by PA educators during the past three decades are presented. The views presented are based on the authors' experiences as PAs participating in PA education from the 1970s to the present. This chapter portrays PA education as a vibrant, creative, and responsive component of professional health care education.

PA education is a powerful force affecting the future of the profession. The influence of education lies in the determination of what knowledge, skills, and attitudes will be presented to PAs during the formative, student stage of their careers. The first responsibility of PA education is to be responsive to the needs of society.

PA education was founded by and resides within universities, which dedicate themselves to responding to the needs of society, not to the needs of a particular profession. For the PA profession to succeed, it must respond to society. This response is most effective when all members of the profession are working toward the same goals.

Four time periods are considered in this chapter discussion: the mid-1960s through the 1970s, the

1980s, the 1990s, and the 2000s. Within each period, four factors are examined, as follows:

- Social forces influencing the period
- Key features of PA education
- Characteristics of PA educators
- Attributes of PA students

THE MID-1960s THROUGH THE 1970s—PIONEER PERIOD

Social Forces

Before the PA profession existed, and thus before PA education was born, society needed improved access to quality medical care. Across the country, a few visionaries responded to this need and dreamed of creating a new type of medical provider who could extend the service of physicians. Working with physicians, these new providers would perform the most fundamental yet complex tasks in medicine—the diagnosis, treatment, and prevention of a wide array of diseases and disorders—not commonly done by nursing or allied health professionals. They would improve access to medical care and make care available to rural and underserved populations. They would counsel and educate patients and their families. They would provide the same quality of services performed by physicians. The new providers would begin work after about 2 years of medical education. They might or might not have any previous health care education or experience. It was quite a set of dreams.

To understand how these dreams originated, a historical perspective is necessary. The forces for change in society during the 1960s were as great as at any time since the Great Depression. Hundreds of thousands of people openly demonstrated for equal rights, equal economic opportunities, personal recognition, and a better place in society. Tens of millions more quietly hoped for these changes. Millions of others resisted change. Fears that the fabric of American society was being rent were repeated daily by news commentators and civic leaders. A mix of fear and hope was visible on faces across the strata of society. Among the many responses of the state and federal government was the declaration of war—a war on poverty and inequality.

Within this context of broad social change came a dramatic expansion of health care delivery. Medicare and Medicaid were born. These two programs provided the means by which millions could obtain health care, which previously had been out of reach. Millions of new patients entered this health care nonsystem. An already stretched medical profession could not meet the demand. Many of the newly enfranchised people resided in rural and inner city areas, the very areas with the fewest physicians.

The dreamers were compassionate, creative individuals who sought answers to society's needs. For every PA program, there was at least one visionary founder. By 1971, the U.S. Department of Health, Education, and Welfare reported that 80 institutions were pursuing the development of PA programs.[1] Some of these institutions did not open programs; others opened and closed them after only a few years of operation. By the end of the 1970s, the number of programs had stabilized at about 50.

It was one thing to dream the dreams. It was another to bring them to reality. For this, the dreams were entrusted to educators.

Education

The designers of PA educational programs required answers to a number of key questions:

- What segments of the population would this new type of provider serve?
- What would be the mission, values, and identity of the new providers?
- What would be the role of these new providers?
- What would be their relationship with physicians?
- How does an educational program teach a physician-PA relationship for which no role models exist?
- What should be the depth, breadth, and priorities of the curriculum?
- What should be the length and intensity of the curriculum?
- What backgrounds and characteristics of applicants would be associated with successful students?
- What methods of teaching would be most successful?
- How do educational programs create markets to employ graduates?
- What factors would lead students to choose positions in specialties and geographic areas that would meet the needs of the targeted portions of society?
- How could educational programs create acceptance for the new role among patients, physicians, and other health care professionals?

Although the answers to many of the questions seem apparent now, there was no clarity at the time. The manner in which the educational features were combined and implemented resulted in new approaches to medical education. These approaches were based on a philosophy of educating people to meet a specific societal need, increased availability of quality health care. The values that the early program leaders projected on PA education and subsequently on the profession were strongly service oriented.

Although programs shared a fairly consistent set of goals, they chose a variety of methods to achieve them. Thus, there were different models for PA programs. Even programs sharing the same basic model created variations to meet local needs or to use different resources. This created significant individuality between programs tempered by an equally strong camaraderie.

Given the breadth of their responsibilities, early educators needed vast amounts of energy and a broad set of skills. In addition to persuading universities and medical communities to start a program and participate in this experiment, they had to find the people and funding to make it happen. They designed and implemented curricula that had never been attempted. Before PAs existed, these early educators were frequently called on to describe the PA role to legislators and health policymakers. As meager numbers were educated, it fell to the educators to convince physicians and other employers to hire the newly graduated PAs. Before sufficient PAs became available to lead the profession, the early educators were responsible for establishing methods to ensure the quality of PA education. They did this by forming a national network of PA educational programs that eventually developed into the Association of Physician Assistant Programs (APAP) and by participating in the development of a national accrediting body for PA educational programs, the Committee on Allied Health Education and Accreditation (CAHEA) of the American Medical Association.

As with many new educational endeavors, PA programs went through an initial period of development that was largely experimental. As with most experiments, not all elements proved successful. However, several early features remain prominent within PA education today.

Compact Curriculum

A commonly heard description of PA education is that it is 75% of medical school in 50% of the time. This intensity is necessary to keep educational costs down. Many students also were coming out of the workforce to return to school and sought to reenter the workforce as soon as possible. Several factors made compactness possible:

- All elements of the curriculum had to contribute to meeting the mission of the program. Mission statements identified the role of graduates and the populations the program intended to serve.
- PAs were educated to make professional judgments involving the health and well-being of others. The breadth and depth of the curriculum ensured a foundation in the arts and sciences sufficient to support understanding of the scientific and behavioral components of the medical information.
- Every course was examined to eliminate superfluous content, reduce redundancy, and maintain practicality. Topics were integrated between courses that were offered simultaneously and those sequenced throughout the curriculum.
- The outcome-based philosophy of the program mission was applied to clinical rotations and didactic courses. Courses were designed and students were evaluated against competency-based outcomes delineated in the learning objectives for every course, often for every lecture and clinical experience.
- Practicality was achieved by coursework that required the same processes and skills that would be necessary after graduation. Lecture topics were frequently presented in a case-based format.
- Community participation in PA education increased practicality. Community-based clinicians presented a large portion of the medical lectures. Many programs required clinical rotations away from teaching hospitals and in community settings where students were assigned to precepting physicians whose only teaching responsibility at the time was one PA student. This one-on-one approach increased the intensity of learning and the weight of decision-making for the student. It also allowed the student to perform in all the settings he or she might experience as a graduate, such as an office, a hospital, or a public health clinic.
- Programs used standardized patients to help instruct students in interviewing techniques, history-taking, physical examination, and clinical problem-solving. By the late 1970s, videotaping students to critique their interviewing skills was widespread.
- The utilization of instructors from a wide variety of disciplines exposed students to the multidisciplinary nature of clinical practice.

Diversity of Education

One danger of a compact, intense curriculum was that programs would all adopt identical curricula. Such “sameness” was contrary to the philosophy of

PA education. Several factors guarded against this possibility, as follows:

- With its first set of accreditation standards published in 1971, the accrediting agency firmly established a competency-based approach for PA education.[2] Promotion of diverse educational approaches among programs with insistence on basic standards became a hallmark of PA education. This has continued to breathe vitality and experimentation into PA programs.
- The practice of programs being sponsored by different types of institutions—general universities, hospitals, colleges, and medical schools—helped to ensure a diversity of educational approaches that fostered creativity and expansion of the profession in a multitude of directions.

Psychosocial Emphasis

Many of the early leaders of programs were not physicians. They viewed medical care from a consumer's perspective. They were critical of what they judged to be a lack of interpersonal skills on the part of many physicians. By including strong psychosocial components in the curriculum, they ensured that PA education would not suffer from this deficit.

- Curricula were evaluated and lecturers were chosen to ensure a patient-centered focus.
- Interviewing and counseling skills were given strong emphasis.
- Programs selected students who already had well-developed interpersonal skills.
- This people-centered philosophy was reinforced by example as programs developed extensive support systems to help students cope with the pressures inflicted upon them by the compact, intense educational system.

Devotion to Underserved Populations

This value was part of the foundational philosophy of many programs. It manifested itself in several ways, as follows:

- It was widespread in program mission statements.
- Several programs were specifically designed to educate PAs who would work with inner city, rural poor, or American Indian populations.
- Many programs made strong efforts to recruit and select students from underserved populations in the hope that they would return there to practice.
- A number of programs concentrated the clinical education of students in clinics, hospitals, and public health services devoted to serving the underserved.

Educators

Initially, the PA profession lay in the hands of educators, none of whom were PAs and many of whom were not clinicians. There was, however, some commonness to their sense of mission—determination to make a difference in health care delivery. They did not set out to establish a new profession, but to respond to the needs of society and to actualize the vision of the founders of each program.

These early PA educators came from a variety of backgrounds, including medicine, social work, nursing, biology, and chemistry. Some had been primarily educators, whereas others were clinicians. Although their educational and professional backgrounds varied considerably, some personal characteristics were important to their success. They had a pioneering spirit—strong on conceptualization, doggedly determined to succeed, willing to take personal risks, eager to experiment, and boundless in energy. They were creative people, as well as skilled team builders, with substantial powers of persuasion.

Students

The diversity of both the mission and the educational approach among PA programs resulted in the admission of groups of students with a wide variety of academic and experiential backgrounds. Nonetheless, some generalizations seem relevant.

Because PA was a new profession, it opened new avenues for people already working in health care but looking for a role with greater decision-making responsibility or more direct work with patients. Although many early students had been military corpsmen, PA programs also attracted large numbers of nurses, medical technologists, radiology technologists, respiratory therapists, and others with substantial prior experience who were looking for added knowledge and responsibility.[3] Students with no prior clinical experience were also admitted. Case Study 3-1 provides examples.

Well into the 1970s, most states did not have laws governing the practice of PAs. Students attracted in the early years were risk takers. As they entered PA programs, they knew there was no guarantee that they would be allowed to practice following graduation.

Students in this era often relished the opportunity to serve as pioneers. Following graduation, many established state and national PA organizations addressed professional issues such as quality assurance, worked for passage of legislation enabling practice, and fought for reimbursement. Some became the first generation of PAs to educate other PAs.

1960s: INNOVATIONS IN PHYSICIAN ASSISTANT EDUCATION

- Concepts of assistants doing physician-type tasks are born
- General medicine and specialty education models arise
- A variety of educational approaches are initiated
- Intense, year-around education model is widely used
- Competency-based educational philosophy is adopted
- Programs meet to collaborate

1970s: INNOVATIONS IN PHYSICIAN ASSISTANT EDUCATION

- Use of actors as standardized patients for student training is introduced
- Curricula are designed for both first-career and career-change students
- Multimedia education methods are widely adopted
- Condensed curricula succeed with small-group, seminar-format instruction
- Clinical instruction uses community health sites, home visits, nursing homes, and so forth
- An undergraduate degree in "medicine" is introduced
- National educational standards and accreditation are instituted
- The national Association of Physician Assistant Programs is founded
- The Physician Assistant National Certifying Examination is first administered
- Federal funding for PA education spurs innovation and growth of programs
- A national test bank to assist faculty is initiated

CASE STUDY 3-1

Miriam was 32 years old when she heard about the PA program in her city. She knew it was the right career for her. After 4 years at a liberal arts college, Miriam had joined the Peace Corps and worked in family planning in the South Pacific for 2 years. She returned to the United States and became active as a health educator in the women's community for several years. Miriam wanted to do more in health care but did not want to be a physician or a nurse. With the goal of working in obstetrics and gynecology, Miriam applied to the PA program and was accepted.

John came to the PA program at age 30 with 6 years of experience as a Navy corpsman, including one tour of duty in Vietnam. John was 19 years old when he was drafted, and he gained considerable medical experience in the service, which was not transferable into civilian jobs. After 5 years of occasional college courses and a variety of short-term jobs, John realized that he missed patient care, and he found out about the PA profession from a physician friend. He applied but was told that his college grades were too erratic. He spent a year bringing up his grade point average and was accepted the following year, with the goal of working in a rural family practice setting.

Maria was 20 years old and had 1 year of college when she applied to the PA program. Maria had been the primary caregiver for her mother for 5 years until her death a year before. Caring for her mother and getting involved in advocacy for patients with multiple sclerosis had convinced Maria that she wanted a medical career with a focus on patient education. Although she was by far the youngest student in her class, with the least formal medical experience, Maria was very successful in the PA program.

Fred was a 45-year-old medical technologist who had risen through the ranks to become the director of laboratory services at the local hospital. Fred had dreamed of becoming a physician but never had the financial resources. When the first PA was hired in the hospital, Fred discovered the PA profession. After several long conversations, Fred realized that he might have a chance to work in medicine as a PA with direct patient contact and make his dream come true. He took a few science courses to brush up on his study skills and began the PA program with the goal of returning to his community hospital as the second PA in the department of medicine.

THE 1980s—MATURATION PERIOD

Social Forces

The 1980s witnessed a strong resurgence of business values in society. It was widely proclaimed that everything from churches and government to universities, medical practice, and health care delivery could be vastly improved if they operated on the profit-based principles of modern business. The early 1980s saw the enrollment of large numbers of students in graduate programs at business schools across the land. By the mid-1980s, many business graduates had found their way into health care. It was the time of development and expansion of health maintenance organizations (HMOs), preferred provider organizations (PPOs), and diagnosis-related groups (DRGs). Health care was to be "managed" as a business for the welfare of society and for the benefit of investors and stockholders.

The PA profession was well positioned to benefit from some aspects of this environment. PA was establishing itself as a profession of cost-effective, high-quality medical care providers. PAs were steeped in the concepts of team practice. As those in charge of health care corporations sought to expand their businesses, keep costs under control, and raise earnings, they discovered PAs. The demand for PAs grew throughout the decade.

As the health care industry developed new systems, it created positions with new foci such as expanded geriatric care, a return to medical care home visits, broader patient education, case management, and more comprehensive occupational medicine. While searching for people with broad-based, primary care education and flexible attitudes to fill the new positions, it discovered PAs.

Within these developing health care systems, employers were looking for multiskilled individuals who combined a medical background with a background in areas involving business, law, education, management, and finance. They discovered PAs. Because PA education is brief compared with physician education, it attracts people with extensive backgrounds and conversely allows practicing PAs to pursue further education in complementary fields.

Physician specialists also discovered PAs. During the decade, virtually every medical specialty came to include PAs.

Hospitals were faced with several problems. Some teaching hospitals faced reductions in the number of physician residents available to them. Others experienced monthly fluctuations in the quality of care as residents rotated to new services. Still others needed to provide additional support to attending physicians to prevent them from straying to competing hospitals. In looking for solutions, hospitals discovered PAs.

By the 1980s, the profession had grown sufficiently to become a visible part of the health care system.

Education

PA education came of age during the 1980s. Growth in the number of practicing PAs and in the diversity of employment situations for PAs resulted in changes in education. Because of variations within the institutions sponsoring PA programs, changes were not uniform across all programs or regions. However, several trends seem apparent.

Acceptance of Programs

The number of operational PA programs stabilized at around 50. Educational institutions began to view PA programs less as educational experiments and more as permanent units. Universities began finding homes for programs within the administrative structure. For some institutions, this meant elevation of programs to departmental status. For others, it involved deciding whether the PA program should be a component of medical or allied health education. The creation of regular, tenure-track positions for PA faculty members began a trend toward graduate-degree requirements for faculty positions. The commitment to attain graduate degrees led many PA faculty members to decide on education as the primary component and clinical practice as the secondary component of their career.

Curriculum Development

Through the use of incentives in training grant programs, the federal government prompted changes in the education of primary care providers. PA programs were induced to incorporate additional health promotion and disease prevention topics in their curricula and to improve student knowledge and skill in serving specific patient populations, such as the aging, racial and ethnic minorities, and those affected by HIV.

Postgraduate Programs

The rise in the percentage of PAs working in medical specialties led to a number of efforts. With the exception of three entry-level programs that prepared students to work in general surgery, entry-level PA programs became limited to a primary care focus. Entry-level programs in orthopedics, urology, radiology, and other specialties closed. Postgraduate programs appeared in a variety of specialties, including occupational medicine, emergency medicine, general surgery, neonatology, and geriatric medicine. Most were 1 year in length and were modeled on residencies in medical education. Most offered a certificate of completion as the credential. A few offered academic master's degrees as the graduation credential.

Issues of Standardization

Debate over the minimum academic degree for entry into the PA profession occurred sporadically throughout the 1980s. In general, the debate took place among practicing PAs and within the American

Academy of Physician Assistants (AAPA). It was focused on whether or not the baccalaureate level should be adopted as the minimum degree. However, while that question went unresolved, events within some of the programs took a different turn.

A small but increasing number of programs began offering master's degrees as the entry-level credential. They did so in response to several factors. As some universities began requiring PAs to hold at least a master's degree to accept a faculty position, it was readily apparent that few PAs held master's degrees. Second, as institutions reviewed the curricula of their PA programs, some determined that the length of college education and the level of learning inherent in PA education were more compatible with the master's degree than with the baccalaureate degree. Finally, factors in the job market began to demonstrate that the responsibility level of PAs was akin to that of other health care professions that awarded master's degrees.

There were also reasons not to offer the master's degree. Extending the length and cost of PA education would limit the people who could attend PA programs and would reduce the cost effectiveness of the profession. It would reduce the pool of people from rural and inner-city backgrounds who could qualify for admission, and thus would negatively influence the distribution of PAs to these areas of need. The competency-based rather than degree-based philosophy of the accrediting body also weighed against adoption of a uniform entry-level degree. Although there was no final resolution of the issue, the percentage of programs offering a master's degree as entry into the profession would gradually increase.

Educators

The shift toward business values in medical care, specialization for PAs, and competition for PAs with other health care professions were widely discussed in PA education circles. As is often the case, educational institutions moved more slowly than the general society. PA programs continued to adhere to the service values upon which they were founded, resisting the move to new values. Likewise, they were slow to respond to the expansion of the job market late in the decade. This slow response created a backlog of pressure that would result in the rapid expansion of programs in the 1990s.

Perhaps the most consequential developments in PA education in the 1980s were linked to gradual changes in the makeup of the faculty. During the 1960s and 1970s, most directors of PA programs were not PAs. Likewise, the array of instructors and preceptors included few PAs. As more PAs became available in the 1980s, the percentage of PAs in education rose dramatically. Eventually, the majority of directorships were held by PAs, and virtually all programs had a core of full-time PAs serving as faculty. Physicians and other clinicians continued to be heavily involved as guest lecturers, clinical preceptors, and medical directors.

The new educators had been students in PA programs during the pioneer period of the 1970s. Often, they had created the first clinical positions they held. Many were the first to work in a particular town, county, hospital, or clinic. They were creative, determined people with an overwhelming sense of ownership of the PA profession. They brought these values and energies to PA education. This shift of personnel at the center of PA education had a number of consequences, as follows:

The PAs came with solid clinical credentials. They also had professional connections with many physicians in the medical community. The medical director was no longer the only person in the program qualified to judge the quality and appropriateness of the medical component of the curriculum. Medical director roles generally became more collaborative or diminished in scope and prominence.

The teaching styles of PAs were less traditionally academic and more clinical. They converted patient-centered clinical practice to student-centered faculty practice. They developed personal commitments to each student and felt obligated to provide intervention strategies for every educational problem that occurred. This led to an educational approach that was heavily student centered.

These educators had been socialized into the service values of the profession when they were trained as PAs. When they found themselves on the admission committees of programs, they exercised their influence and continued to search for candidates with an altruistic or service orientation. PA educators were trying to create new PAs in their own image.

The heavily student-centered approach taken by faculty provided a great deal of support for students who were often struggling to meet the demands of the most intense education they had ever experienced.

As programs were granted departmental status, PA teaching positions often were converted to formal faculty positions. PAs were now faced with meeting the standard requirements of university faculty to teach, perform service, do research, and hold a terminal degree, preferably a doctorate. Because PA instructional positions often did not fit the usual university faculty mold, a period of adjustment was required for programs and faculty. Teaching and performing service were not generally problems. However, most faculty did not hold doctorates and had not been trained to do research. Through the 1980s and to the present, some programs still struggle to design and maintain faculty positions that meet the needs of PAs, the programs, and the universities.

The fact that universities encouraged and often supported faculty to perform professional service proved to be a boon to many state and national PA organizations. Faculty often had the skills, the connections, and the time to devote to these activities.

Students

As was true for most helping professions, the 1980s were marked by fluctuations in the number of people applying to PA programs. The decade began with a sufficient pool, but there was a dip in the size of the pool by the mid-1980s. Finally, the late 1980s saw a rise in numbers that became dramatic in the 1990s.

A shift also occurred in the characteristics and motivations of the applicants. The initial wave of applicants in the 1960s and 1970s consisted predominantly of people with substantial prior clinical experience and a pioneering or altruistic career focus. This ratio continued into the early 1980s. With the climate in the country moving away from altruism toward job security and personal income, the characteristics of applicants changed. The number of applicants seeking PA as a first career rose, although this group still did not predominate. A shift of motivation placed greater value on career income, status, and security. In keeping with these values, more graduates gravitated toward higher-paying specialties in middle and upper middle class practices. Fewer went to rural and underserved areas.

1980s: INNOVATIONS IN PHYSICIAN ASSISTANT EDUCATION

- Early use of distance learning is employed by some programs
- Problem-based and case-based types of education are used
- Early use of active, computer-based learning and instructional design
- Adoption of curriculum-wide learning through objectives
- National workshops for faculty development become readily available
- Widespread integration of diversity training
- Publication of First Annual Report on PA Education in the United States
- National focus on geriatric assessment

THE 1990s—BOOM OR BUST TIME

Social Forces

At work for decades, the social energy for health care reform realized its greatest impact in the 1990s. Years of steadily rising health care insurance costs provided a strong incentive for large corporate employers to find a more affordable solution. Health care experienced steady movement toward larger delivery systems. Mergers and buyouts continued to be the mode of operation. Many small rural hospitals closed, forcing patients to travel to distant centers for care. Likewise, many physician practices were owned or managed by hospitals or large provider organizations. This diminished the presence of service-oriented values at the table of corporate decision-making. The focus shifted toward serving the stockholder and away from the consumer and the provider.

Despite substantial reform, health care in the United States could not be characterized as a system. Rather, it consisted of a patchwork quilt of many local, regional, and national systems. Although there were benefits to this situation, it also created problems of access and availability for people with special or expensive problems, the poor, the working poor, and those living in physically or culturally remote corners of society. The rapid growth of large managed care systems and the rising influence of insurance providers dominated the 1990s.

Simultaneously, growth also occurred in another segment of society. The medically underserved portion of the population expanded.

Another focus of change was the building of primary care services. Efforts were made to reverse the ratio of primary care to specialty physicians and to create a majority of primary care providers. With government funding supporting this change, primary care became the watchword of many health care professions. Competition between professions for the primary care niche increased.

By the 1990s, the PA profession enjoyed high demand, and salaries rose. Early in the decade, the number of positions available for PAs significantly outdistanced the supply. The variety of positions also continued to increase as health care delivery underwent dramatic developments. National publications pointed to PA as a hot career that would not cool down for years to come.[4]

Although early in the decade the number of clinical positions available for PAs was reportedly high nationwide, by the mid- to late 1990s, the situation seemed less clear. Rapid changes in health care delivery seemed to be simultaneously creating surpluses and shortages of positions on a regional or local basis.

Education

Expansion, proliferation, and growth were the hallmarks of PA education in the 1990s. Never had change been so dramatic for PA education. Although slow to respond to the increasing demand for PA jobs in the late 1980s, universities expanded programs in the 1990s. The decade began with 51 accredited PA programs[5]; by 1999, there were 120.[6] Established programs also increased capacity. The average number of applicants per program was fairly stable at 85 to 100 per year from 1984 through 1989. The number rose dramatically between 1990 and 1995, peaking at about 420, and then fell steadily to a low of about 240 by the end of the decade. During this period, the average number of students enrolled per annual class per program rose from 24 (1984) to a high of 43 (1995 and 1998) and then dropped off to 39 by 1999.[6] Between 1983 and 1999, the percentage of minority students increased from 13.8% to 22%. In 1995, there were 9.8 applicants on average for each student enrolled.[7] By 1999, the ratio was reduced to 5.6:1.[6]

This rapid growth in educational programs was not restricted to PAs. Nurse practitioner programs also expanded. Simultaneously, community-based medical education, pioneered for more than 20 years by PA educators, was recognized as an effective method of increasing the distribution of graduates to rural and underserved areas. Success is not always a plus. Government funding incentives requiring that students of health professions perform some of their clinical education in underserved areas created competition among programs and between professions for community-based clinical education sites.

Growth created significant problems for PA education in the 1990s, but they were problems of success. Not the least was the challenge of maintaining the quality of education in the face of significant shortages of program faculty and leadership. Competition among programs, new roles for PAs, and proportionately diminishing government support also occurred. These seemingly negative forces were more than offset by new energy and initiatives to meet the challenges and by an influx of new educators bringing fresh ideas, new skills, and an enthusiastic spirit. Individually and collectively, programs responded with a number of initiatives, including the following examples:

- Faculty recruitment was addressed jointly by the APAP and the AAPA through presentations at the national spring meetings. These informational and skill-building sessions were aimed at getting practicing PAs involved on a part-time or full-time basis with local PA programs.
- Faculty/staff development projects enhanced the skills of clinical PAs coming into programs as clinical coordinators and classroom teachers. Other projects focused on assisting faculty members to develop the research skills needed in their positions. These efforts included sessions at national meetings, independent workshops of several days' duration sponsored by APAP with support from the federal government, and other projects mounted by groups of educators.
- With support from the federal government, APAP conducted studies on the recruitment and retention of minority faculty.
- Leadership development also included annual independent workshops, as well as sessions at national meetings.
- Excellence in education was addressed through a set of services called PATH (Program Assistance and Technical Help) offered by APAP. Services included confidential consultation, annual national workshops, and publication of written materials.
- Networking, perhaps the most valuable tool for educators, was fostered by APAP and aided by new communication technologies.
- Educators created an annual, comprehensive, self-assessment examination (PACKRAT) to provide both students and programs with indicators of the educational preparation of students.
- The Accreditation and Review Committee on Education for the Physician Assistant revised the standards for PA educational programs.[8] The committee also spearheaded a process for reviewing developing programs prior to admission of students. This provided a level of quality assurance to the initial students.
- The National Commission on Certification of Physician Assistants continued to update and improve the certification examination for those entering the profession.
- AAPA, with the support of APAP, initiated a major project to explore the changing roles of PAs by comparing what students were taught with what PAs did in practice. The project was intended to lead to refinements in both entry-level and continuing education for PAs.
- The number of new programs offering a master's degree, coupled with the addition of older programs converting to a master's degree, continued to drive the discussion about establishing an entry-level degree.

It is clear from this brief list that PA education responded vigorously to the challenges presented in the dynamic decade of the 1990s.

Educators

The growth of PA education saw the incorporation of many new people. Doubling the number of programs stressed the pool of available talent for faculty positions. This stimulated institutions to broaden the faculty by including non-PAs with more diverse backgrounds. The increase in diversity strengthened the education offered. Programs also used a greater number of clinically based PAs as guest lecturers, mentors, and preceptors, thus reducing reliance on full-time PA faculty.

Students

Larger applicant pools in the beginning of the decade caused increased competition for admission. Although presumably this led to students who were better qualified, it is too early to determine whether it resulted in PAs who practice "better" medicine. Case Study 3-2 provides examples of PA students in the 1990s.

1990s: INNOVATIONS IN PHYSICIAN ASSISTANT EDUCATION

- Early use of "professional" actors as patients for skills training
- Expanded use of distance learning methods
- Expansion of programs well ahead of national recognition of shortage of clinicians
- Availability of a national program of technical assistance for new and expanding programs
- National focus on recruitment and retention of minority faculty and students
- Launch of a national tool for assessing student knowledge and program curricula

CASE STUDY 3-2

Lisa first heard about the PA profession in high school, when her older brother, Curtis, became a PA. He lived at home while attending school, so Lisa met his classmates and heard stories about his rotations. When Curtis got a job in a local hospital emergency department, he encouraged Lisa to start volunteering. Lisa continued to volunteer and completed an emergency medical technician (EMT) course while in college. She started college as a pre-med major with the goal of becoming a physician but became discouraged by the competitive attitude of the other pre-med students. She enjoyed her time with the local ambulance squad and dropped out of college after her sophomore year to work full time in pre–hospital care. After 2 years, Lisa decided to become a PA to work in emergency medicine, but with a broader scope of practice. She applied to several programs and was accepted on the waiting list of one program. She continued working and took additional college courses while applying again. Upon applying for a second time, Lisa was accepted to the PA program that Curtis had completed.

Luis had been a police officer for 15 years before being disabled by a knee injury. While in the police department, he had completed 2 years of college toward a degree in political science. Throughout his police career, Luis had been an active volunteer in a variety of health-related community groups; he had cared for homebound elders and people with AIDS. After completing his rehabilitation, Luis decided to pursue his lifelong interest in medicine. He worked as a security guard at night to support his family while taking science and other prerequisite courses. After 2 years of taking courses and continuing his community service, Luis was accepted into a PA program. His goal upon graduating was to work in primary care in the urban community where he grew up.

Janice was a high school teacher for 4 years and started a peer-counseling program at her high school for students with alcohol and drug problems. Through this project, Janice became interested in health care and started volunteering at a residential community center for homeless and runaway teens. She met a PA student who was doing a community service project at the teen home and started to learn about the PA profession. After 2 years of volunteering and taking additional science courses, Janice was accepted at a PA program with the goal of working in adolescent medicine.

David was an emergency department nurse for 5 years. While working alongside PAs and physicians in the emergency department, David realized that he was interested in diagnosing and treating patients and found himself drawn to the PA profession. He admired the competence and compassion of the PAs and decided to apply to PA programs. David's grades in nursing school had been mediocre, although his performance evaluations and recommendations were outstanding. After being rejected once, David took courses on a part-time basis for 2 years to improve his academic credentials and was accepted. Although he had always enjoyed emergency medicine, David's goal was to find a family practice position in which he could follow patients and their families over time and provide continuity of care.

THE 2000s—MOVING FORWARD

Social Forces

This period has been shaped by powerful national and international events. Terrorist attacks in New York City and Washington, D.C., in September 2001 introduced a decade marked by ensuing wars in Iraq and Afghanistan, as well as additional terrorist attacks in major cities in Europe. Wars traditionally bring advances in medical care on the battlefield and strains on the health care systems devoted to the treatment and rehabilitation of the injured. Restoring health care to the civilian populations devastated by war also creates great challenges. In addition to these new forces in the decade, many older problems have persisted. Health care in the United States has continued to fail to meet the needs of an increasing number of uninsured citizens, now well over 40 million people. Economic stresses have continued to threaten to reduce care for those covered by Medicaid and Medicare. The post–World War II baby boom generation has begun to retire. During the next 20 to 30 years, this will have two major effects on health care: the large percentage of current health care workers who belong to this generation are beginning to leave the workforce as they retire; simultaneously, the older portion of society that consumes the greatest percentage of health care services is increasing dramatically. This creates a rising shortage of health care workers. It strains the systems that pay for health care. It creates serious problems with access to quality, affordable, available health care. In an effort to address these issues, federal health care reform laws have been enacted. The extent of impact of this reform remains to be seen.

Education

There have been four developments in PA education that merit discussion. All have begun to change PA education. One has the potential to change the profession to a greater degree than it has altered education.

First, in May of 2000, the AAPA adopted two resolutions concerning the level of academic degree that it thought should characterize PA education.

Standard Professional Degree, 2000-B-16a

The American Academy of Physician Assistants believes that a graduate degree, professional or academic, should be awarded by all accredited PA programs to students who successfully complete the program.

Standard Professional Degree, 2000-B-16b

The Speaker communicates to the AAPA and the Accreditation Review Commission for PA Education (ARC-PA) representatives the Academy's desire to make a graduate degree, professional or academic, a requirement represented in the *Standard* (AAPA House of Delegates, May 2000).

In October 2000 at its annual meeting, APAP adopted the following policies:

> The Association of Physician Assistant Programs (APAP) recognizes that PA education in accredited programs is conducted at the graduate level and recommends that PA programs grant students a credential reflective of this level of curriculum.
>
> The credential granted should reflect the institutional mission and needs of the local and regional communities served by the program, and maintain the academic integrity of the curriculum and the competency of students. The Association shall . . . assist programs with conversion to granting a graduate credential (Minutes, APAP Business Meeting, October 26 and 29, 2000, Washington, D.C.).

Although these actions established no requirement for PA programs to offer graduate degrees and set no date by which such a requirement would take place, they captured the existing mood of many programs that had or were converting to master's degrees and accelerated the process for many other programs.

In 1987, there were 48 PA educational programs in the United States. Only 4.2% awarded a master's degree. By 1990, the number of programs had risen to 55, and the percentage of programs awarding a master's degree had nearly doubled to 9.1%. By 1995, the number of programs was 80, and the percentage awarding a master's degree had doubled again to 18.75%. By 1999, the percentage had nearly doubled again to 35.83% of the then 120 PA programs. By 2001, there were 126 PA educational programs in the United States, and 42.86% offered a master's degree.[9,10] As of 2012 the number of programs had reached 169, and 94% awarded master's degrees.[11,12]

In 2003, the membership of the Physician Assistant Education Association (then the Association of Physician Assistant Programs) charged the board of directors to commission a group to define the content and configuration of PA graduate preparation. The Graduate Education Commission (GEC) examined the structure, content, and patterns of PA graduate education and curricula and developed recommendations for educational institutions and the PA Education Association.[13]

The GEC reviewed available literature on graduate education in the PA profession and other professions, surveyed PA program directors, and conducted qualitative analyses. The final report chronicled the history of the transition to graduate (master's degree) PA education, an overview of current trends, and results of the data collected and offered a model for PA graduate education.[13]

The move to graduate-level degrees for entry into the PA profession has many consequences. It affects the qualifications for entrance into programs and the cost of education. This in turn alters the accessibility of PA education to segments of the population. It places the impression of the depth and breadth of PA education on a plane with other professions making similar changes—nurse practitioners, physical therapists, and occupational therapists. It may increase the cost of health care to the consumer as it raises the cost of education. Ongoing analyses of the impact of graduate-level education on the PA profession and PA education are essential.

The second development occurred in 2001, when the APAP introduced the Centralized Application Service for Physician Assistants (CAPSA). This service, which is now used by more than two thirds of programs, has made the application process more efficient for applicants. It facilitates application to multiple participating programs. It has also begun to provide extensive data on the national applicant pool. Analysis of this information assists individual programs and PA education in general to make wiser decisions about recruitment and selection of students. These efforts in turn may lead to a more diverse and more talented student body that is better suited to meet future challenges that the profession will face.

The third factor under way since the early part of the decade has been the internationalization of PA education. This is evidenced by a rise in the number of U.S. programs and students participating in international placements for clinical rotations as part of the educational process. Although this option has been exercised by a handful of programs and students for many years, recent years have seen increased interest and implementation. Aside from the benefits to the individual students, this raises the visibility of the profession in other countries. Indeed, a few PA educational programs have now been founded in other countries, rekindling the hope of many PAs and PA educators that the positive effect of the PA profession on accessibility to quality, available health care may be afforded to many other countries, especially those with high numbers of medically underserved citizens. PA programs in other countries will undoubtedly look much different from programs in the United States because they are designed to meet the health care needs in different societal systems. Nevertheless, the basic concepts of intense, high-quality education leading to widespread distribution of primary care–educated clinicians working as team members with physicians and other providers could greatly expand the availability and accessibility of health care in areas with great need.

The fourth factor is the growth in the number of PA programs. In March 2000 there were 120 accredited PA programs.[14] By March 2012 there were 169 programs.[12] The number is likely to exceed 200 by 2014 and may reach 250 by 2017. This rapid growth is currently creating shortages of two critical resources in the education of PA students, qualified PA faculty members and qualified preceptors for clinical education. These shortages will become more severe in coming years because dramatic growth is occurring not only in the education of PA students but also in the number of medical students, nurse practitioner students, and physician residents. These professions compete with each other for qualified clinical instructors.

Educators

The growth of PA education in the 1990s created the need for a significant increase in the number of PA educators. The response to this need brought many PAs from clinical practice into PA education. The challenge of the 2000s has been to retain them in PA education and equip them with the credentials and skills to have rewarding careers in academia.

2000s: INNOVATIONS IN PHYSICIAN ASSISTANT EDUCATION

- Availability of a centralized application service to assist candidates and programs
- Increasing uses of new classroom technologies to assist evermore condensed curricula
- Expansion of graduate level PA education
- Teaching evidenced-based medicine at the bedside by use of new electronic technologies
- Integration of service-learning into education more widespread
- Incorporation of disaster preparedness training into many programs' curricula
- Greater educational emphasis on health literacy, health financing, and patient rights
- Bioinformatics and genetics are widely added to curricula
- Development of competencies for physician assistants that span initial education and lifelong learning

THE FUTURE—WHAT WILL PA EDUCATION LOOK LIKE BEYOND 2010?

Social Forces

The first aspect to investigate is what society will look like. The social forces described for the first decade of the 2000s will stretch far into the future. Ecologic changes currently well under way, such as global warming and increasing pollution, will change where people live, the dynamics of agriculture, the prevalence of diseases, and the economic centers of society. The focus of health care will change as several factors play out, as follows:

- Advances in the application of genetics to health care will bring sweeping benefits to diagnosis and treatment, along with potential pitfalls.
- As technologies provide tools to fight diseases, they will also continue to facilitate the international spread of disease among both plants and animals.
- Nuclear proliferation and the ongoing global social struggles currently characterized as the global war on terror, along with the rise of fundamentalism, may bring dramatic changes that will alter the focus of health care forever.
- The need to care for large numbers of wounded from current wars will focus technology on evermore sophisticated prosthetic devices.

We hear much about the age of technology, rapid communication, the plethora of information available to consumers, medical advancements in prevention and treatment, the maturing of managed care, and more. Some not-so-startling changes to look forward to include the following:

- The Internet will continue to keep patients better informed, and it will allow them to consult with clinicians around the world, independent of their personal providers.
- The Internet will create more opportunities for clinicians to educate their patients and the public at large.
- Patients will have access to an increasing array of kits for home laboratory tests.
- The clinician-patient relationship will change as patients are better informed and have access to better communication with a larger number of clinicians from coast to coast.
- Selected office visits, especially follow-up visits, will take place via technology, decreasing the need for patients to reside near their clinicians.
- Managed care will mature and become more competitive, better balancing quality care and profit.
- Population shifts that increase the number of people with minority backgrounds, advanced years, and languages other than English will create the need for new skills among clinicians.
- Managed care may change the PA profession by narrowing its scope of practice and weakening its unique bond with the physician.
- As clinicians from many professions vie for larger shares of the primary care arena, PAs may experience a relative shift toward specialty care, as was seen in the 1980s and was reversed in the 1990s. This is a reflection of the breadth and depth of PA education.
- PAs working in primary care may continue to serve rural and underserved populations to a greater extent than other professions.
- Alternative modalities of medical care will increase in appeal to the public, competing for the primary care arena.
- The move to graduate degrees for entry-level PAs may move the profession away from its traditional niche of cost-effective care. As PA vacates that claim, other professions will be started or expanded to fill the niche.

All of this and more will probably come to pass for those with the money, societal class, and education to participate. However, if current trends continue, there will also be greater separation within society, that is, a widening gap between the "haves" and the "have nots." The number of citizens without access to health care in our country has been increasing since the 1990s. This will continue unless other forces intervene. If this continues, it will provide challenges and opportunities for the PA, a profession that takes pride in its ability to adapt to new opportunities.

- National health care reform will affect the volume and scope of services to be provided to patients. As the health care system changes, it will alter the roles of PAs and other clinicians. It will likely increase the demand for PAs and others. Changing roles may affect job satisfaction and in turn the recruitment of students to the profession.

Education

The future for PA education may include the following:

- PA education will be exported to an increasing number of other countries, where its methods for intense medical education will be adapted to meet the needs of other cultures.
- Programs in the United States will lengthen as they find it impossible to include more complex technologic skills with the already compact medical curricula.

- The trend toward requiring a baccalaureate degree for admission to a PA program will decrease the number of rural and minority students in programs as the applicant pool falls.
- The lengthening of programs and the requirement of awarding graduate degrees may lead to the fulfillment of at least one early PA visionary. Namely, medical education may become stepped so that people with bachelor's, master's, and doctoral degrees may be able to practice at different levels and proceed to the next educational level without going back to step 1.
- The continuing inflation of entry-level doctoral degrees in other health professions will lead to the development of a doctorate in PA, which will become the entry-level degree for the profession.
- PA faculty will continue to be challenged to maintain their clinical acumen while acquiring advanced degrees and participating in scholarly endeavors.
- A terminal degree for PA faculty and competencies of PA educators may be required, especially as they relate to eligibility for promotion and tenure in higher education.
- Large health care delivery systems will continue to view the cost of educating physicians, PAs, nurses, and other providers as detrimental to profits. This will pressure programs and ultimately students to pay these systems for providing clinical sites for the education of health professionals.
- Programs paying for supervision by clinical preceptors will significantly increase the cost of education and the financial burden of students. It may also set up a struggle between universities and health care systems for control of the direction of the education of health professionals.

In 1996, APAP hosted a meeting on the future of PA education. Some of the previously mentioned items were drawn from the report of that project.[11] Whether some, all, or none of these opinions come to pass, it is clear that the future will be filled with challenges for the next generation of PA educators. If the past is an indication, it is also apparent that they will face the challenges with creativity, energy, and vision.

Educators and Students

Who will be the educators of PAs in the future? What characteristics will describe them? They will not come from the vision of PA educators of today. Rather, those currently considering a career in PA education will shape them.

FACULTY ROLES

Although students frequently see PA program faculty members as primarily involved with their specific program's educational activities, most faculty members also have major investments in state and national PA educational activities. All these activities are viewed as not only opportunities to represent the program but also personal growth and networking opportunities for the individual faculty member. Typical volunteer assignments and activities of PA program faculty members might include the following:

1. Site visitor for the Accreditation Review Committee.
2. Test item writer for the NCCPA test item committees for the PANCE or recertification examination.
3. Test item writer for the e-PACKRAT.
4. Elected officer, committee chair, or committee member for PAEA activities.
5. Member of the Accreditation Review Committee-PA Commission.
6. Grant writer or grant reviewer (e.g., Health Resources and Services Administration [HRSA] training grants or other federal primary care initiatives).
7. Elected officer, committee chair, committee member, or House of Delegates representative for state PA academies.
8. Nationally elected AAPA officer or appointee to councils, committees, or task forces.
9. Special appointments to federal and state councils and boards.
10. Member or advisor to hospital or health delivery system credentialing and privileging committee.

CONCLUSION

In the 1960s, it began with a simple concept, that people with or without medical experience could be educated to perform many of the tasks previously reserved for physicians; this education could be offered in a format that was briefer than medical school, and the new graduates would assist overworked physicians and extend services to underserved patients. More than 40 years later, these ideas have led to a nationwide network of more than 160 PA programs that admit over 7000 new students annually. PA education and the PA profession have grown and prospered because they have been responsive to society's need for available, cost-effective, quality medical care. These remain strong needs in society. To continue to prosper, the PA profession must position itself as a leader in solving these societal problems.

From its infancy to the present, the educational network of PA programs has continued to provide broad-based medical education that graduates could apply to a wide spectrum of medical areas. PAs provide medical services to all segments of the population.

Programs have offered this foundation through innovative curriculum designs that rely on collaboration with educators from other disciplines and with community-based clinicians. This collaboration accounts for much of the energy, flexibility, and continuous renewal that is common to PA education. PA education is currently growing in many ways: more programs, larger programs, more students, new waves of clinicians becoming faculty members, and new curriculum elements. There are new challenges from society requiring new responses—an increasing number of medically underserved citizens, a rising population of older citizens, new health care environments such as managed care, and new practice models created by the explosion of communication technologies.

PA education will continue to prosper to the extent that it resists the temptation to become static and to simply provide an educational base for a profession. PA education must look for future direction in the place where it has found direction in the past, namely, in the needs of society. It must continue to dream dreams and see visions. It must actualize the dreams with energy, innovation, and determination.

CLINICAL APPLICATIONS

1. Explore the history of your PA program.
   - Who were the founders?
   - What was the founding mission of the program?
   - If your program was created within the past 5 years, find out the basis and assumptions for the curriculum design (both didactic and clinical). If your program has a long history, find out how the curriculum has changed across time in both the didactic and clinical phases.
2. Interview at least one graduate from your program's first class.
   - What were that person's motivations for enrolling in the initial class of a new program?
   - What were the selection criteria for the first class?
   - What were the barriers to practice and utilization for new graduates?

KEY POINTS

- Major social issues at the time included limited access to health care services, health workforce shortages, new legislation creating Medicare and Medicaid, and Civil Rights legislation forcing the restructuring of the U.S. hospital system. In addition, the return of well-trained military corpsmen from the Vietnam War resulted in an available workforce of individuals who were ideal for pioneering a new career.
- PA education is based on the medical education model of general medical didactic knowledge first, followed by application through full-time clinical rotations. Although there have been several successful variations on the medical education model, high-speed, high-volume medical education has been a hallmark of PA education. The PA profession's ability to work in many specialties and settings rests on the breadth and depth of the PA curriculum.
- Early PA education leaders came from many professions. Eventually PAs themselves became the leaders of PA programs and created a stability within PA programs that was not initially seen in the early days of PA education. Since then, PA education has undergone several periods of rapid growth in the number of programs.
- Federal support was instrumental in the early development of many programs. Currently, with cutbacks in federal funding for medicine, nursing, and dentistry, few programs receive federal funding as an incentive for developing and maintaining primary care initiatives.

ACKNOWLEDGMENTS

We would like to thank Glen Combs, MA, PA-C; Christopher J. Daly, MD, FACS; Laurie Dunn-Ryznyk, MPAS, PA-C; Ken Harbert, PhD, CHES, PA-C; Patricia R. Jennings, DrPH, PA-C; Theresa Johnson, MS, PA-C; Patrick Knott, PhD, PA-C; Anthony Miller, MEd, PA-C; Colleen Patton, MMS, RN, PA-C; Allan Platt, PA-CF, MMSc; Bradford W. Schwarz, MS, PA-C; and Michel Statler, MLA, PA-C.

References

1. Selected Training Programs for Physician Support Personnel, U.S. Department of Health, Education and Welfare. Bethesda, MD: National Institutes of Health; 1971.
2. American Medical Association Council on Medical Education. Essentials of an approved educational program for the assistant to the primary care physician. In: Sadler AM, Sadler BL, Bliss AA, (eds). The Physician's Assistant Today and Tomorrow. New Haven, CT: Yale University, 1972.
3. Sadler AM, Sadler BL, Bliss AA. The Physician's Assistant Today and Tomorrow. New Haven, CT: Yale University, 1972.
4. Brindley D, Bennefield RM, Danyliw NQ. 20 hot job tracks. US News 1997;123(16):98.
5. Sixth Annual Report on Physician Assistant Education Programs in the United States, 1989-1990. Alexandria, VA: Association of Physician Assistant Programs; 1990.
6. Sixteenth Annual Report on Physician Assistant Educational Programs in the United States, 1999-2000. Alexandria, VA: Association of Physician Assistant Programs; 2000.
7. Twelfth Annual Report on Physician Assistant Educational Programs in the United States, 1995-1996. Alexandria, VA: Association of Physician Assistant Programs; 1996.
8. Commission on Accreditation of Allied Health Education Programs. Standards and Guidelines for an Accredited Educational Program for the Physician Assistant. Marshfield, WI: Accreditation Review Committee on Education for the Physician Assistant; 1997.
9. Fourth, 7th, 12th, 16th, 17th Annual Reports on Physician Assistant Education Programs in the United States. Alexandria, VA: Association of Physician Assistant Programs.
10. 2001 Physician Assistant Programs Directory. Alexandria, VA: Association of Physician Assistant Programs; 2001.
11. Miller AA. Proceedings: Defining the Future Characteristics of Physician Assistant Education. Alexandria, VA: Association of Physician Assistant Programs; 1996.
12. Physician Assistant Education Association. Program Directory. Degrees awarded. *www. paeaonline.org/index.php?ht=d/contentDir/searching/1/nocrit/1/pid/34340;* Accessed March 28, 2012.
13. Joslin V, Cook P, Ballweg R, et al. Value added: Graduate-level education in physician assistant programs. J Physician Assist Educ 2006;17(2):16.
14. Jacques PF, Snow C, Dowdle M, et al. 2000 Physician Assistant Education Association. Program Directory. 18th ed Alexandria, VA: Association of Physician Assistant Program; 2000.

The resources for this chapter can be found at www. expertconsult.com.

CHAPTER 4

Credentialing: Accreditation, Certification, Licensing, and Privileging

Constance Goldgar • Dan Crouse

CHAPTER CONTENTS

Credentialing is a process of establishing qualifications for groups of professionals or organizations that assesses their background and legitimacy for providing services and grants them the right, through a title or credit, to provide specific services. Credentialing affects physician assistant (PA) students initially while they are enrolled in their programs of education and subsequently when they graduate and enter the health care marketplace. The right to exercise the power to perform or provide services with credentialing is a significant responsibility that must be understood and accepted by both PA students and the institutions charged with educating them. In this chapter, we discuss two separate and distinct credentialing procedures: the credentialing of PA programs and the credentialing of individual PAs on the state, national, and institutional levels.

PROGRAM CREDENTIALING

The process of credentialing PA programs takes the form of accreditation, which is defined as official recognition and approval, or vouching that (as in conformity with a standard) a program maintains standards that qualify the graduates for professional practice and provides them with credentials. PA programs have undergone remarkable professional growth that belies the relatively short history (≈45 years) of the profession. In terms of acceptance and privilege to clinically practice, the accreditation process by which PA programs are evaluated is fundamental to the profession's success.

Accreditation Review Commission on Education of the Physician Assistant

Accreditation is a process of external peer review, encompassing evaluation of an institution or education program to determine whether it meets the standards set up by the accrediting body. If the program or institution meets the standards set, the accrediting body grants recognition that established qualifications and educational standards have been met. The Accreditation Review Commission on Education of the PA (ARC-PA) is the recognized accrediting agency that protects the interests of the public and PA profession and the welfare of students by defining the standards for PA education and evaluating PA educational programs within the territorial United States to ensure their compliance with the standards.[1]

Accreditation of PA programs began in 1971, when *Essentials of an Accredited Educational Program for the Assistant to the Primary Care Physician* were developed under the auspices of the American Medical Association's (AMA's) Subcommittee of the Council on Medical Education's Advisory Committee on Education for Allied Health Professions and Services. Many evolutions to PA program accreditation have occurred since that time. On January 1, 2002, the Accreditation Review *Committee* on Education for the Physician Assistant became the Accreditation Review *Commission* on Education for the Physician Assistant. This was a small name change but a monumental step forward as this organization became a freestanding accrediting agency for the evaluation and accreditation of PA educational programs in the United States. The ARC-PA is the sole authority for PA program accreditation.

The role of the ARC-PA is the following:

1. Establish educational standards using broad-based input
2. Define and administer the process for comprehensive review of applicant programs
3. Define and administer the process for accreditation decision-making
4. Determine if PA educational programs are in compliance with the established standards
5. Work cooperatively with its collaborating organizations
6. Define and administer a process for appeal of accreditation decisions

The goals of ARC-PA (Table 4-1) dovetail with its mission to "protect the interests of the public and PA profession, and the welfare of students by defining the standards for PA education and evaluating PA educational programs . . . to ensure their compliance with those standards."[1]

In its role of accreditation of PA programs, ARC-PA encourages excellence in PA education by establishing and maintaining minimum standards of quality for educational programs. The ARC-PA cooperates and collaborates with several organizations to establish, maintain, and promote appropriate standards of quality for educational programs. Endorsed by a broad consensus within the medical community (Table 4-2), the *Standards* represent current, nationally accepted guidelines for all aspects of program operation. The *Standards*, initially adopted in 1971, have been revised many times over the years

TABLE 4-1 Goals of the Accreditation Review Commission on Education for the Physician Assistant

1.	Foster excellence in PA education through the development of uniform national standards for assessing educational effectiveness
2.	Foster excellence in PA programs by requiring continuous self-study and review
3.	Assure the general public, as well as professional, educational, and licensing agencies and organizations, that accredited programs have met defined educational standards for preparing PAs for practice
4.	Provide information and guidance to individuals, groups, and organizations regarding PA program accreditation

TABLE 4-2 Representative Organizations of the National Commission on Certification of Physician Assistants

American Academy of Family Physicians (AAFP)
American Academy of Pediatrics (AAP)
American Academy of Physician Assistants (AAPA)
American College of Emergency Physicians (ACEP)
American College of Physicians (ACP)
American College of Surgeons (ACS)
American Hospital Association (AHA)
American Medical Association (AMA)
American Osteopathic Association (AOA)
Association of American Medical Colleges (AAMC)
Physician Assistant Education Association (PAEA)
Federation of State Medical Boards (FSMB)
U.S. Department of Veterans Affairs

with its most recent revision in 2010. A copy of the most current *Standards* is available in PDF downloadable format at *http://www.arc-pa.org/acc_standards/*. The ARC-PA *Standards* constitute the minimum requirements to which an accredited program is held accountable and provide the basis on which ARC-PA confers or denies program accreditation. The *Standards* are used for the development, evaluation, and self-analysis of PA programs. They reflect the realization that a commonality in the core professional curriculum of programs remains desirable and necessary in order to offer curricula of sufficient depth and breadth to prepare all PA graduates for practice in a dynamic and competitive health care arena.[1] The *Standards* allow programs to remain creative and innovative in program design and in the methods used to enable students to achieve program goals and acquire the competencies needed for entry into clinical practice.

As delineated in the *Standards*, the PA is academically and clinically prepared to practice medicine with the direction and responsible supervision of a doctor of medicine or osteopathy. The physician–PA team relationship is fundamental to the PA profession and enhances the delivery of high-quality health care. Within the physician–PA team relationship, PAs make clinical decisions and provide a broad range of diagnostic, therapeutic, preventive, and health-maintenance services. The clinical role of PAs includes primary and specialty care in medical and surgical practice settings. PA practice is centered on patient care and may include educational, research, and administrative activities.[1]

The role of the PA demands intelligence, sound judgment, intellectual honesty, appropriate interpersonal skills, and the capacity to respond to emergencies in a calm and reasoned manner. An attitude of respect for self and others, adherence to the concepts of privilege and confidentiality in communicating with patients, and a commitment to the patient's welfare are essential attributes of the graduate PA.

The professional curriculum for PA education includes basic medical, behavioral, and social sciences; patient assessment and clinical medicine; supervised clinical practice; and health policy and professional practice issues. The *Standards* encompass current, nationally accepted guidelines for all aspects of PA program operation, including institutional responsibilities, admissions processes, faculty qualifications, curricular components and design, expected competencies for students, supervised clinical practice, classroom laboratory and library facilities, clinical affiliations, student issues, fiscal stability, program publications, record-keeping systems, and administration.

Accreditation Process for Physician Assistant Programs

The accreditation process by which PA programs are evaluated is fundamental to the profession's success. This voluntary process includes a comprehensive review of the program relative to the *Standards*. There are different categories of accreditation, including provisional accreditation (for new programs), continuing accreditation (for established programs that have been accredited), and probationary accreditation (including administrative probationary accreditation). Accreditation can also be withheld from programs seeking provisional accreditation or withdrawn from established programs determined to be noncompliant with the *Standards*.

The ARC-PA accreditation process does the following:

- Encourages educational institutions and programs to continuously evaluate and improve their processes and outcomes
- Helps prospective students identify programs that meet nationally accepted standards
- Protects programs from internal and external pressures to make changes that are not educationally sound
- Involves faculty and staff in comprehensive program evaluation and planning, and stimulates self-improvement by setting national standards against which programs can be measured[1]

PA programs initiate the process of accreditation. The process is a multifaceted one, involving extensive review of the program by the program itself, as well as by the ARC-PA.[2] A crucial part of the process is that a program provides evidence of a continuous critical self-assessment process, whereby it critically assesses all aspects of its operation with outcome data that identify strengths and weaknesses, develop corrective interventions, and evaluate the results of the interventions. Programs must produce a Self-Study Report (SSR) that describes the self-assessment process and complete a detailed accreditation application in advance of an on-site evaluation by ARC-PA site visitors. The site visitors validate, verify, and clarify information supplied in the SSR and application and make observations that are communicated to ARC-PA.

Accreditation decisions are based on the ARC-PA's review of information contained in the accreditation application, the program's self-study report, the report of site visit evaluation teams, any additional requested reports or documents submitted to the ARC-PA by the PA program, and the program's past accreditation history.[2] The ARC-PA meets semiannually to consider applications for provisional, initial, and continuing accreditation. After review by the commission, a formal notice of accreditation status and the time frame for accreditation are sent to the chief executive officer of the institution and to the program director.

Once ARC-PA accreditation is granted, periodic reviews and on-site evaluations by an accreditation team are required for maintenance of accreditation. The educational process is improved frequently as programs make modifications to maintain or exceed the accreditation *Standards* or to build on insights gained from an on-site evaluation.

Graduation from an ARC-PA–accredited program benefits students by providing the following:

1. Assurance that the program meets nationally accepted standards
2. Recognition of their education by their professional peers
3. Eligibility for professional certification, registration, and state licensure

Further information on PA program accreditation can be found at *www.arc-pa.org* or by directly contacting ARC-PA, 12000 Findley Road, Suite 150, Johns Creek, GA 30097; phone 770-476-1224; fax 770-476-1738.

Physician Assistant Education Association

The Physician Assistant Education Association (PAEA), though not a credentialing body, is the association that serves as a resource for individuals and organizations from various professional sectors interested in the educational aspects of the PA profession. PAEA works to ensure quality PA education through the development and distribution of educational services and products specifically geared toward meeting the emerging needs of PA programs, the PA profession, and the health care industry.[3] PAEA is the only national organization in the United States representing PA educational programs. Its mission is to pursue excellence, foster faculty development, advance the body of knowledge that defines quality education and patient-centered care, and promote diversity in all aspects of PA education.[3]

The Association was founded as the Association of PA Programs (APAP) in 1972 by a group of concerned program faculty who saw a need to address the important issues of accreditation, certification, continuing education, role delineation for PAs, and the overall goal of improving the quality and accessibility of health care through the selection, education, and deployment of PAs.[3] In 1973, APAP established a national office with the American Academy of Physician Assistants (AAPA) in Alexandria, Virginia. On May 1, 2006, the Association moved to independent management as PAEA after more than three decades of operating under a management contract with the AAPA. This amicable parting has allowed the Association to better advance its mission and to be increasingly recognized as the organization representing PA education.

The Association's members comprise the 154 currently accredited PA programs in the United States. PAEA is the organization primarily responsible for collecting, publishing, and disseminating information on PA programs. PAEA also serves as a resource for individuals and organizations from various professional sectors interested in the educational aspects of the PA profession. PAEA provides effective representation to affiliated organizations involved in health education, health care policy, and the national certification of PA graduates.

PAEA works to ensure quality PA education through the development and distribution of educational services and products specifically geared toward meeting the needs of PA programs, the PA profession, and the health care industry. To accomplish its mission, PAEA professes that it will do the following:

- Encourage and assist programs to educate competent and compassionate PAs
- Enhance programs' capability to recruit, select, and retain well-qualified PA students
- Support programs in the recruitment, selection, development, and retention of well-qualified faculty
- Facilitate the pursuit and dissemination of research and scholarly work
- Educate PAs who will practice evidence-based, patient-centered medicine
- Serve as the definitive voice on matters related to entry-level PA education, nationally and internationally
- Foster professionalism and innovation in health profession education
- Promote interprofessional education and practice
- Forge linkages with other organizations to advance its mission

PAEA services include two national meetings for PA educators each year—the fall annual Education Forum and the May semiannual meeting associated with the AAPA annual meeting. The Association publishes the *Journal of Physician Assistant Education* (formerly *Perspective on Physician Assistant Education*) and in 2010 was selected to be indexed and included in the National Library of Medicine's MEDLINE database, an important milestone. This peer-reviewed journal takes a broad look at issues in

PA education. It features in-depth research articles authored by PA faculty on such subjects as health care workforce issues, testing, admissions, educational technology, and teaching tips, as well as a legal forum and regular columns on cultural diversity and the art of medicine, among other areas of faculty interest. PAEA also publishes a monthly electronic newsletter, the *Networker*, which reports on PAEA activities, board meetings, conferences, faculty positions, special projects, and topics of interest to the educational community.

Another resource publication is the *Physician Assistant Programs Directory*, the most comprehensive guide to PA educational programs. Each PAEA member program submits information annually on its entrance requirements, admissions procedures, deadlines, fees, institutional affiliations, financial aid, curriculum, credentials awarded, and more. The directory is available only as an online publication. The directory also contains an online search feature that allows users to locate unique aspects of the programs. The *PAEA Faculty Directory* is a complete resource for faculty and is available online. It provides contact information for all PAEA faculty, committees, and board members, along with information on related organizations such as the AAPA and the ARC-PA. This publication is available only to member and institutional colleague programs.

An initiative to assist applicants to PA programs was developed by PAEA as the Central Application Service for Physician Assistants (CASPA). PAEA initiated CASPA in 2001, with approximately 5000 applicants per year; in 2010 alone there were more than 14,000 unique applications through the CASPA service. More than 126 programs have joined CASPA as of 2010, and others are in the process of converting from their own application services to CASPA.[4]

PAEA systematically collects PA program, student, and applicant data through two sources. CASPA collects information annually on applicants to PA programs. Through the *Annual Report on PA Educational Programs in the United States*, PAEA undertakes a comprehensive review of PA programs, their faculty, and students and compiles data that provide a record of every aspect of PA education, including student and applicant demographics, faculty credentials, salaries, and graduate employment data. Since the mid-1980s, this published report has afforded PAs a history of the educational programs and continues to be the basis for statistical analysis of many areas of PA education.

The PAEA Faculty Development Institute (FDI) is the umbrella entity that oversees all of the Association's faculty development initiatives and workshops. The FDI is responsible for workshops to enhance faculty at every level (e.g., basic skills, clinical coordinators, associate directors, directors). A recently launched program, Education Scholar, offers a convenient and affordable way to provide faculty development for member PA program faculty through a series of faculty enrichment modules.

Through its Research Institute (RI), PAEA supports research on PA education through small grant programs. The Small Grants Program, begun in 1998, has funded more than 150 research proposals. The RI oversees research activities, including the annual grant programs, research workshops, and the student writing competition.

PAEA provides member programs access to a continuously reviewed and upgraded student self-assessment examination, e-PACKRAT. It also sponsors an annual exhibit of educational products for PA faculty at its fall Education Forum.

For further information, contact PAEA, 300 N. Washington Street, Suite 710, Alexandria, VA 22314-2544; phone 703-548-5538; fax 703-548-5539; *www.paeaonline.org*.

GRADUATE CREDENTIALING

Credentialing of graduate PAs has three components, all of which the new PA must understand in order to obtain the right to practice:

1. A national system of certification available to graduates of ARC-PA–accredited programs;
2. A myriad of individual state credentialing procedures; and
3. Individual credentialing and privileging processes for specific institutions and third-party payers.

National Certification and Recertification

In contrast to accreditation, a process applied to educational programs, certification is a process involving the individual. Typically, certification involves a nongovernmental agency or association that grants recognition to an individual who has met certain predetermined qualifications specified by that agency or association. In 1971, the AMA House of Delegates directed its Council on Health Manpower to assume a leadership role in sponsoring a national program for certification of the Assistant to the Primary Care Physician. National certification was favored to give PAs geographic mobility, provide the physician employer with some evidence of competency, and permit greater flexibility in employment transition.[5]

National Board of Medical Examiners

Following endorsement by the Federation of State Medical Boards, the AMA's Council on Health Manpower and the National Board of Medical Examiners (NBME) began a collaborative effort to develop a national certification process for PAs. The NBME, with its long history of evaluating the competency of medical providers, was a logical choice for the task, and, in 1972, it accepted responsibility for developing a national certifying examination. The Physician Assistant National Certifying Examination (PANCE) was developed to ensure that individuals achieved minimum standards of proficiency in primary health care delivery. The examination was administered in 1973 and 1974 by the NBME. Subsequent annual examinations have been administered by the National Commission on Certification of Physician Assistants (NCCPA).

National Commission on Certification of Physician Assistants

NCCPA is the only credentialing organization for PAs in the United States. Established as a not-for-profit organization in 1975, NCCPA is dedicated to assuring the public that certified PAs meet established standards of knowledge and clinical skills upon entry into practice and throughout their careers. Every U.S. state, the District of Columbia, and the U.S. territories have decided to rely on NCCPA certification as one of the criteria for licensure or regulation of PAs. Approximately 86,000 PAs have been certified by NCCPA.[5] NCCPA's mission is "to serve the public through exemplary programs that evaluate critical PA competencies and that require the pursuit of life-long learning and improvement."[5] Table 4-2 includes those organizations that are represented with commissioner seats on the NCCPA Board of Directors.[5]

The NCCPA was initially charged with the following functions:

- Determining eligibility criteria for the entry-level examination
- Reviewing applications to take the examination, then registering candidates
- Administering the examination under contract to the NBME
- Determining the standards for the entry-level examination
- Issuing and verifying certificates
- Recertifying PAs through periodic administration of an examination
- Publishing lists, by state, of PAs certified each year
- Serving as a resource to assist state medical boards, at their request, in establishing and modifying PA legislation, rules, and regulations as they pertain to national certification
- Conducting research activities to disseminate information regarding the PA's responsibilities to the government, professional organizations, the general public, and others

This list of responsibilities grew out of the two tasks with which the NCCPA was charged. First, it was to certify and recertify people who would be called PAs to ensure the public that the quality of practitioners met a national standard. Second, the NCCPA needed to ensure the relevance of the examination to the practice engaged in by the PA.[6] Graduates from PA programs accredited by the ARC-PA or its predecessors are eligible to seek NCCPA certification by taking the PANCE.

NCCPA Examinations

To become a certified PA, beyond having graduated from an accredited PA program, graduates must pass a multiple choice generalist examination, PANCE, which assesses basic medical and surgical knowledge. Examinations are rigorously constructed using the highest testing standards and psychometrics. Test questions are written by committees of certified PAs and physicians and then edited by professional examination developers.[5] In 1997, examiners began using a criterion-referenced passing-point strategy to score the PANCE. This content-based strategy is characterized by the selection of an absolute standard; for example, if 50% of examinees meet that standard, 50% pass, or if 100% of examinees meet the standard, 100% pass.[7]

Graduates from accredited programs are eligible to take PANCE for up to 6 years after completing the requirements for graduation from that program. During that 6-year period, the examination may be taken a maximum of six times. When either the six attempts or 6 years is exhausted, whichever occurs sooner, the individual loses eligibility to take PANCE. The only way to establish new eligibility to take PANCE is to enter into and complete an unabridged ARC-PA accredited PA educational program.[5] Currently, PANCE is administered continuously throughout the year (all but 2 weeks) and consists of 360 multiple-choice questions. The examination is administered by computer and consists of three test sections of 120 questions each. Examinees are allotted 2 hours for each session, for a total of 6 hours of testing time. The current cost of the examination is $475, and it is administered through Prometric (Sylvan) Testing Centers throughout the United States.

Maintenance of Certification

The 6-year certificate maintenance cycle is divided into three 2-year periods. During every 2-year period, PA-C designees must earn and log a minimum of 100 hours of continuing medical education (CME) and submit a certification maintenance fee to NCCPA. At least 50 CME hours must be Category I. These are offered in a "lecture/learner" format as seminars and conferences. Category II CME can comprise the remainder of the 100 hours and includes other practice-related, voluntary, self-learning activities. By the end of the sixth year of the certification maintenance cycle, PA-C designees must have also passed a recertification examination (PANRE).[5] PAs who maintain their certification are eligible to take the PANRE when they are in the fifth or sixth year of the PA-C certification maintenance cycle and have two attempts to pass the recertification examination.[5]

From 1998 to 2006, an alternate Pathway II examination had been administered by NCCPA consisting of a web-based, take-at-home examination among other requirements. The NCCPA Board voted, however, to discontinue this option with the 2010 administration cycle. The NCCPA continues to work to modify the PANRE examination to make it more acceptable to graduates practicing in a wide range of clinical situations.

The use of the designation "C" (for "certified") after the acronym "PA" indicates that the individual so designated has taken and passed the initial examination and adheres to the CME requirement set forth by the NCCPA. The title "PA-C" is a registered service mark, and its use is strictly limited to individuals who have met the listed requirements.

In recent years, the NCCPA has instituted random CME audits, assumed the responsibility for all CME logging, required new graduates to become certified within 6 years or six attempts at PANCE, and has enacted a more comprehensive disciplinary policy, including the establishment of a Code of Conduct for Certified and Certifying PAs.[5]

In 2010, NCCPA introduced the certificate of added qualifications (CAQ) program to become available in 2011. This is a voluntary process that allows PAs to achieve recognition for their specialty experience, skills, and knowledge. The CAQ offers PAs a credential to effectively document their specialty experience and expertise. The CAQ is something that PAs earn above and beyond the PA-C, which remains the foundational credential for the PA profession. To qualify for a specialty CAQ, PAs must first satisfy two basic prerequisites: (1) current PA-C certification and (2) possession of a valid, unrestricted license to practice as a PA in at least one jurisdiction in the United States or its territories, or unrestricted privileges to practice as a PA for a government agency. (Note: If a PA holds licenses in multiple states, all of the licenses must be unrestricted.) For PAs meeting those basic prerequisites, the CAQ process includes **four core requirements:** (1) Category I specialty CME, (2) 1 to 2 years of experience, (3) procedures and patient case experience appropriate for the specialty, and (4) a specialty examination. The CAQ reflects the fact that PAs are grounded first in primary care or generalist practice, a base of training and knowledge that is augmented but not replaced through specialization.[8]

To summarize, maintaining certification with the NCCPA is an ongoing process, beginning with successful completion of the PANCE and continuing throughout a career with the periodic passage of a re-certifying examination and the logging of CME credits. Individuals who pass the PANCE receive a time-limited NCCPA certificate, valid for 2 years. To maintain certification beyond the initial expiration date, a PA is required to re-register every 2 years and document 100 hours of CME. In addition, as a part of the process, the PA is required to take a recertifying examination every 6 years. The Physician Assistant National Recertifying Examination (PANRE) is administered twice yearly by the NCCPA in the spring.[6] Case Study 4-1 presents the dilemma of PAs concerning certification and recertification.

The NCCPA has designed a self-assessment practice examination that an individual can take as soon as NCCPA receives PANCE eligibility from the program director. Each practice examination includes 120 multiple-choice questions that have been extracted from the actual PANCE and PANRE item banks and provides an opportunity to view questions similar in format and style to actual examination questions. In addition, the online assessment is designed to reflect the time constraints (1 minute per question) associated with the actual examination, allowing the opportunity to ensure that an individual candidate can effectively manage time. Students who register for the examination will have 180 days during which to complete the 120-minute assessment. Priced at $35, the practice examination is a tool to assist in assessing relative strengths and weaknesses as one prepares for the initial certification examination.[4]

Physician Assistant Core Competencies

The Competencies for the Physician Assistant Profession document was developed jointly by the NCCPA, ARC-PA, AAPA, and the PAEA and was approved by all four organizations in 2005. A website housed by the NCCPA has a copy of the Competencies, a self-evaluation tool for PAs, and a list of resources. The ARC-PA has prepared a tabular comparison of the Competencies to the accreditation *Standards*, 4th edition, showing that many competencies are addressed by PA programs compliant with the *Standards*. The Competencies and the comparison to the *Standards* are available in PDF format from the ARC-PA (see earlier for contact information).

For further information regarding any NCCPA activities, contact NCCPA, 12000 Findley Rd., Suite 100, Johns Creek, GA 30097; phone 678-417-8100; fax 678-417-8135; *www.nccpa.net.*

CASE STUDY 4-1

The following situations reflect some of the difficult issues facing practicing PAs concerning certification and recertification.

Richard has just received notification that he did not pass his entry-level NCCPA examination. Fortunately, his state's temporary licensure provision gives him two additional chances to pass the examination, because it is now given continuously throughout the year. Richard is struggling with the decision of when to retake the examination. If he takes the examination sooner (which would still give him the opportunity to retake it one more time), he might pass, but he also thinks he will be less well prepared. If he waits, he thinks he will be better prepared.

James is a physician assistant in a Midwestern state who has been practicing for 23 years and is now preparing to take his third NCCPA recertification examination. Although he worked in primary care for 19 years, he is now working in the subspecialty of pediatric neurology. The state in which he practices does not require the recertification examination, although it does require documentation of CME. If he chooses not to take the recertification examination, he will no longer be able to use the title "PA-C" after his name. Lack of ongoing certification may also limit his mobility if he chooses to move to a state where ongoing certification is required. He is uncertain what to do.

State Credentialing

Greater recognition of PAs as health care providers has led to the development of state laws and regulations governing their practice. Recognition of PAs in state law and delegation of authority to a state regulatory body that oversees their practice serve two main purposes: to protect the public from substandard practice by PAs and to promote appropriate expanded delegation within the scope of PA practice by assuring consumers, physicians, and others that PAs are competent.[9] In the late 1960s and early 1970s, while the PA concept was beginning to blossom, there was pervasive dissatisfaction with the prevailing method of credentialing health professionals. Sadler and colleagues[10] summed up the mood of the time:

> At a time when the entire licensure scheme for regulating health personnel is under widespread attack as being archaic, inefficient, and destructive of change, a variety of delegation amendments to state medical practice acts have been enacted as a direct result of the physician assistant movement.

Through their willingness to remain legally dependent, to accept delegation from physicians, and to work under the supervision and control of the physician, PAs are able to function under broad and flexible legal umbrellas that allow them to perform to their capacity.[9]

During the early 1970s, a patchwork of approaches was initiated and many states put forth amendments to state medical practice acts that allowed for the delegation of tasks by the physician to an assistant. Such initial amendments typically consisted of a brief paragraph allowing PAs to function. Most states also identified an agency that would assume the responsibility for regulation of this fledgling profession.

Despite the flexibility of the delegation amendments, it became increasingly clear to many state regulatory agencies that they were inadequate to deal with the tremendous growth in responsibility of the PA profession. Today, most states realize the need to reexamine the definition of the scope of physician assistant practice, and most recognize that PAs must engage in clinical decision-making in order to practice effectively. As they rework legislation relative to PA practice, a few states continue to register PAs, thus giving rise to the designation "RPA-C" (the "R" indicating registration in the particular state), whereas most states have adopted licensure laws to govern PAs.

Statutory authority to promulgate rules and regulations to accompany such laws is typically given to an agency, such as a state medical board. Through the Administrative Rule Making Act, the rules and regulations that are developed, although easier to change than statutes, carry the same weight as laws. State statutes, rules, and regulations are as varied as the states they represent. Whatever the arrangement, the two most consistent criteria for practice in a particular state remain successful completion of the NCCPA national certifying examination and graduation from an ARC-PA accredited PA educational program.

PAs are playing an ever-increasing role in the regulation of their own profession. Nine states have regulatory bodies strictly for PAs (Arizona, California, Iowa, Massachusetts, Michigan, Rhode Island,

TABLE 4-3 **Chronology of Development of Physician Assistant (PA) Regulatory Agencies**[11]

Date	Action
1971	The development of the Essentials of an Accredited Educational Program for the Assistant to the Primary Care Physician was undertaken by the American Medical Association (AMA) subcommittee of the Council on Medical Education's Advisory Committee on Education for Allied Health Professions and Services. The subcommittee included representatives from the AAFP, AAP, ACP, ASIM, AMA, and AAMC. The Essentials prepared by the subcommittee were approved by those organizations, except for the AAMC, which declined to approve or endorse the Essentials.
1972	The National Board of Medical Examiners (NBME) and the AMA convened representatives from 14 different organizations, including the AAPA and PAEA, to discuss the need for establishing an independent certifying authority for the PA profession.
1975	Established as a not-for-profit organization, NCCPA is dedicated to assuring the public that certified physician assistants meet professional standards of knowledge and clinical skills.
1976	The AMA House of Delegates voted to delegate its responsibility for adoption of proposed Educational Standards (Essentials) to the AMA Council on Medical Education and authorized the transfer of responsibility for accreditation from the AMA Council on Medical Education to its Committee on Allied Health Education Accreditation (CAHEA). CAHEA was designed to represent communities of interest for which accreditation actions were taken. The committee comprised representatives from allied health professions, medicine, continuing medical education (CME), and the public.
1988	CAHEA was renamed the Accreditation Review Committee on Education for the Physician Assistant (ARC-PA).
1994	CAHEA was dissolved and accreditation activities were transferred to a new, independent agency—the Commission on Accreditation of Allied Health Education Programs (CAAHEP).
1995	The ARC-PA was incorporated.
2000	The members of the ARC-PA voted to "become a freestanding accrediting agency for the PA profession" with the implementation date of January 1, 2001.
2003	One of NCCPA's ongoing projects was initiated as part of a collaborative effort jointly undertaken by four national PA organizations (NCCPA, AAPA, PAEA, and ARC-PA) to establish a profession-wide definition of PA competencies that can be used as a map for further developing and evaluating those competencies throughout a PA's career.

From Physicians Assistants in the Health Workforce, 1994.

Tennessee, Texas, and Utah). Nearly all state medical boards have PA committees. Some of the committees are advisory, but others have significant responsibilities in rule making, review of applications, and discipline. Seats for PAs are available on 18 other medical, osteopathic, or disciplinary boards.[8] The AAPA strongly endorses the authority of designated state regulatory agencies, in accordance with due process, to discipline PAs who have committed acts in violation of state law. Disciplinary actions include, but are not limited to, suspension and revocation of an individual's license or certificate of registration. The Academy also endorses the sharing of information among the state regulatory agencies regarding the disposition of adjudicated actions against PAs (Table 4-3).[8]

Registration

In the few states where PAs are still registered, issues related to PA practice are addressed either by a subcommittee of a state medical board that has been formed to deal with PA practice or by a state medical board that includes a seat (or seats) for PA representation. The medical board most often functions in an advisory capacity to a state governmental agency, such as a department of commerce or department of business regulation. In rare instances, physicians are regulated by a nongovernmental agency, and, in such cases, PAs are generally covered by the same arrangement.

Licensure

An increasing number of states are creating separate PA licensing boards as a result of new PA practice acts that replace the initial delegation amendments to medical practice acts. Such boards are usually composed of practicing PAs and practicing physicians who employ or work with PAs. The boards are typically advisory to a governmental agency, which has ultimate authority in the regulation of PAs. PAs are licensed in 46 states, the District of Columbia, and most U.S. territories.[8] They are certified in two states (Ohio, Vermont) and registered in two states (Massachusetts, New York).[8] Only five states do not have statutes or rules regulating temporary licensure (Montana, New Hampshire, North Carolina, North Dakota, Ohio). Temporary licensure for most states allows for new graduates to start work as a PA before taking their PANCE examinations. The temporary license typically expires after receiving the results of the test. A few states allow continuation of a temporary license under certain circumstances. It is best to review the individual state's statutes and rules before applying for a temporary license.

Institutional Credentialing and Privileging

Unless a PA is practicing exclusively in a private medical practice with no regulation, he or she will also be subject to credentialing by the institution in which he or she practices. The Joint Commission and the National Commission on Quality Assurance mandate a credentialing process for licensed providers working within an institution. Typically, a committee of the medical staff administers this process with the technical support of credentialing professionals. The institutional credentialing process, which is also carried out by some third-party payers, verifies the training and experience of providers who see patients in the institution's delivery system. Hospital practice requires a further step: privileging. This second step, administered by the medical staff, requires that providers document their training and experience with specific procedures before being granted the privilege of performing these activities within the system. Providers typically are given expanded privileges over time as they gain additional training and experience with new procedures.

CLINICAL APPLICATIONS

1. Interview the director of your PA program to review the program's accreditation history.
   - When was it first accredited?
   - What are the current evaluation and growth issues for the program?
   - What experience do the director and other faculty members have as evaluators and site visitors for other PA programs?
   - What changes does your program director foresee in the future accreditation of PA programs in general and your program specifically?
2. Review the past and present PA literature on the issues of initial certification and recertification.
   - What are the commonly held views regarding the advantages and disadvantages of each examination?
   - What has been the history of certification requirements in your state?
   - Would you recommend any changes in your state licensing act regarding certification? Why or why not?
3. Talk with a PA in your community who practices in an institutional setting. Find out about the credentialing and privileging process in his or her institution and discuss how he or she is reviewed periodically for this process.

KEY POINTS

- Currently, all states have enacted laws or regulations recognizing physician assistants.
- The AAPA provides up-to-date summary information on state requirements for PA practice.
- The reader is advised to contact the appropriate state agency for further state specific information.

References

1. ARC-PA website. *http://www.arc-pa.org/about/mission.html.*
2. ARC-PA website. *http://www.arc-pa.org/about/about_acc.html.*
3. PAEA website. *http://www.paeaonline.org.*
4. PAEA website. *http://www.paeaonline.org/index.php?ht=d/sp/i/87253/pid/87253.*
5. NCCPA website. *http://www.nccpa.net.*
6. Schafft GE, Cawley JF. The Physician Assistant in a Changing Health Care Environment. Rockville, MD: Aspen Publications, 1987.
7. New Pass/Fail Standard-Setting Procedures Implemented. Commission Update. Atlanta, GA: Newsletter of the NCCPA; 1997; 1:2, 6.
8. NCCPA website. *http://www.nccpa.net/NewsArticles/NewsArticlesCAQreplacesspecialtycertAug10.aspx.*
9. Physician Assistant State Laws and Regulations. 11th ed. Alexandria, VA: American Academy of Physician Assistants; 2010.
10. Sadler AM, Sadler BL, Bliss AA. The Physician's Assistant Today, and Tomorrow: Issues Confronting New Health Practitioners. 2nd ed. New Haven, CT: Yale University Press; 1972.
11. Physicians Assistants in the Health Workforce, 1994. Final Report of the Advisory Group on Physician Assistants and the Workforce submitted to the Council on Graduate Medical Education (COGME). Health Resources and Services Administration, Division of Medicine, Rockville, MD.

The resources for this chapter can be found at www.expertconsult.com

CHAPTER 5

NATIONAL COMMISSION ON CERTIFICATION OF PHYSICIAN ASSISTANTS SPECIALTY RECOGNITION: CERTIFICATE OF ADDED QUALIFICATIONS

Daniel T. Vetrosky • Ruth Ballweg

CHAPTER CONTENTS

In mid-2011, the National Commission on Certification of Physician Assistants (NCCPA) launched a Certificate of Added Qualification for certified physician assistants (PAs) practicing in the following specialty areas: cardiovascular and thoracic surgery, emergency medicine, nephrology, orthopedic surgery, and psychiatry. The program is voluntary and requires that the PA has met the following requirements:

> (1) Current PA-C certification and (2) possession of a valid, unrestricted license to practice as a PA in at least one jurisdiction in the United States or its territories, or unrestricted privileges to practice as a PA for a government agency.
>
> (Note: If a PA holds licenses in multiple states, all of the licenses must be unrestricted.)
>
> For PAs meeting those basic prerequisites, the CAQ process includes *four core requirements:* (1) Category I specialty continuing medical education (CME), (2) 1 to 2 years of experience, (3) procedures and patient case experience appropriate for the specialty, and (4) a specialty examination.
>
> The first three core requirements may be completed in any order. Once those are complete, PAs are eligible for the examination. The current cost of this program (2011) is $350, including a $100 administrative fee and a $250 examination registration fee.[1]

NCCPA's purpose for instituting the CAQ is expressed as follows:

> In support of a commitment to promote the health and safety of the public, NCCPA will offer Certificates of Added Qualifications to physician assistants who

demonstrate that they meet professional standards of knowledge, skills, and experience.[2]

Although the purpose for initiating a program such as this might seem straightforward, many of the PA organizations such as the NCCPA, American Academy of Physician Assistants (AAPA), Physician Assistant Education Association (PAEA), and Accreditation Review Commission on Education of the Physician Assistant (ARC-PA) have been discussing this issue for many years. This chapter addresses some of the pivotal concerns that have been discussed and examined which have led to the current CAQ program. Some of these concerns include but are not limited to the generalist mission of the PA profession instituted by Dr. Stead and others, professional fragmentation, specialty "certification," PA specialty association needs, and physician specialty associations' input.

HISTORY

Before the mid to late 1970s, the issue of specialty practice and specialty recognition in the PA profession was not being considered on a wide scale. This was mostly due to professional development, becoming established as a new health care profession, and the primary care emphasis that was promulgated by the AAPA and APAP (now PAEA) and supported, through funding, by the federal government. The idea of the PA generalist, who would have maximum flexibility in the rapidly changing health care environment, was built into PA educational models and the accreditation process.

Although there were specialty PA training programs such as The University of Alabama at Birmingham's Surgical PA program and the Child Health Associate program at the University of Colorado, these programs were seen as "unique to their environment" and never became the established model for PA training. In the early days of the PA profession, there were also shorter "specialty" PA programs with a relatively narrow focus on specialties such as orthopedics, pathology, or women's health. Because these shorter programs had difficulty gaining credibility, they soon closed. The passage of time from the late 1970s to the present would see the PA job market widen from mostly primary care practice to encompass many subspecialty practices including surgery and its subspecialties, emergency medicine, nephrology, radiology, gastrointestinal medicine, and psychiatry, to name a few. This "market" expansion was a primary factor that brought the topic of specialty expertise and recognition to the forefront.

The concern over specialty recognition was seriously discussed during the 1980s and 1990s in conjunction with the beginning of the NCCPA recertification process for all PAs. The dialogue occurred because more and more PA graduates were being hired to work in medical and surgical subspecialty areas. One issue that moved the dialogue forward was the PAs who worked in specialty areas feeling the pressure of having to take a primary care–emphasized recertification examination rather than being examined in their particular field of practice/expertise. During this period the AAPA, NCCPA, and many subspecialty organizations considered various dimensions of the specialty recognition issue.

AAPA AND NCCPA

The AAPA Education Council had been addressing the possibility of implementing a "diplomat" program recognizing specialty achievement above and beyond NCCPA's certification since 1990. This program was explored due to the significant concerns being voiced to the AAPA leadership from numerous PAs and PA subspecialty groups. Much discussion occurred both formally and informally during this time, and the Education Council researched the diplomat possibility in depth. Recognizing that to offer a diplomat would in essence be conferring a certification, and understanding the implications both legal and financial, the further development of such a program was dropped in or around 1993.

During this time, AAPA was also addressing the specialty issue from two other perspectives. The first was to afford opportunities for recognition of both medical and surgical subspecialties through the continuation of the Surgical Congress and the creation of the Medical Congress under the auspices of AAPA. This was an effort to identify and determine which groups belonged under which Congress, as well as to afford those new and established groups common grounds for support and representation. The second was the pilot project that began in 1992 for the development of an alternative pathway for recertification in conjunction with the NCCPA. The impetus for this project was to afford those PAs working in specialty areas and those who did not want to take a paper/computerized examination to concentrate their CME in areas of interest and to complete a take-home examination. This led to the establishment of Pathway II, which officially began in 1997 and lasted 14 years.

The last Pathway II examination was administered in late 2010.[3,4]

REMEDIATION AND RETOOLING

Though not directly related to the establishment of the Certificate of Advanced Qualification, the AAPA and the APAP (PAEA) discussed a program of remediation and retooling in the early 1990s for PAs who wanted to change specialties or who had been away from practice and wanted to refresh their knowledge and skills.[4] Over the years, roundtable discussions have taken place at the Annual PAEA meetings related to this subject. Sentiments that postgraduate specialty programs are already in existence and that there is no urgent need to set up remediation and retooling programs has remained the prevailing opinion.

INSTITUTIONAL CONCERNS

As PAs moved into institutional settings—particularly in jobs that emphasized surgical and procedural skills—hospitals began to ask for additional verification of training and experience beyond graduation from accredited PA programs and successful completion of certification or recertification examinations. Although some hospitals were willing to accept logbooks or attestations from previous employers or employing institutions, PAs were beginning to report that they were seen as less competitive than other clinicians who had documentation of formal training or certification programs. Several specialties such as cardiovascular surgery and dermatology began to develop their own certification or recognition programs to respond to institutional credentialing and privileging committees. An additional concern was that eventually the Joint Commission would create requirements for certification or recognition that would negatively affect PA roles in hospitals and other settings.

EXTERNAL THREATS

Although there was recognition within the profession of these growing concerns, external entrepreneurs began to see financial opportunities in the creation of specialty certification processes. The PA organizations might not have agreed on what should be done about the "specialty issue," but they did agree that having external entities creating certification systems without input or involvement from PA organizations, physician specialty organizations, PAs, and sponsoring physicians was not acceptable.

NATIONAL MEETING

In June 2006, the NCCPA sponsored a Forum for PAs Practicing in Specialties that included representatives from 3 physician organizations and 24 PA groups. Not surprisingly, there was little agreement between the specific groups about which path to take. Each group was invited to submit key "take-away" messages from the meeting. The statements included[5]:

No Changes Needed

- The PA profession has been well served by its foundations in generalism, time-limited certification and lifelong learning. (American Academy of Family Physicians)
- There is no support for specialty certification because of its negative impact on the PA profession's ability to remain flexible in order to serve an ever-changing patient population and health care delivery system. (American Academy of Physician Assistants)
- The current system is working. There are some problematic issues that need to be addressed in a thoughtful manner but there is not a crisis. (Association of PAs in Obstetrics and Gynecology)
- PAs have been and continue to be trained as generalists. To create recognition for PAs in various fields will be nearly impossible. (Society for PAs in Pediatrics)

The Roles of Physicians

- The role of the supervising physician remains important in PA practice, and an emphasis on documented training and competency must be preserved. (American Academy of Family Physicians)
- More physician supervision and training is needed in the beginning. Emphasis within the profession should be on helping PAs and employers/physicians to train and educate PAs to work effectively in specialty practice. (Association of Postgraduate PA Programs)
- Collaboration with physician specialty organizations should be central in the identifications of core competencies in specialty practice. (Association of PAs in Cardiovascular Surgery)

Support for a Specialty Process

- The time for recognition of PAs in specialty settings is overdue. Increasing specialization and subspecialization of PAs has occurred as a result of employment opportunities and has been market driven. While PA positions in specialty settings have enjoyed rapid growth in recent years, continued growth is threatened by competing health care providers as a result of perceived lack of education or training in specialty practice. (Association of PAs in Cardiology)
- Our biggest challenge [is] to attaining privileges in hospitals to perform invasive procedures without

formal training in post graduate residency programs or documented specialty training or certification. (Society of PAs in Radiology)

Discussion also included Specialty Certification (replacing the PANRE recertification examination), whether any new process should include an examination component, and whether there should be an education/qualification-based recognition. The Society of PAs in Pediatrics was alone in opposing all options, although this is no longer their position. Everyone was unanimous in opposing specialty certification, thinking that a replacement for the PANRE examination would severely limit PAs' options in the future. Most groups favored specialty recognition, which was modeled on physician structures that had been created within specialties. There was a general lack of enthusiasm for additional formal examinations, however. With the exception of pediatrics, all groups favored education/qualification-based recognition.[6]

NCCPA CONSENSUS POINTS

As a result of the June 2006 meeting, the NCCPA Board approved a series of "consensus points" regarding specialty recognition to guide their continued discussions. These were revised in 2008 to say:

> **Preamble:** NCCPA assures that certified physician assistants meet professional standards of knowledge and skills. Physician assistant practice ranges from primary care to specialty and subspecialty services with all care being provided with physician supervision. In order to fulfill NCCPA's mission to assure that certified PAs meet professional standards of knowledge and skills, NCCPA seeks to create and develop appropriate eligibility criteria and assessment mechanisms for specialty recognition. As with all NCCPA programs, specialty recognition will be a competencies-based process.
>
> 1. Changes in the healthcare system and the clinical diversity of PA practice indicate that it is the appropriate time to pursue specialty recognition.
>   a. There is an increasing number of PAs practicing in specialty areas other than primary care.
>   b. Employers and others are placing heightened emphasis on patient safety and risk management. Patient safety is an integral aspect of NCCPA's mission.
>   c. Complexities and increased demands of current healthcare practice place constraints and increased burdens on the mentoring aspects of the physician-PA relationship.
>   d. Individuals entering PA training programs have more academic and less clinical experience than those from the profession's formative years.
>   e. The profession's growth and increasing visibility has resulted in the need for greater accountability.
> 2. NCCPA will develop and administer specialty recognition according to the following principles.
>   a. Specialty recognition will be voluntary and will be independent of NCCPA's certification and recertification processes.
>   b. Specialty recognition will support and reinforce relationships between PAs and physicians.
>   c. NCCPA will seek input and cooperation from appropriate stakeholders.
>   d. Specialty recognition will support the credentialing process and not create barriers to licensure and practice.[7]

FEEDBACK FROM THE FIELD

The AAPA and state academies were quick to respond. In January 2007, AAPA President Mary Ettari wrote to Randy Danielson, Chair of the NCCPA:

> The [AAPA] board appreciates the thought process that the NCCPA has put into this issue since May, as well as the transparency of your process. . . . The AAPA Board agrees that there is some need for recognition of the individual knowledge and capabilities that a PA has acquired through education and practice. Such recognition is important for Pas, as well as for consumers. . . . However, the Board feels strongly . . . that it is neither necessary nor appropriate to establish recognition activities or programs that in any way would limit entry into areas of practice. . . .
>
> The Board also feels strongly that any recognition activity designed to assess or reflect in any way the basic knowledge or requirements for practice in a specialty area quickly will become a de facto requirement for practice in that specialty. In our view, once the profession starts down the road of specialty certification for practice, there will be no turning back. The AAPA Board would request clarification of your "consensus" principles with regard to these concerns and anything that might be done to help guard against or prevent voluntary standards from becoming de facto requirements for PA practice in any area of medicine or surgery.[8]

A letter from the Tennessee Academy of Physician Assistants is an example of other feedback provided to the NCCPA. On January 3, 2007, Frank Warren, president of the Tennessee Academy wrote:

> The Tennessee Academy of Physician Assistants Board of Directors did meet on November 18th and discussed the issue of "specialty recognition" or "specialty certification" as some fear. We continue to have many concerns and fear this could lead to a dramatic and detrimental change in the PA profession. . . . First, we feel "specialty recognition" would place a large burden on new graduates to focus on a specialty and upon graduation learn they prefer another area, or they may have to

take a job in a different field of medicine due to location, unavailability of job in chosen discipline, economics, or other unforeseen reason. . . . [M]any in our constituency feel "specialty" recognition" or certification may just be "keeping up" with the nurse practitioners in a credential race, and adding more initials/credentials after our names is not necessarily a worthy endeavor for our profession and its flexibility.[9]

CERTIFICATE OF ADDED QUALIFICATIONS SOLUTION

As the discussion continued, NCCPA representatives from Family Medicine suggested a model used by the American Board of Family Medicine (ABFM) to create a mechanism for recognition of experience and training while at the same time retaining generalism and flexibility as key features of the PA career. Certificates of Added Qualification (CAQ), offered by the ABFM in Adolescent Medicine, Geriatric Medicine, Hospice and Palliative Medicine, Sleep Medicine, and Sports Medicine, offer voluntary recognition without replacing generalist certification or recertification. They also can be applied to a wide range of educational experiences, including short fellowships and on-line learning.

Definition: "CAQ stands for Certificate of Added Qualification. A CAQ enables a physician to add to his or her skill set and qualifications, without completing an additional full fellowship-training program. A CAQ consists of additional coursework, clinical education, and testing of a subspecialized technique, procedure or area of medicine within the physician's medical specialty. A CAQ does not take as long as a fellowship, so physicians may complete them midcareer as needed. A fellowship often takes 6 to 9 months, whereas the CAQ could take a few weeks or months, depending on the CAQ. CAQs can help the physician learn a new procedure, surgical technique, or subspecialty area."[10]

The NCCPA voted to begin developing a specialty recognition program with CAQs and to consider the accompanying policies for the CAQ process that had been developed by the ABFM.[11]

Choosing the Specialties

On the basis of the information received from the June 2006 forum with PA specialty organizations and physician groups, the NCCPA considered which specialties it should include in an initial launch, and ultimately it decided to choose five specialties for initial development of the CAQs. A structured set of variables was used to make this judgment, including the size of the specialty group, the support of the PA and physician specialty organization, the criticality of patients served by the specialty, the degree to which the specialty is hospital based, and the degree to which the specialty is procedurally intense. Five specialties were chosen: cardiovascular surgery, emergency medicine, nephrology, orthopedic surgery, and psychiatry.

Specialty Advisory Groups and Policies

The next step was the creation of small advisory groups (five to six individuals) including PAs and MDs from the specialty. Each group was chaired by a PA member of the NCCPA Board and was charged with recommended creating the policies for each specialty-specific components of the process within guidelines established by the NCCPA Board. The process would utilize well-established NCCPA processes including CME verification/attestation, a practice analysis to create an examination blueprint, a test-writing committee, and a standard setting process.

The policy and processes for each examination are available on the NCCPA website:

Cardiovascular Surgery: *http://www.nccpa.net/Cardiothoracicsurgery.aspx*
Emergency Medicine: *http://www.nccpa.net/Emergencymedicine.aspx*
Nephrology: *http://www.nccpa.net/Nephrology.aspx*
Orthopedic Surgery: *http://www.nccpa.net/Orthopaedicsurgery.aspx*
Psychiatry: *http://www.nccpa.net/Psychiatry.aspx*

OUTCOMES—FUTURE PLANS

With the first CAQ examinations given in late 2011, the NCCPA is analyzing data from the first cohort of candidates. This analysis includes not only examination performance but also level of participation and evaluations of the process of itself. The second round of CAQs is scheduled for September 2012. NCCPA announcements and reports will carry information about long-term policy decisions regarding the process and possible decisions to include other specialties in the future. Within the NCCPA, the CAQ process is assigned to the Certification Committee, which is responsible for monitoring and refining the process.

CASE STUDY 5-1

John is a 36-year-old PA who works in an office-based psychiatric practice. He has been with the current practice for 7 years and has established a population of patients he sees on a routine basis. His supervising physician has privileges at the local hospital, where the practice is consulted at least weekly for hospitalized patients with emotional/psychiatric problems. John would be allowed to perform the initial consult evaluation, but the hospital staff office requires that he have some documentation showing he is qualified in the psychiatric specialty above and beyond the years of psychiatric practice and the endorsement of his supervising physician. John recently heard about the NCCPA's CAQ in psychiatric medicine and started the application process.

CASE STUDY 5-2

Jill recently completed the NCCPA's CAQ in cardiothoracic surgery. She sat for the examination for two reasons: (1) to become recognized as having advanced knowledge and skills in her chosen field and (2) to have the advanced qualification should third-party insurance companies require this type of recognized documentation. Her practice endorsed and paid for her CAQ and will require this of all eligible PAs.

KEY POINTS

- History shows that the PA profession is dynamic and changes with the needs of health care environment.
- Since the mid 1970s, specialty care and expertise became a field of interest from the precepting physician's perspective and, subsequently, the PA profession's perspective.
- Specialty training programs at the undergraduate and graduate level evolved from this need.
- AAPA, NCCPA, and PAEA all perceived the need for some kind of recognition for PAs who had specialty expertise and training and investigated the possibilities for recognition.
- The NCCPA convened a meeting of stakeholders to generate consensus points leading to the establishment of a Certificate of Advanced Recognition for PAs in various specialties.
- In the fall of 2011 the NCCPA administered the first CAQ examinations for the following specialties:
  - Psychiatry
  - Cardiothoracic surgery
  - Nephrology
  - Emergency medicine
  - Orthopedic surgery

References

1. Certificate of Added Qualification. *http://www.nccpa.net/SpecialtyCAQs.aspx;* Accessed September 19, 2011.
2. Purpose of the CAQ. *http://www.nccpa.net/PDFs/CAQ%20Policies.pdf;* Accessed September 19, 2011.
3. Hooker RS, Carter R, Cawley JF. The National Commission on Certification of Physician Assistants: History and Role. Perspective on Physician Assistant Education Winter 2004;15(1):8.
4. AAPA Education Council Meeting Minutes; February 28 through March 1, 1992, and July 24–25, 1992.
5. Summary of Key Take-Aways, Needs and Ideas Provided by Specialty Forum Participants—NCCPA document prepared for Task Force on Specialty Recognition, Jacksonville, Florida, January 6–7, 2007.
6. Summary of Needs and Position of Specialty PA Groups NCCPA document prepared for Task Force on Specialty Recognition, Jacksonville, Florida, January 6–7, 2007.
7. NCCPA website. *http://www.nccpa.net/NewsArticles/NewsArticlesPOC08.aspx;* Accessed December 2011.
8. Letter: American Academy of Physician Assistants from M Ettari, MPH, PA-C, President AAPA, January 2, 2007.
9. Letter: Tennessee Academy of Physician Assistants from FD Warren, PA-C, January 3, 2007.
10. About.com health careers website. *http://healthcareers.about.com/od/h/g/CAQ.htm;* Accessed December 2011.
11. American Board of Family Medicine website. *https://www.theabfm.org/caq/index.aspx;* Accessed December 2011.

CHAPTER 6

FINANCING AND REIMBURSEMENT

Michael L. Powe

CHAPTER CONTENTS

Physician assistants (PAs), physicians, and other health care professionals entered the fields of medicine and surgery to improve the health and well-being of patients. Their goal was not to become experts in business management, health care accounting techniques, or contract negotiation strategies. However, it is increasingly apparent that these business skills are becoming essential competencies for successful medical practices as the line between the practice of medicine and the business of medicine continues to blur.

The fundamental challenges of the U.S. health care system are well known. The United States spends more per capita on health care than other countries. Health care spending consumes nearly 18% of annual gross domestic product, and costs are increasing at a pace significantly faster than the overall rate of inflation. More than 45 million residents are without health care coverage, nearly 20% of whom are children. In 2009, a Harvard study found that 45,000 deaths occur annually in the United States due to gaps in insurance coverage.[1] In addition, an aging population that will require more health services combined with the ongoing development of expensive high-tech diagnostic and treatment equipment will only exacerbate resource allocation concerns.

Rather than establishing a systematic structure of coordinated care that bases payments and financial incentives on cost-effective outcomes, the health care financing methodologies used in our current system are based on a piece-meal approach that pays for individual medical services, tests, and encounters with limited focus on overall efficiency and outcomes.

With or without federally mandated health care reform, this country will likely continue to undergo an evolution in the manner in which health care services are delivered and financed. Health care professionals who understand the relationship between patient care, payment policies, and practice management systems are likely to be among those who will most successfully navigate a transformed health care system.

It is obvious to most that reimbursement and payment policies should not, in and of themselves, determine patient care treatment decisions or practice patterns. At the same time it is naïve to believe that payments policies do not have a significant impact on how care is delivered, what type of care is provided, the geographic areas in which health care professionals choose to practice, and patient accessibility to health care.

PHYSICIAN ASSISTANTS DELIVER MEDICAL AND SURGICAL SERVICES

PAs deliver quality medical and surgical services that would otherwise be provided by a physician. Numerous government and private sector research reports and studies have verified that within the PA's scope of practice, the quality of care delivered is similar to that of physicians. In addition, patient satisfaction with care provided by PAs is generally equal to that of physicians when PAs treat patients as part of the physician-PA team concept of delivering health care.

When interacting with public and private payers about the services PA perform, it is beneficial to avoid the term *physician assistant services* because this might be construed as referring to a separate set of services not already included in the patient's health plan benefit package. A better approach is to talk in terms of physician services provided by PAs. Always be clear that services are being delivered by a state-authorized PA working with a physician within state law guidelines.

GOVERNMENT-SPONSORED PROGRAMS

Medicare

Medicare, which provides coverage to more than 47 million people, is a health care program available for the aged (older than 65 years), the disabled who have received cash benefits under Social Security for at least 24 months, and those with permanent kidney failure (e.g., end-stage renal disease). The Medicare program is administered by the federal government and is funded through a combination of Medicare premiums, general fund revenues, and patient deductibles and co-payments.

Medicare's coverage is divided into four parts—A, B, C, and D. Medicare Part A pays for hospital facility, equipment, and supply costs; some inpatient care in a skilled nursing facility (SNF); home health care; and hospice care. Medicare Part B pays for professional services delivered by physicians, PAs, and other health care professionals; durable medical equipment; and other medical services and supplies not covered by Part A.

Medicare Part C is a coverage option available to Medicare-eligible beneficiaries that allows them to receive medical coverage through health maintenance organizations (HMOs) or other types of managed care entities or health care networks. Sometimes known as Medicare+Choice plans, Part C plans typically offer an enhanced benefit package (such as routine physicals, eye glasses coverage, and no deductible visits) as compared with Medicare fee-for-service plans. The trade-off is that Medicare Part C enrollees are required to receive their care from a health care professional in a particular health plan or network, whereas those who choose the Medicare Part B fee-for-service option can receive care from any health care provider that accepts Medicare.

Medicare Part D is a prescription drug plan created by the Medicare Prescription Drug Improvement and Modernization Act of 2003 that covers certain costs related to prescription drugs. The program provides prescription drug coverage for both brand-name and generic drugs. The legislation creating Part D included a coverage gap, often referred to as a *donut hole*, in which prescription drugs generally are not covered. Once the Medicare beneficiary and their Part D drug plan have spent $2840 for covered drugs including the deductible, co-payment, and coinsurance amounts, they will be in the donut hole. Under the original Part D plan, a beneficiary had to pay the full cost of prescription drugs while in the donut hole. However, in 2011, beneficiaries received a 50% discount on covered brand-name prescription medications. The donut hole continues until a beneficiary's total out-of-pocket cost reaches $4550. Everyone with Medicare is eligible for Part D coverage, regardless of their health status or current prescription drug utilization when they first qualify for Medicare enrollment.

Our primary focus is on Medicare Parts A and B because those programs have the most direct impact on reimbursement for medical and surgical services provided by PAs and physicians.

Medicare Part A

Generally, Part A does not pay for professional services delivered by physicians and PAs but rather pays institutions such as hospitals on an all-inclusive rate basis. Hospitals, for example, are paid by Part A for inpatient care based on a patient-specific diagnosis-related group (DRG). This lump-sum DRG payment is intended to cover certain employee costs (e.g., licensed practical nurses, technicians), overhead costs of the institution, and supply costs during the patient's stay in the hospital. This prospectively determined DRG payment is meant to cover all facility-related costs associated with the patient's care for the particular admission. If the hospital can deliver the necessary treatment to the patient for less than the DRG payment amount, the hospital keeps the difference. If the hospital's costs for delivering care are higher than the DRG payment, the hospital loses money. Currently, there are more than 500 DRGs, as determined by the Centers for Medicare and Medicaid Services, the government agency that administers the Medicare and Medicaid programs.

Administratively, payments to hospitals are made by *intermediaries*, who are under contract to the federal government to administer the Part A program in a specific geographic state or region. Intermediaries are typically insurance companies, such as Blue Cross Blue Shield.

Medicare Part B

Medicare Part B pays for professional services provided in hospitals, nursing homes, private offices, or a patient's home. Part B also covers services provided "incident to" the physician's care. As with Part A, Medicare contracts with private insurance companies, such as Blue Shield, to administer the Part B program on behalf of the federal government. The administrators of the Part B program are called *Medicare administrative contractors*.

Most Medicare beneficiaries receive services on what is commonly referred to as a *fee-for-service* basis. Under such an option, if a patient walks into a physician`s office or urgent care facility with a broken arm, the physician takes a radiograph, reads the radiograph, sets and casts the fracture, and bills Medicare for the services provided. The value of the service is determined according to the Resource-Based Relative Value Scale (RBRVS) Medicare fee schedule.

Fee-for-service gives the beneficiary maximum flexibility in selecting the physician or other practitioner of choice. However, the patient's out-of-pocket expenses can be higher under the fee-for-service arrangement.

Medicare beneficiaries must satisfy an annual deductible before Medicare pays for any services they receive. (Some Medicare health maintenance organizations [HMOs] and managed care plans may waive the deductible payment.) Once the deductible has been met, Medicare covers 80% of the fee schedule amount and the patient is responsible for the remaining 20%, after meeting the deductible. Medicare's fee schedule amount is generally less than the medical practice's usual charge for the service. This can be shown by a list of the typical fees assessed for the patient who became dizzy and fell off a ladder, as described in Case Study 6-1.

CASE STUDY 6-1

Patient: Paul Peterson, Anytown, Virginia
Practitioner: James Jones, MD, Anytown, Virginia
Medical problem: Patient was on a ladder changing a light bulb. Patient became dizzy, fell, and is suspected to have a broken arm.

Services Provided	Charge	Fee Schedule
Office visit	$75	$60
Radiograph	$65	$45
Casting	$150	$95
Total	$290	$200

Although the fees the physician normally charges amounted to $290, Medicare's approved fee schedule allowed the physician to charge only $200. The actual Medicare payment to the practice would be $160 ($200 × 80%), with the patient being responsible for the 20% (or $40) difference, assuming that the patient has paid his deductible and the physician participates with Medicare (Table 6-1).

For some time, PAs had been covered for services delivered in offices or clinics, hospitals, skilled nursing facilities, and for first-assisting at surgery. Rates of reimbursement have ranged from 65% to 85%. However, services provided by PAs in nonrural health professional shortage area offices and clinics were covered only when billed under the "incident to" billing method, which required the constant on-site presence of the physician. In 1997, the Balanced Budget Act extended coverage to all practice settings at one uniform rate.[2] As of January 1, 1998, Medicare pays the PA's employer for medical and surgical services provided by the PA at 85% of the physician's fee schedule. This includes the office or clinic setting even when the physician is not physically present, if allowed by state law. PAs may treat new Medicare beneficiaries or established patients with new medical problems when billing the service under their name and Medicare national provider identifier (NPI) number. The office bills at the full physician rate, and Medicare will pay for the service at 85% on the basis of use of the PA's NPI number.

The PA's employer bills for the services delivered by the PA, and payment is made to the employer. The employer is required to accept assignment for services provided by the PA. In all cases, the PA must be supervised by a physician; however, the degree of supervision is determined by state law. Typically,

TABLE 6-1 **Medicare Policy for Physician Assistants**

Setting	Supervision	Reimbursement Rate	Services
Office or clinic when physician is not on-site	State law	85% of physician's fee schedule	All services PA is legally authorized to provide that would have been covered if provided personally by a physician
Office or clinic when physician is on-site	Physician must be in the suite of offices	100% of physician's fee schedule*	Same as above
Home visit or house call	State law	85% of physician's fee schedule	Same as above
Skilled nursing facility and nursing facility	State law	85% of physician's fee schedule	Same as above
Office or home visit if rural health professional shortage area	State law	85% of physician's fee schedule	Same as above
Hospital	State law	85% of physician's fee schedule	Same as above
First-assisting at surgery in all settings	State law	85% of physician's first-assist fee schedule†	Same as above
Federal rural health clinic	State law	Cost-based reimbursement	Same as above
HMO	State law	Reimbursement is on capitation basis	All services contracted for as part of an HMO contract

*Using carrier guidelines for "incident to" services.
†85% of 16% = 13.6% of primary surgeon's fee.
HMO, health maintenance organization.

when billing is submitted under the PA's name and Medicare provider number at 85%, only general supervision is required. General supervision, in most states, simply requires that the physician and the PA have access to electronic (e.g., telephone) communication. The PA's employer can be a physician, physician group, hospital, nursing home, group practice, professional medical corporation, limited liability partnership, or limited liability company. In 2002, the Medicare program expanded the ability of PAs to have an ownership interest in a practice. Rules that became effective in April 2002 allow PAs to own an approved Medicare corporation that is eligible to bill the Medicare program.

"Incident to" Services

Medicare has a long-standing policy of covering medical services provided by PAs in offices and clinics under what is called the "incident to" provision, at 100% of the physician's fee schedule. Even with the expansion of PA coverage at the 85% reimbursement rate in all settings through the Balanced Budget Act of 1997, "incident to" remains an appropriate billing mechanism for PAs as long as Medicare's more restrictive billing requirements are followed. "Incident to" billing allows a PA to treat a patient, bill the service to Medicare under the physician's name, and be reimbursed at 100% of the fee schedule, even though the physician never provided hands-on care to the patient during the encounter in which the PA delivered care.

If a medical service provided by PAs is to be billed under the "incident to" provision, the following criteria must be met:

- "Incident to" billing applies in private offices or clinics and not in the inpatient setting.

The physician must personally examine the patient and establish a diagnosis during the patient's first visit for a particular medical problem; any established patient who presents with a new medical condition must also be treated and diagnosed by the physician to qualify for "incident to" billing.

PAs may provide the follow-up care for the diagnosed medical problem.[3]

The physician must be in the suite of offices (direct supervision) when the PA renders follow-up care. *Direct supervision* does not require that the supervising physician be in the same room with the PA or have any interaction with the patient when the PA delivers care, but he or she must be in the office suite and immediately available to provide assistance and direction, if necessary.

The physician is responsible for the overall care of the patient and should maintain involvement in the patient's care at a frequency that reflects his or her active involvement and participation in the ongoing management of the patient's treatment. That involvement could be reviewing the patient's medical record or having the PA and physician discuss the patient's progress.

Shared Services

When both a physician and a PA deliver an evaluation and management (E/M) service to a hospital inpatient/outpatient or emergency department patient, the physician may bill for the entire service as long as he or she provides any face-to-face portion of the E/M encounter. Payment for the combined service is at 100% of the physician fee schedule. The rules governing the ability to bill a shared visit include the following:

- Only E/M services qualify for shared service billing; procedures or critical care services cannot be billed as a shared service.
- The physician must personally provide some portion of the E/M service in a face-to-face encounter with the patient. The physician's professional service rendered to the patient must be clearly documented in the patient's medical record. Simply having the physician cosign and/or review the patient's chart would not be sufficient to support billing under the shared visit billing guidelines.
- Care delivered by the physician and the PA must occur on the same calendar day, not simply within a 24-hour period of time. (The physician is not required to be in the hospital at the time the PA delivers his or her portion of care.)
- Both the physician and PA must have a common employer or work for the same entity (e.g., same hospital, same group, or solo physician employing a PA).

Certified Rural Health Clinics

In the mid-1960s, the shortage and/or maldistribution of physicians had reached a crisis. The supply of physicians had become insufficient to meet the demands of smaller, rural communities. Although PAs were well accepted by residents in these rural communities, Medicare and Medicaid coverage for their services was not available in most cases.

In 1977, Congress passed the Rural Health Clinic Services Act (Public Law 95-210) in an effort to increase the availability of primary health care services to rural areas of the country. Federal certification as a rural health clinic (RHC) allows the clinic to be reimbursed by means of a cost-based methodology, as opposed to the fee-for-service payment system. Medical care provided by a PA in a certified RHC is covered at the same basic rate as that provided by a physician, as long as the PA is practicing in accordance with state law and state regulatory requirements. Physicians who provide care in designated underserved areas receive a 10% bonus payment. At present, that bonus payment is available only to physicians.

Two types of RHCs exist: independent and provider based. An independent RHC is generally a stand-alone clinic that could be owned by a PA. Provider-based RHCs are typically an integral part of a hospital, nursing home, or home health agency that is already a Medicare-certified provider. Each rural health clinic has a per-patient reimbursement rate generally based on the clinic's overall reasonable costs divided by the number of yearly patient encounters. For independent RHCs there is a maximum per-patient encounter amount that will be paid, which is referred to as a payment limit or cap. Provider-based RHCs affiliated with a hospital with fewer than 50 beds are not subject to the cap.

To be eligible for federal RHC status, the clinic must be located in nonurban rural areas with current health care shortage designations. In addition, the clinic must have either a PA, a nurse practitioner, or a certified nurse midwife on-site and available to patients at least 50% of the time the clinic is open.

Medicaid

Medicaid, authorized by Title XIX of the Social Security Act, is a program jointly funded by federal and state governments that provides medical assistance for low-income individuals, families with dependent children, the aged, and the disabled. Although the federal government sets basic guidelines, establishes a basic set of core benefits, and generally pays 50% to 80% of the cost of Medicaid (depending on the state's per capita income), individual states actually administer the program. The Medicaid program, which began on January 1, 1966, covers more than 60 million people.

In their Medicaid programs, states may cover medical and surgical services provided by PAs. The decision as to whether to cover PAs generally rests with the state, except with respect to federally certified rural health clinics. If a clinic is designated by the federal government as a certified RHC, the state's Medicaid program must cover PA-provided services in the clinic. Presently, all states cover PAs under their fee-for-service or managed care Medicaid plans.

As Medicaid costs rose in the late 1980s and early 1990s, states began to experiment with more cost-effective methods of providing care to beneficiaries; fee-for-service programs were shifted to managed care delivery systems. To make many of these changes, states were required to get permission from the federal government in the form of 1915 and 1115 waivers, which provided states with exemptions from the traditional guidelines of the Medicaid program.

One of the popular concepts that states have used to lower costs, and ideally to improve the quality of care, is to assign Medicaid beneficiaries to a specific health care provider, known as a primary care provider (PCP). The rationale is that beneficiaries will have better continuity of care and will be more likely to access the health care system at the appropriate time and place if one specific provider is responsible for directing their overall care. The PCP can refer the beneficiary to specialist and hospital inpatient care services as required. The federal government allows PAs to serve as PCPs, and some states allow PAs to assume that role.

States have the authority to name PAs as primary care case managers (PCCMs) under the Medicaid program. A PCCM is typically paid a small monthly fee to act as a gatekeeper or coordinator of care for beneficiaries. States may cover PAs at the physician`s rate of reimbursement or on a slightly discounted fee basis. Coverage may apply in all practice settings and for all medical services, or there may be limitations. Table 6-2 shows the most current information on how states cover PAs under their Medicaid plans.

PRIVATE INSURANCE

Almost all private insurance companies cover medical and surgical services provided by PAs. However, with scores of different payers and plans, including preferred provider organizations (PPOs), health maintenance organizations (HMOs), and fee-for-service programs operating in the United States, there may be differences in both how services delivered by PAs are covered and how claim forms should be submitted. Even within the same insurance company, PA coverage policies can change on the basis of the particular plan type, the specific type of service being provided, and the part of the country in which the service is delivered. That being said, in fact there are only two basic variations in PA coverage by private payers. The service is either billed under the name of the supervising physician or under the name of the PA. The key is to determine the particular policy for each insurance company. Although many private payers do not separately credential or issue provider numbers to PAs, that does not negatively affect coverage of services delivered. When plans do not credential or issue provider numbers to PAs, they typically want the service billed under the name of the supervising physician, occasionally with a modifier code attached. As mergers and acquisitions continue to consolidate the health care marketplace, coverage policies for PAs are becoming much more consistent throughout the country.

As of 2011, 14 states had some type of reimbursement mandate in place requiring payment by third-party payers. Those mandates range from mandating coverage for first assisting at surgery, to care delivered in underserved communities, to coverage of all services that would have been covered if provided by a physician.

Many businesses have opted to no longer purchase medical coverage for their employees from managed care organizations (MCOs) and insurance companies. Instead, they are self-insuring (paying out of their company funds the full cost of providing insurance/paying claims) and are using insurance companies only for claims processing and other administrative tasks, also known as *administrative services*. These self-insured companies are free to design their own benefit plans and to decide which health care professionals are eligible to deliver care. Employee health plans for businesses that are self-insured are exempt from state reimbursement mandates.

Because of the potential variation, it is virtually impossible to present a complete picture of specific private insurance plan coverage policies, as has been done with respect to Medicare and Medicaid. Instead, this section attempts to outline basic concepts that can help in the determination of how medical and surgical services provided by PAs are covered. Detailed information on nearly all private payers can be obtained from the American Academy of Physician Assistants (AAPA) members-only website.

Physician Assistants' Recognition

The AAPA occasionally receives calls from PAs who have contacted a particular insurance company and been told that PAs are not reimbursed. Upon closer examination, the medical services provided by the PA were covered, but the insurance company did not pay directly to the PA. Instead, payment for the PA's services was made to the employing physician or employer. The following case study may better explain the potential problem.

TABLE 6-2 **Coverage for Physician Assistants in State Medicaid Programs**

State	PA Covered Provider	Reimbursement Rate (% Physician Fee)	Physician Supervision Requirements*
Alabama	Yes	80%-100%	Same as PA law
Alaska	Yes	85%	Same as PA law
Arizona[†]	Yes	90%	Same as PA law
Arkansas	Yes	100%	Physician on-site
California	Yes	100%	Same as PA law
Colorado	Yes	100%	Same as PA law
Connecticut	Yes	100%	Same as PA law
Delaware	Yes	100%	Same as PA law
District of Columbia	Yes	100%	Same as PA law
Florida	Yes	80%-100%	Same as PA law
Georgia	Yes	90%	Same as PA law
Hawaii	Yes	100%	Physician on-site
Idaho	Yes	85%	Same as PA law
Illinois	Yes	100%	Same as PA law
Indiana	Yes	100%	Same as PA law
Iowa	Yes	Hospital—75% Nursing—85% All other—100%	Same as PA law
Kansas	Yes	75%	Same as PA law
Kentucky	Yes	75%	Same as PA law
Louisiana	Yes	80%-100%	Same as PA law
Maine	Yes	100%	Same as PA law
Maryland	Yes	100%	Physician on-site*
Massachusetts	Yes	85%	Same as PA law
Michigan	Yes	100%	Same as PA law
Minnesota	Yes	65%-90%	Same as PA law
Mississippi	Yes	100%	Same as PA law
Missouri	Yes	100%	Same as PA law
Montana	Yes	90%-100%	Same as PA law
Nebraska	Yes	100%	Same as PA law
Nevada	Yes	65%-87%	Same as PA law
New Hampshire	Yes	100%	Same as PA law
New Jersey	Yes (MCO only)	100%	Same as PA law
New Mexico	Yes	100%	Same as PA law
New York	Yes	100%	Same as PA law
North Carolina	Yes	100%	Same as PA law
North Dakota	Yes	75%	Same as PA law
Ohio	Yes	85%-100%	Same as PA law
Oklahoma	Yes	75%	Same as PA law
Oregon	Yes	100%	Same as PA law
Pennsylvania	Yes	100%	Same as PA law
Rhode Island	Yes	100%	Same as PA law
South Carolina	Yes	100%	Same as PA law
South Dakota	Yes	90%	Same as PA law
Tennessee	Yes	Varies by MCO	Same as PA law
Texas	Yes	92%-100%	Same as PA law
Utah	Yes	100%	Same as PA law
Vermont	Yes	90%	Same as PA law
Virginia	Yes	100%	Physician on-site
Washington	Yes	100%	Same as PA law

TABLE 6-2 **Coverage for Physician Assistants in State Medicaid Programs—cont'd**

State	PA Covered Provider	Reimbursement Rate (% Physician Fee)	Physician Supervision Requirements*
West Virginia	Yes	100%	Same as PA law
Wisconsin	Yes	90%-100%	Same as PA law
Wyoming	Yes	100%	Same as PA law

*In the case of federally certified rural health clinics, the state Medicaid program cannot establish supervisory requirements more stringent than those found in the state PA law. Consequently, the "physician on-site" requirement does not apply to Medicaid reimbursement in rural health clinics unless it is a requirement of the Medical Practice Act.

†Arizona Health Care Cost Containment System (AHCCS).

MCO, managed care organization.

CASE STUDY 6-2

A PA once called the AAPA to say that she was told by a major insurance company that the company would not reimburse for a service provided by a PA. The insurance company was immediately contacted by AAPA staff, and the following question was asked: "Are physician medical services covered when performed by PAs under the supervision of the physician when billed under the physician's name and provider number?" The answer was that yes, of course, those services would be covered. The AAPA staff person indicated that a PA had just called the company and received a response indicating that the service would not be covered. The insurance company representative said that she remembered the call and said that "the person who called had asked if the company paid the PA for providing a medical service. We don't pay the PA, we pay the PA's employer." Was this a simple misunderstanding or an attempt to use semantics to avoid paying a claim? The lesson to be learned is that how you ask the question will often determine the kind of answer you get.

Instead of asking whether PAs can bill for services or whether the insurer will pay to the PA, it may be more useful to ask whether services performed by PAs are covered by a particular plan, as well as how the service should be billed to the company. It is important to keep in mind that PAs are acting as legal agents of the supervising physician. In general, the services performed by a PA are deemed to have been delegated by the supervising physician.

Credentialing, Enrollment, and Recognition

Some confusion may exist regarding terms that describe the relationship between PAs and third-party payers. The issue is how payers recognize PAs and the PAs' ability to deliver and report the care provided to the payers' subscribers. Some payers enroll PAs in their plans, whereas others ask that PAs be credentialed. Not to be confused with the concepts of being credentialed and/or privileged to provide services in a hospital setting, credentialing with payers refers to the collection of basic information such as licensing data and malpractice coverage or claims information.

In general, there is no direct correlation between enrollment or credentialing of PAs and payment for their services, as long as the payer has another method of accounting for and covering the PAs' services.

HEALTH CARE REFORM—NEW MODELS OF CARE DELIVERY

There is a growing recognition that the prevalent reimbursement model currently in use, fee-for-service (FFS) reimbursement, is at least partially responsible for the inefficient system of care delivery. Simply put, FFS reimbursement often rewards uncoordinated, high-volume care with little emphasis on outcomes.

Some of the recent health care delivery models have the potential to achieve improved care delivery while also reducing costs. One of the tenets of these new care models includes correlating reimbursement to patient health care outcomes through entities such as accountable care organizations (ACOs), patient-centered medical homes, and insurance exchanges.

Accountable Care Organizations

An ACO, in general terms, is a local or regional health organization consisting of health care professionals, typically one or more hospitals and related health care entities that have a formal or informal relationship and are jointly responsible for achieving measurable improvements in the quality and cost of health care delivered within a given community. ACOs will have a strong base of primary care professionals but may also provide a wide range of specialty care. ACOs, perhaps with the assistance of public and/or private third-party payers, should have the ability to establish achievable, evidence-based benchmarks for quality and cost for a defined patient population, a formal legal structure allowing them to administer payments, and a system to distribute shared savings, or levy penalties, depending on whether targets are met. In short, an ACO will likely have the capability to impose practice, reporting, and compensation standards on all participating professionals and health care organizations. If the ACO concept becomes widely accepted, it will fundamentally change how PAs, physicians, and other health care professionals interact with hospitals, as well as how practices are clinically organized and paid for delivering medical and surgical services.

Patient-Centered Medical Home

The goal of an effective patient-centered medial home (PCMH) is to establish a primary care model of care that improves the value and quality of health care for patients. Conceptually, a PCMH transforms the manner in which health care in general, and primary care in particular, is delivered. The PCMH is responsible for providing and coordinating a patient's total health care needs and, as needed, arranging care with other qualified professionals and health care organizations. A medical home provides comprehensive and integrated care that is patient and family centered, culturally appropriate, committed to quality and safety, cost-effective, affordable, and provided by a health care team led by a physician, PA, or other qualified health care professional.

The PCMH seeks to alter the paradigm of the fractionalized, episodic health care approach that is so prevalent in this country. The belief is that coordinated care leads to better outcomes for patients at a lower cost.

Insurance Exchanges

One of the central components of the Patient Protection and Affordable Care Act (PPACA) is the creation of health insurance exchanges. These primarily state-regulated programs will provide an assortment of health insurance plans to uninsured individuals, those who purchase individual health policies, and small group employers. The exchanges will provide an opportunity for consumers to review and compare health coverage options on the basis of the plan's benefit structure, as well as on pricing information such as premiums, deductibles, and coinsurance.

Simply put, an insurance exchange is the formation of a competitive state or regionally based marketplace offering certain consumers an opportunity to purchase health insurance policies, presumably at a more competitive price than that which is available in the current marketplace. In theory, the exchanges will have bargaining power with hospitals and health care systems that rival some of the largest employer group plans. How states choose to implement exchanges and whether the overall concept will work falls back on that well-worn idiom—the devil is in the details.

The PPACA requires that each state establish an American Health Benefit Exchange by January 1, 2014. States are expected to establish exchanges, with the federal government maintaining the authority to establish an exchange if a state fails to do so. States can create multiple exchanges, as long as only one exchange serves a specific geographic area. States can also work together to form regional exchanges.

The plans offered by the exchange will have to meet minimum essential benefit standards developed by the federal government.

Some of the expected benefits of an insurance exchange include the following:

- Increased selection: Consumers will have access to a choice of health plans.
- Portability: Health insurance coverage will not be linked to employment, making it easier for individuals to maintain coverage even when they change employers.
- Information: Consumers will be able to more directly compare plans and potential government subsidies, making it simpler for them to determine if they qualify for financial assistance.
- Nondiscrimination: Insurers will not be able to discriminate or deny coverage on the basis of health history.
- Competitive pricing: Health plans within the exchange will disperse risk in a manner similar to large group plans, causing premiums to be more competitive.

Pay for Performance

Pay for performance is an emerging health care concept that is being rapidly adopted by segments of federal government and by private payers. Pay for performance is known by a number of different names, such as *value-based purchasing*, *quality-based purchasing*, or *P4P*. P4P is an attempt to use financial incentives to elicit specific types of treatment patterns from health care professionals and/or medical outcomes for patients. The intent is to improve the quality of care for patients while reducing overall health care costs by encouraging the utilization of the most effective and current treatment regimens. Financial incentives may take the form of lowering payments or creating financial disincentives (penalties) when certain goals are not met, increasing reimbursement, or adding a bonus payment when those goals are achieved. In reality, P4P and the qualitative reporting measures associated with it are in their early stages with limited evidence of their practical application.

The Medicare program has been involved with several P4P programs for hospitals, nursing homes, and physician offices. One of the larger Medicare P4P programs is known as the Physician Quality Reporting System (PQRS). This program is open to physicians, PAs, and other health care professionals. The PQRS will pay a bonus on a practice's total Medicare billing if the practice reports up to three quality measures at least 80% of the time those measures are applicable to Medicare patients that are being treated in the practice. A list of quality measures have been developed by Centers for Medicaid and Medicaid Services for use in the program. The quality measures have been developed with input from health care professionals. Examples of reporting measures include ensuring that a diabetic patient (type 1 or type 2) has had his or her hemoglobin A_{1c} checked during the reporting period and ordering an antibiotic for a patient at least 1 hour before beginning surgery, if applicable.

Concerns about the number of medical errors, a lack of adherence to the most up-to-date standards of care, and a desire to reduce costs through early intervention would suggest that P4P activities are here to stay. It is essential that the measures being developed have appropriate collaboration and buy-in from the health care professional who will ultimately implement the measures.

CONCLUSION

The PA profession has proven its ability to deliver quality medical and surgical care to patients. As this country continues to search for solutions to increasing health care costs, the growing availability of expensive technologies and treatment options, and millions of uninsured individuals, even more payers and health care–related organizations should realize the important role that PAs play in the health care system. One must not forget, however, that to a large extent health care is a business. In addition to delivering physician-quality medical care, PAs must be cognizant of their responsibility to understand their value to their employers and more broadly to the health care system. A better understanding of both the financing and payment mechanisms of the health care system are important steps in achieving that goal. While acknowledging that an understanding of the financial aspects of health care is important, the most important quality that PAs bring to the health care system has, and will continue to be, a focus on what is best for the patient.

Any health care system that has as its goal increased access to cost-effective care should recognize that PAs, working in a team with physicians, are an indispensible part of the solution. It should also be recognized that logic has not always been the driving force in health care policy decisions. All PAs and PA students must understand the importance of being advocates for the profession as health care continues to transform at both the state and national levels.

CLINICAL APPLICATIONS

1. What are the potential problems with a fee-for-service reimbursement system?
2. What is the difference between Medicare Part A and Medicare Part B?
3. Define Medicare's "incident to" and shared billing concepts, and list the criteria that must be met for reimbursement for services provided by PAs under these two reimbursement methodologies.
4. What potential benefits do ACOs and patient-centered medical homes offer to patients?
5. Define the method by which payment is made to certified rural health clinics.

KEY POINTS

- Although clinicians do not like to think of themselves as "business experts," today's health care environment requires that MDs and PAs be well informed about a patient's health care coverage in order to ensure that they receive optimum care.
- Although Medicare provides for reimbursement for services provided by PAs, there are stringent rules to avoid submission of duplicate bills by the PA and his or her supervising physicians. This can be particularly confusing in academic health centers where there are separate rules for residents.
- Medicaid reimbursements vary widely from state to state—both for types of providers who are reimbursed and for covered services.
- Private fee-for-service insurance companies must comply with state laws for reimbursement of PAs. In addition, a specific insurance company may have a wide range of contracts for different "plans" for individual employers. Knowledge of these contracts may be an important consideration in negotiating employment contracts.
- New systems of care created by the Accountable Care Act are intended to create clearer reimbursement policies that are designed to increase efficiency, improve quality, and decrease costs.

References

1. Wilper AP, Woolhandler S, Lasser KE, et al. Health insurance and mortality in US adults. Am J Pub Health 2009;99:2289–2295.
2. Medicare Transmittal 1764, August 28, 2002.
3. Medicare Program Memorandum, Transmittal No. AB-98-15, April 1998.

The resources for this chapter can be found at www.expertconsult.com.

CHAPTER 7

The Political Process

Ann Davis

CHAPTER CONTENTS

Please do not skip this chapter just because you never intend to become involved in politics. You have entered medicine during a period of rapid and profound changes in health care delivery. Where there is change, there is politics. You *are* involved in politics. Although sometimes politics is described in disparaging tones, being involved in politics is nothing to be ashamed of because, in its truest sense, politics is the art of getting things done—and physician assistants (PAs) are masters at getting things done!

This chapter is not written for professional lobbyists, policy wonks, or pundits. It is written for the rest of us. Because it deals with the political process of making laws and regulations, you will find frequent use of words such as *most* and *usually*. Just as there can be a good deal of ambiguity in law, there can be a good deal of it in the making of laws. This lack of predictability can be difficult for PAs because it may seem unscientific. After you work with the process for a while, however, you will be able to predict some outcomes that initially seemed unpredictable, and, as in medicine, you will become comfortable with some level of uncertainty. The chapter is divided into five parts:

- Individual responsibilities
- The role and importance of professional organizations
- The legislative process
- The regulatory process
- Case studies

Because state processes are generally structured along the lines of federal processes, the description of the federal system precedes the description of state mechanisms. In the discussion of state activities, where and how you can exert influence is integrated into the text.

The word *you* is used frequently. Please do not interpret this to mean that anyone expects or wants you to take on the entire government single-handedly. Although individualism is highly valued in our society, the fact is that government responds best to group influence. You can and should be an important part of the PA group.

This chapter aims to engage you in advocacy as a PA and presents this activity as a two-step process: become informed and become involved.

INDIVIDUAL RESPONSIBILITIES

As a PA, you have a personal responsibility to understand the political process and to use that knowledge to advance the interests of patients. There are many levels of involvement. At minimum you should stay abreast of current issues and trends in health care by reading journals, newspapers, and professional publications, and you should vote. You can also provide moral or financial support for the efforts of others who work on your behalf by becoming a member of a PA organization or advocacy group. You can become one of those workers yourself, participating in the government-related activities of PA and other health care organizations. You can seek appointment to a licensing board or run for public office at the local, state, or national level.

If running for public office is not for you, consider supporting a candidate whose positions on health care and other issues are compatible with your own. There are dozens of ways to support a candidate: becoming a campaign manager or an issues coordinator, hosting a fundraiser, canvassing for votes, working on a phone bank to solicit supporters, organizing a committee of "Physician Assistants for Candidate N," speaking at community functions in support of the candidate, distributing campaign materials, working to "get out the vote" on election day, and, of course, voting.

If campaign work is not attractive or feasible, consider volunteering your services to individuals already elected to federal or state office. One valuable function you can perform is to advise elected officials about health care issues affecting your community. All legislators are called on to make decisions on a wide variety of topics. Having a constituent health care expert as a resource is a great asset.

Make friends before you need them. If legislators and others in government know you and understand the valuable role that PAs play in health care delivery, they will be more likely to come to your assistance when you need help. Your credibility will have been enhanced if, in the past, you were involved with issues that were not self-serving, such as bicycle safety measures, support for prevention programs, or health care for the homeless. If you know someone has introduced legislation in one of these areas, offer your personal support. Historically, PAs have been interested in the broader health care issues because resolving these issues has benefited patients. If you maintain a genuine interest in patient welfare, rather than speaking up only when someone threatens your professional "turf," you will earn genuine respect.

You can do several things to influence the legislative and regulatory processes, even when no issues in which you are interested are awaiting legislation. In fact, if you do these things routinely, you will enhance your credibility, which is like money in the bank.

The first thing to do is to maintain contact with your elected representatives. The idea is to have them smile, instead of groan, when they see you coming. When you meet with an elected official, it is best to make an appointment and be prepared to discuss a specific issue. Of course, you will not wait until the busiest days of the legislative session, when everything is in turmoil, to make your visit. Personal contact with legislators when they are at home in the district or between sessions is most productive.

A personal visit is not the only option. You may read something about your representative's pet project and write him or her a letter of support (if, in fact, you are in support). Such letters are read and often remembered. If you receive an interesting piece of information on health care that you think might be useful, pass it along.

You may also do this with regulators. Remember, regulators are all people who are trying to develop or maintain a level of expertise. They need information, so provide it. A good relationship with a legislator, a legislator's staff person, or a regulator is invaluable.

Finally, support your state and national PA organizations. This suggestion is not just another pitch for membership; it is a tactical imperative. When any organization testifies before a governmental body, one of the first questions asked is, "How many people does your society represent?" The larger the number, the more credibility the organization is given. It is also important to know where your professional organizations stand on an issue before you go to your representative's office to voice your opinion. If you are an active member, you may have already influenced the organization's policy-making process. Even if you disagree with the group's final determination, at least you will understand how and why it reached its decision and you may choose to remain silent rather than undercut its efforts.

Remember the value of belonging to a professional organization. There is a symbiotic relationship between an organization and its members. Organizations need you, and you need them. They know the legislative and regulatory processes, as well as what issues are under consideration. You know the issues from a personal perspective because you confront them daily. Your personal professional perspective is essential and should be conveyed to lawmakers or regulators, particularly when your association says it is time to call, write, or visit them.

One of the first things you must know about government is that it regulates almost every aspect of your professional life. The most important law affecting you as an individual PA is one passed by the state and implemented by a state licensing board or agency—the PA practice act.

PRACTICE LAWS

Occupational regulation is the prerogative of the state, rather than the federal government. Each state licenses, certifies, or registers a number of different professions and occupations, everyone from physicians and architects to barbers and plumbers. The goal of occupational regulation is to protect public health and safety. This is done by granting licenses only to individuals who meet minimum standards of education and skill, by defining a scope of practice, and by disciplining those who break the law or fail to uphold certain professional standards. A licensing or regulatory agency can seek an injunction and ultimately revoke a license to prevent the public from being harmed by a negligent or incompetent practitioner. Lawbreakers may also face civil or criminal penalties.

PAs belong to a regulated profession. In broad terms, this means that an individual seeking to work as a PA must first obtain permission from the state and then abide by any conditions of practice that the state has established. The requirements for securing this permission, which is called *licensure*, or rarely *state certification*, or *registration*, vary from state to state. As a result of efforts by the American Academy of Physician Assistants and state PA associations, there is growing uniformity in the laws that govern PAs. Total uniformity is an unrealistic goal because each state writes its laws slightly differently and cherishes its prerogative to do so. The differences in style and content are problems with which every regulated occupation and profession must cope.

The basis for regulation of PAs is found in the language of the PA practice act. The law may be included in the medical practice act, which governs doctors, or it may be a separate section of the state statutes. The law is further amplified by regulations issued by the licensing board. Every PA should have a copy of the current state law and regulations governing his or her practice, which may be obtained from the licensing board or found on the licensing board's website. Ignorance is no excuse if you are ever accused of breaking the law.

Who is responsible for licensing and regulating PAs? In most cases, the regulatory agency is the Board of Medical Examiners, the same entity that licenses physicians. A small number of states have separate PA boards. A handful of states have departments of education or professional regulation that regulate all health practitioners. A list of PA state regulatory agencies is available on the American Academy of Physician Assistants website.

In the law and regulations, you will find details about qualifications; applications and fees for licensure; scope of practice, or what physicians may delegate to PAs; supervision requirements; prescribing and dispensing privileges; criteria for license renewals, protection of the title "physician assistant"; and what constitutes a violation of the law and the disciplinary measures that can be invoked, as well as information about administrative procedures and due process. You may also find information on the composition, terms of appointment, and other powers of the regulatory board, allowing you to determine what role PAs play in the state's regulatory system. Most medical boards have PA advisory committees that provide PAs with a way to participate in, and contribute to, the regulatory process, and a growing number of states include PAs as medical board members.

The two universal requirements for obtaining state credentials (best referred to as "licensure") as a PA are:

1. Graduation from an accredited PA educational program
2. Passage of the Physician Assistant National Certifying Examination (PANCE), administered by the National Commission on Certification of Physician Assistants (NCCPA)

The NCCPA examination, though part of a voluntary, private sector certification process, functions as the national licensing examination for PAs. Every state requires that potential licensees have passed it. Although a few states may test PAs on their familiarity with state law, no state administers its own examination to test clinical knowledge.

Your state license must be renewed on a regular cycle, every 1, 2, or 3 years. Some jurisdictions require that you provide evidence that you have maintained your NCCPA certification or that you have completed a minimum number of continuing medical education (CME) credits and you will need to pay a renewal fee. Keep in mind that the NCCPA certification system must be dealt with separately; do not confuse it with your state license, certification, or registration. To maintain certification by the NCCPA, you must pay NCCPA a fee and register 100 hours of CME every 2 years. It is also necessary to recertify every 6 years by taking an examination. You may use the letters "PA-C" after your name only if you are currently certified by the NCCPA.

The PA law and regulations also include criteria for physician supervision. Most states include in their definition of supervision the ability of the physician and the PA to be in contact with each other by telecommunication. More details may be specified if the PA will be practicing in an office or clinic separate from the supervising physician. Although no state allows a PA to work without a supervising physician, no state requires that a supervising physician must always be on site while a PA is providing care. The most effective state laws allow the specific requirements for supervision, including the number of PAs that a physician may supervise and requirements for chart co-signature, to be determined at the practice level.

All U.S. states have authorized PAs to sign prescriptions if the supervising physician delegates this authority. The law or regulations may place restrictions on which kinds of medications a PA may prescribe. The authority to dispense medications is also regulated by the state. Pharmacists vigorously protect this privilege and make good arguments for a separation of the prescribing and dispensing functions. Therefore a physician's or PA's ability to provide patients with medications from a supply maintained in the office or clinic is often more easily justified in rural areas or other locations without pharmacy services. Some states do not permit anyone other than a pharmacist to dispense drugs. In nearly all jurisdictions, giving patients drug samples that have been supplied by a pharmaceutical company is not the same as dispensing and is not subject to the same restrictions.

Regulation of the PA profession has been evolving since the first practice act was passed in the late 1960s. The founders of the profession made a conscious, political decision to establish a system in which PAs were recognized under the licenses of their supervising physicians. Changes in health care delivery and greater numbers of PAs, as well as the need for administrative efficiency, have persuaded most states to modify this approach. The more modern system, advocated by the AAPA, is one in which licensure is granted to a PA on the basis of his or her credentials (i.e., on proof of meeting the educational and examination requirements of the law). A licensed PA can practice once he or she has established a physician-PA relationship with one or more licensed supervising physicians. Such systems greatly facilitate rapid deployment of the PA workforce and diminish administrative burden for licensees and for the state.

A good state law is one that allows physicians to delegate to PAs any task or responsibility within their scope of practice that the PA is competent to perform. However, a PA's scope of practice can be limited by a law, a regulation, or even a licensure application that contains a list of tasks that physicians may delegate. It can be limited by a system in which licensing board members are allowed, when reviewing PA practice descriptions, to arbitrarily delete certain procedures on the basis of their personal biases. It can also be limited by legislators who do not understand the depth and breadth of PA education and training.

SIX KEY ELEMENTS OF A MODERN PA PRACTICE ACT

- Licensure as the regulatory term
- Adaptable supervision requirements
- Full delegated prescriptive authority
- Chart co-signature requirements determined at the practice level
- Scope of practice determined by physician delegation
- No restriction on the number of PAs a physician may supervise

From American Academy of Physician Assistants, 2008.

INDIVIDUALS: PART OF THE WHOLE

This section provides you with information on the structure and mission of your professional organizations: the AAPA and the state PA academies. Many PAs also find great value in belonging to a PA specialty society.

The AAPA, established in 1968, is the national professional society for PAs. At the headquarters in Alexandria, Virginia, a full-time staff carries out the organization's major activities: advocacy and government relations, research and data collection, public education, publications, continuing medical education and professional development, employment, and other member services. One of the Academy's most important functions is to speak for the profession before the U.S. Congress and federal agencies. Even in a representative democracy such as the United States, it is difficult for one person to single-handedly affect the shape of laws and regulations. It is generally true that legislators and bureaucrats are more responsive to organizations that convey the interests of a large group than they are to individuals. Efficiency, accountability, and credibility come into play here. Therefore, the Academy performs an important role when it voices the PA profession's views on federal legislation and regulations.

Lobbying is done daily by the professional staff of the AAPA. At congressional hearings or during appointments with lawmakers and their aides, the staff may be accompanied by PAs who are elected officers of the Academy or who have special expertise or established relationships with the legislators. The Academy also has a congressional visit program that facilitates individual meetings between PAs and their senators and representatives. Legislative alerts and Academy publications are used to inform AAPA members about important issues or to request that they contact their congressional representatives or a federal agency about a particular subject. Biennially, the AAPA invites members to attend a government affairs conference in Washington that includes a day on Capitol Hill.

On the state level, PA interests are represented by state PA associations. These associations are chartered constituent chapters of the AAPA. Among its other projects, each state academy must advance the interests of the profession before the legislature, the licensing board, and other state agencies. A majority of PA state societies employ professional association management staff. Many have lobbyists and legal counsel. However, even in the chapters with a significant number of paid employees, the most substantive work is done by the members themselves. The AAPA advocacy and government affairs staff helps chapter leaders with these projects by providing information, technical resources, and consultation services. For example, the AAPA can supply copies of other state laws, model language, fact sheets, and demographic data, as well as analyses of proposed rules and legislation. The Academy can also assist state chapters by sending statewide e-mail "legislative action alerts" on behalf of the chapter. The Academy's goal is to promote uniformity and maximize the ability of PAs to provide care through appropriate state laws and regulations.

FEDERAL LEGISLATIVE PROCESS: HOW A BILL BECOMES LAW

The legislative processes in the U.S. Senate and the House of Representatives are similar, although each chamber has its own rules and traditions. With only 100 members, the Senate seems flexible and informal compared with the 435-member House, in which a strict hierarchy and rigid system of rules are necessary to expedite business.[1]

Legislative proposals may be introduced by senators or representatives when Congress is in session. The bill—prefixed with *HR* when introduced in the House of Representatives and *S* when introduced in the Senate—is given a number that is based on the order of introduction. It is then referred to a committee that has jurisdiction over the bill's subject matter.

The committee is the heart of the legislative process because it is here that a bill receives its sharpest scrutiny. Professional staff expedites the committee's business by researching issues, identifying supporters and opponents, and designing politically acceptable options and compromises. When a committee decides to act on a legislative proposal, it generally conducts hearings to provide the executive branch, interested groups, and individuals an opportunity to formally present their views on the issue. After hearings have ended, the committee meets to "mark up" the bill (i.e., decide on the language of amendments). When a committee votes to approve a measure and send it to the floor, it justifies its actions in a written statement called a *report*, which accompanies the bill. The committee report is useful because it describes the purpose and scope of the bill, explains the committee amendments, indicates proposed changes in existing law, and frequently includes instructions to government agencies on how the language of the new law should be interpreted and implemented.[1]

Most bills never make it out of committee. The enormous volume of legislation (≈25,000 measures in each 2-year Congress) makes it impossible for every bill to be considered. In addition, many are duplicative, lack sufficient support, or are purposefully ignored in an effort to "kill" them. Only a small percentage of all bills introduced are enacted into law.

The route to a vote by the full House of Representatives usually lies through the Rules Committee, which sets guidelines for the length and form of the debate. The Senate, on the other hand, calls up a bill by voting on a motion to consider it or by "unanimous consent," in which the bill comes up for a vote if no one objects. In both houses, bills may be further amended on the floor before the vote on passage. However, because lawmakers rely heavily on the committee system to ensure that issues are carefully and expertly assessed, amendments on the floor need considerable support in order to be approved.

When a bill has been passed, it is sent to the other chamber for action, where the entire legislative process starts over. Often, the House and Senate consider similar bills. If the measures passed by the two bodies are identical, the resultant bill is sent to the White House for the president's signature. Usually, the measures are not identical, and unless the chamber that first passed the bill agrees to the changes made by the second, a House-Senate conference is arranged to resolve the differences.

Conference committees comprise members of the committees that originally considered the bills. Theoretically, the conferees are not authorized to delete provisions or language that both the House and the Senate have agreed to, nor are they supposed to draft or insert entirely new provisions. In practice, however, they have wide latitude. When agreement is reached, a conference report is written that includes a final version of the bill with the conferees' recommendations. Each chamber must then vote on the report. If no agreement is reached by the conferees, or if either chamber does not accept the conference report, the bill dies.

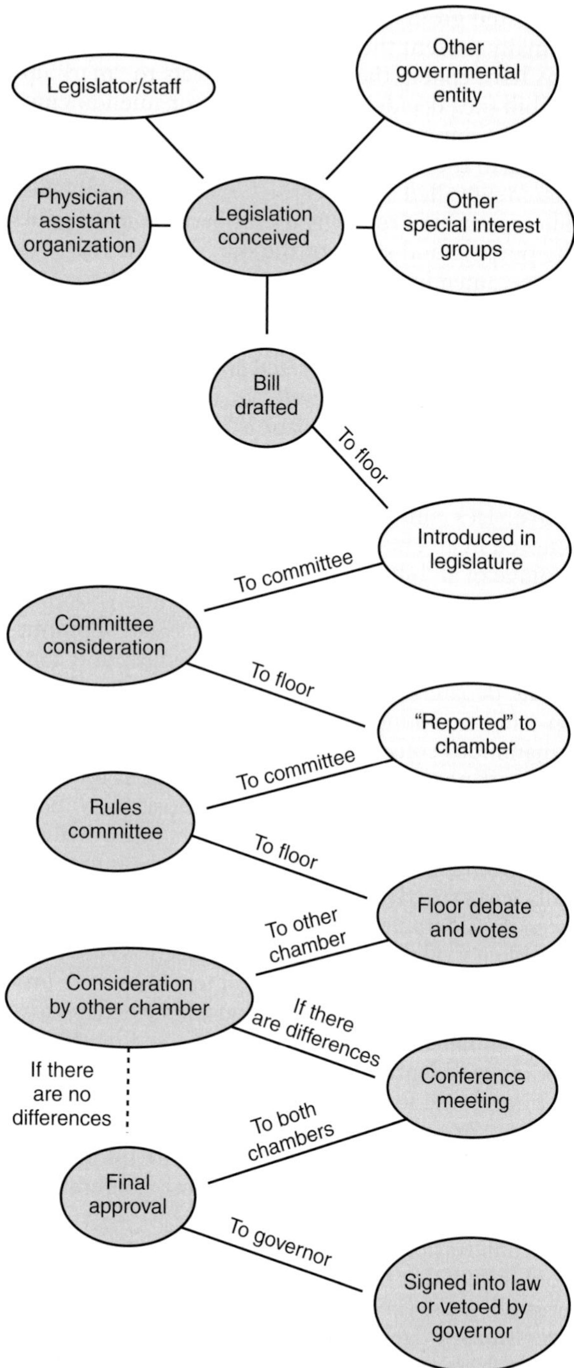

FIGURE 7-1 ■ The legislative process, or "How a Bill Becomes Law," designates points in the process at which your involvement is necessary.

A bill that has been approved by both chambers of Congress is sent to the White House. If Congress is in session and the president does not sign the bill within 10 days, it becomes law automatically. If the president favors the bill, he may sign it into law. If he does not like it, he may veto it by returning it to Congress without signature. To override the president's veto, a two-thirds vote in both the House and the Senate is required.[1]

Interested individuals can monitor congressional activity by watching televised floor proceedings or by reading various government documents. Copies of bills, as introduced, reported, and passed, are available from the House and Senate document rooms and may be accessed electronically. The document rooms also have the committee reports that accompany the bills and copies of "slip laws," the first official publication of newly enacted statutes. Hearing transcripts are frequently published by committees. Proceedings on the floor of both chambers are reported daily in the *Congressional Record*, which is available electronically.

STATE LEGISLATIVE PROCESS

Like the federal legislative process, the state process is set into motion when a condition is perceived to require change. For example, if a state lacks legislation permitting physicians to delegate to PAs the authority to prescribe controlled medications, the need for change would be great. As the solution to the problem or to a situation requiring change begins to crystallize, it is put down in writing and becomes a bill or, in some states, a resolution (Figure 7-1). Although writing a bill is usually considered the legislator's job, sometimes the best way to get what you need is for your state chapter to work closely with the legislative staff in this initial phase. Most legislatures employ professional staff to draft bills requested by senators and representatives.

The next step is sponsorship. If a representative has written the bill, he or she will usually sponsor it. If your state chapter has written the bill, a sponsor will have to be found. You may select your personal representative, one who is known to be sympathetic to your cause, or a member or chairperson of the committee to which the bill is expected to be referred. Bipartisan sponsorship is a good idea, particularly if different political parties control the state house, the state senate, or the governorship.

Once the bill is printed, it is placed on the legislative calendar and "introduced." The introduction is a reading of the bill before all the members of the chamber in which it is introduced (all states except

Nebraska have bicameral legislatures, i.e., two chambers). In most states, there is a gatekeeper committee, usually the rules or finance committee. If you want to influence when (or whether) a bill is introduced, you need to know which committee performs this function and, ideally, you must know someone who is assigned to the committee. Alternatively, having a good relationship with the clerk or staff of the committee is invaluable if you want to know when a particular bill is to be introduced. Once introduced, the bill is referred to committee for study. It is here that you and your state chapter become a crucial part of the process. Given the diversity of issues with which legislators are faced, it is impossible for them to know everything about every subject. In the area of medicine, you know more about PAs than your legislator does. Therefore, when your bill is referred to committee, write to or visit your personal representative, the members of the committee to which it has been referred, and the chair of that committee. Do not wait for the actual committee meeting at which your bill will be considered because that may be too late! Committees often publish calendars, but calendars can arrive on short notice and it may be impossible to rearrange your schedule so that you can make a 1 PM meeting the same day in a city 3 hours away. Even if you do get there, the rules of the committee may preclude your speaking. Once again, regular contact with a legislative staff person can be vital.

If you go to the Capitol, you may not meet with the actual representative, but with one of the staff instead. Do not feel slighted. Staff members usually concentrate their activities in particular subject areas to develop considerable specific expertise. The staff member will have some knowledge about the issue and will welcome an opportunity to learn more.

You should remember a few things about making legislative visits. First, they are only the first step. Rarely does one isolated visit send a bill sailing through the legislature. Do not feel compelled to "win the battle" here. Keep your visit short and to the point. Second, keep it pleasant. This does not necessarily mean you will agree on everything. That is all right. Offer to send additional information to clarify your position. You may want to leave a one-page statement or data sheet behind. Also, leave your name, address, and phone number. Finally, remember to follow up. Always send a prompt note thanking the legislator or staff person for his or her time. Emphasize your areas of agreement, and send along any material you promised. If you met with a staff person whom you found particularly pleasant or well informed, a note to the boss never hurts.

Going to visit a legislator requires preparation. Even the best professional lobbyists rarely walk into an office and start talking "off the cuff." Do your homework. What are the pros and cons of the bill? Too many people go into a legislative visit without considering both sides of an issue. That is fine if the legislator agrees with you, but it leaves you in a fix if he or she does not. Think of the questions the opposition might raise, and have nonconfrontational answers ready. Consider how this bill is going to affect the legislator's constituents. Does the legislator represent a medically underserved area in which allowing PAs to write prescriptions for controlled medications, for example, would improve the quality of health care that the constituents are receiving? How does the bill fit into the legislator's personal health care agenda?

Attending a committee meeting can be a revealing experience. Find out in advance whether you and other PA association representatives will be allowed to speak while the meeting is in session. Often you will not, but by watching the give and take during the meeting, you can decide who needs to be targeted for a special visit. In some committees, there is no give and take. The clerk reads off the bill numbers and the committee members vote. All discussions have been held and all decisions have been made before the meeting, which is why it is so important to visit all the committee members as soon as you found out which committee was going to handle your bill.

Once a committee approves a bill, it goes to the full chamber. Another series of visits or e-mail or phone contact may be necessary before that vote. You recall that when the bill was introduced, that was its first "reading." Although most states require three separate readings on 3 separate days, some do not. In some states, the only requirement is that the legislators have possession of the bill for a given number of days, commonly as few as 3. This is particularly important to remember at the end of the legislative session, when everything is chaotic and a bill that legislators have had in hand for months may advance from the first to the third reading and a final vote in 30 seconds. In states in which many bills are introduced each session, it is important to remember that the legislative calendar is dynamic. It is often perfectly acceptable to do tomorrow's bills in addition to today's.

States now post legislative calendars and bill scheduling information on the state legislature's website. The bill's text, including amendments to the introduced version, can be found there, too.

For the most part, the full House follows a committee's recommendation on a particular bill. If you do not consider that recommendation wise, then you can contact everyone again and express your concerns. You may be able to get two or three sympathetic legislators to orchestrate the floor debate so that those concerns are brought to the attention of the full chamber.

A bill that passes the first chamber must then be introduced in the second. Everything you did in the first chamber must be repeated: visits, thank you notes, committee meetings, more visits. The process may be conducted slightly differently in the two chambers, so be sure you learn the rules.

Once a bill has passed both chambers, it must be signed by the governor before it becomes effective. It is perfectly legitimate to attempt to influence the executive chamber. Action here must be planned in advance because the governor may sign the bill the moment it crosses his or her desk. In some states, agencies that will be implementing the bill (e.g., the Health Department) may write memoranda to the governor recommending signature or veto of a particular bill. If you can talk to the person who will be writing the memorandum, you may be able to influence its content. Know what the "vest-pocket veto" provisions are in your state. In some states, if the governor does not sign the bill within a fixed period, it is automatically vetoed.

If your bill is vetoed, there is always the outside chance that two thirds of the members of each house can be persuaded to override the veto. It is a long shot, but veto overrides sometimes happen.

This process is described as if it is your organization alone that will have an impact on your bill. Of course that is not the case. Legislators cannot possibly be experts in all of the areas in which they are asked to cast a vote, so in general they look to stakeholder groups to help them develop their response to legislation. State PA organizations that have repeated success at the legislature generally report that having the support of key stakeholder groups before the introduction of legislation is key to positive results.

STAKEHOLDERS TO WORK WITH BEFORE DRAFTING LEGISLATION

- State medical society
- State association of family physicians
- State association of emergency physicians
- Rural health association
- Primary care association
- Hospital association
- Other organizations with a particular interest in the topic of your legislation

FEDERAL REGULATORY PROCESS

The legislative branch of government makes laws that typically contain policy statements and directives. It then delegates to the executive branch—the agencies of the federal government—the authority to implement them. This has been a normal feature of American government since 1790, when the first Congress declared that traders with the Indians should observe "such rules and regulations as the President shall prescribe."[2] Federal regulations generally describe how a program is to be administered. The federal Administrative Procedures Act (APA) guides agencies in their rule making. The APA procedure has four fundamental elements. First, it guarantees that notice of proposed rule making is published in the *Federal Register*. Second, it gives "interested persons," which really means everyone, the opportunity to comment on the proposal through at least written submissions. Third, it requires the agency to create a "statement of basis and purpose," justifying and explaining the final rule. Last, it requires publication of the final rule and creates a 30-day gap between publication and the effective date.[2]

Therefore, when a new law is passed, an existing law is amended, or a policy requires clarification, the affected federal agency publishes a notice of proposed rule making in the *Federal Register*. The notice includes the proposed rules and their statutory basis; provides background on their content; invites participation from the public through the submission of written comments, data, or arguments; and sets a deadline for the receipt of such comments. Comments must generally be submitted within 30, 60, or 90 days. On the federal level, hearings are seldom held.

Federal agency staff members analyze the comments and may make revisions in the rules on the basis of the information received. When final rules are published in the *Federal Register*, they are prefaced by a discussion of the comments, accompanied by the agency's response to them. For example, in 1989, the Health Care Financing Administration published final rules that changed the Medicare system for certification of nursing homes.[3] The preamble to the rules contained the following discussion:

> Paragraph (e): Physician Delegation of Tasks
>
> *Comment:* In proposed section 483.40(e), we would permit physician delegation to physician extenders, that is, physician assistants and nurse practitioners, of tasks that the regulations do not otherwise require to be performed by the physician personally. An overwhelming majority of commenters expressed general support for permitting the delegation of tasks to physician extenders.

> *Response:* We believe that, to the extent feasible, the regulations should be written in a manner that allows for the effective utilization of physician extenders in the nursing home setting. For this reason, we are withdrawing our proposed requirement in section 483.40(b) that all orders be signed by the physician personally. This means that under sec. 483.40(e)(2), requirements concerning physician signature or countersignature of orders are determined by individual State law and facility policy. . . .

There are exceptions to this procedure (some based in law, others in politics), but it represents the most common method of federal rule making.

General and permanent rules published in the *Federal Register* by the executive departments and agencies of the federal government are codified in the *Code of Federal Regulations*. The *Code* is divided into 50 titles that represent broad areas subject to federal regulation, such as "public health." Each title is further divided into chapters, and the chapters into parts covering specific agencies and regulatory areas.[4] The *Code* is always changing, in response to either acts of Congress or agency revisions of regulations. The *Federal Register*, published daily, is available in most public libraries, by subscription, and on the Internet. The *Code of Federal Regulations* is sold by the Superintendent of Documents and may also be viewed online.

STATE REGULATORY PROCESS

Agencies, boards, and departments are the regulators at the state level, and they touch what every citizen does every day. They are responsible for inspecting food, keeping the costs of utilities at a given rate, and of course, governing the practice of medicine.[5] Although almost everyone knows when it is time to contact elected representatives, few know when, let alone how, to interact with agencies. This is crucial because "the rise of administrative bodies has probably been the most significant legal trend of the last century and perhaps more values are affected by their decisions than by those of all the courts. . . . They have become a veritable fourth branch of the Government, which has deranged our three-branch legal theories as much as the concept of a fourth dimension unsettles our three-dimensional thinking."[6] Agencies are here to stay, and it behooves us to learn how to deal with them.

Agencies (the inclusive term used in this chapter for regulatory bodies) are set forth in the Constitution, are created by legislatures, or are created by executive order and sanctioned by the legislature. The powers of the agency come from the body that creates it.[5] The work of agencies and legislatures is intertwined, but the players and processes are different.

First, consider the players. Legislators are elected by the people of the state and stay in office only as long as their work satisfies the voters, unless the length of time they may serve is limited by law. Top-level agency personnel are usually appointed by the governor (with confirmation by one or both houses of the legislature) and serve at the pleasure of the governor. Midlevel agency staff members are generally civil service employees, although some political appointments exist at this level as well. Many of these people are career civil servants; they intend to make the government their life's work. Contrast this time frame with that of a legislator, who must think in terms of 2 or 4 years, depending on when he or she is up for reelection. Commissioners or department secretaries, the top-level personnel, may be career civil servants or they may have aspirations for elected office. As such, their thinking is hybrid: They need to think of the long-term policy implications of their actions, as well as how such actions may influence the governor's reelection in a few years. So legislators and agency personnel think in different time frames and at different paces.

Legislators and bureaucrats also think differently in terms of content. A legislator is elected to represent all the interests of his or her district—the schools, the environment, the businesses. Legislators must also keep overall interests of the state in mind when involved in policy matters or budget negotiations. It is somewhat unrealistic to expect any one person to become expert in all these areas, particularly within 2 or 4 years. Add to that the need to balance the competing interests, and you have an almost impossible task. Contrast this situation with agencies. The subject matter is limited and specific—education, environment, *or* business, not all three. Agency personnel who work with an agency over a long period become quite expert in their specific subject areas. Because of their expertise and the fact that they do not depend on the good will of voters to keep their jobs, agency personnel may be the people who can answer your questions accurately and in great detail—even if they do not give you the answers you want to hear.

But what is it that agencies do? For this discussion, the focus is on the agency's function in creating rules and regulations. Like Congress, state legislatures pass laws (also known as statutes) whose language provides only a skeleton for a given policy. It is the agency's job to flesh out this skeleton by promulgating detailed rules and regulations.[7] The legislature may pass legislation for PAs that says, "A physician assistant is anyone who is licensed by the State Board of Medicine as a physician assistant." But how does one get licensed? This is the sort of thing that will be detailed in state regulations. For example, to be licensed as a PA, one must submit an application documenting that he or she is a graduate of a PA program, has passed an examination, and is of good moral character. Regulations, in most cases, have the force of law.

Just as you can influence the legislative process, you can affect the regulatory process. The process is quite well defined in most states. With a few exceptions, states follow the 1981 modifications of the Model State Administrative Procedures Act (MSAPA), which sets forth a specific rule-making process that includes public notification and public comment. Your elected representative should be able to refer you to the agency in your state that is charged with enforcing your state Administrative Procedures Act. If you anticipate a protracted exchange on a regulatory level, it is wise to review the provisions of this act with the help of an attorney who knows administrative law.

Once a law has been passed, an agency (or agencies) is charged with developing the regulations necessary for its implementation (Figure 7-2). Usually,

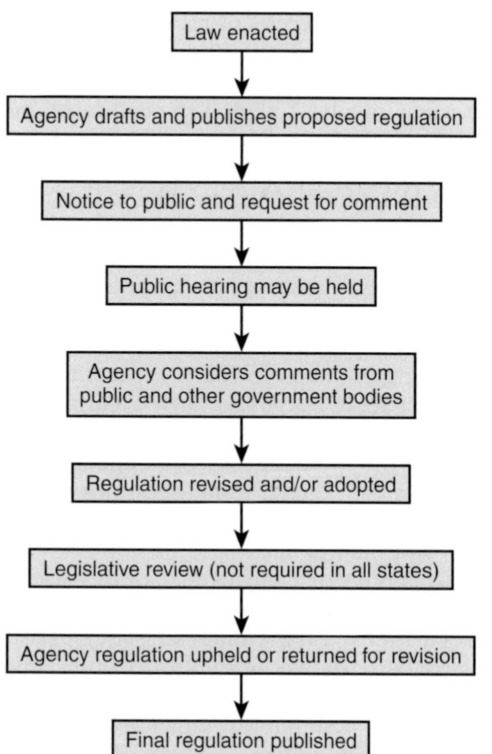

FIGURE 7-2 ■ Procedures for state rule making.

the staff of a bill's sponsor can tell you who is going to be writing the regulations. This is the time to get involved; it is much easier to influence what gets written than it is to change what has been written. Your initial contact with the regulator should focus on gathering and giving information. Are there any special concerns the agency needs to address in writing these regulations? What outside pressures (e.g., budgetary implications) might be brought to bear on the drafting? When does the agency intend to promulgate the regulations?

Unless you know the political atmosphere in which the regulator is operating, you cannot supply really useful information. You know the language of PA practice, and the regulator knows the language of regulation. You need to work together. If you disagree with the regulator, fine; there are ways to deal with that. Over time, you will find that being helpful and reasonable with regulators will help to create an atmosphere in which public protection and reasonable regulation of the profession find common ground.

Once the initial regulations are written, the MSAPA requires that interested parties be notified. Notification can take many forms. In larger states, the proposed regulations can be published in a register or some other regular publication that includes nothing but proposed regulations. In smaller states, they might be published in a newspaper that has statewide circulation. Agencies also generally post proposed regulations on their websites. In states that have adopted MSAPA, if you have notified the agency in advance that you want to know about any rules it promulgates, your name is added to its mailing list. If you have not made such a request, do not assume that just because the agency personnel know that you are interested in PA issues, they will notify you. Although it is the agency's responsibility to notify the public, that responsibility does not extend to personal notification. It is also unwise to rely on your agency "contacts" to inform you of a proposed rule. Their primary responsibility is to the agency. If they know your organization is going to make the rule-making process more complicated, they might not notify you in advance.

A comment period follows notification, during which anyone may submit written feedback to the agency. Like all other written communication with government, comments should be succinct and unemotional. Your state PA organization may also be submitting comments, so you should try to express your ideas in concert with theirs. "In concert" does not mean using a form letter or parroting what the organization says. Your own thoughts and insights will be more persuasive.

Depending on the statute that was passed and on the particular state administrative procedures act, public hearings may be required. During the public hearing, interested individuals may comment on the proposed regulations. Individual testimony is usually limited to 5 or 10 minutes, including questions and answers. The agency will ask you to submit a written copy of your testimony. When you testify, it is best not to read from your written copy. Paraphrase what you have written and answer any questions the regulators may have. Some people find public testimony intimidating. You might find it useful to watch testimony before state or federal agencies before presenting testimony yourself. It is much easier if you are well prepared and remember that the regulators work for you. In some cases, you may wish to bring in experts from the AAPA or another organization that has had experience with the issue.

After the comment period and hearings, the regulation as initially drafted or a modification of the proposed regulation is published and subsequently adopted. Some states have a time frame within which a regulation must be adopted or the process terminated.

In many states, the legislatures have not welcomed the rise of the administrative agencies just described. In an effort to curb what they saw as usurping of legislative mandates, they have adopted sunset laws and legislative oversight procedures. In a sunset law, the statute authorizing the existence of a regulatory agency expires in a fixed number of years unless it is reviewed and reauthorized by the legislature. In states with legislative oversight provisions, a committee of the legislature reviews all proposed regulations. State PA organizations have used these opportunities successfully to achieve needed change.

As you might expect, the regulatory process just described is somewhat neater than the reality. Some variations on the theme follow. All of the steps in the process have time limits. Perhaps the proposed rule needs to be published in only two consecutive weekly issues of the newspaper. Any PA group should make sure that one of its members is reading proposed rules on a regular basis. Most states have emergency adoption provisions that allow an agency to circumvent the time limits.[5] It only makes sense that if the state health department detects an increase in tuberculosis cases in August, it is not going to want to wade through the entire process, which may take 90 days, before requiring tuberculosis skin testing for students entering preschool. Usually, emergency rules are effective for only 120 days, with the option of one extension, after which time the agency must go through the notification and comment process.

CASE STUDIES

Examples of the political process, advocacy and the "get informed, get involved" strategy are presented in the following case studies of actual events.

CASE STUDY 7-1

UPGRADING THE PA PRACTICE ACT IN OREGON

Oregon was one of the first states to authorize PA practice, and PAs in Oregon became integrated into the state's workforce in both rural and urban areas over a four-decade span. The Oregon Society of Physician Assistants (OSPA), the state's PA professional society, developed strong ties to the state medical society with PAs serving on key medical society committees and a stable legislative leadership group.

OSPA paid close attention to trends in professional regulation and to laws that had an impact on PA practice. Oregon laws were amended to change PAs to "licensed" rather than "certified" by the state, to authorize PAs to sign forms that patients commonly bring to a practice, and to allow physicians to delegate full prescriptive authority to PAs.

However, as PAs moved into specialty practice problems began to emerge. Practices, physicians, and PAs themselves would contact the medical board to ask if certain procedures or types of services could be performed by PAs. Because the PA statute authorized the board to approve PA scope of practice, this was seen by the medical board as a legitimate role for the state board.

The board staff sought to create a list of tasks that all PAs could perform so that staff could answer the question of "Can a PA do that?" when queried. This created predictable conflicts. Requests from physicians to delegate nonlisted procedures required creation of a process. Eventually physician-PA teams were required to send documentation and sometimes appear in person at a board meeting to support a request for a PA to perform a specific procedure. The board's Physician Assistant Committee would review the request and make a recommendation to the full board. Then the full medical board would make a final determination.

Over the course of years it became common for the PA Committee to recommend approval, only to have the full board vote to deny the request. There was also inconsistency. Some years procedures would be approved but the next year denied on the basis of the board membership. Sometimes high acuity procedures would be approved while low acuity but high visibility procedures (e.g., the injection of Botox) were denied.

The Oregon Society of Physician Assistants decided that the law needed to be changed to place scope determinations with the physician-PA team and any facility that grants practice privileges. Knowing that they would seek legislation in 2011, the OSPA leadership began planning in 2009.

OSPA leaders began by presenting the problem and its solution to the medical board itself. They documented that PAs were leaving Oregon because practice was so difficult. The OSPA team strategized with AAPA state advocacy staff, and the AAPA team drafted a bill, supporting documents, a *Microsoft PowerPoint* presentation, and comparison information.

OSPA educated its members, sought and obtained the full support of the medical association, and upgraded its lobbying team. Legislation was introduced by a state senator who had worked with OSPA in the past and considered the PA bill to be a high priority. Through the legislative process OSPA met repeatedly with the medical society and medical board and continued to be open to reasonable amendments to address stakeholder concerns.

SB224, the Oregon Physician Assistant Modernization Act, was signed by Governor Kitzhaber, an emergency physician, on August 4, 2011.

CASE STUDY 7-2

A Comprehensive Upgrade in Hawaii

When a PA on the Big Island of Hawaii began working with a local group concerned about access and workforce adequacy on the island, he wondered what laws that affect PA practice might be improved to ensure that physician-PA teams were functioning most efficiently. After discussing the issue with a PA on the medical board's Physician Assistant Committee and the president of the Hawaii Academy of Physician Assistants, the PAs sought AAPA's assistance in evaluating all the laws that affect PA practice in Hawaii.

The PA practice act itself was already fairly progressive. PAs could not be delegated the ability to prescribe Schedule II medications, but this was not seen as a significant local problem. A chart co-signature requirement and ratio restriction were identified, but again, these were not perceived as issues that were current barriers to efficient practice.

The group did identify a number of laws that fall outside of the PA practice act that were a problem. For example, PAs were not included in the definition of "health care provider" in many sections of Hawaii health law. In addition, PAs were not authorized to order physical or occupational therapy.

Working closely with the AAPA, the Hawaii Academy took the lead. A physician Senator who chaired the Senate Health Committee understood the issue clearly and agreed to sponsor the Senate version of the legislation, and a former Navy nurse representative sponsored the bill in the House. HAPA activated grassroots support through the AAPA's Legislative Action Center, and PAs, physicians, and clinics sent letters of support to legislators at critical times in the legislative process. Although the legislation was lengthy, HAPA developed this clear and concise description of the bill:

> SB 1142 removes archaic barriers to full utilization of PAs. This legislation does not change PA scope of practice, but rather adds PAs to numerous specific sections of statute that govern reporting of gunshots and stab wounds, provision of health care in disasters, care for school children, testing for blood alcohol levels, and other measures that PAs are commonly delegated to do, but that outdated laws have not specifically authorized.

The legislation proceeded through the process without any opposition. However, as the end of the session approached, the bill appeared to be in danger of not being brought up for critical votes in time to meet key deadlines. The Hawaii Academy consulted with AAPA, and a decision to hire a lobbyist was made. A contract lobbyist who also advocated for the Hawaii Medical Association was retained to be on site at the Capitol and ensure that the bill made it through all required processes on time.

The bill was passed by the state legislature and was signed into law by Governor Linda Lingle in June 2009.

CONCLUSION

Contrary to what we hear every day about the failure of government, the system does work. It works because individuals and organizations keep doing their part to make it work. We hope this chapter will make it easier for you to be effective and even excited about your part in advocacy. The goal of this chapter was to help you "get informed." Take the next step—get involved!

CLINICAL APPLICATIONS

1. You are a PA living in a state that does not have prescriptive privileges for controlled medications for PAs. You have been asked by the state chapter to become politically active on behalf of your profession to improve health care in the state. Compose a sample letter that could be directed to a state legislator, expressing your support of controlled medication prescriptive privileges for PAs. Prepare information and handouts that you might use in visiting a state legislator's office. Discuss other activities that you might propose to the state chapter leadership that could help in this legislative effort.
2. Examine the health care needs of your local community. Discuss ways in which legislation and regulations could improve the health status of your community.

KEY POINTS

1. You do not need a huge number of people or a large war chest to win a legislative battle. What was crucial in these cases was that individual s and the state chapters considered it their responsibility to effect a legislative change.
2. You need to mobilize the membership. Although in each case only a small number of people were actually "working" the legislature, the membership was behind them. They sent e-mail, wrote letters, and made telephone calls. Membership input is crucial. If you choose to be a chapter leader, give the membership the information they need to write an intelligent letter. If you choose not to be a chapter leader, write intelligent letters when asked.
3. You do not have to be a professional lobbyist to win. Professional lobbyists are great—they know the system and when to pull which strings—but you can do much of what they do. Legislators want honest information. Deliver it with enthusiasm, and you are halfway home.
4. Look for windows of opportunity in both timing and alliances. Sometimes the best strategy is to wait until a powerful opposing force is moved out of the way by an election or expiration of a term of office.
5. There is no need to "go it alone." Both organizations worked closely with the AAPA. Alliances with physician organizations can be extremely helpful in making both legislative and regulatory changes.
6. You must be persistent. Do not be discouraged if your efforts require multiple legislative sessions to complete. Keep at it.
7. The most important lesson: Keep patients first. When you focus your advocacy message on how it will have a positive impact on patient care, you will keep a firm foundation.

References

1. Congressional Quarterly's Guide to Congress. 6th ed. Washington, DC: Congressional Quarterly; 2007.
2. Koch CH Jr. Administrative Law and Practice. St. Paul, MN: West, 1997.
3. 54 Federal Register 5342. Washington, DC: U.S. Government Printing Office.
4. 42 CFR § 61.1. Washington, DC: U.S. Government Printing Office.
5. Breyer S, Stewart R, Sunstein C, Vermeule A. Administrative Law and Regulatory Policy: Problems, Text, and Cases. New York, NY: Aspen; 2006.
6. Jackson JR (dissenting). Federal Trade Commission v Ruberoid. 343 US 470 487 (1952).
7. Christoffel T. Health and the Law: A Handbook for Health Professionals. New York: Macmillan; 1982.

The resources for this chapter can be found at www.expertconsult.com.

SECTION II

MEDICAL KNOWLEDGE

CHAPTER 8

EVIDENCE-BASED MEDICINE

Anita Duhl Glicken

CHAPTER CONTENTS

The dawning of the information age has had a major impact on society, giving rise to a cultural and technologic revolution that has dramatically changed the delivery of health care. Rapid availability of information from across the world has transformed medical decision-making. Although practitioners are still likely to seek consultations from colleagues down the hall, they now also draw on the opinions of international panels of experts. As physician assistants (PAs) continue to search for treatments that yield the best outcomes for their patients, we increasingly rely on a growing body of literature that critically evaluates current standards of care and emerging treatments. Evidence-based medicine (EBM) provides a paradigm for practice that applies the best available evidence to the decision-making process of patient care.

HISTORY OF EVIDENCE-BASED MEDICINE

The evolution of EBM can be traced back to the early 1970s. During this period, a strong debate existed about medicine's shortcomings. In 1972, Archie Cochrane received international recognition when he published his reformist views in "Effectiveness and Efficiency."[1] According to Cochrane, evidence from randomized controlled trials (RCTs) was essential to inform rational choices made by practitioners, patients, and health care policy experts. In 1979, he published an additional paper criticizing the medical profession for its repeated failure to conduct timely systematic reviews of accumulating clinical evidence. Cochrane lived to see the first organized response to his efforts with the 1988 publication of a database of neonatal randomized controlled trials by Ian Chalmers and colleagues. This was followed in 1989 by the release of an important book titled *Effective Care in Pregnancy and Childbirth*.[2] For the first time at the conclusion of this book Chalmers, Enkin, and Keirse included their personal perspectives on the reported treatments, on the basis of conclusions they formed from the preceding articles. The authors concluded that although some strategies and forms of care were useful, others were of questionable value. Moreover, some interventions commonly thought to be useful were, in fact, of little benefit or even harmful to patients. In 1992, a similar publication, *Effective Care of the Newborn Infant*, provided a compilation and review of all existing neonatal RCTs.[3]

Several developments in medicine in the late 1970s and early 1980s stimulated this early effort. The demand for health care increased due to an aging population, new technology and knowledge, and increased expectations on the part of professionals and their patients. However, the growth of available resources for health care did not rise at the same rate as the increase in demand. As a result, there was increasing pressure on health care organizations and professionals to demonstrate that procedures and practice were both clinically and cost effective. EBM became an important thread in the fabric of the health care industry, ensuring that available resources are allocated effectively and the services provided are of high quality.

In 1991, the National Health Service (NHS) launched an evaluative culture through the establishment of a Research and Development Program. In 1992, this program developed two important centers for evidence collation, The United Kingdom (UK) Cochrane Center at Oxford and the NHS Center for Reviews and Dissemination, where certain forms of evidence are synthesized to produce systematic reviews and meta-analyses. The Cochrane Center conducts the meta-analysis of randomized controlled trials. The Collaboration represents a global community whose role is to collaborate with others in building and maintaining a core database of systematic up-to-date reviews of randomized controlled trials of health care and to arrange for these reviews to be readily accessible through various electronic media. Many of the reviews focus on specific questions of importance to the NHS, principally in areas of effectiveness and cost-effectiveness of health care interventions, management, and organization of health services.

In 1992, EBM developed further with the publication of an article entitled "Evidence-Based Medicine: A New Approach to Teaching the Practice of Medicine" in the *Journal of the American Medical Association*.[4] This paper, published by the newly formed, EBM working group, was the precursor to many subsequent articles describing the process and practice of EBM.[5] By 1998, more than 850 articles had been published. Now specific search engines are dedicated to finding articles using an EBM methodology, and there are more hundreds of EBM-related websites including centers for EBM, child health, dentistry, emergency medicine, mental health, nursing pathology, and pharmacotherapy. In 1998, EBM became a focus of major curriculum reform for medical schools as both the Liaison Committee for Medical Education and the Medical Schools Objectives Project identified it as a priority. One of the first known EBM curricula in PA education was launched at the University of Colorado in 1995, and most PA programs now teach EBM as part of their core curriculum.

WHAT IS EVIDENCE-BASED MEDICINE?

EBM is the application of the best available evidence to patient care. Most practitioners recognize that the ideas underlying EBM are not new; clinicians have always consulted literature. However, for decades the gap between research and practice has grown larger, leading to expensive, ineffective, or harmful decisions. The term *evidence-based medicine* was coined at McMaster Medical School in Canada in the 1980s to label a specific clinical learning strategy, which had been under development there for more than a decade.[6]

FOUR CORE SKILLS OF EVIDENCE-BASED MEDICINE

Typically, evidence-based practice is recognized as having four core skills:

1. Formulating a clear, researchable question for a clinical problem
2. Searching the literature for relevant clinical articles
3. Evaluating (critically appraising) the evidence for its validity and usefulness
4. Implementing useful findings in clinical practice

The new paradigm of evidence-based practice was designed to enhance clinical judgment, not replace it. Where practitioners of the past relied heavily on expert opinion and testimonial evidence, the clinician of today has an opportunity to explore a high grade of evidence in rigorous research, thereby generating a new standard for medical practice.

Core Skill 1: Formulating a Question

As an exercise, think about the patients you have seen in your clinic over the past week. Take 5 minutes to brainstorm about questions you had regarding these patients. Typically, it does not take long to generate a long list of questions from clinical practice. Alternatively, consider the following case scenario:

CASE STUDY 8-1

Mary P., a 75-year-old white woman, presents to the office with complaints of fatigue and cough, which she has had for 2 weeks. She was last seen 3 months ago for a follow-up visit for stable hypertension.

Many questions might be generated from this case. Consider the following lists of questions in Table 8-1. Notice that the first list of questions is typical of beginning PA students. Students might ask general questions about the disorder, acute bronchitis, attempting to find what can be called "background" knowledge.[7] Well-built clinical questions about background knowledge usually have three components: a question **root** (who, what, when, where, why, and how), a verb (causes), and an aspect of the health condition at hand (disorder, syndrome, finding, concern). "What are the causes of pneumonia?" from Table 8-1 is an example of a background question.

The second column of questions is typical of those asked by practitioners with more experience. They are specific questions about how to best care for this patient with bronchitis, seeking what can be called foreground knowledge. Well-built questions about foreground knowledge usually have three or four components. These include the following:

- The patient or problem
- The intervention of interest
- The comparison intervention, when relevant (such as for questions about therapy or diagnostic tests)
- The clinical outcomes of interest

Review the questions you created at the beginning of this section to determine whether they were background or foreground questions. If they were background questions, how might you change them to make them a foreground question? The distinction between types of questions is an important one because answers to different types of questions are often found in different places. Textbooks often answer background questions, whereas foreground questions are typically answered in medical journals and places where information can be updated routinely as new data emerge.

Core Skill 2: Searching the Literature

EBM clinicians face two major challenges in accessing medical knowledge: (1) finding the most relevant and reliable information to address a clinical problem at hand and (2) keeping abreast of important new developments in the expansive mass of published research. Both of these rely on skills of searching the Internet for literature. Mastering appropriate and efficient searching techniques is the second step in becoming an EBM practitioner.

The goal of a search strategy is to retrieve the most reliable information in as short an amount of time as possible. Priority is given to sites that are most likely to yield valid information and cover large amounts of research on a topic. Therefore, we first search for reliable sources of integrative literature. If these time-saving resources do not contain the information we seek, we next search MEDLINE, which is the "gold standard" but is a more time-consuming database. MEDLINE is a service of the U.S. National Library of Medicine (NLM) and is an acronym for its online Medical Literature Analysis and Retrieval System. This comprehensive database has cataloged more than 10 million journal articles since 1966. Most of the information a clinician needs can be found in this database. The challenge is understanding how the information is cataloged so that it can be accessed efficiently. If we are still unsuccessful in finding what we need, then specific medical information searches are performed. Finally, if we have still not found the required information, we may dredge the Internet by putting any related search term into a general search engine, remembering to be cautious with respect to the quality of data. Many excellent EBM textbooks[8] or your local medical librarian can familiarize you with the mechanics of navigating your search if you are unfamiliar with the particular search engines and databases available to you. Most search engines use some form of "MeSH terms"—medical subject headings or keywords. Some of these are not intuitively obvious. Others are menu driven, allowing you to select from a range of topics and modifiers for your search.

Searching for High-Grade Sources of Integrative Literature. As previously noted, in EBM we frame the clinical question, identify and retrieve all relevant information, appraise it, and integrate it so that we can apply it to our patient. This often takes a great deal of time, more than allowed in a brief

TABLE 8-1 **Questions from Practice**

What are the causes of pneumonia?	In patients presenting with fatigue and cough, with possible pneumonia, which test more accurately confirms the diagnosis, a chest radiograph or oxygen saturation levels?
What physical examination findings would be expected from acute bronchitis?	In patients with acute bronchitis, does use of a bronchodilator in aerosol form relieve symptoms of cough and wheezing as compared with placebo?
What information would help differentiate acute bronchitis from bacterial pneumonia?	In patients with acute bronchitis, do β-agonists reduce the duration of cough compared with placebo or erythromycin?
What treatments are available for acute bronchitis?	In patients with acute bronchitis, do antibiotics prevent nonsuppurative complications of β-hemolytic streptococcal pharyngitis?

office visit. A number of sites present information in which this sequence of steps has already been done. Integrative literature provides summary findings or recommendations in the form of overviews, meta-analysis, and/or practice guidelines of consensus statements.

Just because the literature has been integrated does not guarantee it is valid. As responsible readers, we need to be certain that each step has been rigorously performed. Critical appraisal takes time, but groups that assemble many reviews or guidelines often use a uniform methodology that is available as a supporting document. Reading the group's supporting article once enables us to assess their entire body of work. If we are satisfied that their method of assembling literature is rigorous, we can use the review with confidence. We typically assume that the review or guideline is evidence based and that its host site is likely to be an efficient and reliable location for us in the future.

Some examples of sites you may find useful in your search for valid integrative literature include the following:

- Cochrane Collaboration (Cochrane Database of Systematic Reviews [CDSR]) is a rapidly growing collection of updated systematic reviews. The Cochrane Collaboration is a worldwide group with more than 50 Collaborative Review Groups whose members prepare, maintain, and disseminate systematic reviews primarily based on the results of RCTs. These reviews are published electronically in the Cochrane Library, which contains the CDSR (*http://www.cochrane.org/cochrane-reviews/about-cochrane-library*), along with editorial comments on these reviews. Comments come from an international group of individuals and institutions dedicated to summarizing randomized controlled trials relevant to health care. Their process of compiling reviews is rigorous, focusing on a particular clinical question. All available trials are critically appraised. Studies that meet specific quality criteria are summarized quantitatively, using meta-analysis. Summary findings are also presented qualitatively.
- The Database of Abstracts of Reviews of Effectiveness (DARE) (*http://www.crd.york.ac.uk/crdweb/*), a collection of international reviews including those from the Cochrane Collaboration. Reviewers at the National Health Service Center for Reviews and Dissemination at the University of York, England, provide quality oversight including detailed structured abstracts that describe the methodology, results, and conclusions of the reviews. The quality of the reviews is discussed along with implications for health care. Of particular note is that this vast database is indexed not only by keywords but also by the official Medical Subject Headings, or MeSH terms of the MEDLINE database, which can improve the specificity of our search.
- NIH: Health Services Technology Assessment Text. The National Library of Medicine provides documents useful in health care decision-making. This site has many guidelines and references for clinicians sponsored by the Agency for Health Care Policy and Research. This site also contains the complete U.S. Preventive Health Series Task Force Guidelines from 1996, as well as consensus documents and research sponsored by the National Institutes of Health.
- National Guidelines Clearinghouse (*http://www.guideline.gov/browse/index.aspx?alpha=A*), maintained by the U.S. Department of Health and Human Services, Agency for Health Care Research and Quality (AHRQ), in partnership with the American Medical Association (AMA) and the American Association of Health Plans (AAHP). This site provides a wide range of clinical practice guidelines from institutions and organizations. Structured abstracts facilitate critical appraisal, and abstracts on the same topic can be compared on a side-by-side table, allowing comparisons of relevance, generalizability, and rigor of research findings. Links also are provided to the full text of each guideline, when available. The site allows you to display comparable guidelines on a table, enabling you to compare issues of relevance, rigor, and generalizability. The site also links to the full text of the guidelines.

Although the sites described earlier may provide the data you need to answer your specific clinical question, often the information required is so new that it is not yet available in these sources. Additional sources are available to help you obtain the most recent information. These sources will also help you stay up to date as an EBM practitioner with emerging trends and new data. Many major journals have websites. Most provide free access to the abstracts; some also provide free access to full text and figures. They can often be found using a search engine like MEDLINE and the name of journal. If the journal has an electronic site, it will also typically be found at *e.journal*. Sites are updated before or on the day of publication. Information may be available here before the articles are indexed in MEDLINE. Most good electronic journal sites have their own search engines (e.g., *Annals of Internal Medicine*, *British Medical Journal*, *Journal of the American Medical Association*, *Lancet*, and *The New England Journal of Medicine*.)

Reviewing summaries of key articles excerpted from journals is another way to view current research findings. Reading prereviewed summaries from publications that have scanned many journals for quality articles can be an efficient use of time when looking for the latest research on common clinical issues. Many such publications are available to PAs. The three publications discussed next pay particular attention to the rigor and validity of the articles reviewed:

Published bimonthly, the *American College of Physicians Journal Club* (ACPJC) abstracts key articles from a number of "core" internal medicine journals (e.g., *American Journal of Medicine, Annals of Internal Medicine, Archives of Internal Medicine, BMJ, JAMA, Lancet, The New England Journal of Medicine, Journal of Internal Medicine*). Articles are selected according to their perceived importance and rigor, judged by specific criteria on the basis of the *User's Guide to the Medical Literature*. A content expert reviews each article. A commentary follows each summary describing any significant methodologic problems and providing a context of previous literature, as well as recommendations for clinical applications of the study findings. A select group is available for free; the entire list is available with payment or through a library.

Evidence-Based Medicine is generated using identical procedures, is published bimonthly, and also requires a subscription fee but may be available at no charge through your local medical library. *EBM* has a broader focus than *ACPJC*, reviewing more than 100 journals covering family practice, surgery, psychiatry, pediatrics, obstetrics, and gynecology. *EBM* also publishes about 50% of the abstracts reviewed in *ACPJP*.

Best Evidence is an electronic presentation of all issues of *ACPJC* (1991-) and *Evidence-Based Medicine* (1995-). *Best Evidence* also includes editorials from *ACPJC* and notes from *Evidence-Based Medicine*.

Core Skill 3: Critical Appraisal of the Evidence

The following section of this chapter builds on the principles discussed in Chapter 9. Before continuing, it is suggested that the reader review the distinction between research articles and clinical review articles. The critical appraisal skills outlined as follows refer only to medical research articles, not clinical review articles.

Medical research is often categorized as either studies or integrative literature. Descriptive studies "describe" individual variables (i.e., incidence or qualities of a disease). Analytic studies present an analysis of the association between two or more variables (i.e., an intervention and morbidity). Most of the studies we use to determine the efficacy of treatment are the analytic type. Analytic studies are further commonly divided into four basic study designs: experimental, cohort, case-control, and cross-sectional. Detailed descriptions of the various study types can be found in any research methods textbook.

Integrative literature "integrates" information from individual studies using a specified framework to provide a conclusion or recommendation. Overviews, practice guidelines, and meta-analysis are all examples of integrative literature. Meta-analysis is a statistical method of combining data from independent studies.

The Evidence-Based Medicine Working Group (EBMWG) has published a series of articles, "User's Guide to Medical Literature," describing an approach to systematically evaluating various types of published medical research. These guides provide relevant questions used when critically evaluating various types of studies (therapy, diagnosis, prevention, harm) and integrative literature (e.g., overview, practice guidelines). This chapter follows the basic framework of these publications, evaluating a study's validity and results as they relate to patient care. The approach presented here differs, however, in two ways:

First, the EBMWG approach individualizes evaluation across different types of studies. The approach below uses one set of questions for all studies, including diagnostic tests, interventions, risk, and prognosis. Also, the current approach emphasizes the context of other relevant knowledge to assist the clinician in estimating the posttest probability and/or believability of a given outcome.

The following discussion focuses primarily on the evaluation of analytic studies because analytic studies provide much of the emerging information needed for practice. This model is adapted from a discussion by Daniel Friedland in his book entitled *Evidence-Based Medicine: A Framework for Clinical Practice*,[9] in which he described five steps for systematic analysis of a study including the following:

- Step 1. Do I want to evaluate the study?
- Step 2. Outline of the study
- Step 3. Is the study finding believable?
- Step 4. What is the clinically relevant finding?
- Step 5. Will the study help me in caring for my patient?

Each step is addressed individually. The format in Table 8-2 is provided to assist the reader in organizing an evaluation of a research study.

Step 1: Do I want to evaluate the study? You must have a motivation to evaluate a study. By developing a habit of browsing the literature, you will soon recognize the factors that interest you. Typically, clinicians are looking for information that extends previous knowledge about the topic. You will want

TABLE 8-2 Matrix for Critical Appraisal

Citations	
STEP 1. DO I WANT TO EVALUATE THE STUDY? (INTERNATIONAL NORMALIZED RATIO)	
Is the study: Interesting? Novel? Relevant?	
STEP 2. WHAT IS THE STUDY OUTLINE/METHOD?	
Research question Subjects/target population Predictor variable defined Outcome variable defined Findings	Temporal and geographic characteristics Intended follow-up Sampling
STEP 3. IS THE STUDY FINDING BELIEVABLE?	
Do the subjects and variables accurately represent the research question?	Subjects: Predictor variable: Outcome variable:
Are findings attributable to other factors? (chance, bias, confounders)	Possible chance Possible bias Bias in selecting study subjects Biases in following up on the study subjects Biases in executing or measuring the predictor variable Biases in measuring the outcome variable Biases in analyzing the data Possible confounders
Are the findings believable within the context of other knowledge?	Possible consistency with other literature Possible biologic plausibility Possible analogy
STEP 4. WHAT IS THE CLINICALLY RELEVANT FINDING?	
(Likelihood ratios [LRs] for diagnostic tests; disease-specific mortality [DSM]; patient-specific mortality [PSM] and/or life expectancy [LE] for prognosis; absolute risk reduction [ARR]; number needed to treat [NNT]; discounting for therapy) Weighing costs and benefits	
STEP 5. WILL THE STUDY HELP ME IN CARING FOR MY PATIENT?	
Are the subjects adequately described and applicable to my patient? Is the predictor variable adequately described and applicable to my patient? Will the finding result in an overall net benefit for my patient?	

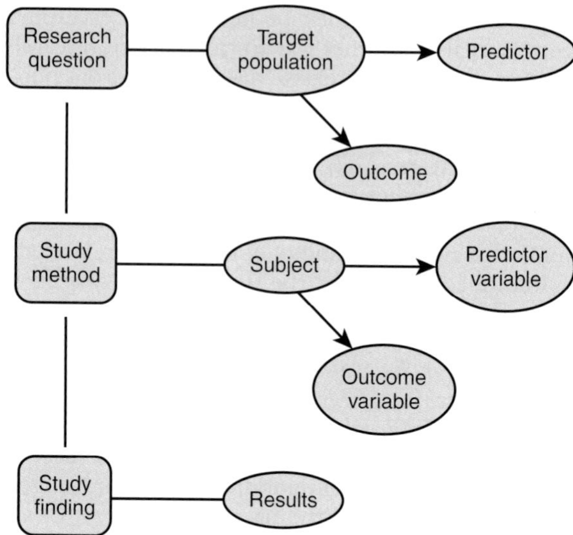

FIGURE 8-1 ■ Outline of a research study.

to evaluate studies that are relevant for your practice and determine whether study questions will have clinical importance for your patients. In other words, do the outcomes have short-term or long-term impact on patients? Much of this information can be found in the article's abstract, which will help you identify whether or not you want to evaluate the study further (Figure 8-1).

Step 2: Outline of the study. The outline of the study consists of the research question, the study method, and the findings. The **research question** represents knowledge we are seeking and considers the association between a given predictor and outcome in a given population. A predictor is something that precedes, affects, or tests for an outcome. Therefore, predictors might be a risk, a diagnostic test, a therapeutic intervention, or a prognostic factor. The outcome is whatever is being affected by the predictor or whatever we are diagnosing. For example, consider the following question:

CASE STUDY 8-2

We are familiar with the drug fluoxetine, a selective serotonin-reuptake inhibitor (SSRI), in treating depression. In a patient with type 2 diabetes, what is the efficacy of fluoxetine in improving glycemic control, as evidenced by decreased fasting blood glucose levels, decreased HbA_{1c} levels, and weight loss? In this example, fluoxetine would be the predictor. Glycemic control, as evidenced by decreased fasting blood glucose levels, decreased

HbA_{1c} levels, and weight loss, would be the outcome in a target population of patients with type 2 diabetes.

When outlining the **study method,** one should take note of the type of study design, the subjects, and the variables. As mentioned earlier, analytic studies analyze the association between predictor and outcome variables. Analytic studies are classified as one of four study designs: **experimental, cohort, case-control,** and **cross-sectional**.

The double-blind, randomized, controlled trial is considered the model **experimental** design. Subjects are randomly assigned to either an intervention or control group. "Double-blinding" means that neither the researcher nor the patient is aware of which group they are in. Single masking implies that only the patient is unaware of which therapy is being received.

In the **cohort** study the researcher collects data about patients over a period of time, and associations are made between the predictor and outcome variables. In **case-control** studies, associations are made between the predictor and outcome variables by selecting groups on the basis of whether the outcome is observed or absent. The researcher then looks within each of these groups to identify whether the predictor variable occurred. In **cross-sectional** studies, one identifies a single point in time and a group of study subjects are evaluated at that time looking for associations between predictor and outcome variables. Additional information on these study designs is available in Blessing's *A Physician Assistant's Guide to Research and the Medical Literature.*[9] Friedland has identified three questions to help differentiate between these analytic study designs[9] (Figure 8-2).

Because it is typically not feasible to study all of the subjects in a population, a group is chosen that is representative of the problem through a selection process. **Subjects** are described according to several descriptive factors, which frequently identify inclusion or exclusion criteria. These include **temporal characteristics,** such as the dates of the recruitment period or the length of follow-up. Other information may include **geographic characteristics,** which detail where the study took place or whether it was a multicenter trial. One of the most important pieces of information related to subjects is the **sampling strategy** used to select the representative population. For example, were the subjects a **random** sample, or were they enrolled **consecutively**? Some mention of **attrition** tells us how many of the subjects dropped out of the study before completion.

The **variables** in a study tell us how the predictor and outcome were defined, measured, and/or implemented by the researchers. For example, consider the following question:

CASE STUDY 8-3

Do females between the ages of 15 and 30 who receive medroxyprogesterone acetate injections (Depo-Provera) have decreased bone mineral density (BMD) compared with females using no hormonal contraception? If you were evaluating this study, you would note in your outline how the variables define the predictor and outcome. The predictor variable would be how the authors defined and measured the use of Depo-Provera. Similarly, the outcome variable, decreased BMD, can be expressed as a percentage of bone loss as determined by dual x-ray absorptiometry (DEXA).

A description of the **study finding** completes the outline. This is the association between the predictor and outcome variables in the study. The level of statistical significance is typically presented along with the magnitude of the outcome (typically presented as a *P* value or confidence interval). Outlining the study in your mind or using the matrix in Table 8-2, or both, will help you decide whether the study you found is likely to yield the information you are seeking. In addition, you will use the outline to organize your thinking as you proceed with a critical appraisal of the study.

Step 3: Is the study finding believable? The first question to be considered when exploring the validity of any study is whether the **subjects** and **variables** accurately reflect the research question. For example, we have already determined that the target population is defined by a set of inclusion and exclusion criteria. We need to be sure that the subjects in the study actually meet these criteria.

CASE STUDY 8-4

A randomized clinical trial of a new acne medicine released for adolescents was conducted by randomizing 100 adolescents with severe acne to the new medicine and 100 with severe acne to a placebo.

Ninety percent of the adolescents randomized to the new medication experienced "very satisfying" results with a decrease in the number of facial lesions. The placebo group had no apparent improvement. How would it affect the study if it was later determined that up to 50% of the adolescents in the treatment group had only moderate or intermittent skin problems or that 24% of the participants were older than 25 years of age? In either of these cases, the study would not answer the intended question and instead would be testing a different association.

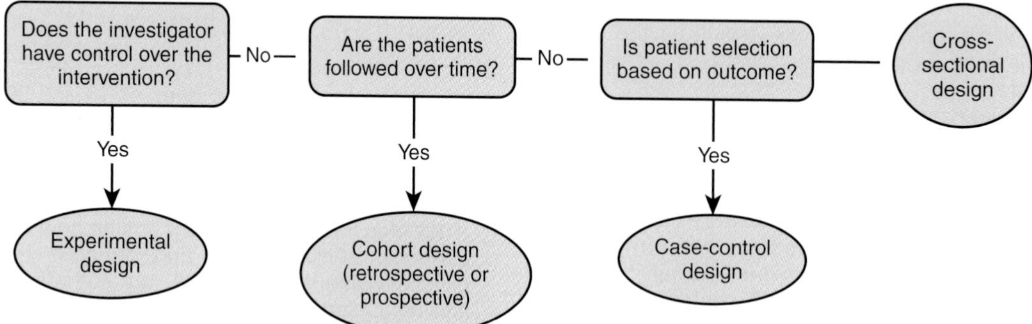

FIGURE 8-2 Differentiating study designs.

The **variables** of the study also must accurately represent the predictor and outcome; we must therefore consider how each of these is measured. If the measurement of the variables is inaccurate, the association between the variables will not be believable, no matter how much the researchers attempt to limit other confounding variables. If, however, we determine that the patients and variables accurately represent the research question, we go on to explore whether the association between the predictor and outcome is valid and credible, given what is known about other research and information on this topic.

To determine if the association between the predictor and outcome variable is valid, we need to determine whether the predictor was responsible for the finding or whether the finding is due to other factors. Two things help determine whether the finding can be explained by other things: study design and study source. First we consider whether the **study design** is descriptive or analytic. If there is no comparison or control group, the study can only describe an occurrence in a given population and cannot analyze associations between outcomes.

CASE STUDY 8-5

For example, consider a study of children with otitis media and antibiotic therapy. If the study does not include a control group and only describes the population of children taking antibiotics, we cannot conclude anything about the association between the antibiotics and resolution of the otitis media. If, however, the study does include a comparison group, the study is analytic and can determine whether the antibiotics might have cured the otitis media. With a comparison group, we can determine whether the outcome is due to the predictor variable, rather than the natural resolution of the illness.

The **strength of an analytic study design** is directly related to its susceptibility to chance, bias, and other confounding factors. The experimental study design is typically considered the strongest design and least susceptible to bias, followed by the cohort study, case-control study, and cross-sectional study design. Another factor that affects the strength of the study design is whether the study is prospective or retrospective. Prospective studies are considered stronger. This study design identifies a predictor variable and then tracks the subjects forward over time looking for an observable outcome. With this methodology, we can be pretty certain that the predictor preceded the outcome. Retrospective studies look backward at the predictor and the outcome. This makes it less clear that the predictor caused the outcome because the outcome could have caused the predictor.

The **source of the study** is another piece of information that helps us determine how comfortable we are in accepting the validity of the study at face value. This consideration includes who sponsored the study, whether it was published by a known and respected author, and the overall reputation of the journal. Pharmaceutical companies are likely to fund original research on new drugs; however, they may also be less likely to publish research that sheds unfavorable light on their products. Clearly, if the journal and author have a known reputation, one feels more comfortable with the appraisal process that has gone on before publication.

Three additional major factors also affect the credibility of the findings: **chance, bias,** and **confounding factors** (Figure 8-3).

The researcher considers the effect of **chance** when presenting the power of the study, the *P* value, and confidence interval. The power of a study dictates the probability of finding a specific magnitude of association between the predictor and outcome variables, if such an association exists. This is calculated before a study takes place and takes into

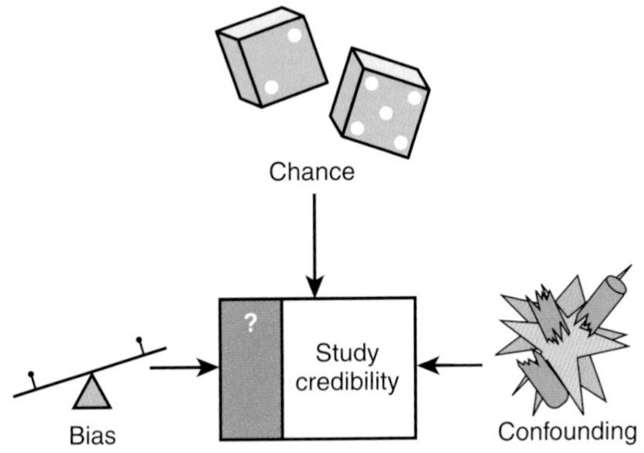

FIGURE 8-3 Chance, bias, and confounding factors.

consideration the number of subjects, the estimated magnitude of effect, and the precision of the measures that are being used. A power of 0.8 (80% probability) is typically used and is considered satisfactory in detecting a specific effect size that has been determined before the study. (A review of common statistical terms and tests is included in Chapter 9.)

The ***P* value** is the probability that the association between the predictor and outcome variables could have occurred strictly by chance when in reality there was no association between predictor and outcome. If the *P* value is less than 0.05 (<5% chance of finding an association when no association exists), the finding is considered statistically significant and unlikely to be due to chance alone.

Just as the power statistic informs the design of a study, the width of the **confidence interval** helps us determine whether more precise variables or a greater number of subjects might have allowed the researcher to find a particular association. The confidence interval (CI) represents the range of values that are statistically compatible with the estimate of the study result. When using 95% confidence intervals, we can determine whether or not the reported data are statistically significant with a *P* value less than or equal to 0.05. For example, a study that reports symptom reduction of 10% (95% CI, 7-20) implies that the data are statistically compatible with an effect as small as 7% or as large as 20% at a significance level of 0.05. Typically the CI is expressed as a span for an odds ratio to the patient. (Remember that the odds ratio represents the proportion of subjects with the event divided by the proportion of subjects without the event.) For odds ratios, 1 represents the point at which the odds of disease are the same whether or not the risk factor is present. Therefore, an odds ratio of 1 is actually the same as the null hypothesis, which states that the risk for having the disease is the same whether the risk factor is present or absent. If a 95% CI around the observed odds ratio does not extend beyond 1, you conclude that the odds ratio is statistically significant with a *P* value less than or equal to 0.05. The same strategy applies to relative risks. Consider the following study.

CASE STUDY 8-6

Imagine a study in which the odds ratio of skin cancer and sun exposure was 8(6,10). The 8 indicates the odds ratio for the sample, which means that the odds of having skin cancer are increased eightfold for those with sun exposure. An odds ratio of 1 would mean that there are the same odds of having skin cancer if you had sun exposure as there are if you had none. The CI on this odds ratio tells us with 95% confidence that the odds ratio in the larger population is between 6 and 10. The lower confidence limit is 6, much greater than 1, and this allows us to be quite sure that a substantial odds ratio is present not only in our sample, but also in the larger population from which our sample was obtained. Consider an odds ratio for the same problem with an odds ratio of 8(–2,9). In this case, the observed odds ratio is greater than 1; however, the lower limit of our 95% confidence interval extends below 1, indicating that we should be uncertain about whether sun exposure actually increases the risk for skin cancer.

Bias in a study is often a matter of judgment. Unlike the confidence interval, there is no statistic that indicates bias is present in the study. Bias can be defined as "any process which tends to produce results or conclusions that differ systematically from the truth."[9] There are exhaustive lists of potentially biasing factors available in most research textbooks. The reader should review Chapter 9 for screening tests used in evaluating the medical literature. You can identify some of the most significant sources of bias by using your study outline and reviewing the study method and study findings. In this way you can explore the issue of bias with respect to the selection and follow-up of study subjects, executing and measuring the predictor variable, measuring the outcome variable, and analyzing the data.

For example, in studying a new diagnostic procedure, the investigator must convince us that an appropriate spectrum of patients is represented in the data. If the diseased patients all have more advanced illness than the nondiseased patients, we are more likely to find a false-negative test result in the diseased population. The nondiseased subjects are similarly less likely to have a false-positive result.

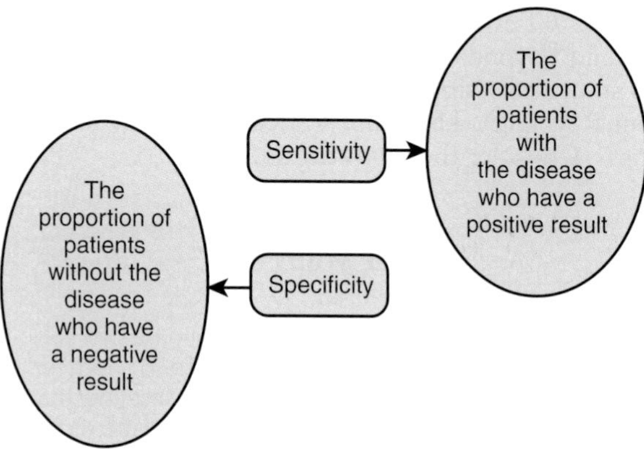

FIGURE 8-4 Sensitivity and specificity.

This type of sampling would overestimate the sensitivity and specificity of the test in a population with a broader spectrum of the disease (Figure 8-4).

When critically appraising the study population for an experimental randomized controlled trial, it is important that both the study and control group are equally likely to have the identified outcome. For example, in a study of a new treatment for preventing high blood pressure, if the patients in the comparison group are all overweight, the comparison group is more likely to have the outcome than the study group patients. That might lead us to believe that the intervention was more successful than it actually was. Alternatively, in a case-controlled study, the presence of the predictor variable should not influence the process of group selection.

Additional bias may occur when following up on study subjects. Consider what happens to the data analysis when some patients drop out or are lost to follow-up. Consider a study designed to test the efficacy of a new, noninvasive treatment for carpal tunnel syndrome in a population of factory workers who do repetitive tasks. How would the findings be affected if this population typically leaves the workplace to seek other opportunities when affected by this problem?

Bias can also be present in the **predictor variable.** Consider the effect on the magnitude of the finding if some people did not really receive the intervention as planned or received an additional therapy or different therapy. For example, in a study evaluating the effects of a new medication on depression, what would happen if some of the patients also enrolled in an outside exercise program? We would have a difficult time determining which intervention actually caused an effect. Bias also could occur in measuring the predictor variable. This is a particular concern in case-controlled studies where the subjects and controls are selected on the basis of outcome variable. Retrospective interview data from these subjects may be compromised by the subject's memory of the exposure, or the data may be inaccurate due to the researcher's ability to accurately and completely locate data in charts or medical records. Investigator bias might also occur if the researcher is not blind to the outcomes. For example, if the researcher's hypothesis is that the outcome variable is attributable to a particular predictor variable (e.g., lung cancer is attributable to exposure to electromagnetic waves) the investigator may be unconsciously more persistent in eliciting a history of exposure from patients with lung cancer.

Measuring the **outcome variable** is also subject to bias from both the subject and investigator. If blinding is not present and subjects are aware that they have received an intervention, they may change their behavior or fail to report negative findings. For example, if patients receive a new homeopathic treatment for headaches, they might also modify their diet or exercise routine or fail to report some minor headaches that were not as severe as those that they were experiencing before the intervention.

Most clinicians assume that reputable journals have individuals in the peer review process who evaluate whether an appropriate statistical test was used in analyzing the relationship between the predictor and outcome variables. However, one particular issue that does not relate to the test itself but rather the process of analysis in randomized-controlled trials warrants further mention. Many studies fail to indicate whether an **intent-to-treat** analysis was used. Intent-to-treat means that groups are analyzed according to their original assignments, despite the fact that some members of the control group may have, for whatever reason, ended up receiving the intervention and members of the treatment group did not. Intent-to-treat analysis is important for preserving the random allocation assigned to the study subjects. For example, consider what would happen if patients in the treatment group got well before the intervention and therefore did not receive it. If they were then analyzed as part of the control group, it would bias the results of both groups because the control group would be healthier than the treatment group at the outset of the intervention. This would introduce bias in the results in favor of the control group.

Bias can occur during the design, implementation, or analysis phase of a study through intrinsic errors in the process such as those previously outlined. **Confounded** results emerge from an extrinsic cause. A confounder causes a skewed result in the outcome variable and is related to the predictor variable. For example, referring back to Case Study 8-1, what if an

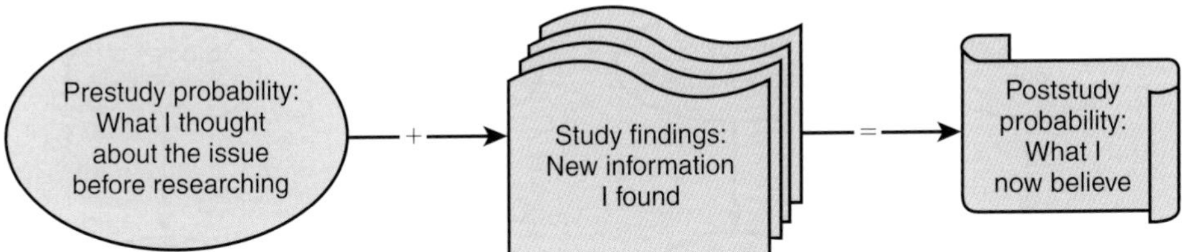

FIGURE 8-5 Clinical decision-making.

author conducts a study of the use of fluoxetine for weight loss in type 2 diabetes, and some of the population under study is also diagnosed with comorbid depression? The author can limit the effect of confounders on the study population by excluding subjects with the particular confounder from the study population. Alternatively, subjects and controls in the study can be matched based on the confounder. If these strategies are not implemented at the front end of the study, researchers can also attempt to control for confounders in the data analysis process, either through stratification of the data or by using multivariate analysis. In a critical appraisal, the important determinant related to confounders is whether the author of the study has attempted to control for these.

As a clinician, you will consider all of these issues as you evaluate a study's validity. However, you should also ask how the study's findings relate to other knowledge you may already have or may find in the literature. If the finding is not believable within the context of other knowledge, you may be reluctant to integrate this new information into your practice. Any time we read a new study finding, we consider what we knew before. We consider this information in light of what was known and reevaluate or review what we now believe about the issue[10] (Figure 8-5).

We weigh several factors as we qualitatively assess this issue. We may look to the information's consistency with other literature. Is there literature that would support the present finding? For example, because we are exploring the use of fluoxetine for weight loss in type 2 diabetes in Case Study 8-1, does other literature report this outcome from fluoxetine use in other populations? We also would consider the biologic plausibility of our findings. Does the pathophysiology that we already know make sense in terms of the study? Are there analogous situations where this intervention has been shown to be an effective treatment? These factors influence our judgment about the validity of new study findings. In conjunction with our consideration of the potential impact of chance (*P* value, confidence intervals); bias (systematic, intrinsic factors); and confounding factors (extrinsic factors), we can make a reasonable judgment about whether the outcomes reported are truly associated with the predictor variable. If we determine that this is the case, we proceed to consider whether this information will help in caring for the patient.

Core Skill 4: Implementing Useful Findings

Step 4: What is the clinically relevant finding? An understanding of a limited number of key concepts and statistical calculations will help a clinician recognize the clinically relevant finding. Most statistical calculations are presented in a journal article; however, it is important for clinicians to understand what the statistics mean for the patient and how to interpret these findings in the context of clinical practice. Figure 8-6 presents a selection of these calculations, and in Chapter 9 statistics are discussed as well. Because most of the clinical studies we used involve interventions in patient care, we review these in greater detail.

As clinicians, we select the treatments to use with our patients. This selection is often based on a qualitative evaluation in which we weigh the risks and benefits of a particular therapy to the patient. We can also assess the relative value of an intervention quantitatively. Studies of intervention may report the benefit of a given therapy as a relative risk reduction (RRR). This may not represent the true impact on our patient population. A better way of expressing the benefit of an intervention may be the **absolute risk reduction (ARR)** and the number **needed to treat (NNT)**.

CASE STUDY 8-7

Two studies of cardiac arrest were undertaken with different populations. Both studies used the same therapy and same follow-up for 4 years. Study A's intervention group had a 5% cardiac event rate, with a control group event rate of 10%. Study B's treatment group had a 10% cardiac event rate, with a control group rate of 20%. In both cases the therapy reduced the relative risk for cardiac arrest by 50%.

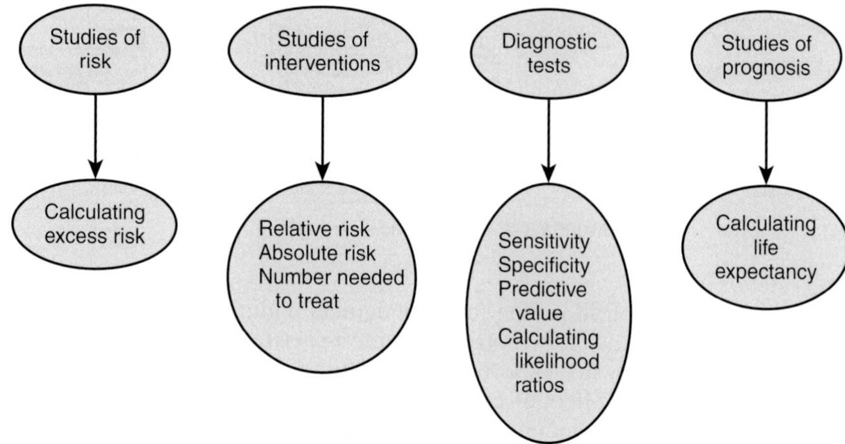

FIGURE 8-6 ■ Statistical calculations.

$$R = \frac{\text{incidence of outcome control group} - \text{incidence of outcome study group}}{\text{incidence of outcome control group}}$$

INCIDENCE OF OUTCOME CONTROL GROUP

In Study A, the RRR={10−5}/10=50%; in Study B, the RRR={20−10}/20=50%. It would seem that the therapy had the same impact on both study populations. The absolute risk reduction (AAR) would indicate, however, that the impact on the populations is actually very different.

ARR = incidence of outcome control group − incidence of outcome study group

For Study A, the ARR over 10 years equals 10 − 5 = 5%; in Study B the ARR = 20 − 10 = 10%. This means that for every 100 patients treated during a 10-year period, 5 cardiac arrests were prevented in Study A and 10 cardiac arrests were prevented in Study B. The number needed to treat (NNT) follows from this. This represents the number of patients we need to treat to prevent one outcome event. This is the inverse of the ARR if the ARR is in the form of a fraction or is 100 divided by the ARR, if the ARR is displayed as a percentage.

In the Study A, the NNT = 100/5 = 20 and for Study B, the NNT = 100/10 = 10. Therefore, in Study A, 20 patients were treated to prevent 1 cardiac arrest, whereas in Study B, 10 patients were treated to prevent 1 cardiac event. The impact of the intervention is obviously greater in Study B. The NNTs for these studies were calculated over a 4-year period. Therefore, for Study A, the NNT of 20 over 4 years is equivalent to treating 80 patients to prevent 1 cardiac arrest per year (NNT = 20/4 = 80 per year). This is why it is important to make sure that studies you compare follow patients for comparable lengths of time. In general, the less time patients are followed, the less opportunity to see an effect. This would result in a smaller ARR and a larger NNT.

We perform the same steps if the intervention is harmful. We calculate the **absolute risk increase (ARI).** The inverse of the ARI is the **number needed to harm (NNH).** This would tell us the number of patients we would need to treat to observe a single adverse event. For clinicians it is particularly important to remember that your patient may be sicker or healthier than the one in the study you are reading. In that case, you would adjust the NNT for your particular patient. The amount of the adjustment would depend on your assessment of your patient's anticipated risk relative to the study population. For example, if the NNT for a study is 15 and you estimate that your patient's risk of outcome without intervention would be three times that of the study group, the NNT for your patient is 15/3 = 5.

New models, which incorporate ethical decision-making, weigh costs and benefits and can be completed at the patient's bedside. These models incorporate the probabilities of various outcomes of a treatment and the outcome probabilities of no treatment in addition to a consideration of patient preferences for treatment. Although these models are quite complex, it is important to recognize that the patient's perspective is a critical piece in clinical decision-making that should not be overlooked. Another way of saying this is to consider a process known as **discounting.** In discounting, we consider that future life may be "discounted" over present life. In other words, a patient might value his or her present life over a future life. This implies that a patient may not want to take a risk today for the promise of a health benefit in the future. Informing patients of up-front risks is essential in reaching a mutual decision regarding treatments and outcomes.

Step 5: Will the study help me in caring for my patient? The final question clinicians must ask in evaluating studies is whether the information reported would assist them in caring for a particular patient. First, we refer to the information we reviewed in Step 2. We explore the target population and determine if it was adequately described so that we can compare our patient to the study group. Similarly, we determine whether the predictor variable or intervention, or both, were adequately described and comparable with treatments under consideration for your patient. We may also want to consider whether local resources are available to implement the intervention or test. Finally, we consider whether the finding will provide the patient with an overall net benefit. If we have determined in Step 3 that the findings were valid and that the study subjects and predictor variables relate to our patient, we can determine that the clinically relevant result will be useful information for our clinical decision-making.

CONCLUSION

The guidelines in this chapter will help busy PAs and PA students separate the "wheat from the chaff" and focus attention on those published articles that have direct clinical application to patients. Clinicians must continue to exercise caution, however, as they embrace new medical literature for the "truths" it contains. Even the best quality literature may be filled with discrepancies with respect to an individual patient's situation. For example, what if the literature describes a daily treatment for a condition that your patient can only access weekly, or the literature describes efficacy in a population older or younger than your patient? Clearly, clinical judgment remains the predominant factor in determining patient care. So why bother with peer-reviewed research when making clinical decisions, particularly when so many clinicians remain appropriately uneasy about this element of the medical process? The more we know in medicine, the more questions we seem to be asking, including what to do with the new information we have gained. Probably one of the strongest arguments for mastering EBM skills is that it challenges us to continually attempt to find better solutions for our patients. Discrepant literature will continue to be an important force in medicine, promoting additional research and dialogue on the efficacy of practice and the quality of care.

CLINICAL APPLICATIONS

- Pretend you are interviewing for a position with a practice where several of the providers are at the end stage of their career. They tell you that they have practiced together for 40 years and feel that they know what is best for patients. They have interviewed other students who are keen on changing their practice to include more "evidence-based" approaches. What would you say?
- Your patient brings you an article from an Internet website that indicates he or she can send away for a new treatment that will cure _________. How would you respond to your patient?
- When treating your patient, what do you feel is more important, clinical judgment or systematic reviews of the literature about the patient's clinical problem?
- What are the advantages and disadvantages to relying on the findings of a randomized controlled trial for decision-making about your individual patients?

KEY POINTS

- EBM is the application of the best available evidence to patient care.
- Four key skills of EBM are the following:
  - Formulating a clear question for a clinical problem
  - Searching the literature for relevant clinical articles
  - Evaluating the evidence for validity and usefulness
  - Implementing useful findings in clinical practice
- Clinicians should exercise caution as they apply the "best evidence" to an individual patient's care.
- EBM challenges us to continually look for better solutions for our patients.

References

1. Cochrane AL. Effectiveness and Efficiency. Random Reflections on Health Services. London: Nuffield Provincial Hospitals Trust; 1972, (Reprinted in 1989 in association with the BMJ; Reprinted in 1999 for Nuffield Trust by the Royal Society of Medicine Press, London [ISBN 1-85315-394-X]).
2. Chalmers I, Enkins M, Keirse M. Effective Care in Pregnancy and Childbirth. New York: Oxford University Press; 1989.
3. Sinclair JC, Bracken MB. Effective Care of the Newborn Infant. New York: Oxford University Press; 1992.
4. Evidence-Based Medicine Working Group. Evidence-based medicine. A new approach to teaching the practice of medicine. JAMA 1992;268:2420.
5. Guyatt G, Rennie D, Meade M, Cook D. User's Guides to the Medical Literature: A Manual for Evidence-Based Clinical Practice. 2nd ed. New York: McGraw Hill Medical, JAMA Archives; 2008.
6. Straus SE, Glasziou P, Richardson WS, Haynes RB. Evidence-Based Medicine: How to Practice and Teach It. 4th ed. Edinburgh: Churchill Livingstone; 2011.
7. Greenhalgh T. How to Read a Paper: The Basics of Evidence Based Medicine. 4th ed. London: BMJ Publishing Group; 2010.
8. Friedland D, Go AS, Davoren JB, et al. Evidence-Based Medicine: A Framework for Clinical Practice. Stamford, CT: Appleton & Lange; 1998.
9. Blessing JD. A Physician Assistant's Guide to Research and the Medical Literature. Philadelphia: FA Davis; 2001.
10. Sackett DL. Bias in analytic research. J Chron Dis 1979;32:51.

CHAPTER 9

RESEARCH AND THE PHYSICIAN ASSISTANT

J. Dennis Blessing • Vasco Deon Kidd

"If we knew what it was we were doing, it would not be called research, would it?"
ALBERT EINSTEIN

CHAPTER CONTENTS

Even though the term *research* invokes fear in most people, it is an integral part of society and affects every industry, from the person developing a business plan for a start-up company, to the clinician providing evidence-based medicine. Undoubtedly, research is all round us. Research has been the impetus for the science of medicine and how health professionals provide care across the continuum of health. Research has created an environment that directly or indirectly governs almost all that physician assistants do in patient care. Research today is far more than spending countless hours in a laboratory crunching numbers and reviewing data; it is common threat that connects all health care.

Research is a tool to use. Primarily, research is a process (Figure 9-1). It is a process born in curiosity and a need to know. From the simple parental admonition to "Look it up!" to a tightly controlled environment with specific rules and requirements, research answers our tough questions. For example, when we need to review clinical guidelines or best practices for improving patient care, we look to research.

As a physician assistant (PA) or a student, you cannot escape research. It is part of the educational process. Most students are required to engage in some type of research activity. Student research can range from a thesis to a community-based project or other related activities as part of academic and professional development. PA educators have the dual responsibility of educating and training future clinicians and contributing and advancing scientific knowledge. Many unknowns about our profession need exploration. Advancement is achieved only through research.

Clinically practicing PAs, at a minimum, must understand how to critically appraise and apply research to improve medical decision-making and patient outcomes. Additionally, clinical investigations have become a part of many practices and a primary responsibility for some PAs. As our profession grows, its members must expand their contributions to the social, mental, and physical knowledge base of humankind. Research is the primary tool with which these contributions will come to fruition. We must be scientists and clinicians.

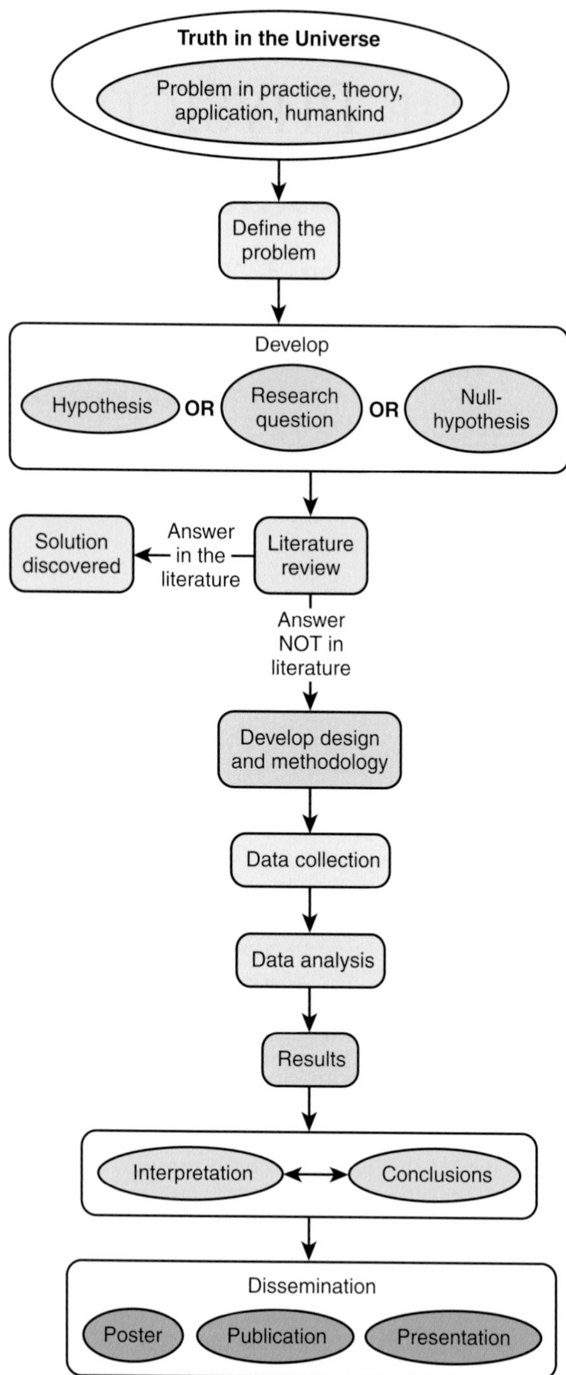

FIGURE 9-1 ■ **The Scientific Process.** (Reproduced by permission from Blessing JD (ed). Physician Assistant's Guide to Research and Medical Literature, 2nd ed. Philadelphia: FA Davis, 2005.)

Our intent is for this chapter is to provide a basic overview of research that will provide an outline and format for interpreting the medical literature. Many voluminous tomes are written on these subjects. So let this chapter be a guiding resource as you develop your understanding of research. Consider the possibility that at some point in your career, you may become involved with research. For example, you may be called on to answer the question about the care you provide and how your approach improves patient outcomes and satisfaction. You will have to do some form of research to answer that question. Research should become part of who we are as professionals if we are to advance scientific knowledge and broader professional goals.

DEFINING RESEARCH

Webster's New World College Dictionary defines research as "careful, systematic, patient study and investigation in some field of knowledge, undertaken to discover or establish facts or principles."[1] From this basic definition, the world of research springs to life: from simple (a person at the mall with a clipboard) to complex (the human genome). What research means may vary among professions. For example, attorneys review cases and judgments for legal precedence (legal research). This is entirely different from the process and approach that a clinical investigator who is interested in the outcomes of drug A versus drug B in a patient population would use. Of course, both are different from the basic scientist working in a laboratory. More examples and types of research are available. Physician assistant involvement with research and as researchers has been limited, but that cannot continue in the era of health care reform and evidence-based medicine. We must become more knowledgeable of what research can do for us. As PAs, we must advance the fund of knowledge for the benefit of society, medicine, and our profession. This chapter serves as a brief introduction to the concepts of research and is not intended to be an all inclusive discussion of research techniques, statistics, or methodology.

The purposes of research are (1) to develop new theories or philosophies; (2) to discover new knowledge; (3) to explain relationships; (4) to reexamine, confirm, or modify what is known; and (5) to develop understanding of our world (universe?, existence?). These purposes of research are achieved by employing the *scientific method* (Figure 9-1). The scientific method is a system of exploration and discovery that allows us to advance our knowledge of the universe and to validate, correct, or repudiate conventional wisdom. This involves identifying a problem, gathering data, analysis, and interpretation while limiting bias and controlling extraneous variables.

Categories of research can be defined as follows:

Applied—designed to answer practical questions; may or may not involve human subjects

Clinical—human subject investigations performed in the "real world"

Descriptive—defining phenomena related to a group or situation

Laboratory—performed in a controlled environment, usually not involving human subjects; basic science research

Pure—abstract and general intended to generate new theory

Experimental—manipulation of a variable (independent variable) for effect on another variable (dependent) while controlling influences (confounding) variables. Subjects are assigned randomly.

Quasi-experimental—has the elements of experimental design, but subject assignment is not random[2,3]

Definitions

As a starting point, here are some brief working definitions, purposely limited in number by the authors. These are common terms found in many investigations. Many more exist. The *Dictionary of Statistics and Methodology*[4] is an excellent resource for definitions.

Quantitative Research—research that uses continuous, ordinal, categoric data to describe phenomena

Qualitative Research—research that involves non-numeric data to describe phenomena

Phenomenon (phenomena, pl.)—something that can be observed and therefore measured

Population—the group we want to study

Sample—a chosen number of a population that represents that population

Subject—an individual in the sample

Methodology—the way (or method) that a research study is conducted, often called *research design*

Literature—the published body of knowledge on a subject

Confidence interval—the range of values where a population parameter is estimated to fall

Confidence level—the estimated probability that a population parameter lies within the confidence interval

Power analysis—a process to establish sample size that allows sample analysis to be applied to a population

Probability—a level of significance used to determine if a study result occurs by chance; often referred to as a *P* value and expressed as a number (example: $P < .05$); using $P < 0.5$ as an example, if our statistical analysis yields a value less than .05, then we can state that the likelihood the result occurring by chance is less than 5%. Also referred to as the *level of significance*

Data—observations, information, measurements

Continuous data—numeric data (numbers) where the distance between values is the same (i.e., the distance between 5 and 6 is the same as for 18-19 is the same for 993-994 and so on); there are two types:

Interval—continuous data that have no "0" value

Ratio—continuous data that have a value of "0"; zero (0) does not necessarily mean the total lack of, but rather is one value on the scale. An example is Fahrenheit temperature; "0°" does not mean a total lack of temperature; rather, it is one value on the scale.

Nominal data—data that categorize a subject, sample, population such as age, gender, ethnicity, occupation, marital status, education, etc.; typically produces demographics

Ordinal data—data that have order or rank but no defined interval between values

Verbal frequency scales—used in survey research in which a subject may respond to a statement by "Strongly Agree," "Agree," "Neutral," "Disagree," "Strongly Disagree," or a similar set of words

Hypothesis—a statement to be tested by an investigation or study; written as a directed or positive statement, usually a predictive statement

Null-hypothesis—a statement that asserts no differences exist between tested variables; written as a negative statement

Research question—a statement of the problem to be investigated written as a question

Parametric—refers to data that have a normal distribution; continuous data are always initially considered to have a normal distribution

Nonparametric—refers to data that do not have a normal distribution; ordinal and nominal data are considered nonparametric

Variable—phenomenon; an observable characteristic that can be identified, observed, measured, and analyzed

Independent variable—a variable that is manipulated in an investigation

Dependent variable—the variable that is measured for change that occurs from manipulation of the independent variable

Confounding variable—a variable that influences the dependent variable, but it cannot be controlled

Regression—a statistical analysis used to establish the relationship between variables

Reliability—the degree to which a test or instrument produces the same results on repeated uses or measurements

Validity—the degree to which a test or instrument measures or tests what it purports to test or measure

Bias—anything that unduly influences or produces an error in a research project; can occur at any point in the design of the project; in subject selection/assignment; procedures or instrumentations; design; analyses, etc.

Components of a Research Report

We are going to approach our introduction to research by a somewhat different manner than what is usually done. We develop our understanding by following the outline for chapters used in theses and dissertations. Variations exist, but most theses and dissertations have five chapters: Chapter 1—Introduction; Chapter 2—Review of the Literature; Chapter 3—Methodology (or Methods); Chapter 4—Results; Chapter 5—Discussion. References (or bibliography) follow the five chapters. An abstract is the lead-in for the manuscript. Each chapter may have a number of subchapters and section headings. Journal publications generally have the same components for their manuscripts but are more concise and shorter in length. As you read about each component in the following sections, consider how you would evaluate them as part of your interpretation of the medical literature.

Introduction

The Introduction to the research report presents the reader with the background to the investigation. This opening chapter should also capture the reader's interest and desire to read the study. This is where the importance of the investigation is driven home to the reader. Along with the introductory material, this is where you define the problem(s) to be studied and frame those problems as a *hypothesis*, *null-hypothesis*, or *research question* (see definitions). Everything that follows in the research report is designed to answer or explain the hypothesis, null-hypothesis, or research question. See Box 9-1 for examples of a hypothesis, null-hypothesis, and research question. Although these formats are similar, they are different and some forms may be better than others for some types of studies, particularly for data analysis.

Where do research questions or problems come from? For most of us, problems originate in our environment. Questions may arise from your practice or training; there may be controversy in the literature; there may be a need to identify the best treatment or practice; almost anything that arouses your curiosity or interest can be a source of a research project. Many times, there is a need to replicate studies to support or refute reported findings. Ultimately, if you are looking for a research project, it must be something in which you have an interest and something that you have the capability to do. As you begin to define your research statement, break the problem down into its simplest components. You should try to keep your research down to one or a small number of problems. The more items to investigate, the more complicated the study becomes. Each investigation should deal with one or two problems. For each point you want to investigate, you should ask yourself these questions[5]:

1. What is the significance of the study?
2. Has the issue been addressed in whole or part?
3. How important is the issue and its timeliness?
4. What is the cost in time, effort, and dollars?
5. What is the contribution to our fund of knowledge?

If you can answer these questions to your satisfaction and believe that an investigation is indicated, you are ready to move forward.

BOX 9-1 EXAMPLES OF A HYPOTHESIS, NULL-HYPOTHESIS, AND RESEARCH QUESTION

Problem	You have noted in your practice that patients who take hypertension medication "A" in the morning have better control than patients who take the medication at bedtime. This investigation problem could be framed in the following ways.
Hypothesis	Patients who take medication "A" in the morning have better blood pressure control than patients who take the medication at bedtime.
Null-hypothesis	There is no difference in blood pressure control between patients who take medication "A" in the morning and patients who take the medication at bedtime.
Research question	Is there a difference in blood pressure control in patients who take medication "A" in morning versus those who take it at night?

Review of the Literature

Sometimes called *literature review*, this is where you present what is known about the problem or issue being studied. The literature review must be a systematic exploration and analysis of the medical literature. The review can include almost any source including personal communication. One must remember that when you make statements about your subject, those statements must be referenced to the source. This allows the reader to go to the same sources for information or to verify your interpretation. You do not have to include everything published on your topic, but you must provide a substantive background that will allow the reader to understand what is currently known and how the research project will lead to further understanding. This will allow the reader to develop an appreciation for the questions being asked and, hopefully, answered by the study.

This is why it is important to be concise rather than broad or excessive with research questions. If the reader understands the background or issues involved, then a better understanding of how your investigation will affect our knowledge will be possible. By understanding what is known, the reader will have a better understanding of the problem and how you intend to address it.

For example, suppose a PA wants to know whether cortisone injections improve knee pain in patients with severe knee arthritis. The first thing is to conduct a literature review of all relevant material on the basis of inclusion and exclusion criteria developed for the search. By narrowing the search criteria, the best evidence on the subject of interest is collected. The answer may be in the literature and, if not, a study is warranted. However, if you are not familiar with how to conduct a literature review, then consult a medical librarian in your hospital or a resource librarian at a local university.

Proper referencing is extremely important in your literature review. A number of style manuals can assist you with referencing. When preparing an article for journal submission, follow the style required by the journal. All journals have an "Information for Authors" section or guidelines. If you are writing a thesis or dissertation, your institution will have a preferred style. Usually, this is published in the catalog or by the graduate school.

It is important to give credit where credit is due. In the research world, plagiarism is the unpardonable sin and should be avoided at all cost. As a rule, generally accepted and well-known concepts and theories do not have to be referenced. For example, "The sky is blue" does not need referencing. However, a theory about why the sky is blue would need a reference.

BOX 9-2 REFERENCE EXAMPLES FROM THE *JOURNAL OF PHYSICIAN ASSISTANT EDUCATION*

Journal	Hudson CL. Expansion of medical professional services with nonprofessional personnel. *JAMA*. 1961;176:839-841.
Book Chapter	Jones T. Ethical decision making and ethical principles. In: Cassidy BA, Blessing JD, editors. Ethics and professionalism; A guide for the physician assistant. Philadelphia: FA Davis; 2008. p. 19-34.
Book	Hooker RS, Cawley JF, Asprey DP. Physician assistants: Policy and practice. 3rd ed. Philadelphia: FA Davis; 2010.
Website	American Medical Association. *AMA Code of Medical Ethics.* Available at: http://www.ama-rg/ama/pub/category.html. Accessed February 2, 2005.
Agency or Institutional Report	US Department of Health and Human Services. Surveillance for selected public health indicators affecting older adults—United States. *MMWR Morb Mortal Wkly Rep.* 1999;48:33-34.
Unpublished Material	Statler M, Sullivan D. The impact of promotion and tenure on physician assistant faculty. Paper presented at: Association of Physician Assistant Programs Annual Education Forum; November 4, 2005; Fajardo, Puerto Rico.

In addition, if you reproduce word for word more than three consecutive words from a source, a reference is required. In some instances, quotation marks may also be necessary to delineate exact statements. Box 9-2 contains some examples of the style format required by the *Journal of the American Academy of Physician Assistants.*[6] The American Academy of Physician Assistants (AAPA) requires references in the form describe in the *American Medical Association Manual of Style* or the *Uniform Requirements for Manuscripts Submitted to Biomedical Journals.*

A key component of your literature review is keeping a record of your references. You should have a full copy (not just an abstract) of all articles, book chapters, interviews, books (if possible), and all other resources used in your research. You should keep a record of all your electronic searches, even if you do not use some of the material that you find. It is important to save these resources in a format you can retrieve. Back up everything!

Electronic medical and research databases (e.g., Ovid-Medline, EMB reviews, EBSCO, ERIC, CINAHL) are a boon to students, novices, and expert investigators. Large volumes of information can be searched using key words, authors, journals, and titles. Often, full text articles are available online. Using an electronic database takes some time and skill to navigate; however, training is available through online resources and, as stated earlier, many academic institutions have librarians to help you.

Methodology

This is where you describe your study in detail so that the reader will understand explicitly what you did and how you did it. The description of the project methodology should be detailed to a level that anyone who wants to replicate your work could do so. The type of study dictates the methodology in many instances. There are true experimental designs, quasi-experimental designs, other quantitative designs, and qualitative designs. A complete description of research methodology is far beyond the scope of this chapter. A plethora of books and other resources cover research methodology in great detail. It is also beneficial to consult a statistician about the statistical analysis for your research. The type of statistical analyses depends on the type of data collected and the intent of analyses. Numerous qualitative and quantitative textbooks are available.

At a minimum, the description of your methodology should include (1) a description of the subjects and how they were selected or assigned; (2) the instrumentation used (including surveys) and when used; (3) procedures (if any) carried out or used; (4) how the data were analyzed.[7]

A project must be conducted as it is described in the methodology. You cannot and should not change what you are doing on the basis of results or data collected as the investigation proceeds. Do what you said you were going to do and follow your design protocol.

Results

This is often the shortest chapter or section of the manuscript. This is where the reader will see the results of the analyses. The presentation of the data should be direct, to the point, and done so without commentary. The results are the results. This is not the place to try to explain or interpret the data. That comes in the next chapter.

Often the best way to present data is in the form of charts, graphs, and tables. Many different types of charts graphs, and tables exist. Your choice is made with the intent to give readers a clear understanding of outcomes. Remember, a picture is worth a 1000 words; this adage is even more true when you are trying to meet a journal's word limit. Charts, graphs, and tables save space and may shorten the length of a manuscript, which is important to editors who may publish your work. Every chart, graph, or table should be appropriately labeled and easy to read. Data presented in a chart, graph, or table should also be grouped by similar themes or concepts with properly defined unit values (e.g., grams vs. pounds; Celsius vs. Fahrenheit; months vs. years; percent vs. percentile).

You should present the results from every analysis. Your results should match the analyses you described in the methodology section. Failure to report results because they do not support your beliefs, wishes, or hypotheses is dishonest and unethical. If the methodology (process) is sound, then the results are sound. Again, the results are the results and speak for themselves. It is your responsibility to make sense of them.

Discussion

This is the section of the paper where you present your interpretation of the study. Answers to the original questions are also presented. The discussion section may have several subsections such as limitations, implications, conclusions, and recommendations for further or additional research. You should be precise in your explanations, carefully explaining how your findings contribute to the body of knowledge, support or disapprove other research findings, or provide new or novel findings. You must make logical connections between your research questions (hypotheses or null-hypotheses) via the methodology and analyses to the results AND your interpretations. You also want to discuss or explore any bias (intentional or not) in the study. Recognizing the limitations of your investigations and any possible bias is important in the discussion. This will help readers understand the results in light of problems or issues that may have affected the investigation or outcomes. It will also limit the appearance that you may be trying to hide something or exaggerate findings known as *publication bias.*

The bottom line is that the discussion is your interpretation of the results and what they mean. Your interpretation should be reasonable in light of the study and make sense of what you have done. You may find that your investigation has created more questions than it answered. Bring those questions to light and discuss them. New or unanswered questions allow additional research opportunities for you and the people who read your manuscript. Remember, few of us will make earth-shattering discoveries. Be happy with adding a small (usually a very small) piece to our understanding and knowledge.

RESEARCH ETHICS AND HUMAN SUBJECTS

The protection of human subjects and their data is an important aspect of research. The actions of Nazi scientists during World War II and the Tuskegee syphilis experiment are egregious examples of what can happen when there are no checks, balances, or restrictions on what researchers can do. Since the latter half of the 20th century, efforts to protect human subjects from unfair, unethical, and unsafe research practices have been increasing.[8] Every institution has a committee (Research Ethics Committee) or board, often called the Institutional Review Board (IRB), that reviews and approves studies involving human subjects. The IRBs operate under rules developed and mandated by the federal government. The purpose of the IRB is to protect human subjects and to ensure that human studies are ethical and meet established standards. Almost all research that involves human subjects is covered by IRB regulations and review.

If you are an employee or student of an institution of any type, you must have approval of the IRB to conduct your investigation. There are three classifications of investigations: *exempt*, *expedited*, and *full review*. Exempt studies (those with no or minimal risk) such as systematic reviews or surveys must be approved as such by the IRB. Full reviews involved everything from informed consent, study methodology, subjects selected, data analyses, and even the advertisement used to recruit subjects. To learn more about an IRB, check your institution's website or research department for information. Many IRBs will have local requirements for research in addition to the mandated requirements. As a side note, it is important to obtain IRB approval because many journals will request this information before considering your manuscript for review or publication. It is the responsibility of every investigator to familiarize himself or herself with local institutions' IRB requirements. Failure to follow IRB requirements can lead to corrective action and possible litigation against an investigator. If it involves a person at any level, the IRB must be consulted.

MEDICAL LITERATURE

Interpretation

How are you going to keep up? More than 2 million new research articles are published in biomedical and scientific journals each year.[9] It is unlikely that you will be able to read them all, but every one of them, theoretically, could be important to your practice and care of patients. You will have a huge number of journals and medical resources at hand. Deciding what is important to your practice is a skill that every PA must hone, develop, and use. Although there are many books written on interpreting medical and research articles, we cover the basics in this last part of the chapter. We also introduce more terms that will help further your understanding of research.

Most medical organizations, including the American Academy of Physician Assistants, produce a professional journal. If you add these to other journals produced by a variety of groups (learned societies) and professional publishers, you have a lifetime of reading. So how do you decide what to read and how do you make decisions about what is important to you and the care of your patients?

1. First, Internet browsers are not the place to look for medical information. Use medical databases. Use professional literature. This can include web publications, but be sure of the source.
2. Choose journals that deal with your specialty or with the problem at hand. For example, you may work in family medicine and use PA and medical journals that deal with primary care but need to go to a source that deals with endocrinology for a patient with a thyroid problem.
3. Is there "peer review?" See Box 9-3. Quality journals have a peer review process. Be careful, though, because not everything in a "peer-reviewed" journal may be peer reviewed.
4. What is the subject of the material? Is it specific for your problem? You do not have a lot of time for reading material that is not pertinent to your problem. Read the abstract and use it as a guide to whether or not you should read further.
5. Is it a report of an investigation or an overview of a problem (a clinical review)? You will evaluate original research slightly differently

BOX 9-3 PEER REVIEW

A review process for manuscripts, presentations, grants, posters, and other materials intended for dissemination in some format. Peer review is a process that allows experts in a field to scrutinize, critique, evaluate, and make recommendations on a piece of work before its publication and dissemination. These reviewers make recommendations to the editor on the fate of the manuscript. The work may be accepted as is; returned for major or minor revision; or rejected. The purpose of peer review is to attempt to ensure that published materials meet the accepted standards of a discipline and the scientific process.

from a clinical review. Typically, most of the articles in the PA journals are clinical reviews or reviews and summaries of a disease entity.

6. If you are reading a report of a research study, then you have to identify the following and ask if all are relevant to what you are seeking.
   A. The population represented by the sample
      i. How was the sample selected and assigned?
   B. What is the design of the study?
      i. What type of study is reported?
   C. Is the methodology of the study appropriate to investigate the problem?
      i. Are the data analyses sound?
   D. What are the results?
      i. Are the results clear?
      ii. Are results presented or accounted for from all statistical analyses?
      iii. Do the results seem valid?
   E. Are the authors' interpretations of the results sound?
      i. Are the interpretations consistent with the intent of the analyses?
      ii. How do the results compare with what is known and accepted?
   F. How can you apply the results in your practice?

Over past 10 to 15 years, the advancement of statistical techniques and analyses has led to outcomes measurements known as *evidence-based medicine* (EBM). EBM is defined as "the conscientious, explicit, and judicious use of current best evidence in making decisions about the care of individual patients."[10] There are many levels of evidence from expert opinion to meta-analysis of random controlled trials to systematic reviews. As we move forward in the 21st century, there will be even more EBM to help guide us in the care of our patients. As policy makers look to improve patient care, lower health care costs, and reduce abuse, EBM will become the standard by which care is judged.

Clinical Review

As stated earlier, the most common type of article appearing in the PA literature is the clinical review. Clinical reviews are likely the most common type of capstone for PA students. They are the most likely type of manuscript to be done by practicing PAs. Of course, this makes perfect sense for a profession that is clinically oriented and whose members are primarily in medical practice. For this reason, we are going to cover some of the basics in writing a clinical review.

Clinical reviews can be loosely separated into four general categories: (1) general review of a clinical topic (an overview); (2) summative review of a clinical topic (narrower in focus); (3) systematic review of the literature on a specific topic (review of all evidence); and (4) case or case series report (a case report with literature review to explain).[11] The clinical review is, basically, a summary of the assessment and management of a disease, injury, or medical problem. The clinical review may bring medical information into a concise format that aids to update the reader or present a completely new understanding or approach. The case study is just that, a study of a case. Case studies (or review of a series of related cases) usually deal with common problems presenting in an atypical fashion or uncommon progression of disease.

Keys to a successful clinical review follow:

1. Choose something you are interested in. As a student, a patient problem that you encounter may be an excellent starting point
2. Make your initial literature searches wide ones. Go back as far as you can because there may be important historical points or considerations that need to be included in your review
3. Narrow your search to more recent time. How far back in time is considered "recent"? There is no answer. If there are a large number of publications on a subject, perhaps you need to look at 2 or 3 years of literature. If there is not much or there is a timeline of progress in the development of our understanding of the problem, then you may need to go back several years. Our usual rule is 5 years, but we have no data to support that decision. A big thing to remember is that a textbook will give you the basics on a condition, but its information will not be the most recent or up to date.
4. Before you begin to construct your report, summarize in outline form what you have learned.
5. As you construct your report, remember your goal is to bring the reader up to date on the disease or condition. You want to help the reader improve his or her ability to assess and manage that disease or problem.
6. As you write your paper, you want to be concise, clear, and to the point. Length and reading time are important.
7. Although the sections or components of a clinical review will vary among journals or publication types, the following are generally expected in some format:

- Introduction; present the problem or condition
- Anatomy, physiology, pathophysiology involved with the disease, injury, or condition
- Presenting history, physical examination, laboratory, radiologic, features, etc.

- Assessment and management
- Discussion/Conclusion

When writing your review, it is best to use short sentences. No report is written correctly on the first try. You need to work on it, walk away for a while, and then work some more. Grammar and spelling are important. Have two people proofread the report when you are near completion. One person should be someone in medicine who will have some idea about your subject. The other person should be someone not in medicine. If the report makes sense to both, then you are ready to complete the final draft. When you ask someone to critique your work, ask them to be as severe a critic as possible. Do not take the criticism personally; take it as the opportunity to improve your manuscript.

CONCLUSION

In this chapter we have only begun the exploration of research and what it means to society, medicine, and the PA. Certainly, you will need additional resources and references to further any research effort you undertake. Additionally, there is no doubt that research will play a major part in what you do as a PA. You may also become involved with research in your practice. It may be as simple as documenting patient problems or case complexity by provider all the way to participating in clinical investigations and outcome studies, which more and more practices are doing. At a minimum, you will have to stay up to date with the medical literature and must have some basic understanding of research in order to do that. Develop a process for reviewing the literature and set time aside every day or at least every week for reviewing the literature. If you do not, you will fall behind. You can be certain that your patients are on the web, watching TV, listening to the radio, and reading. Direct-to-the-consumer advertisements and claims of miracles are pervasive. Your patient will be informed (misinformed), so you need to be up to date.

CLINICAL APPLICATIONS

Why is research important to medical practice?
- What is *level of significance*, and why is it important?
- What is the purpose of an *Institutional Review Board* or *Research Ethics Committee*?
  - Why are they important?
- What are the key points to consider when interpreting a research article?
- What is *evidence-based medicine*?

KEY POINTS

- Research provides the basis for the practice of medicine.
- Research provides the best evidence for practice.
- A basic understanding of research is necessary for the interpretation of the medical literature.
- Many practices are becoming involved with clinical investigations.
- The profession needs PA researchers.

References

1. Neufeldt V, Guralnik DB, (eds). 3rd ed. Webster's New World College Dictionary. MacMillin USA: Cleveland; 1997. p. 1141
2. Bailey DM. Research for the Health Professional: A Practical Guide. 2nd ed. Philadelphia: FA Davis; 1997, xxii.
3. Campbell DT, Stanley JC. Experimental and Quasi-experimental Designs for Research. Boston: Houghton Mifflin Company; 1963, p. 34.
4. Vogt WP. Dictionary of Statistics and Methodology. 3rd ed. Thousand Oaks: Sage Publications; 2005.
5. Ayachi S. The Research Problem in Blessing JD. Physician Assistant's Guide to Research and Medical Literature. 2nd ed. Philadelphia: FA Davis; 2005. p. 21.
6. American Academy of Physician Assistants JAAPA Submission Guidelines. Available at *http://www.jaapa.com/jaapa-submission-guidelines/section/508/*; Accessed June 20, 2011.
7. Bork CE, Jarski RW. Methodology in Blessing JD. Physician Assistant's Guide to Research and Medical Literature. 2nd ed. Philadelphia: FA Davis; 2005. p. 33.
8. Dunn Cm, Chadwick G. Protecting Study Volunteers in Research: A Manual for Investigative Sites. Boston: CenterWatch; 1999, p. 8.
9. Lee KP, Schotland M, Bacchetti P, Bero LA. Association of journal quality indicators with methodological quality of clinical research articles. JAMA 2002;287:2805–2808.
10. Sackett DL, Richardson WS, Rosenberg W, Haynes RB. Evidence Based Medicine: How to Practice & Teach EBM. New York: Churchill Livingstone; 1997, p. 2.
11. Dehn RW. The Clinical Review in Blessing JD. Physician Assistant's Guide to Research and Medical Literature. 2nd ed. Philadelphia: FA Davis; 2005. p. 83.

The resources for this chapter can be found at www.expertconsult.com.

CHAPTER 10

SAFETY IN CLINICAL SETTINGS

Darwin Brown

CHAPTER CONTENTS

This chapter provides information to prepare physician assistant (PA) students for safe clinical experiences. Health professional students are typically required to hone many skills by working and practicing on real patients. Students are sometimes placed in "educational" situations with minimal supervision and asked to perform procedures for which they are not adequately trained. Such circumstances place the student at risk for injuries ranging from needlestick to more substantial injuries.

All PA programs require students to provide basic health information when they are admitted. The only confidential student health information that can be disclosed to the program involves immunizations and results of tuberculosis screening. Programs do not have access to other types of health information on students. Students usually complete a "health status" form describing any medical concerns or significant items in their medical history. In addition, programs require an immunization record with special emphasis on the currency of rubeola, rubella, and tetanus booster. Most, if not all, programs require students to obtain the hepatitis B vaccine prior to enrollment. Tuberculosis testing is also performed on entry into the program and is repeated annually. The Accreditation Review Commission for the Education Physician Assistant directs these basic requirements as part of the PA program's accreditation process and by the educational institution with which the program is affiliated.

Before enrollment or at orientation, many programs require students to undergo background checks and/or drug screening. These procedures help to ensure a safe environment within the educational institution.

Students may receive required information on sexual harassment, bloodborne pathogens, safety, and the Health Insurance Portability and Accountability Act (HIPAA). PA programs cover those topics to ensure a level of student health and safety. The greatest potential for exposure to risk starts when students begin clinical rotations. The exposures may include infectious agents (hepatitis, human immunodeficiency virus [HIV], tuberculosis [TB]), physical injury (needlestick, lacerations, latex allergy, physical attack by a patient), and emotional abuse (verbal abuse, belittlement, sexual harassment). Programs differ in the ways they educate, prevent exposures, and protect students. In the following sections, safety issues important to the clinical portion of a PA training program are explored.

ROTATION SAFETY

To maintain your safety on clinical rotations, common sense is the rule. Be aware of your surroundings at all times, especially when at a new location. Ask your preceptor to review clerkship safety policies. Ask questions regarding who has access to the clinic space, whether chaperones are required for male and female examinations, what to do in case of an emergency, and what to do if you sustain an injury.

TABLE 10-1 **Universal Precaution Requirements**

Universal Precautions Required	Universal Precautions Do *Not* Apply
Semen	Feces
Vaginal secretions	Nasal secretions
Synovial fluid	Sputum
Cerebrospinal fluid	Sweat
Pleural fluid	Tears
Peritoneal fluid	Urine
Pericardial fluid	Vomitus, unless contaminated with blood
Amniotic fluid	Saliva, unless contaminated with blood

From Centers for Disease Control and Prevention (CDC). 2007 Guideline for Isolation Precautions: Preventing Transmission of Infectious Agents in Healthcare Settings, 2009. http://www.cdc.gov/hicpac/2007IP/2007ip_tables.html. Accessed June 12, 2012.

Remember to have your needlestick injury protocol available on rotations.

Universal Precautions

One area often neglected by students is the consistent use of universal precautions. Universal precautions are infection control guidelines designed to protect health care providers from exposure to diseases spread by blood and certain body fluids.[1] Implemented in the 1980s as HIV infection became more prominent, universal precautions eliminated concerns about which patients might require precautions because of infection and which patients were not infected. Simply put, universal precautions require that you assume everyone may be able to transmit hepatitis B, HIV, or other infectious agents, and, therefore, the same precautions are used for all patients. The types of exposures for which universal precautions should be used and for which they are not necessary can be found in Table 10-1.

Universal precautions involve the use of personal protective equipment such as gloves, gowns, masks, and protective eyewear, which can reduce the risk of bloodborne pathogen exposure to the health care student's skin or mucous membranes. As a student and future professional, it is incumbent on you to utilize universal precautions whenever appropriate. If you are performing phlebotomy, suturing a laceration, or performing a punch biopsy, these precautions are in place to protect you from exposure to infectious agents, but they are effective only if you use them consistently.

INTERNATIONAL TRAVEL

Increasing numbers of health care students travel outside the United States as part of their clinical experience. International rotations are frequently seen as exciting and exotic adventures. These types of experiences provide students with a unique appreciation of diverse cultures, intensive language development, and an opportunity to observe uncommon diseases. Most traveling students have a wonderful experience, bringing back lifetime memories and a desire to return to these areas in the future. However, to enjoy this type of clinical experience, you must consider your safety a priority and devote a portion of your preparation time toward this goal.

Many international clinical destinations are in developing countries that may pose safety concerns. Before you leave the United States, participate fully in the planning of your trip. Check with your medical insurance company to determine if you are covered for emergency care while abroad. Evacuation back to the United States can easily cost $10,000 or more, depending on your location and medical condition. If you are not already covered by such insurance, purchase a policy that provides medical coverage and evacuation if necessary. The U.S. Department of State (*http://www.state.gov/travel/*) is an excellent resource for information on traveling to foreign countries, including facts on medical emergencies and evacuation.

NEEDLESTICK AND SHARPS INJURIES

Needlestick and sharps injuries are the most efficient method of transmitting bloodborne pathogens between patients and health care providers, and, therefore, they pose a significant risk to health care workers and students. According to the Centers for Disease Control and Prevention (CDC), approximately 385,000 needlestick and other sharps-related injuries occur each year in hospital-based situations.[2] Needlestick and sharps injuries are primarily associated with transmission of hepatitis B, hepatitis C, and HIV, but other types of infections can also result.[3] Health care students are at especially high risk for needlestick injuries because of their relative inexperience; exposure rates have been reported as between 11% and 50% of students.[4] One PA program found that 22% of its students had some type of exposure, 60% of which were percutaneous injuries.[5]

The most important points of this discussion of student safety are prevention of needlestick injuries and reporting of an injury if one should occur.

Prevention of needlestick and sharps injuries has improved significantly through the adoption of safer needles, protocols on handling sharps, and improved provider education on safety techniques. It is incumbent on PA educational programs to train their students in safe procedures and to establish a comprehensive response process for handling expected injuries.

PA students must take advantage of their programs' training opportunities in areas of phlebotomy, initiation of IVs, suturing, and other procedures that involve needles and sharps. Usually, training in these techniques takes place far in advance of actual clinical experience. Students should be closely supervised to ensure that they are performing appropriate procedures for which they have been trained, and that they are doing so correctly. It is natural to want to impress the supervisor or preceptor, which can lead students to perform procedures for which they are not yet qualified. To remain safe, students must be aware of these behaviors and understand their roles in caring for patients.

PA programs are required to provide students with a process for reporting and seeking medical care in the unfortunate event of a needlestick injury. Current recommendations call for the student to be evaluated and given appropriate postexposure prophylaxis within hours after an exposure.[6] PA programs provide this information; however, it is imperative that you keep it readily available so that you can make appropriate contacts when the need arises. Exposures that occur in a training hospital are usually handled quickly, but injuries in a rural site without access to appropriate prophylactic medications can be a challenge. Any student who will be in a rural clinical location needs to be familiar with the program's needlestick reporting process.

A troubling concern identified in the medical literature is the failure of health care workers and students to report needlestick and sharps injuries.[7,8] Reasons for not reporting include fear of losing insurance or employment, concerns about effectiveness of postexposure prophylaxis, and a tendency to deny personal risk.[7,9] Failure to report even what is considered an inconsequential exposure can have a significant impact on future ability to practice. Although it may seem inconvenient, reporting provides several benefits to both the student and the health care entity. Reporting an incident may be useful for future insurance and disability claims. It typically results in the student being evaluated medically and helps the institution assess internal systems that may prevent similar exposures for other health care workers.

CASE STUDY 10-1

During a busy Saturday morning in the emergency department (ED) of a rural community hospital, a senior PA student was busy suturing a laceration on the scalp of a male patient. The patient was being held by local law enforcement for drug dealing. He had been in a fight at the jail that resulted in his laceration. The patient was somewhat uncooperative, and while the PA student was placing a suture, the patient moved suddenly, causing the bloody needle to deeply puncture the student's gloved right middle finger. The student called for a nurse to assist him and to monitor the patient while he spoke with the family physician covering the ED. He asked the physician what he should do and was told to thoroughly clean the puncture site and then contact his program for advice. The student remembered he had been given a needlestick emergency contact card with a toll-free telephone number to call in case of an injury. After cleaning the site, he called the appropriate number and was given information about testing, follow-up, and postexposure prophylaxis, as well as points to discuss with the patient about having his blood tested for infectious diseases. The patient refused to consent to testing for HIV and hepatitis B and C. The student underwent baseline testing and decided to begin HIV prophylaxis medication. He was counseled on the risk for developing HIV, the need for safe sexual practices, and length of time for follow-up. He completed the postexposure prophylaxis without incident, and his HIV test remained negative 1 year later.

TUBERCULOSIS SCREENING

As part of any type of formal health care training, students are required to be screened for tuberculosis annually.[10] For PA students, this is required as part of a PA program's accreditation. Tuberculosis is still a significant disease process for which health care workers are at increased risk. According to the Centers for Disease Control and Prevention (CDC), in 2003 health care workers accounted for 3.1% of reported TB cases nationwide.[11] The rate of health care student conversion while in training is unknown, but because of increased risk for exposure, all health care workers and students are screened annually.

The CDC recommends that groups considered to be at high risk undergo targeted tuberculin testing using the purified protein derivative (PPD) tuberculin skin test for latent tuberculosis infection. Three cut points have been recommended for defining a positive tuberculin reaction: ≥5 mm, ≥10 mm, and ≥15 mm of induration. For individuals at the highest

TABLE 10-2 **Criteria for Tuberculin Positivity, by Risk Group**

Reaction ≥5 mm of Induration	Reaction ≥10 mm of Induration	Reaction ≥15 mm of Induration
Human immunodeficiency virus–positive persons	Recent immigrants (i.e., within the past 5 yr) from high-prevalence countries	Persons with no risk factors for tuberculosis
Recent contacts of tuberculosis case patients	Injection drug users	
Fibrotic changes on chest radiograph consistent with prior tuberculosis	Residents and employees† of the following high-risk congregate settings: prisons and jails, nursing homes, and other long-term facilities for the elderly, hospitals and other health care facilities, residential facilities for patients with acquired immunodeficiency syndrome, and homeless shelters	
Patients with organ transplants and other immunosuppressed patients (receiving the equivalent of 15 mg/day of prednisone for 1 mo or more)*	Mycobacteriology laboratory personnel	
	Persons with the following clinical conditions that place them at high risk: silicosis, diabetes mellitus, chronic renal failure, some hematologic disorders (e.g., leukemias and lymphomas), other specific malignancies (e.g., carcinoma of the head or neck and lung), weight loss of ≥ 10% of ideal body weight, gastrectomy, and jejunoileal bypass	
	Children younger than 4 yr of age or infants, children and adolescents exposed to adults at high risk	

Modified from Screening for tuberculosis and tuberculosis infection in high-risk populations: recommendations of the Advisory Council for the Elimination of Tuberculosis. MMWR Recomm Rep 1995;44(No.RR-11):19.

*Risk of tuberculosis in patients treated with corticosteroids increases with higher dose and longer duration.

†For persons who are otherwise at low risk and are tested at the start of employment, a reaction of ≥15 mm induration is considered positive.

risk for developing active TB, ≥5 mm of induration is considered a positive result. For groups with the lowest risk for contracting TB, a skin reaction is considered positive if it is ≥15 mm of induration (Table 10-2).[12] You will undoubtedly learn more about tuberculosis during your training; however, it is important to have an understanding of the rationale for your annual tuberculin skin testing.

LATEX ALLERGY

Latex is ubiquitous in the health care system. It has been used in all facets of medicine for several decades. The use of latex soared during the 1980s and 1990s as latex gloves were recommended as protection against bloodborne pathogens, including HIV.[13] As use of latex products increased, so did the incidence of allergic reactions associated with latex proteins. Commonly, latex gloves are coated with cornstarch powder as a dry lubricant. The latex protein particles easily stick to the powder and aerosolize when the gloves are removed, resulting in latex allergy reactions, which can be local (skin), respiratory, or both.

The actual prevalence of latex allergy is difficult to pinpoint. Data on occupational health care subgroups range from 0.5% to 24%. This wide range can be attributed to several issues related to the quality of the research studies and inconsistencies in the definition of "latex allergy."[14]

Three types of clinical syndromes are associated with latex exposures. The majority of reactions involve an irritant dermatitis caused by the rubbing

CASE STUDY 10-2

During routine annual testing for tuberculosis, a senior PA student was noted to have 17 mm of induration on her tuberculin skin test. Records showed that she had tested negative for tuberculosis at entry into the PA program and again after completing her first year in the program. She had spent the past 12 months in clinical rotations locally, regionally, and internationally. She denied any known exposure to anyone with active TB, although she had spent 4 weeks in Guatemala within the previous 3 months. She denied any suspicious symptoms, weight loss, night sweats, or cough. Her chest radiograph was interpreted as normal. She was counseled by student health personnel on the need to begin isoniazid and pyridoxine. She agreed to take the state-provided medications for the recommended 9 months. She tolerated the medications well without adverse effects and completed the regimen without incident.

of gloves on the skin. This type is not immune mediated and is not associated with allergic symptoms.

A second form is the result of a delayed (type IV) hypersensitivity reaction, causing a contact dermatitis within 24 to 48 hours after exposure. Individuals with a history of atopic disease are at greater risk for this type of reaction. The most serious and least common presentation is the immediate (type I) hypersensitivity reaction. This is mediated by immunoglobulin E response specific to latex proteins. As the process escalates, histamine and other systemic mediators are released, possibly resulting in anaphylaxis.

Since awareness of latex allergies has grown, so too has the replacement of latex examination gloves with powder-free, low-protein gloves and latex-free gloves. If you have a latex sensitivity or allergy, you should carry a medical alert bracelet that can identify your allergy for health care providers. Avoid latex gloves and other products, and notify your supervisor and/or preceptor of your condition. Finally, if your reaction is severe, obtain a prescription for an epinephrine self-injection pen for use in an emergency.

STUDENT MISTREATMENT

Health care students are intelligent, compassionate, and excited and eager to learn. However, as Silver[15] wrote in 1982, medical students become "cynical, dejected, frightened, depressed, or frustrated" over time. He noted these changes were similar to those found in abused children, which may result from enduring unnecessary and harmful abuse. The term "medical student abuse" is now commonly referred to as "student mistreatment."

Knowledge of medical student mistreatment dates back to the 1960s. Several studies have explored the phenomenon and provided a better understanding of what constitutes mistreatment.[16-19] Students who reported mistreatment had more anxiety, depression, difficulty with learning, thoughts of dropping out, and drinking problems.[17-19] These data suggest that mistreatment can have significant negative effects on students.

Since 1992, the Association of American Medical Colleges (AAMC) has included the topic of medical student mistreatment on its annual questionnaire to graduating medical students. The questionnaire covers mistreatment related to the following areas: general, sexual, racial/ethnic, and sexual orientation. In 1998, the AAMC reported 51% of students believed they were publicly humiliated or belittled during their training.[20] In the 2011 AAMC Medical School Graduation Questionnaire, 81% of graduates believed they were humiliated or belittled at some point during their education, which is at its lowest level of report since 2007 (89.4%).[20] A recent study by Frank[18] found that 84% of medical students reported having been belittled or harassed, although only 13% reported the incident as severe.

Only recently have data been gathered about the mistreatment of PA students. Asprey[21] surveyed a group of senior PA students regarding mistreatment in six categories (Box 10-1). Although conclusions were limited by low response rates, a total of 79% of students admitted to having experienced at least one form of mistreatment during their training. Interestingly, Asprey's findings were consistent with those in medical students, in that the PA students reported similar rates of general mistreatment. However, PA students reported sexual mistreatment (50.4%) as the most common form of abuse, closely followed by verbal mistreatment (47.5%). In addition, those responsible for the mistreatment were physicians (33%), followed by PA program faculty (17.7%).[21]

An important distinction concerns the perception of mistreatment. Do students and preceptors agree on what constitutes mistreatment? In a study that used five video vignettes depicting potentially abusive situations, the authors surveyed physicians, resident physicians, nurses, and students to determine their perceptions.[22] They found good agreement regarding abuse in the belittlement, ethnic insensitivity, and sexual harassment scenarios. This study suggests that authority figures and students often agree on what constitutes mistreatment in a clinical situation.

A large proportion of mistreatment appears to go unreported. Studies have identified several reasons for students not reporting: They did not recognize the experience as mistreatment at the time that it happened, did not think reporting would make a difference, feared the reporting could adversely affect their evaluation, and believed that reporting would be more trouble than it was worth.[16,19,23]

Reporting an episode of mistreatment is an individual decision. Students often think that their position does not allow them to report behavior by a superior because of possible repercussions. However, in the current health care climate, most organizations have well-defined procedures for handling disruptive providers. These policies are primarily directed at physicians but include anyone within the organization who receives a formal complaint.

SEXUAL HARASSMENT

One form of student mistreatment that deserves special attention is sexual harassment. Federal law protects students from sexual harassment by instructors, staff,

BOX 10-1 PHYSICIAN ASSISTANT SURVEY QUESTIONS BY CATEGORY OF MISTREATMENT

VERBAL MISTREATMENT

Have you been belittled, humiliated, or denigrated verbally?
Have you been verbally threatened with harm?

PHYSICAL MISTREATMENT

Have you been physically abused (hit, pushed, slapped, kicked, etc.)?

SEXUAL MISTREATMENT

Have you been subjected to unwanted or inappropriate verbal comments, such as slurs, lewd comments, or sexual jokes?
Have you been subjected to unwanted sexual advances (repeated requests for sexual interactions or activities)?
Have you been physically touched in an unwanted sexually oriented manner (groped, fondled, kissed, etc.)?
Have you been sexually assaulted (raped, forced to perform sexual acts, etc.)?
Have you been asked for sexual favors in return for grades, positive evaluations, recommendations, etc.?
Have you been subjected to unwanted or inappropriate verbal comments, such as slurs, lewd comments, sexual jokes, etc. on the basis of your sexual orientation?
Have you been denied educational or training opportunities solely on the basis of your sexual orientation?
Have you been assigned lower evaluations or grades solely on the basis of your sexual orientation?

GENDER-BASED MISTREATMENT

Have you been denied educational or training opportunities on the basis of your gender?
Have you been assigned lower grades or negative evaluations solely on the basis of your gender?

RACE-ORIENTED MISTREATMENT

Have you been subjected to unwanted or inappropriate verbal comments on the basis of your race or ethnicity?
Have you been denied educational or training opportunities on the basis of your race or ethnicity?
Have you been assigned lower grades or negative evaluations solely on the basis of your race or ethnicity?

RELIGIOUS-BASED MISTREATMENT

Have you been subjected to unwanted or inappropriate verbal comments on the basis of espoused religious beliefs?
Have you been denied educational or training opportunities solely on the basis of your espoused religious beliefs?
Have you been assigned lower grades or evaluations solely on the basis of your espoused religious beliefs?

From Asprey DP. Physician assistant students' perceptions of mistreatment during training. J Phys Assist Ed. 2006;17:5. Reprinted by permission of the Physician Assistant Education Association.

and other employees of an educational institution. As with any other form of student mistreatment, consequences of sexual harassment can be far-reaching.

Inappropriate sex-based behaviors in all areas of higher education have been well documented. The types of sexual harassment behaviors reported include offensive body language, flirtation, unwelcome comments on students' dress, outright sexual invitations, propositions, sexual contact, sexual bribery, and sexual assaults.[23] In addition, exclusion from educational opportunities based solely on gender and discriminatory grading has been reported.[24,25]

The U.S. Department of Education's Office of Civil Rights 2001 guidelines define two types of sexual harassment: quid pro quo and hostile environment.[26] Quid pro quo sexual harassment occurs when an employee of the school explicitly or implicitly applies conditions to a student's participation in an educational program or activity on the basis of the student's submission to unwelcome sexual advances, requests for sexual favors, or verbal, nonverbal, or physical contact of a sexual nature.[26] Hostile environment can be further defined to include persistent, severe, or pervasive unwelcome sexual conduct that limits a student's ability to participate in or benefit from an educational program or activity or that creates a hostile or abusive educational environment.[26] The statistics describing the extent of sexual harassment in medical training are based primarily on experience from medical schools and resident training programs. In 2011, the AAMC's Medical School Graduation Questionnaire found, specific to sexual mistreatment,

Harassment

On the basis of race, color, gender, age, national origin, disability, gender orientation, genetic information, veteran status and religion is prohibited.

Hostile work environment is created by severe and pervasive conduct, which may include the following:

- Jokes with sexual, racial, or inappropriate content;
- Epithets, slurs, profanity, and name calling;
- Demeaning or sexually suggestive pictures (whether real or virtual), objects, writings, e-mails, or faxes;
- Unwelcome love letters, gifts, or requests for dates;
- Unwelcome behavior that any "reasonable person" would find offensive.

Misuse of power to gain sexual favors is a form of sexual harassment.

How to address harassing behavior ...

- Notifying your supervisor
- Contact the Affirmative Action Office in Human Resources—Employee Relations
- Faculty may report complaints directly to the Chair of the Faculty Senate Grievance Committee

Factors to note ...

- A single incident can be enough to be harassment
- Harassers may include supervisors, co-workers, faculty, students and non-employees
- We expect students and employees to be free from harassment whenever or wherever individuals are engaged in activities on behalf of the university, including off-site events
- We will take immediate action to eliminate harassment
- We will not permit retaliation against any individual who in good faith complains of harassment

If you have questions about harassment, you may contact:

FIGURE 10-1 Sexual harassment bookmark. (Courtesy Carmen Sirizzotti, MBA, at UNMC.)

12.8% reported having been denied opportunities for training or rewards because of their gender on one or more occasions; 8.0% had been subjected to unwanted sexual advances by school personnel on one or more occasion; 19.8% had been subjected to offensive sexist remarks or names on one or more occasion; and 16.6% believed they had received lower evaluations or grades solely on the basis of their gender rather than performance.[20] The good news is that although the numbers are impressive in total, the overall percentages have declined over the past 4 years. Other researchers have found that a larger number of students are sexually harassed during their medical education, ranging from 11% to 21% of male students and 35% to 64% of female students.[27,28] In addition, the effects of sexual harassment may be profound for the individual student, affecting performance; inducing feelings of anger, fear, and guilt; and leading to personal and professional dissatisfaction.[28]

Few data exist specific to PA students and sexual harassment experiences. Asprey's survey of 22 PA programs regarding mistreatment among soon-to-be graduates found that 50% of senior PA students experienced some type of sexual mistreatment during their training.[19]

The surprising conclusion to be drawn from these data is that sexual harassment continues to be a problem in professional graduate education. PA students, male and female, should be aware of their programs' policies on mistreatment and sexual harassment. Legal protections are in place that provide for a nonhostile educational environment in which students can feel safe. In addition, students should be aware of what constitutes sexual harassment (Figure 10-1).

If you have concerns about an experience, speak with a PA program faculty member, the school's ombudsman, or the school's human resource department. PA program faculties have a responsibility to develop professional attitudes and behaviors in their students as much as expanding their medical knowledge. Failure to enforce program policy may perpetuate sexism within our profession and result in producing PAs who treat their patients and colleagues with disrespect.

KEY POINTS

- Entering the clinical phase of training is an exciting time; however, the practice of medicine and surgery is an inherently dangerous activity.
- PA students must be properly immunized, educated about safety concerns, and vigilant about their own safety when starting clinical rotations.
- PA students must be aware of their own limitations and lack of experience, especially when volunteering to learn new skills.
- Locate and review your program's needlestick and blood and body fluid exposure policy. Make sure you have a copy of the emergency contact information with you at all times.
- Students should report any type of injury sustained during clinical training immediately and complete appropriate paperwork in a timely fashion.
- Students are encouraged to report any type of mistreatment that may occur during their training to program faculty or other appropriate resources in their institutions.

References

1. Siegel JD, Rhinehart E, Jackson M, Chiarello L. The Healthcare Infection Control Practices Advisory Committee, 2007. Guideline for Isolation Precautions: Preventing Transmission of Infectious Agents in Healthcare Settings. *http://www.cdc.gov/hicpac/2007IP/2007isolationPrecautions.html;* Accessed December 28, 2011.
2. Panlilio AL, Orelien JG, Srivastava PU, et al., the NaSH Surveillance Group, and the EPINet Data Sharing Network. Estimate of the annual number of percutaneous injuries among hospital-based healthcare workers in the United States, 1997-1998. Infect Control Hosp Epidemiol 2004;25(7):556.
3. Collins DH, Kennedy DA. Microbiological hazards of occupational needlestick and other 'sharps' injuries. J Appl Bacteriol 1987;62:385.
4. Cervini P, Bell C. Brief report: Needlestick injury and inadequate postexposure practice in medical students. J Gen Intern Med 2005;20:419.
5. LaBarbera D. Accidental exposures of physician assistant students. J Phys Assist Educ 2006;17:40.
6. Panlilio AL, Cardo DM, Grohskopf LA, et al. U.S. Public Health Service. Updated U.S. Public Health Service guidelines for the management of occupational exposures to HIV and recommendations for postexposure prophylaxis. MMWR Recomm Rep 2005;54(No. RR-9):1.
7. Sharma GK, Gilson MM, Nathan H, Makary MA. Needlestick injuries among medical students: incidence and implications. Acad Med 2009;84(12):1815.
8. Makary MA, At-Attar A, Holzmueller CG, et al. Needlestick injuries among surgeons in-training. N Engl J Med 2007;356(26):2693.
9. Osborn EHS, Papakakis MA, Gerberding JL. Occupational exposures to body fluids among medical students, a seven-year longitudinal study. Ann Intern Med 1999;130:45.
10. Screening for tuberculosis and tuberculosis infection in high-risk populations: recommendations of the Advisory Council for the Elimination of Tuberculosis. MMWR Recomm Rep 1995;44(No.RR-11):19.
11. CDC. Reported tuberculosis in the United States, 2003. Atlanta, GA: US Department of Health and Human Services, CDC; 2004.
12. CDC. Targeted tuberculin testing and treatment of latent tuberculosis infection. Am J Resp Crit Care Med 2000;161: S221.
13. Behrman AJ, Howarth M. Latex allergy. eMedicine. *http://emedicine.com/emerg/topic814.htm;* Accessed December 28, 2011.
14. Statham BN. Epidemiology of latex allergy. In: Chowdhury MMU, Marbach HI (eds). Latex Intolerance: Basic Science, Epidemiology, and Clinical Management. New York: CRC Press; 2005.
15. Silver HK. Medical students and medical school. JAMA 1982;247:309.
16. Komaromy M, Bindman AB, Harber RJ, Sande MA. Sexual harassment in medical training. N Engl J Med 1993;328:322.
17. Silver HK, Glicken AD. Medical student abuse. Incidence, severity, and significance. JAMA 1990;263:527.
18. Frank E, Garrera JS, Stratton T, et al. Experiences of belittlement and harassment and their correlates among medical students in the United States: longitudinal survey. BMJ 2006;333:682.
19. Nagata-Kobayashi S, Sekimoto M, Koyama H, et al. Medical student abuse during clinical clerkships in Japan. J Gen Intern Med 2006;21:212.
20. Association of American Medical Colleges. 2011 Medical School Graduation Questionnaire. *https://www.aamc.org/download/256776/data/gq-2011-rm.pdf;* Accessed on December 29, 2011.
21. Asprey DP. Physician assistant students' perceptions of mistreatment during training. J Phys Assist Ed 2006;17:5.

22. Ogden PE, Wu EH, Elnicki MD, et al. Do attending physicians, nurses, residents, and medical students agree on what constitutes medical student abuse? Acad Med 2005;80(Suppl):S80.
23. Balwin Jr DC, Daugherty SR, Rowley BD. Residents' and medical students' reports of sexual harassment and discrimination. Acad Med 1996;71(Suppl. 10):S25.
24. Cook DJ, Liutkus JF, Risdon CL, et al. Residents' experiences of abuse, discrimination and sexual harassment during residency training. CMAJ 1996;154:1657.
25. Rees CE, Monrouxe LV. A morning since eight of just pure grill: a multischool qualitative study of student abuse. Acad Med 2011;86(11):1374.
26. Revised Sexual Harassment Guidance. Harassment of Students by School Employees, Other Students, or Third Parties, Title IX. 2001. *http://www2.ed.gov/about/offices/list/ocr/docs/shguide.html;* Accessed November 28, 2011.
27. Lubitz RM, Nguyen DD. Medical student abuse during third-year clerkships. JAMA 1996;275:414.
28. Richman JA, Flaherty JA, Rospenda KM. Perceived workplace harassment experiences and problem drinking among physicians: broadening the stress/alienation paradigm. Addiction 1996;91:391.

CHAPTER 11

Clinical Procedures

Edward M. Sullivan

CHAPTER CONTENTS

The ability to perform clinical procedures is a necessary skill for practicing physician assistants (PAs) and PA students alike. Procedures often provide valuable information that may aid in the diagnosis and treatment of a patient's disease. No matter how routine and uncomplicated a clinical procedure may seem to a health care provider, it must always be regarded as a unique and personal experience for the patient.

Preparing the patient for the procedure both mentally and physically remains a challenge to all health care providers. Preparation skills must be developed and applied often. The PA must have a complete understanding of the procedure to be performed, including the indications and contraindications; a command of the anatomy involved; an attention to detail; and an awareness of the goal that is to be accomplished by each procedure.

A majority of all clinical procedures are painful in some way to the patient. Many times, the patient's ability to cope with a procedure lies in the sure hands of the clinician. A positive, gentle manner combined with thoroughness in the explanation will instill confidence in the patient, as well as in the other health care providers assisting with the procedure. A patient who has a complete understanding of what is to be accomplished is much more likely to cooperate with specific requests and is better prepared to handle any difficulties that may be encountered. Finally, no matter how many times a PA or PA student may have performed a clinical procedure, he or she must keep in mind that it may be the first time for the patient, and that the better prepared the patient is, the more satisfying the outcome will be.

CASE STUDY 11-1

Mr. W., a 29-year-old man, was in a pedestrian crossing when he was struck by a car. He was transported to the emergency department (ED), where the PA evaluated his injuries. During the primary survey, his vital signs were as follows: blood pressure (BP) 80/50 mm Hg, pulse 110 per minute, and respirations 24 per minute. He was alert and oriented to name, place, and date; the airway was patent; and there was no evidence of respiratory distress. A venipuncture was performed to obtain a complete blood count and electrolyte panel. A peripheral intravenous (IV) line was started to provide fluid resuscitation to correct the hypotension. A Foley catheter was inserted to monitor his urinary output.

During the secondary survey, the lungs were clear bilaterally, heart sounds were normal, and the abdomen was soft and nontender. Bowel sounds were hypoactive but present in all quadrants. His speech was fluent, and he was able to follow commands. There were several abrasions of the left leg and arm, as well as a 4-cm laceration on the left lower leg and a large hematoma on the upper left thigh. Subsequent radiographs of the left leg revealed a compound fracture of the left femur. Cervical spine, chest, and pelvis films were unremarkable.

The abrasions were cleaned and covered with sterile dressings. The lower leg wound was irrigated and closed primarily. The patient also received an injection of tetanus toxoid because his last immunization was more than 7 years ago. Throughout his evaluation and treatment in the ED, the PA explained each intervention to the patient. Following stabilization in the ED, Mr. W. was admitted to the hospital for definitive care of his femur fracture.

WOUNDS AND THEIR TREATMENT

Any consideration of an invasive clinical procedure must begin with an understanding of wounds and their healing process. This chapter provides only a brief overview of wounds because a detailed explanation of the pathophysiology is beyond the scope of this discussion. The resource list at the end of the chapter provides sources for more comprehensive study and an in-depth discussion of specific types of wounds.

Definitions

A *wound* can be defined as any break in the normal anatomic relationship of tissues. Wounds can be classified as *internal* (those inside the skin) and *external* (those involving the skin). This chapter concentrates on external wounds because of their relationship to the performance of clinical procedures.

Wounds caused by any clinical or surgical procedure are classified, according to degree of contamination and risk for infection, as clean, clean-contaminated, contaminated, or dirty, as follows:

- *Clean:* A clean wound is typically a surgical incision made under sterile conditions. Clean wounds are generally considered to be relatively new wounds, meaning that they are less than 12 hours old. For the most part, wounds caused by clinical procedures are performed under sterile conditions and therefore can be considered clean.
- *Clean-contaminated:* A wound that begins as a clean wound but has experienced a potential source of contamination is clean-contaminated. One example is the opening of the colon during a bowel anastomosis. In this case, special precautions should be initiated to prevent spillage.
- *Contaminated:* A contaminated wound may have begun as a clean wound or may have been made under nonsterile conditions and has a greater incidence of infection. Some examples are a knife or glass laceration, the bowel opened during an operation with spillage of the contents into the surrounding sterile tissue, and the opening of an abscess, whether accidentally or by design, without containment of the enclosed infected material.
- *Dirty:* A dirty wound presents with an established infection—for example, a soft tissue abscess.

Wound Healing

Wounds heal by forming scars. The process of forming scars is traditionally divided into three main phases:

1. Inflammatory or exudative phase.
2. Fibroplastic or proliferative phase.
3. Maturation phase.

Inflammatory or Exudative Phase

Wound healing begins immediately after an injury has occurred to otherwise normal tissue. The inflammatory phase, which usually lasts 2 to 4 days, serves to cleanse the wound of dead tissue and foreign objects by a sequence of physiologic and biochemical events, beginning with an immediate vasoconstriction to minimize blood loss. This vasoconstriction is brief and is followed by a histamine-induced vasodilatation and a migrating of leukocytes into the wound. The polymorphonuclear neutrophils (PMNs) and mononuclear leukocytes are the source for many of these mediators of the inflammatory response. The primary role of the PMNs and monocytes is to débride the wound of any foreign material. Serum enters the wound from gaps between endothelial cells, aiding the activation of platelets, kinin, complement, and prostaglandin components of the clotting cascade.

Hemostatic Factors

The hemostatic factors of wound healing are all activated immediately following the injury. One of the first is the *activation of platelets*, which adhere to one another and to the edges of the wound, forming a plug that attempts to cover the wound. This plug or clot soon retracts and stops the loss of blood. The kinins are a group of polypeptides that influence smooth muscle contraction, which may induce hypotension. Additionally, they increase the permeability of small blood capillaries, serving to increase the amount of blood flow, which in turn increases the amounts of other hemostatic factors previously mentioned.

Complements are other hemostatic factors whose main job is to produce bacteriolysis and hemolysis by accumulating fluid within the cells, causing them to eventually rupture. *Prostaglandin* acts to increase vasomotor tone, capillary permeability, smooth muscle tone, and the aggregation of platelets. *Fibronectin* aids in the migration of neutrophils, monocytes, fibroblasts, and endothelial cells into the wound and also promotes the ability of these cells to adhere to one another, creating a framework of fibrin fibers. Fibronectin is found in abundance within the first 48 hours, gradually decreasing as protein synthesis begins to produce the collagen fibers that will eventually be the scar. The wound appears red and swollen and is painful and warm to the touch during the inflammatory phase, which typically lasts about 4 days. Accordingly, it is difficult to distinguish from an early wound infection at this time.

Fibroplastic or Proliferative Phase

The second phase of wound healing can begin only when the wound is covered by epithelium. This phase begins on or about the fourth day after an injury and continues alongside the maturation phase. An injured patient must have a normal amount of circulating calcium (Ca), platelets, and tissue factor before the second phase can begin. If these three substances are present as blood is exposed to air, prothrombin will be converted to thrombin. Thrombin acts as a catalyst in the conversion of fibrinogen to fibrin fibers, which stabilize the clot.

Fibroblasts are normally located in the perivascular tissue, and once they get into the wound, they produce several substances essential to wound repair, ending with the formation of collagen fibers. *Collagen* is the principal structural protein found in tendons, ligaments, and fasciae. Arranged in bundles, it strengthens and supports these tissues. Collagen levels rise continuously for approximately 3 weeks and have a negative feedback mechanism related to the number of fibroblasts found in the wound. As collagen increases, the number of fibroblasts decreases, eventually causing a decrease in the production of collagen. The rapid gain in tensile strength during this phase is directly related to the remodeling of collagen from a randomly arranged fiber mesh to a more organized formation of fibers that respond to the local stress found at the wound site.

At this stage, although it is less swollen, inflamed, and painful, the wound may look its worst. The scar may appear beefy red and may feel hard and raised. This is normal and should be expected. If the wound remains painful and inflamed at this stage of the healing process, however, some foreign material may have been retained, and reexploration may be warranted.

Maturation Phase

During this third phase of wound healing, metabolic activity remains high, but there is no increase in collagen production. This phase is sometimes referred to as the "remodeling phase" because of the rearrangement of the collagen fibers from their initial haphazard appearance after production to one of more organization. This pattern is determined by the anatomic location of the wound and the amount of stress placed on the skin and the scar at that location.

This phase usually begins at 3 weeks and can be active for 9 to 12 months, depending on the health status of the person. The appearance of the scar becomes less conspicuous as it begins to flatten out and fade and gradually begins to resemble normal skin tissue. The scar becomes more supple and more permanent as the cross-links of collagen are reorganized.

Factors That Affect Wound Healing

The health of an individual can greatly affect the time involved in the healing of a wound. Proper wound closure is paramount to the successful healing of an injury, but many other factors influence this process. The surgical technique, the type of injury, the degree of contamination, and the health status and biochemical makeup of the patient all play important roles in the final outcome of an injury. Suturing and other techniques of wound closure are discussed later in the chapter, but first, some consideration of the biochemical factors and the health status of an individual with a wound is warranted. Some of the factors that directly relate to the healing process are as follows:

- *Oxygen:* Fibroblasts are closely related to the partial pressure of oxygen (Po_2) in the circulating blood. A Po_2 of less than 30 mm Hg severely retards the healing process by lowering the production of collagen in the cytoplasm of the fibroblast. Disease processes such as small vessel atherosclerosis, chronic infection, and diabetes mellitus can be greatly affected by the oxygen delivery system.

- *Hematocrit:* There must be an adequate supply of hemoglobin in the blood to carry oxygen to the tissues.
- *Steroids (antiinflammatory):* Steroids slow the inflammatory phase of the healing process by inhibiting macrophages and fibrogenesis. Anabolic steroids and vitamin A, on the other hand, can reverse the effects of antiinflammatory drugs by restoring the monocytic inflammation process of the wound.
- *Vitamin C:* Vitamin C is important to the maturation process of fibroblasts.
- *Vitamin E:* In large doses, vitamin E can decrease the tensile strength of a wound by lowering the accumulation of collagen.
- *Zinc:* Epithelial and fibroplastic proliferation is slowed in patients exhibiting a low serum zinc level.
- *Antiinflammatory agents:* Aspirin and ibuprofen decrease collagen synthesis in a dose-related fashion.
- *Age:* Both tensile strength and wound closure rates decrease as a person ages.
- *Mechanical stress:* Wounds involving the skin over joints, where the stresses are greatly increased by normal usage, take longer to heal. The delay is due to the constant stretching and tearing of the collagen mesh, which results in reinitiation of the entire wound-healing process.
- *Nutrition:* Poor nutrition results in absence of the essential building blocks of protein for collagen production, prolonging the inflammatory phase and inhibiting fibroplasia. Glucose supplies energy for leukocytes to function. Fats are necessary for synthesis of new cells.
- *Hydration:* A well-hydrated wound, not a wet wound, epithelializes faster than a dry wound. Keeping a wound covered by a dressing enhances the humidity of the wound and speeds the healing process.
- *Environmental temperature:* Wound-healing time is shortened by environmental temperatures greater than 30°C. Wound-healing time can increase by as much as 20% in temperatures of 12°C or less, owing to vasoconstriction and lowering of the capillary blood supply.
- *Denervation:* Denervated skin is less susceptible to local temperatures and more prone to ulceration. Paraplegics develop massive, rapidly destructive ulcers that can be five times worse than those in the patient with an intact nervous system.
- *Infection:* The ability of local tissue defenses to cleanse the wound is greatly diminished by a larger number of pathogenic organisms. Infection prolongs the inflammatory phase of the healing process.
- *Idiopathic manipulation:* Overhandling and rough handling of tissue by health care providers along with tight sutures can result in tissue ischemia and poor healing.
- *Chemotherapy:* Anti-cancer drugs decrease the fibroblast proliferation.
- *Radiation therapy:* Acute radiation injury is manifested by stasis and occlusion of small vessels, resulting in the formation of ulcers at the point of ischemia.
- *Diabetes mellitus:* Defective leukocyte function and microvascular occlusion may occur secondary to hyperglycemia in diabetes mellitus. High glucose levels interfere with the ability of cells to transport ascorbic acid, resulting in a decrease in the production of collagen.

Tensile Strength

All the factors just described can affect the tensile strength of a wound during the healing process. *Tensile strength* is defined as the greatest force a substance can bear without tearing apart. The tensile strength of a wound is directly related to time and is low for approximately the first 3 weeks following an injury and a primary closure. Extreme care must be taken to protect the newly formed scar from reinjury at this time. The strength of the wound increases rapidly during the early stages of the maturation phase as the collagen fibers are rearranged and simplified according to the mechanical stresses applied to the scar. Although the wound needs 9 to 12 additional months of maturing before the final cosmetic result should be evaluated, the scar no longer gains strength after the maturation phase.

Wound Anesthesia

Injection of a local anesthetic for painless clinical and minor surgical procedures is an important tool that is readily available and easy to use. The ability to remove the pain whenever a clinical procedure is warranted not only provides a sense of relief for the patient but also gives the practitioner the option to perform the procedure at his or her own pace. This option minimizes the cost and time commitment and usually results in a more favorable outcome for both the patient and the clinician. Local anesthetic agents have redefined the "office procedure," making it a significant alternative to hospitalization. Suturing of minor lacerations and the performance of office-based clinical procedures are the hallmark of PA practice. Therefore, a good understanding of these agents and their properties is an important aspect of PA education. The practicing PA should have the knowledge and ability to perform clinical procedures wherever and whenever possible, thus enabling the physician to concentrate on the more seriously ill patients.

Anesthesia is used in a number of different ways. The most common is *local*, whereby just the area around the wound is anesthetized. A *hematoma block* is local anesthetic injected directly into a hematoma. This is primarily used in fractures where there is some internal bleeding around the fracture site. The anesthetic is allowed to filter throughout the surrounding tissue and fracture site. Once an adequate amount of anesthesia has been achieved, the fracture can be set. A *field block* is the injection of an anesthetic around a given surgical operative site. A *nerve block* targets a specific nerve at a distant site from the area of the proposed surgery. A *digital block* administered at the base of the involved finger or toe is used to numb an entire digit. This is especially useful when a laceration of a finger or toe is massive and a local infiltration would result in increased swelling and a more difficult closure. Injection of the anesthetic on both sides of the affected digit will provide effective anesthesia to the area. Lastly, a *regional block* is used to anesthetize a large specific area; for instance, an epidural block (regional) allows the parturient patient to remain awake during the delivery of her child. A digital block may be referred to as a regional block in some instances. Regional blocks may affect the motor activity of the affected area.

The properties of the ideal local anesthetic are few and simple. It must be easy to administer and have a rapid onset. Its effect must last as long as needed for a given procedure, and it must dissolve completely, with no adverse effects or toxic effects either locally or systemically. Local anesthetics work by blocking depolarization of a nerve impulse. Of the numerous anesthetic agents available on the market today, lidocaine is probably the most widely used for local anesthesia. It is manufactured in a variety of solutions, but the two most commonly used for local anesthesia are 1% and 2%. One percent lidocaine works well in blocking pain stimuli while leaving the sensations of touch and pressure relatively intact. Two percent lidocaine usually blocks all stimuli from a wound area.

Two other agents, procaine hydrochloride (Novocain) and bupivacaine hydrochloride (Marcaine), are well known and warrant some discussion. Novocain has a rapid onset, usually about 4 to 7 minutes, and lasts approximately 1 hour. Lidocaine has an equally rapid onset but may last approximately 3 hours. Marcaine takes longer to reach its anesthetic level but lasts up to 10 hours. Choosing the right anesthetic for the wound takes a significant amount of skill that is developed with years of wound evaluation and experience. The clinician must also be aware of the possible complications involved in the use of these agents. Some general rules to avoid any complications are of value, and the safety of the patient should always be of primary concern, as with the use of any medication.

Use the least amount of local anesthetic to gain the maximum amount of anesthesia for a given wound.

Almost all the local anesthetic agents give the patient a sensation of burning on injection. Before injecting, explain to the patient that this is a normal response. When injecting, go slow and wait for some of the anesthetic effects of the agent to begin working before continuing.

Always aspirate when attempting to inject an agent into the body. If there is a blood return, remove the needle and apply local pressure to ensure hemostasis.

Be aware of the signs of an allergic reaction, such as wheezing, hives, and hypotension. Always be prepared to support the airway with ventilations if necessary. Although a true allergic reaction to lidocaine is rare, extra precautions should be taken if the patient reports any history of this type of allergy.

Be aware of the maximum dosages allowable for local anesthetic medications. The toxic dose of plain lidocaine is 7 mg/kg when it is administered over an hour. The common side effects that are associated with lidocaine toxicity include blurred vision, tinnitus, and tremors. Cardiac side effects can also occur, including heart block and a decrease in cardiac output.

The last area for potential complications concerns those local anesthetics that contain a vasoconstrictive agent. Epinephrine, in concentrations of 1:100,000 or 1:200,000, is most commonly used to prolong the effects of the local anesthetic. Because of its vasoconstrictive action, it may also be used to control or decrease bleeding. It is this use for which the potential for complications arises. The local anesthetics that contain epinephrine should *never* be used in areas of the body that have terminal vasculature, such as the ears, tip of the nose, fingers, penis, and toes. The vasoconstricting action can lead to tissue death and gangrene in such areas. There is also a higher potential for wound infection because prolonged vasoconstriction delays the highly effective cleansing agents from entering the wound. Adherence to meticulous hemostasis is also important under these conditions to control the potential for increased bleeding once the effects of epinephrine wear off.

The anesthetics mentioned in this discussion are easy to use and readily available. The resource list at the end of this chapter provides in-depth studies of these agents.

Sutures

Numerous types and sizes of suture materials are available. A variety of different sutures may be used to adequately repair any given wound. The selection of suture material depends on the type of wound (clean vs. contaminated), the location of the wound (face vs. arm or leg), as well as the personal preference of the clinician. The following discussion provides some general principles to help in the selection of a dependable suture for a specific area of the body and a specific type of wound.

Suture Types

Sutures can be divided into two categories—absorbable and nonabsorbable. Absorbable sutures may be either *natural* (e.g., plain catgut, chromic catgut) or *synthetic* (e.g., polyglycolic acid [Vicryl or Dexon], polydioxanone [PDS]). Nonabsorbable sutures may be either *multifilament* (e.g., silk, cotton) or *monofilament* (e.g., nylon, polypropylene [Prolene], stainless steel wire).

When evaluating a wound for primary closure, the clinician must keep in mind the ideal qualities of a suture and must choose the most appropriate suture for each particular wound. The ideal suture:

- Maintains adequate tensile strength until its purpose is served.
- Causes minimal tissue reaction.
- Does not serve as a nidus for infection.
- Is nonallergenic and noncarcinogenic.
- Is easy to handle and tie.
- Holds knots well.
- Is inexpensive.
- Is easily sterilized.

Absorbable sutures should be used when the suture needs to function for a short time and cannot be recovered when its use is completed, as for the inner layer of a bowel anastomosis. The suture serves only to approximate the mucosa and to assist in temporary hemostasis until the body's hemostatic mechanism can secure permanent hemostasis and wound closure. The suture used most often for this type of anastomosis is catgut. Absorbable catgut sutures, which are obtained from the small intestine of cattle or sheep, generate an inflammatory response within the wound that eventually leads to their absorption. Plain catgut sutures lose approximately 50% of their initial tensile strength in just 7 days. Chromic tanning of plain catgut (chromic catgut), on the other hand, prolongs the absorptive time and the life of this suture to about 3 weeks. The synthetic absorbable sutures (Vicryl, Dexon) do not generate as extensive an inflammatory response as catgut suture material. Their chief advantage is their uniform loss of tensile strength. Research has shown that these sutures lose their strength at a steady rate for about 21 days, at which time they have no residual benefit.

Silk, throughout the years, has been the most commonly used nonabsorbable suture. It is easily obtained at a lower cost than the monofilaments and is comfortable to work with. Additionally, it holds knots securely. The major disadvantages of using silk include the following:

1. The tissue reaction it stimulates, which, although less than that produced by catgut sutures, is more than that of the synthetic monofilaments.
2. It is a multifilament suture that may be associated with an increased risk for inflammation.[1]

A multifilament suture is made of many filaments or fibers intertwined, producing numerous interstices (spaces between the fibers) that, when contaminated with bacteria, serve as a continuous nidus for infection. The interstices are small enough to deter body host defenses but large enough for bacteria to multiply. Cotton suture has the same advantages and disadvantages as silk; however, cotton is slightly weaker than silk initially but maintains its tensile strength in the tissue for a longer period.

Monofilament sutures (nylon, polypropylene [Prolene], poliglecaprone [Monocryl] stainless steel wire) share the advantages of prolonged high tensile strength, low tissue reaction, and lack of interstices. Their chief disadvantages are difficulties for the clinician in handling and tying knots. More throws (seven or eight) are required in a single knot in order to maintain its security. The monofilaments are also more expensive and are less readily available than silk and cotton.

Suture Sizes

Suture sizes are graded by a number or a zero (e.g., 2, 1, 0, 00 [2-0], 000 [3-0], 0000 [4-0], 00000 [5-0], and so forth); the more zeros, the smaller the size of the suture material. The larger sizes (2, 1) are used for heavier work (i.e., closing fascial layers or placing retention sutures in the abdomen), whereas the smallest sutures (9-0 or 10-0 and smaller) are used exclusively in microvascular surgery.

Choice of Suture

The question still remains: What type of suture should be used? Because of the numerous types and

TABLE 11-1 Suture Size and Type According to Wound Location

Location of Wound	Suture Size	Suture Type
Skin		
Face	5-0, 6-0	Nylon
Hands	4-0, 5-0	Nylon
Scalp	3-0, 4-0	Nylon
Extremities, abdomen	3-0, 4-0	Nylon
Subcutaneous tissue	3-0, 4-0	Vicryl, Dexon
Fascia	0	Prolene
	2-0	Stainless steel wire
	0	Surgilon
Peritoneum*	2-0, 3-0	Vicryl, Dexon
Bowel anastomosis		
Inner layer	3-0, 4-0	Catgut
Outer layer	3-0, 4-0	Silk, propylene

*The peritoneum is usually included with fascial suture but may be closed separately.

sizes of sutures available to the clinician, the choice of sutures for each specific purpose reverts to personal preference and wound closure experience. Because many possible different sutures can be used to close a wound, Table 11-1 is supplied as a general guide for the novice in choosing the type of suture according to the anatomic location of the wound. Multifilament sutures (silk) should not be used on the skin. The skin contains an overabundance of bacteria, and the interstices of the multifilament greatly increase the incidence of wound infection. Accordingly, monofilament sutures are a better choice for skin closures.

Retention Sutures

A special type of suture that needs to be mentioned is the *retention suture*, which is placed as noted in Figure 11-1. Observe that the retention suture encompasses all of the abdominal wall layers. After placement, the retention sutures are tied over a skin bridge—usually a plastic, red rubber catheter—to prevent the suture from cutting into the skin and causing areas of skin necrosis. This type of suture is used to decrease the tension and prevent dehiscence on a healing fascial wound. A heavy (2, 1), nonabsorbable, monofilament suture is chosen and then removed after an adequate period of healing, usually 3 to 4 weeks. Obviously, most wounds heal without retention sutures, and the judgment of the clinician dictates closure of the wound with this type of procedure. Patients at high risk for wound dehiscence are those with poor

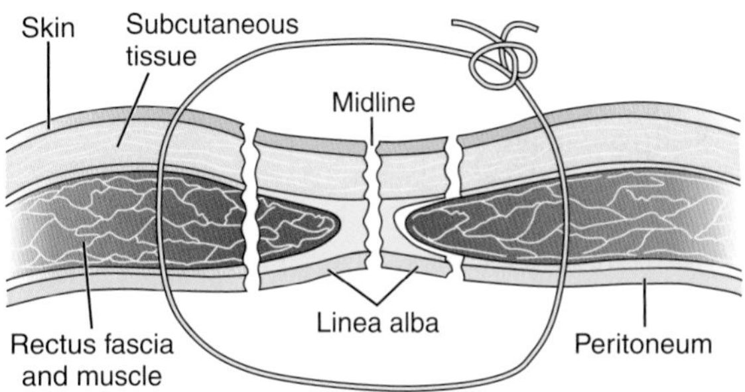

FIGURE 11-1 A retention suture must contain all layers of the abdominal wall from the peritoneum to the skin.

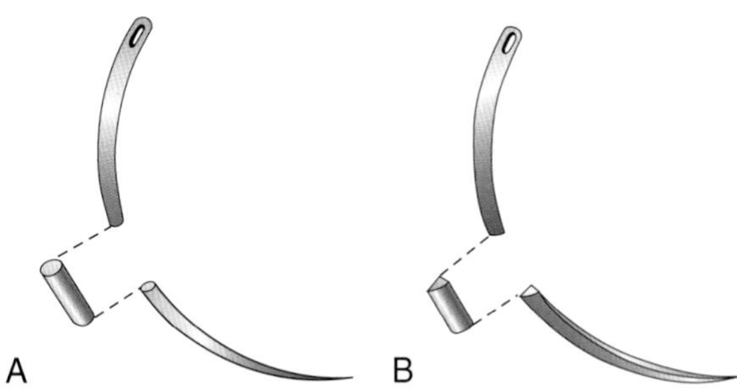

FIGURE 11-2 **A,** Tapered needle. **B,** Cutting needle.

nutrition, cancer, diabetes, obesity, massive trauma, or long-term systemic steroid ingestion, as well as those in whom contamination occurs during surgery with a high likelihood of wound infection. In these patients, retention sutures are most often considered.

Suture Needles

Two basic types of needles are used with suture material in surgery—tapered and cutting (Figure 11-2). A *tapered needle* has a sharp point and a round body. Tapered needles are less traumatic to the tissues than cutting needles. *Cutting needles* are beveled and have sharp, knifelike edges that make them well suited for skin sutures. A general rule is that cutting needles are used for skin suturing and tapered needles are used for most other tissues.

Sutures come prepackaged with a label indicating the size, type, and length of the suture and the type and size of the suture needle. Labels are usually color-coded according to the type of suture material contained.

Skin sutures should be removed when they have fulfilled their purpose. The longer sutures remain, the more inflammatory the response they generate, which ultimately results in a larger, more noticeable scar. The clinician must weigh the odds of creating an unsightly scar against the chance of a wound dehiscence if the sutures are removed prematurely.

The following is a guideline for when to remove sutures according to location:

Face 3–4 days
Scalp 5–7 days
Trunk 6–8 days
Extremities 7–14 days; longer for areas under maximal tension

Wound Closure

Wounds, however they are created, require proper and timely attention to facilitate the best possible outcome. As the clinician approaches a wound, whether it is a result of trauma or a specifically designed surgical incision, a few general principles can aid in deciding on the best approach to closure. The history plays an important role in determining the cause of the wound and, moreover, the possibility of contamination. The history also reveals valuable information about the health status of the patient, which may influence the final decision on how the wound should be treated. Surgical wounds are almost always closed primarily because of the controlled atmosphere in which they are created. Acute, accidental wounds need much more evaluation prior to treatment. Often the decision focuses on the size and shape of a wound and the degree of contamination suspected.

Historically, there are three methods of treating wounds, and timing is the most critical aspect to consider when choosing among them.

Primary Closure

The immediate suturing, stapling, or taping of a wound yields the best possible outcome with minimal scarring (Figure 11-3). Two factors to consider in deciding whether a wound can be closed primarily are the amount of tissue loss and the degree of contamination. Clean, surgical wounds fall into this category, as well as lacerations from sharp objects, such as a glass, knife, or sharp piece of metal, in which there is almost no tissue loss and contamination is minimal. Generally, an accidental wound is not closed primarily if it is more than 8 hours old. In instances in which the wounds are in areas with a good vascular supply (i.e., the face and scalp), wounds can still be closed if more than 8 hours old, although each patient needs to be evaluated on an individual basis to determine whether it is appropriate to close primarily.

Delayed Primary Closure

The wound is left open, usually because of a significant amount of bacterial contamination. Through a process that is not fully understood, the wound develops a resistance to infection over the next 4 to 5 days (Figure 11-4). This development occurs only if the wound is cleansed of all foreign material and is loosely packed with a sterile dressing. The wound is then closed by reapproximation of the two sides using as little suture as possible.

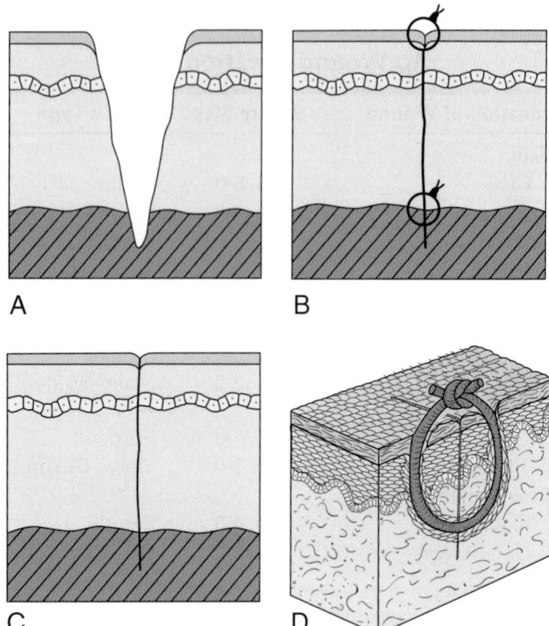

FIGURE 11-3 ■ Primary wound closure. Closing a wound primarily—within the first 8 hours—will yield the least possible scarring. **A,** Simple laceration. **B** and **D,** Correct placement of a simple interrupted stitch. **C,** The best possible result of a laceration closed primarily. (**A** and **C** from Westaby S. Wound Care. St Louis: CV Mosby, 1986; **D** from Schultz BC, McKinney P. Office Practice of Skin Surgery. Philadelphia: WB Saunders, 1985.)

Healing by Secondary Intention

A wound treated by secondary intention typically involves a large amount of tissue loss or heavy contamination by bacteria. In this case, the wound closes by the process of epithelialization and contraction rather than any type of suturing (Figure 11-5). The wound is carefully observed throughout the healing process, which may take weeks or months. To promote healing, the wounds are packed with sterile dressings that are changed daily to promote débridement of the wound. All wounds heal in this manner if they can remain free of bacteria and no fistula or sinus tract develops. The cosmetic result of this type of closure is extremely poor, however, and may require consultation with a plastic surgeon to improve the cosmetic result.

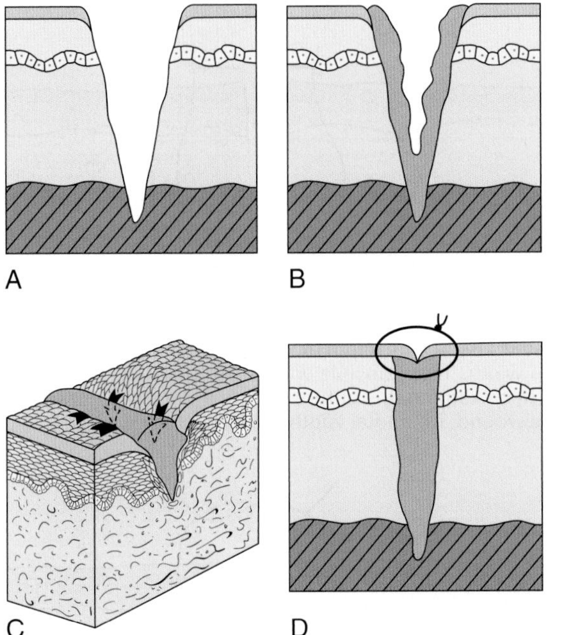

FIGURE 11-4 Delayed primary closure results in a larger and more noticeable scar. **A,** Simple laceration. **B** and **D,** The laceration is allowed to granulate. **C,** Correct placement of a simple interrupted stitch on the fourth or fifth day with the absence of any sign of infection. (**A, B,** and **D** from Westaby S. Wound Care. St Louis: CV Mosby, 1986; **C** from Schultz BC, McKinney P. Office Practice of Skin Surgery. Philadelphia: WB Saunders, 1985.)

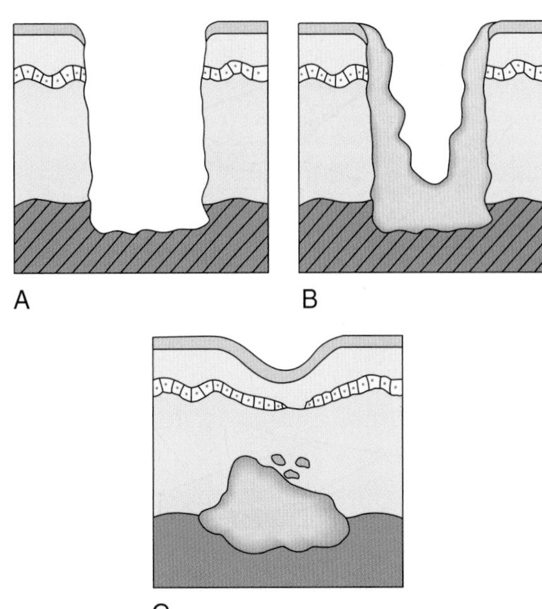

FIGURE 11-5 Allowing a wound to heal secondarily is usually done if there is a large amount of tissue loss or an overabundance of bacterial contamination. **A,** Wound with a large amount of tissue loss. **B,** The wound is allowed to granulate completely until epithelialization **(C)** covers the entire area, which may take weeks or months. (From Westaby S. Wound Care. St Louis: CV Mosby, 1986.)

Wound Suture

The principles of wound suturing are few and simple. Ideally, when the clinician is evaluating a wound for primary closure, he or she wants to produce the best possible result with the least amount of pain by using the most appropriate material with the least financial cost to the patient. A person's skin is his or her showcase to the world, and wounds and scars create physical changes that often affect self-image. The psychological aftermath of scars can be deeper than the wound itself. Every health care provider must be aware of how an injury has affected the patient. Clinicians can maximize cosmetic results by perfecting their techniques as much as possible. A referral to a plastic surgeon is appropriate for more complicated wounds, especially those involving the face and hands.

Two things make scars visible—color and shadows. The clinician has little control over the color of the patient's skin, but the smaller the scar, the less likely it is that a color change will occur. Shadows, however, are created by a centralized light source catching a subject at an angle. Even the smallest elevation or indentation of a scar makes it visible (Figure 11-6). This problem is expertly addressed by good portrait photographers in their use of multiple lighting sources to obliterate all possible shadows. The only way for the clinician to address this concern is to make the scar as flat as possible because a flat scar leaves no shadow.

First Principle

The first principle of wound repair is to close the wound in layers, making sure that each layer of skin, from the deep fascia to the epidermis, butts up against its counterpart on the other side. Perfect epithelium-to-epithelium matching and a technique called "everting of the skin edges" give the best possible result (Figure 11-7). The key is to remove tension from the outer wound edges by placing absorbable sutures inside deep lacerations and matching them layer to layer. This arrangement will support the skin and remove any underlying abnormal pull on the skin. Correctly placed layered stitches can result in a closure that may not even need skin sutures. The skin edges can be everted by making sure that (1) the depth of the stitch is greater than the width and (2) the stitch reaches the bottom of the wound.

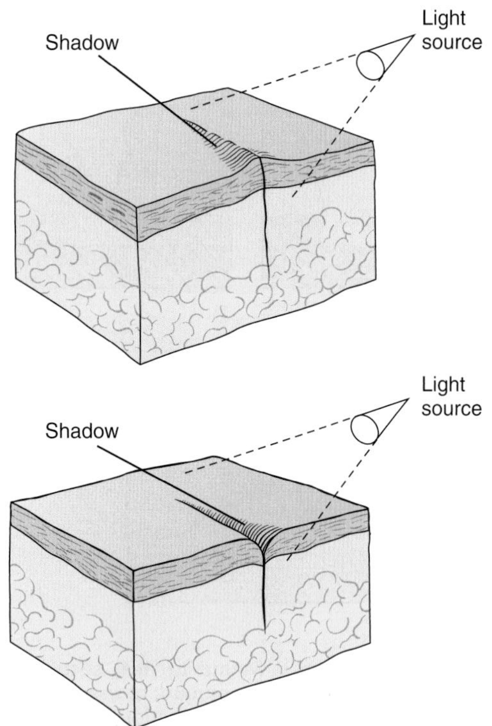

FIGURE 11-6 ■ A single centralized lighting source creates a visible shadow. The least amount of scar elevation or indentation can cause a shadow.

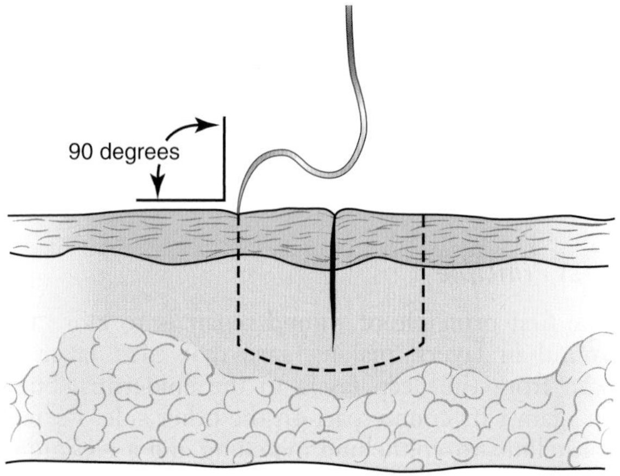

FIGURE 11-7 ■ The suture needle should enter the skin at a 90-degree angle to the surface.

Adherence to this principle automatically everts the skin edges (Figure 11-8). As the suture needle is placed in the skin, it should follow a direction that is oblique, back, and away from the wound edge. This creates the desired bottleneck effect of the stitch in the wound (Figure 11-9). In a wound that has been closed with this technique, the tissue will fall back into place when the sutures are removed, and the scar will eventually flatten.

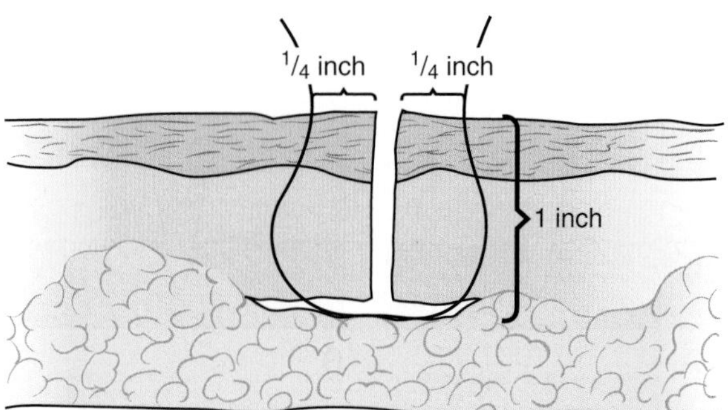

FIGURE 11-8 ■ The depth of the stitch should be greater than the width. This principle will help evert the wound edges. In this example, the suture enters and leaves ¼ inch from the wound, for a total width of ½ inch; the depth is 1 inch.

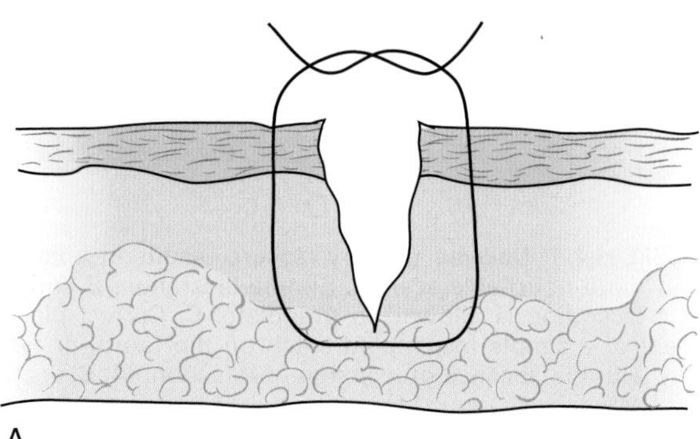

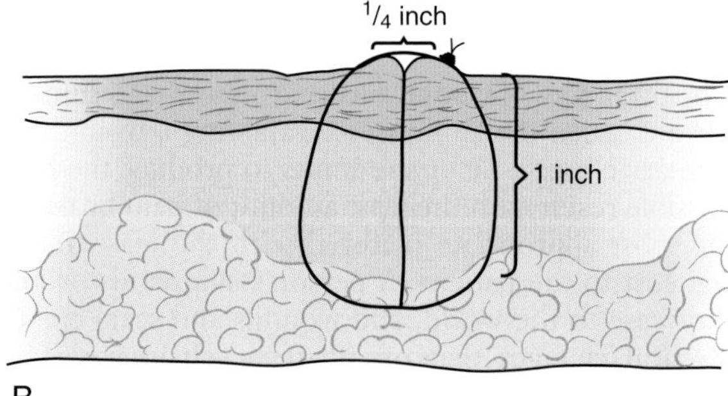

FIGURE 11-9 ■ Gathering more tissue within the stitch at the base of the wound **(A)** will create the desired bottleneck effect **(B)** and aid in everting the wound edges.

Second Principle

The second principle of wound repair is to match any landmarks that are readily identifiable. Before the first stitch is placed, the wound should be inspected for the location and identification of landmarks (e.g.,

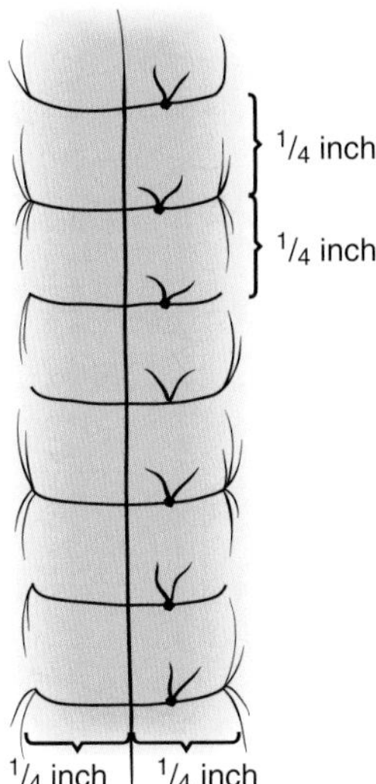

FIGURE 11-10 The "quarter-inch rule." Consistency in the spacing between sutures (¼ inch) and the distance of the suture from the wound edge (¼ inch) greatly enhances healing of the wound.

creases or wrinkles, birthmarks, old age spots, tan lines, hairlines, the vermilion of the lip, eyebrows, eyelids, tattoos). The first stitch should be placed in the landmark or as close to it as possible to match it precisely. Stair-step effects in linear lines, especially on the face, are visible, and extreme caution should be taken to avoid this result.

Third Principle

The third principle is the need for proper placement of the sutures. In the majority of the lacerations seen in the ED, one side of the wound is longer than the other. Care must be taken in attempting to correct this imbalance. Taking more tissue between stitches on one side than on the other will create what is known as a dog-ear. To avoid a dog-ear effect, it is essential to place the sutures at the same distance along each side of the wound. In the absence of landmarks, measuring may be necessary. A good rule to follow is to measure ¼ inch down one side of the laceration from the apex, to place the stitch in the skin about ¼ inch from the wound edge (Figure 11-10), and then to repeat the procedure on the other side. This method gives the most accurate closure possible.

Wound Tension

Wound tension is another aspect of suturing that must always be considered. The amount of tissue captured within a suture loop, no matter how little, creates a potential for ischemia by the overzealous use of force when the knot is tightened. The reduced capillary blood flow within the suture loop can result in tissue necrosis, prolonging the inflammatory response and potentially leading to a breakdown in healing that can result in a dehiscence of the wound. The wound edges should be brought together so that they merely touch because edema created by the inflammatory response increases the amount of tension in the suture loop. This could be disastrous if the suture line is already compromised by an overzealous tightening of the sutures. Approximating the edges so that dead space is eliminated and tension is minimal should be the goal in each wound closure.

Dèbridement

Occasionally, a wound may need débridement before primary closure. *Débridement* is the careful removal of dead or damaged tissue in addition to any unwarranted foreign material from the wound. This procedure should be considered when wounds, such as crush injuries, create jagged edges that have obliterated any previously existing landmarks. The goal of the clinician at this point is to create a more manageable wound that will produce a better cosmetic result and minimize the opportunity for any bacterial growth. Occasionally, the margins of a wound will be ragged and contused. The wound can be converted into a nicely incised surgical wound by excision of a 2- to 3-mm wound margin. This can be most easily accomplished by using a No. 15 surgical blade on a scalpel to cut into the dermis along a predetermined line that is safe to excise. Cut along the line created by the scalpel with a pair of surgical cutting scissors, excising the margins of the wound in a perpendicular fashion. Following débridement of the wound, especially if the skin edges are involved, the wound may require undermining of the skin to bring the skin edges together without tension on the wound (Figure 11-11). Do not excise tissue on the scalp or the eyebrows. This will create a prominent, hairless scar.

Dead Space

Dead space occurs when a suture placed in the skin does not encompass the entire wound (Figure 11-12). Hematomas often develop in the dead space. Hematoma is historically a great culture medium for bacteria. This happens in deep wounds in which the skin suture has not reached the full depth of the wound. In this case, deep sutures using absorbable suture material should be used to eliminate the dead space (Figure 11-13). However, caution should be

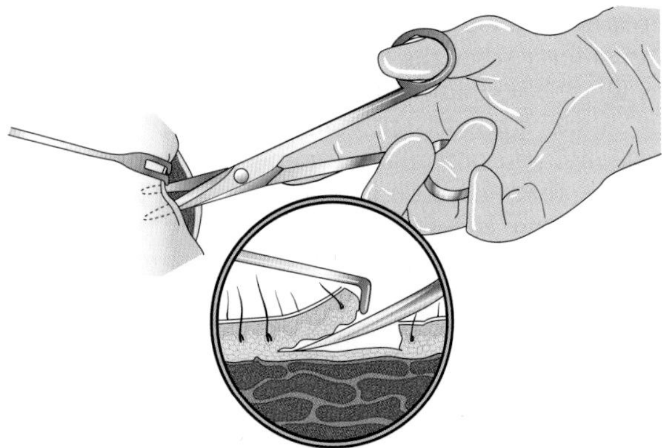

FIGURE 11-11 ■ Undermining the skin at different levels releases tension on the entire wound and can give a better result.

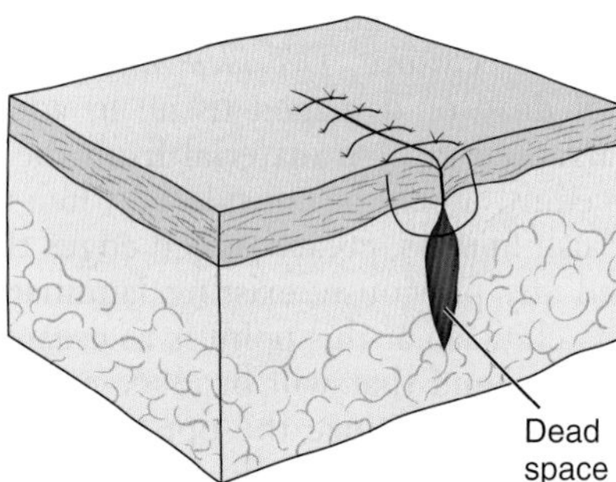

FIGURE 11-12 ■ Dead space occurs when the stitch fails to reach the base of the wound. The shallowness of the stitch leaves an open area that is an ideal nidus for bacterial growth, leading to infection. Absorbable synthetic sutures are ideal for placement in the base of the wound to eliminate any dead space.

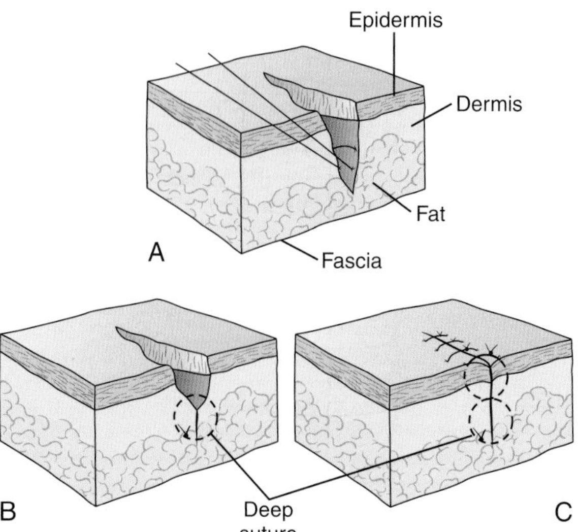

FIGURE 11-13 ■ **A-C,** Proper placement of a deep, internal absorbable suture. Absorbable synthetic sutures are ideal for placement in the base of the wound to eliminate any dead space **(B)**. The wound is then closed primarily **(C)**.

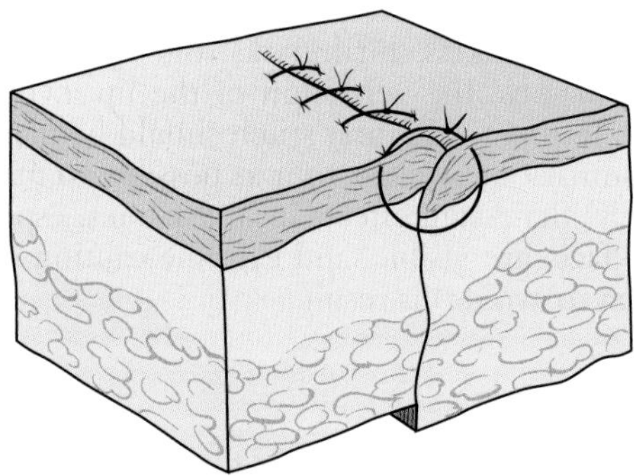

FIGURE 11-14 ■ Poor technique can result in rolling of one wound edge over the other. Care must be taken to ensure that equal amounts of tissue on either side of the wound are enclosed within the stitch. The scar resulting from wound edge rolling is readily avoidable if care is taken to match the internal levels of tissue.

taken to avoid the overuse of deep absorbable sutures because these sutures act as foreign objects, and the inflammatory response around them may result in prolonged healing or wound dehiscence. A few well-spaced, deep sutures can remove the dead space and lessen the tension on the outermost layers of the wound, resulting in a minimal "good" scar that will not require revision. Additionally, use of deep sutures should be avoided in grossly contaminated wounds. In an obviously contaminated wound, any additional foreign material, whether in the form of a hematoma or a suture, can serve as a nidus for infection and can delay the healing process.

Poor Technique

What causes "bad" scars? Understanding how poor technique may cause bad scarring gives the clinician insight as to what to avoid when closing a wound. Speed is one of the most notorious culprits in the poor results of a wound. The clinician must never sacrifice a good cosmetic result for speed. Rolling one of the wound edges is also a result of poor technique (Figure 11-14). When one edge of epithelium is rolled under the other, the raw wound edge lying on top of the normal epithelial skin surface will not heal. When the sutures are removed, that portion of the wound will open, resulting in a much bigger scar. With proper eversion of both skin edges, scarring can be minimized. Occasionally, although diligent and adhering to these principles, the clinician will find the remains of a dog-ear at the end of a procedure. Plastic surgeons use a procedure to remove the

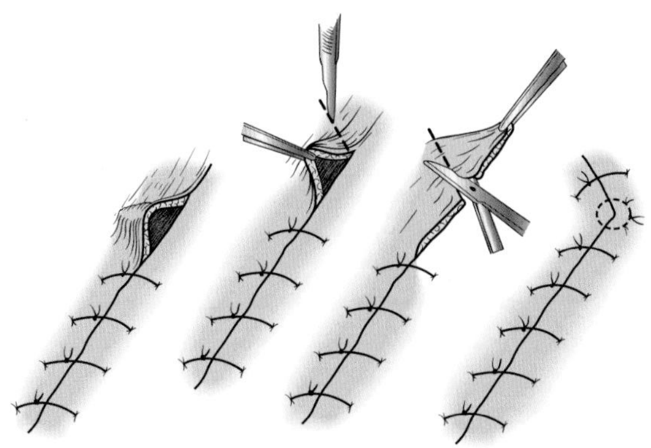

FIGURE 11-15 Procedure for eliminating a dog-ear. See text for explanation.

excess tissue, called a "dog-ear maneuver" (Figure 11-15), as follows:

1. Undermine the area involving the dog-ear, using blunt dissection (see Figure 11-11), between the dermal layer and the fascial layer of the skin.
2. Cut a straight line away from the apex of the dog-ear, at an angle of 45 to 55 degrees, just the length of the dog-ear.
3. Measure the resulting triangular piece of excess skin on that side.
4. Redrape the excess skin to determine just how much of the dog-ear should be removed.
5. Cut and remove the excess tissue, and close the new wound primarily.

The basic technique of instrument-assisted wound closure is shown in Figures 11-16 and 11-17. The key here is to be certain that the first knot laid down on the wound is a square knot. A minimum of six throws, or three knots (two throws equaling one knot), should be used with each suture placed in the wound. These principles are crucial to all wound closures. They can be improved and altered as a student becomes more sophisticated in suturing. When wounds are large or have a great amount of tissue loss, however, even the most respected plastic surgeons return to these basics for initial wound closure with difficult wounds.

Special Considerations and Problems in Wound Closure

Triangular Flaps

A commonly encountered problem is a triangular flap with a sharp point. With a triangular flap, care must be taken to protect the distal-most portion of the flap, which has the most compromised blood supply.

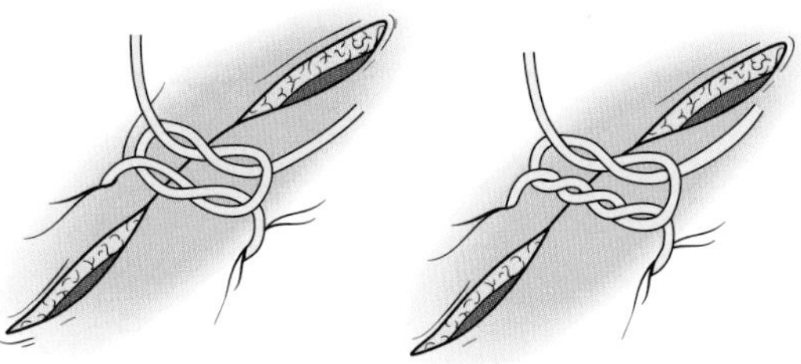

FIGURE 11-16 *Left*, Square knot. *Right*, Surgeon's knot.

Accordingly, sutures should not be placed through the skin at the distal-most point. Rather, a stitch is placed transversely under the dermis at the tip of the flap to avoid ischemia, which could develop if sutures are placed over the skin surface. This technique is demonstrated in Figures 11-18 to 11-21.

Poor Skin Quality

The elderly and those who have been long-term steroid users create a special situation that does not occur in the general population. Their skin is thin and fragile, and it is common to see large, avulsed flaps of this type of skin from relatively minor trauma. It is difficult to close these flaps normally because the sutures will tear through the skin, which is friable. Steri-Strips and tincture of benzoin work well. Paint the flap and surrounding skin with benzoin and allow it to dry, being careful not to get any benzoin in the wound itself. Then place the Steri-Strips on the wound, drawing the wound edges close together, and allow them to remain in position for about 3 weeks.

Contaminated Wounds

Some wounds should not be closed primarily. *Grinder injuries* are notorious for getting infected, despite the amount of brushing and irrigating of the wound that is done. Lacerations of the lower leg caused by objects thrown by a *lawn mower* nearly always get infected. *Human bites* are heavily contaminated with bacteria. *Dog bites* usually involve crush injury and bacterial contamination. A dog's tooth is a blunt instrument, and the biting mechanism is such that the bite does not create a sharp incision. The first effect is to crush the tissue and then puncture it. Because of the angle of closure of the dog's jaw, a bottle-shaped defect in the tissue is created, and there is usually a tearing of the tissue as the bite is completed. Calcareous plaques from the dog's teeth may be deposited deep in the wound and act as foreign bodies. *Wounds more than 12 hours old* are frequently heavily contaminated with bacteria and should not be closed primarily.

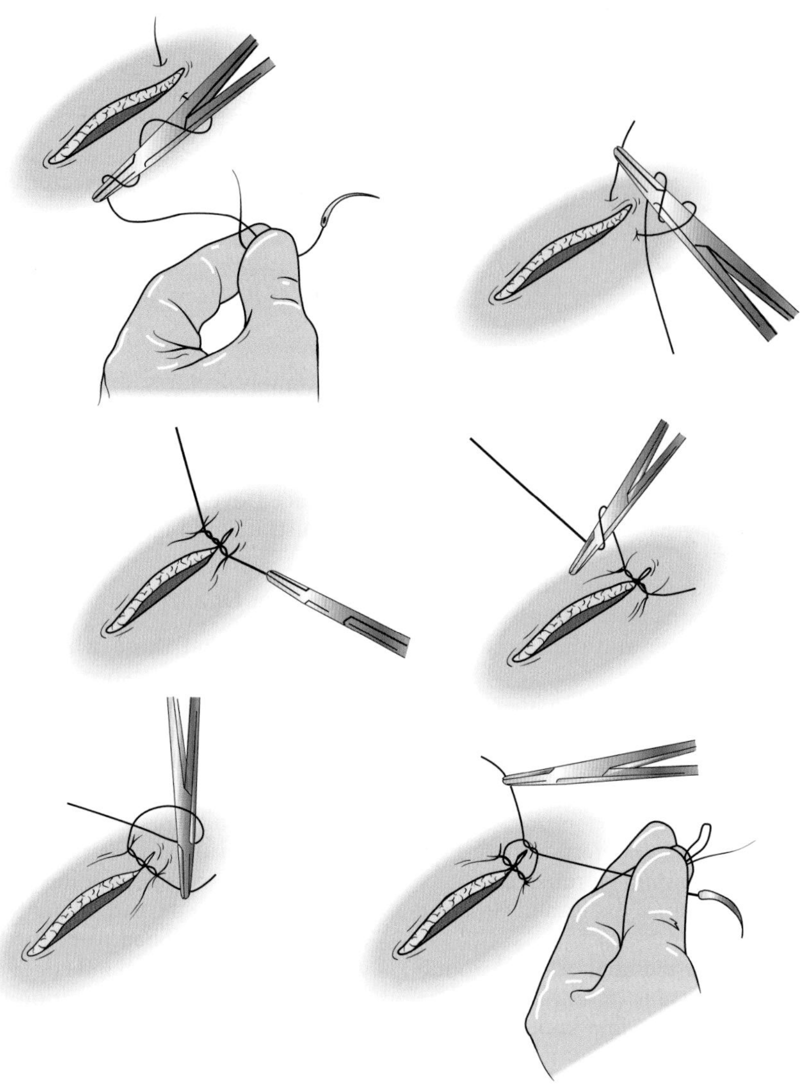

FIGURE 11-17 ■ The technique of surgical instrument wound closure.

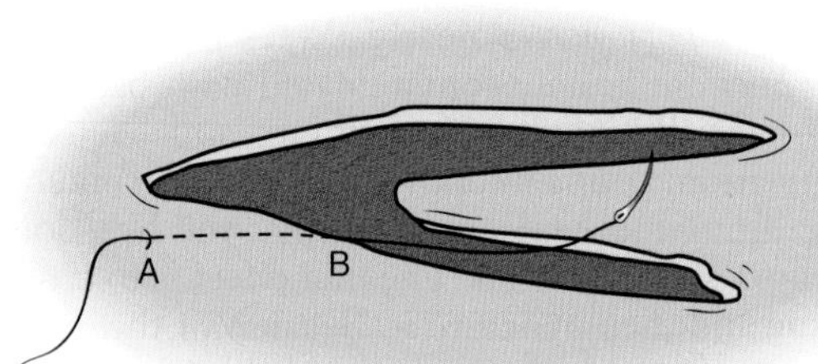

FIGURE 11-18 ■ For closure of a triangular flap wound with a sharp point, pass the needle through the skin at point *A* and exit through the dermis at point *B,* which is inside the wound.

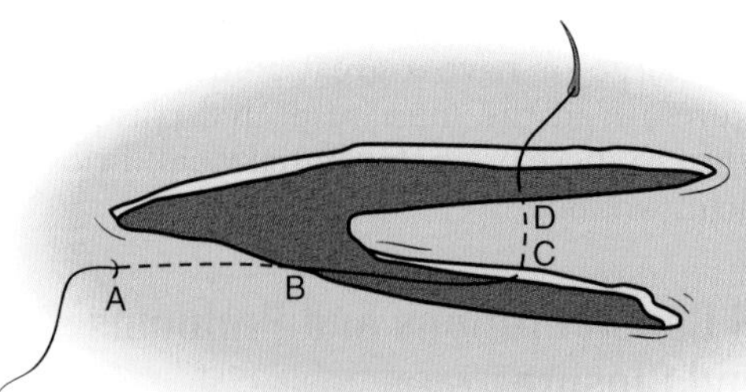

FIGURE 11-19 ■ After following the procedure shown in Figure 11-18, pass the needle transversely through the dermis at the tip of the wound flap from point *C* to point *D,* being careful to maintain the same depth of the suture on both sides of the wound.

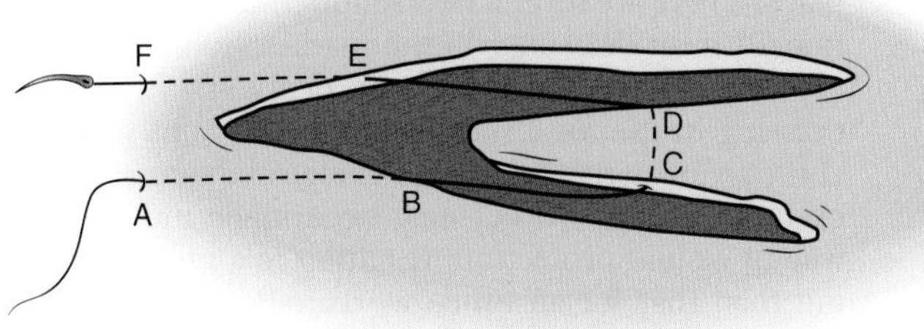

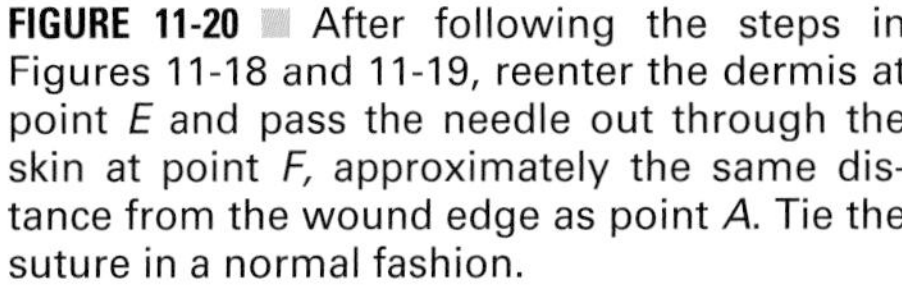
FIGURE 11-20 ■ After following the steps in Figures 11-18 and 11-19, reenter the dermis at point *E* and pass the needle out through the skin at point *F*, approximately the same distance from the wound edge as point *A*. Tie the suture in a normal fashion.

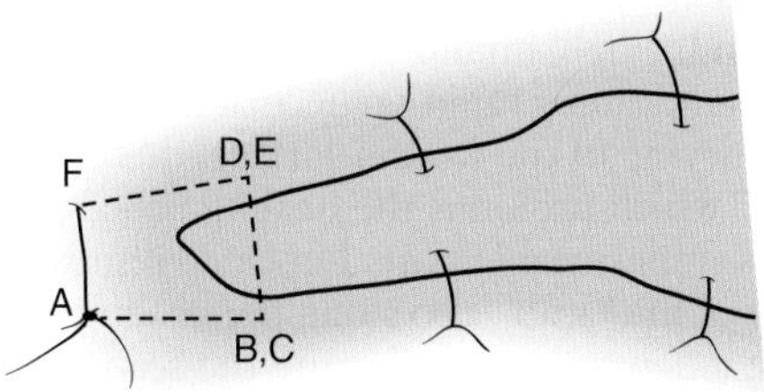

FIGURE 11-21 ■ After the steps shown in Figures 11-18 to 11-20 are completed, the entire wound is sutured closed.

The "golden period" for all wounds to be closed primarily is within the first 6 hours of injury.

There are two ways to deal with contaminated wounds. The first is to let the wound heal by secondary intention. This is satisfactory if the wound is small. Most grinder injuries, injuries caused by objects thrown by lawn mowers, and many dog bites fall into this category. The second option is to perform a delayed primary closure, as described previously in this chapter. These types of wounds should be anesthetized, irrigated and cleansed profusely, and then dressed. The dressing should be changed every day, and antibiotic treatment should be initiated. After 4 to 5 days, the wound should be reassessed; if there is no evidence of an infection, the wound may be reanesthetized and closed primarily. Avoid the use of absorbable sutures in a wound that is at high risk for infection because they will act like foreign bodies and decrease the resistance of the wound to infection.

The preceding guidelines can be adjusted for facial injuries because the face, with its rich vascular supply, has a high resistance to infection. The major concern here is getting the best cosmetic result. For this reason, most dog bites and wounds more than 12 hours old on the face are closed primarily. Always use antibiotic coverage in these cases.

Dermabond

Dermabond is a topical skin adhesive put out by Ethicon (Cornelia, Georgia); it can be thought of as superglue for the skin. It is easy to use and will leave an airtight, hard coating over the wound when applied correctly.

Dermabond is intended for topical application only to hold closed easily approximated skin edges from surgical incisions, including punctures from minimally invasive surgery, and simple, thoroughly cleansed, trauma-induced lacerations. It can be used in conjunction with, but not in place of, subcuticular sutures. Dermabond should not be used on any wound with evidence of active infection or gangrene, or on wounds of decubitus etiology. It should not be used on any mucosal surfaces or across mucocutaneous junctions (e.g., oral cavity, lips) or on skin that may be regularly exposed to body fluids or with dense natural hair (e.g., scalp). It should not be used on patients with a known hypersensitivity to cyanoacrylate or formaldehyde, and great care must be taken if it is used near the eye. Other areas to avoid with this material are high–skin tension areas such as knuckles, elbows, and knees, unless the joint will be temporarily immobilized during the healing period. This superglue for the skin is fast drying and can adhere to just about any surface, including stainless steel. There is no need for a dressing when Dermabond is used. (See Figure 11-22, *A* to *D*.)

PROCEDURE FOR WOUND CLOSURE WITH DERMABOND ADHESIVE

The procedure will require two people.

1. Make sure the wound is clean, dry, and hemostatic.
2. Using two pairs of Adson forceps with teeth, each person should grasp the skin approximately 2 mm from the corners of the wound and retract away from each other, pulling the skin edges as close together as possible.
3. Apply the Dermabond liquid over the approximated wound edges, covering the wound completely.

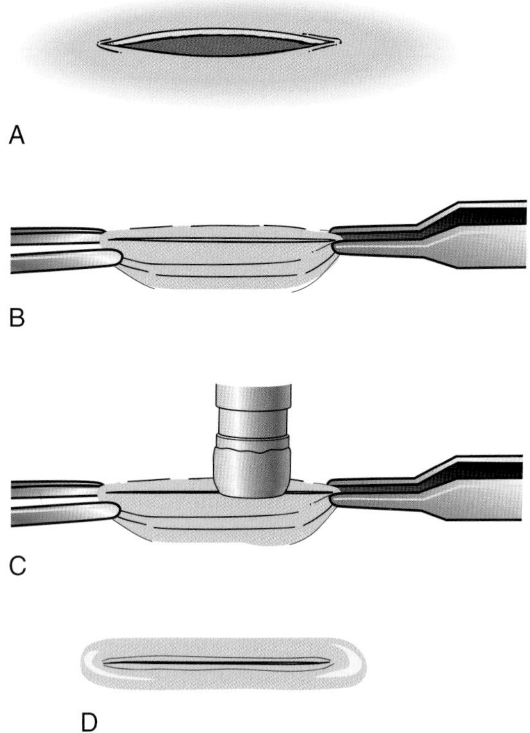

FIGURE 11-22 Dermabond wound closure technique. **A,** Clean open wound. **B,** Wound edge approximated by retraction with Adson forceps. **C,** Dermabond is applied to the closed wound surface. **D,** The wound is closed, and Dermabond is in place.

4. Remove excess liquid from any area wider than 5 mm around the wound before it has a chance to dry.
5. Maintain tension until the liquid has dried and become adherent to the skin.
6. Remove the forceps.
7. The Dermabond will peel away naturally in 7 to 10 days, after the wound has healed.

Dressings

A basic wound dressing consists of four parts. The first part is a nonadherent base that allows the wound to breathe while maintaining a high level of humidity over the wound. The second part is an absorbent gauze sponge that allows the wound to drain and does not obstruct the gaseous exchange that aids in wound healing. An obstructive sponge may result in the drying of the exudate, creating a new wound each time the dressing is changed. The third part is a gauze wrapping that allows free movement of gases through the dressing and holds the first two parts in place. The last part is some sort of adhesive to hold the entire dressing in place. There are several new semipermeable, occlusive, nonadherent dressings on the market. Some are more expensive than others, and the decision as to which dressing to use for a specific wound remains with the clinician's experience and knowledge of the patient. For example, a farm worker may need much more in the way of wound protection, resulting in a bulkier dressing than that for an office worker. Petrolatum-based antibacterial ointments (e.g., bacitracin, polymyxin B sulfate, silver sulfadiazine, neomycin sulfate) may be applied to the surface of the closed wound often. This aids in maintaining a moist environment over the wound. High humidity between the wound and the dressing causes rapid epidermal healing and helps prevent drying of the wound surface, thereby avoiding a "scab," which prolongs the healing process by creating a gas-impermeable state. Repeated removal and recreation of the "scab" also slows the healing process by creating a new wound each time the scab is removed, thereby reinitiating the inflammatory phase of healing and resulting in a bigger and less cosmetic scar.

The dressing also maintains the heat of the wound by providing a thermal insulator between the wound and the environment. The heat of the wound must remain as close to body core temperature as possible. Phagocytic and mitotic activity decreases greatly in temperatures below 30°C. Removing the dressing from a wound that has high humidity can drop the temperature of the wound to as low as 12°C, and the resulting recovery to full mitotic activity can take up to 3 hours. Every attempt should be taken to shorten the time involved in changing a dressing and to maintain the temperature of the wound at or above a 30°C environment. A dressing must also be impermeable to airborne microorganisms. Wounds that are infected despite the available phagocytic processes do not heal. In *strike-through*, an overabundance of exudate produced by the wound results in soaking of the dressing through to the outer layer. This provides a wet pathway from the surface of the dressing to the wound for any airborne microorganisms. Strike-through can take as little as 6 hours, and the resulting infection can drastically prolong the healing process.

The optimum dressing for any wound has the following characteristics:

- Is sterile.
- Is big enough to cover and protect the wound.
- Has enough absorptive qualities for wound drainage.
- Is comfortable and has good handling capabilities, both wet and dry.
- Maintains a good shelf-life (remains sterile in storage).
- Is easily disposable.

In summary, the objectives of a dressing are simple and, when they are met, the healing process can be shortened by days. These objectives are as follows:

- To maintain a high humidity between the wound and the dressing.
- To remove excess exudate and toxic compounds.
- To allow gaseous exchange.
- To provide thermal insulation to the wound surface.
- To be impermeable to bacteria.
- To be free from particles and toxic wound contaminants.
- To allow removal without causing trauma during dressing change.

Universal Precautions

In 1987, the Centers for Disease Control and Prevention (CDC) published guidelines outlining the steps to take to guard against blood and other body fluid from patients. These guidelines, which were created to decrease infection, are known as *universal precautions.* Universal precaution guidelines address handwashing and the use of gloves, eyewear, and gowns when caring for patients. When performing clinical procedures, it is especially important to keep these guidelines in mind to protect the patient, as well as the clinician. Gloves are required whenever there will be direct contact with blood or other bodily fluids. Similarly, masks and protective eyewear (i.e., goggles or face shields) should also be used whenever there is a risk for exposure to blood or other fluids during a procedure. If a clinician anticipates an even greater exposure, wearing a gown is recommended in addition to the gloves and protective eyewear.[2]

COMMONLY PERFORMED CLINICAL PROCEDURES

This section describes some of the clinical procedures most commonly conducted in the delivery of health care. As the clinician becomes more confident and sophisticated in the ability to perform these tasks, he or she may refine or streamline individual procedures and develop preferences. Each description is simply one proven way to complete a given procedure and obtain the desired results.

Injections

Injections are used to deliver a variety of substances, including drugs, vaccinations, and skin test antigens, through the skin by means of a needle. The types of injections most commonly used are intramuscular, subcutaneous, and intradermal.

Intramuscular Injections

PROCEDURE FOR INTRAMUSCULAR INJECTION

1. Verify the patient and the medication.
2. Fully expose and palpate the anatomic landmarks. The muscle being injected should be at rest and should be non–weight bearing.
3. Prepare the skin with an alcohol wipe, starting at the injection site and extending outward in a circular motion, using the bull's-eye method, for about 5 cm. Allow the skin to dry completely before injection to avoid burning.[2]
4. Fill the syringe with the desired amount of fluid to be injected. (Recommended use of 3–5 mL syringe with an 18- to 22-gauge 1-inch needle.)
   a. Wipe the rubber stopper of the vial of medication with an alcohol wipe.
   b. Pull the plunger of the syringe back to the mark signifying the amount of medication to be withdrawn from the vial, filling the syringe with air.
   c. Insert the needle through the center of the rubber stopper of the vial.
   d. Invert the vial.
   e. Inject air into the vial.
   f. Withdraw the desired amount of medication into the syringe, making it as free of air bubbles as possible.
   g. If medication to be administered is in an ampule: Tap the neck of the ampule to ensure that all of the medication is in the bottom of the ampule. Wrap the neck of the ampule with gauze and carefully break the neck of the ampule. Aspirate the medication from the bottom of the ampule and then remove any air from the syringe. Dispose of the ampule in the appropriate container.[2]
5. Pull the subcutaneous tissue slightly to one side.
6. Rapidly plunge the needle perpendicular (a 90-degree angle) into the surface of the skin.
7. Insert the needle to a depth of 1 inch.
8. Aspirate to ensure that the needle is not in a blood vessel. If blood returns, do not inject at this site, but withdraw the needle and apply pressure to encourage hemostasis. Repeat steps 5 and 6.
9. Inject the medication slowly.
10. Withdraw the needle and dispose in an appropriate chamber.
11. Massage the area briefly with a gauze sponge to promote absorption.
12. Apply a self-adhesive bandage, if necessary.

Indications. Intramuscular injections are used for drugs that are not easily absorbed orally, when an intermediate rate of onset and duration of action are preferred, and when parenteral delivery is necessary.

Contraindications. Intramuscular injections should not be given at any site where a dermatitis or cellulitis exists.

Equipment. The following equipment should be assembled:

- Alcohol wipes.
- Syringe of appropriate size depending on the volume to be injected.
- Needle. Selection of needle depends on the depth of insertion and the viscosity of the drug. In general, adults require a 19- to 22-gauge, 1½- inch needle. An obese patient may require a longer needle.
- Medication to be injected.
- Sterile gauze sponge.
- Self-adhesive bandage.
- Needle disposal container.

Injection Sites

Deltoid Muscle. Use the main body of the deltoid muscle, which lies lateral and a few centimeters below the acromion. Large volumes (greater than 2 mL) and irritating solutions should not be given at this site.

Gluteal Muscle. The gluteal muscle is the most common and preferred site of injection in adults and in children older than 2 years. A large volume of solution can be injected into the muscle, and the skin over the area is thin and easily pierced. The site for injection into the gluteal muscle should always be in the upper outer quadrant of the buttock, to avoid injury to the sciatic nerve and superior gluteal muscles.

Vastus Lateralis Muscle (Lateral Thigh). The vastus lateralis is the preferred injection site in infants. Although it may be used in adults, it is painful due to the firmness of the underlying fascia lata. The injection should be given into the bulk of the muscle.

Possible Complications. The following complications may occur with intramuscular injections:

Injection into blood vessels may cause a toxic reaction, injury to the vessel, or a hematoma.

Injection into a deep nerve may cause pain, paresthesias, and possible permanent damage to the nerve.

The needle may break off and become embedded in the muscle.

Sterile and septic abscesses at the injection site may occur if equipment is not sterile, the injection site is not properly cleansed, or a site is overused.

Follow-up. No special follow-up is required.

Subcutaneous Injections

PROCEDURE FOR SUBCUTANEOUS INJECTION

1. Verify patient and medication.
2. Fully expose the area.
3. Prepare the skin with an alcohol wipe, starting at the injection site and extending outward in a circular motion, using the bull's-eye method, for about 5 cm. Allow the skin to dry completely before injection to avoid burning.[2]
4. Fill the syringe with the desired amount of medication to be injected, usually 2 to 3 mL (see instructions for preparing medication under "Intramuscular Injections"). (Recommended use of 3 mL syringe with 24- to 26-gauge, 1-inch needle.)
5. Pinch up the subcutaneous tissue into a roll between the thumb and the forefinger to pull subcutaneous tissue away from the muscle.
6. Insert the needle with one quick motion at a 45-degree angle to the skin at the midpoint of the roll.
7. Advance the needle about three fourths of its length.
8. Release the roll of skin.
9. Aspirate to ensure that the needle is not in a blood vessel. If blood returns, do not inject at this site; withdraw the needle and repeat steps 4 through 7.
10. Inject the medication slowly.
11. Withdraw the needle and dispose in an appropriate chamber.
12. Apply gentle pressure with a gauze sponge over the site.
13. Apply a self-adhesive bandage, if necessary.

Indications. Subcutaneous injections are to be used for small volumes of drugs that require slow absorption and long duration of action, such as heparin or insulin.

Contraindications. Subcutaneous injections should not be given at any site where a severe dermatitis or cellulitis exists.

Equipment. The following equipment should be assembled:

- Alcohol wipes
- Syringe of appropriate size, depending on the volume to be injected
- Needle: 25- to 27-gauge, ¾ to 1 inch
- Medication to be injected
- Sterile gauze sponge
- Self-adhesive bandage
- Needle disposal container

Possible Complications. Local reactions can occur with repeated injections over the same site.

Follow-up. No specific follow-up is required.

Intradermal Injections

PROCEDURE FOR INTRADERMAL INJECTION

1. Verify patient and medication.
2. Fill the syringe with the desired amount of solution, usually 0.1 to 0.2 mL. (Recommended use of 1-mL tuberculin syringe with 27-gauge, ½-inch needle.)
3. Clean the ventral surface of the forearm with an alcohol pad using the bull's-eye method. Allow the skin to dry completely before injection to avoid burning.[2]
4. Hold the skin taut between the thumb and the index finger.
5. Hold the needle bevel up and angle it about 10 to 15 degrees (almost parallel) to the skin.
6. Insert the needle into the dermis for about two thirds of its length.
7. Inject the solution. A wheal should form immediately.
8. Withdraw the needle. Discard the needle and gauze in an appropriate container.
9. Do not rub the injection site.[2]
10. Record the following information on the patient's chart: type of test, date and time done, and exact location of each test injection mode.

Indications. Intradermal injections are used to test for hypersensitivity to extrinsic allergens and for infection by tuberculosis, nontuberculous mycobacteria, and certain fungal infections.

Contraindications. Intradermal injection should not be given at any site where dermatitis or infection exists. Patients with a previous positive tuberculin skin reaction should not be retested.

Equipment. The following equipment should be assembled:

- Alcohol wipes
- Tuberculin syringe
- Needle: 27-gauge, ½ inch
- Medication to be injected
- Sterile gauze sponge
- Needle disposal container

Injection Sites. The ventral forearm is the most common site used. The back may be used for extensive allergen testing.

Possible Complications. Severe local skin reactions may develop in hypersensitive patients.

Follow-up. Patients should be instructed about when to return to have the skin reaction read, usually in 48 to 72 hours. If the skin reaction is positive, the diameter of the cutaneous induration should be measured and recorded.

Venipuncture

Venipuncture is one of the most frequently performed clinical procedures. It is a skill that can be learned and perfected through frequent practice to minimize patient discomfort. Venipuncture, or phlebotomy, is used to obtain blood samples for diagnostic analysis.

Phlebotomy

PROCEDURE FOR PHLEBOTOMY

1. Wash hands first. Verify patient and labs to be drawn.
2. Position the patient in a sitting or supine position to ensure comfort.
3. Inspect the patient's arms for the optimal venipuncture.[2]
4. Apply the tourniquet 2 to 3 inches above the antecubital fossa (or other venipuncture site) so that it may be removed quickly with one hand. Do not apply the tourniquet too tightly, to avoid causing patient discomfort and blood stasis. The tourniquet should be removed if cyanosis is observed in the arm. In general, it should not remain on for longer than 1 minute.
5. Select the vein site. Palpate and trace the path of the vein with the index finger, or use one of the methods previously described.
6. Cleanse the skin with the alcohol pads and allow the area to dry.

7. Put on gloves.
8. Grasp the patient's arm firmly with the nondominant hand and stabilize the vein, using the thumb to anchor the vein by drawing the skin taut.
9. Insert the needle, bevel up, under the skin at an angle of 15 to 30 degrees with a quick motion. A sensation of resistance will be felt, followed by ease of penetration as the vein is entered.
10. Transfer the blood as required by equipment chosen.
    a. If using a syringe, withdraw the desired amount of blood into the syringe.
    b. If using a Vacutainer system, hold the Vacutainer needle and unit steady with the hand used to do the venipuncture. Push the vacuum tube forward onto the needle, and look for the inflow of blood into the Vacutainer. Allow the tube to fill until the blood flow ceases. Remove the tube from the holder. If multiple tubes are needed, insert the next tube into the holder and repeat the procedure. The shutoff valve automatically covers the butt end of the needle, stopping blood flow until the next tube is inserted.
    c. If using a butterfly catheter, remove the cap at end of the tubing and attach a syringe. Withdraw the required amount of blood into the syringe.
11. Release the tourniquet.
12. Place a sterile gauze pad just above the venipuncture site.
13. Remove the needle quickly and smoothly, and slide the gauze down to the site with a moderate amount of pressure. Maintain pressure until bleeding has ceased.
14. Apply a self-adhesive bandage.
15. If a syringe was used, fill the appropriate tubes by puncturing the rubber stopper of the tube with the needle and allowing vacuum to fill the tubes.
16. If using tubes containing an additive, mix them immediately by gently inverting them 10 to 12 times each.
17. Make sure all tubes are properly labeled.
18. Used needles should not be recapped but should be disposed of directly into an appropriate needle disposal container, which should be readily available.

Indications. Phlebotomy is used to obtain blood samples for laboratory analysis and to remove blood in the treatment of polycythemia.

Contraindications. Phlebotomy should not be performed if there is evidence of phlebitis, cellulitis, lymphangitis, scarring, recent venipuncture, or venous obstruction at the proposed site of venipuncture. Phlebotomy should not be performed in the same arm in which an intravenous line is positioned because the intravenous fluids may dilute the specimen and interfere with the laboratory results.

Equipment. The following equipment should be assembled:

- Tourniquet.
- Alcohol pads.
- Disposable latex gloves.
- Vacutainer needle holder or syringe (5, 10, or 20 mL).
- Vacutainer needle or a 20-gauge needle for the syringe. If a large amount of blood is to be drawn, it is best to use an 18-gauge needle. Needles smaller than 22-gauge should be avoided because the blood sample tends to hemolyze in the small bore. A butterfly needle may be necessary for small veins.
- Properly labeled Vacutainer tubes.
- Sterile gauze pads.
- Self-adhesive bandage.
- Needle disposal container.

Important: Know which specific tests are to be collected so that the proper tubes are available.

Site Selection. The arm is the best site for phlebotomy, especially in the antecubital fossa (Figure 11-23). The superficial veins of the arm are more easily observable and accessible, distinct, and palpable. Size, elasticity, and distance below the skin determine vein selection. In general, the most easily palpable vein, even though it may not be the most visible, should be selected for phlebotomy. To aid in selection of a vein, the clinician can:

- Apply the tourniquet first to observe for a suitable vein.
- Have the patient open and close the fist to help pump blood from muscles into the superficial veins.
- Lower the extremity to a dependent position.
- Apply warm, wet towels over the area to encourage venous dilation.
- Gently tap repeatedly over the vein with the tips of the fingers to cause reflex dilation of the veins.
- When a suitable vein cannot be found in the forearm, one of the superficial veins on the dorsal surface of the hand may have to be used. These veins are small and collapse easily, so they should not be used to draw large amounts of blood.

Patient Preparation. The procedure should be explained to the patient to help reduce anxiety and elicit cooperation. The patient should be positioned comfortably with the arm resting on an even, solid surface.

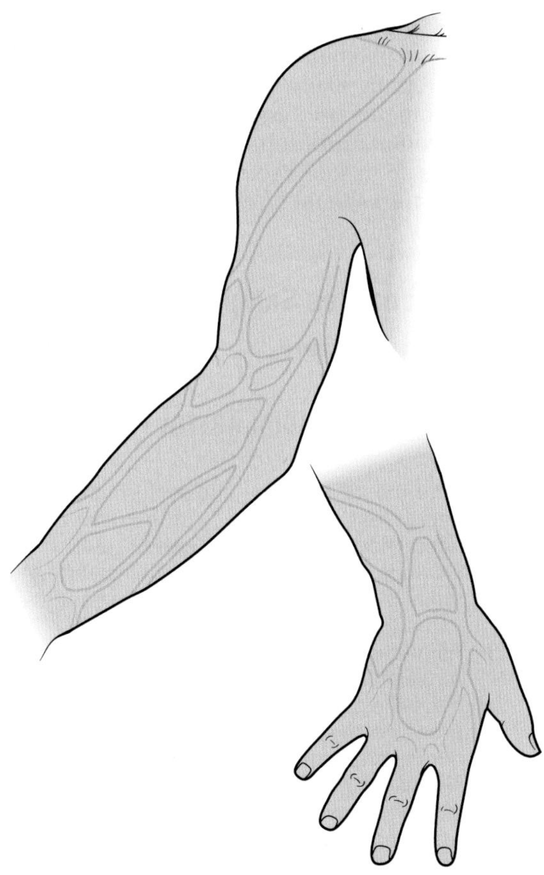

FIGURE 11-23 ■ Arm and hand anatomy most commonly used for venipuncture.

Peripheral Intravenous Catheterization

PROCEDURE FOR PERIPHERAL INTRAVENOUS CATHETERIZATION

1. Verify the patient and the need for intravenous fluid.
2. Assemble and prepare the intravenous fluid and tubing. Run the fluid through the tubing to flush all air from the system, and recap the end of the tubing.
3. Apply a tourniquet 4 to 6 inches above the proposed site in a way that allows quick removal. The tourniquet should be tight enough to stop venous flow, but not arterial flow.
4. Select the vein to be used. The techniques used for phlebotomy can be used to help palpate and visualize a suitable vein for catheterization.
5. Palpate the course of the vein. Make sure it is long enough to accept the catheter to be used.
6. Put on gloves.
7. Cleanse the skin around the insertion site with the antiseptic sponges (i.e., alcohol or povidone-iodine).
8. Inspect the catheter-over-needle unit to ensure that the beveled tip of the metal needle is well beyond the tip of the catheter and that the catheter slides easily.
9. Anchor the vein by gently applying pressure and pulling distally with the thumb of the non-dominant hand.
10. Insert the needle, bevel up, through the skin at an angle of 15 to 30 degrees, either on top or to the side of the vein. Insert the needle and the catheter into the vein. A "pop" will be felt, and blood will flow back into the hub of the needle or the "flash" chamber.
11. Advance the needle and the catheter a few millimeters until both have entered the lumen of the vein.
12. Gently and gradually advance the catheter into the vein while withdrawing the needle. Palpate the catheter through the skin as it is advanced inside the vein. Applying gentle pressure just proximal to the end of the catheter prevents blood from leaking back through or around the catheter.
13. Never reinsert the needle into the catheter because this can cause shearing of the catheter.[3]
14. Make sure the entire length of the catheter is inside the lumen of the vein.
15. Release the tourniquet and remove the needle.
16. Attach the intravenous tubing, and check for leakage along the entire system.
17. Secure the catheter in place with tape, and apply an antiseptic or antibiotic ointment to the puncture site. Apply the transparent sterile dressing. Loop and tape the IV tubing onto the forearm to prevent accidental dislodgment of the IV catheter.
18. Label the insertion site with the catheter gauge, date and time of insertion, and initials of the person performing the procedure.

Indications. Peripheral intravenous (IV) catheterization is used to administer fluids, medications, blood, and blood products. In most cases, catheter placement into the vein is preferred over needle placement because a catheter lasts longer and is better tolerated by the patient. The catheter-over-needle unit (Angiocath) is the most common type used. A butterfly intravenous line may be preferred for patients requiring brief venous access and immediate removal of the line.

Contraindications. Catheters should never be placed where there is cellulitis, phlebitis, lymphedema, or pitting edema of the extremity. Previous mastectomy or other axillary surgery by which ipsilateral venous drainage may have been impaired is another contraindication. Hyperosmolar fluids and agents known to cause chemical phlebitis should not be administered through peripheral veins. Arteriovenous shunts should never be used for placement of routine intravenous lines.

Equipment. The following equipment should be assembled:

- Tourniquet.
- Povidone-iodine (Betadine) antiseptic skin preparation sponges.
- Tape to secure the intravenous line. Prepare two 4-inch lengths of ½- inch-wide tape.
- Catheter-over-needle (Angiocath) unit or butterfly needle of appropriate diameter for the rate and type of fluid to be infused (see "Catheter Selection").
- Bag of IV fluid or blood products with appropriate connecting tubing.
- Disposable latex gloves.
- Transparent sterile dressing, antiseptic or antibiotic ointment, and labels.

Catheter Selection. Considerations in selecting the correct catheter include the size and condition of the vein and the viscosity of the fluid to be infused. The following guideline can be used:

14–16 gauge: Trauma or major surgery
16–18 gauge: Blood and blood products, administration of viscous medications
20–22 gauge: Most patient applications
24–gauge: Pediatric patients and neonates

Site Selection. The veins most suitable for intravenous therapy are found at the dorsum of the hand, the volar aspect of the proximal ulnar forearm, and the radial aspect of the forearm just proximal to the wrist (see Figure 11-23 for venous anatomy). In general, the principles below should be followed:

- Use distal veins first.
- Use patient's nondominant arm when possible.
- Avoid veins at areas of flexion, such as the antecubital fossa.
- Select a vein that will not interfere with the patient's daily living activities.
- Select a vein that has not been used previously and is relatively straight.
- Avoid veins in the legs because there is an increased risk for complications, such as thrombophlebitis.

Patient Preparation. Explain the procedure fully to the patient to minimize anxiety and elicit cooperation. The patient should be in a comfortable position with the extremity to be used resting on a solid surface.

Possible Complications. Hematoma formation, extravasation, phlebitis, cellulitis, bacteremia, and sepsis may occur. Daily inspection of the site and aseptic technique are essential to minimize the chances of complications. Intravenous sites should be changed every 3 to 4 days to reduce the probability of phlebitis, or they should be changed at the first signs of phlebitis or infection.

Arterial Blood Gas Sampling

Radial Artery Puncture

PROCEDURE FOR RADIAL ARTERY PUNCTURE

1. Palpate the radial artery, and perform the Allen test to assess the adequacy of the ulnar artery collateral flow to the hand (Figure 11-24).
   a. Occlude both the radial and ulnar arteries while the patient makes a tight fist and elevates the arm.
   b. Allow the hand to blanch, and lower the arm to waist level.
   c. Have the patient open the hand. Release the pressure over the ulnar artery while maintaining pressure over the radial artery.
   d. Normal skin color should return to the ulnar side of the palm within 6 seconds, with color returning to the whole palm quickly. Failure of the hand to regain color within 6 seconds signifies inadequate ulnar collateral circulation, and radial artery puncture is contraindicated.
2. Extend the patient's supinated wrist to about 30 degrees by placing a rolled towel under the wrist to bring the radial artery closer to the surface.[3]
3. Palpate the artery to determine where the pulsation is most prominent.
4. Cleanse the skin over the puncture site with the antiseptic sponges (i.e., alcohol or povidone-iodine).
5. Put on sterile gloves.
6. Anesthetize the skin over the puncture site with the 1% lidocaine. Care should be taken not to inject into the circulation.
7. Relocate the point of maximal impulse with the nondominant hand. Facing the patient, hold the syringe with the dominant hand like a pencil, bevel up.
8. Gently insert the needle through the skin at an angle of 45 to 60 degrees (Figure 11-25). Advance the needle toward the point of maximal impulse until arterial blood returns into the syringe. The needle and syringe may be advanced until the periosteum of the radius is encountered. If blood returns, allow the syringe to fill itself.

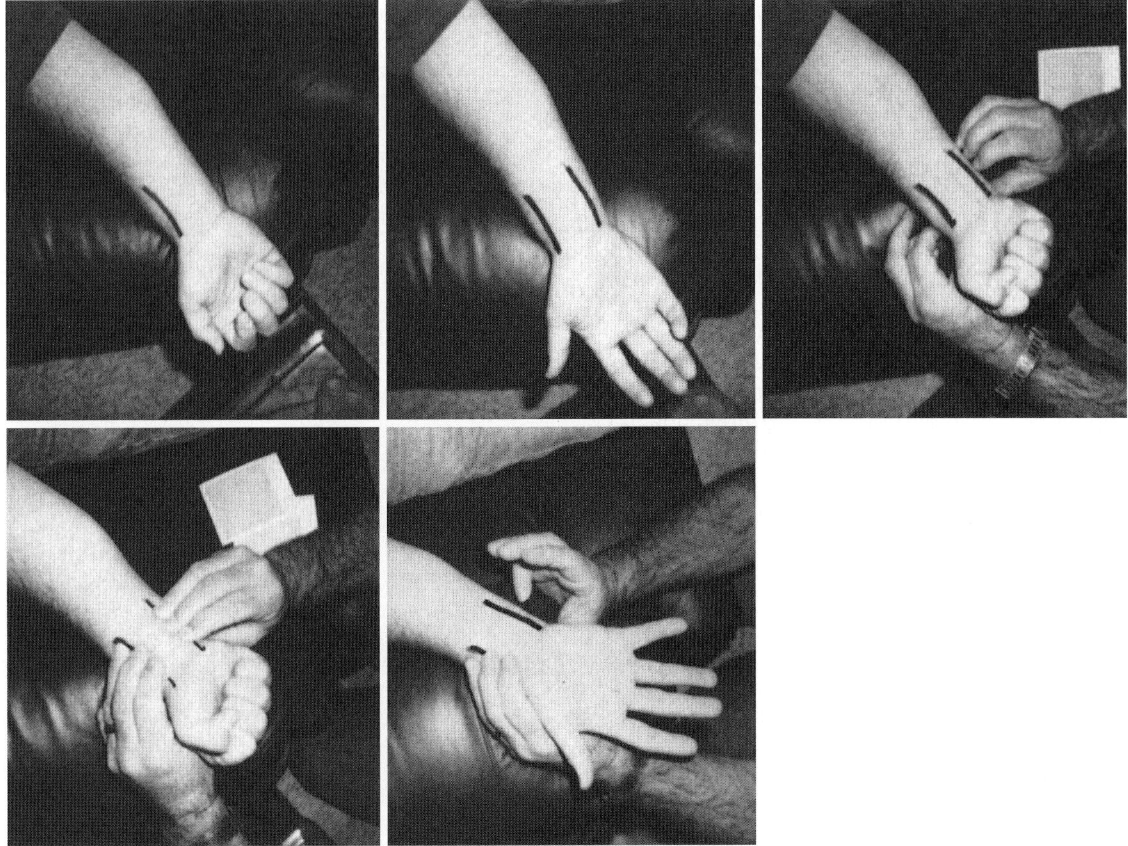

FIGURE 11-24 ■ Allen test. See text for explanation. (Photographs by Christopher Sullivan.)

PROCEDURE FOR RADIAL ARTERY PUNCTURE—CONT'D

9. If no blood is obtained, slowly withdraw the needle and syringe and continue to observe for blood return. If this is still unsuccessful, withdraw the needle to a position just under the skin and repeat the attempt, redirecting the needle toward the point of maximal impulse.
10. Collect the desired amount of blood and remove the needle quickly. Immediately apply direct pressure with a gauze sponge over the puncture site for 10 minutes.
11. Expel all air bubbles from the syringe. Gently roll the syringe between the fingers to mix the blood with the anticoagulant, remove the needle, and dispose of in the appropriate container. Embed the needle in a rubber stopper or place a cap on the end of the syringe, and place the syringe on ice.[3] Make sure the syringe is properly labeled and transported to the laboratory immediately.

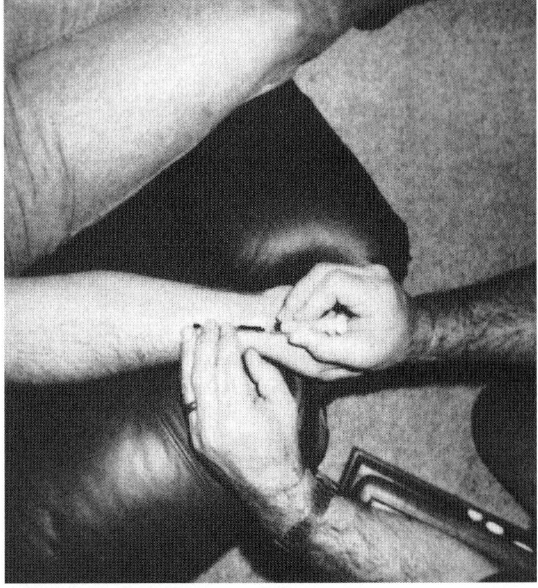

FIGURE 11-25 ■ Technique for obtaining an arterial blood gas sample from the radial artery. The needle should enter the skin, bevel up, at an angle of 45 to 50 degrees. (Photograph by Christopher Sullivan.)

Indications. Arterial blood gas (ABG) levels, used in a variety of clinical problems, such as an acute exacerbation of asthma or a suspected pulmonary embolus, may be determined using samples of arterial blood. ABG sampling has become an important and commonly used procedure. The most common site is the radial artery; alternative sites are the brachial and femoral arteries.

Contraindications. Poor collateral circulation in the hand, as determined by the Allen test, or no palpable pulse in the radial artery, is an absolute contraindication. The Allen test should always be done before a radial arterial puncture (see procedure for the Allen test in box) (see Figure 11-24). Arterial puncture should not be done over areas of cellulitis or local infection. It is relatively contraindicated in patients with bleeding disorders and patients on anticoagulant and thrombolytic therapy. When essential to management, arterial puncture should be done into the radial artery, with careful monitoring and prolonged postpuncture compression.

Equipment. A prepackaged blood gas sampling kit may be used, or assemble the following:

- Glass or plastic syringe, 3 to 5 mL
- Plastic syringe, 3 to 5 mL, containing 1% lidocaine without epinephrine
- Two needles, 25 gauge, ½ inch
- Heparin, 10,000 U/mL solution, 1 mL
- Povidone-iodine (Betadine) skin preparation sponges
- Rubber stopper or a cap for the syringe
- Rolled towel
- Crushed ice
- Sterile gauze sponges
- Sterile gloves

If not using a prepackaged blood gas sampling kit, the syringe to collect the specimen should be heparinized first.[3]

Preparation of the Syringe. To heparinize one 5-mL glass (or plastic) syringe and 25-gauge needle, withdraw 0.5 mL heparin into the syringe. Hold the syringe with the needle up, pull the plunger to the end of the syringe, and expel all the heparin through the needle. This procedure leaves an adequate amount of heparin in the syringe and needle. Too much heparin left in the syringe gives an artificially low pH.

Patient Preparation. Explain the procedure to the patient to facilitate patient cooperation and reduce anxiety. Tell the patient to expect some discomfort and pain. It is important that the patient keep as still as possible.

Possible Complications. Hemorrhage or hematoma may occur at the puncture site, causing vascular compromise. Hematoma formation can be avoided by providing pressure on the puncture site for 10 minutes following the procedure. Transient spasm may also occur. Thrombosis at the puncture site can lead to ischemia or gangrene of the hand or fingers. Accordingly, the patient should be instructed to notify the physician or PA if the hand becomes numb, painful, cold, or blue. A consultation with a vascular surgeon should be arranged immediately if arterial flow is compromised in any way.

Brachial Artery Puncture

PROCEDURE FOR BRACHIAL ARTERY PUNCTURE

1. Fully extend the patient's arm, with the forearm supinated.
2. Palpate the brachial artery at the medial side of the antecubital fossa.
3. Prepare the skin with antiseptic sponges.
4. Anesthetize the area with the 1% lidocaine, taking care not to inject into the circulation.
5. Locate the point of maximal pulsation, face the patient, and hold the syringe with the dominant hand like a pencil, bevel up.
6. Insert the needle through the skin at an angle of 60 to 90 degrees, and advance the needle slowly toward the point of maximal pulsation. Watch for return of arterial blood into the syringe. If no blood is obtained, withdraw the needle to just under the skin and attempt again.
7. Once the amount of blood needed is collected, withdraw the needle. Immediately apply direct pressure with a gauze sponge over the puncture site for 10 minutes.
8. Expel all air bubbles from the syringe. Gently roll the syringe to mix, embed the needle in a rubber stopper, and place the syringe on ice. Make sure the syringe is properly labeled and transported to the laboratory immediately.

The use of the brachial artery should be reserved for situations in which the radial artery cannot be used. Potential complications from the brachial artery are more common, and the procedure is often more painful. The contraindications, equipment, syringe preparation, and patient preparation are the same as for radial arm puncture.

Possible Complications. The possible complications of brachial artery puncture are essentially the same as for radial artery puncture. Any signs of arterial compromise seen in the forearm, hand, or fingers should prompt an immediate consultation with a vascular surgeon.

Femoral Artery Puncture

Although many believe that femoral artery puncture is the easiest to obtain, it should still be used only when radial arterial blood cannot be obtained. The close proximity of the femoral vein makes inadvertent venous sampling common. There is also a risk for embolization to the distal extremity. Postpuncture bleeding that is undetected can occur. The technique used for femoral artery puncture is similar to that for radial and brachial artery puncture, except for anatomic considerations. The differences in procedure are as follows:

- The patient should be in a supine position with the hip extended and slightly externally rotated. The femoral artery can be palpated just distal to the inguinal ligament in the groin.
- The needle should be inserted perpendicular to the skin surface.

Possible Complications. The possible complications in femoral artery puncture are essentially the same as for radial artery puncture. Any signs of vascular compromise seen in the leg, foot, or toes should prompt an immediate consultation with a vascular surgeon.

Lumbar Puncture

PROCEDURE FOR LUMBAR PUNCTURE

1. Put on the mask, protective eyewear, and sterile gloves and prepare all equipment. Assemble the manometer and stopcock, and have the specimen tubes ready for use.
2. Position the patient on his or her side with the knees flexed upwards and the neck flexed forward toward the chest. Palpate both superior iliac crests; draw an imaginary line between the two to identify the L4-5 interspace. Mark the spot with your fingernail or by holding pressure over the site with a pen to mark the spot.
3. Draw up the 1% lidocaine into the 5-mL syringe with the 25-gauge, ½-inch needle.
4. Cleanse and prepare the skin with the iodine solution, starting at the needle site and working outward until a wide sterile field has been prepared. Drape the back.
5. Locate the needle site and administer the 1% lidocaine. First raise a skin wheal, and then infiltrate into the deeper tissues between the spinous processes anticipating the intended track for the spinal needle.[4] Aspirate for blood return before injecting the lidocaine.
6. Hold the spinal needle between the index and middle fingers with one thumb over the stylet and the other thumb stabilizing the needle. Avoid touching the tip and shaft of the needle.
7. Introduce the needle perpendicular to the skin, and advance the needle at an angle of 15 to 20 degrees, directing the needle toward the umbilicus. The bevel of the needle should be up if the patient is in the lateral decubitus position or to the side if the patient is in the sitting position.
8. As the needle is slowly advanced, a distinct "pop" is felt as the needle penetrates through the ligamentum flavum and the arachnoid membrane. If no pop is felt, the stylet should be removed after frequent small advancements to look for CSF return. Advancement too far through the subarachnoid space will result in piercing of the ventral epidural venous plexus, with a subsequent traumatic tap.
9. If bony resistance is encountered, withdraw the needle to the subcutaneous tissue, redirect the needle more caudally, and try again.
10. Once CSF begins to flow, observe the first few drops of fluid. If the CSF is bloody, but it clears after a few drops, the tap was most likely traumatic. If the CSF does not clear the blood clots, replace the stylet, withdraw the needle, and reattempt at a different level. If the CSF does not clear or clot, the patient may have had a subarachnoid hemorrhage and the CSF needs to be checked for cell counts and the presence of xanthochromia.[4] Do not aspirate because a nerve root might become trapped against the needle and cause injury.
11. Measure the opening pressure.
    a. Have the patient carefully straighten the legs to decrease intraabdominal pressure.
    b. Attach the three-way stopcock to the manometer, remove the stylet, and attach the stopcock and manometer to the hub of the needle. The lever of the stopcock should be toward the patient.
    c. Rotate the lever back toward the clinician. The CSF will fill the manometer, and the opening pressure can be measured. Normal pressure is 65 to 195 mm H_2O. If the pressure is elevated, check the patient's position to make sure it is not causing jugular or abdominal compression. CSF pressure should decrease with inspiration and increase with expiration.
12. Fill the specimen tubes with 0.5 to 2 mL per tube. Drain the CSF from the manometer into the first tube. Remove the manometer, and collect the remaining samples.
13. The first tube should be labeled for cell count and differential; the second tube for Gram staining and bacterial culture, the third for glucose and protein tests, and the fourth tube for a repeat cell count and differential or special studies. If further information is necessary, more samples should be obtained.

Continued

PROCEDURE FOR LUMBAR PUNCTURE—CONT'D

14. If therapeutic injection is necessary, inject the solution slowly over 30 seconds after removing at least an equivalent volume of CSF.
15. Replace the manometer and measure the closing pressure.
16. Replace the stylet and remove the needle.
17. Remove residual iodine from the skin, and cover the puncture site with a self-adhesive bandage.

Lumbar puncture (LP) is an important diagnostic procedure that provides cerebrospinal fluid (CSF) from the lumbar subarachnoid space. It is used diagnostically in both emergency and nonemergency situations and is used therapeutically to give medication intrathecally.

Indications

Lumbar puncture is indicated for the following situations:

- Suspected meningitis
- Follow-up of meningitis therapy
- Suspected subarachnoid hemorrhage
- Aid to diagnosis of neurologic diseases (e.g., multiple sclerosis)
- Diagnosis and staging of neoplastic disease
- Intrathecal administration of antimicrobial or antineoplastic agents
- Administration of spinal anesthesia
- Therapeutic reduction of CSF pressure (i.e., pseudotumor cerebri)

Contraindications

Lumbar puncture is contraindicated by the presence of the following:

- Unexplained increased intracranial pressure (papilledema)
- Suspected intracranial mass lesion (e.g., tumor, abscess, hematoma)
- Suspected spinal cord mass lesion
- Local skin infection over the lumbar area
- Bleeding coagulopathy, thrombocytopenia (platelet count <50,000/cm^3) or anticoagulation therapy (relative contraindication)

Equipment

Prepackaged lumbar puncture kits contain all the equipment needed to perform the procedure. The kits should include the following essential items:

- Spinal needles, 22 and 25 gauge, with stylet
- 25-gauge, ½-inch needle
- 22-gauge, 1½-inch needle
- 5-mL syringe
- 1% lidocaine with epinephrine
- Three-way stopcock and manometer
- Sterile collection tubes (minimum of four)
- Sterile towel and barrier
- Sterile gauze sponges
- Mask, protective eyewear, and sterile gloves
- Povidone-iodine solution and materials for skin cleansing
- Self-adhesive bandage

Patient Preparation

Informed written consent is usually required, unless the procedure is an emergency and the patient is confused or lethargic. To reduce anxiety and elicit cooperation, the procedure should be explained fully to the patient before it is begun.

Patient Positioning

Patient positioning is the most important step in performing a successful lumbar puncture. In most cases, the lateral decubitus position should be used. In patients with scoliosis, marked obesity, or ankylosing spondylitis, the sitting position may be more beneficial.

Lateral Decubitus Position

1. Place the patient on his or her side as close to the edge of the bed as possible.
2. The patient should lie in a fetal position with the knees pulled up toward the abdomen and the head flexed forward toward the chest. Forward flexion allows greater access to the interspaces between the spinal processes. An assistant can help support the patient in this position.
3. Put a pillow under the patient's head to keep the spinal axis parallel to the bed.
4. The patient's spine should lie along the edge of the bed, with the bed raised until the spine is at midchest level for the seated clinician.

Sitting Position

1. Have the patient sit on the edge of the bed facing away from the clinician.
2. Have the patient bend over a bedside table with the arms resting on the table and the head, knees, and hips flexed.
3. Raise the bed until the lower lumbar spine is at midchest level for the seated clinician.
4. The sitting position is preferable for obese patients.

Site Selection

The safest site to perform a lumbar puncture is at the L4-5 interspace because the spinal cord terminates between L1-2 for most adults. The L4-5 interspace is also the easiest to identify by drawing an imaginary line between the iliac crest. Although the L4-5 interspace is used most commonly, the L3-4 and L5-S1 interspaces can also be used.

To facilitate locating the landmarks before prepping the skin, mark the skin with a ballpoint pen or an impression from a fingernail. The location of needle entry should be the exact midpoint of the interspace between the spinous processes.

Possible Complications

Several complications of lumbar puncture may occur, such as cerebral herniation, bloody CSF, and spinal headache.

Cerebral Herniation. A mass lesion, cerebral abscess, or increased intracranial pressure could result in cerebellar herniation through the foramen magnum upon removal of CSF. An increase in the intracranial pressure is associated with a change in the patient's mental status and evidence of focal neurologic findings (i.e., a cranial nerve III palsy). When these conditions are suspected, lumbar puncture should be deferred until a more definitive evaluation can be undertaken with a neuroimaging study to avoid precipitating cerebral herniation.

Bloody Cerebrospinal Fluid. Bloody CSF may occur from a traumatic tap or a subarachnoid hemorrhage. A traumatic tap occurs when the spinal needle passes through the subarachnoid space into the ventral epidural plexus. Features that may signify a traumatic tap rather than a previous intracranial bleed are as follows:

- Normal cerebrospinal pressure
- Decline in amount of blood after several tubes have been obtained
- Decline in the red blood cell count in successive tubes
- Absence of xanthochromia
- Subsequent lumbar puncture at higher interspace, showing clear CSF

Spinal Headache. Spinal headaches are the most common complication associated with lumbar punctures and can be seen in approximately 20% of patients. The headache usually develops in the first 24 hours following the procedure. This usually occurs as a result of persistent CSF leakage through the dura, or following the removal of large amounts of CSF. Using the smallest spinal needle possible and prescribing bed rest for 6 to 12 hours after the procedure usually can minimize the risk for headache. Analgesics, bed rest, and oral hydration usually relieve the symptoms.

Follow-up. The patient should be instructed to remain prone for 1 to 3 hours after lumbar puncture to minimize the risk for postpuncture headache. If headache develops, bed rest, oral analgesics, and adequate hydration are indicated. The patient should be instructed to contact a physician if the headache persists. If the headache persists beyond 24 hours despite conservative measures, a blood patch can be performed by an anesthesiologist. A blood patch is performed by slowly injecting 10 to 20 mL of the patient's blood into the epidural space at the original puncture site, effectively sealing any CSF leak. If a therapeutic agent was injected, the patient should be placed in the Trendelenburg position for 30 to 60 minutes after the procedure.

Urethral Catheterization

PROCEDURE FOR URINARY CATHETERIZATION IN MALES

1. Place the patient in a supine position.
2. Put on the mask, protective eyewear, and sterile gloves, and drape the genital area with the sterile towels.
3. Use the antiseptic solution to moisten the cotton swabs with povidone-iodine. Grasp the shaft of the penis with the gloved, nondominant hand, hold it at a 90-degree angle, and retract the foreskin if the patient is uncircumcised. Cleanse the glans from the meatus to the corona of the glans with downward strokes, using a new cotton swab with each stroke.
4. Lubricate the end of the catheter tip with the sterile lubricating jelly. Holding the penis at a 90-degree angle to the body, advance the catheter into the meatus; using gentle pressure, pass the catheter through the urethra and into the bladder until urine returns.
5. If the bladder is markedly distended, it should be drained gradually; generally no more than 1000 mL of urine should be drained at a time.
6. Inflate the balloon with the sterile water. Pull on the catheter gently to ensure that the balloon is in place.
7. For uncircumcised males, be sure to replace the foreskin after the catheter is inserted to avoid constriction.[3]
8. Connect the catheter to the drainage bag. Tape the distal catheter to the inner aspect of the patient's thigh.

Continued

PROCEDURE FOR URINARY CATHETERIZATION IN MALES—CONT'D

9. For patients with an enlarged prostate secondary to benign prostatic hypertrophy, direct instillation of lubricant into the urethra can facilitate passage of the catheter. Additionally, viscous lidocaine may be used to minimize discomfort. Be sure to allow a minimum of 5 minutes after injecting the lidocaine into the urethra for the benefit of the anesthetic.[3]

PROCEDURE FOR URINARY CATHETERIZATION IN FEMALES

1. Place the patient in a supine position with the soles of the feet together.
2. Put on the mask, protective eyewear, and sterile gloves, and drape the genital area with sterile towels.
3. Use the antiseptic packet to moisten the cotton swabs with povidone-iodine. Separate the labia with the gloved, nondominant hand. Cleanse the outside of the labia and the urethral meatus with the swabs. Stroke from anterior to posterior in a downward stroke, using a new cotton swab each time.
4. Lubricate the tip of the catheter with the sterile lubricating jelly. Insert the catheter into the urethral meatus until urine returns, and then advance the catheter another 4 to 5 cm.
5. Collect a urine specimen in the sterile cup, and let the rest of the urine drain into the basin.
6. If the bladder is markedly distended, it should be rained gradually; in general, no more than 1000 mL of urine should be drained at a time.
7. Inflate the balloon with the sterile water. Pull on the catheter gently to ensure that the balloon is in place.
8. Connect the catheter to the drainage bag. Tape the distal catheter to the inner aspect of the patient's thigh.

Indications

The insertion of a Foley catheter through the urethra to the bladder for urinary drainage is a common bedside procedure indicated for treating urinary retention, monitoring urinary output, and performing diagnostic studies.

Contraindications

Urethral disruption secondary to trauma and inability to pass the catheter through the urethra into the urinary bladder are contraindications to the procedure. Suspect a disruption to the urethra with a history of pelvic trauma and evidence of blood at the urethral meatus, the presence of perineal ecchymosis, or if the prostate is nonpalpable on examination.

Equipment

Disposable Foley catheter trays are generally available for use. The essential items are as follows:

- Foley catheter of proper size. Most adults tolerate a 16-French (Fr) or 18-Fr rubber catheter with a 5-mL balloon. (The larger the French number, the larger the diameter.)
- Drainage bag and connecting tube.
- Sterile specimen cup.
- Sterile syringe containing 5 mL of sterile water.
- Sterile lubricating jelly.
- Antiseptic cleansing solution (povidone-iodine) and cotton swabs.
- Emesis basin or small tray to catch urine.
- Sterile towels to drape the area.
- Sterile gloves, mask, and protective eyewear.

Types of Catheters

Robinson Catheter. Also known as a straight catheter, these catheters are designed to be used once for an "in and out" catheterization.

Coudé Catheters. This type of catheter is bent at the distal-most end to allow smoother insertion in patients who have false passages in the urethra.

Foley Catheters. This type of catheter has an inflatable balloon at the end to keep the catheter in place in the bladder.

Patient Preparation

The necessity for catheterization and the procedure itself should be explained to the patient. The female patient should be supine with both legs raised (lithotomy position). The male patient should be supine with legs flat.

Possible Complications

Infections such as cystitis, pyelonephritis, and bacteremia from long-term indwelling catheters can occur. Traumatic catheterization may cause hematuria, as can occur upon creation of a false urethral passage.

Follow-up

Routine Foley catheter care is important. Keep the urethral meatus area clean, and keep the bag below the level of the bladder to prevent gravity drainage of contaminated urine from the tube into the bladder. Removing the catheter as soon as possible will reduce the risk for infection. Make sure to deflate the balloon before removing the catheter.

Nasogastric Intubation

PROCEDURE FOR NASOGASTRIC INTUBATION

1. Put on the gloves, protective eyewear, and gown.
2. Determine the tube length needed by measuring from the patient's ear to the umbilicus, and mark the length on the tube.
3. Lubricate the distal end of the tube with the water-soluble lubricant.
4. With the patient's neck slightly flexed, insert the tube into one of the nostrils, along the nasal floor, and toward the posterior pharynx. When the tip of the tube reaches the back of the throat, resistance is met, and the patient may gag.
5. Have the patient drink small sips of water through a straw, and every time the patient swallows, advance the tube. If the tube slips into the trachea, violent coughing and gagging will occur. Pull the tube back to the level of the pharynx, and repeat the attempt. Do not pull the tube entirely out of the nose. The most important step is timing the advancement of the tube with swallowing.
6. Advance the tube into the stomach. Entry into the stomach can be determined when the measured mark on the tube reaches the opening of the patient's nasal passage.
7. Check for the tube's placement in the stomach by aspirating for stomach contents. Inject air down the tube while listening over the epigastrium for the sound of air bubbling into the stomach. If no sound is heard, reposition the tube and inject more air. Obtain a chest radiograph to confirm correct tube placement.
8. Secure the tube to the nose with tape and benzoin. Avoid pressure to the ala of the nose to prevent skin irritation.[3] The tube should not exert pressure or traction on the nostril when the patient moves.

The insertion of a nasogastric (NG) tube is common in both hospital and ED settings. It is an uncomfortable procedure for most patients.

Indications

NG tubes are inserted to facilitate gastric lavage, for gastrointestinal bleeding, or for treatment of drug overdose, as well as for gastric decompression in association with an ileus or an obstruction.

Contraindications

In semiconscious or fully unconscious patients, NG tube insertion should not be attempted without inserting an endotracheal tube first to prevent aspiration. Massive facial trauma or head trauma with the potential for a basilar skull fracture contraindicates NG intubation. When there is evidence of head or neck injury, obstruction of the nose, throat, or esophagus should be ruled out first. Esophageal burn, such as from the ingestion of corrosive acids or alkali, and esophageal atresia or stricture will also contraindicate insertion of an NG tube.

Equipment

The following equipment should be assembled:

- NG tube of proper diameter. Two types of NG tubes are in common use—the single-lumen tubes (Levin) and the double-lumen sump (Salem's sump) tubes. The single-lumen tubes are best for decompression, and the double-lumen sump tube is best for continuous lavage or irrigation of the stomach. Both may be used for either purpose. Although sizes of catheters range from 10 to 18 Fr, most adults require a 16- to 18-Fr tube. The limiting factor is the size of the nostril or any deviation of the nasal septa.
- Suction syringe (30 mL) with a catheter tip.
- Suction tube and suction device (wall or portable suction).
- Sterile lubricating jelly.
- Glass of water and a straw.
- Emesis basin.
- Disposable latex gloves, goggles, and gown.
- Hypoallergenic tape and benzoin.

Patient Preparation

The procedure should be explained to the patient, especially the fact that introduction of the tube will produce gagging. Ask patients if they have any symptoms of nasal obstruction, and check for nasal patency to determine which side is the most open. The patient should be in a comfortable sitting position and leaning on a backrest. If the patient is unconscious, position supine with the head slightly elevated. It is important that the patient maintain cervical flexion, to enable the entrance to the trachea to be closed when the patient swallows and to allow the tube to enter only the esophagus.

Possible Complications

Accidental placement of the tube into the tracheal airway, aspiration pneumonia, gastric erosion with hemorrhage, and nasal mucosa erosion or alar necrosis may occur with NG intubation. Sinusitis may develop secondary to obstruction of the sinus ostia from the NG tube; not typically seen unless the NG tube has been in place for a prolonged time.

Follow-up

The tube should be checked to ensure proper functioning and should be removed as soon as possible. The tube should be kept lower than the nose. Avoid taping the tube to the forehead because this will cause pressure against the ala of the nose, potentially leading to skin breakdown. Proper taping of the tube and frequent monitoring of the tube placement can prevent this complication. If the tube is left in for an extended period, the nostril should be monitored periodically for signs of necrosis.

CLINICAL APPLICATIONS

1. List the factors that affect wound healing.
2. List the causes of "bad" scars that can result from poor suturing technique.
3. List the equipment needed for each of the following clinical procedures:
   - Phlebotomy
   - Peripheral intravenous catheterization
   - Arterial blood gas sampling
   - Lumbar puncture
   - Urethral catheterization
   - NG intubation

If you were entering a rotation or new job situation in which you would be performing the procedures listed in item 3, how would you develop a reminder system for the equipment needed and the steps of each procedure?

KEY POINTS

- A clear management plan for treating wounds must be in place.
- Wounds, whether intentional (as in a surgical procedure) or accidental, have common attributes and in most cases can be treated the same way.
- Knowing the anatomy before performing any invasive clinical procedure is paramount for the provider and can directly affect the outcome.

References

1. Chen H, Sonnenday CJ. Manual of Common Bedside Surgical Procedures. 2nd ed. Philadelphia: Lippincott Williams & Wilkins, 2000.
2. Dehn RW, Asprey DP. Clinical Procedures for Physician Assistants. Philadelphia: WB Saunders, 2002.
3. Gomella LG, Haist SA. Clinician's Pocket Reference. 11th ed. New York: McGraw Hill, 2007.
4. Lawrence PF. Essentials of General Surgery. 4th ed. Philadelphia: Lippincott Williams & Wilkins, 2006.

The resources for this chapter can be found at www.expertconsult.com.

CHAPTER 12

GENETICS IN PRIMARY CARE

Constance Goldgar • Michael Rackover

CHAPTER CONTENTS

In the "omics" era, expectations are mounting that advances in human genomics and related fields (e.g., transcriptomics, proteomics, metabolomics) will lead to enhanced patient-centered health care and disease prevention (Box 12-1).[1] These discoveries will increasingly have an impact on clinical medicine with important implications for primary care practice. Patients hear about genetic testing in the media and elsewhere and turn to their primary care provider with concerns about their risk for diseases and the appropriateness of genetic testing.[2] Because there are not enough geneticists and genetic counselors to address the burgeoning needs of patients, primary care providers, including physician assistants (PAs), will need to develop skills in case recognition and risk assessment. PAs will also need to assess the value of genetic tests for their patients and be able to communicate risks, benefits, and limitations of genetic tests to enable patients to make informed choices.

For many PAs, the impact of this transformation on medicine is already being experienced and may seem daunting. Given the rapid pace of genomic discovery and the complex nature of the science, we may not think we have adequate knowledge and training to apply these advances to the care of patients and their families. The divide between up-to-date genetics knowledge and practice is extensive for many PA and other providers. The incorporation of genetics into PA educational programs, parallel to what is also seen in medical school and resident training, has lagged behind the advent of genetic applications into clinical practice. And often, when incorporated into curricula, genetics is sidelined as a specialty that still emphasizes Mendelian transmission of disease. Some health professional groups perceive genetics as "science" and "difficult," and anticipation of a scientific rather than a practical, clinical approach can put people off.[6] Genetics literacy among primary care providers needs to be improved to enable their participation in the debate on the hopes and hypes of genomic medicine and to distinguish between useful and useless practical applications in health care.[7]

The Accreditation Review Commission on Education for Physician Assistants (ARC-PA) recognized this education gap in 2006 and mandated teaching "the genetic and molecular mechanisms of health and disease" in all PA programs. This dictum may help our PA students, but what about currently practicing PAs? How do we become genetics savvy? What do we need to know?

The National Coalition for Health Professional Education in Genetics (NCHPEG) has developed tools, resources, and core competencies for all health professionals. NCHPEG[8] has declared that at a minimum, each health care professional should be able to do the following:

- Examine one's competence of practice on a regular basis, identifying areas of strength and areas where professional development related to genetics and genomics would be beneficial
- Understand that health-related genetic information can have important social and psychologic implications for individuals and families.
- Know how and when to make a referral to a genetics professional

BOX 12-1 DEFINITIONS

Transcriptomics—the transcription of genes to produce ribonucleic acid (RNA) is the first stage of gene expression. The transcriptome is the complete set of RNA transcripts produced by the genome at any one time.[3] Unlike the genome, which could be considered "fixed" for a given cell line (excluding mutations), the transcriptome can vary with external environmental conditions and reflects the genes that are being actively expressed at any given time. The transcriptomes of stem cells and cancer cells are of interest to researchers studying carcinogenesis and potential drug targets.

Proteomics—Proteomics studies the structure and function of proteins and refers to all the proteins produced by an organism, much like the genome is the entire set of genes. Proteomic technologies will play an important role in drug discovery, diagnostics, and molecular medicine because of the link among genes, proteins, and disease. Understanding how defective proteins cause particular diseases, for instance, will help development of new drugs that may alter the shape of a defective protein or mimic a missing one.[4]

Metabolomics—Metabolomics detects and quantifies low-molecular-weight molecules, known as metabolites (e.g., antibiotics, carbohydrates, fatty acids, amino acids), produced by active, living cells under different conditions and times in their life cycles.

Metabolic profiling can give an instantaneous snapshot of the physiology of that cell. It is beginning to be used for a variety of health applications: pharmacology, preclinical drug trials, toxicology, transplant monitoring, and newborn screening.[5]

The PA profession, with the help of NCHPEG and the National Human Genome Research Institute, published initial core competencies specific to our profession in 2008.[9] These competencies, which have been further refined by using the structure of the six overarching PA competencies, can be found at the Genetic Genomic Competency Center or G2C2 (see *http://www.g-2-c-2.org/*). The G2C2 is an interprofessional resource that provides links to curricular materials and resources for PA educators, though many of the resources are also applicable to ongoing self-education in genetics for practicing PAs.

GENETIC SKILLS NEEDED IN PRIMARY CARE

Family History

Understanding how to take and interpret a family health history is essential to providing patient care in the era of genomic medicine and has been incorporated into many competency recommendations.[8] The family history has long been used to detect familial transmission of single-gene disorders, but its use in uncovering genetic, environmental, and lifestyle attributes shared within a family has made it a critical tool for risk assessment of common multifactorial disorders such as cardiovascular disease, cancer, and mental illness. A properly taken family history helps to inform diagnosis, ascertain risk status, and change management (e.g., determine who might benefit from genetic testing, make a referral, or institute preventive measures). The family history has other important clinical attributes that augment patient-centered care—it helps build rapport with patients; family relationships and dynamics graphically emerge; and family education, support, and service needs become more apparent. Its role is recognized as being so important that public service announcements have been created, aimed at engaging the U.S. public in understanding how their family history can be used to guide health care decision-making.[10]

Among the ways to collect a family history, the most efficient is a pedigree. This graphic representation of the family history can be a time-saving, inexpensive diagnostic and screening tool. Many clinicians write out the family history in various levels of depth and detail in textual form. However, once a clinician is used to taking a pedigree, it usually requires less time than writing out text, is easier to review later, and is often more concise and specific.[11] The pedigree allows patterns of disease, if they exist, to be identified more readily. It is a record that can be easily updated or built on over several visits. Pedigrees have internationally standardized symbols that have been in use since 1995. Figure 12-1 displays common pedigree symbols and nomenclature.

A comprehensive family history includes at least three generations. One usually begins the family history with the patient's health history and then extends to questions about siblings, parents, and children. If the patient is young, grandparents should be included. Questions about relatives should include information found in Tables 12-1 and 12-2. NCHPEG has developed a Microsoft PowerPoint slide set (*http://www.nchpeg.org/*) to assist health care providers in creating a standardized pedigree, identifying

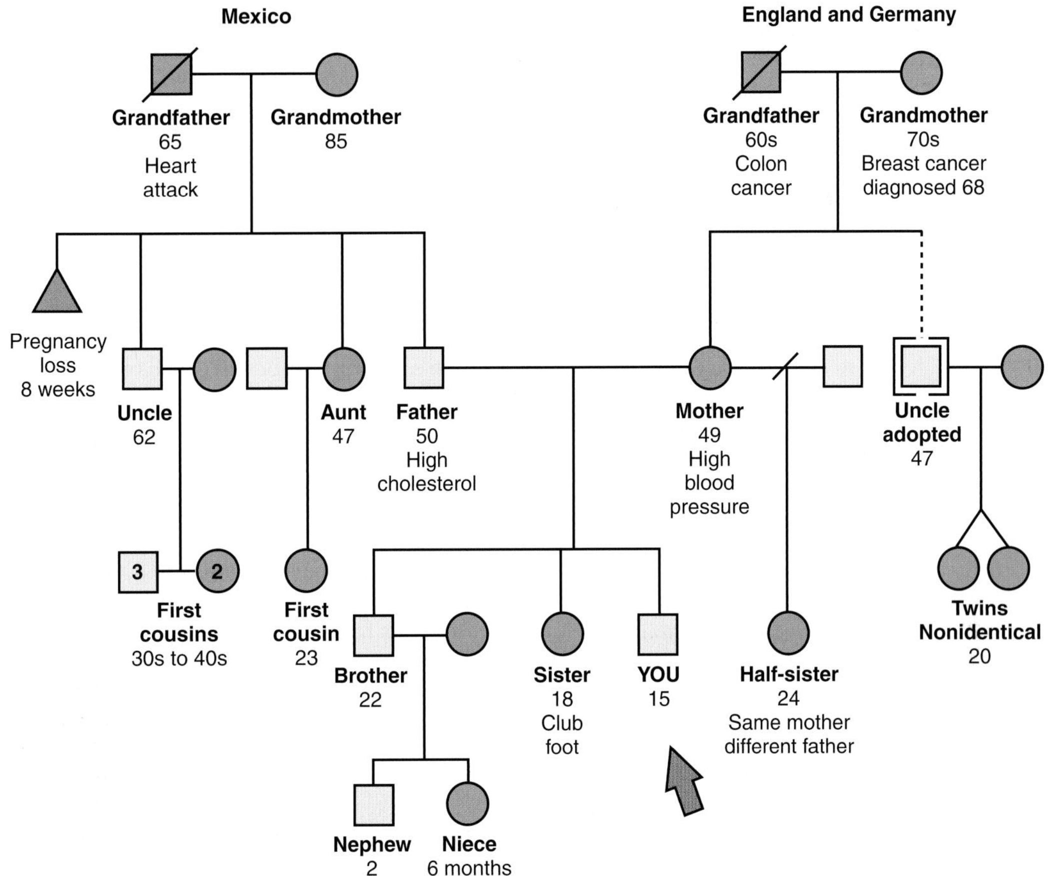

FIGURE 12-1 Example of pedigree with standardized symbols.[19]

risk in a pedigree, and also provides other practical family history tools.[12]

Barriers do exist to taking and recording a family pedigree. Limited training, comfort level in genetics, and lack of time and reimbursement may limit its use. Providers are also hesitant to incorporate family history assessment into clinical decision-making because there are questions about clinical utility and reliability of the information.[13] Some of these barriers are currently being addressed with different solutions.

To promote the use of family history as a screening tool for disease prevention and health promotion, several initiatives, including those from the U.S. Surgeon General, have called for the use of self-administered family history collection tools to help clinicians interpret and apply family history information to patient care. The U.S. Surgeon General's website for family history, My Family Health Portrait (MFHP, *https://familyhistory.hhs.gov*), has been updated several times since its launch in 2004. It is

TABLE 12-1 Typical Information Obtained in Three-Generation Pedigree

Name
Age or year of birth (date of birth is preferable, if known)
Age at death and cause of death
Ethnic background of each grandparent
Relevant health information (see Table 12-2)
Relevant symptoms and/or diagnoses and age at diagnosis (if known)
Information regarding pregnancies including infertility, spontaneous abortions, stillbirths, and pregnancy complications
Developmental delay and learning disabilities
Dysmorphic features/congenital anomalies
Consanguinity issues
Date and write your name legibly on the pedigree together with an explanation of any abbreviations.

From Rich EC, Burke W, Heaton CJ, et al. Reconsidering the family history in primary care. J Gen Intern Med 2004; 19:273.

TABLE 12-2 **Relevant Health Information to Inquire about When Collecting Family History Data**

Alcohol abuse	Drug abuse
Allergies	Emphysema
Alzheimer disease or dementia	Epilepsy or seizurs
Anemia	Glaucoma
Asthma	Hearing loss
Arthritis	Heart trouble
Birth defects or malformations	Hemochromatosis or "iron overload"
Any cancer	High blood pressure
Breast cancer	Infertility
Ovarian cancer	Kidney trouble (renal disease)
Uterine cancer	Memory loss/Alzheimer disease
Lung cancer	Mental illness
Colon or rectal cancer	Mental retardation
Prostate cancer	Multiple miscarriages
Thyroid cancer	Neurofibromatosis
Brain cancer	Obesity
Melanoma	Osteoporosis or "hip fracture"
Other cancer	Phenylketonuria or "metabolic" disease at birth
High cholesterol	Sickle cell anemia
Chronic infections	Smoking
Clotting or bleeding problems	Stillborn/Infant death
Depression	Stroke
Diabetes mellitus	Violence/Domestic abuse
Down syndrome	Other:_____________

From March of Dimes "Genetics and Your Practice." Family History. *http://www.marchofdimes.com/gyponline/.* Accessed July 28, 2011.

designed to make family health information easy to gather, easy to share, and ready for enhanced use in an electronic health record (EHR) environment. The 2009 version allows information to be shared electronically by the consumer with family members and providers, creating a more robust family health history record.[14]

Facio and colleagues[15] recently assessed the ability of MFHP to collect accurate family history data for six common heritable disorders. The study validated use of MFHP for four common conditions: diabetes and colon, breast, and ovarian cancer. The tool performed less well for coronary artery disease and stroke. The data suggest that MFHP is a valid tool for the initial collection of family history information, which then can be incorporated into the EHR to aid busy primary care clinicians interested in more efficiently identifying and managing risk of common chronic conditions.

In addition to the MFHP, structured questionnaires for patients to complete before a visit may make family history collection more efficient and useful. Several websites (Table 12-3) provide validated questionnaires for various types of clinical encounters. For example, the March of Dimes and American Medical Association sites have separate forms for adult, pediatric, and prenatal visits.

Other efforts are under way to help address providers' concerns. The EHR should allow family history information to be incorporated more efficiently. Optimally, pedigree construction and family history risk assessment will be part of EHR software development. Understanding the scientific foundation of family history is important if clinical decision aids (based on the information) are to be useful to clinicians and persons in typical practice settings and in improving clinical outcomes.[13] There remains a need for tools that automate and streamline the acquisition and interpretation of family history data because increased use of this information will help define health risks for patients.

A pedigree is an important instrument for genetic diagnosis and research. It can be used to establish possible patterns of inheritance and diagnosis of a condition. It may also be useful in demonstrating familial variation in disease expression (e.g., variable age at onset, variable disease severity). The pedigree will also help the provider determine who might benefit from genetic testing. Its usefulness will continue to develop in tandem with the growing spectrum of molecular, bioinformatics, and proteomic tools.[16]

Table 12-3 provides useful websites for family history and pedigree construction for the patient and the clinician. Self-administered forms still need to be reviewed with the patient to verify information, clarify the data recorded, and allow an opportunity for questions.

Risk Assessment

The systematic collection and interpretation of family history information is still the most appropriate screening approach to identify increased genetic risk or susceptibility. A comprehensive family history can reveal increased risk factors for common disorders that may not have been suspected. Specific cancers, heart disease, and type 2 diabetes mellitus are examples of common conditions identified in a family history. The pedigree may indicate increased risk of disease (e.g., by showing a single affected first-degree relative). If multiple family members are affected in several generations or have common disease with earlier than expected onset, this may indicate a "red flag" for significant genetic contribution to a disease

TABLE 12-3 Websites That Aid Pedigree Construction for Clinicians and Patients

Website	Tools Available
U.S. Surgeon General's Family History Initiative *http://www.hhs.gov/familyhistory/*	Patients can use tool to organize family history information to print out or to be saved on their own computer. Available in English or Spanish versions.
March of Dimes *http://www.marchofdimes.com/gyponline/index.bm2*	Provides guidelines for collecting and recording family history. The "Family Health History Form" is downloadable (pdf), as are the AMA forms.
American Medical Association *http://www.ama-assn.org/ama/pub/category/2380.html*	Three downloadable forms (pdf) are available for adult, pediatric, and prenatal clinic encounters.
Centers for Disease Control and Prevention (CDC) *http://www.cdc.gov/genomics/famhistory/resources/tools.htm*	Contains links to multiple sites for family history resources and tools.

All sites active and accurate as of July 2, 2012.

TABLE 12-4 Recognizing Familial Risk (Genetic Red Flags)

- Family history of known genetic disorder
- Multiple affected family members with same or related disorders
- Developmental delay or mental retardation
- Features suggestive of a genetic or chromosome syndrome
- Unexplained infertility or pregnancy losses
- Significant family history of cancer
- Earlier age at onset of disease than expected
  - Breast, ovarian, and endometrial cancer <50 yr (premenopausal)
  - Colon and prostate cancer <50 yr
  - Stroke and noninsulin-dependent diabetes <50 yr
  - Dementia <60 yr
  - Coronary artery disease <55 yr in males and <65 yr in females
- Sudden cardiac death in a person who seemed healthy
- Multifocal or bilateral occurrence in paired organs
- More severe phenotype including multifocal disease
- Ethnicity associated with certain genetic disorders
- Disease in the less-often-affected sex (e.g., breast cancer in a male)

TABLE 12-5 General Guidelines for Risk Stratification

High Risk

- Premature disease in a first-degree relative (sibling, parent, or child)
- Premature disease in a second-degree relative (coronary artery disease only)
- Two affected first-degree relatives
- One first-degree relative with late or unknown disease onset and an affected second-degree relative with premature disease from the same lineage
- Two second-degree maternal or paternal relatives with at least one having premature onset of disease
- Three or more affected maternal or paternal relatives
- Presence of a "moderate-risk" family history on both sides of the pedigree

Moderate Risk

- One first-degree relative with late or unknown onset of disease
- Two second-degree relatives from the same lineage with late or unknown disease onset

Average Risk

- No affected relatives
- Only one affected second-degree relative from one or both sides of the pedigree
- No known family history
- Adopted person with unknown family history

Modified from Scheuner MT, Wang SJ, Raffel LJ, et al. Family history: a comprehensive genetic risk assessment method for the chronic conditions of adulthood. Am J Med Genet 1997;71:315.

with possible high risk for other family members. Red flags that may indicate increased genetic risk are numerous and may vary according to the age and need of the patient. The March of Dimes "Genetics and Your Practice" website resource divides red flags into prenatal, pediatric, and adolescent/adult.[17] Table 12-4 lists commonly recognized genetic red flags across the lifespan.

Once the provider determines that the family history shows an individual to be at risk for a genetic or familial condition, can the provider assign a degree of risk (Table 12-5)? The next steps are to decide what genetic testing or screening, preventive or surveillance measures, or other medical management options are available to help the patient (Table 12-6). At this time it is crucial that the provider understand his or her limitations with regard to clinical genetic applications. At any step along the process, the provider needs to self-assess abilities to know when to seek help or refer.

For instance, if the provider determines that an individual's genetic risk for health complications or disease is moderate to high, it is crucial for the provider to

TABLE 12-6 **Actions to Take on the Basis of Genetic Risk Stratification**

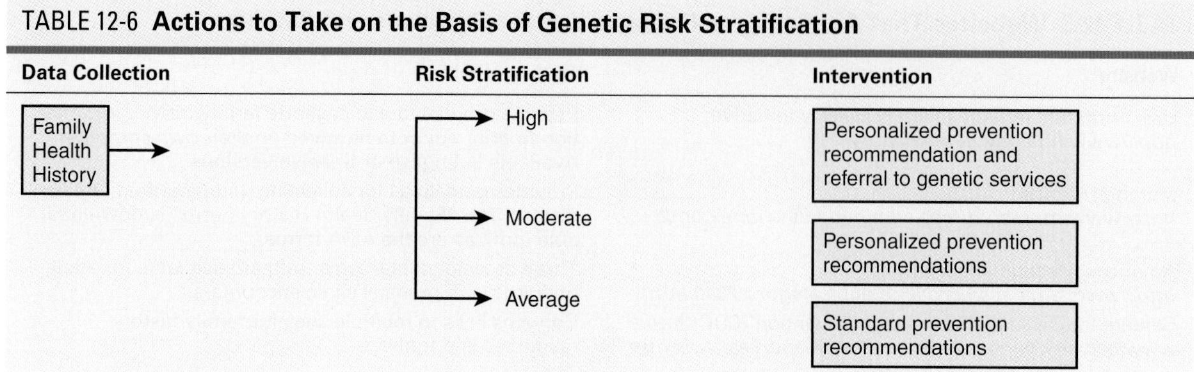

Modified from Scheuner MT, Wang SJ, Raffel LJ, et al. Family history: a comprehensive genetic risk assessment method for the chronic conditions of adulthood. Am J Med Genet 1997;71:315 and Khoury MJ, Gwinn M, Yoon PW, et al. The continuum of translation research in genomic medicine: how can we accelerate the appropriate integration of human genome discoveries into health care and disease prevention? Genet Med 2007;9(10):665.

understand how to communicate that information to the patient so that it is understood. The information could be as simple as the nature or results of a biochemical test for cholesterol or as complex as informed consent for genetic testing for neurofibromatosis in a toddler. With the communication and testing of genetic risk comes the potential for additional risk (and the need for confidentiality) for other family members, including minors, who may share that genetic heritage. It is important to be mindful of the psychosocial and legal implications of such information (e.g., anxiety, depression, relief, discrimination, stigmatization, preservation of family integrity, undisclosed adoption, nonpaternity, duty to warn, duty to recontact). There will likely be a need for referral to genetic services for further education and counseling or for consideration of genetic testing or evaluation.

The clinician should use knowledge of the patient's risk to guide management, including preventive recommendations and surveillance that may reduce the occurrence of premature illness and death. Evidence-based guidelines have begun to emerge that help direct providers to specific evaluation modalities and interventions, as well as potential surveillance, based on identified genetic risk. Failure to identify clinically significant family histories denies patients access to specialty and support services for those at risk or affected by a disease that has genetic components. In addition, failure to consider other at-risk relatives limits this tool's potential benefits and impact on public health.

Resources for information about genetic tests and genetic counselors is available in many reliable and valid resources (Table 12-7). It is most advantageous for primary care providers to develop relationships with genetic professionals in their area for ease of consultation.

Referral and Counseling Process

The clinician may consider referral to a genetic specialist or genetic counselor at many points along the continuum of patient management, depending on the comfort and knowledge level of the provider. Trained genetics practitioners include medical geneticists, genetic counselors, and genetic nurses. Genetic specialists help to identify the appropriate tests to order (genetic or additional laboratory tests), consider the family history in detail, and provide information about the treatment and long-term outcomes for patients diagnosed with a genetic disorder, including recommendations to other medical specialists. Often, the role of the genetic counselors/genetic nurses is to provide the bulk of information gathering, risk assessment, and counseling. Medical geneticists make the diagnoses. Genetic services are most often offered as part of a multidisciplinary evaluation in a specialty clinic and often are located in large academic medical centers.

Diagnosis of a genetic disorder can have a profound impact on the patient and the family members. It is clear that aside from the need for medical and genetic information, families affected by genetic disorders often need help coping with the emotional, psychologic, medical, social, and economic consequences of the diagnosis. In particular, psychologic issues such as denial, anxiety, anger, grief, guilt, or blame are addressed and, when necessary, referrals for in-depth counseling are offered. Comprehension, retention, and personal perception of the detailed level of information communicated about a genetic diagnosis are often overwhelming tasks for patients. Genetic services, therefore, generally are better provided over a series of visits.

TABLE 12-7 **Reliable and Valid Electronic Genetic Resources for Clinicians**

Database	Description
GeneTests GeneReviews *http://www.genetests.org/*	Comprehensive information on genetic testing and genetic counseling; includes educational materials on genetic testing, genetics consultation, genetic cases, etc.
March of Dimes *http://www.marchofdimes.com/gyponline*	Many resources for providers, as well as patient education materials; offers an interactive online genetics information website (Genetics & Your Practice)
Centers for Disease Control and Prevention (CDC) *http://www.cdc.gov/genomics/famhistory/index.htm*	Many genetic/genomic resources for patients and providers including links to other resources; public health genomics
Genetic Alliance *www.geneticalliance.org*	Offers information on genetic conditions and issues related to genetic conditions, including support services for families
Online Mendelian Inheritance in Man (OMIM) *www.ncbi.nlm.nih.gov/entrez/query.fcgi?db=OMIM*	An electronic catalog of human genes and genetic disorders; a comprehensive though complex source of information
National Human Genome Research Institute (NHGRI) *www.genome.gov*	Provides information on human genome project, genetic and/or rare diseases research, genetic/rare conditions, patient support groups, etc.
Genetics Home Reference *http://ghr.nlm.nih.gov/ghr/template/Home.vm*	A service of the National Library of Medicine that provides consumer-friendly information about the effects of genetic variations on human health

All sites active and accurate as of July 2, 2012.

Attempts to help families cope with these varied needs created a model of genetic education and counseling—genetic counseling. Genetic counselors work as part of a health care team, providing information and support to families affected by or at risk of a genetic disorder. They help to identify families at possible risk of a genetic disorder, gather and analyze family history and inheritance patterns, calculate risks of recurrence, and provide information about genetic testing and related procedures. In particular, genetic counselors can help families understand the significance of genetic disorders in the context of cultural, personal, and familial situations. Genetic counselors also provide supportive counseling services, serve as patient advocates, and refer individuals and families to other health professionals and community or state support services. They serve as a central resource of information about genetic disorders for other health care professionals, patients, and the general public.[18] For more information about genetic counseling or to find a genetic counselor in your area, please see the National Society of Genetic Counselors website at *http://www.nsgc.org*.

Genetic Testing

A PA may decide to evaluate a patient with a suspected genetic disorder by using evidence-based guidelines to order a genetic or biochemical test. Alternatively, depending on the complexity of the case, genetic testing may be done after referral to genetic services.

Genetic testing includes a variety of methods used to analyze human DNA, RNA, chromosomes, proteins, or certain metabolites. Genetic testing may be classified as molecular, biochemical, cytogenetic, or some combination of these techniques[19] (Table 12-8).

Genetic testing can be applied in a variety of contexts, including clinical diagnosis in individuals with symptoms and prognosis, population screening, determination of future disease risks in asymptomatic individuals, prenatal diagnosis and screening, tissue analysis for acquired mutations, pharmacogenomic testing, forensic testing, toxicogenomic testing, research, and heritage testing.[20]

Special consideration is required when ordering genetic tests, beyond that of other laboratory tests. For example, genetic tests can be used in asymptomatic individuals to identify a future risk of disease, a mutation that confers a potential risk to an unborn child, or the presence of an active disease process. Genetic testing may disclose information that has significance for both the individual and other members of the family.

As genes and genetic factors are identified for a growing number of inherited disorders, common disorders, and drug-related responses, genetic testing will become more realistic and play an increasingly important role in medicine.

TABLE 12-8 Genetic Testing Techniques

Type	Definition	Example
Molecular Testing		
Direct deoxyribonucleic acid (DNA) testing (mutation and sequence analysis)	Detects specific DNA mutations (mutation analysis); most informative when there are a limited number of disease-causing mutations existing in the gene being studied	Cystic fibrosis, *BRCA1*, fragile X
Linkage analysis	Traces markers physically close to the gene of interest in a family; requires testing multiple family members; costly and time consuming	May be used preliminarily; hemophilia B
Chromosome Analysis		
Karyotype	An organized microscopic profile of a person's chromosomes that is used to evaluate their size, shape, and number	Trisomy 21 (aneuploidy) or Williams syndrome (deletion)
Fluorescence in situ hybridization (FISH)	Involves applying DNA probes to a chromosome spread; the labeled probes can be used to identify different chromosomes or targeted chromosome regions to help recognize abnormalities	Trisomies, translocations, or deletions not visible with use of a microscope
Biochemical		
	Evaluate the products of gene function, such as metabolites or enzymes; usually chemicals that circulate in plasma, urine, or amniotic fluid	Phenylketonuria (PKU), familial hypercholesterolemia
Protein Product Testing		
Gene product analysis	Analyze the product of a specific gene that may be the translated protein (or transcribed RNA); measurement of enzyme activity addresses functionality of the gene producing the enzyme	Tay-Sachs, Gaucher disease

Types of Genetic Testing

Prenatal testing is performed to provide information about the fetus. This type of testing includes multiple marker screening, fetal nuchal translucency measurement, fetal ultrasound, chromosome evaluation from amniocentesis, chorionic villus biopsy, or fetal blood sampling. Quadruple screening is usually performed between 15 and 17 weeks' gestation to assess risk for fetal anomalies, including open neural tube defects, abdominal wall defects, Down syndrome, and trisomy 18.

Newborn screening is done to detect specific disorders whose associated morbidity and mortality can be reduced if detected and treated early. Every state screens for or will soon be screening for at least 30 conditions, and some states screen for up to 57. When a screening test result is positive, diagnostic testing is usually required to confirm or specify the results, and counseling is offered to educate the parents. Phenylketonuria (PKU) is an example: It occurs at relatively high frequency in some populations, is easily detectable, and is readily treatable by dietary modification.

Diagnostic testing is performed when a fetus, child, or adult has clinical findings suggestive of a genetic disorder. The purpose of testing is to confirm or rule out a diagnosis in a symptomatic individual, similar to any other diagnostic laboratory study. An example would be hemoglobin electrophoresis in the evaluation of a sickle cell diagnosis.

Predictive testing is used to identify asymptomatic individuals who are at increased risk to develop a particular genetic disorder at some point later in life. Most commonly, predictive genetic testing is undertaken because there is a known or suspected family history of an adult-onset condition. Huntington disease, an autosomal dominant condition with adult onset, is an example of where predictive testing could be used.

Presymptomatic testing (also called *susceptibility* or *predispositional testing*) is for diseases where subsequent development of symptoms is likely, but not certain, when the gene mutation is present. Results from predictive testing do not always indicate that the disease will definitively occur (even with a positive result) or remain absent (even with a negative result). This type of testing does not provide a yes-or-no answer for developing a disease, but rather a change of the initial risk. For example, a woman who tests positive for a *BRCA1* gene mutation has a 55% to 85% risk for developing breast cancer by age 70.[21] In contrast, 7% of all women in the United States will develop breast cancer by the age of 70. Thus, a woman with a *BRCA1* mutation would have a 15% to

45% chance of *not* developing breast cancer by age 70 despite having this mutation. This information may be useful in a patient's decision about treatment choices and lifestyle adjustments.

Preimplantation testing is performed on early embryos resulting from in vitro fertilization to assess whether a particular serious genetic condition exists in the fetus; it provides an alternative to prenatal diagnosis and termination of affected pregnancies.

Carrier screening is used to identify individuals who are at increased risk to have a child with a genetic disorder because the individual carries a mutation for a recessive disorder. Individuals who are carriers of recessive conditions are generally unaffected themselves because they have one normally functioning copy of a gene and one copy that carries the mutation (genes typically come in pairs, with the exception of genes carried on the sex chromosomes in males). Carriers are most commonly unaware of their status.

Pharmacogenomic testing is available for portions of the population who carry genetic variants (polymorphisms) that affect their response to various drugs. Many relevant polymorphisms have been identified, and tests for some of them are available. Warfarin is but one example of drugs affected by the cytochrome p450 enzyme system. Warfarin is metabolized by the CYP2C9 enzyme. More than 100 therapeutic drugs are metabolized by CYP2C9, including drugs with a narrow therapeutic index such as warfarin, where the relationship between drug dosage and a patient's genetic status for the *CYP2C9* gene can affect metabolism by either inhibiting or inducing the enzyme. This can lead to either toxicity or, alternatively, lack of response at normal therapeutic doses for a plethora of important common medications (e.g., losartan, glipizide, phenytoin). The p450 system includes a "superfamily" of CYPs, the major enzymes involved in drug metabolism, and accounts for approximately 75% of the total Constantin metabolism.[22]

Besides being familiar with the unique nature and types of genetic testing, there are several questions the clinician needs to address before ordering genetic tests (Table 12-9). Haddow and Palomaki[23] developed a rubric, further refined by the Centers for Disease Control, to help clinicians determine the validity and reliability of genetic testing as the evidence base for clinical genetic applications develops. The ACCE framework, which takes its name from the four main criteria for evaluating a genetic test—Analytic validity, Clinical validity, Clinical utility, and associated Ethical, legal, and social implications (ELSI)—is a model process that includes collecting, evaluating, interpreting, and reporting data about DNA (and related) testing for disorders with a genetic component in a format that allows policy makers to have access to up-to-date and reliable information for decision-making.

Direct-to-consumer (DTC) genetic testing looks at individual single nucleotide polymorphisms, or SNPs (pronounced "snips"), to detect whether the individual who requested the test is at increased risk for a number of diseases. DTC tests are typically advertised and sold over the Internet without the involvement of an independent health care provider. After the company performs the test, it sends a test report to the consumer, informing him or her of the risk for a number of conditions. DTC genetic testing is controversial despite its having gained prominence over the past several years. Proponents of DTC testing cite benefits that include increased consumer access to testing, greater consumer autonomy and empowerment, and enhanced privacy of the information obtained. Critics of DTC genetic testing have pointed to the risks that consumers will choose testing without adequate context or counseling, will receive tests from laboratories of dubious quality, and will be misled by unproven claims of benefit.[20] The American Society of Human Genetics has recommended transparency, provider education, and increased regulation of test and laboratory quality, as well as additional research to protect consumers from potential harm.[24]

Advances in genetic research and expansion of genetic tests currently available place increased responsibility on the provider's shoulders. To meet this challenge, providers will need to consider the range of uses of genetic testing, including diagnosis in symptomatic and asymptomatic people (predictive testing), risk assessment, reproductive decision-making, and population screening. The number of

TABLE 12-9 Practical Steps for Critically Using Genetic Tests in Clinical Practice

1. Clearly define the information you hope to obtain from the test.
2. What is the most appropriate test for this clinical situation?
3. Is a reliable test available?
4. What information does the laboratory need?
5. Is the client fully informed about the benefits and limitations of the test?
6. What do you do with the results?

Modified from Constantin CM, Faucett A, Lubin IM. A primer on genetic testing. J Midwifery Womens Health 2005;50:197.

CASE STUDY 12-1

Diane is a 28-year-old female who presents for a first appointment and inquires about a prescription for oral contraceptives. She states that she read an advertisement about a birth control pill that helps "control acne."

The patient's past medical history is remarkable for an allergy to penicillin and a tonsillectomy at age 5. The patient smokes "socially" and has a 5-pack-year history.

The patient's past medical history is remarkable for a sister who had a "blood clot" while she was pregnant and a maternal aunt who had a "DVT" (deep vein thrombosis). Additionally, the patient's mother has adult-onset diabetes mellitus and has had three miscarriages, but medical information about these occurrences is not available. The patient's maternal grandmother is alive and well and in her late 80s. The patient's maternal grandfather died in his late 70s of congestive heart failure. The patient's father is 65 years old and in good health. Medical information about his family is not available.

The patient was advised that she was not a candidate for oral contraceptives because of her family history of "blood clots." Further evaluation revealed that the patient carried one factor V Leiden gene. This family history is an example of an inherited thrombophilia that follows an autosomal dominant pattern of inheritance (Figure 12-2).

common conditions for which predictive genetic tests are available is increasing rapidly. Some of these are valid and useful in carefully selected circumstances (e.g., several cancer syndromes, hemochromatosis, or factor V Leiden–associated thromboembolism). Other tests may be clinically available, but clinical utility and predictive value have been generally poor (e.g., ApoE analysis for Alzheimer disease). Most problematic are the laboratories that offer predictive genomic panels (often directly to the consumer) to assess risk for such outcomes as cardiovascular disease, osteoporosis, poor nutritional status, and mental health conditions, without an appropriate evidence base.

Ultimately, the clinical value of testing will depend on interventions that are both effective and sufficiently safe to merit use in reducing risk. Otherwise, knowledge about genetic susceptibility would create a potential stigma without compensatory health benefit and might even produce harm by reducing the motivation to pursue risk-reducing measures.[25]

FUTURE

Genomic medicine promises predictive, preemptive, participatory, and personalized health care.[26] To achieve this goal, it must be translated into the mindset and daily routine of health care delivery on the

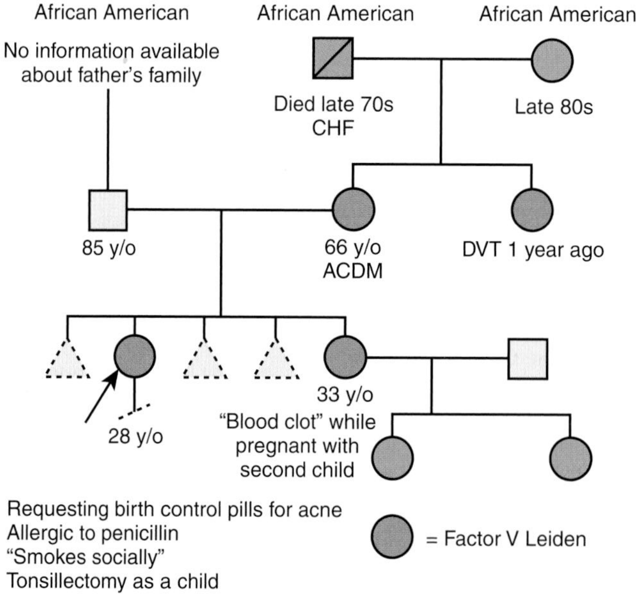

FIGURE 12-2 Patient pedigree for Case Study 12-1.

part of patient and provider.[27] As genetic information becomes a more integral part of medical practice, primary care providers will play an increasing role in the demand of managing genetic information. We must not miss the opportunity to be on the vanguard in preparing to meet this demand and to help predict and mitigate the effects of medical predispositions for the individual and for their future generations.

Discussion

Forty percent of individuals younger than the age of 50 who are admitted for a thrombotic episode have an identifiable, inherited thrombophilia. Factor V Leiden is one of several inherited thrombophilias. An individual who carries one copy of the factor V Leiden gene (heterozygote) has a seven-fold greater increase of having a thrombotic episode than an individual in the general population. If an individual carries two copies of the factor V Leiden gene (homozygote), then he or she has an 80 times greater chance of having a thrombotic episode. Factor V Leiden disorder exhibits a *gene dosage* effect, which means that one copy of the gene may cause clinical problems, and two copies of the gene are even more likely to cause clinical problems. Although testing for Factor V Leiden, either for that mutation alone or in concert with other inherited thrombophilias, was done on this patient, the family history alone provides sufficient significant information for management.

Knowing that an individual has a genetic risk or predisposition means that environmental factors can be modified. In this instance, the patient can be advised not to use oral contraceptives, not to smoke, and to seek medical advice before becoming pregnant.[28]

CASE STUDY 12-2

Mark is a 42-year-old male whom you have seen for several urgent care visits over the past 2 years. He presents at this visit for a routine history and physical examination. He has no current complaints, and his personal medical history is significant for an arthroscopy of his right knee at age 23 for "torn cartilage." He has a remote 10-pack-year history of smoking but quit 9 years ago. He drinks alcohol moderately. He has begun jogging only recently because of gradual weight gain over the past few years. A family history reveals that his father had a "heart attack" and died in his early 50s. He has one sibling, a brother aged 47, who was diagnosed with angina this year. The patient's paternal grandmother, in her late 80s, is alive and well. The paternal grandfather died in his mid-60s of "a heart condition." His mother, aged 69, has moderate osteoarthritis but is otherwise healthy (Figure 12-3).

On physical examination, his height is 5′11″ and weight is 190 lb (body mass index [BMI] 26.5). His blood pressure is 140/90. Laboratory evaluation shows that his total cholesterol is 242; LDL 164, HDL 42, and triglycerides 180. On the basis of the data you have collected, you determine Mark's Framingham Risk Score (FRS) to be 8.3% (without factoring in a strong family history of premature coronary artery disease [CAD]). Using the QRISK2 Cardiovascular Risk Score from the United Kingdom,[29] which incorporates family history, ethnicity, comorbidities, and other factors, a risk calculation of 13% is shown. You decide to search for an evidence-based guideline to determine potential further evaluation and primary prevention for your patient.

Discussion

This case demonstrates a significant and premature history of CAD. Most notable are the facts that the patient's father had a fatal myocardial infarction (MI) in his early 50s and his brother was diagnosed with angina at age 47. Although we may not know the cause of his father's MI, the pattern of transmission in this family is consistent with an autosomal dominant pattern of CAD, but shared environmental factors would certainly be factors to consider in counseling the patient.

A search of the National Guideline Clearinghouse using the term "coronary artery disease" yielded a joint evidence-based guideline from the American College of Cardiology Foundation/American Heart Association Task Force (2010) on assessment of cardiovascular risk in asymptomatic adults.[30] See Tables 12-10 and 12-11 for excerpted recommendations pertinent to this patient case.

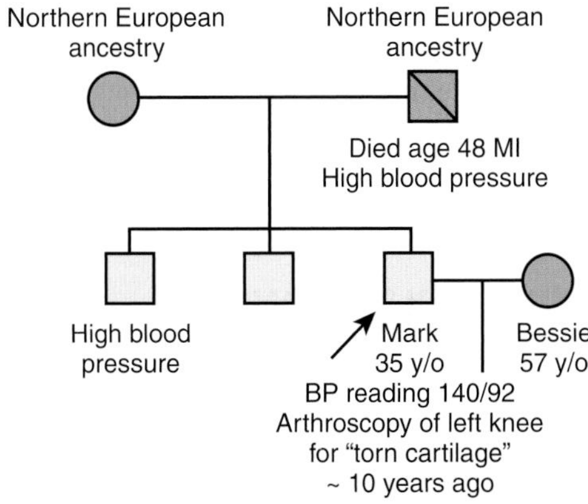

FIGURE 12-3 Patient pedigree for Case Study 12-2.

TABLE 12-10 **Recommendations for Further Assessment of Cardiovascular Risk in Asymptomatic Adults**

Recommendation	Level of Evidence
Evaluation with global risk scores (e.g., FRS) to target preventive interventions	B
Gathering family history of atherothrombotic cardiovascular disease (CVD) for cardiovascular risk assessment in all asymptomatic adults	B
Measurement of a standard fasting lipid profile, but measuring lipid parameters, including lipoproteins, apolipoproteins, particle size, and density is *not* recommended	C
Genotype testing for coronary heart disease risk assessment in asymptomatic adults is *not* currently recommended	B
Measurement of natriuretic peptides (e.g., brain natriuretic peptide) is *not* recommended	B
In asymptomatic high-risk adults, measurement of CRP is *not* recommended for cardiovascular risk assessment	B

Adapted from Greenland P, Alpert JS, Beller GA, et al. American College of Cardiology Foundation, American Heart Association. 2010 ACCF/AHA guideline for assessment of cardiovascular risk in asymptomatic adults: a report of the American College of Cardiology Foundation/American Heart Association Task Force on Practice Guidelines. J Am Coll Cardiol 2010;56:e50.

As you problem solve Mark's case, you consider the benefit/harm/cost of the recommendations for determining his baseline risk and potential surveillance according to current evidence. The patient is counseled that because of his family history, he should pay close attention to this condition and work with the health care team to address lifestyle factors that will help decrease his risk. Mark is asked to find out the exact cause, if possible, of his father's MI because this information may affect his treatment.

This case demonstrates that even when genetic testing is not available or necessarily recommended, family medical history is useful in helping ascertain risk and management for primary prevention of CAD.

CLINICAL APPLICATIONS

1. Research and write your family pedigree. Would analysis of your pedigree result in changes in your own health risk behaviors?
2. If you were the PA in Case Study 12-1, how would you counsel Diane about the risks of oral contraceptives? What alternatives could be offered?
3. If you were the PA in Case Study 12-2, how would you counsel Mark about his risk of cardiovascular disease? What modifications in his lifestyle would be recommended? What baseline risk measurements and surveillance would you use?

TABLE 12-11 **Recommendations for Cardiac and Vascular Tests for Risk Assessment in Asymptomatic Adults**

Recommendation	Level of Evidence
A resting electrocardiogram (ECG) is reasonable for cardiovascular risk assessment in asymptomatic adults with hypertension or diabetes.	C
Measurement of carotid intima-media thickness (IMT) on ultrasound is reasonable in asymptomatic adults at intermediate risk.	B
Measurement of Ankle-Brachial Index (ABI) is reasonable in asymptomatic adults at intermediate risk.	B
An exercise ECG may be considered in intermediate-risk asymptomatic adults.	B
Stress echocardiography is *not* indicated in low- or intermediate-risk asymptomatic adults.	B
Measurement of computed tomography for coronary calcium (CAC) is reasonable for asymptomatic adults at low to intermediate risk (i.e., 6%-10% and 10%-20% 10-year risk).	B
Stress myocardial perfusion imaging (MPI) may be considered for advanced cardiovascular risk assessment in asymptomatic adults with diabetes or asymptomatic adults with a strong family history of coronary heart disease	C
Coronary computed tomography angiography (CCTA) is *not* recommended.	C
Magnetic resonance imaging (MRI) for detection of vascular plaque is *not* recommended.	C

Modified from Greenland P, Alpert JS, Beller GA, et al, American College of Cardiology Foundation, American Heart Association. 2010 ACCF/AHA guideline for assessment of cardiovascular risk in asymptomatic adults: a report of the American College of Cardiology Foundation/American Heart Association Task Force on Practice Guidelines. J Am Coll Cardiol 2010;56:e50.

Take-Home Points

1. It is our responsibility as PAs to become more genetically literate so that we can provide quality health care to our patients.

2. For the primary care provider, the construction and use of the patient pedigree is a critical first step in assessing risk.
3. Identification of risk and the indications for referral to genetic services are critical to providing optimal patient care.
4. Accurate self-assessment of genetic knowledge and appropriate use of valid Internet databases are necessary in lifelong learning for all providers.

KEY POINTS

- PAs need to understand basic concepts in genetics/genomics as they affect clinical practice from preventive care through management of most conditions.
- Students must be able, at a minimum, to take and record a family history, preferably in the form of a pedigree, as well as interpret and assess genetic risk for their patients.
- It is critical to know when to refer a patient for specific genetic testing or genetic services and incorporate resulting information into the patient's care after they have received such services.
- Genetic testing includes a variety of methods and types of testing, and it also requires special considerations for the patient because results affect not only the patient but potentially family members.

References

1. Khoury MJ, Gwinn M, Yoon PW, et al. The continuum of translation research in genomic medicine: how can we accelerate the appropriate integration of human genome discoveries into health care and disease prevention? Genet Med 2007;9(10):665.
2. Telner DE, Carroll JC, Talbot Y. Genetics education in medical school: a qualitative study exploring educational experiences and needs. Medical Teacher 2008;30:192.
3. The Human Genome. Wellcome Trust website. See *http://genome.wellcome.ac.uk/*; Accessed August 4, 2011.
4. Proteomics. American Medical Association. See *http://www.ama-assn.org/ama/pub/physician-resources/medical-science/genetics-molecular-medicine/current-topics/proteomics.page*; Accessed August 6, 2011.
5. Tyagi S, Raghvendra US, Taruna K, Kavita M. Application of metabolomics—a systematic study of the unique chemical fingerprints: an overview. Int J Pharm Sci Rev Res 2010;3:83.
6. Farndon PA, Bennett C. Genetics education for health professionals: strategies and outcomes from a national initiative in the United Kingdom. J Genet Counsel 2008;17:161.
7. Houwink EJF, van Luijk Henneman L, van der Vleuten C, et al. Genetic educational needs and the role of genetics in primary care: a focus group study with multiple perspectives. BMC Family Practice 2011;12:5. See *http://www.biomedcentral.com/1471-2296/12/5*; Accessed July 20, 2011.
8. National Coalition for Health Professional Education in Genetics. Core Competencies in Genetics for Health Professionals. 3rd ed. 2007, September. See *http://www.nchpeg.org/index.php?option=com_content&view=article&id=94&Itemid=84*; Accessed December 9, 2011.
9. Rackover M, Goldgar C, Wolpert C, et al. Establishing essential physician assistant clinical competencies guidelines for genetics and genomics. J Physician Assist Educ 2007; 18(2):48.
10. Secretary's Advisory Committee on Genetics, Health, and Society, 2010. Genetics Education and Training of Health Care Professionals, Public Health Providers, and Consumers, February, 2011 See *http://oba.od.nih.gov/SACGHS/sacghs_documents.html#GHSDOC_005*; Accessed July 23, 2011.
11. Bennett RL. The family medical history. Prim Care 2004;31:479.
12. Family history educational aids. National Coalition for Health Professional Education in Genetics (NCHPEG). See *http://www.nchpeg.org/index.php?option=com_content&view=article&id=145&Itemid=64*; Accessed August 6, 2011.
13. Berg AO, Baird MA, Botkin JR, et al. National Institutes of Health State-of-the-Science conference statement: family history and improving health. Ann Intern Med 2009;151:872.
14. Office of the Surgeon General and the National Human Genome Research Institute. My Family Health Portrait. "About My Family Health Portrait." See *https://familyhistory.hhs.gov/fhh-web/home.action*; Accessed July 14, 2011.
15. Facio FM, Feero G, Linn A, et al. Validation of My Family Health Portrait for six common heritable conditions. Genet Med 2010;12(6):370.
16. Bennett RL. Genetic family history, pedigree analysis, and risk assessment. Encyclopedia of Genetics, Genomics, Proteomics and Bioinformatics, published online. November 2005. *http://onlinelibrary.wiley.com/doi/10.1002/047001153X.g106402/abstract?systemMessage=Wiley+Online+Library+will+be+disrupted+on+7+July+from+10%3A00-12%3A00+BST+%2805%3A00-07%3A00+EDT%29+for+essential+maintenance&userIsAuthenticated=false&deniedAccessCustomisedMessage*.
17. March of Dimes "Genetics and Your Practice." Red Flags. See *http://www.marchofdimes.com/gyponline/*; Accessed July 23, 2011.
18. Genetic Alliance and the New England Public Health Genetics Education Collaborative Understanding Genetics. A New England Guide for Patients and Health Professionals. Chapter 5: Genetic counseling. *http://www.geneticalliance.org/understanding.genetics*; Accessed July 2, 2012.

19. Genetic Alliance and the New England Public Health Genetics Education Collaborative. Understanding Genetics: A New England Guide for Patients and Health Professionals. Chapter 3: Pedigree and family history. *http://www.geneticalliance.org/understanding.genetics*; Accessed July 2, 2012.
20. Botkin JR, Teutsch SM, Kaye CI , et al. on behalf of the EGAPP Working Group, Outcomes of interest in evidence-based evaluations of genetic tests. Genet Med 2010;12(4):228.
21. Antoniou A, Pharoah PD, Narod S, et al. Average risks of breast and ovarian cancer associated with *BRCA1* or *BRCA2* mutations detected in case series unselected for family history: a combined analysis of 22 studies. Am J Hum Genet 2003;72(5):1117.
22. Cytochrome p450. Published August 1, 2011. Genetics Home Reference. See *http://ghr.nlm.nih.gov/glossary=cytochromep450*; Accessed August 5, 2011.
23. Haddow JE, Palomaki GE. ACCE: a model process for evaluating data on emerging genetic tests. In: Khoury M, Little J, Burke W, eds. Human Genome Epidemiology: A Scientific Foundation for Using Genetic Information to Improve Health and Prevent Disease. Oxford, England: Oxford University Press. Cited by: Office of Genomics and Disease Prevention. Evaluation of genetic testing. ACCE: a CDC-sponsored project carried out by the Foundation for Blood Research. 2003. Available at: *http://www.cdc.gov/genomics/gtesting/ACCE*; Accessed December 9, 2011.
24. Hudson K, Javitt G, Burke W. Byers P and the ASHG Social Committee. Statement on Direct-to-Consumer Genetic Testing in the United States. Am J Hum Genet 2007;81:635.
25. Burke W. Genetic testing in primary care. Annu Rev Genomics Hum Genet 2004;5:1.
26. Cheng TL, Cohn RD, Dover GJ. The genetics revolution and primary care pediatrics. JAMA 2008;299(4):451.
27. Lose EJ. The emerging role of primary care in genetics. Curr Opin Pediatr 20:634.
28. Wu O, Robertson L, Twaddle S, et al. Screening for thrombophilia in high-risk situations: systematic review and cost-effectiveness analysis. The Thrombosis: Risk and Economic Assessment of Thrombophilia Screening (TREATS) study. Health Technol Assess 2006;10(11):1.
29. Patient UK. Primary Cardiovascular Risk Calculator. See *http://www.patient.co.uk/showdoc/40026126/*; Accessed August 2, 2011.
30. Greenland P, Alpert JS, Beller GA, et al. American College of Cardiology Foundation, American Heart Association. 2010 ACCF/AHA guideline for assessment of cardiovascular risk in asymptomatic adults: a report of the American College of Cardiology Foundation/American Heart Association Task Force on Practice Guidelines. J Am Coll Cardiol 2010 14;56(25):e50.

CHAPTER 13

CHRONIC CARE PERSPECTIVES

Virginia Hass • Mindy G. Milton

CHAPTER CONTENTS

Chronic conditions are the leading causes of illness, disability, and death in the United States today. More than 145 million people in the United States have one or more chronic conditions such as diabetes, heart disease, and asthma.[1] Almost 50 million Americans are disabled by a chronic condition.[2] By 2030, this is expected to grow to 171 million people. In addition to the personal burden of disease, the costs to the U.S. health care system are staggering. Total health care spending in 2007 was 16.3% of the U.S. gross domestic product ($2.2 trillion). It is projected that by 2017, health care spending will rise to 19.5% of the U.S. gross domestic product ($4.3 trillion).[3] The direct and indirect costs of diabetes care alone totaled $174.4 billion in 2007.[4] In 2007, chronic illness accounted for more than three fourths of U.S. health care expenditures.[5] In 2007, 17.5 million Americans were diagnosed with diabetes.[4] This is projected to grow to 48.3 million by 2050.[6]

Although chronic illnesses affect individuals of all ages, they are most prevalent in older people.[7] There are almost 40 million people aged 65 and older in the United States. This population is expected to double by 2030, representing almost 20% of the U.S. population.[7] The average person in this age range suffers from two or more chronic conditions, many of which are associated with physical and/or mental disability. A threefold or greater increase in the disabled elderly population is predicted by the year 2050.[8] The burden of chronic illness falls disproportionately on the poor, educationally disadvantaged, and ethnic minorities.[9] *REACH 2010* reported a substantially higher prevalence of health-risk factors (e.g., obesity, cigarette smoking) and selected chronic conditions (diabetes, cardiovascular disease, hypertension, hyperlipidemia) among ethnic minorities in the United States compared with national estimates.[10] Additionally, age and socioeconomic stress factors interact synergistically to increase risk.

CURRENT CARE SHORTFALLS

These figures highlight the need for high-quality care of chronic disease and conditions. Today's health care system in the United States is organized primarily to address patients with acute, episodic care needs; it is poorly organized to meet the challenges of chronic illness care. As described in the 2001 Institute of Medicine report, *Crossing the Quality Chasm: A New Health System for the 21st Century*, the "current health care system cannot do the job" and "merely making incremental improvements in current systems of care will not suffice."[11] Patients experience care that is uncoordinated and unsupportive, which often leaves them feeling incapable of meeting the day-to-day challenges of living with a chronic condition. In fact, "over 50% of people with chronic illness do not receive modern, evidence-based care."[12]

A NEW MODEL OF CARE

Beginning in the mid-1990s, a number of organizations around the country started addressing these challenges. The MacColl Institute of Healthcare Improvement, under the direction of Ed Wagner, MD, MPH, developed a new systematic model for chronic illness care. This model has been widely introduced into a variety of clinical settings nationwide, including several hundred community health centers funded by the Bureau of Primary Health Care. From evaluation of these efforts, there is a growing body of research documenting that a more systematic, proactive, patient-centered, and evidence-based approach to care can keep patients with chronic illnesses healthy for a longer period of time.[13-15] By addressing the educational needs of both patients and clinicians, the Chronic Care Model (CCM) has direct application to the stated objectives of *Healthy People 2020* to reduce morbidity and mortality related to chronic illnesses, including but not limited to diabetes, cardiovascular disease, asthma, and depression.

CHRONIC ILLNESS CARE CREATES A PARADIGM SHIFT: THE PATIENT-PROFESSIONAL PARTNERSHIP

This partnership involves collaborative care, self-management education, and self-efficacy. Self-efficacy, the confidence to carry out a plan necessary to reach a desired goal, is essential to the concept of an "informed, activated patient."[13] Patients are active members of the teams that manage their chronic illness. Effective chronic illness care demands clinicians who can provide effective self-management support and improved communication among all members of the health care team. This will require innovative solutions such as "interdisciplinary eHealth teams,"[16] in which information is shared between clinicians and patients via resources such as the Internet. Health care providers now routinely use such resources (e.g., electronic medical records, electronic patient registries).

To change outcomes requires fundamental practice changes. These are difficult to achieve in the current health system. The CCM identifies six essential elements needed to improve chronic care within the community and health system. Community factors include resources and policies; health system factors include health care organizations, patient self-management support, delivery system design, decision support tools, and clinical information systems.[13] The goal of the model is "promoting effective change in provider groups to support evidence-based clinical and quality improvement across a wide variety of health care settings."[1] This goal is accomplished through "productive interactions" between a "prepared, proactive practice team" and an "informed, activated patient," which in turn will lead to improved health outcomes.[13-15] The CCM was developed to promote integrated change with components directed at the following:

- Influencing provider behavior
- Better use of nonphysician team members
- Enhancement of information systems
- Planned encounters (interactions linked through time to achieve specific goals)
- Patient self-management
- Modern self-management support

The CCM incorporates additional themes within the context of the Model elements: (1) patient safety (Health System); (2) cultural competency (Delivery System); (3) care coordination (Health System and Clinical Information Systems); (4) community policies (Community Resources and Policies); and (5) case management (Delivery System Design).[1] Figure 13-1 illustrates the relational concepts of the model.

ELEMENTS OF THE CHRONIC CARE MODEL

The *community* creates the context in which health care is delivered. Community programs can support or expand a health system's ability to care for chronically ill patients. The health care system can enhance care for its patients by forming partnerships to support and develop interventions that fill gaps in needed services and by avoiding duplication of effort.[1]

Health systems can create an organizational culture and mechanisms that promote safe, high-quality care. Ideally, this culture "(1) visibly supports improvement at all levels of the organization, beginning with

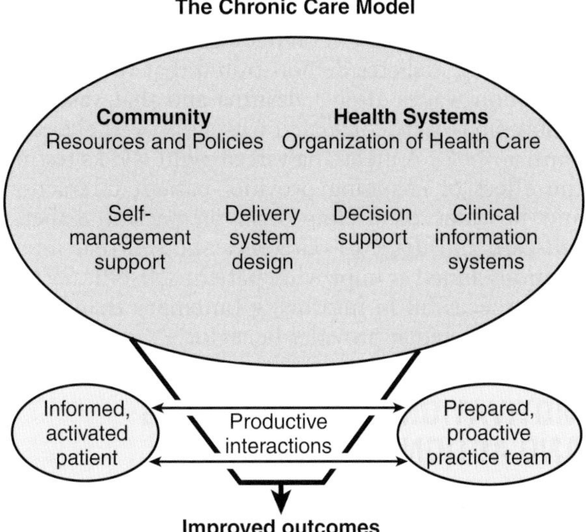

FIGURE 13-1 The Chronic Care Model. (Developed by the MacColl Institute and reproduced with the permission of the American College of Physicians.)

the senior leader; (2) promotes effective improvement strategies aimed at comprehensive system change; (3) encourages open and systematic handling of errors and quality problems to improve care; (4) provides incentives based on quality of care (e.g., pay-for-performance, provider incentives); and (5) develops agreements that facilitate care coordination within and across organizations."[1]

All people make decisions and engage in behaviors that affect their health, and this is no less true for people with chronic illness. It is these behaviors that constitute *self-management*. The outcomes of chronic illness depend largely on the self-management decisions patients make. Effective *self-management support* prepares patients and their caregivers to manage their health and health care by (1) emphasizing patients' central role in managing their health; (2) using strategies that include assessment, goal setting, planning, problem-solving, and follow-up; and (3) organizing resources to provide sustainable self-management support.[1]

Improving the health of people with chronic illness requires the creation of a system that is proactive and focused on promotion of health. This objective is accomplished through design of *delivery systems* that ensure effective clinical care and self-management support. This design increases the use of nonphysician team members by defining roles and distributing tasks on the basis of the efficient use of team members' skills. In a proactive delivery system, there are planned interactions that support evidence-based care. Approaches to these interactions may include (1) longer visits (not necessarily more frequent); (2) an agenda; (3) regular follow-up by the team; and (4) clinical case management services for patients with complex needs. Health literacy and cultural competency are two important concepts in health care. Effective delivery system design includes the ability to respond effectively to the diverse cultural and linguistic needs of patients.[1]

Decision support is essential to the delivery of high-quality, evidence-based care that incorporates patient preferences. In a delivery system with effective decision support, evidence-based guidelines are embedded into daily clinical practice through reminders, feedback, standing orders, and other methods that increase their visibility at the time that clinical decisions are made. Furthermore, these guidelines and information are shared with patients to encourage their participation. For more complex patient care, specialist expertise is integrated into the delivery of primary care.[1]

Effective chronic illness care requires information systems that ensure access to vital data on both individual patients and patient populations. *Clinical information systems* may be electronic or paper based and are used to organize patient and population data to facilitate care. At the individual level, information systems provide reminders to patients and providers and facilitate individual care planning. At the population level, information systems identify related subpopulations for targeted care and aid monitoring the performance of providers, the practice team, and the care system.[1]

These six elements combine to support *productive interactions* that are the core of chronic illness care. Note that "interaction" is used deliberately to move away from the idea that all encounters are clinical visits. Phone calls, e-mails, self-management classes, and support groups are all examples of strategies demonstrated to be effective in improving patient-clinician communication.[17-20] To have productive interactions, we need a different kind of team than we have in the acute care–driven system. Half of the productive interaction is a *prepared, proactive practice team*. This means that, at the time of the interaction, the team has decision support tools, clinical information systems available at the point of service, and the resources necessary to deliver high-quality care. The other half of the productive interaction is an *informed, activated patient (and caregiver)*. An informed, activated patient has the knowledge, skills, confidence, and motivation to self-manage care. This requires more than the traditional patient teaching and is discussed later in this chapter. There is evidence that, with appropriate self-management support, almost any patient can become a relatively effective self-manager.[21-24] So, how do we recognize productive interactions? In the interaction there would be (1) assessment of self-management skills and confidence, as well as clinical status; (2) collaborative definition of problems; (3) collaborative setting of goals and problem-solving; (4) the development of a shared care plan; (5) tailoring of clinical management by stepped protocols and guidelines; and (6) planned, active, and sustained follow-up.[1]

Self-Management and Self-Management Support

Self-management and self-management support are at the core of the clinician-patient encounter. All patients manage their day-to-day life and health, whether they do it effectively or otherwise. In the context of chronic illness, self-management becomes particularly important. Research regarding the effectiveness of patient education tells us that providing information alone is not enough. That is, providing information in the absence of self-management support does not change health outcomes.[17,25,26] This has been described by Bodenheimer[22,24] as the "50% rule": half of patients are unable to repeat back what they are told by a physician, half do not understand how to take their medications and take them incorrectly, and half of patients leave a clinical visit without understanding what the physician said.[27-29] The lifelong work of patients managing chronic illness encompasses three sets of tasks. The first set entails medical management of the illness, such as diet, medications, regular follow-up, and laboratory tests. The second set includes adaptation of life roles and behaviors, such as modification of work or recreational activities to fit functional capacity. Finally, the third set involves coping with the emotional aspects of chronic illness, which can include depression, anger, and fear. Self-management programs, therefore, must include all three sets of tasks required to effectively manage chronic illness.[30]

The components of effective self-management support include (1) providing information; (2) intensive, disease-specific skills training; (3) encouraging healthy behavior change; (4) teaching patients both action-planning and problem-solving skills; (5) assisting patients with the emotional aspects of having a chronic illness; (6) encouraging patients to become "informed and activated"; and (7) providing ongoing and regular follow-up.[31] Current evidence demonstrates that follow-up has the greatest impact on health outcomes, and that follow-up need not be a clinic encounter. Strategies such as web-based programs, e-mail, telephone calls, and peer support are all effective.[18,20] A meta-analysis of 31 randomized controlled trials (RCTs) testing the effect of self-management education on hemoglobin A_{1C} in adults with type 2 diabetes demonstrated that the effect of education wanes after 3 months and that sustained follow-up closely correlated with improved glycemic control.[18,19,32] A meta-analysis of eight RCTs testing the effect of changing provider-patient interaction and provider counseling style on patient diabetes self-care and diabetes outcomes showed that interventions aimed at improving patient self-efficacy was more successful in improving outcomes than interventions aimed at provider behavior.[23]

MOTIVATIONAL INTERVIEWING AND ACTION PLANNING

Miller and Rollnick[33] define motivational interviewing as "a directive client-centered counseling approach for initiating behavior change by helping clients to resolve ambivalence." It is beyond the scope of this chapter to instruct the reader in all the aspects of motivational interviewing. For further information, the reader is referred to *Motivational Interviewing: Preparing People for Change*, 2nd ed. (p. 325). Motivational interviewing is a philosophy in which a blend of patient-centered and coaching strategies, combined with understanding of what triggers behavior change, is used to guide clinician-patient interactions. The key principles of motivational interviewing are summarized in Table 13-1. Two key concepts of motivational interviewing are addressing ambivalence and recognizing resistance as a cue to the need for changing *clinician* behavior. Ambivalence can be defined as a conflict between two courses of action, each of which has potential advantages and disadvantages. Ambivalence may derive from (1) not knowing what to change; (2) not knowing how to change; (3) not believing a change needs to occur; (4) not understanding why a change needs to occur; and/or (5) doubt in the ability to be successful in making the change. Resistance occurs because the person is unwilling to make the change or perceives the costs associated with the change (e.g., giving up smoking) as outweighing the benefits (e.g., possibly avoiding future lung disease). The principles of motivational interviewing are best described as an interpersonal style that can be used in a variety of therapeutic encounters, rather than a prescribed set of techniques. Table 13-2 compares clinician behaviors that facilitate motivational interviewing with those that impede the process. Physician assistants (PAs) are in an excellent position to identify patients at risk for poor health outcomes and to use the patient-centered communication method

TABLE 13-1 Key Principles of Motivational Interviewing

1. Express Empathy
   - Reflective listening is used to *understand* the patient's feelings *without judging.* Accurate empathy is acceptance of the patient's perspective as valid within their framework. It is *not* agreement or approval.
   - Acceptance facilitates change.
   - Ambivalence is normal.
2. Develop Discrepancy
   - Develop and magnify, from the patient's point of view, the discrepancy between the behavior and their long-term or larger goals.
   - The goal is to aid the patient in moving past ambivalence toward change.
   - The patient, not the health care provider, should present arguments for change.
3. Roll with Resistance
   - Resistance is a signal to respond differently. Resume asking questions rather than offering answers.
   - The patient, not the provider, generates solutions.
   - An analogy is to "dance with" rather than "wrestle with" the patient.
   - Respectful of autonomy.
   - Avoids arguing for change by not directly challenging resistance.
4. Support Self-Efficacy
   - The patient's belief that change is possible is an important motivator.
   - The patient, not the provider, chooses and brings about the change.
   - Self-efficacy (confidence) is a good predictor of outcomes.

Modified from Miller WR, Rollnick S. Motivational Interviewing: Preparing People for Change, 2nd ed. New York: The Guilford Press, 2002.

of motivational interviewing to actively engage them in a successful behavior change process. The role is not to tell patients what to do, but to listen, provide empathy, alleviate ambivalence, provide information, and serve as a change agent. Motivational interviewing strategies provide a framework for this effort, as demonstrated in Case Study 13-1. Respect of autonomy and self-determination and support of self-efficacy are key elements that contribute to success.

SUPPORT SELF-EFFICACY

Self-efficacy is a patient's confidence that he or she can make life changes. Self-efficacy is an important motivator for behavior change, and supporting self-efficacy is a key skill of motivational interviewing.[33] Look for opportunities to praise the efforts patients

TABLE 13-2 Comparison of Clinician Behaviors Impact on Motivational Interviewing

Clinician Behaviors That Facilitate Motivational Interviewing	Clinician Behaviors That Impede Motivational Interviewing
• Use reflective listening to understand the patient's perspective • Express acceptance and affirmation • Elicit and selectively reinforce the client's own self-motivational statements, self-efficacy, and resolution of ambivalence • Assess the patient's readiness to change • Avoid resistance by not moving forward faster than the patient • Respect and acknowledge the patient's autonomy and freedom of choice	• Argue that the patient must change • Offer direct advice without the patient's permission • Direct behavior change without actively encouraging the person to make his or her own decisions • Use the "expert" role to keep the patient in a passive role • Control the conversation by doing most of the talking • Behave punitively or coercively • Use "motivational techniques" as a means to manipulate the patient

make toward positive behavior change. For example, Mr. S. comes in for a planned visit and tells you, "I've cut down on my smoking." A supportive response would be, "That's an important step to improve your health; tell me more about how you did it." Such a response congratulates and reinforces the positive change the patient has made and facilitates the discussion of any difficulties he is encountering. In this conversation, he has accepted the fact that behavior change might decrease his risk for early death and disability. As Mr. S. continues to direct the conversation, he begins to believe he can continue cutting down on his smoking and develops ideas for other ways to reduce his stress. This is the time to actively engage him in action planning. In the end, Mr. S. elicited his own arguments for change and set goals for action.

The goal of motivational interviewing is to elicit "change talk"[33] and thus facilitate goal setting. Action planning is a proven strategy for building self-efficacy while working toward goals.[34-36] The "5 A's"—Assess, Advise, Agree, Assist, and Arrange—adapted from the Agency for Healthcare Quality Research (AHQR) clinical practice guidelines,[31,32,37-39] are a patient-centered model of behavioral counseling that is congruent with the CCM. They have been frequently used to enhance self-management support

CASE STUDY 13-1

USING MOTIVATIONAL INTERVIEWING STRATEGIES IN SMOKING-CESSATION COUNSELING

S.S. is a 50-year-old Vietnamese man with a recent diagnosis of chronic obstructive pulmonary disease (COPD). He has a 36-pack-year history of cigarette smoking. He works as a computer programmer. He has been happily married for 27 years, with three children, ages 25, 22, and 14. The youngest child lives at home; the older two live nearby. He has lived in the United States since age 15. He has a large extended family also living in the area. Family history is significant for gastric cancer in his mother and early death due to lung disease in his father. Both of his parents smoked. S.S. is here today for a planned visit to follow up on his COPD. He also has a chief complaint of productive cough. As his primary care PA, your role is to provide information and support for health behavior change related to his lung disease and smoking.

EXPRESS EMPATHY

Empathy expression is accomplished by being nonjudgmental, with a genuine concern for the patient's well-being, allowing him to set the agenda while you ask necessary questions.[33] You can begin to raise awareness about COPD by asking him about the symptoms he is having, his tobacco use, and previous attempts to quit smoking. Encouraging the patient to talk is respectful and builds autonomy. Asking open-ended questions facilitates information gathering and explores his feelings. Reflective listening demonstrates to him that what was said is actually being heard. As the conversation continues, the goal is to develop discrepancy. Mr. S. stated he knew that his smoking was making his cough worse; and he is concerned that he will die early, as did his father, and "miss knowing my grandchildren." He has tried to quit twice before but "just couldn't do it." Cigarettes help him relax when his work pressures "build up." Empathy is the objective identification with the affective state of another, not their experience. Empathy is the primary interpersonal skill for expressing caring and understanding. For example, Mr. S. wants to quit smoking but enjoys the relaxation he gets from smoking. We do not have to smoke ourselves to understand these conflicting desires. An empathic response would be, "It would be difficult to quit smoking when it helps you relieve stress." Strategies such as affirming and elaborating further explore and reinforce self-efficacy.

DEVELOP DISCREPANCY

Developing discrepancy is a means of creating cognitive dissonance,[33] the psychological discomfort that arises from holding two conflicting thoughts in the mind at the same time. Cognitive dissonance is a powerful motivator of change. Discrepancy may be developed by asking the patient to list the benefits versus the costs of the behavior or behavioral change they are contemplating and then reflecting on the pros and cons while highlighting inconsistencies. Asking the patient to elaborate on discrepancies between stated goals and present behaviors that contradict those goals is a powerful means of developing discrepancy and motivating change. For example, Mr. S. continues to smoke. You state, "Mr. S., I see that you continue to smoke. What are your thoughts about how this affects your goal to live long enough to know your grandchildren?" The question is nonjudgmental and draws on Mr. S.'s own conclusions. Although it creates dissonance, it does not present an argument for change. The question is designed to facilitate the patient's "change talk" or arguments for change on the basis of examining his risks, recognizing them, and foreseeing potential consequences.

AVOID ARGUMENT

Avoiding argument means not eliciting resistance by forcing patients to defend the behaviors they are trying to change. By avoiding argument, it is more likely that patients will see you as an ally.[33] For example, Mr. S. states, "I've tried quitting smoking before and couldn't do it. There's no point in trying again." Resistance is a cue to change your approach; use open-ended questions to get the patient talking. Rather than tell him many patients have to try more than once, you state, "It sounds as if you're frustrated by your previous attempts to quit smoking. What problems did you have?" This response is empathic, addresses the patient's emotional state, and asks for additional input.

ROLL WITH RESISTANCE

Rolling with resistance means going with what the patient is willing to do. This sometimes means doing nothing at that time.[33] For example, Mr. S. states, "I'm okay. My breathing isn't nearly as bad as my father's was." Rather than arguing with this statement by responding, "If you continue smoking, you will probably get worse," you can roll with the resistance by saying, "I hope that your health continues to stay good. However, keep getting regular checkups because that may change. I'm here to help if you want to quit smoking as time goes on." In this way, you have followed the direction set by the patient, as well as created a discrepancy. You have not scolded him and have left the door open for future conversations.

TABLE 13-3 **Five A's**

ASSESS	Patients' beliefs, behavior, and knowledge.
ADVISE	Patients by providing specific information about health risks and benefits of change.
AGREE	On a collaboratively set of goals based on patients' confidence in their ability to change the behavior.
ASSIST	Patients with problem-solving by identifying personal barriers, strategies, and social and environmental support.
ARRANGE	A specific follow-up plan.

Modified from Agency for Healthcare Quality Research. Three brief clinical interventions. *http://www.ncbi.nlm.nih.gov/books/NBK18002/.* Retrieved July 8, 2011.

0	1	2	3	4	5	6	7	8	9	10
Not important										Very important

FIGURE 13-2 Importance scale.

0	1	2	3	4	5	6	7	8	9	10
Not sure										Very sure

FIGURE 13-3 Confidence scale.

and linkages to community resources. Table 13-3 outlines the "5 A's." Readiness scales measure two concepts: (1) How important is the change to the patient? and (2) How confident is the patient that he or she can do what is necessary? Importance and confidence levels of "7" or higher correlate to higher probability of success. See Figures 13-2 and 13-3 for examples of these scales. The "5 A's" and readiness scales are a quick and effective way for eliciting discussions on change and determining what else needs to happen for the patient to make an even greater commitment to change. Case Study 13-2 illustrates the use of readiness scales.

CASE STUDY 13-2

Using Readiness Scales

In Case Study 13-1, you sense some ambivalence or resistance on the part of Mr. S. about quitting smoking. You decide to use the readiness and confidence scales to explore his ambivalence. Ask, "On a scale from zero to ten, where zero is not at all important and 10 is very important, how important is it for you to quit smoking?" Mr. S. answers, "Four." Rather than responding, "Why a four and not a ten?" which would cause him to talk about why he does not want to quit smoking, ask, "Why a four and not a zero?" This response elicits "change talk" because it allows Mr. S. to state reasons why he thinks it is important to quit smoking. Let him respond, and then ask, "What would it take to make your answer five or six?" This elicits motivating factors from Mr. S. and encourages him to think about incremental change. If he cannot come up with an answer at this moment to raise his response to 5 or 6, ask him to think about it and let you know at a follow-up visit. You are planting the seeds of dissonance to create change. The same steps are used with the confidence scale. Ask Mr. S. how confident he feels that he can quit smoking at this time.

Once the patient's priorities and confidence level are identified, the next step is to facilitate action planning. Successful action plans build self-efficacy by breaking larger, long-term goals into manageable pieces. They have five basic characteristics: (1) The action to be taken is something the *patient* wants to do; (2) the goal is reasonable (can be accomplished in 1 week); (3) they are behavior specific; (4) they answer the questions—what? how much? when? and how often?; and (5) the patient's confidence level is 7 or more.[40] The steps of action planning are listed in Table 13-4. Case Study 13-3 illustrates a patient's use of the steps.

CASE STUDY 13-3

Action Planning

Ms. T. is a 47-year-old woman who is morbidly obese and has not exercised in years. During a clinic visit, she identifies two goals for improving her health: losing 60 lb. and exercising daily, which she defines as walking around the park with her friend who is "very fit."

Step 1. Decide what she wants to accomplish.

Ms. T.'s list includes the goal, "I want to be able to walk around the park with my friend." The perimeter of the park is 1 mile, and she currently can walk 1 block before stopping to rest.

Step 2. Look for alternatives to accomplish the goal, and identify barriers.

A barrier Ms. T. identifies is that she is concerned that she will not be able to get home if she walks too far. Options for reaching the goal include driving to the park before walking, taking her cell phone on her walk, and walking in front of her house.

TABLE 13-4 Patient Steps for Action Planning

1. *Decide* what you want to accomplish.
   - These are the long-term goals—they will be broken into "do-able" chunks later.
   - Make a list of goals; put a star next to the one you want to work on first.
2. Look for *alternative ways* to accomplish this goal. Think about barriers you might encounter and include ideas for overcoming them.
   - List the options you might use to reach the goal. Ask family and friends for ideas if you are having difficulty with this.
   - Thoroughly explore each option before discarding it as unworkable.
3. Start making *short-term* plans by making an action plan or agreement with yourself.
   - This is the action plan; it should be a specific, measurable *behavior or set of behaviors* that can be accomplished in 1 week and will help you move toward your goal.
   - Decide *what* you will do *this week.* The plan should contain five parts:
     a. Exactly what will you do?
        Start where you are, or start slowly. For example, "I will walk up and down the sidewalk in front of my house."
     b. How much will you do?
        Be specific. Continuing the above example, "for 5 minutes."
     c. When will you do it?
        Connecting the new activity to a favorite old one is a good way to make sure you do it. Continuing the above example, "before watching the evening news."
     d. How often will you do it?
        Setting a goal that is less than your ideal (e.g., 3 to 4 times per week, rather than daily) decreases the pressure to perform. It also gives you some time off. Continuing the above example, "3 times a week."
     e. Assess your confidence level on a scale of 0-10. If your confidence that you can accomplish the plan is less than 7, consider modifying the plan.
4. *Carry out* your action plans.
   - This is usually the easy part, if the action plan is well written and realistic.
   - Keep track of your progress by noting your activities; both when the activity was accomplished and when it was not. This record is used in the next step.
   - In the example, this might include making a log for recording activity or noting on the calendar both the days you walked and the days you did not. Be sure to note the factors that helped you accomplish your activity or that prevented you from doing it.
5. *Check* the results against the plan.
   - At the end of the week, review the action plan. Did you complete it? Are you farther along toward your goal?
6. Make *changes* as needed.
   - This is the problem-solving step. If you did not accomplish all the parts of your action plan, *do not give up.*
   - Identify the barriers that prevented you from achieving the steps.
   - List possible remedies to the problem (much as you did in step 2). Then pick *one* to try.
   - Repeat steps 3 to 6, modifying your action plan so that the steps are easier to achieve.
   - Note that not all problems are solvable. If several honest attempts to work out a problem are not successful, it may be advisable to move on to another goal at present.
7. Remember to *reward* yourself.
   - Accomplishing your goals is a reward and builds confidence (self-efficacy). But do not wait until you reach your goal to reward yourself!
   - Rewards do not have to be expensive or elaborate. Think about healthy pleasures you can add to your life.

Modified from Lorig K, Holman H, Sobel D, et al. Living a Health Life with Chronic Conditions, 3rd ed. Palo Alto, CA: Bull Publishing, 2006.

Step 3. Develop short-term plan.

Ms. T.'s action plan reads, "I will walk up and down the sidewalk in front of my house for 5 minutes, before watching the evening news, three times per week; and my confidence level is '7'." This is a specific, measurable statement of the behavior change, with a reasonable probability of success.

Step 4. Carry out the plan.

Ms. T. recorded her activity on a wall calendar with large date areas for writing. She noted the days she walked and the days she did not, with the reasons for not walking.

Step 5. Check the results.

Ms. T. walked for 5 minutes in front of her house on 2 days during the week.

Step 6. Make changes as needed.

As part of her problem-solving, Ms. T identified that it was rainy and cold on 5 of 7 days during the week; she was concerned about being out in the weather. She decided to purchase a treadmill so that she could walk indoors on rainy days.

Step 7. Reward yourself.

Ms. T. decided that she would drink a 4-oz. glass of her favorite red wine only after she had completed her walking. This turned a glass of wine into her reward.

POPULATION-BASED MANAGEMENT OF CHRONIC DISEASE

Population-based disease management evolved from single-payer systems in Europe and staff model HMOs in the United States as a strategy to improve the cost-effectiveness and quality of care to high-risk populations.[41] Population-based care is a structured approach to a subset of patients who share a particular characteristic or medical condition. Clinical information systems, such as patient registries, are used to collect outcome data. Evaluation of these data enables tracking of health outcomes.[42] Population-based care facilitates the delivery of targeted interventions to improve health outcomes within the population. Third-party payers and employers also use population data to monitor the performance of providers and health care systems. The National Committee for Quality Assurance (NCQA) developed and maintains the Health Plan Employer Data and Information Set (HEDIS). HEDIS is a set of standardized performance measures used by health care purchasers and consumers to compare the performance of managed health care plans. In turn, third-party payers use HEDIS measures to evaluate health systems and providers. Health care providers also use HEDIS measures to self-evaluate the care they provide. HEDIS measures relate to many chronic conditions, such as heart disease, diabetes, and smoking, and include consumer satisfaction, as well as health outcomes measures.[42] These measures give health care consumers and purchasers the ability to evaluate and compare the quality of health plans and providers. The ability to obtain and apply information about patient populations and the larger population from which they are drawn allows the PA to implement practice-based learning and improvement. Case Study 13-4 illustrates an approach to population-based care.

CASE STUDY 13-4

POPULATION-BASED CARE TO IMPROVE DIABETES OUTCOMES

A PA working in a community health clinic is concerned about the rate of complications among the patients who have diabetes. She knows that addressing individual health behaviors is an important part of chronic illness care, and she uses strategies such as motivational interviewing and action planning with her patients. However, she wonders if there is a systems-based problem that is affecting health outcomes and whether a more collaborative approach to care would improve outcomes.

The PA works with the clinic staff and her supervising physician to develop a list of the patients seen at the clinic who have diabetes. Having read about the CCM, the PA investigates the Improving Chronic Illness Care website *(www.improvingchroniccare.org)* and finds a wealth of resources for implementing the CCM into practice *(http://www.improvingchroniccare.org/index.php?p=Toolkit&s=244).* On this site, she searches the CCM Implementation Tools and finds a link to a variety of public domain electronic chronic disease registry tools. She selects the Chronic Disease Electronic Management System [CDEMS] *(http://www.cdems.com).* Using this tool, she can develop and customize a registry to share with her colleagues. The clinic does not have an integrated electronic medical record (EMR); therefore, data are pulled from paper charts, as well as the computerized scheduling and laboratory reporting systems. Although the task appears daunting, the team works together to create a registry database for each patient that includes key health outcome measures for diabetes: (1) date of last foot examination; (2) date of last eye examination; (3) last blood pressure and date; (4) last $HgbA_{1C}$ and date; (5) last low density lipoprotein (LDL) and date; and (6) latest self-management goal and date.

The PA and her supervising physician analyzed the data they had collected, compared the results with HEDIS[42] targets for those measures, and identified the following trends in the clinic's population of patients with diabetes:

- 103 (76%) have a foot examination documented within the past year
- 45 (33%) have an eye examination documented within the past year
- 121 (89%) have last BP at or below the target of 130/80 mm Hg
- 75 (55%) have last $HgbA_{1C}$ of <9.0%
- 82 (60%) have last LDL of ≤100
- 56 (41%) have a documented self-management goal

They realize that four of the six measures have room for improvement. As with action planning and behavior change with patients, systems change is best broken into manageable, achievable steps toward a goal. The entire clinic staff meets as a team to prioritize the list of goals. They elect to work on self-management goal setting with patients first because they see this as the indicator likely to have the biggest impact. The steps identified in reaching this goal were (1) training all clinic staff in the CCM, emphasizing self-management support and action planning. They also decide to explore community resources to facilitate access to eye examinations for their patients to improve this health measure.

This scenario illustrates a constructive process for a health care provider to follow in implementing population-based care:

1. Observe and verify the existence of important patterns of disease.
2. Use published resources and/or conducts a literature review to identify health outcome goals and tools for change.
3. Identify the community resources available to facilitate health access for populations.
4. Serve as a facilitator for the communication of ideas and systems change.

ROLE OF THE PA IN CHRONIC ILLNESS CARE: AN INTEGRATION OF THE PHYSICIAN ASSISTANT CORE COMPETENCIES

At the foundation of the CCM is the use of a population-based approach to care and of interdisciplinary teams in the coordination of care. Research suggests that people with chronic illnesses can be risk stratified, with interventions tailored to the risk level of individual patients and populations.[14,15] In applying such tailored interventions, the use of an interdisciplinary team plays a central role. Clearly, PAs can play a key role in such an interdisciplinary team. Depending on the practice setting, the PA will provide care in group visits for patients who are in reasonable control of their condition and provide regular, planned chronic care visits for patients who are newly diagnosed or in poor control. The PA will also play an important role in providing self-management support for patients with chronic illnesses, ensuring that care fits with the patient's cultural background.

Whether caring for patients with diabetes, hypertension, congestive heart failure, asthma, or a combination of several chronic diseases, the PA, as a member of the prepared practice team, is instrumental in improving patient outcomes. To change, and in that we mean to improve, outcomes requires fundamental practice changes. The integrated practice changes that are necessary to shift into a chronic care collaborative approach, as identified by Edward Wagner, MD, MPH, and his team at the MacColl Institute for Healthcare, are directed at influencing physician behavior, using PAs and other nonphysician team members better, enhancing information systems, and using planned encounters.

Incorporation of the CCM is a systematic method to decrease variation in quality of care between practitioners. Interesting to point out is that research has shown that this variation of quality of care delivered is greater within a single practice than between health care systems.[12] This means that individual providers can indeed have a profound effect in changing practice to improve health outcomes in their patient population. With that in mind, there are six aims of the CCM: patient safety, effective evidence-based medicine treatment, patient-centered, timely, efficient, and equitable. The PA's role and the competencies for the PA profession integrate nicely into this model of care.

Before a discussion of how PA competencies relate to the CCM, a historical perspective in their development is warranted. In 1995, the American Academy of Physician Assistants (AAPA) initiated the first of three studies to identify the "core competencies" of the PA profession. This was in response to many calls for an increased focus on competency, one of which first occurred in the same year, when the Pew Health Professions Commission released its report, *Reforming Health Care Workforce: Policy Considerations for the 21st Century*.[43] They concluded that workforce regulation could be responsive to public expectation (safe, high-quality health care) if practice acts for the health professions focused on "demonstrated initial and continuing competence."[43] From 1999 to 2003, the Institute of Medicine (IOM) released a series of reports concerning quality of health care and patient safety. The first, *To Err Is Human: Building a Safer Health System*,[44] captured the public's attention with its estimate that as many as 98,000 people die annually in hospitals from preventable medical errors. The IOM suggested that patient safety could improve if licensing, certification, and accreditation agencies were to develop and implement specific patient safety standards.[44] In 2001, the IOM released a follow-up report, *Crossing the Quality Chasm*,[11] in which it recommended that change was necessary at all levels of the health care system if quality of care was to improve. The IOM advocated for training and ongoing certification to ensure the continued competence of health care providers. In their 2003 report, *Health Professions Education: A Bridge to Quality*, the IOM advocated for a shift to a competency-based approach to education and ongoing certification.[45]

As already mentioned, in the mid-1990s, with support from the Robert Wood Johnson Foundation, Ed Wagner, MD, MPH, and the MacColl Institute of Healthcare developed an innovation, the CCM. This model was created as a response to the same marketplace pressures: (1) chronic disease emerging as the dominant health problem; (2) health care systems poor performance measured by outcomes; and (3) societal expectation to receive safe, high-quality health care. Chronic disease is now the principal cause of disability and consumes 78% of health expenditures in this country.[46] It is understandable that because the Accreditation Council for Graduate Medical Education (ACGME) and PA profession core competencies and the CCM are driven by the same desire to improve health care outcomes for patients, they would share the same vision and principles.

The *Competencies for the Physician Assistant Profession*,[47] adopted in 2005, was based on the 1999 general list of competencies for medical residents from the ACGME. This list was modified collaboratively by the national leadership within the American Academy of Physician Assistants (AAPA), the Accreditation Review Commission on Education for the Physician Assistant, Inc. (ARC-PA), the National Commission on Certification of Physician Assistants (NCCPA), and the Physician Assistant Education Association (PAEA), a collaboration of clinicians, accreditation and certification bodies, and educators representing the PA profession. These four organizations have taken the first step to answer the public's demand for improved quality and accountability in health care and ultimately enhance the PA profession. So, too, can the individual PA, by seeking opportunities to enhance personal development in these competencies.[48] Learning and implementing the CCM to improve chronic disease management of patients requires the same knowledge and many of the skills listed as important tenets in the competencies for the PA profession.[47]

The clinical role of PAs includes primary and specialty care in medical and surgical practice settings. Professional competencies for PAs include the effective and appropriate application of medical knowledge, interpersonal and communication skills, patient care, professionalism, practice-based learning and improvement, and systems-based practice, as well as an unwavering commitment to continual learning and professional growth. The physician-PA partnership works for the benefit of patients and the larger community being served. For an individual PA, these competencies are demonstrated within the scope of practice as defined by the supervising physician and appropriate to the health care setting.[47]

PAs can use their medical knowledge and communication skills in the context of the CCM to provide appropriate care to patients with chronic conditions. To accomplish this, PAs:

- Incorporate evidence-based medicine guidelines into their management of patients.
- Obtain and apply information about their population of patients and the larger populations from which their patients are drawn.
- Are proactive by scheduling follow-up appointments, using planned encounters versus reactive encounters when a patient is in crisis or ill.
- Implement modern self-management support. *Modern* in the sense that there is research that shows improved outcomes when using certain surveys or motivational interviewing techniques.

With the patient at the center of care, motivational interviewing is important to assess the patient's knowledge, skills, and confidence to establish measurable goals that are achievable through an action plan. Effective self-management support increases the patient's knowledge, skills, and confidence to set goals and achieve a healthier state and perhaps reduce further risk or consequences of an uncontrolled chronic condition. As an example, the physician–PA team, along with their staff, can improve a diabetic patient's health outcome by (1) offering *knowledge support:* regarding the etiology of diabetes, how diet and exercise for weight loss and medication works to counter the high sugar state, and consequences of poor control; (2) offering *skills support:* teaching how to perform a finger stick, use a glucometer, inject insulin and count calories, and (3) encouraging *goal setting with confidence assessment support*, through motivational interviewing. Patients may set goals to achieve a certain LDL level or $HgbA_{1C}$ level or state they want to exercise five times weekly. The key to goal setting is that it must be achievable, and the patient must have high enough confidence that they will succeed. The PA needs to give emotional support to patients with chronic conditions, focusing on care versus cure, and improving patients' function and comfort. This requires interpersonal and effective listening skills. Case Study 13-1 demonstrates the motivational interview process.

Within the context of practice-based learning, PAs, along with their supervising physicians and health care managers, "should assess, coordinate, and improve the delivery of health care and patient outcomes."[46] In the CCM, using clinical information systems and participating in quality improvement work are tied directly to delivery system design and health system organization. It is important for PAs to understand not only their role within the health care team but also how their practice and their patients fit into the larger health care system and the community as a whole. Accessing community resources will improve patient care and reduce duplication of effort, which will reduce costs. Table 13-5 illustrates

TABLE 13-5 Comparison of Competencies for the Physician Assistant Profession and the Chronic Care Model

Competencies for the Physician Assistant Profession (Excerpted from AAPA)	Concepts within the Chronic Care Model
Medical Knowledge • Demonstrate core knowledge of established and evolving biomedical and clinical sciences and apply it to patient care • Provide appropriate care to patients with chronic conditions • Demonstrate an investigatory and analytic thinking approach to clinical situations	**Decision Support** • Promote clinical care that is consistent with scientific evidence and patient preferences • Embed evidence-based guidelines into daily clinic practice • Integrate specialist expertise and primary care
Interpersonal and Communication Skills • Apply an understanding of human behavior • Appropriately adapt communication style and messages to the context of the individual patient interaction • Effective listening skills, nonverbal, explanatory, questioning, and writing skills to elicit and provide information	**Self-Management Support** • Empower and prepare patients to manage their health and health care • Negotiate self-management action plans with patients • Offer proven programs that provide basic information, emotional support, and strategies for living with chronic disease. • Use effective self-management support strategies that include assessment, goal setting, action planning, problem-solving, and follow-up • Emphasize the patient's central role in managing his or her health • Use a collaborative approach; providers and patients work together to define problems, set priorities, establish goals, create treatment plans, and solve problems
Patient Care • Effective, patient centered, timely, efficient, and equitable care • Make informed decisions partially on the basis of patient information and preferences • Work effectively with physicians and other health care professionals to provide patient-centered care • Develop and carry out patient management plans • Counsel and educate patients and their families	
Professionalism • Understanding the appropriate role of the physician assistant • Knowing professional and personal limitations • Respect, compassion, and integrity • Sensitivity and responsiveness to patients' culture, age, gender, and disabilities • Responsiveness and accountability to needs of patients and society	**Delivery System Design** • Define roles and distribute tasks among the team • Incorporate concepts of health literacy and cultural sensitivity; effective responsiveness to diverse cultural and linguistic needs • Give care that patients understand and that fits with their cultural background
Practice-Based Learning and Improvement • Analyze practice experience and perform practice-based improvement activities using a systematic methodology in concert with other members of the health care delivery team • Obtain and apply information about patient population and the larger population from which patients are drawn	**Clinical Information Systems** • Organize patient and population data to facilitate efficient and effective care • Use patient registry and clinical information systems to share information with patients and providers to coordinate care • Monitor performance of practice team and care system
Systems-Based Practice • Cost-effective health care and resource allocation • Improve the delivery of health care and patient outcomes • Responsible for promoting a safe environment for patient care	**Health System** • Create a culture, organization, and mechanisms that promote safe, high-quality care; advocate for policies to improve patient care, community resources • Encourage open and systematic handling of errors and quality problems to improve care

Modified from Improving Chronic Illness Care. The Chronic Care Model. Retrieved July 8, 2011, from *http://improvingchroniccare.org/change/index.html*, and AAPA Special Article, Competencies for the physician assistant profession. JAAPA 2005;18:14, 15, 18.

how the PA competencies interrelate and overlap with the concepts and framework of the CCM.

By embracing the CCM approach, which encompasses the societal, organizational, and economic environments in which health care is delivered, and applying it to their practice, each PA will exhibit and demonstrate the competencies laid out for the profession.

CLINICAL APPLICATIONS

1. Interpersonal and Communication Skills
   a. Identify a patient in your practice for whom health behavior change would decrease health risk(s) or improve control of a chronic illness.
   b. Schedule a planned encounter to discuss the health behavior.
   c. Practice the techniques of motivational interviewing and self-management support outlined in this chapter.
   d. Evaluate yourself. How did the conversation go? If you encountered resistance, consider how you could change your approach the next time. If you were successful in "rolling with resistance," keep up the good work!
2. Practice-Based Learning and Improvement
   a. Create a registry for subpopulations in your clinical practice. These may be patients with any chronic illness.
   b. Research the HEDIS measures for the chronic illness you have identified.
   c. Analyze the health outcomes of your population on the basis of the HEDIS guidelines.
   d. Collaborate with your colleagues and supervising physician to develop a plan for improvement that is based on the results of your analysis.

KEY POINTS

- The demand for health care providers who can provide systems and population-based chronic illness management, as well as individual care, will continue to grow as the U.S. population ages.[2,5,8-10]
- Disparities in health outcomes persist, especially in vulnerable, high-risk populations. The CCM model has been demonstrated to be cost-effective, improve quality of care, improve quality of life, and reduce morbidity and mortality associated with diabetes, asthma, arthritis, and depression.[13-15]
- PAs are logical collaborators as we build solutions to what seem to be intractable problems in caring for chronically ill patients. These solutions can include developing patient registries, taking ownership for a population of patients, and creating plans to improve the care for specific groups of patients.
- PAs must be able to analyze the health systems within which they work, design quality improvement plans and delivery systems that support chronic disease management, and evaluate the outcomes of such plans. Critical to the success of such projects is the ability to partner with patients and motivate behavior change.[13,14,33]
- PAs must be ready to practice within the new paradigm of the CCM. In doing so, PAs will aid the achievement of the goals of *Healthy People 2020:* (1) attain high-quality, longer lives free of preventable disease; (2) achieve health equity and eliminate disparities; (3) create social and physical environments that promote good health; and (4) promote quality of life, healthy development, and healthy behaviors across life stages.[9] Attainment of these goals will reduce the burden and costs of chronic disease.
- Since the mid-1990s, the CCM has been implemented widely. Evidence demonstrates the model's effectiveness in improving health outcomes for patients with chronic illness.

References

1. Improving Chronic Illness Care. The Chronic Care Model. Accessed November 27, 2011, from *http://improvingchroniccare.org/change/index.html*.
2. Centers for Disease Control and Prevention. Measuring Healthy Days. Atlanta: Centers for Disease Control and Prevention, 2000.
3. Keehan S, Sisko S, Truffer C, et al. Health spending projections through 2017: the baby-boom generation is coming to Medicare. Health Affairs;27, (no. 2)2008; w145. Accessed November 27, 2011, from *http://content.healthaffairs.org/content/27/2/w145.full.html*.
4. Dall TM, Mann SE, Zhang Y, et al. Distinguishing the economic costs associated with type 1 and type 2 diabetes. Popul Health Manag 2009;12:103.

5. Vogeli C. Shield AE, Lee TA, et al. Multiple chronic conditions: prevalence, health consequences, and implications for quality, care management, and costs. J Gen Intern Med 22(Suppl. 3):391.
6. Narayan KM, Boyle JP, Geiss LS, et al. Impact of recent increase in incidence on future diabetes burden, U.S., 2005-2050. Diabetes Care 2006;29:2114.
7. He W, Segupta M, Velkoff VA, DeBarros KA. 65+ in the United States: 2005. Curr Popul Rep; Accessed November 26, 2011, from *http://www.census.gov/prod/2006pubs/p23-209.pdf*.
8. Jackson SA. The epidemiology of aging. In: Hazzard WR, Blass JP, Ettinger WH, et al (eds). Principles of Geriatric Medicine and Gerontology. New York: McGraw-Hill, 1999.
9. U.S. Department of Health and Human Services. Healthy People 2020. November, 2010; Accessed November 25, 2011, from *http://www.healthypeople.gov/2020/topicsobjectives2020/default.aspx*.
10. Liao Y, Tucker P, Okoro CA, et al. REACH 2010 Surveillance for Health Status in Minority Communities—United States, 2001–2002. Morb Mortal Wkly Rep Surveill Summ 2004;53(6):1.
11. Committee on Quality Health Care in America. Institute of Medicine. Crossing the quality chasm: a new health system for the 21st century. Washington, D.C.: National Academy Press, 2001.
12. Wagner E. The Chronic Care Model. Presentation; Accessed November 27, 2011, from *http://www.improvingchroniccare.org/index.php?p=The_Model_Talk&s=27*.
13. Wagner E. Improving Chronic Illness Care: The Chronic Care Model: Model Elements; Accessed November 28, 2011, from *http://www.improvingchroniccare.org/index.php?p=Model_Elements&s=18*.
14. Bodenheimer T, Wagner EH, Grumbach K. Improving primary care for patients with chronic illness. JAMA 2002;288:1775.
15. Bodenheimer T, Wagner EH, Grumbach K. Improving primary care for patients with chronic illness: the chronic care model, part 2. JAMA 2002;288:1909.
16. Wiecha J, Pollard T. The interdisciplinary eHealth team: chronic care for the future. J Med Internet Res 2004;6(3):e22; Accessed November 27, 2011, from *www.jmir.org/2004/3/e22/*.
17. Haynes RB, Yao X, Degani A, et al. Interventions for enhancing medication adherence. Cochrane Database of Systematic Reviews 2005; Issue 4. Art. No.: CD000011. DOI: 10.1002/14651858.CD000011.pub2.
18. Lorig KR, Ritter PL, Laurent DD, Plant K. Internet-based chronic disease self-management: a randomized trial. Med Care 2006;44:961.
19. Norris SL, Lau J, Smith SJ, et al. Self-management education for adults with type 2 diabetes: a meta-analysis of the effect on glycemic control. Diabetes Care 2002;25:1159.
20. Lorig KR, Laurent DD, Deyo RA, et al. Can a back pain e-mail discussion group improve health status and lower health care costs? Arch Intern Med 2002;162:792.
21. Lorig K, Holman H. Self-management education: history, definition, outcomes, and mechanisms. Ann Behav Med 2003;26:1.
22. Bodenheimer T. Self-management support: is it evidence based? Presentation to the California Academic Chronic Care Collaborative, February 21, 2007.
23. van Dam HA, van der Horst F, van den Borne B, et al. Provider-patient interaction in diabetes care: effects on patient self-care and outcomes. A systematic review. Patient Educ Couns 2003;51:17.
24. Bodenheimer T, Lorig K, Holman H, Grumbach K. Patient self-management of chronic disease in primary care. JAMA 2002;288:2469.
25. Gibson PG, Powell H, Coughlan J, et al. Limited (information only) patient education programs for adults with asthma. Cochrane Database of Systematic Reviews 2002; Issue 1. Art. No.: CD001005. DOI: 10.1002/14651858.CD001005.
26. Riemsma RP, Kirwan JR, Taal E, Rasker JJ. Patient education for adults with rheumatoid arthritis. Cochrane Database of Systematic Reviews 2003; Issue 2. Art. No.: CD003688. DOI: 10.1002/14651858.CD003688.
27. Schillinger D, Piette J, Grumbach K, et al. Closing the loop: Physician communication with diabetic patients who have low health literacy. Arch Intern Med 2003;163:83.
28. Schillinger D, Wang F, Rodriguez M, et al. The importance of establishing regimen concordance in preventing medication errors in anticoagulant care. J Health Comm 2006;11:555.
29. Roter DL, Hall JA. Studies of doctor-patient interaction. Ann Rev Public Health 1989;10:163.
30. Griffin S, Kinmonth AL. Systems for routine surveillance for people with diabetes mellitus. Cochrane Database of Systematic Reviews 1998; Issue 1. Art. No.: CD000541. DOI: 10.1002/14651858.CD000541.
31. Shilts MK, Horowitz M, Townsend MS. Goal setting as a strategy for dietary and physical activity behavior change: a review of the literature. Am J Health Promotion 2004;19:81.
32. Cullen KW, Baranowski T, Smith SP. Using goal setting as a strategy for dietary behavior change. J Am Dietetic Assoc 2001;101:562.
33. Miller WR, Rollnick S. Motivational Interviewing: Preparing People for Change. 2nd ed. New York: The Guilford Press, 2002.
34. Anderson R, et al. Patient empowerment: results of a randomized control trial. Diabetes Care 1995;18:943.
35. Bodenheimer T, Lorig K, Holman H, Grumbach K. Patient self-management of chronic disease in primary care. JAMA 2002;288:2469.
36. Lorig K, Sobel D, Stewart A, et al. Evidence suggesting that a chronic disease self-management program can improve health status while reducing utilization and costs: a randomized trial. Med Care 1999;37:5.
37. California Academic Chronic Care Collaborative. Self-Management Support. Unpublished manuscript from the California Academic Chronic Care Collaborative Learning Session 1, February 21-22, 2007.
38. Agency for Healthcare Quality Research. AHCPR Supported Guide and Guidelines [Internet]. Rockville (MD): Agency for Health Care Policy and Research (US); 1992-2008. Three brief clinical interventions; Accessed November 1, 2011, from *http://www.ncbi.nlm.nih.gov/books/NBK18002/*.
39. The Tobacco Use and Dependence Clinical Practice Guideline Panel. Staff, and Consortium Representatives. A clinical practice guideline for treating tobacco use and dependence: A US Public Health Service report. JAMA 2000;283:3244.
40. Lorig K, Holman H, Sobel D, et al. Living a Health Life with Chronic Conditions. 3rd ed. Palo Alto, CA: Bull Publishing, 2006.
41. Lasker RD. The Committee on Medicine and Public Health. Improving the quality and cost-effectiveness of care by applying a population perspective to medical practice. Medicine and Public Health: The Power of Collaboration. New York: The New York Academy of Medicine, 1997.
42. Bell D, Brandt Jr EN. National Committee on Quality Assurance (NCQA). HEDIS—Health Plan Employer Data and Information Set. Volume 1. Narrative. Washington, D.C.: NCQA; 2011.
43. Mudge C, Price CA. Pew Health Professions Commission. Reforming Health Care Workforce Regulation; Policy Considerations for the 21st Century. Report of the Taskforce on Health Care Workforce Regulation December 1995.

44. Kohn LT, Corrigan JM, Donaldson MS, (eds). To Err Is Human: Building a Safer Health System. Washington, D.C: Committee on Quality of Health Care in America, Institute of Medicine, 2000.
45. Greiner AC, Knebel E, (eds). Health Professions Education: A Bridge to Quality. Washington, D.C: Committee on Health Professions Education Summit, Institute of Medicine, 2003.
46. Holman HR. Patient self-management: essential to solving the health care crisis. Presentation at University of California, Davis, Health System; May 16-17, 2005.
47. AAPA Special Article. Competencies for the physician assistant profession. JAAPA 2005;18:14; 15, 18.
48. Kohlhepp B, Rohrs R, Robinson P. Guest editorial: charting a course to competency. JAAPA 2005;18:16.

The resources for this chapter can be found at www.expertconsult.com.

CHAPTER 14

Pharmacology: The Use of Medications

Lawrence Carey

CHAPTER CONTENTS

The prescribing of sophisticated drugs is unquestionably one of the most important and powerful tools in modern medical practice. The statutory authority to prescribe is increasingly being extended to physician assistants (PAs), nurse practitioners, and pharmacists. The responsible, safe, and effective use of this privilege is an essential element of practice and a serious responsibility for PAs as professionals.

To the student or new graduate PA, the thought of choosing from a bewildering array of drugs, using them effectively and safely, dealing with a competitive industry, and, in general, managing this new responsibility is intimidating indeed. In this chapter the legal basis of prescribing is described, general principles for choosing drugs are outlined, some specific suggestions on communicating with the pharmacist and the patient are discussed, and some of the ethical and practical implications of prescribing are presented. With solid grounding in these basic principles, the fledgling prescriber can approach therapeutic decisions appropriately and with relative confidence. It is the purpose of this chapter to serve as an introduction to the thought processes and communication skills essential for conscientious prescribing. PA training program curricula contain significantly more detail. This chapter should serve as a basis for further discussion. Information on specific drugs, such as indications, side effects, and dosage, is available in several excellent resource works, some of which are described at the end of the chapter.

LEGAL BACKGROUND

The authority to prescribe medications in the United States is determined by state law. In 1973, North Carolina enacted legislation allowing PAs to prescribe from a limited formulary developed by the

State Board of Medical Examiners.[1] Several other states followed suit, and in 1978, the Washington State Supreme Court upheld this authority when it was challenged by a suit from the State Nursing Association.[2] The legal principle on which this decision was based is that of "agency" (i.e., that the PA is an "agent" of the physician and that orders from the PA are equivalent to those from the physician).[3]

Research on PA prescribing has revealed three important patterns that have strengthened the case for expanded authority. First, prescribing habits of PAs are similar to those of physicians in terms of appropriateness and safety. Second, few PAs have been disciplined for misuse or abuse of the privilege. Finally, states that allow physicians to delegate prescribing have a higher percentage of PAs practicing in rural areas.[4]

As of 2007, all 50 states allow some form of prescriptive authority for PAs. There is wide variation among state laws as to the specific requirements of and restrictions on PA prescribing. Some states use a "formulary" approach, by which the Board of Medical Examiners has a list of specific drugs from which PAs may prescribe. Other states take a more general delegatory approach and allow the physician/PA team to develop its own prescribing protocols. It is the responsibility of all prescribers to know and comply with the laws of the state in which they practice.[5] In recent years, electronic prescribing (e-prescribing) has become increasingly important, as national health care reform has been studied. Many organizations, including the American College of Physicians and the American Medical Association, have authored guides to help the prescriber transition from a paper-based system to one that is solely electronic. It is also important for practices to have awareness about e-prescribing because monetary penalties may be incurred from nonadoption of this method. AAPA has also participated in awareness campaigns to assist PAs into adopting e-prescribing in their everyday practices.

DRUG CLASSIFICATION AND REGULATION

Approval and regulation of therapeutic agents is the domain of the U.S. Food and Drug Administration (FDA). The FDA classifies drugs as either over-the-counter, that is, available without a prescription, or legend, meaning that they bear the legend statement, "Caution: Federal law prohibits dispensing without a prescription." These determinations are based on drug safety, the conditions for which it is indicated, and in some cases, the strength or dosage form. The FDA determines the conditions or indications for which a drug may be advertised, labeled, or otherwise marketed. This determination does not, however, limit the manner in which a physician (or other prescriber) may use an approved drug. Accepted medical practice, in other words, often includes use of drugs that is not reflected in package labeling that shows FDA-approved uses. For example, many angiotensin-converting enzyme inhibitors such as enalapril or lisinopril are used in the management of diabetic proteinuria, although only captopril is FDA approved for this use. Unfortunately, non–FDA-approved uses of drugs are not published in the commonly used *Physicians' Desk Reference (PDR)* or the PDA application ePocrates, but they are included in some other references, such as the online text *UpToDate or Essential Evidence Plus* (see Resources).

The FDA also categorizes drugs according to their safety in pregnancy or potential for harm to the fetus. Owing to the ethical problem in performing controlled studies on pregnant women, the human data for most drugs are incomplete and these ratings are largely based on animal studies. The difficult decision to prescribe any drug for a pregnant woman must be made on an individual basis with a clear understanding of the risk-benefit ratio (Table 14-1).

Drugs that have the potential for abuse or addiction are further regulated by the U.S. Drug Enforcement Agency (DEA). These include opiate and synthetic narcotics, sedatives, stimulants, and hallucinogens, which are collectively referred to as "controlled substances." Controlled substances are classified into one of five categories or schedules according to their potential for abuse or addiction (Table 14-2), and for this reason they are sometimes referred to as "schedule" drugs. Providers who are legally authorized to prescribe controlled substances, including PAs in most states, must comply with DEA rules and sometimes with additional state regulations regarding prescription format, refills, and record keeping.

GENERAL PRINCIPLES OF DRUG THERAPY

The decision to implement drug therapy and the choice of appropriate drugs are complex undertakings. Careful consideration of host factors, suspected or known causes of disease, and the properties and actions of available drugs are always required. In addition, the clinician should remember that drugs are not always the best solution to a clinical problem. Often, a nonpharmacologic therapeutic plan is the best choice for the patient. The following case will be used in the discussion that follows, to illustrate the process of deciding to use drug therapy and choosing from available agents.

TABLE 14-1 **Key to FDA Use-in-Pregnancy Ratings***

Category	Interpretation
A	Controlled studies show no risk. Adequate, well-controlled studies in pregnant women have failed to demonstrate risk to the fetus.
B	No evidence of risk in humans. Either animal findings show risk but human findings do not, or if no adequate human studies have been done, animal findings are negative.
C	Risk cannot be ruled out. Human studies are lacking, and animal studies are either positive for fetal risk or lacking as well. However, potential benefits may justify the potential risk.
D	Positive evidence of risk. Investigational or postmarketing data show risk to the fetus. Nevertheless, potential benefits may outweigh the potential risk.
X	Contraindicated in pregnancy. Studies in animals or humans, or investigational or postmarketing reports, have shown fetal risk that clearly outweighs any possible benefit to the patient.

From Gara N. Physician Assistants: Presenting and Dispensing Summary. Alexandria, VA: American Academy of Physician Assistants, 1992.

*The Food and Drug Administration's Pregnancy Categories are based on the degree to which available information has ruled out risk to the fetus balanced against the drug's potential benefits to the patient. Ratings range from "A," for drugs that have been tested for teratogenicity under controlled conditions without showing evidence of damage to the fetus, to "D" and "X," for drugs that are definitely teratogenic. The "D" rating is generally reserved for drugs with no safer alternatives. The "X" rating means there is absolutely no reason to risk using the drug in pregnancy.

TABLE 14-2 **Key to Controlled Substances Categories***

Category	Interpretation
C I	High potential for abuse. No accepted medical use.
C II	High potential for abuse. Use may lead to severe physical or psychological dependence. Prescriptions must be written in ink or typewritten and must be signed by the practitioner. Verbal prescriptions must be confirmed in writing within 72 hr and may be given only in a genuine emergency. No renewals are permitted.
C III	Some potential for abuse. Use may lead to low-to-moderate physical dependence or high psychological dependence. Prescriptions may be oral or written. Up to 5 renewals are permitted within 6 mo.
C IV	Low potential for abuse. Use may lead to limited physical or psychological dependence. Prescriptions may be oral or written. Up to 5 renewals are permitted within 6 mo.
C V	Subject to state and local regulation. Abuse potential is low. A prescription may not be required.

Modified from Gara N. Physician Assistants: Presenting and Dispensing Summary. Alexandria, VA: American Academy of Physician Assistants, 1992.

*Products listed with the symbols shown here are subject to the Controlled Substances Act of 1970. These drugs are categorized according to their potential for abuse. The greater the potential, the more severe are the limitations on their prescription.

CASE STUDY 14-1

Ms. C, a 45-year-old woman with a history of asthma, comes to the clinic with a 3-day history of upper respiratory infection (URI) symptoms—an increasingly productive cough, burning substernal chest pain, mild wheezing and shortness of breath, and a fever. Careful history and physical examination, peak flow measurements, and an abnormal chest radiograph lead to a diagnosis of community-acquired pneumonia and an exacerbation of her asthma.

RISK-BENEFIT RATIO

Given that virtually all drugs carry some degree of risk, whether to the patient, society, or the biosphere, all decisions to prescribe drugs should be predicated on evidence that the potential benefit will outweigh this risk. Often, the expectations of patients can make this point a challenge to the provider—it takes less time to write a prescription than to persuade the patient that a medication is not necessary! By the same token, once the decision has been made to use drug therapy, the choice of drugs often rests on consideration of the risk-benefit ratio. In this respect, the guiding principle, as always, is "First, do no harm."

DRUG ALLERGIES

Hypersensitivity reactions, or drug allergies, are allergic reactions to chemicals that occur after previous sensitization to that compound or to other compounds with structural similarities. The clinical effect of hypersensitivity reactions can range from mildly bothersome to life threatening and even fatal. Comprehensive medication histories should be taken on all patients because a missed allergy can be fatal, and because patients frequently but erroneously label adverse effects of medications as allergies. A complete history includes asking about any medications to which the patient is "allergic," along with the specific untoward effects the medications had in that particular patient. This type of history will provide the practitioner with a great deal more information than a simple list of drugs under the rubric of allergy. For example, many patients will state an allergy to codeine—nausea—which is not usually a true allergy but is a simple adverse effect of opiate narcotics.

The clinician should understand that an allergic response to a compound increases the likelihood of an allergic response to compounds with similar molecular structures. For example, a patient who has an allergic response to penicillin is also more likely to be allergic to antibiotics in the cephalosporin category than is a patient with no allergic history. Because of chemical similarities between sulfonamides and sulfonylureas, patients who are allergic to sulfonamide antibiotics may also be allergic to sulfonylurea hypoglycemic agents. Cross-reactivity exists among several categories of medications.

Allergic responses may be divided into four discrete categories by immunologic mechanism.[6] Type I reactions are mediated by immunoglobulin (Ig) E antibodies. During this type of reaction, several mediators, including histamine, leukotrienes, and prostaglandins, are released, causing vasodilation, edema, and a general inflammatory response. This type of allergic response can affect the gastrointestinal tract (food allergy), the respiratory system (rhinitis and bronchoconstriction), the vasculature (shock), and the skin (urticaria and atopic dermatitis). Penicillin-induced anaphylactic shock, which can be fatal, is an example of a type I reaction. Type II, or cytolytic, reactions are mediated by IgM and IgG antibodies and the subsequent activation of the complement system. Cells in the circulatory system are most frequently affected by type II reactions. Methyldopa-induced hemolytic anemia and quinidine-induced thrombocytopenia are examples of type II reactions. Arthus reactions, serum sickness, or type III reactions are mediated primarily by IgG and the deposition of antigen-antibody complexes in vascular endothelium. Certain anticonvulsants, sulfonamides, and other drugs have been linked to type III reactions. Delayed hypersensitivity, or type IV, reactions are mediated by macrophages and sensitized T lymphocytes. Contact dermatitis caused by poison ivy is an example of a type IV reaction.

CASE STUDY 14-1—CONT'D

Although pneumonia in an otherwise healthy patient is usually an uncomplicated condition that will resolve with rest, symptomatic therapy, and antibiotics, Ms. C's asthma puts her at increased risk for complications. Her dyspnea and wheezing also suggest the need for a bronchodilator. In response to further questioning, Ms. C states that she had a prescription for an albuterol inhaler but allowed it to lapse due to lack of money. She also has a prescription for theophylline tablets for her asthma. She is supposed to take 200 mg twice a day, but she says she often forgets. She is not currently sexually active, her last menstrual period was 2 weeks ago and normal, and she denies any possibility that she might be pregnant. Ms. C is a waitress with no health insurance and must pay for her medications herself. She knows of no drug allergies.

LIMITING THE ARMAMENTARIUM

A helpful and practical suggestion for the neophyte prescriber faced with the bewildering array of available products is this: Strive to know a few drugs in each therapeutic class well. With careful choices based on proven efficacy and safety, the beginner will gradually become comfortable with them and will rarely find it necessary to diverge from the chosen list. Until PAs reach this level of comfort, it is well worth their time to look up a drug each time they prescribe it.

The usual offending organisms in community-acquired pneumonia include *Streptococcus pneumoniae*, *Mycoplasma pneumoniae*, *Haemophilus influenzae*, and viruses. Classes of antibiotics covering this spectrum (excluding viruses) that are appropriate to use in this situation include macrolides (e.g., azithromycin or clarithromycin), tetracyclines (e.g., doxycycline), and antipneumococcal quinolones (e.g., levofloxacin). Alternatives include extended-spectrum penicillins (e.g., high-dose amoxicillin or high-dose amoxicillin/clavulanic acid), and second- and third-generation cephalosporins (e.g., cefuroxime, cefpodoxime, cefdinir). Effective bronchodilation for acute asthmatic symptoms is often achieved with any of several beta-agonist sympathomimetics (e.g., albuterol). Theophylline is an older methylxanthine drug that can be used as a long-acting bronchodilator, either alone or as an adjunct to other drugs. It is effective and inexpensive, but it has some significant disadvantages, as we discuss later. Newer drugs, such as montelukast, may help the asthmatic whose disease process is thought to be driven via an allergic response.

ROUTES OF ADMINISTRATION

The next decision to be addressed is how to get the drug into the patient. With the current marketing of new "delivery systems" (designed for patient convenience and compliance), this is an increasingly complex choice because we must consider available dosage forms and routes of administration. Dosage form is the physical form in which the drug is administered. Tablets, capsules, solutions, suspensions, gases, and ointments are all examples of dosage forms. The physical properties of a given dosage form can have a significant effect on how rapidly and completely the drug is delivered to the target tissue. For example, drugs taken orally must be in solution if they are to be absorbed into the circulation. Drugs that are already in solution or suspension are obviously absorbed faster than tablets or capsules, which must first dissolve. Development of newer dosage forms, such as orally disintegrating tablets (ODTs), have helped patients who may have difficulty in swallowing because these drugs melt in the mouth on ingestion.

The traditional routes of administration are oral (taken by mouth and absorbed by the gastrointestinal tract), topical (applied directly to the skin or mucous membranes), and parenteral (any route that bypasses the gastrointestinal absorption system). Parenteral injection choices are the direct intravenous route, intramuscular and subcutaneous routes, and intra-arterial and intrathecal (into the spinal column) routes for special applications. Other parenteral routes are inhalational (via the lungs), sublingual (absorbed by the oral mucosa), transdermal (placed on the skin for absorption into the circulation), and rectal.

The previously mentioned antibiotic classes and the xanthines are all available in a variety of oral and parenteral dosage forms. Sympathomimetics are most often inhaled using a metered-dose inhaler or nebulizer, although oral and parenteral preparations of some are available.

PHARMACOKINETICS AND PHARMACODYNAMICS

The study of how drugs are absorbed, distributed, metabolized, and excreted is known as *pharmacokinetics.* The study of how drugs produce an effect on the body is pharmacodynamics. Although a detailed discussion of these fields is beyond the scope of this chapter, it is critical that the prescriber understands some basic principles and considers their implications for therapy and patient education.

The first principle to consider is that of bioavailability, the fraction of the drug taken that actually reaches the systemic circulation. Bioavailability of an orally administered drug is influenced by two major factors: absorption of the drug by the gastric mucosa and metabolism of the drug as it passes through the liver from the portal system (the first-pass effect). These in turn are influenced by the properties of the drug itself, as well as by host factors such as other gastric contents, gastric motility, and the state of liver enzymes. Although ampicillin itself is not well absorbed orally, an alternative, amoxicillin, is well absorbed. As is often the case, variations in bioavailability of the other antibiotics are compensated for by the dosage schedule. Xanthines are variably absorbed and, as will become apparent, must be dosed carefully. Inhaled sympathomimetics are rapidly absorbed directly from the lungs to the systemic circulation. Proper use of the inhaler, however, is essential to ensure delivery of the desired dose to the lungs.

The distribution of a drug to various body tissues is primarily influenced by its relative solubility in water and by the degree to which it becomes bound to plasma proteins. The important thing to remember is that it is the free (unbound) drug that is dissolved in the plasma that is available to produce an effect. Drugs that are hydrophobic, such as barbiturates, are largely distributed to fat and muscle tissue, whereas some drugs, such as warfarin, have a high affinity for plasma proteins. In both cases, a small fraction of the originally absorbed drug is left freely dissolved and therefore able to produce an effect. Competition for protein-binding sites is one of the major mechanisms of drug-drug interactions.

CASE STUDY 14-1—CONT'D

None of the drugs being considered for Ms. C is protein bound to a clinically significant extent.

The third major pharmacokinetic variable is the rate of excretion from the body, or clearance. The major routes of drug excretion are the kidney, liver (through the bile or cytochrome P450; CYP-450 is an important group of enzymes that break down or metabolize drugs), gastrointestinal tract, and lungs. Small amounts of drugs may also be excreted in saliva, sweat, and breast milk. (This may be significant for a nursing infant.) The most important concepts of clearance for the prescriber are those of half-life and steady state. Simplistically speaking, the half-life of a drug is the time it takes for 50% of a dose of that drug to be cleared by the body. A steady state is achieved when the rate of administration of a drug is equal to the rate of clearance, thereby keeping the plasma concentration constant. Although drug half-lives are often given or estimated, we must use these with caution because many host factors, such as age, disease states, and drug interactions, influence the actual clearance. In some cases in which relatively toxic drugs are being used (e.g., theophylline), serum concentrations can be measured to ensure that the drug concentration is within the therapeutic range. Additionally, patient-specific pharmacokinetic parameters (i.e., clearance, half-life, and volume of distribution) may be calculated with pharmacokinetic equations using drug concentration data and patient characteristics. Most often, these calculations are done on request by a clinical pharmacist and can be of great assistance in the assessment of compliance, efficacy, toxicity, and future dosing regimens.

For antibiotic therapy of pneumonia, the route of excretion is not a major issue. For a urinary tract infection, however, it may be, because the drug would have to concentrate unchanged in the urine. In addition, the desired effect of most antibiotics does not depend on a constant plasma concentration, but rather on adequate peak levels. On the other hand, steady state is important when one is considering the xanthine bronchodilators. Theophylline has a narrow therapeutic window, which means that the therapeutic plasma concentration is close to the toxic plasma concentration.

Pharmacodynamics is a complex field, and this chapter is too limited to explore it. The reader should remember, at least, that no drug has just one effect, and that there are always going to be desired (or therapeutic) effects and undesired (or toxic) effects associated with a drug. Perhaps the most important knowledge a prescriber must have is what the potential toxic effects of a prescribed drug are, how to monitor for them, and what action to take should they appear. Patient education plays a major role in this respect, as is explored later (see Chapter 19).

CASE STUDY 14-1—CONT'D

Antibacterial drugs generally act either by causing the death of the organism (bactericidal activity) or by simply inhibiting its reproduction (bacteriostatic activity). If the host immune system is impaired for any reason, or if the condition is resistant to immune mechanisms (as in bacterial endocarditis), the bactericidal effect may be necessary to prevent a relapse. Amoxicillin, cephalosporins, and quinolones are bactericidal, whereas erythromycin seems to be either bactericidal or bacteriostatic, depending on the dose. Tetracyclines are bacteriostatic. Other than an allergic reaction, the only significant toxic effect among the agents being considered in this case is the well-known gastrointestinal upset associated with erythromycin. The two classes of bronchodilators both work by increasing the supply of cyclic adenosine monophosphate (cAMP) in smooth muscle cells, but they do so by different mechanisms. Ms. C is taking her theophylline inconsistently, so her level is probably subtherapeutic. In this case, an argument can be made for reinforcing her compliance with the theophylline, discontinuing the theophylline altogether, or adding a sympathomimetic. To minimize cardiac side effects when using sympathomimetics, a beta$_2$-selective agent such as albuterol or levalbuterol is preferred.

DRUG INTERACTIONS

Another vastly complex area is how drugs interact with one another in vivo. Most interactions occur by one of three major mechanisms:

1. Pharmacokinetic interference with absorption, distribution, metabolism, or excretion
2. Pharmacodynamic mechanisms such as additive or competitive receptor binding
3. Combined toxicity

Most prescribers become familiar with a few well-known and common drug interactions over time; therefore, they must consult reference books or electronic aids and trust that their patients' pharmacists will detect potential interactions among the drugs they supply.

CASE STUDY 14-1—CONT'D

It is well known that macrolide antibiotics (excluding azithromycin) can inhibit the metabolism of theophylline, thereby increasing theophylline's effect. Because theophylline has a narrow therapeutic window, administration of macrolides may, in fact, cause theophylline toxicity. However, the most appropriate management of Ms. C's asthma would be to discontinue the theophylline and replace it with an inhaled corticosteroid. This would remove the issues of drug interactions and toxicity associated with theophylline. In this case, the most appropriate choice of antibiotic is a macrolide, doxycycline, a fluoroquinolone, or a second-generation cephalosporin. The only other interaction to consider is the potential combined toxicity of theophylline and a sympathomimetic, which in this case will probably not be clinically significant, especially if the theophylline is discontinued.

SAFETY IN PREGNANCY

Pregnancy should be considered a possibility in all women of reproductive age. In Ms. C's case, her history makes pregnancy unlikely. If she were pregnant, FDA Use-in-Pregnancy Ratings would need to be consulted before final antibiotic choice. For the antibiotics under consideration, amoxicillin would be the safest (Category B) and doxycycline would be excluded (Category D) because of its potential adverse effects on the fetus.

COST-EFFECTIVENESS

With all other therapeutic considerations being equal, the choice of a specific agent may be a question of relative cost. With the current public focus on rising health care costs and the advent of managed health care systems, relative cost of prescribed drugs is an increasingly important and complex issue.

One major factor that influences drug costs is whether a drug is produced under patent or is available in a generic form. The pharmaceutical company that develops a new drug is allowed an exclusive patent on it for 20 years. When the patent has expired, other companies are free to produce and market the drug under its generic, or chemical, name, while the original company maintains the proprietary name and often continues to sell the agent at a higher price. In nearly all cases, the generic preparations are therapeutically equivalent to the brand name product. Many insurance companies and professional organizations are developing policies on generic prescribing, and in some systems, a pharmacy and therapeutics committee or a formulary committee may have input on these decisions. In addition, public third-party payers such as Medicare and Medicaid have specific restrictions on what drugs they will pay for. It is our bias that with a few notable exceptions, generic preparations, when available, should be used.

Another factor related to cost is variability in price among retail outlets. Especially with medications taken on a long-term basis, patients can realize significant savings by doing some comparison shopping. This is not only a direct benefit for them, but it may affect compliance as well. On the other hand, it is safer for a patient who is taking multiple medications to purchase them all at one pharmacy.

Azithromycin is chosen for Ms. C because it is well tolerated, has no significant drug interactions in this case, and is usually effective in uncomplicated pneumonia. Although it is not the cheapest antibiotic available for her illness, it is available generically, is reasonably priced, and comes in a convenient dosing regimen that will enhance patient adherence to therapy. The decision was made to discontinue her theophylline therapy. Additionally, she will be given a new prescription for an albuterol inhaler and a corticosteroid inhaler. Steroid inhalers should always be used with a spacer to minimize local adverse effects from the steroid. The next step is to decide what communication is necessary to accomplish this goal.

COMMUNICATION WITH THE PHARMACIST

A pharmacist is a professional member of the health care team who is trained and authorized by law to stock and dispense medications on the order of an authorized prescriber. A pharmacist completes 5 to 8 years of education and is knowledgeable about the actions and side effects of drugs. Pharmacists can be a valuable resource to the prescriber by assisting in choosing medications, dosing medications, reviewing regimens for drug interactions, and counseling patients regarding their medication.

THE PRESCRIPTION

Once the PA has evaluated a patient, arrived at a diagnosis, and determined that drug therapy is indicated, he or she must communicate the order to the pharmacist. This is done with the prescription. A prescription for noncontrolled substances may be written on a preprinted form or any blank paper. A prescription may also be transmitted over the telephone by speaking directly to a licensed pharmacist or pharmacy intern. Although it is common practice for this duty to be delegated to the prescriber's office personnel, this practice may lead to communication errors and should probably be avoided. Schedule II controlled substances may not be prescribed over the telephone, and some states require specially numbered, duplicate forms. The prescription for any controlled substance must contain a valid DEA number.

However the order is transmitted, it must contain certain legal elements. Incomplete or sloppily written prescriptions are the source of many dangerous medication errors, much patient confusion leading to poor compliance, and hours of wasted time for the pharmacist. Some states now require all prescriptions to be typed or printed; cursive writing is not allowed for anything except the prescriber's signature.

In 2008, the federal government required all prescriptions for Medicaid patients to be written on tamper-resistant prescription pads. The Centers for Medicare and Medicaid Services require the following to be in place to qualify as industry-recognized features for tamper-resistant prescriptions: a design that prevents unauthorized copying of the prescription; a design that prevents "the erasure or modification" of the written information on the prescription; and a design meant to prevent the use of counterfeit prescription forms. The new rules will apply to "all outpatient drugs including over-the-counter drugs in states that reimburse for prescription for such items." These requirements will not apply when the prescription is communicated by the prescriber to the pharmacy electronically, verbally, or by fax. The following list describes all of the elements of a complete prescription, with suggestions for accuracy in each:

- The date the prescription was written.
- Prescriber identification: Name, professional degree, office address and telephone number, and DEA number if required.
- Patient identification: Name and at least one other point of identification, such as date of birth (DOB), address, age, or gender. Weight is often added to pediatric prescriptions to facilitate correct dosing.
- Superscription: Rx, an abbreviation of a Latin phrase meaning "take thou."
- Inscription: The name of the drug and the strength. This should be the strength of each dosage unit, not the total dose to be taken by the patient. Abbreviations for drug names should be used only if the prescriber is certain that they will be clearly understood by the pharmacist.
- Subscription: Instructions to the pharmacist regarding the dosage form and the number of dosage units to dispense. Instructions should be specific about the dosage form (i.e., tablets, capsules, suspension), and a quantity must be specified if it is a liquid or semisolid (e.g., 120-mL suspension or 30-g tube). For controlled substances, quantities should be written in words and numbers to guard against alteration, such as "Dispense: thirty (30) tablets."
- Signa: Instructions to the patient. These should be as simple, complete, and specific as possible and should include how much to take, when to take it, and why it is being taken. "As directed" and "usual directions" should be avoided; such instructions are confusing and dangerous and are even illegal in some states.
- Refill information: The number of times (or time period) that the patient may renew the prescription without authorization from the prescriber. Prescriptions for schedule II controlled substances may not be refilled, and schedule III to V controlled substances have a five-refill or 6-month limit.
- Container information: Unless the prescriber specifies otherwise, medications will be dispensed in childproof containers, which may create problems for elderly or arthritic patients.
- Generic substitution: In most cases, the pharmacist may substitute a generic preparation for a prescribed brand, unless the prescriber specifies "dispense as written" on the order. Several phrases can be used to indicate generic substitution, which can differ between individual states.
- Warnings: The prescription should specify what, if any, warning labels should be attached to the medication vial. "May cause drowsiness" and "Do not take with alcohol" are examples.
- Prescriber's signature.

The use of abbreviations and symbols in prescription writing is unavoidable but increasingly discouraged to reduce medication errors. The Joint Commission, for example, has published a "Do Not Use" list of dangerous medical abbreviations that member organizations are expected to prohibit within their settings.[7] The prescriber should make every effort to ensure that any abbreviations used are clear and standard to avoid confusion. A common technique is the use of lowercase Roman numerals for numbers (e.g., "iii tabs PO tid" to specify three tablets by mouth three times daily). Table 14-3 lists standard prescription abbreviations, including some that should no longer be used.

CASE STUDY 14-1—CONT'D

The decision is made to treat Ms. C with azithromycin, 500 mg, to be taken by mouth on day 1, then 250 mg to be taken once daily for the next 4 days. In addition, she is to be given an albuterol inhaler to use four times daily and fluticasone inhaler (with a spacer), two puffs twice a day. Figure 14-1 shows complete prescriptions, legibly written, for this treatment.

ELECTRONIC MEDICAL RECORDS IN PRESCRIBING

Many clinics are converting their charting systems to computer-based electronic medical records. Depending on the system used, some of these include prescription templates that will automatically generate dosing regimens and other elements of the prescription as soon as a drug is chosen. Although the

TABLE 14-3 **Standard Abbreviations Used in Prescriptions, Including Some That Should No Longer Be Used**

Abbreviation	Meaning
Dose	
dr	Teaspoonful (do not use—always write "5 mL")
g, gm	Gram
gr	Grain
gtt	Drops
μg	Microgram (do not use —always write "microgram" or "mcg")
mcg	Microgram
mg	Milligram
Route	
AD	Right ear (do not use—always write "right ear")
AS	Left ear (do not use—always write "left ear")
AU	Each ear (do not use—always write "both ears")
OD	Right eye (do not use—always write "right eye")
OS	Left eye (do not use—always write "left eye")
OU	Each eye (do not use—always write "both eyes")
PO	By mouth
Susp	Suspension
supp	Suppository
PR	Per rectum
vag	Vaginally
Frequency	
ac	Before meals
ad lib	Freely, at pleasure
bid	Twice a day
h	Hour
hs	At bedtime
pc	After meals
prn	As needed
q	Every
qd	Every day (do not use—always write "once daily")
qid	Four times a day
qod	Every other day (do not use—always write "every other day")
stat	At once, immediately
tid	Three times a day
ut dict	As directed (do not use—always write out the instructions for use)
Miscellaneous	
cap	Capsule
c	With
Disp	Dispense
qs ad	Add a sufficient amount to make
ss	One half
sig	Directions for use
tab	Tablet

Modified from Katzung BG. Basic and Clinical Pharmacology, 10th ed. New York: McGraw-Hill/Lange, 2007.

Rain City Medical Clinic

1234 Main Street
Hometown, WA 99999
PH 509-123-4567
FAX 509-123-5678

Allergies
☒ NKMA

☐ No Drug Product Selection Allowed If Checked Here

NAME Jane Coper DOB ##
ADDRESS DATE ######

℞ Azithromycin 250 mg
Disp: #6
Sig: 2 tabs PO on day one, then 1 tab daily until gone, for pneumonia

Practitioner's Signature *John Doe, PA-C*

PRINT OR STAMP
Practitioner's Name John Doe, PA-C

DEA # Refill None times

A

Rain City Medical Clinic

1234 Main Street
Hometown, WA 99999
PH 509-123-4567
FAX 509-123-5678

Allergies
☒ NKMA

☐ No Drug Product Selection Allowed If Checked Here

NAME Jane Coper DOB ##
ADDRESS DATE ######

℞ Albuterol 90 mcg/spray MDI
Disp: 1 (one)
Sig: 2 puffs INH q4-6 hr PRN for wheezing

Practitioner's Signature *John Doe, PA-C*

PRINT OR STAMP
Practitioner's Name John Doe, PA-C

DEA # Refill 6 (six) times

B

Rain City Medical Clinic

1234 Main Street
Hometown, WA 99999
PH 509-123-4567
FAX 509-123-5678

Allergies
☒ NKMA

☐ No Drug Product Selection Allowed If Checked Here

NAME Jane Coper DOB ##
ADDRESS DATE ######

℞ Fluticasone 44 mcg INH
Disp: 1 (one)
Sig: 2 puffs bid for asthma maintenance

Practitioner's Signature *John Doe, PA-C*

PRINT OR STAMP
Practitioner's Name John Doe, PA-C

DEA # Refill 6 (six) times

C

FIGURE 14-1 ■ Sample prescriptions for azithromycin **(A)**, albuterol **(B)**, and fluticasone **(C)**.

convenience and potential of such systems to reduce medication errors is impressive, the PA is still responsible for reviewing all computer-generated prescriptions for accuracy and appropriate dosing. Similarly, prescription applications, such as ePocrates, can provide a wealth of drug information in a compact portable device and reduce the PA's reliance on memory or whatever print resource can be found at the time of need. However, no electronic aid can substitute for background knowledge, clinical judgment, and attention to detail when prescribing safely and appropriately.

INPATIENT ORDERS

Inpatient orders differ only slightly from the preceding description. Because they are usually written in the patient's chart on a preprinted, duplicate order form that is stamped with the patient's identifying data, the prescriber does not have to supply this information. In addition, medications are generally continued until the provider writes a discontinue order or the patient is discharged, or unless an expiration policy exists for that medication. Therefore, the elements of the hospital order are the same as the "body" of the outpatient prescription-inscription, subscription, and signa.

DISPENSING

Some states have specific laws allowing PAs to dispense medications under certain circumstances. The purpose of these rules is generally to serve the patient's best interest when the services of a pharmacist are not available or in emergency situations. In some cases, they also allow the dispensing of office samples. In most states, the laws specify that the PA must comply with labeling regulations when dispensing.

CASE STUDY 14-1—CONT'D

Ms. C is finally ready to receive her prescription. What information should the PA discuss with her before she leaves?

PATIENT EDUCATION

It is tempting, in a busy office setting, for the clinician to simply hand the patient the prescription and send him or her to the pharmacy. It is critical to the success and safety of the treatment, however, that the provider gives careful instructions about what to do with the prescribed drug. Although most pharmacists repeat the instructions when dispensing the drug, good patient education by the provider influences the outcome of treatment to a great extent. The principal areas to reinforce with the patient include the following:

- The reason for the treatment
- The expected outcome and how and when to take the medication
- The side effects to be alert for
- What to do if side effects should appear
- Any precautions to take

Every patient has the right to a full explanation of his or her condition, the rationale and risks of drug therapy, and what other options, if any, exist. With this explanation and the guidance of the provider, the patient becomes a fully consenting participant in his or her care rather than simply a consumer of service. As part of this process, a discussion of what toxic effects are commonly encountered is essential. Because the required listing of reported side effects in drug package inserts is often intimidating, it is the provider's role to put the important side effects in perspective and to give specific instructions about what to do if they should appear. Preprinted summaries of this information for common conditions and medications written at an appropriate educational level can be helpful to have on hand in the office to give to patients at the time of their visit.

The provider should confirm that the patient will be able to obtain the medicine and comply with instructions. Often, the involvement of a spouse or other caregiver is valuable at this point to enhance compliance. Specific suggestions about when to take the medication and how to remember to do so are helpful, for example, "Keep it in the kitchen and take it when you start to fix each meal," and "Keep it by your toothbrush so that you'll remember to take it at bedtime." In addition, care should be taken not to assume that the patient knows even something that may seem obvious. Therefore, instructions such as "Be sure to take the foil off the suppository before you insert it" are often not unreasonable. In addition, the duration of therapy should be explained, and the patient should be encouraged to take the medication until it is gone.

With long-term drug therapy, it is important to review instructions at each visit and to reinforce and monitor compliance. Repeated instruction on the proper use of inhalers, for example, can greatly enhance the success of this therapy.

CASE STUDY 14-1—CONT'D

The PA gives Ms. C her prescription for azithromycin. She confirms that she can pay for it and will go straight to the pharmacy next door. She is told to take two tablets on the first day with water, then one tablet per day for the next 4 days. The PA explains that some antibiotics are better absorbed on an empty stomach, but this one can be taken with or without food. The PA also gives her an albuterol inhaler from office samples, along with thorough instructions and a demonstration of its proper use. Additionally, the PA gives a sample of a fluticasone inhaler with a spacer. Ms. C was told to use this inhaler 5 minutes after she completes her albuterol inhalations. She is told to be alert for any side effects of the azithromycin, especially abdominal pain, diarrhea, or vaginitis, and to stop the medicine and call the clinic immediately if anything serious should appear. The PA also alerts Ms. C to the fact that the bronchodilator may make her feel a little "shaky" and dry in the mouth.

As with many elements of PA practice, a final critical consideration in prescribing is that of documentation. The patient's office chart should contain complete treatment information, including dosages, precautions, and follow-up. All medications approved for refill should also be noted in the chart. Attention to detail in this respect is a matter of good medical practice and can only help PAs and their patients overall.

PHARMACEUTICAL INDUSTRY

The production and sale of therapeutic drugs in the United States represents a huge industry worth many billions of dollars. Even a small market share of a single drug can mean millions in profit to a company. It is no wonder that drug manufacturers have large marketing departments dedicated to encouraging the prescribing of their products. The individual prescriber encounters such encouragement through advertisements in professional journals and through contact with company representatives, or "detailers." These representatives make routine calls to providers' offices and often have displays at professional meetings. Although pharmaceutical industry support of educational meetings and materials is a valuable contribution, prescribers must exercise care to avoid any potential conflict of interest. Professional organizations, including the American College of Physicians and the American Academy of Physician Assistants, have developed guidelines for interaction with this industry.[8]

Industry representatives often give free samples of their products to prescribers. Many providers consider accepting these samples useful to patients who could not otherwise pay for medications. Often, however, such samples are of more expensive, brand name products, so starting patients on these can be more costly in the long run. Although detail visits can be good sources of information about new products and community trends, the PA should have access to unbiased references on medications and their uses. Evidence-based newsletters such as *The Medical Letter*, *Prescriber's Letter*, or online references such as *UpToDate* or *Essential Evidence Plus* can provide valuable comparison data and advice about new and old drugs.

In the final analysis, the new prescriber would do well to consider two suggestions about dealing with the pharmaceutical industry. The first is to examine all product claims with as critical an eye as he or she would any piece of medical literature. The second is that it may not be the best policy to be among the first to use a new drug. Conversely, one should probably not stubbornly refuse to change an old habit in the face of convincing evidence that there is something better. Keeping these caveats in mind, PAs can achieve a mutually beneficial relationship with the pharmaceutical industry.

ETHICAL AND PRACTICAL CONSIDERATIONS OF PRESCRIBING

As has been mentioned, the prescribing of potentially dangerous drugs is a tremendous responsibility. Although it is often referred to as prescriptive authority, the ability to do so is best considered a privilege and treated with care. Perhaps extra considerations for PAs reflect the dependent nature of the practice and the necessity of close coordination with the supervising physician. A consistent approach to the following issues among the health care team can prevent misunderstandings.

It is not uncommon for a friend or family member who knows of a PA's skills and training to ask informally for information or medical advice. Although this occurrence is often a boost to the ego, it is fraught with danger and should be carefully planned for. The difficulty involved in maintaining professional objectivity when dealing with family members or friends is well known. One must also consider that the legal authority (in most states) to treat patients extends only to those who have an established relationship with the supervising physician. Finally, it may be helpful to consider the potential consequences, both legal and emotional, of a complication or bad outcome.

By the same token, a PA might be tempted to treat himself or herself by taking from office samples rather than making the effort to see another health care provider. To that temptation, one can simply answer by quoting Voltaire: "He who is his own physician has a fool for a doctor." In many states, prescribers are legally prevented from prescribing controlled substances for themselves.

A prescriber faces another difficult situation when he or she knows or suspects that a patient is seeking to obtain drugs for other than therapeutic use. The PA should be alert to this possibility but should not be too quick to label someone as a drug seeker simply because his or her pain is not convincing. Perhaps taking a philosophical approach can be helpful: That drug-seeking behavior is itself the problem for which intervention is indicated. On the other hand, the PA does not want to become known as an "easy mark." Reasonable caution includes protecting prescription pads and DEA numbers from theft, protecting prescriptions from alteration, and being alert to common ploys, such as lost prescriptions, uncommon allergies, and inconsistent stories. In addition, local knowledge of the resources available for referral and help with problems of substance abuse and addiction can be useful.

CONCLUSION

The authority to prescribe medications is a privilege extended to PAs in many states. When exercising this authority, it is incumbent on the practitioner to understand the rules and regulations regarding the prescribing of medications. The choice of medication used in each situation must be tailored to the individual patient and the disease being treated. Considerations should include the risk-benefit ratio, drug allergies, the most appropriate route of administration, pharmacokinetics and pharmacodynamics, possible drug interactions, and cost. Pharmacists are a readily available source of information and should be used. Prescriptions should be accompanied by patient education to ensure compliance. When used in an appropriate fashion, pharmacologic therapy can be one of the most effective tools clinicians have at their disposal.

CLINICAL APPLICATIONS

1. Interview pharmacists from a large health care system (e.g., managed care organization, academic health center, hospital system) that use a closed formulary for its providers. Discuss how drugs are chosen for, or excluded from, the formulary. Who makes the decisions? What are the criteria? Is there a research component to the decision-making (evidence-based)? What is the role of pharmaceutical companies in influencing these decisions?
2. Interview practicing pharmacists to whom you may refer patients. Find out what type of relationship they ideally would like to have with a PA. Describe typical patterns of communication between pharmacists (or PharmDs) and prescribers in your community, and recommend strategies for providing optimal patient care through maximizing this communication.

KEY POINTS

- The prescribing of drugs in unquestionably one of the most important and powerful tools in modern medical practice.
- As all 50 states extend prescribing privileges, safeguarding this responsibility is an essential element of practice for PAs as medical professionals.
- An ongoing review of current prescribing practices, along with the assessment of new drugs coming into the marketplace, is critical to provide safe and effective pharmacotherapy for patients.
- This information can be bewildering at times, but armed with a strong background in pharmacology and other related disciplines such as pharmacokinetics and pharmacodynamics, you can make sound therapeutic decisions.
- With exploding health care costs crippling the United States, cost-effective decisions, made in collaboration with other health care professionals such as pharmacists, become vitally important.
- Ethically based prescribing and practice of medicine is paramount to a successful career as a PA.

ACKNOWLEDGMENTS

This chapter was originally written by John Yerxa and revised by John R. White, Jr. for the second and third editions. Minor revisions for the fourth edition were made by Henry Stoll, with appreciation for the previous efforts of Yerxa and White. Minor revisions were made for the fifth edition by Lawrence Carey, with appreciation for the previous efforts of all three predecessors.

References

1. NC Gen Stat § 90 (1973).
2. Washington State Nurses Association v Board of Medical Examiners, 93 Wash 2d 117, 605 P2d 1269 (1980).
3. Creighton H. Law for the nurse supervisor: physician's assistant medication orders. Superv Nurse 1981;12:46.
4. Willis JB. Prescriptive practice patterns of physician assistants. J Am Acad Physician Assist 1990;3:39.
5. Where Physician Assistants Are Authorized to Prescribe. American Academy of Physician Assistants. *http://www.aapa.org/the_pa_profession/federal_and_state_affairs/resources/item.aspx?id=756&terms=prescribing*; Accessed December 2, 2011.
6. Brunton L, Lazo J, Parker K, (eds). Goodman and Gilman's The Pharmacological Basis of Therapeutics. 12th ed. New York: McGraw-Hill, 2010.
7. The Official "Do Not Use" List. Joint Commission. *http://www.jointcommission.org/assets/1/18/Official_Do_Not_Use_List_6_111.PDF*; Accessed December 2, 2011.
8. Position Paper. Physician-Industry Relations. Part 1: Individual Physicians. American College of Physicians. *http://www.annals.org/cgi/reprint/136/5/396.pdf.* Guidelines for Ethical Conduct for the Physician Assistant Profession. American Academy of Physician Assistants. *http://www.aapa.org/your_pa_career/becoming_a_pa/resources/item.aspx?id=1518&terms=Guidelines%20for%20Ethical%20Conduct.* Accessed December 2, 2011.

The resources for this chapter can be found at www.expertconsult.com.

CHAPTER 15

COMPLEMENTARY AND ALTERNATIVE MEDICINE

Emily WhiteHorse

CHAPTER CONTENTS

Complementary and alternative medicine (CAM) refers to the use of approaches, therapies, and treatments that are not considered part of the biomedical (conventional) model of medicine. CAM also encompasses a broad range of philosophies and beliefs regarding the nature of health, healing, illness, and disease different from those on which our health care system is based. Other terms such as *integrated* or *holistic* medicine have also been used.

By definition, *complementary* refers to those approaches or therapies that are used in addition to conventional medicine treatments, such as the use of acupuncture with physical therapy and medications in patients with chronic pain syndromes. *Alternative* refers to those approaches or therapies that are used instead of or in place of conventional medicine (e.g., the use of homeopathy and homeopathic remedies instead of pharmaceutical medications). In everyday use this clear distinction is lost.

The biomedical model is based on clearly defined philosophies and approaches to health and illness that are based on the beliefs and values of the Western scientific culture. Many complementary and alternative approaches represent philosophies, beliefs, values, and approaches of health care systems from other cultures and other countries, such as the use of the meridian system and the concept of *Qi* in the diagnosis and treatment of illness in traditional Chinese medicine. In addition, some CAM approaches emerge from visionary ideas and experimentation initiated by individuals within a given culture (e.g., homeopathy).

Every health care system in the world is based on the dominant beliefs, values, and expectations of the people it serves. This is known as the *explanatory model.* Because of the vast and growing ethnic diversity in the United States, understanding CAM is intimately connected to cultural sensitivity, awareness, and competency. For the nature and uses of CAM to be understood, it is important to understand the culture and/or explanatory model from which the therapy originated. This makes the study of CAM a daunting task. Although it is not possible or necessary to know all the modalities or systems of healing encompassed in CAM, it is possible for physician assistants (PAs) to develop the skills needed to navigate the use of CAM by their patients.

This chapter does not present detailed information on specific CAM therapies and treatments; rather, it discusses broad categories, suggests approaches, and provides resources. Its main focus is to offer guidelines and suggestions to help PAs learn how to interact and communicate effectively with patients regarding both their beliefs about health, healing, and disease and their use of CAM. It is imperative that PAs gather the tools and learn the skills to support open and honest communication with the goal of providing the best care possible for each patient, which in today's society means asking about a person's belief system and about CAM.

HISTORY

The existence, use, and popularity of CAM are not new phenomena in the United States. CAM has been part of our history since the early colonial days, and its prevalence has waxed and waned throughout the centuries. The seeds for the most recent resurgence of interest in approaches other than conventional western medicine began in the 1960s and have continued to gain momentum up to the present day.

The most recent rise in the use of CAM has been influenced by several factors: (1) the social and civil rights movements of the 1960s; (2) the growing cost of health care; (3) the emergence of the field of psychology and the role of the mind in relationship to illness and disease; (4) the uncovering of the debilitating and sometimes fatal side effects of medications previously thought safe; (5) the emergence of resistant strains of bacteria; (6) the human immunodeficiency virus/acquired immunodeficiency syndrome (HIV/AIDS) epidemic; and (7) a world that has become smaller through technology.

Over the past 50 years many events have led to the erosion of faith and trust that the American people have had regarding our health care system's ability to treat, cure, and/or prevent illness. The increasing prevalence of chronic diseases and the general unsatisfactory progress in the multimillion dollar "war on cancer" have caused many to wonder if the range of modern medicine's effectiveness has reached its limits. In addition, there is a heightened awareness of the public to the constant growing number of studies that demonstrate unnecessary, counterproductive, and dangerous practices in our medical system, including prolonged use of addictive drugs, unnecessary surgeries, and increased numbers of iatrogenic diseases. The most recent event that illuminated the limitations of biomedical medicine despite its vast advances in technology was the beginning of the AIDS epidemic in the 1980s.

Additional factors that have greatly influenced the reemergence and use of alternatives in this country are the explosion of communication technology and the vast political changes that have occurred in other countries. These factors have allowed for the open flow and exchange of cultural and religious customs, as well as exposure to the health care systems of other countries. Today's patients are better educated and more aware of the existence of other ways to manage their health or illness beyond that of the biomedical model. In addition, as our country grows richly diverse and moves away from the *melting pot* philosophy, many immigrants are maintaining and using their country of origin's cultural and/or religious traditions concerning health and healing.

The reasons for choosing alternatives today are not much different than they were more than 200 years ago. Patients are once again looking for a kinder, gentler, more personal approach to health and healing. They are also looking for more choices and more control in their health decisions, and they are less likely to accept the debilitating side effects of biomedical treatments.

GOVERNMENT RESPONSE

Because of the rising use of alternative approaches, a Congressional mandate established the Office of Alternative Medicine (OAM) within the National Institutes of Health (NIH) in 1991. The purpose of this office was to facilitate the evaluation of alternative medical treatment modalities and their effectiveness through research and other initiatives. The initial financial budget for this undertaking was $2 million.

In 1999 the Omnibus appropriations bill resulted in the change of title and status of the OAM from an office to a center, the National Center for Complementary and Alternative Medicine (NCCAM) within the NIH. This change provided for a more expansive role to include establishing a clearinghouse to provide information to providers and patients, conducting and funding research, disseminating health information and other programs with regards to the investigation, and validation of CAM treatments.[1] The budget for this expanded role was $68 million in 2000 and has increased to $128 million in 2010.[2] Today the NCCAM is the federal government's leading agency for scientific research on CAM with a newly defined strategic plan, which includes a focus on research regarding mind-body interventions, modalities, and disciplines and research on the safety and efficacy of CAM products, particularly herbal and botanical medicines and supplements.[3,4]

The NCCAM loosely divides CAM into four broad-based categories to include natural products, mind-body medicine, manipulative and body-based practices, and other CAM practices. However, some may fit into more than one category. Natural products include herbal medicine, vitamins, and minerals, most of which are sold as dietary supplements. Examples of natural products include *Echinacea*, antioxidant vitamins, and probiotics. Mind-body medicine anchors its approach in the physiologic and emotional connection between the body and the mind to effect physical change and promote health. Practices such as meditation, yoga, acupuncture, guided imagery, and tai chi are considered in this category. Manipulative and body-based practices are based on the use of techniques and approaches that focus on the physical body, such as joints, bones, soft tissue, and the lymphatic system to enhance and affect both functional and structural capacity in both the physical and emotional realms. Examples include chiropractics, various forms of massage, and craniosacral therapy. Other CAM practices encompass a broad range of approaches, some based on health care belief and delivery systems from other countries and cultures such as traditional Chinese medicine or Ayurvedic medicine or practices used by traditional healers such as Native American medicine men. This category also includes approaches that involve the use or manipulation of energy fields such as Reiki and Qi Gong and those that use movement as a means to promote physical and emotional well-being such as Pilates, Trager, and Alexander techniques. Homeopathy and naturopathy are also considered under this category.[5]

PREVALENCE OF USE OF CAM IN THE UNITED STATES

In the first of two landmark research studies done by David Eisenberg, MD,[6] regarding the use and prevalence of CAM in the United States, he found that 33.8% of Americans used alternative medicine in 1990. Americans spent more than $13 billion for alternatives with an estimated $10 billion spent out of pocket, and visits to alternative practitioners (425 million) exceeded visits to primary care physicians (388 million). The most commonly used CAM modalities in 1990 included relaxation techniques, chiropractic, and massage. An alarming finding was that only 39.8% of patients disclosed this use to their primary care providers.[6]

In the follow-up study done in 1997, the usage of CAM increased to 42.1%, and for adults ages 35 to 49 it was estimated that one of every two adults used some form of alternatives. Spending also increased to $21 billion with $12 billion paid out of pocket, and there was a 47.3% increase in total number of visits to alternative practitioners (425 billion to 629 million). While relaxation techniques, chiropractic, and massage continued to be popular, the use of herbal medicine, self-help groups, folk remedies, energy healing, and homeopathy had also increased.[6,7] However, the disclosure rate to primary care providers remained relatively unchanged at 38.5%.[7]

In a study published in the *Southern Medical Journal* in 2000, the use of CAM was found to be 44% of those who responded to the survey. The overall disclosure rate of alternative modality use to a conventional practitioner was 43%, and there was a 25% disclosure rate specifically for the use of herbs and/or vitamins. Speculation regarding the reasons for this lack of disclosure by patients included fear of disapproval, patient perception that such information is not important, lack of time during the quick office visit, or doubt the conventional provider would understand.[8]

In a 2001 study in the *Annals of Internal Medicine*, 79% of patients surveyed who admitted use of both conventional and CAM providers perceived the combination of both treatments to be superior to either treatment alone. However, their reported disclosure rate to the conventional provider regarding their CAM use was only 37%. The main reason offered by patients for the lack of disclosure was concern about their conventional provider's inability to understand or incorporate CAM therapy into their overall management.[9]

In 2004, the Centers for Disease Control and Prevention's (CDC) National Center for Health Statistics (NCHS) released the results of one of the most comprehensive surveys to date regarding the use of CAM among the American population. They surveyed more than 31,000 adults in the United States in 2002 and found that 36% of adults in America used some form of CAM therapy during the past 12 months.[10]

A follow-up study was conducted by the CDC and NCHS in 2007. This study was expanded for the first time to include the use of CAM in children (age: birth to 17 years) and adults in the United States. More than 75,000 adults and more than 9000 children were surveyed regarding their use of CAM over the past 12 months, with the data showing about 4 out of every 10 (38.8%) adults and 1 out of every 9 (11.8%) children indicating some use (Figure 15-1).[1]

TRENDS

The use of CAM spans people of all backgrounds. Black adults were more likely than white or Asian adults to use CAM. When prayer is included, use among Asian, black, Hispanic, and white populations was 61.7%, 71.3%, 61.4%, and 60.4%, respectively.[10] Puerto Rican (29.7%), Dominican (28.2%), and Mexican Americans (27.4%) were the highest users of CAM within the Hispanic subpopulations (Figure 15-2).[1] Consistent with earlier studies, CAM continues to be used more by women, in adults between the ages of 30 and 69, in people with higher

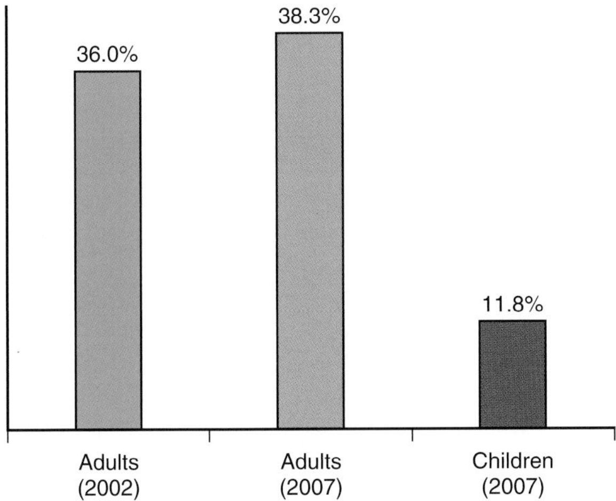

FIGURE 15-1 Complementary and alternative medicine use by U.S. adults and children. (From Barnes PM, Bloom B, Nahin R. CDC National Health Statistics Report #12. Complementary and Alternative Medicine Use among Adults and Children: United States 2007. December 2008.)

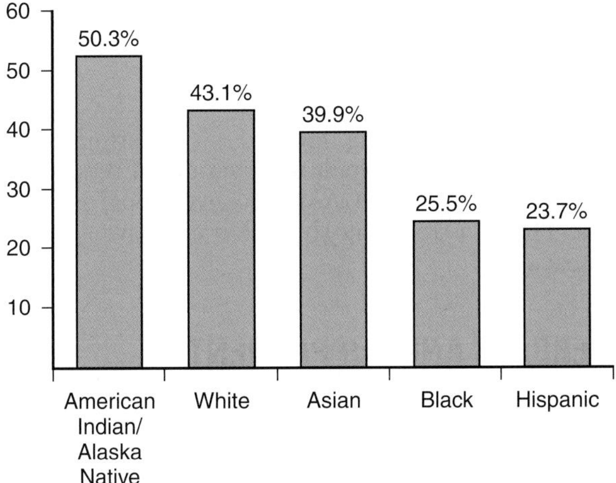

FIGURE 15-2 Complementary and alternative medicine use by race/ethnicity among adults: 2007. (From Barnes PM, Bloom B, Nahin R. CDC National Health Statistics Report #12. Complementary and Alternative Medicine Use among Adults and Children: United States 2007. December 2008.)

education levels, people who have been hospitalized in the past year, those living in urban areas, and former smokers.[1,10,11]

The overwhelming majority of patients who use CAM therapies do so to complement conventional care, rather than in lieu of it.[1,7,12] Additional reasons for using CAM include failure of conventional medical treatments and/or unacceptable side effects from those treatments or no conventional treatment available.[13] Those who use CAM tend to want more autonomy in their health care choices and treatments; tend to have a more holistic philosophic orientation, believing in the importance of mind, body, and spirit; and value environmentalism, spirituality, and personal growth. They also tend to seek health promotion and health prevention and are more likely to have had a transformation experience that changed their worldview.[12]

In the 2002 CDC/NCHS study, 54.9% of adults believed that the use of CAM combined with conventional medicine would be helpful, 50% did so because they were curious, 26% used CAM because they believed conventional medicine would not help them, and 13% of adult CAM users did so because they felt conventional medicine was too expensive.[10] Consistent in both the 2002 and 2007 CDC/NCHS studies, adults were more likely to use CAM when the cost of conventional medical care was a concern or simply unaffordable.[1,10] Keep in mind that these are general patterns observed, and it is inherently the responsibility of the PA to explore a patient's reason for the use of CAM.

In the early studies conducted in the 1990s, conditions for which CAM treatments or providers were most commonly used included back problems, allergies, fatigue, arthritis, hypertension, insomnia, lung problems, skin problems, digestive problems, depression and anxiety,[6,7] cancer, and HIV. In the 2002 and 2007 CDC/NCHS reports, the most common conditions for which CAM therapies were used continued to include back and neck pain or problems, anxiety, and depression (Figure 15-3).[1,10] Today, certain commonly used CAM modalities such as massage, acupuncture, and relaxation/stress management have moved more into mainstream biomedical medicine. However, factors such as geographic location, ethnicity, and socioeconomic status all influence the popularity and use of CAM modalities within a given patient population.

In the 2002 CDC/NCHS study, the top three most commonly used CAM therapies (excluding prayer) were natural products (18.9%), deep breathing (11.6%), and meditation (7.6%). Therapies such as chiropractic care, yoga, and massage were 7.5%, 5.1%, and 5.0%, respectively.[11]

The three most commonly used CAM therapies in 2007 were natural products (17.7%), deep breathing exercises (12.7%), meditation (9.4%), chiropractic (8.6%), massage (8.3%), and yoga (6.1%) (Figure 15-4). There was an increase in the use of some mind-body therapies from 2002 to 2007, specifically deep breathing exercises, meditation, and yoga. Other areas of increase include use of acupuncture, massage therapy, and naturopathy.[1]

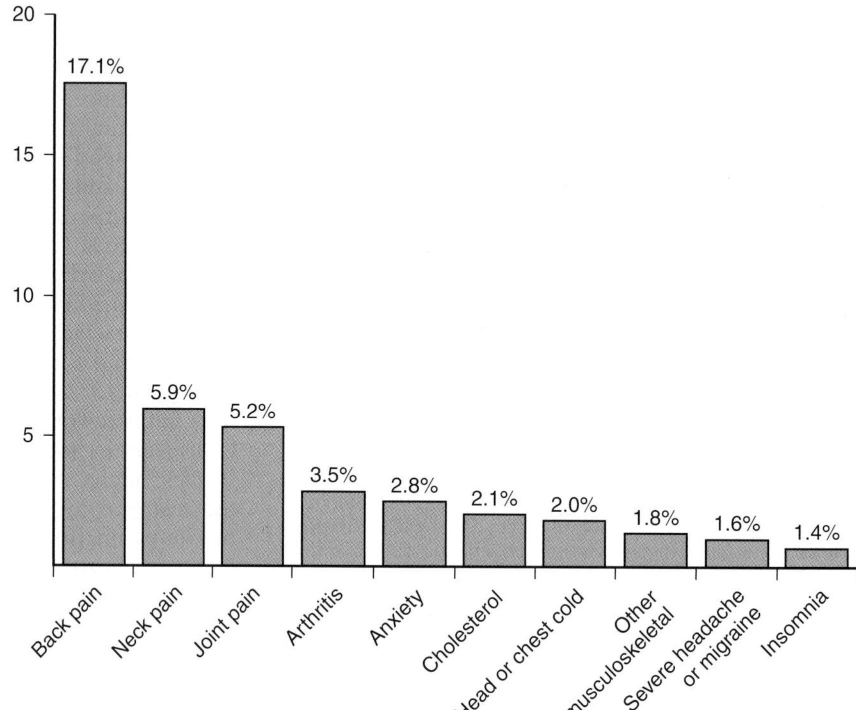

FIGURE 15-3 Diseases/conditions for which CAM is most frequently used among adults: 2007. (From Barnes PM, Bloom B, Nahin R. CDC National Health Statistics Report #12. Complementary and Alternative Medicine Use among Adults and Children: United States 2007. December 2008.)

With the first look into the use in children age 17 or younger, those whose parents used CAM were twice as likely to use CAM as well. Adolescents who were 12 to 17 years old were more likely to use CAM than younger children, and white children were twice as likely as black children and 1.5 times as likely as Hispanic children to use CAM. Similar to adult use, when the cost of care was a concern or unaffordable, CAM use was more likely.[1]

The most common therapies used in those 17 years and younger were natural products (3.9%), chiropractic (2.8%), deep breathing (2.2%), yoga (2.1%), and homeopathic treatments (1.3%) (Figure 15-5). The most common medical conditions treated with CAM in children were back or neck pain, head or chest colds, anxiety or stress, other musculoskeletal problems, and attention deficit hyperactivity disorder (Figure 15-6).[1]

Over the past 14 years, studies continue to demonstrate that the use of CAM by people in the United States is here to stay. Unlike some changes within our health care system that originate from within the system itself, this movement originated and has been sustained by those outside the system—the patients. This use of other health care models, methods, systems, and treatments in addition to or in lieu of conventional medicine is not showing any signs of slowing or reversing. However, it is alarming that patients are still reluctant for a variety of reasons to disclose their use of CAM to conventional providers. This is a trend on which PAs can have a direct impact.

HERBALS AND SUPPLEMENTS

The use of natural products such as herbals and supplements continues to grow. It rose from 12.1% admitted usage by adults in 1997 to 18.6% in 2002.[14] Between 1990 and 1997 the use of herbal remedies increased 380%, and the use of high-dose vitamins increased 130%, so that one in five Americans were taking prescription medications along with herbs, vitamins, or both.[7] In a study done by Kaufman and colleagues[15] in 2002, researchers found that 80% of Americans take at least one type of medication, herb, or supplement, and 16% use these substances concomitantly.

In 2007, natural products were the most popular form of CAM used among adults and children.[1] The most commonly used natural products for adults included fish oil/omega 3s (37.4%), glucosamine (19.9%), *Echinacea* (19.8%), flaxseed (15.9%), and

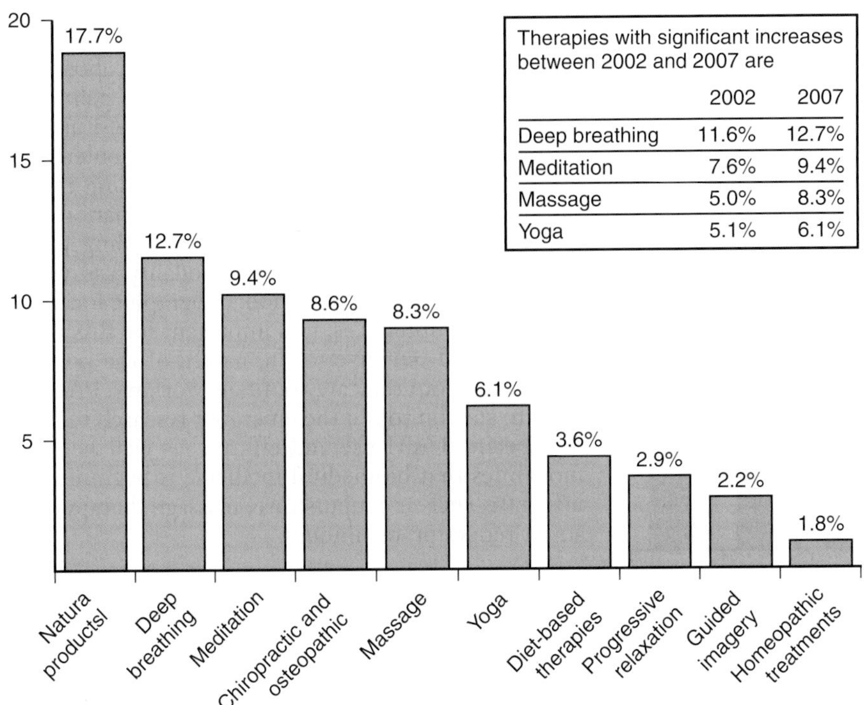

Therapies with significant increases between 2002 and 2007 are	2002	2007
Deep breathing	11.6%	12.7%
Meditation	7.6%	9.4%
Massage	5.0%	8.3%
Yoga	5.1%	6.1%

FIGURE 15-4 ■ Ten most common complementary and alternative medicine therapies among adults: 2007. (From Barnes PM, Bloom B, Nahin R. CDC National Health Statistics Report #12. Complementary and Alternative Medicine Use among Adults and Children: United States 2007. December 2008.)

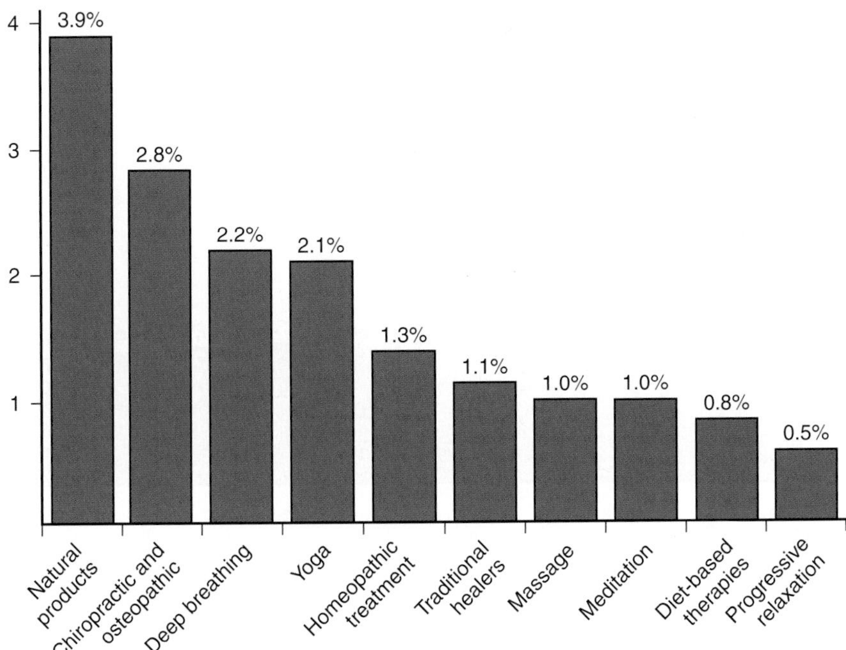

FIGURE 15-5 ■ Ten most common complementary and alternative medicine therapies among children: 2007. (From Barnes PM, Bloom B, Nahin R. CDC National Health Statistics Report #12. Complementary and Alternative Medicine Use among Adults and Children: United States 2007. December 2008.)

ginseng (14.1%) (Figure 15-7). For children, those most commonly used were *Echinacea* (37.2%), fish oil/omega 3s (30.5%), combination herb pill (17.9%), and flaxseed (16.7%).[1] In 2002, the top herbs or supplements used included *Echinacea* (40.3%), ginseng (24.1%), *Ginkgo biloba* (21.1%), garlic (19.9%), and glucosamine (14.9%).[10] In 2001 the herbs that saw the greatest increase in use included soy, valerian root, milk thistle, green tea, and black cohosh. In 2000, *Gingko biloba*, St. John's wort, saw palmetto, *Echinacea*, ginseng, and garlic saw the highest use.[16]

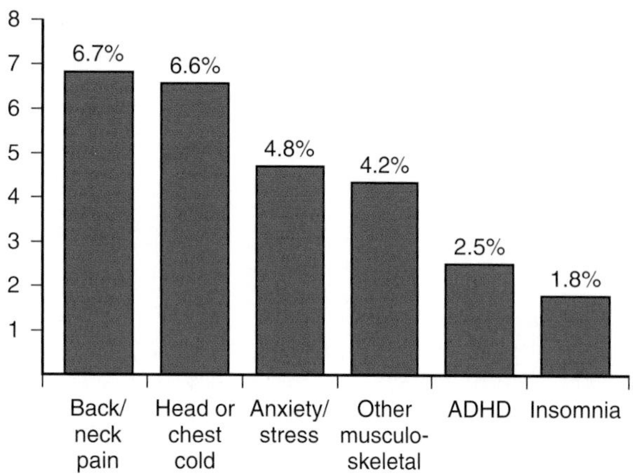

FIGURE 15-6 Diseases/conditions for which complementary and alternative medicine is most frequently used among children: 2007. *ADHD,* Attention deficit hyperactivity disorder. (From Barnes PM, Bloom B, Nahin R. CDC National Health Statistics Report #12. Complementary and Alternative Medicine Use among Adults and Children: United States 2007. December 2008.)

The changing nature of herbs and supplements use is influenced by several factors including media information and emerging research information that either supports or refutes the herbs' healing properties. Because trends of CAM modality use varies on the basis of the time period, geographic location, and cultural influences, it is important for PAs to be aware of and sensitive to the nature of the population with whom they are routinely working. PAs also need to stay on top of the emerging research regarding specific CAM use and efficacy, as well as those modalities that biomedical medicine is beginning to integrate, such as acupuncture, massage therapy, and stress-reduction techniques.

IMPLICATIONS FOR PHYSICIAN ASSISTANTS

In 1999, AAPA passed a resolution that PAs need to become more knowledgeable about CAM practices. Although most PA programs include education about

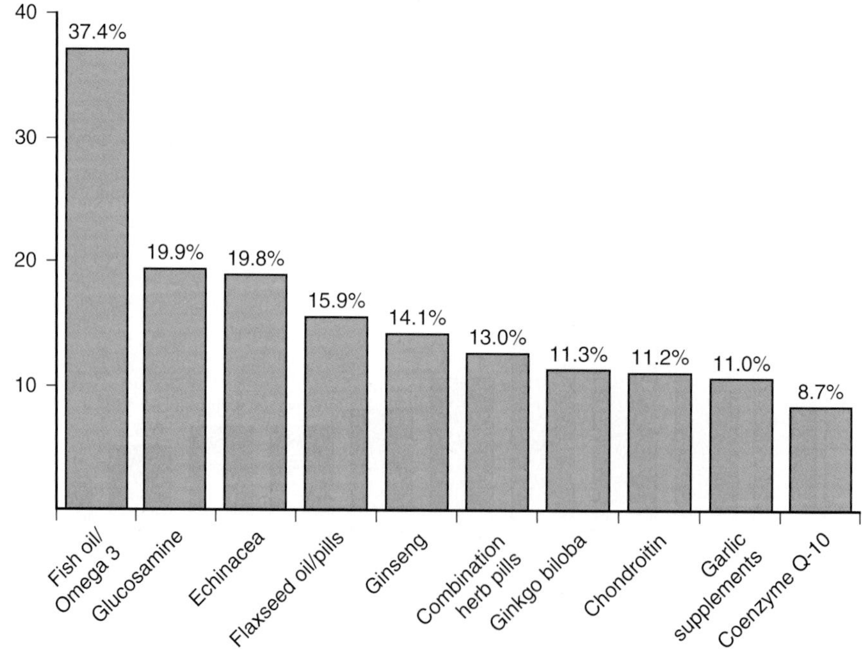

FIGURE 15-7 Ten most common natural products among adults: 2007. (From Barnes PM, Bloom B, Nahin R. CDC National Health Statistics Report #12. Complementary and Alternative Medicine Use among Adults and Children: United States 2007. December 2008.)

CAM, the main responsibility of learning about these approaches rests with each PA.

Therefore it is important for PA students and practicing PAs to begin to educate themselves regarding CAM, especially those approaches or modalities that are being used by their current patients. The continued prevalence and use of CAM in the country indicates that to be successful in today's health care arena, knowledge about CAM is vital. A growing number of reputable conferences, journals, coursework, and Internet sites offer a wide variety of accurate and up-to-date information about the changing face of medicine and the integration of CAM modalities into everyday practice. It is imperative that PAs begin to use these resources.

WHAT PAs SHOULD KNOW WHEN MANAGING PATIENTS AND CAM USE

Most of what is necessary for PAs to comfortably navigate patients who are interested in or already using CAM is an open mind, good communication skills, the willingness to spend some time researching and learning about CAM, and the need to ensure patient safety. PAs need to ask every patient about the use of CAM and be open, supportive, and nonjudgmental when patients share things that may at first seem incomprehensible (e.g., believing that an illness is caused by an evil spirit when the PA is confident it has been caused by bacteria). The patient may want to go to a community healer to remove the evil spirit, so the role of the PA is to support the patient in going to the healer and also negotiate with the patient the added benefit of taking the antibiotic. In this way the PA acknowledges the power of the patient's belief regarding what has caused the illness and what must be done to cure it, the patient learns to trust the PA, and the treatment reflects a plan acceptable to both.

At the core of a PA's work with patients using CAM is to ensure the overall health and well-being of the patient. This is achieved through evaluating a CAM modality for its safety and efficacy. In today's environment, many reputable scientific sources are available to assist a PA in determining the safety and efficacy of a therapy. Just as PAs use evidence-based medicine to aid in guiding their conventional treatment of disease, so too can evidence-based medicine be used to evaluate the safety and efficacy of a CAM modality. Practical recommendations for clinicians regarding whether or not to recommend or support CAM treatments or modalities or referral to CAM providers include the following:

1. It is acceptable to use or recommend those CAM modalities for which safety and efficacy have been demonstrated through research.
2. It is safe, but caution must be used for a CAM modality that has been established to be safe; however, its efficacy is inconclusive.
3. Significant caution must be used for those CAM modalities for which either safety or efficacy are inconclusive.
4. Avoid use or recommendation of those modalities for which there is no evidence to support safety and/or efficacy.

Decisions must be made on evidence-based research. If the decision to recommend or support the use of CAM by a patient is exercised, the sources from which the information was found regarding safety and efficacy should be documented, along with documentation of the discussion with the patient regarding the use of the CAM modality. Monitoring and patient follow-up are also a must. It is important for the patient to know that even if he or she goes against medical advice and uses a CAM modality, the PA will continue to be available to them as a place to turn should the CAM modality not work or the patient changes his or her mind and wants to use Western approaches.

With such a high prevalence of the use of herbs or supplements, there is some basic knowledge that all PAs should know that will be helpful in educating and guiding their patients with selection and use of these products. Herbal medicinal products are defined as "medicinal products containing as active ingredients exclusively plant material and/or vegetable drug preparations."[17] An example of an herbal medicinal product would be St. John's wort, which is derived from constituents of the plant by the same name. Herbal products may come in one or more of the following preparations: liquid extract, liquid tincture, dry extract (pill or capsule), and teas. These preparations have varying potency. Liquid extracts are the most potent form of the herb and contain the highest concentration of the herb within liquid, usually a 1:1 ratio. Liquid tinctures are slightly more dilute than extracts, usually a 1:5 or 1:10 ratio and thus slightly less potent. Dry extracts in pill or tablet format are generally at a potency ratio of 4:1 (herb to dry fillers). Teas are usually the less potent form of herbs, especially commercial preparations. However, teas created by traditional healers or herbalists may be much more potent.[18]

As defined by Congress in the Dietary Supplement Health and Education Act of 1994, a dietary supplement is a product (other than tobacco) that is intended to supplement the diet and contains one or more dietary ingredients including vitamins, minerals, herbs, or amino acids.[19,20] An example of a supplement would be glucosamine, which is derived from fish cartilage.[21]

When counseling a patient about the use of herbs or supplements, all PAs need to know several practical recommendations to ensure patient safety.

1. Herbs and/or supplements are not inherently safe. Side effects and toxicities are possible, as are potential drug-herb interactions. Patients should understand the importance of using herbs as one would a medication in terms of indications, dosage, and frequency. Inappropriate use could lead to harm.
2. Treatment effects have a slower onset. Often it will take 4 to 6 weeks before the effects of the herb are realized. Thus it is important to educate the patient so that he or she continues treatment long enough to determine efficacy.
3. Do not combine herbs, supplements, or pharmaceuticals with similar effects because this may have a synergistic or toxic effect. Thus it is critically important to ask in the history about the use of herbs or supplements before prescribing any medication. Many times patients have tried self-treatments before seeking the advice of a medical provider.
4. If an herb or supplement is going to be used, it is best to advise the use of a single ingredient product rather than combined products. For example, *Echinacea* is commonly combined with goldenseal. The concern with combined products is that if the patient has a reaction, it is more challenging to determine which substance in the product caused the reaction.
5. Recommend that products be purchased from a reputable source. A number of independent and governmental organizations provide both the public and the medical community with information regarding products that have been tested and are deemed safe.
6. Avoid use of herbs in pregnant or nursing women. Because most of the studies done have been on nonpregnant adults and not children, there are simply not enough data to ensure safety of use for these patients.

ROLE OF THE PHYSICIAN ASSISTANT

Given this knowledge that many patients are using some form of CAM on a regular basis, many times along with conventional therapies, and that this information is not necessarily being provided by the patient, PAs have the responsibility to open the door to communication. It is no longer acceptable to wait for the patient to disclose. There is the growing concern that without disclosure, the course of patients' treatment may have an unexpected or undesired effect, such as a drug-herb interaction. To effectively navigate the changing face of medicine in today's environment, PAs need to incorporate some adjustments in their approach to *all* patients. The following six recommendations should be considered in every patient encounter:

1. **Ask Your Patients.** The disclosure rate of the use of CAM by patients to their conventional providers is an alarming statistic that PAs can easily change. The most important thing practicing PAs and PA students can begin to do immediately is to routinely ask *all* their patients about use of CAM. This can easily be integrated into history-taking in several areas. First, when asking patients what they have tried to make the symptom better or worse, listen to the patient's response and then follow up with additional questions, such as, "*Other patients have tried alternative approaches such as herbs or massage or another practitioner. Have you tried any of those?*" If the patient's response is affirmative, then the PA needs to ask a few more questions, such as, "*Did the treatments help? Whom did you see? What did the treatments consist of? How long did you use the treatment?*" It is not uncommon for patients to have used or visited a number of alternative providers before making an appointment with a conventional provider.

   Another opportunity to explore patients' potential use of CAM, as well as gaining insight into their explanatory model, is in the social history. In order to better understand patients, it is important that providers know more about their belief systems. These questions should be asked of *all* patients, not just those who are obviously from a different culture or country. Questions could include, "*What do you do to stay healthy emotionally, physically, and spiritually? What is most important to you in your life? What do you think might be causing your symptom?*"

   The final opportunity to ask about CAM use, which is of critical importance, is when asking about medications. PAs should not be providing a prescription without having asked *every* patient not only about prescription or over-the-counter medication use but also about the use of herbs, remedies, vitamins, and/or supplements. If the patient is taking an herb or supplement for which the PA is not familiar, it is the PA's responsibility to find out more about what the patient is using before combining it with a pharmaceutical. Merely telling the patient to stop the herb or supplement is not acceptable to many patients. The PA's communication skills play an important role here to work with the patient in negotiating the treatment plan and to ensure safety. Sometimes patients can offer information about why they are using a particular herb or remedy; however, this information may not be accurate even though it provides insight into the patient's reason for its use. Fortunately, there are abundant scientific and reliable resources now available to find out more about a product the patient is using and any potential interactions. Because of to the large number of patients using pharmaceuticals and herbs, remedies, vitamins or supplements, asking this question has become a vital one, as more research uncovers potential synergetic, antagonistic, or neutralizing effects of such combinations.

2. **Become Knowledgeable.** The Guidelines for the Ethical Conduct for the Physician Assistant Profession and the American Academy of Physician Assistants emphasize the importance of staying up to date and knowledgeable regarding all health care issues, including CAM. There are a growing number of opportunities to learn about CAM, such as conferences and continuing medical education (CME) activities, by talking with or experiencing the work of CAM practitioners, and by attempting to locate those practitioners in your area should you decide to refer patients. More and more insurance companies are providing some coverage of CAM, so it is also important to find out which modalities or practitioners may be covered. Locate CAM practitioners in your area and learn about their practice and modality.
3. **Be nonjudgmental, be open-minded, and make no assumptions.** Health care systems in other countries are commonly different than those in the United States. In fact, 75% of the world's population uses folk or lay healers in approaches that include physical and nonphysical components, as well as using aspects of family or ceremony not common to the biomedical model.[22] Although some of these aspects may seem unfamiliar or bizarre, these beliefs and customs have significant and powerful meaning to the patient. Therefore all inquiries regarding the use of CAM must be asked in an open-minded, open-ended, nonjudgmental way. Patients are sensitive to and perhaps overly cautious about a conventional provider's negative judgment or disapproval. If a PA dismisses or devalues these in front of the patient, irreparable damage can result in the patient-provider relationship. Therefore, PAs need to be sensitive and compassionate to these differences.
4. **Work toward a mutually acceptable treatment plan.** Being open, sensitive, and compassionate regarding a patient's beliefs concerning health, healing, and disease allows for the conventional provider to work more closely with the patient in creating a treatment plan that incorporates and respects the patient's needs and wishes. Whatever treatment plan is decided on, it is imperative that follow-up with the patient occurs on a regular basis, especially if the plan includes only alternative modalities or a combination of the CAM and conventional. This enhances and maintains the patient-PA relationship so that if the CAM treatments should be unsuccessful and the patient wants to try a conventional approach or make some adjustment in the treatment plan, the doorway has been left open to do so. Unfortunately, many times patients think that if they do not do what the conventional provider recommended, they cannot go back, should they decide later to enlist the help and support of that practitioner.
5. **Be willing to communicate directly with CAM providers.** It was not until 1980 that the American Medical Association lifted its statement regarding the interaction between conventional and alternative providers. It has become essential for PAs to interact and communicate with CAM providers that patients are seeing. This bridge building serves several functions. First, it allows patients to create health care teams that truly reflect and support their needs in their healing process. Second, it provides a resource and possible future relationship from which the PA can learn about a specific CAM modality or provide a referral for other patients. Third, it supports the emerging new health care model of integrated medical approaches and treatments.
6. **Lastly, do not omit or negate your required responsibilities such as making a diagnosis, ordering laboratory or diagnostic studies, using prescriptions or recommending surgery, and documentation.** Just because a patient states he or she is using CAM, that does not negate or relieve you of your duty to meet and carry out your role and responsibility in the manner in which you have been trained.

Working with patients who are using or interested in using CAM should not be viewed as an "either-or" perspective: either it is the biomedical approach or the alternative approach. Rather, consider the perspective of "both-and." It is possible for a patient's treatment to use *both* biomedical *and* alternative, and it appears this is what patients want.

CASE 15-1

A 53-year-old man with a history of coronary heart disease is approaching the point of needing surgical intervention despite treatments with medications and diet changes. During his most recent visit, you review your concerns regarding the progression of his disease and you discuss the inevitable need for surgical intervention in the near future. He expresses significant concern and fear regarding surgery. He has just learned that his only child is pregnant with their first grandchild, and he wants to make sure he will be around to see this grandchild and any others. He states that his father died on the operating table during surgery and asks if there is anything else he can do or any other options.

This case describes a common situation when patients are uncomfortable with the proposed course of treatment yet aware that something needs to be done. In this case, as in many situations, the diagnosis of a serious illness provides an opportunity and the motivation for patients to significantly change those aspects or behaviors that may have contributed to the illness in the first place. When patients ask, *"Is there anything else I can do?"* they are communicating an important message that PAs need to hear. This may be that they are deeply uncomfortable or fearful of the proposed treatment or they do not agree with it because it creates a conflict within their own beliefs (explanatory model) about health, healing, and illness. PAs need to recognize and explore these possibilities with the patient.

In addition, if the PA is knowledgeable about CAM, he or she can in fact offer more information and options. For example, recent studies have revealed that more and more surgeons and/or hospitals are offering patients CAM modalities before and during surgery that helps to reduce both the mental and physiologic stress of surgery. Such modalities presently being used include hypnotherapy, guided imagery, and Reiki. Studies have reported that by decreasing preoperative stress and postoperative pain, complications have been significantly reduced and patients are discharged sooner.[18,19] Another option is the Dr. Dean Ornish's Opening Your Heart Program, which was specifically designed for patients with coronary artery disease (CAD) who want to try to manage their disease from a nonsurgical approach. This is the first program of its kind that scientifically documented the reversal of CAD without surgery. The program is located in many cities and is also covered by some insurance plans. The components include techniques of stress management, such as yoga and meditation, a low-fat and low-cholesterol diet, cessation of smoking and other addictions, using group therapy and support groups, and exercise.[23]

Finally, in any patient for whom surgery is recommended, it is imperative to find out if that patient is taking any herbs, supplements, or vitamins. Studies are beginning to document that certain supplements interfere, potentiate, or negate anesthetic agents or have effects on blood coagulating properties. For example, the properties of commonly used herbs such as *Gingko biloba,* garlic, and Asian ginseng all increase the risk of bleeding. Therefore, it is important to know this and, if possible, have the patient stop the herb at least 2 weeks before surgery.[24,25] Conversely, some herbs taken preoperatively have been found to be beneficial to the healing and recovery period postoperatively, such as vitamins A and C, zinc, and aloe vera.[25,26]

CASE 15-2

Evaluation of a slender, active, 52-year-old woman complaining of right knee pain reveals moderate osteoarthritic changes of joint narrowing and minimal spurring on radiograph. She has a history of peptic ulcer disease and has been using acetaminophen for pain relief; however, she reports it is only minimally effective.

The drugs of choice for osteoarthritis are the nonsteroidal antiinflammatory medications, but due to her history of peptic ulcer disease this class is not recommended. Other possible medications include the use of topical creams containing capsicum and opioid analgesics; however, the side effects of opioids may include sedation and drowsiness.

At this point, many conventional providers have little else to offer, and the patient may leave the office feeling disappointed. This is one of the motivations for patients seeking alternatives. In this case, the PA did ask the appropriate questions and learned that the patient has made significant changes to her eating and lifestyle habit since her diagnosis of peptic ulcer disease, including losing weight and exercising regularly. She meditates regularly and is vegetarian. She also states she just started yoga to see if this might help with her knee pain and is more interested in working with her body from a more natural approach. She also takes a combination of antioxidant vitamins.

If the PA is unsure of what other options are available for osteoarthritis, a follow-up appointment should be scheduled, which will give the PA time to review the research, consult with colleagues or alternative practitioners or other reliable resources to begin to develop a treatment plan. In this way the patient-provider relationship is maintained even though the patient may not use conventional approaches.

The PA learned that additional options may be more acceptable for this patient and provide a mutually acceptable treatment plan. For example, research has shown that the use of glucosamine sulfate reduces the pain of osteoarthritis without the side effects of nonsteroidal antiinflammatory drugs and less adverse effects overall. A trial period using glucosamine sulfate may be more acceptable for this patient because of the lack of side effects. However, as with recommending or prescribing any medications, attention is warranted about potential adverse or unwanted interaction or side effects. Glucosamine sulfate should be used with caution in patients who are allergic to shellfish or those on sodium-restricted diets because glucosamine sulfate is made from shellfish and tends to have high sodium content. The PA also learned that yoga is known to have beneficial effects on flexibility and strength, both of which are important for patients with osteoarthritis, and the patient was encouraged to continue with the yoga.[27]

As with any treatment plan, follow-up should be scheduled to document the progress of the patient. It is important to educate the patient that many CAM approaches may take weeks to months before they take effect, which is another reason to maintain regular follow-up appointments.

CONCLUSION

This chapter serves as an introduction to the complexity of CAM and the present issues facing practitioners trained in the biomedical model, including PAs. Today, patients come from diverse belief systems regarding health and healing, and they are better educated and are seeking additional options in lieu of or in combination with conventional medicine. As the health care system of this country attempts to navigate these changes, which includes finding ways to integrate different health care systems, philosophies, and treatments, PAs must also begin to integrate some basic changes in their approach to every patient, including asking about the patient's belief systems and the use of alternatives. In addition, PAs need to take advantage of the emerging research and educational opportunities regarding CAM to better educate themselves and their patients about the use of alternatives. Doing so will serve to enhance and deepen the PA-patient relationship and will play a vital role in the integration of a health care system that honors, recognizes, and respects the validity and viability of different approaches to health and healing.

CLINICAL APPLICATIONS

1. Take a moment to reflect on the following. What were your beliefs about illness when you were a child? Where did those beliefs come from? What did your family of origin believe about the causes of illness, and how they should be treated? What are your beliefs now?
2. Have you ever used some form of CAM? Think about the reasons why you did. What CAM modality did you choose, and why that particular one? What was your experience? Did the existence of quantitative research play a role in your decision to use the alternative? Did you or would you share this information with your health care provider? Why or why not?

KEY POINTS

- It is every PA's responsibility to become knowledgeable about CAM modalities, as well as where to locate reliable research and information.
- It is imperative that PAs are able to establish open and effective provider-patient relationships that will enable patients to freely discuss CAM usage, questions, and concerns.
- Be nonjudgmental, be open-minded, and make no assumptions concerning CAM, the patient's use of CAM, and CAM providers.

References

1. Barnes Patricia, Bloom B. Complementary and Alternative Medicine Use among Adults and Children: United States. 2007; CDC National Health Statistics Reports, December 10, 2008 Number 12. Available from *http://nccam.nih.gov/news/2008/nhsr12.pdf*; Accessed June 10, 2011.
2. National Center for Complementary and Alternative Medicine. NCCAM Funding: Appropriations History. National Center for Complementary and Alternative Medicine. Available from *http://nccam.nih.gov/about/budget/appropriations.htm*; Accessed November 26, 2011.
3. National Center for Complementary and Alternative Medicine. Facts at a Glance and Mission. Available from *http://nccam.nih.gov/about/ataglance*; Accessed November 26, 2011.
4. National Center for Complementary and Alternative Medicine Exploring the Science of Complementary and Alternative Medicine. Third Strategic Plan: 2011–2015. Available from *http://nccam.nih.gov/about/plans/2011/*; Accessed November 26, 2011.
5. What Is Complementary and Alternative Medicine? National Center for Complementary and Alternative Medicine. Available from *http://nccam.nih.gov/health/whatiscam/*; Accessed November 26, 2011.
6. Eisenberg DM, Kessler RC, Foster C, et al. Unconventional medicine in the United States: prevalence, costs and patterns of use. N Engl J Med 1993;238:246.
7. Eisenberg DM, Davis RB, Ettner SL, et al. Trends in alternative medicine use in the United States. JAMA 1998;280:1569.
8. Oldenkick R, Coker Al. Usage of complementary medicine among patients of mainstream physicians. Southern Med J 2000;93:375.
9. Eisenberg DM, Kessler RC, Van Rompay MI, et al. Perceptions about complementary therapies relative to conventional therapies among patients who use both: results from a national survey. Ann Intern Med 2001;135:344.
10. Barnes P, Powell-Grier E, McFann K, Nahin RL. Complementary and alternative medicine use among adults: United States. CDC Advance Data from Vital and Health Statistics; 2002, May 27, 2004, Number 343 (online), *http://nccam.nih.gov/news/report.pdf*; Accessed February 12, 2007.
11. The Use of Complementary and Alternative Medicine in the United States. 2004 (online), *http://nccam.nih.gov/sites/nccam.nih.gov/files/news/camstats/2002/report.pdf*; Accessed February 4, 2007.
12. Astin JA. Why patients use alternative medicine. JAMA 1998;279:1548.
13. Eisenberg, David. Advising patients who seek alternative medical therapies. Ann Intern Med 1997;127:61.
14. News Release, Harvard Medical School Office of Public Affairs. Complementary and Alternative Medicine Use by One Third of U.S. Adults Unchanged from 1997. Boston. 2005.
15. Kaufman DW, Kelly JP, Rosenberg L, et al. Recent patterns of medication use in the ambulatory adult population of the United States: the Slone Survey. JAMA 2002;287:337.
16. Blumenthal Mark. Herb sales down 15 percent in mainstream market. Herbalgram 2001;51:69.
17. Blumenthal Mark. The Complete German Commission E Monographs Therapeutic Guide to Herbal Medicine. Texas: American Botanical Council, 1998.
18. Kligler Benjamin, Roberta Lee. Integrative Medicine Principles for Practice: McGraw Hill, 2004.
19. U.S. Food and Drug Administration Dietary Supplement Health and Education Act of 1994, Public Law 103-417, 103rd Congress. October 1994.
20. NIH Office of Dietary Supplements, Background Information. April 12, 2006 *http://ods.od.nih.gov/factsheets/DietarySupplements.asp*; Accessed November 26, 2011.
21. Glucosamine, Medline Plus. January 2007. *http://www.nlm.nih.gov/medlineplus/druginfo/natural/patient-glucosamine.html*; Accessed November 26, 2011 .
22. Helman, Cecil G. Culture, health and illness. 3rd ed. Oxford: Butterworth- Heinemann, 1994.
23. Ornish Dean. Program for Reversing Health Disease. New York: Ballantine; 1990.
24. Ang-Lee MK, Moss J, Yuan C-S. Herbal medicine and perioperative care. JAMA 2001;286:208.
25. Pribitkin ED, Boger G. Surgery and herbal therapy: essential guidelines on bleeding, skin reactions, and wound healing. Comp Health Pract Rev 2000;6:29.
26. Petry Judith. Surgery and complementary therapies: a review. Altern Ther 2000;6:64.
27. Glucosamine, One Medicine [database on-line] (Newton, Mass: Integrative Medicine Communications). *http://www.healthandage.com/Home/gm-20*; Accessed March 2002.

The resources for this chapter can be found at www.expertconsult.com.

SECTION III

INTERPERSONAL AND COMMUNICATION SKILLS

CHAPTER 16

COMMUNICATION ISSUES

Shani D. Fleming

CHAPTER CONTENTS

"When you give everyone a voice and give people power, the system usually ends up in a really good place. So, what we view our role as, is giving people that power."[1]

MARK ZUCKERBERG, FACEBOOK CREATOR

Communication between humans is a complex interplay of many integrated parts. Successful communication must incorporate a level of comprehension and literacy. When a concept or thought needs to be articulated, concerns including the audience, education level, language, and ethnicity must be considered to communicate the message in a concise and easy-to-understand manner. The receiver then interprets that information through his or her cultural, emotional, and individual perspective and creates a meaning on the basis of what they heard. Linguistics, literacy, and pragmatics are highly complicated processes well beyond the reach of this chapter; however, this simple description allows a small insight into the complexities of communication and comprehension. Many external variables provide other layers of intricacy into this process, such as medical terminology, health literacy, and language barriers.

Historically, information has been transmitted primarily through oratory. Only fairly recently has the written word transformed the vehicle of communication by providing permanency of thought and the ability to reach an exponentially larger audience. In the current technologic era, the oral and written word has been integrated within a multimodal digital storm that has transformed the transmission and reception of information. Current technology has provided an intersection of both oral and written techniques through e-mail, text messaging, telemedicine, and social networking. These media modalities have increased access for many, bridging the communication gap that often exists between providers and patients. When technology becomes universally affordable and therefore universally accessible, it will be a positive step toward closing a communication gap that currently exists.

The Internet provides a means to broadcast health information to facilitate interaction between and among patients and health care providers. Studies suggest that close to 80% of adults have used the Internet for health care purposes.[2] One of the initial goals of health information technology was to bridge the gap between individuals and providers when services were simply out of reach. This continues to be a slow process, and until we address other disparities that continue to leave a segment of the population behind, the technology push will further divide the haves from the have-nots.

SOCIAL NETWORKING

Social networking has transformed the way that information is used by millions of users. The modalities that fall under the umbrella of this dynamic machine appear to morph on a daily basis. The intersection of written, oral, art, and technology is depicted within the multiple modalities that encompass social networking. Physician assistants (PAs) and other health providers have used social networking to connect with other providers, educate the public, and promote wellness. The ability to reach the public with speed over great distances has transformed public health announcements, dissemination of information and warnings, and marketing strategies. The Centers for Disease Control publishes the *Morbidity and Mortality Weekly Report* on Facebook, and the Department of Health and Human Services used Twitter to disseminate information about the H1N1 pandemic.[3] Public health broadcasts regarding drug and product recalls are propagated instantly to millions of users. Podcasts and YouTube videos are being used by more health care providers to provide continuing medical information within the medical community, as well as educating their patient populations. Politicians now use "social media" campaigns in which electronic petitions and appeals for legislation are leveraging forces exemplified through the recent health care reform political process.

The speed by which information is now transmitted to a huge network of people was beyond our imagination several years ago. When looking at the reach of many of these Internet sites, it is clear how health promotion and disease prevention has a global span. Here are examples of various social networks and the users for each site.

- Twitter
  - 140-character text-based posts
  - 200 million users[4]
- Facebook
  - Recreational peer-to-peer social network[5]
  - 800 million users[6]
- YouTube
  - Video sharing
  - 490 unique users
  - 3 billion views daily[7]
- Blogs
  - Internet web diary that allow non-experts to build easily updatable online journals[8]
  - 156 million blogs[9]
- LinkedIn
  - Professional peer-to-peer networking
  - 120 million users[10]
- Wikis
  - A collaborative software that allows users to add and edit content
  - 47% of surveyed Americans have used Wikipedia[5]
- Forums and discussion boards
  - Online locations to post questions and receive community replies
  - 20% of surveyed Americans have posted on bulletin boards[5]
- Peer-to-peer social network
  - Organization's own social network, which includes profiles of its members
  - 47% of surveyed American adults report using a peer-to-peer social networking site[5]
- Examples of health social networks: Sermo, PatientsLikeMe, MedHelp, CureTogether, DailyStrength, FacetoFace Health.[5]

Patients create communities allowing discussion of their health conditions, evaluation of health care experiences, and researching medical conditions.[5] During medical conferences, health care providers are able to tweet, provide podcasts, and blog about the latest research instantly. It is important to frame social networking as a source to allow information exchange globally, discuss latest developments, and not to simply pass on information.[11] According to many, we are currently only at the tip of the social software iceberg.[8] Social networkers empower patients and build communities of practice.[3]

ONLINE COMMUNICATION IN HEALTH CARE OFFICE SETTINGS

Patients can search on the Internet through their insurance company website or through various search engines to locate health care facility websites. These websites provide an array of information concerning the providers, services, insurances accepted, and hours of information of the facility. Many health care providers place registration forms, health history forms, and Health Insurance Portability and Accountability Act (HIPAA) forms for completion before the actual medical appointment. Patients may use the website to sign on to an individual account, which may provide laboratory or imaging results. Depending on the literacy of the patient, these tools can be time-saving measures in an already time-constrained medical environment.

Studies have shown that few clinicians report communicating with their patients through direct e-mail correspondence.[12] Considering the amount of e-mail that currently fills our inboxes, having every patient with access to us certainly seems overwhelming. Clinicians sorting through urgent versus non-urgent e-mails and the concern over possible delay responding to a potentially urgent condition are liabilities that most clinicians would be hesitant to take on. Reimbursement from the time spent responding to e-mails is not clearly defined by insurance companies. Direct e-mail communication with patients has the potential of being a major burden in an already administrative paperwork–filled medical environment. Sending information to a wrong e-mail address, patients blind carbon copying (BCC) individuals, and e-mail hacking continue to make confidentiality a major concern with online e-mail correspondence.

E-mail consultations for preventive health care, health education, and managing nonurgent conditions can serve to be mutually beneficial for the patient and provider.[13] Cost savings for patients when considering time off work versus the convenience of e-mailing questions for nonurgent complaints is a real benefit. Cost savings for providers can be associated with missed appointments if patients are able to still have access for nonurgent complaints.[13] Health care centers and patients may benefit from e-mail prompt s that can include appointment reminders, directions, important phone numbers, and parking information.[13] There is an increased use of smartphones and tablets, so patients are able to access these e-mails virtually anywhere.

Health care centers may consider triaging medical complaints and scheduling appointments via instant messenger or chat features. Health care staff can use e-mail correspondence to encourage medication adherence, as well as solicit responses about side effects of prescribed medication.[13] Automated e-mail reminders can also promote health maintenance and prevention tools.

TELEMEDICINE

PAs are participating in telemedicine health teams throughout many health care systems. Telemedicine is "the use of electronic information and communications technologies to provide and support health care when distance separates the participants."[14] The Health Resources and Services Administration estimates a shortage of internal medicine clinicians over the next decade, largely as a result of the aging population.[15] Although there is some discrepancy within studies to demonstrate the clinical benefit of telemedicine and hospital mortality, this is an area that will continue to grow and be used within the health care settings.[16] The benefit of telemedicine can be seen in pediatric intensive care unit settings (e.g., it allows parents to be able to monitor their children from a distant location).[14] Radiology has also benefited greatly from accessing and reading images remotely.

The home health setting will continue to explore the advantages of using telemedicine for consultations and limiting visit travel time. There is some concern about the relatively slow growth and various uses of telemedicine. Potential state licensure issues are associated with interstate transmission of health care services.[14] High costs may also be associated with data transmission. Finally, some encounters may have variability between states regarding reimbursement. Overall, telemedicine offers increased access to services and providers that may have been otherwise unattainable.

PATIENT-PROVIDER COMMUNICATION

Successful patient-provider communication is a key ingredient to achieve positive health outcomes. Communication establishes rapport, encourages patient compliance, increases patient satisfaction, and averts medical errors. There is an inherent power difference that takes place within patient-provider communication. Providers should promote a trust and mutual respect that will empower patients and give them a more active voice.

Time constraints within busy clinical practice will definitely lead clinicians to be more creative with communication approaches. The patient who presents with Internet print outs and a long laundry list of questions, although demonstrating a great sense of interest in his or her health, can also be a challenge within the constraints of a 15-minute office visit. Clinicians must always remember how important it is to establish rapport as the first step within any encounter. This is accomplished through self-reflection before entering the room, sitting down, shaking hands, offering a smile, and calling the patient by name. All of these things can encourage open, honest, and impartial discussion. Patients should feel connected when providing the necessary components of their health history. Interrupting the patient within 18 to 23 seconds of the encounter must be a thing of the past.[17]

LISTEN[18]

When I ask you to listen to me
And you start giving me advice,
You have not done what I asked.
When I ask you to listen to me
And you begin to tell me 'why' I shouldn't feel that way,
You are trampling on my feelings.
When I ask you to listen to me
And you feel you have to do something to
Solve my problems,
You have failed me, strange as that may seem.
Listen! All I ask is that you listen;
Not talk, nor do—just hear me.

Advice is cheap:
Twenty-five cents will get you both Dear Abby
And Billy Graham
In the same newspaper …
… So please listen, and just hear me, and if you
Want to talk, Wait a minute for your turn,
And I'll listen to you.

ANONYMOUS

HEALTH LITERACY AND INTERCULTURAL COMMUNICATION

Health literacy specifically refers to the degree to which a person can obtain, process, and understand basic health information and services needed to make appropriate health care decisions.[19] PAs are serving diverse populations, and the demographics are changing at a rapid pace. It is thought that within a decade the current majority will become the new minority. This shift has already occurred within many states regarding the youth population.[20] It is the hope that in the next few years the health care system will receive 30 million more individual users who will be able to be insured. Culturally competent providers who are linguistically competent will be a necessity to address health literacy within a diverse patient population. The National Center for Cultural Competence defines linguistic competence as follows:

> The capacity of an organization and its personnel to communicate effectively, and convey information in a manner that is easily understood by diverse audiences, including persons of limited English proficiency, those who have low literacy skills or are not literate, and individuals with disabilities.[21]

Healthy People 2020 outlines a series of objectives to address health communication and health information technology. These interventions will assist in bridging the health disparities gap that exists among many cultures.

CONCLUSION

There is much to be said, especially in the health care arena, about personal connection through communication. Are we moving further away from the "healing touch" offered by providers with more and more interaction through electronic means? Is the connection lost by not looking into your patient's eyes while gathering the components of the health history versus staring at the electronic medical record, or reviewing the form presented by the patient already completed from being downloaded from the health center website? We must ensure that the quality of health care provided through potential reduction in medical errors, increased patient safety, and medical advancements is not at the detriment of human-connected care as technology integrates within the health care milieu.

As we continue to expand our capacity in communication, PAs cannot lose sight of why this profession was initiated: to serve the underserved. Studies indicate that less educated and geographically remote individuals may use the Internet at a slower rate.[12] Health literacy among our minority population continues to play a significant role as a continuing source of health care disparities. Our geriatric population is one of the largest cohorts who will be using our services at greater rates. We need to ensure that everyone has equal access to the benefits of this technologic boom and may achieve improved health outcomes as a result of such access. PA students can have outstanding board scores, and practicing PAs can log hundreds of continuing medical education hours. However, we must remember communication is a skill that requires lifelong development and continuous effort. PAs have a unique position as a link between the patient and supervising physician/health care practice. Similar to Mark Zuckerberg's reasoning for the creation of Facebook, patients have a voice and through communication can be empowered to manage their health and have better outcomes.

CLINICAL APPLICATIONS

1. Take time to complete the following self-assessment[22]:
   How comfortable are you doing the following?
   a. Performing a physical examination on a Muslim woman who wears a veil
   b. Working effectively with a professional interpreter
   c. Discussing a patient's religious preferences and constraints regarding his treatment
   d. Asking questions and giving information to the spouse of a patient, if requested
   e. Communicating about various components of sexual activity within the lesbian, gay, bisexual, and transgender community
2. An adolescent social circle has been discovered within a community that is culturally different from your own. These adolescents gather in abandoned homes, friends' homes, and school basements engaging in drinking, drug use, and unprotected sex. There has been an outbreak within the community of syphilis, which has been traced to several of the teenagers

attending these parties. In addition, two of the adolescents have been recently arrested for armed robbery in a drug deal sting operation. As a PA serving adolescents within the local health department, you have been asked to attend a local community health fair in which many of the neighborhood adolescents will be in attendance.

a. What are the health concerns within this case?
b. What are your personal values, judgments, and assumptions regarding this case?
c. Is communication at this community event necessary? Why?
d. Who is the audience, and what is the message?
e. Which communication modalities would you use for message delivery? Why?
f. Would the message or modality change if the adolescents had a different sexuality status, race, religion, or economic status?
g. What barriers to the delivery of this message exist?
h. How will you know whether the audience receives the message?

KEY POINTS

- Communication is a complicated process, and the methods by which messages are delivered continue to evolve.
- Social networking is still in its early stages and has already transformed the way individuals connect and information is disseminated and marketed.
- Online forms and e-mail may serve a vital role as we continue to improve efficiency and promote health.
- The patient-provider relationship must include connectivity through establishing rapport within the time constraints and technologic environment.
- Health literacy and intercultural communication are areas that all clinicians must learn more about as our population changes before our eyes.
- We must continue to fight for equal access to the achievement of improved health outcomes.

References

1. All Great Quotes. *http://www.allgreatquotes.com/facebook_quotes.shtml*; Accessed September 25, 2011.
2. Baker L, Wagner T, Singer S, Bundorf K. Use of the Internet and e-mail for health care information: results from a national survey. JAMA 2003;289:2400.
3. Miller EA, Pole A. Diagnosis blog: checking up on health blogs in the blogosphere. Am J Public Health 2010;100:1514.
4. Twitter. *http://en.wikipedia.org/wiki/Twitter*; Accessed September 25, 2011.
5. Deloitte Center for Health Solutions. Social networks in health care: communication, collaboration and insights. 2010. *https://www.deloitte.com/assets/Dcom-UnitedStates/Local%20Assets/Documents/US_CHS_2010SocialNetworks_070710.pdf*; Accessed September 25, 2011.
6. Facebook. *http://en.wikipedia.org/wiki/Facebook*; Accessed September 25, 2011.
7. YouTube. *http://en.wikipedia.org/wiki/YouTube*; Accessed September 25, 2011.
8. Kamel Boulos MN, Wheeler S. The emerging Web 2.0 social software: an enabling suite of sociable technologies in health and health care education. Health Info Libr J 2007;24:2.
9. Blog. *http://en.wikipedia.org/wiki/Blog*; Accessed September 25, 2011.
10. LinkedIn. *http://en.wikipedia.org/wiki/LinkedIn*; Accessed September 25, 2011.
11. McNabb C. What social media offers to health professionals and citizens. *http://www.who.int/bulletin/volumes/87/8/09-066712/en/* Bull World Health Organization 2009;87:566.
12. Miller E, West D. Where's the revolution? Digital technology and health care in the Internet age. J Health Polit Policy Law 2009;34:261.
13. Car J, Sheikh A. Email consultations in health care: 2—acceptability and safe application. Br Med J 2004;329:439.
14. Field M, Grigsby J. Telemedicine and remote patient monitoring. J Am Med Assoc 2002;288:423.
15. Tran B, O'Gowan R. Extending the PA role with telemedicine. Adv NPs PAs 2009;17:46.
16. Kahn J. The use and misuse of ICU telemedicine. J Am Med Assoc 2011;305:2227.
17. Marvel MK, Epstein RM, Flowers K, Beckman HB. Soliciting the patient's agenda: have we improved? JAMA 1999;282:942.
18. Long V. Facilitating Personal Growth in Self and Others. Pacific Grove, California: Brooks/Cole Publishing Company, 1996.
19. Health Literacy Policy Brief. *http://www.ahrq.gov/research/healthlit.htm*; Accessed September 25, 2011.

20. Morello C, Mellnik T. Minorities become a majority in Washington region. August 31, 2001. *http://www.washingtonpost.com/local/minorities-become-a-majority-in-washington-region/2011/08/30/gIQADobxqJ_story.html*; Accessed September 25, 2011.
21. National Center for Cultural Competence. Conceptual Frameworks/Models, Guiding Values and Principles. *http://nccc.georgetown.edu/foundations/frameworks.html*; Accessed September 25, 2011.
22. Hudelson P, Perron NJ, Perneger T, et al. Self-assessment of intercultural communication skills: a survey of physicians and medical students in Geneva, Switzerland. BMC Med Educ 2011;11:1.

The resources for this chapter can be found at www.expertconsult.com.

CHAPTER 17

ELECTRONIC HEALTH RECORD

Roy H. Constantine

CHAPTER CONTENTS

Health informatics (also known as *health care informatics*, *healthcare informatics*, *medical informatics*, *nursing informatics*, or *biomedical informatics*) is a discipline at the intersection of information science, computer science, and health care. It deals with the resources, devices, and methods required to optimize the acquisition, storage, retrieval, and use of information in health and biomedicine. Health informatics tools include not only computers but also clinical guidelines, formal medical terminologies, and information and communication systems.[1]

Health information technology (HIT) includes electronic methods used to manage people's health and health care.[2] Legislation requires the use of certified electronic health record (EHR) technology for exchange of health information to improve the quality of health care.[3] The terms *EMR* and *EHR* are frequently interchanged.[4] However, there is a difference. The electronic medical record (EMR) is simply an electronic version of the paper chart. The EHR shares health information across the continuum of services (e.g., physicians and laboratories). Information can follow the patient through different health care settings (e.g., clinics, hospitals, nursing homes, catastrophic events). Hurricane Katrina is an example of a catastrophic event after which medical information of displaced patients was retrievable.

The personal health record (PHR) extends the capabilities of what is being called the *virtual chart*. The PHR can stand alone or be interconnected to the EHR. Capabilities include prescription refills, appointments, insurance information, and patient education.[2] Sharing of medical data in the PHR can be influenced by patients' willingness to share their condition and sociodemographic variables, which include age, education, and severity of health and public health emergencies. Although safety-monitoring mechanisms are being implemented, patient trust will ultimately facilitate support sharing.[5]

DEVELOPMENT

The 2000 Institute of Medicine (IOM) report estimated 44,000 to 98,000 deaths occur annually due to error in the United States. The IOM's report "Crossing the Quality Chasm" emphasized that a redesign in health care should include a focus on information technology.[6] The Leapfrog Group,[7] a voluntary program focusing on the safety, quality, and affordability of health care, and The Joint Commission,[8] an accrediting body for organizations and programs, promote the implementation of EHR. However, they also agreed with the Food and Drug Administration that "consistency, reliability, and accuracy needed to be evaluated."[9]

In 2008, only 2% of the nonfederal general acute care hospitals had a comprehensive EHR, whereas 7.6% had a basic EHR.[10] Larger hospitals and teaching hospitals had higher utilization of electronic record systems.[11] Adoption rates did not differ among high and low indigent patient populations in hospitals known as the Disproportionate Share Index Hospitals (DSH).[10]

Regional Health Information Organizations (RHIOs) were designed to enhance clinical data availability and provide Health Information Exchange (HIE).[2] A federal initiative from the Office of the National Coordinator of Health Information Technology (ONCHIT) included the development of a functional health information infrastructure.[6] The ONCHIT funded Health Information Technology Regional Extension Centers (RECs). The RECs provided assistance to primary care physicians, physician assistants (PAs), and nurse practitioners in the United States to develop their EHR system.[12] The Health Information Technology Economic & Clinical Health Act (HITECH) provided an opportunity to expand the use of HIT with grants, loans, and financial assistance.[10] HITECH funds mostly supported primary care and critical-access/rural hospitals with fewer than 50 beds.[12]

Recent federal initiatives include the American Reinvestment and Recovery Act (ARRA), for which "meaningful use" incentives were applied. ARRA focused on standards, quality needs, functionality, communication, and government program links to enhance financial incentives. Requirements for meaningful use requirements include transmitting prescriptions to the pharmacy electronically and demonstrating the capability of the EHR to electronically exchange key information.[10] The intent was to enhance the distribution of health information between organizations.[13]

Lewis[14] notes that the decision to switch his office to an electronic system provided fantasies of a streamlined, technologically efficient, and almost functionless setting, which in reality was not the case. Practices and organizations are starting to use the EHR now to avoid penalties, but it is important not to rush. Improved outcomes occur when emphasis is placed on better technology, integration, and privacy concerns.[15] One should consider the implementation of an EHR system in an institution with 200 or more beds to take the same time as completion of construction on a new hospital building.[9]

IMPLEMENTATION

Major EHR market vendors include Cerner, Eclipsys, EPIC, iMD Soft, McKesson Provider Technologies, MediTech, Misys Healthcare Systems, Philips Medical Systems, Picis, and Siemens.[9] In 2004, the military implemented the Armed Forces Longitudinal Technology Application (AHLTA), which is the Department of Defense's global health record.[16]

When choosing a system, it is important to look at the success of the system in the marketplace. Ideally, you would speak with other institutions that have implemented the same system and discuss customer satisfaction. Workflow implications differ for various stakeholders within institutions.[17] Approximately 30% of EHR implementations fail due to steep learning curves and loss of productivity. The development of a flexible navigation system, enhanced functionality, and the ability to complement your work will enhance usability.[18]

It is essential there is organizational commitment when EHR implementation is going to occur. A broad group of extrinsic and intrinsic stakeholders needs to be involved in the implementation process. Change is not an easy concept. Therefore, the existence of a change management organizational culture is essential. Intentional planning that is clear and consistent with the vision and principles of the organization must be present.[19]

It is important that PAs become incorporated early in the process of EHR development. Factors that go beyond technology can hinder HIE.[13] The cultural change is even more important than the challenge with technology. Work sessions need to be created to enhance training, develop workflows, and limit complaints during the process.[20]

Many clinicians think that EMR is a direct extension of computerized physician order entry (CPOE) and that improvements in functionality, performance, learning curves, and technology have resulted.[21] A selected group of subject matter experts (SMEs) should develop order set content. Integrating general admission order sets with disease-specific order sets improves outcomes.[22] Selected PAs with subject matter expertise strengthen the integration process. PAs who use specific order sets can incorporate evidence-based links to enhance core-measure compliance. Development of order sets will increase utilization, time, and compliance, in addition to eliminating discrepancies with handwriting, signature, dating, and timing in the EHR (Figure 17-1).

Mandatory elements in the EHR include a problem list, a medication list, vital signs, allergies, a smoking record, discharge documentation, a discharge summary, CPOE for medications, drug-to-drug and drug-to-allergy checks, the ability to electronically exchange key clinical information, decision support, security, laboratory test results, patient list of conditions, patient-specific education sources, and medication reconciliation. Additional functions include advanced directives, electronic surveillance, and the ability to submit electronic data to public health organizations.[11]

Functionality is incorporated across services and commonly occurs in laboratory data, radiology images, and radiology reports.[10,23] Laboratory data and reports are considered to be passive, whereas writing progress notes and CPOE are considered to be active.[9] Clinical information and data should be handled at "point of care," or in "real time."[6] The use

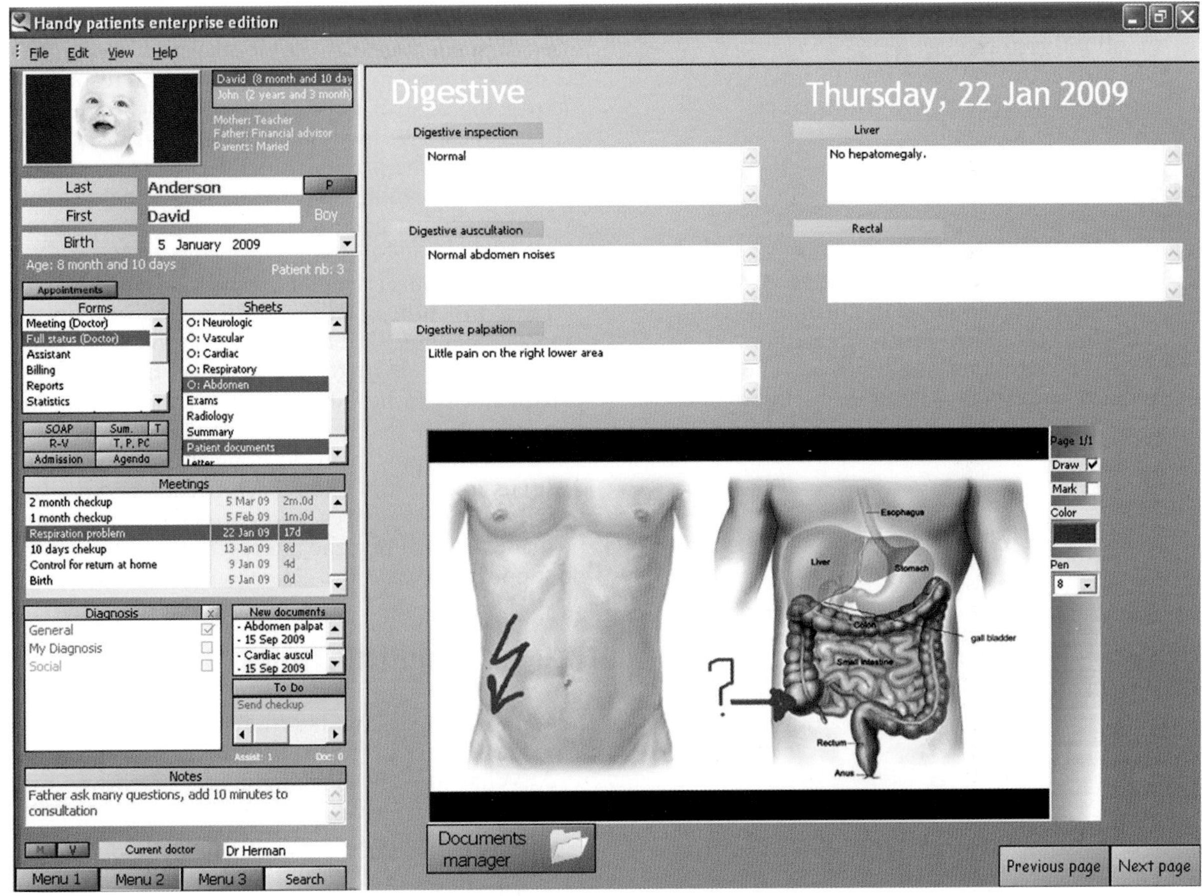

FIGURE 17-1 Sample of an electronic medical record. (From the Creative Commons website. *http://creativecommons.org/licenses/by-sa/3.0/us/*. Accessed May 13, 2012.)

of bar coding and the integration of hemodynamic measurements from devices can be converted into data and incorporated.[6,9]

PA "champions" are integral in the necessary training and reinforcement during the EHR initiative. If hospital-wide implementation follows a big-bang initiative, then administrative recommendations are made to be 100% paperless. Other hospitals may want to start slowly with one service at a time being integrated into the paperless process. System failures have been noted where a paper backup is required. The prevention of workarounds is essential with both approaches to minimize safety flaws and incident.

BENEFITS TO IMPLEMENTING ELECTRONIC HEALTH RECORDS

- Reduction of errors
- Improvement in clinical decision-making during encounters
- Universal access to information in real time
- Integration of patient information
- Increase quality across a wide range of patient populations[24]
- Legibility
- Billing efficiency
- Ease
- Quality of personal performance[25]

BARRIERS TO IMPLEMENTING ELECTRONIC HEALTH RECORDS

- Cost
  - Purchasing, implementation, and maintenance[2,26]
  - Who should pay for EHR usage?
- Time
  - Considerably more time for electronic versus traditional medical record keeping is necessary.[27]
- Poor planning

- Poor technical expertise
- Cultural factors
- Reluctance to embrace new technology[24]
- Belief of garbage in and garbage out[25]

SECURITY

The Health Insurance Portability and Accountability Act (HIPAA) focuses on unauthorized access to patient data or improper disclosure of health information.[2] Sole providers are becoming a rarity with authorized disclosure of this information being available to the workplace or insurance companies. Therefore disclosure of health information is considered to be beyond the boundaries of the "Hippocratic Oath."[28] Hospitals will need to create new relationships to control the medical record and increase this control. Legal issues include who views the medical record as multiple clinicians and institutions are involved. The privacy of the data must be secured at all times. Warnings and alerts in the record should not be overridden, and if a safety issue occurs, appropriate reporting is necessary.[29] The incorporation of passwords and logouts is helpful (Figure 17-2).[9]

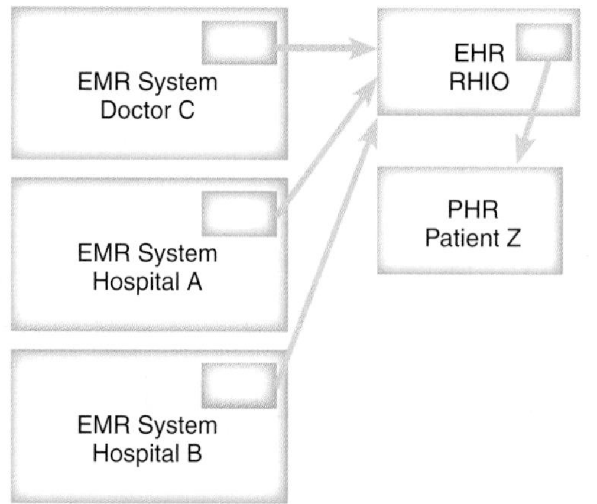

FIGURE 17-2 An electronic health diagram. (From ed. informatics.org website. *http://ed-informatics.org/healthcare-it-in-a-nutshell-2/emr-vs-ehr-vs-phr/*. Accessed May 13, 2012.)

Layman[30] notes that the EHR must maintain the ethical elements of beneficence, autonomy, fidelity, and justice. If there is a breach in the EHR, the patient needs to be informed about the breach and potential harm that can occur. Ethical procedures for disclosure must be made along with a time frame. A discussion on how the breach occurred, what was breached, consequences, and corrective action must be made. At all times, the interest of the patient must be supported.[31]

CLINICAL APPLICATIONS

1. How would you determine the best electronic health record (EHR) for your organization?
2. What are the meaningful use incentives that you would strive to meet?
3. Discuss budget requirements, device selection, staffing, and training for your organization's EHR.
4. Discuss the importance of the Health Insurance Portability and Accountability Act (HIPAA) in the development of your organization's health information security policy.

KEY POINTS

- Health informatics globally focuses on information science, computer science, and health care.
- Health information technology uses electronic methods that maximize health care.
- PAs are savvy and passionate teachers who provide testing, training, and end-user support.
- PAs are subject matter experts who are integral in template development, clinical content, and workflows.
- In addition to the mandatory elements of the electronic health record, PAs have expertise in the integration of performance indicators, handoff communication, and the development of the legal chart.
- Remember, you are an important member of the clinical systems planning team.

References

1. Wikipedia website. *http://en.wikipedia.org/wiki/Health_informatics*; Accessed July 4, 2011.
2. Health Information Technology in the United States—Where We Stand. 2008. Robert Wood Johnson Foundation, Massachusetts General Hospital and The George Washington University.
3. Murphy EM, Oxencis CJ, Klauck JA, et al. Medication reconciliation at an academic medical enter: implementation of a comprehensive program from admission to discharge. Am J Health System Pharm 2009;66:2126.
4. Ong K. Medical Informatics—An Executive Primer. Chicago: Healthcare Information and Management Systems Society, 2007.
5. Weitzman E. Sharing medical data for health research: the early personal health record experience. J Med Internet Res 2010;12:e14.
6. Palacio C, Harrison JP, Garets D. Benchmarking electronic medical record initiatives in the US: a conceptual model. J Med Syst 2010;34:273–279.
7. The Leapfrog Group website. *http://www.leapfroggroup.org/about_us*; Accessed July 6, 2011.
8. The Joint Commission website. *http://www.jointcommission.org/about_us/data_mart.aspx*; Accessed July 6, 2011.
9. Friedman L, Halpern N, Fackler J. Implementing an electronic medical record. Critical Care Clinics 2007; 23:347.
10. Health Information Technology in the United States—On the Cusp of Change. 2009. Robert Wood Johnson Foundation, Massachusetts General Hospital and The George Washington University.
11. Jha AK, DesRoches CM, Kralovec PD, Joshi MS. A progress report on electronic health records in U.S. hospitals. Health Affairs (Millwood) 2010;29:1951–1957.
12. Maxson E, Jain S, Kendall M, et al. The Regional Extension Program Center program: helping physicians meaningfully use health information technology. Ann Intern Med 2010;153:666.
13. Vest J. More than just a question of technology: factors related to hospitals' adoption and implementation of health information exchange. Int J Med Inform 2010;79:797.
14. Lewis S. Brave new EMR. Ann Intern Med 2011;154:368.
15. Abraham S. Technological trends in health care. Health Care Manag 2010;29:318.
16. Rand Corporation website. *http://www.rand.org/topics/electronic-medical-records.html*; Accessed May 9, 2011.
17. *portal.ahrq.gov/portal/server.pt/gateway/PTARGS_0_898095_0_0_18/Electronic Health Records Overview.pdf*; Accessed on May 9, 2011.
18. Smelcer J, Miller-Jacobs H, Kantrovich H. Usability of electronic medical records. International Journal of Usability Studies 2009;4:70.
19. McGrath D. The sociology of change. J Med Pract Manage 2009;25:105.
20. Devore S, Figlioli K. Lessons premier hospitals learned about implementing electronic health records. Health Aff 2010;29:664.
21. Vishwanath A, Singh SR, Wnkelstein P, et al. The impact of electronic medical record systems on outpatient workflows: a longitudinal evaluation of its workflow effects. Int J Med Inform 2010;79:778.
22. Munasinghe R, Arsene C, Abraham TK, et al. Improving the utilization of admission order sets in a computerized physician order entry system by integrating modular disease specific order subsets into a general medicine admission order set. J Am Med Inform Assoc 2011;18:322.
23. Health Information Technology in the United States—Moving Towards Meaningful Use. 2010. Robert Wood Johnson Foundation, Massachusetts General Hospital and The George Washington University.
24. Harrison J, Palachio C. The role of clinical information systems in health care quality improvement. Health Care Manag 2006;25:206.
25. Holden R. Physicians' beliefs about using EMR and CPOE: in pursuit of a contextualized understanding of health IT use behavior. Int J Med Inform 2010;79:71.
26. Jha A, DesRoches CM, Campbell EG, et al. Use of electronic health records in U.S. hospitals. N Engl J Med 2009;360:1628.
27. Tevaarwerk G. Electronic medical records. Can Med Assoc J 2008;178:1323.
28. Rothstein M. The Hippocratic bargain and health information technology. J Law Med Ethics 2010;38:7.
29. Sitting D, Sing H. Legal, ethical and financial dilemmas in electronic health record adoption and use. Am Acad Pediatr 2011;124:31042.
30. Layman E. Ethical Issues and the Electronic Health Record. Health Care Manag 2008;27:165.
31. American Medical Association website. *http://www.ama-assn.org/resources/doc/hod/a-09-ceja-opinons-reports.pdf*; Accessed May 10, 2011.

The resources for this chapter can be found at www.expertconsult.com.

CHAPTER 18

Using Consultants and Community Resources

Albert Simon • Daniel T. Vetrosky • Ernest L. Stump

CHAPTER CONTENTS

The process of seeking consultation and community referral is an integral part of every practitioner's practice pattern. Since the beginning of medical practice, health care providers have sought counsel about difficult patients. As the complexity of medical practice increases, it is logical that one would seek expert advice about the treatment and management of conditions out of the realm of one's expertise or resources.

Physician assistants (PAs), as dependent practitioners, consult with other health care practitioners as a routine portion of their daily practice. This is especially true for the consultation that goes on between PAs and their supervising physicians. Every PA uses some form of consultation with the physician-supervisor. There is a great deal of latitude as to the form that process of consultation takes. For some PAs, the supervising physician is on-site and acts as a consultant for review of elements of every case. Other PAs practice in locations remote from their supervisors and tend not to consult as frequently. Most PAs also use individuals other than their supervisory physicians for consultation. The primary reason for consultants is the need for expert opinions when decisions are made regarding patient care.[1] In addition, consultants expand the knowledge base for a PA in areas related to the PA's practice.

Providers today are confronted with a host of process rules that result from the changes in an ever-evolving health care system. PAs need to understand the process rules concerning referrals that govern many interactions for specialty consultation so that the patient may be channeled to the proper care in the most expedient fashion without encountering roadblocks. Issues that may pose an obstacle for effective patient referral include the lack of ability of the patient to self-refer, criteria that may exist for the use of special testing referral (e.g., use of magnetic resonance imaging in cases of low back pain), and constraints of cost. These types of rules have added complexity to the provider/patient interaction, as well as new responsibility. As a patient's primary care provider, the PA must have the ability to appropriately guide the patient though this complex system and act as an advocate on the patient's behalf.

Technology has also entered the referral arena. Telemedicine is increasingly used as a method of providing access to specialty consultation services. This technology also provides access to services that were previously unavailable in certain remote areas or in areas that could not support certain services because of a small population base. Even social networking is changing the way individuals seek medical care and form opinions about what type of treatment they should receive.[2] These are powerful influences that may play to the patient's advantage when used properly.

Finally, by having a clear understanding of how to make an effective referral for consultation, the PA can help to ensure that the patient's time and monetary resources will be used most effectively and that the patient will receive the most appropriate care in the proper timeframe.

When a referral or consultation is necessary, the PA must be cognizant of the resources available in the community. These include human resources, in the form of other health care providers, as well as helping organizations. This chapter discusses methods used in seeking consultation and the appropriate use of community resources through patient referral.

USING CONSULTANTS

For patients to make their way to specialty services, they must have a means of moving along the medical hierarchy. This pathway has been dubbed the "referral chain."[3] Patients may enter the referral chain from a number of starting points and may be referred by a general practitioner to a specialist, by a specialist to a specialist, or by a specialist to a general practitioner. Each of the providers along the chain may be used as a consultant. The goal of the referral chain (and thus the use of consultants) is to guide patients to the appropriate level of medical care.

Primary care practitioners often initiate the entry of the patient into the realm of specialists. Indeed, in countries with nationalized health care systems, primary care providers are looked upon as gatekeepers to the more expensive and scarce specialist care.[4] The following two cases illustrate the types of situations in which consultations typically occur.

CASE STUDY 18-1

A 42-year-old female presents with a history of headache and slurred speech. These symptoms have been progressive over the past month or two. On examination, the PA finds cranial nerve deficits and refers the patient for immediate computed tomography (CT) scan. The examination reveals a cerebral tumor. The patient is referred for immediate neurosurgical consultation.

CASE STUDY 18-2

A 63-year-old woman with advanced degenerative joint disease has been under the care of a general practitioner for several years for management of the arthritis. She now needs specialty referral to an orthopedist for hip replacement.

Both of these cases depict patients moving from primary care situations to the use of specialists or subspecialists. Referral in the other direction, from specialist to primary care provider, is also appropriate, as is shown in the following case.

CASE STUDY 18-3

Mr. W is a 65-year-old white man with a number of medical problems. During each 6-month period, Mr. W sees a cardiologist, a pulmonologist, and a neurologist. Each of the specialists involved in this case has prescribed at least one medication. On the last visit, the neurologist refers the patient to a family practitioner.

Mr. W's situation is not uncommon. This patient is involved with multiple specialists, each providing quality medical care but focused from a specialty perspective. In these cases, consultation with colleagues in family medicine or general internal medicine is entirely appropriate. The inclusion of primary care providers serves to help coordinate the patient's overall treatment. It is easy for a patient (usually an older patient) receiving care from multiple specialists to be "lost in the shuffle," with no one to coordinate care from the broader perspective.

Another aspect of the consultation that should not be neglected is its role in the process of medical education.[5] In the past, consultations between specialists and primary care providers occurred at the bedside. Currently, this exchange more often occurs via written correspondence. Even without personal contact between the health care providers, an opportunity for teaching still exists in the consultation process. The detailed information about the patient (e.g., personal and family history, reaction to treatment to date) possessed by the primary care provider can provide valuable insight to the consultant. The consultant obviously has detailed expertise to pass on to the primary care provider relative to specific disease processes and their management. For this education to be substantive, communication must be effective as characterized by clear communication between all parties and well-coordinated care. With the appropriate use of the consultative process, the patient, the referring provider, and the consultant all may benefit.

Consultants are used in any situation in which special skills are necessary. Referral to a consultant may be to a specialist, a subspecialist, or a primary care provider, as the situation dictates. The referral chain can be considered effective if the patient reaches the appropriate health care provider within a time that is not detrimental to his or her medical condition and effective, coordinated care is rendered.

Choosing a Consultant

After the decision to make a referral has been made, the PA must choose the consultant. What attributes are desirable in a consultant? First, a consultant must be *qualified*. This usually means being board certified in the area of practice. Board certification certainly speaks to competence on one level. The "fit" of the consultant in the referral chain may extend beyond board certification. A visit to the consultant's practice allows the PA the chance to talk at length with the consultant. The visit also serves to showcase the consultant's facilities, making the PA aware of the range of services he or she may provide. The PA may then develop a sense of the consultant's approach to patient care and his or her perspectives and priorities as they pertain to practice. With the advent of changes in the health care system, the provider may be limited in the consultants who may be used, unless the patient wants to go "out of the system" and pay out of pocket for the service. A consultant should also be *available*. This availability should extend to both the provider and the patient. The consultant should be available for inquiries via telephone and for "bedside consults" in the hospital. The patient should also benefit from the consultant's availability by not having to wait unduly for an appointment with a referral. It may also be important to know what forms of payment are accepted by the consultant.

Making the Referral

For the consultant to adequately perform his or her job, appropriate information must be transmitted. In a patient referral, it is customary to send a formal communication that contains a synopsis of the history of current illness, the medical history, pertinent physical findings, and current medications, including the current form of treatment and the results. Most important, the reason for requesting the consultation must be included. This last statement may seem self-evident, but a review of the literature reveals that such may not be the case. In a study of 500 nonurgent referrals to the Manchester Royal Eye Hospital by general practitioners and ophthalmic opticians, many of the baseline data were found to be lacking. In only 27.5% of cases was an adequate medical history provided, and in only 13% was any drug information provided. Fully 43.7% of patients' referral records to this specialty eye hospital from general practices contained no evidence that an ocular examination had been performed.[6] Other studies have reviewed referral letters from general practitioners and found that a high percentage (59.4%) were barely adequate or were poor.[7] The following is recommended information to be included in a request for consultation or referral:

- Introductory sentence (identifies patient)
- Synopsis of history of present illness
- Pertinent medical history and review of systems
- Social or personal history as it relates to the case
- Physical examination findings
- Statement of why the consultation is being initiated
- Follow-up instructions the patient has received

In the outpatient setting, referral information can be dictated in a short letter (usually one or two pages) and sent directly to the consultant via the mail or electronically. Occasionally, this letter is sealed and given to the patient to carry by hand. The office staff at the referring practice usually phones to make the appointment with the consultant's office for the patient. The contact from the referring office staff should ensure that the patient has an appointment within a reasonable time. A sample referral letter is shown in Figure 18-1.

In the institutional setting, a standardized form is usually provided for requesting consultations. This form (either paper or digital) can be obtained from the unit manager or ward secretary. Once the form is completed, ward staff members generally process the request and notify the consultant. One may elect to designate the consultation as *emergent*, in which case the consultant is called immediately; as *urgent*, whereby the consultant is notified within a couple of hours; or as *routine*, by which the patient is generally seen in the next day or two. A word concerning emergent consultations may be appropriate here. An emergent consultation implies the need for immediate intervention necessary to prevent the patient's condition from deteriorating. This type of consultation is generally expensive for the patient and stressful for the consultant. Many practitioners have witnessed the abuse of this designation. People are called in from home to see a patient and perform diagnostic studies, only to realize that by the time the studies are finalized, the requesting practitioner is no longer available to act on the information generated.

In cases that are complicated or emergent, the provider usually elects to call the consultant and discuss the case personally. This allows the provider to

Deborah R. Jones, M.D.
Family Practice
Suite C Benlo Place
Altoona, PA 16601

June 1, 2012

David Smith, M.D.
Neurology
501 Howard Avenue
Altoona, PA 16601

Dear Dr. Smith:

Please allow me to introduce Mr. James Walker. Mr. Walker is a 37-year-old white male who has been a patient in our practice for the last five years. Mr. Walker presented to my office earlier this week with a complaint of photopsia in his right eye. The photopsia has occurred two times during the past month. Each time the photopsia occurs, it lasts approximately fifteen minutes. The patient states that at the conclusion of the photopsia, he feels somewhat washed out. On the last occasion, Mr. Walker reported a mild headache located over the left frontal area. The photopsia is not associated with any other symptoms; particularly, I note a lack of nausea, vomiting, or other sensations of aura, such as unusual smells. Mr. Walker denies any history of vertigo, dizziness, or paresthesia. He denies any ataxia or problems with coordination. A similar episode occurred approximately one-and-a-half years ago, at which time he sought attention from his optometrist. The optometrist examined Mr. Walker's fundus and advised him to return should this particular problem occur again. He had no further episodes until this month. He presented to our practice at this time because of the increased frequency of the episodes.

He is in generally good health, with the following ongoing medical problems: Mild hypertension that has been well controlled by Lisinipril, 10 mg q d at HS. He is mildly obese and struggles to maintain his weight at a reasonable level; I have recommended that he lose approximately 20 pounds. Finally, we have found on one occasion that his serum cholesterol was elevated to 232. I have recommended a level one diet. His cholesterol will be rechecked within six months. There is no history of migraine headache or other neurological maladies in his past or family history. Mr. Walker is a chairman of a medium-sized corporation here in Altoona and indicated that he feels that he is under quite a bit of stress in his job. He does admit to difficulty sleeping, particularly in falling asleep, and sometimes has early morning awakening. He also indicates that he suffers from bruxism.

Physical examination reveals a mildly obese, well-developed, well-nourished white male in no acute distress. Skin is warm and dry. **HEENT**—benign bilaterally, no evidence of embolic phenomenon or hypertensive retinopathy. The thyroid is not enlarged. **Thorax and lungs**—clear to auscultation and percussion. **Cardiovascular system**—heart rate at 86 with regular rate. II/VI systolic ejection murmur located at Erb's point without radiation. No clicks or heaves are present. Pulses are all equal at 2/4; no bruits are heard at the carotid, aortic, or renal areas. **Abdomen**—soft without tenderness or organomegaly. **Musculoskeletal**—full range of motion without deformity; strength is 5/5 and equal at all. **Neurological**—cranial nerves 1 through 12 are intact. Motor—gait and station are intact. Romberg is negative. Coordination and rapid alternating movements are performed well. Sensory—intact to touch and sharp/dull through all major dermatomes. Stereognosis and graphesthesia are intact bilaterally. Reflexes— +2/4 and equal bilaterally, no clonus noted. Mental status—affect is appropriate, recent and remote memory are intact.

My thought at this point is that these phenomena represent the onset of ocular migraines; perhaps the stress is playing a role. I am interested in getting your opinion relative to the photopsia. Could this represent early multiple sclerosis or other neurological processes? Please evaluate Mr. Walker and relay your impression to me. I have instructed Mr. Walker to make an appointment to see me 2 weeks after your examination and diagnostic workup are complete. I am also sending Mr. Walker for ophthalmological referral to rule out primary retinal disease.

Thank you for seeing this patient in consultation.

Sincerely,

John Williams, PA-C

FIGURE 18-1 Sample referral letter.

establish a clear sense of the case with the consultant and to be informed about additional initial management or laboratory studies needed before the consultant sees the patient.

Many providers forget that one of the most frequent referrals is to the radiologist. Yet often a patient is sent for an abdominal ultrasound or other radiologic procedure without the radiologist's being notified of the history and physical findings. Each consultant needs adequate information on which to base recommendations. Some consultants do not have the advantage of seeing the patient, and few have the background knowledge of the case that the referring practitioner has. The responsibility of the referring provider is to transmit as much of the essence of the case to the consultant as possible in a clear and succinct form. Consultants should also be obliged to inform the referring health care provider of their findings, recommendations, and treatments. This is usually accomplished by a follow-up communication sent to the referring provider shortly after the consultation has been completed. Failure of the consultant to engage in this practice is a common source of dissatisfaction for referring providers.[8]

Referral Rates

In today's climate of practice comparisons and nonanalytic data, a provider may wonder how many patients should be referred. Is the PA referring too many or too few patients? The literature provides little clear guidance on these points. Referral rates vary by practitioner, by location, and by specialty. It seems clear, however, that consultations are requested for a variety of personal and medical reasons.[9]

Although health care system changes are affecting referral rates, it is not clear exactly what impact it is having or whether it is appropriate. Gomez and colleagues[10] studied residents' behavior in connection with a managed care curriculum presented during their residency experience. A lower rate of referrals was one outcome of this experience. The investigators indicated that the lower rates of referral might have been due to the intimidation of scrutiny of these behaviors by colleagues. The authors go on to warn against undercare that may result from this trend. At present, it seems prudent to recommend that a referral be made when the circumstances dictate. These parameters include the personal characteristics of the practice. Scientifically, no clues currently exist as to whether practitioners in general practice refer too few or too many patients.[11]

Patient Considerations

The referral situation holds the potential for great benefit for the patient but also for the patient to become alienated from the primary care provider. Should the referral to a consultant be made without a proper explanation, the patient may feel "dumped off" or perhaps lost in the "doctor shuffle."

A good way to avoid disgruntled feelings is to rely on good basic patient interaction techniques. The patient who is involved in the decision-making and consideration of treatment options is apt to be more accepting of the notion of the referral. The idea and reasons for the referral should be introduced to the patient. The provider should point out that the consultant will indicate preferences for treatment, but that through the process of negotiation, the patient will have a role in approving which treatment option is chosen. The primary care provider may then reassure the patient that he or she will be available to help discuss any treatment options, should the patient desire.

The primary care provider must be sure to follow up with a referred patient, inquiring about how the patient perceived the consultant. The provider should try to evaluate the level of the patient's satisfaction with the consultant visit. Patient dissatisfaction can rank high as a reason for treatment failure. In these situations, basic skills become quite important. In a study of patients needing a second opinion, a group of dissatisfied patients indicated that the physician had not spent enough time with them, even though 90% of this group indicated that the physician had asked appropriate questions and 60% believed that their questions were answered adequately.[12] By having a good working knowledge of the personalities and styles of the consultants that one uses, one may choose to provide the patient with some expectations of what they will experience when they attend the consultation with that specialist. These expectations may help to improve patients' satisfaction with their visit. When a choice of consultants is available, one may be able to match patients with consultants who will not only meet their medical needs but also blend with their personality, perhaps improving compliance.

The provider should also review the consultant's recommendations with the patient and put them into a workable perspective relative to the practice orientation. Again, it is important for the patient to be an active participant in deciding on a treatment plan. If the patient is not invested in the process, he or she cannot relate to following medication regimens or making behavioral changes critical to the management of the illness.

Nontraditional Consultants

The United States has experienced a dramatic increase in the number of immigrants arriving over the past 2 decades. Before 1980, most immigrants coming to the United States were from European nations. Since that time, the demographics have shifted and now the vast majority of immigrants are from non-European nations. Along with their values and culture, patients from other countries bring experiences in health care systems different from traditional Western medicine. In attempts to provide culturally competent patient care to this diverse population, consultations with traditional healers from these various cultures are increasingly common. Originally dismissed as nonscientific, curanderos, shamans, santiguadoras, and other traditional healers are now increasingly acknowledged as powerful allies to Western medicine. Although they may be accessing care within the U.S. health care system, many people hold deep-seated beliefs in methods of treatment rooted in their culture and values. The recommendations in the following provide strategies for working with patients who use traditional healers.

Negotiate the treatment plan with the patient and discuss how you are willing to work with the traditional healer for the patient's benefit. Encourage the patient to continue on the necessary course of Western therapy and keep you informed about additional treatments employed by the traditional healers. Use the LEARN model to assist in reducing cultural barriers and increasing patient compliance in your culturally diverse patients[13]:

- **L** Listen with understanding to the patient's perception of the problem.
- **E** Explain your perceptions and strategy for treatment.
- **A** Acknowledge and discuss differences in perceptions.
- **R** Recommend treatment with respect to the patient's cultural perceptions.
- **N** Negotiate agreement, keeping in mind the patient's conceptual framework of disease.

Employing traditional healers in the treatment plan for these patients can often assist in the patient's recovery. During the patient interview, it is helpful to inquire what the patient believes is causing the illness. This line of questioning may reveal that the patient believes an evil spirit or other entity is at the root of the problem. When patients hold these beliefs, it may be helpful to consult with traditional healers.

In many areas of the United States, traditional healers may be located by contacting local religious leaders in the community. Often, these individuals can help to provide insight about the culture and values of your patient, and they will usually be aware of what traditional healers are available in the area. Other contacts that may be helpful include ethnic organizations and alternative therapy units of larger hospitals.

If your practice has a large culturally diverse population, it may be wise to establish relationships with local nontraditional healers to facilitate future referrals. Most traditional healers are willing to work with Western practitioners to assist in the patient's recovery.

CASE STUDY 18-4

Mr. W is an 86-year-old Hispanic male who is unable to drive because of vision problems secondary to his diabetes. He and his wife live on a small ranch just outside of town. Mrs. W drives, but her vision is also failing and she is uncomfortable driving farther than about 10 miles from their home. She is unable to drive at night. Mr. W is in need of a specialty consultation that is available only in a large community about 160 miles away (3 hours by automobile). The couple does not want to make the drive, but the PA needs to have the consultant see the patient.

USING COMMUNITY RESOURCES

Case of the S Family

Before the discussion of community resources begins, let us consider the following case. It will help the reader understand how a PA becomes involved in referrals to community resources.

CASE STUDY 18-5

The S family has been coming to a general practice for years. The previous PA worked with them for several years. Mr. S is 48 years old, and Mrs. S is 46. They have five children: Mary (17), John (15), Sean (11), David (9), and Beth (1). Mrs. S is a diabetic and has been treated for depression in the past. Mr. S has struggled for years with control of his hypertension. The new PA notes from the chart that Mr. and Mrs. S have both had drug and alcohol problems in the past. Mr. S is in the office today for his regular appointment.

After introducing herself and explaining her transition into the practice, the new PA mentions the fact that Mr. S's blood pressure is 170/100 mm Hg. Mr. S indicates that he sometimes forgets to take his medication because he has many other things on his mind these days. When the PA asks for details, Mr. S describes his current situation.

Mr. S has worked in the local automobile plant for years. That plant is now closing, and in 6 months he will be out of a job. Mrs. S has never worked outside the home, choosing to stay home with the children. Mrs. S has become depressed and has called the local mental health center for services. Her name has been added to its waiting list. Mr. S has tried desperately to pull his wife out of this depression but has been unsuccessful. He states that she has alluded to thoughts of suicide. A great deal of the responsibility for the care of the children has now fallen to Mr. S. He seems able to manage fairly well with Beth and David. David presents difficulty sometimes because his borderline mental retardation makes it difficult for him to understand his mother's disinterest. John and Sean, according to Mr. S, are doing okay at home. However, he states that he has had calls from the school informing him that John has been getting into fights and that Sean refuses to socialize, appearing withdrawn. The most recent family upset has come with Mary's announcement that she is pregnant. Mrs. S blames Mr. S for letting this happen because he should have taken more responsibility for the family when she became depressed. Mrs. S claims he is a poor father, and she has proposed divorce.

Mr. S remarks that it feels good to tell someone about all of this. He then asks whether there is any further help the PA can suggest.

At first glance, this scenario may seem overwhelming to approach. The practitioner at any level of experience who has a sound knowledge of community resources could, however, use a systematic approach to assist this patient. In fact, it would be considered a clear opportunity for community involvement integrated with a realistic treatment and prevention plan for the patient. The reader should remember this scenario while reading the section on community resources. At the conclusion of the chapter, a discussion of one approach to Mr. S's problems is presented.

Community resources vary widely, and there are often crossover relationships and duplicate services within a single community. A particular community service agency, such as a family service agency, may have services for families, individuals, and groups. A mental health center in the same community may also have services for families, individuals, and groups. These agencies may use one another's services and refer patients back and forth, depending on the nature of a client's needs, the agency's ability to serve that client at that particular time, and the desires of the client or the family. The novice soon discovers what the experienced user of community resources knows, namely, that no matter how many services a community resource provides, there are often waiting lists, or it may be difficult to find the appropriate resource for a particular patient.

These situations may overwhelm the PA. It would seem easier to simply ignore this part of the differential diagnosis and eliminate it completely from the treatment plan. Experienced practitioners are aware, however, that community resource referral is an essential part of the differential diagnosis and treatment plan. There are simply times when no physical reason can be found for a patient's complaint. Patients may believe that they must have a physical complaint in order to see the practitioner. Consider the following case.

CASE STUDY 18-6

A patient comes to the office for her regular prenatal check. She is 25 weeks pregnant. The PA notices that she is wearing heavier makeup than usual and seems to avoid eye contact. When the PA inquires about her behavior, the patient begins to cry and says that her boyfriend hit her after consuming a lot of alcohol. She explains that her boyfriend feels pressured to provide for the baby and to get married. He is young, she says, and had different plans for his future.

To simply treat this situation as a routine prenatal visit would be an act of negligence on the part of any clinician. Recognizing that this patient needs a different kind of treatment plan fulfills the patient's needs, as well as the clinician's obligation to treat and heal. There are many potential referral sources for this particular scenario, such as:

- A family service agency to assist with the relationship difficulties, that is, to enable the patient's boyfriend to deal with his feelings about the pregnancy, to provide counseling for abusive behavior, and to assist the patient in making decisions about the relationship.
- Possible drug and alcohol assistance services for the patient's boyfriend.

The clinician in this scenario must act as the catalyst and facilitator by identifying services for the patient. The patient must ultimately determine what assistance she will or will not accept. It is the responsibility of the clinician to be knowledgeable about the assistance available, to facilitate referral by discussing the idea with the patient and significant others, and to make the initial referral to the appropriate community service agency.

OVERVIEW OF TYPICAL COMMUNITY SERVICES

As has been discussed previously, there is overlap of services among community service agencies. For the purposes of this chapter, five specific *areas* have been identified as problem categories for the family—personal/social, financial/employment, addiction, legal, and health. Examples of each category, along with the possible community service responses available for each identified family problem, are listed in Tables 18-1 through 18-5 and discussed in this chapter. The brief explanation of each community service listed serves as a helpful reference for the reader. The lists of services shown, however, are not to be viewed as all-inclusive; in fact, they fall far short of that. They are also not to be viewed as representative of any particular agency's services.

PAs must recognize that it is necessary to become knowledgeable about the network of community services available in their particular practice areas. They must also be aware of individual agency resources; many communities now have a human service directory that can be of invaluable assistance in helping the practitioner discover these resources. Finally, PAs must be aware of community services that are not available. Ultimately, it is the PA's responsibility to integrate all three of these areas of knowledge into the treatment plans for their patients.

Personal and Social Problems and Needs

Table 18-1 shows which of the community resources discussed here are generally available for personal and social problems.

Family service agencies are probably the most generic of all community service providers. Counseling for individuals and families is often the core of services offered by this type of agency. Many family service agencies use a sliding fee scale for payment, which makes them ideal for people with limited incomes.

Mental health services and centers provide evaluation, diagnostic, and treatment services for people of all ages who are experiencing emotional or mental health difficulties. A sliding fee scale is usually applied. Crisis intervention services are usually available on a 24-hour basis.

Family planning centers offer educational, screening, and testing services for women regarding pregnancy and gynecologic problems. A sliding fee scale is usually applied.

Psychiatrists, psychologists, and social workers in private practice are valuable to the community. Their services include individual psychotherapy, marital and family counseling, and psychological testing. Provision of service is based on ability to pay.

Child welfare agencies provide protective, adoptive, foster care, and institutional services for children (18 years of age and younger) in the community. These agencies are mandated service providers for situations of physical, emotional, and sexual abuse and exploitation of children. Many child welfare agencies have direct working relationships with governmental juvenile parole and probation departments.

Services for mentally handicapped services and centers are sometimes directly tied to mental health services in a community and sometimes are private services. They offer vocational assistance, advocacy, and supervision to mentally retarded community members. Services are also provided to anyone caring for a mentally retarded family member in the home.

Senior citizen centers are the central providers of services to the elderly in a community. Their services range from in-home care, adult day care, services, transportation, and employment to volunteer programs. Protective services for the abused or exploited elder family member are also available.

In *Big Brothers* and *Big Sisters* programs, same-sex companionship is provided to children from single-parent families. Emphasis is placed on assisting a child in his or her development through contact with a positive role model.

Private and public day care centers furnish child care to parents interested in entering or remaining in the workforce. Educational programming and development for children are emphasized in many of these centers.

Personal care boarding and nursing homes offer care to people who are no longer able to maintain themselves in their own homes. Nursing homes provide a range of nursing and medical care needs to the elderly person in poor health.

In *adult day care* arrangements, elderly individuals unable to take responsibility for themselves are supervised and monitored while their primary caregivers are at work or otherwise unable to care for them.

Special services for exceptional children are often provided through the local school district. Mentally challenged, socially or emotionally disturbed, learning disabled, physically handicapped, speech handicapped, and mentally gifted students are eligible for such services.

In community *adult education centers*, interested adults can obtain a high school graduate equivalency certificate or receive special training.

Centers for special learning provide assistance to children with developmental difficulties. *Head Start*

TABLE 18-1 **Community Resources Available for Specific Personal and Social Problems and Needs***

Community Resource	Adolescent Pregnancy	Adult and Elder Care	Adult Physical and Sexual Abuse	Anxiety	Child Physical and Sexual Abuse	Child Care and Companionship	Child and Adult Education	Depression
Family service agencies	X		X	X			X	X
Mental health centers			X	X	X		X	X
Family planning centers	X						X	
Private practice psychologists and social workers			X	X	X			X
Child welfare agencies					X		X	
Mental retardation centers and services		X	X				X	
Senior citizen centers		X	X				X	
Big Brothers and Big Sisters						X		
Private and public care centers and homes		X				X		
Employee-assisted day care						X		
Professional care boarding and nursing homes		X						
Adult day care								
School special services for exceptional children	X					X		
Adult education centers						X	X	
Centers for special caring								
Head Start programs								
Religious communities								

*An X indicates that assistance is available from the resource for the problem.

programs prepare low-income children and children with special needs to enter kindergarten.

An often-overlooked community resource is the *religious community* (e.g., church, synagogue, temple). Many religious leaders are trained in both pastoral and personal counseling.

Financial and Employment Assistance

Table 18-2 shows which services from the community resources discussed here are generally available for financial and employment problems.

The *department of public welfare* is a state agency providing cash assistance, assistance for medical care, and similar services to low-income or needy people.

Many community service resources, such as family service agencies and agencies affiliated with particular religious denominations, provide one-time *emergency financial assistance* to persons in need.

Budget and credit counseling are available both publicly and privately to people needing help with money management.

State or local *offices of employment security* (unemployment offices) assist people with job placement, job testing, and other employment services, in addition to processing unemployment insurance claims.

People who need financial support for children from the legally responsible parent who is unwilling or reluctant to meet his or her financial care responsibilities are assisted in obtaining such support by *domestic relations resources*.

Housing authorities and *resource groups* help low-income and moderate-income people of all ages obtain housing.

American Rescue Workers and the *Salvation Army* offer emergency shelter on a temporary basis for people in need.

Both *Goodwill Industries Skills Training* and *Employment Programs* provide employment and training for mentally retarded and mental health consumers.

Assistance for Addiction Problems

Table 18-3 shows which services from the community resources discussed here are generally available for addiction problems.

Alcoholics Anonymous is a self-help group composed of recovering alcoholics who help one another maintain their sobriety and help others attain it. *Al-Anon* and *Alateen* are related self-help groups that assist adults or teens in coping with alcohol dependence in a family member or friend.

TABLE 18-2 **Community Resources Available for Specific Financial or Employment Problems***

Community Resource	Unemployment	Housing	Transportation	Budgeting	Cash Assistance	Discrimination
Departments of public welfare	X	X	X	X	X	X
Emergency financial services					X	
Budget and credit counseling	X			X		
Offices of employment security	X					
Domestic relations resources					X	
Housing authorities and resource groups		X				
American Rescue Workers		X				
Salvation Army		X		X		
Goodwill Industries and Skills Training and Employment Programs	X					
Equal Employment Opportunity Commission and human relations commissions	X	X				X

*An X indicates that assistance is available from the resource for the problem.

Another self-help group, *Narcotics Anonymous*, is composed of individuals who are recovering from dependency on drugs.

Drug and alcohol clinics provide outpatient services to individuals dealing with drug and alcohol problems. Group therapy and counseling are usually offered. An *inpatient rehabilitation facility* offers a battery of treatment services for addicted persons judged to require intensive treatment.

Relapse programs offer services on an outpatient basis. Group sessions are intended to assist individuals who have abstained from drugs and alcohol but have had a recent relapse of use.

Legal Assistance

Table 18-4 shows the services available for legal problems from the community resources discussed here.

Adult probation and parole departments are responsible for the supervision of all adult parolees and probationers from the prison and court systems.

Juvenile probation departments are responsible for the supervision of juvenile offenders who have been either put on probation or institutionalized.

Legal Aid services help eligible people who cannot afford to hire a private attorney deal with civil legal matters such as divorce, landlord and tenant matters, and bankruptcy.

Through *victim/witness* programs, victims of or witnesses to crimes obtain compensation or referral to community social service agencies for counseling or other appropriate services.

Assistance with Health Care and Related Problems. Table 18-5 shows resources available for specific health problems and needs.

Food banks give food to individuals and families on a limited basis in times of emergency and crisis when other services, such as food stamps, are not available or eligibility for them has not yet been determined.

Vast arrays of support groups are available to individuals, particularly in the health field. Groups for health-related concerns and diseases such as cancer, diabetes, Parkinson and Alzheimer diseases, and epilepsy have been formed in many communities. Other support groups offer help to single parents dealing with a delinquent teenager or to victims of sexual assault or other crimes.

Hospital social services and *case management services* help patients and their families cope with the stress accompanying hospitalization. Follow-up referrals to community service agencies and medical facilities are also provided.

Associations for the blind and visually handicapped offer preventive programs and educational services to minimize the incidence of loss of vision. They also assist impaired individuals by furnishing special equipment, transportation, and counseling.

A *community nursing services* agency supplies nursing care, physical therapy, nutrition education, prenatal services, hospice home services, and counseling to patients in their own homes.

The *Easter Seals Society* offers an extremely broad range of assessment and treatment services to people of all ages and varying economic status in the community. Its services include speech and language, orthopedics, hearing evaluations, equipment rentals, summer camps, psychological testing, and day care.

TABLE 18-3 Community Resources Available for Specific Addiction Problems and Needs*

Community Resource	Drugs	Alcohol
Alcoholics Anonymous		X
Al-Anon		X
Alateen		X
Narcotics Anonymous	X	
Drug and alcohol clinics	X	X
Inpatient rehabilitation facilities	X	X
Relapse programs	X	X

*An X indicates that assistance is available from the resource for the problem.

TABLE 18-4 Community Resources Available for Specific Legal Problems and Needs*

Community Resource	Incarceration	DUI	Legal Aid Services	Juvenile Delinquency
Adult probation and parole, including DUI programs	X	X		
Juvenile probation offices	X	X		X
Legal aid services			X	
Victim/witness programs			X	

*An X indicates that assistance is available from the resource for the problem.
DUI, driving under the influence.

TABLE 18-5 Community Resources Available for Specific Health Problems and Needs*

Community Resource	Aging	Handicapped (Physically or Educationally Disabled)	Hospitalization	Home Health Needs	Immunizations and State Health Laws	Nutrition	Cancer
Food banks	X	X				X	
Support groups	X	X	X	X			X
Hospital social services		X	X	X		X	X
Associations for blind and visually handicapped		X	X				
Community nursing services	X	X	X	X	X	X	X
Easter Seals Society		X	X	X			
Vocational rehabilitation		X	X				
March of Dimes		X		X			
State health centers	X				X	X	
Associations and services for learning disabled		X					
American Cancer Society							X

*An X indicates that assistance is available from the resource for the problem.

The primary focus of the *March of Dimes* is prevention of birth defects through educational programming. Prenatal patients, for example, may be referred for education services.

Vocational rehabilitation agencies formulate programs to increase the employability of people with learning, physical, mental, or addictive problems.

State health centers provide immunizations and health guidance to individuals. Community health education is also a priority.

Associations for learning disabilities assist children and adults with developmental disabilities to gain referral and information for services, legal rights, tutoring, and advocacy.

The American Cancer Society offers information, support services, and advocacy for people and families living with cancer.

CONCLUSION: HELP FOR THE S FAMILY

In Case Study 18-6, Mr. S has already given the PA one clue as to his needs. He needs someone with whom to discuss his situation and to sort out and develop alternatives to his circumstances. Although this counseling component is well within the realm and abilities of the PA, it must be carefully weighed with the time such an undertaking would require and how that would fit with a busy practice. Even if the time is available, a community referral for this patient and his family should address the need for family and marital counseling. The S family appears to be a prime candidate for referral to a family service agency, where a multiservice approach could be taken. The PA could continue to see Mr. S for support and coordination of the community resources, either as part of his regular medical appointments or as separate appointments. The PA might also consider meeting with the S family to discuss the need for referral to a family service agency. This would lend support to Mr. S's efforts to help his family and could almost be seen as a prescription for this dysfunctional family. The PA, acting as community resource coordinator, could also help by contacting the local mental health center to facilitate assistance for Mrs. S. Other community resources for this family would include mental retardation services for David, to help him understand what is happening at home, and a contact with the school system to discuss John's and Sean's behavior. All of this, of course, would be done with the S family's permission.

CLINICAL APPLICATIONS

1. You are the family practice PA caring for Mr. W in Case Study 18-3. What is your role, and how can you help to coordinate Mr. W's health care?
2. You are the PA seeing Ms. Q in Case Study 18-4. How will you describe your function to

Ms. Q and explain why she cannot self-refer to a neurologist?
3. On the basis of your history and physical examination findings, you believe that Ms. Q needs a neurologic consultation. Her managed care plan refuses this referral. How will you handle this situation?
4. You are the PA caring for Mr. S in Case Study 18-6. How will you present the array of community resources available to your patient and his family? What will you say that will educate Mr. S about the usefulness of these resources, while making sure that he knows that you want to continue as his PA?

References

1. Braham RL, Ron A, Ruchlin HS, et al. Diagnostic test restraint and the specialty consultation: original articles. J Gen Intern Med 1990;5:95.
2. Eisenbach G. Medicine 2.0: Social networking, collaboration, participation, apomeditation, and openness. J Med Internet Res 2008;10(3):e22. *http://www.ncbi.nlm.nih.gov/pmc/articles/PMC2626430*; Accessed July 8, 2012.
3. Jones RB, Larizgoita I, Casado I, Barric T. Clinical audit: how effective is the referral chain for diabetic retinopathy? Diabet Med 1989;6:262.
4. Wilkin D, Metcalfe DH, Marinker M. The meaning of information on GP referral rates to hospitals. Community Med 1989;11:65.
5. Langley GR, Tritchler DL, Llewellyn-Thomas HA, Till JE. Use of written cases to study factors associated with regional variations in referral rates. J Clin Epidemiol 1991;44:391.
6. Jones NP, Lloyd IC, Kwartz J. General practitioner referrals to an eye hospital: a standard referral form. J R Soc Med 1990;83:770.
7. Westerman RF, Hull FM, Bezemer PD, Gort G. A study of communication between general practitioners and specialists: original papers. Br J Gen Pract 1990;40:445.
8. Eaglstein WH, Laszlo KS. Patient referrals to a dermatologist: the referring physician's perspective. Arch Dermatol 1996;132:292.
9. Bienia R, Heuser G, Bienia B. Consultation patterns in an urban hospital setting. Va Med 1989;116:371.
10. Gomez AG, Grimm CT, Yee EF, Skootsky SA. Preparing residents for managed care practice using an experienced-based curriculum. Acad Med 1997;72:959.
11. Roland MO, Green CA, Roberts SOB. Should general practitioners refer more patients to hospitals? J R Soc Med 1991;84:403.
12. Sutherland LR, Verhoef M. Patients who seek a second opinion: are they different from the typical referral? J Clin Gastroenterol 1989;11:308.
13. Berlin EA, Fowkes WC. Teaching framework for cross-cultural care: application in the family. West J Med 1983;139:934.

The resources for this chapter can be found at www.expertconsult.com.

SECTION IV

PATIENT CARE

CHAPTER 19

HEALTH PROMOTION, DISEASE PREVENTION, AND PATIENT EDUCATION

Walter A. Eisenhauer • Anna Mae Smith

CHAPTER CONTENTS

Historically, a disease-centered, provider-driven model of health care delivery has been pervasive in the United States. Medical education models and health care delivery systems have developed around disease treatment and chronic disease management rather than individual health and the prevention of disease. The United States spends a larger proportion of its gross domestic product annually on health care than any other nation, at 16% annually compared with 8% to 10% in most major industrialized countries.[1] Analysis of global health systems by the World Health Organization ranks the U.S. health care delivery system 37th out of 191. The ranking was based on equity of distribution, preventable deaths, and utilization of existing health resources.[2] Expenditures of health care resources in the United States are predominantly directed at the treatment of late-stage disease. Treatment of end-stage disease in the last year of life accounts for 30% of all Medicare expenditures, and approximately 40% of these expenditures are consumed in the last 30 days of life. Logically, health-promotion and disease-prevention activities have the potential to decrease the individual and societal burden of suffering from acute and chronic diseases and can effectively decrease the overall cost of health care delivery.[3]

So many of our health problems can be avoided through diet, exercise, and making sure we take care of ourselves. By promoting healthy lifestyles, we can improve the quality of life for all Americans and reduce health care costs dramatically.

Tommy G. Thompson, Secretary, DHHS

During the past 2 decades, awareness of the importance of public health measures, health promotion, and disease prevention have been illuminated through evidence-based research and have demonstrated both the economic and noneconomic value of seeking the root cause of, and prevention of, disease. This chapter provides an approach for physician assistant (PA) students and practicing PAs to address health-promotion and disease-prevention (HPDP) strategies within their respective practices. The generalist curriculum and underlying philosophy, found in most PA educational programs, is well suited to provide PAs entering the medical workforce with a foundation in HPDP. PAs in all health care settings should take every opportunity to evaluate a patient's HPDP status and implement interventions wherever possible, thereby avoiding lost opportunities to improve the quality and quantity of health.

Practicing PAs must take into consideration the entire spectrum of factors that are known to influence health outcomes. The health model outlined by Dahlgren and Whitehead (Figure 19-1) provides a snapshot of the multitude of factors that influence health. Traditionally in the United States, HPDP interventions have been implemented only from within the clinical setting. Community health care models that attempt to implement HPDP efforts by drawing on community resources, as well as leaders known to be influential within their communities, have proved to significantly improve outcomes over those that are implemented by the traditional health care system. Community leaders tend to have a greater appreciation for the nonbiologic factors that influence health. Strategies to improve health behaviors must be implemented in the home, schools, places of employment, places of worship, and other social settings where individuals actively participate in their communities.

Health promotion is defined as "any combination of educational, organizational, economic, and environmental supports for behavior and conditions of living conducive to health."[4] Disease prevention encompasses primary, secondary, and tertiary prevention. Primary prevention attempts to remove or modify the risk factors or causes of disease in patients, thus preventing the disease process from occurring in the first place. Encouraging use of bicycle safety helmets, water fluoridation, and recommending immunizations are considered primary preventive measures. Secondary prevention detects a condition in its earliest stage while it is still asymptomatic and provides an opportunity to intervene to cure or stop the progression of that condition. This may involve the regular use of Pap smears and mammograms, as well as prescribing beta-blockers to prevent a second myocardial infarction. Tertiary prevention is aimed at the treatment of an existing symptomatic disease or condition to prevent complications. The goal of tertiary prevention is to limit disability/morbidity or prevent premature death and/or to rehabilitate the patient. Examples of tertiary prevention would include control of asthma or diabetes mellitus, physical therapy following a stroke, or postmyocardial infarction cardiac rehabilitation. Frame[5] has extensively evaluated preventive measures aimed at infectious disease, atherosclerotic disease, cancer, metabolic diseases, and behavioral conditions and deemed interventions useful if they meet the following conditions:

- The disease or condition has a significant impact on the quality or quantity of life.
- Acceptable methods of treatment must be available.
- The disease or condition must have an asymptomatic period during which detection and treatment significantly reduces morbidity and mortality.

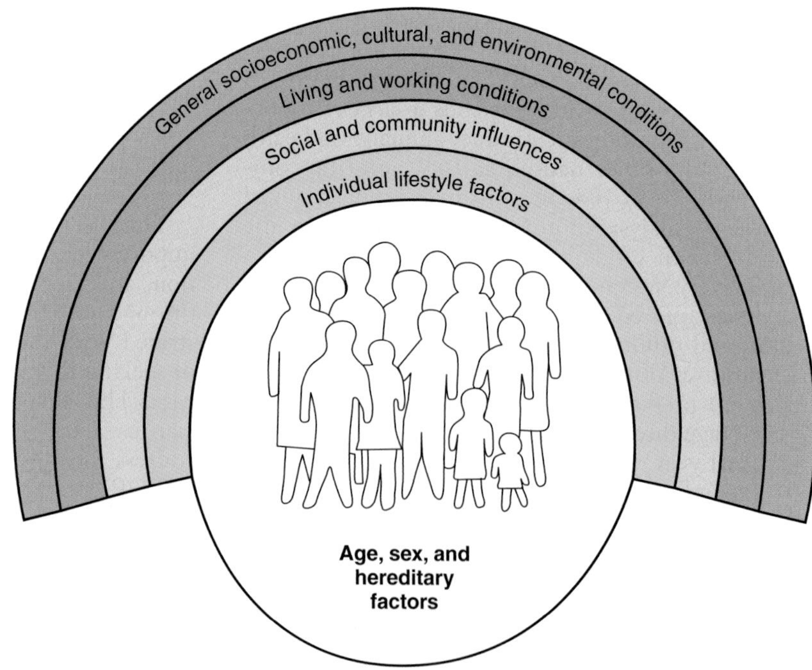

FIGURE 19-1 (From Dahlgren G, Whitehead M. Policies and strategies to promote social equity in health. Stockholm: Institute of Futures Studies, 1991. Retrieved from *http://www.planningcouncil.org/PDF/LIHF_Milw_CAP_final_w_cover.pdf*)

- Treatment in the asymptomatic phase must yield a therapeutic result superior to that obtained by delaying treatment until symptoms appear.
- Tests that are acceptable to patients must be available at a reasonable cost to detect the condition during the asymptomatic period.
- The incidence of the condition must be significant enough to justify the cost of screening.[5]

Most clinicians suffer from information overload when they attempt to grapple with the myriad of recommendations made by various health care entities. At any given time, recommendations from various physician specialty groups and nonprofit organizations may be in conflict due to biases that exist within these organizations. The U.S. Preventive Services Task Force (USPSTF) is an independent panel of experts in primary care and prevention that systematically reviews the available evidence and develops recommendations for clinical preventive services. The scientific basis for each recommendation is evaluated in the following areas: "burden of suffering" (incidence, prevalence, morbidity, and mortality); "efficacy of screening tests" (sensitivity, specificity, predictive value, and reproducibility); and "effectiveness of early detection" (availability of "clinical interventions that can prevent or delay the disorder"). The work of the task force is ongoing and considered to be the gold standard for recommendations regarding screening and preventive services. Opinions afforded by the panel are free from bias and represent scientific and evidence-based opinion regarding available screening and preventive services. Task Force recommendations are categorized into the five classifications identified in Table 19-1. PAs should routinely do the following:

- Discuss services with **"A" and "B" recommendations** with eligible patients and offer them as a priority.
- Discourage the use of services with **"D" recommendations** unless there are unusual additional considerations.
- Give lower priority to services with **"C" recommendations;** they need not be provided unless there are individual considerations in favor of providing the service.
- For services with **"I" recommendations,** carefully read the Clinical Considerations section for guidance and help patients understand the uncertainty surrounding these services.

A listing of selective recommendations is available in Table 19-2.

HISTORY AND PHYSICAL EXAMINATION

The role of genetic and environmental factors on a patient's risk for disease is increasingly being understood through the work of the Human Genome Project. PAs should routinely include a family pedigree in their patient history to establish risk for genetically acquired diseases. Identification of an increased genetic risk for disease may necessitate a change in prevention strategies to minimize the likelihood of partial or full genetic expression of the disease

TABLE 19-1 **USPSTF Recommendations and Ratings**

The USPSTF grades its recommendations according to one of five classifications (A, B, C, D, or I) reflecting the strength of evidence and magnitude of net benefit (benefits minus harms).

A	The USPSTF strongly recommends that clinicians routinely provide [the service] to eligible patients. The USPSTF found good evidence that [the service] improves important health outcomes and concludes that benefits substantially outweigh harms.
B	The USPSTF recommends that clinicians routinely provide [the service] to eligible patients. The USPSTF found at least fair evidence that [the service] improves important health outcomes and concludes that benefits outweigh harms.
C	The USPSTF makes no recommendation for or against routine provision of [the service]. The USPSTF found at least fair evidence that [the service] can improve health outcomes but concludes that the balance of benefits and harms is too close to justify a general recommendation.
D	The USPSTF recommends against routinely providing [the service] to asymptomatic patients. The USPSTF found at least fair evidence that [the service] is ineffective or that harms outweigh benefits.
I	The USPSTF concludes that the evidence is insufficient to recommend for or against routinely providing [the service]. Evidence that [the service] is effective is lacking, of poor quality, or conflicting, and the balance of benefits and harms cannot be determined.

USPSTF, U.S. Preventive Services Task Force.

TABLE 19-2 **Selected Recommendations from the USPSTF***

Intervention	Recommendation	USPSTF Category
Aspirin chemoprophylaxis	Discuss daily aspirin use with men 40+, women 50+, and others at increased risk for heart disease for the prevention of cardiovascular events	A
Tobacco use screening and brief intervention	Screen adults for tobacco use, provide brief counseling, and offer pharmacotherapy	A
Colorectal cancer screening	Screen adults 50+ routinely with FOBT, sigmoidoscopy, or colonoscopy	A
Hypertension screening	Measure blood pressure routinely in all adults and treat with antihypertensive medication to prevent the incidence of cardiovascular disease	A
Problem drinking screening and brief counseling	Screen adults routinely to identify those whose alcohol use places them at increased risk and provide brief counseling with follow-up	B
Vision screening—adults	Screen adults aged 65+ routinely for diminished visual acuity with the Snellen visual acuity chart	B
Cervical cancer screening	Screen women who have been sexually active and have a cervix, within 3 yr of onset of sexual activity, or age 21 routinely with cervical cytology (Pap smears)	A
Cholesterol screening	Screen routinely for lipid disorders among men aged 35+ and women aged 45+ and treat with lipid-lowering drugs to prevent the incidence of cardiovascular disease	A
Breast cancer screening	Recommends screening mammography, with or without clinical breast examination (CBE), every 1-2 yr for women aged 40+	B
Chlamydia screening	Screen sexually active women younger than age 25 routinely	B

*A full listing of current recommendations is available at *http://www.ahrq.gov/clinic/uspstfix.htm#Recommendations%20recommendations.*

FOBT, fecal occult blood test; USPSTF, U.S. Preventive Services Task Force.

in question. A thorough preconception history is likewise essential to tailor prevention strategies at decreasing poor birth outcomes including preterm and low-birth-weight deliveries.

In the early 1900s, life insurance companies implemented the "screening" physical examination as a standard practice to establish the presence of risk factors for disease. Current evidence has recently questioned the value of the complete screening physical examination in terms of time spent and cost to the patient. It is imperative that the PA clearly understands the difference between a comprehensive screening history and physical in the asymptomatic patient and the need for a comprehensive physical examination in the patient who presents with a new medical or surgical condition. Individuals presenting with new conditions obligate the PA to perform an exhaustive search for the etiology of the current medical problem, risk factors, or the presence of comorbid disease and to implement HPDP strategies that are appropriate for the patient's age and gender. Scheduled visits for screening examinations in asymptomatic individuals should be limited to those who have demonstrated clinical effectiveness in detecting diseases that are treatable or identifying risk factors that are modifiable. Examples of history and physical examination components that meet these criteria are body mass index determination, blood pressure measurement, tobacco and alcohol screening, and brief intervention.

IMMUNIZATIONS

Immunoprophylaxis has been demonstrated to be a highly efficacious strategy in the primary prevention of disease. The Advisory Committee on Immunization Practices (ACIP) of the Centers for Disease Control and Prevention (CDC) meets biannually to consider updates and new recommendations to practice. The implementation of a vaccine preventing *Haemophilus influenzae* type B infection has dramatically decreased the incidence of this once life-threatening infection. Recent advances in vaccine development, such as conjugation, have significantly improved the efficacy rates of vaccines against *Streptococcus pneumoniae* and *Neisseria meningitidis* by improving the human immune response to the polysaccharide coating of these organisms. Routine immunization against influenza and *S. pneumoniae* are recommended for high-risk groups including children, adults older than age 65, and those with chronic disease. The most recent ACIP recommendations include routine childhood immunization against hepatitis A and result from a three-stage effort to decrease the burden of hepatitis A in the United States. Stages 1 and 2 were directed at immunizing high-risk individuals and decreasing the burden of disease in endemic regions of the United States. Similarly, in 2008, the CDC pursued an effort to recommend that all individuals be immunized against meningococcal disease. The first vaccine (quadrivalent human papillomavirus [types 6, 11, 16, 18] recombinant vaccine) with the potential to prevent the majority of cases of cervical cancer is now available and recommended for females beginning at age 9. Recent outbreaks of *Bordetella pertussis* infections among adolescents and young adults in the United States, coupled with the availability of acellular pertussis vaccine, have prompted the recommendation for a single acellular pertussis booster for individuals between the ages of 11 and 65. This booster should be routinely incorporated with tetanus/diphtheria boosters that are required every 10 years. Guidelines for immunization of children have been established by ACIP and endorsed by the American Academy of Pediatrics. A summary of current childhood and adult recommendations is provided in Tables 19-3 and 19-4.

TABLE 19-3 **ACIP Childhood Immunization Schedule 2011**

Age	Vaccine
Birth	Initiate hepatitis B series
2 mo	Initiate tetanus, diphtheria, acellular pertussis, HIB, pneumococcal, inactivated polio, and rotavirus vaccine series
4 mo	Tetanus, diphtheria, acellular pertussis, HIB, pneumococcal, inactivated polio, and rotavirus vaccine series
6 mo	Tetanus, diphtheria, acellular pertussis, HIB, pneumococcal, inactivated polio, and rotavirus vaccine series; influenza annually
12 mo	MMR, varicella, hepatitis A

From Centers for Disease Control website. Recommended immunization schedule for persons age 0 through 6 years—United States, 2011. *http://www.cdc.gov/vaccines/recs/schedules/downloads/child/0-6yrs-schedule-pr.pdf.* Accessed October 17, 2011.

HIB, *Haemophilus influenzae* type B; MMR, measles, mumps, and rubella.

BARRIERS TO IMPLEMENTATION

Successful implementation of any health promotion requires that the PA considers a multitude of barriers. Frequently, providers view the implementation of behavior modification strategies and preventive services as futile and therefore expend minimal effort implementing them into practice. The section of this chapter dedicated to patient education discusses the importance of understanding stages of change and motivational interviewing as effective strategies resulting in behavioral change. PAs must convey a positive attitude toward a patient's ability to implement behavioral change and serve as a champion for the patient's efforts to implement these changes. Time and monetary costs are often dependent on the practice setting and the patient's insurance coverage. Language and cultural issues increasingly require providers to develop an understanding of cultural attitudes toward health and implementing strategies aimed at improving compliance with required lifestyle modifications. PAs in all settings should incorporate HPDP strategies into their practice routines. The use of tools to easily identify HPDP interventions is valuable and serves as a reminder of required services and educational interventions. Continuity of logging information must exist to ensure that all routinely scheduled interventions are conducted and reinforced. Computerized logging systems or paper flow sheets in medical records serve as a valuable tool

TABLE 19-4 **ACIP Adult Immunization Schedule, 2011**

	16-49	50-59	>60
All persons	Td q 10 yr (substitute 1 dose Tdap for Td), MMR (or 2 doses), varicella (2 doses), HPV	Td q 10 yr (substitute 1 dose Tdap for Td), influenza annually	Td q 10 yr (substitute 1 dose Tdap for Td), influenza vaccine, pneumococcal vaccine, zoster
Recommended if some other risk factor present	Pneumococcal vaccine (1-2 doses), influenza vaccine annually, hepatitis A, hepatitis B meningococcal vaccine	Pneumococcal vaccine (1-2 doses), influenza vaccine annually, hepatitis A, hepatitis B meningococcal vaccine	Hepatitis A, hepatitis B meningococcal vaccine

From Centers for Disease Control and Prevention website. Recommended adult immunization schedule—United States, 2011. *http://www.cdc.gov/vaccines/recs/schedules/downloads/adult/mmwr-adult-schedule.pdf.* Accessed October 17, 2011.

ACIP, Advisory Committee on Immunization Practices; HPV, human papillomavirus; Td, tetanus diphtheria toxoid; Tdap, tetanus, diphtheria, pertussis.

to remind clinicians and ensure documentation of routine HPDP practices.

PATIENT EDUCATION AND COUNSELING

One of the most common challenges faced by PAs is encouraging patients to change their behavior to improve their health. Every patient has the capacity to change behavior that will lead to a positive health outcome. PAs must be able to transcend cultural differences, educational level, social and occupational influence, as well as attitudes and beliefs, to effect a change in behavior. One must have empathy, be genuine and respectful, and develop mutual trust to have a positive impact on behavioral change.

Several behavioral change models that are currently in use have proved highly successful. They start with interviewing skills that allow a relationship to develop between the patient and the provider. Motivational interviewing (MI), first introduced by William Miller and Stephen Rollnick in the early 1990s, is a brief, nonconfrontational way of developing a safe and supportive rapport with a patient to facilitate thinking about behavior and ways to make changes. Choice is a critical aspect of motivational interviewing, and a patient must take ownership for the decision and responsibility for behavior and change. The PA must be able to assess the patient's readiness for change.

One method for assessing readiness to change is based on Prochaska's Transtheoretical Model, which integrates a patient's readiness to effect change by understanding the cycle/continuum of behavioral modification. PAs can facilitate a patient's self-change rather than treating to effect change. The patient enters the cycle at the precontemplation stage and goes on to contemplation, preparation, action, maintenance, and termination. These six stages suggest a temporal relationship between desire to change a behavior and actual change. Precontemplation stage relates to ambivalence in which advice and assistance is generally futile in regard to behavior change, but the opportunity to provide information and raise awareness must not be ignored. An example of this is the alcohol abuser who does not see that drinking a bottle of wine every evening is a problem because he is able to perform his daily job. An additional tool that may be helpful at this stage is seen in Table 19-5, the Readiness to Change Ruler.[6]

The contemplative stage may come and go quickly. PAs may get a glimpse into the problem while the patient is being seen for a totally unrelated complaint. For example, a patient may visit the office with a respiratory complaint, and tobacco abuse increases the severity of the symptoms. Once the patient identifies the problem and takes responsibility for change, the PA must use motivational interviewing techniques that enable the patient, as the agent of change, to understand the problem and offer individual solutions. The patient's inner resources may be revealed by reflective listening through empathy, legitimizing feelings, respect, support, optimism, and partnership.

The action stage of behavioral changes involves resisting temptation by avoiding triggers, remaining realistic, and remembering the prize. PAs can help the patient develop an action plan by providing encouragement, maintaining focus on goals, circumnavigating roadblocks, and using tools such as daily logs and behavioral contracts.

The maintenance stage encourages frequent follow-up and follow-through by the patient and the provider. This stage also involves setbacks and relapses. Tools that can be used to combat these behaviors include talking back to negative urges and thoughts, coping with pressures from others to engage in negative behaviors, and, most importantly, focus on lifestyle enhancement. Once the behavior becomes learned and automatic, the cycle can be terminated.

CASE STUDY 19-1

Almeda is a 49-year-old paralegal who has been smoking one pack per day for the past 30 years. She knows that she should quit and has made a few unsuccessful attempts. She has come into the office for her yearly mammogram and Pap smear. This visit is the perfect time to assess Almeda's readiness for change by using motivational interviewing techniques. The PA can help her by discussing behaviors and ways to alter long-standing habits, as well as exploring ways to decrease potential resistance to change. By setting realistic goals and with close follow-up via telephone calls, e-mails, and office visits, Almeda may reach her goal and her new behavior is learned. These visits are also a great opportunity to educate, deliver appropriate educational materials, and discuss screenings and tests that she should undertake to ensure a healthy lifestyle.

PAs are becoming more involved with patient education. As such, PAs need to be able to deliver educational materials that allow the best comprehension, and therefore compliance, for the greatest number of

TABLE 19-5 Changing Your Health[6]

1. On the line below, mark where you are now on this line that measures change in behavior. Are you not prepared to change, already changing, or someplace in the middle?

   0 1 2 3 4 5 6 7 0 9 10

   Not prepared to change ... Already changing

2. Answer the questions below that apply to you.
   - If your mark is on the left side of the line:
     How will you know when it is time to think about changing?
     What signals will tell you to start thinking about changing?
     What qualities in yourself are important to you?
     What connection is there between those qualities and "not considering a change"?
   - If your mark is somewhere in the middle:
     Why did you put your mark there and not farther to the left?
     What might make you put your mark a little farther to the right?
     What are the good things about the way you are currently trying to change?
     What are the not-so-good things?
     What would be the good result of changing?
     What are the barriers to changing?
   - If your mark is on the right side of the line:
     Pick one of the barriers to change and list some things that could help you overcome this barrier.
     Pick one of those things that could help and decide to do it by ____________________ (write in a specific date).
   - If you have taken a serious step in making a change:
     What made you decide on that particular step?
     What has worked in taking this step?
     What helped it work?
     What could help it work even better?
     What else would help?
     Can you break that helpful step down into smaller pieces?
     Pick one of those pieces and decide to do it by ____________________ (write in a specific date).
   - If you are changing and trying to maintain that change:
     Congratulations! What is helping you?
     What else would help?
     What are your high-risk situations?
   - If you have "fallen off the wagon":
     What worked for a while?
     Do not kick yourself—long-term change almost always takes a few cycles.
     What did you learn from the experience that will help you when you give it another try?

3. The following are stages people go through in making important changes in their health behaviors. All the stages are important. We learn from each stage. We go from "not thinking about it" to "weighing the pros and cons" to "making little changes and figuring out how to deal with the real hard parts" to "doing it!" to "making it part of our lives."
   Many people "fall off the wagon" and go through all the stages several times before the change really lasts.

The Readiness to Change Ruler can be used with patients contemplating any desirable behavior, such as smoking cessation, losing weight, exercise, or substance-abuse cessation.

patients. The average reading level is at the eighth- to ninth-grade reading level. One out of five patients reads at the fifth-grade level or below. Adults and children read at or slightly below the greatest educational grade obtained. Adults with limited literacy are less likely to use screening procedures, keep medical appointments, follow treatment plans, or seek help at earlier stages of disease. Patient education materials should aim for the sixth-grade reading level.

CONCLUSION

HPDP and effective patient education are essential components of practice for PAs in all settings. Providers should perceive all interactions with patients as potential opportunities to implement positive behavioral change of unhealthy behaviors. Starting with a meticulous history and physical examination that identify an individual's risk or evidence of preventable disease, PAs should develop a strategy to implement all recommended interventions that are appropriate for the patient's age and gender. Behavioral modification and patient education should consider unique circumstances and the patient's readiness to adopt healthier lifestyles within a continuum of change. Motivational interviewing strategies should be implemented to improve behavioral change outcomes. Health-promotion and disease-prevention strategies should be directed at not only individual patients but also the community as a whole. Working with community groups and organizations to help provide a consistent message to the public on health promotion topics will provide reinforcement to the individual patient. Increasing exercise, appropriate diet, and smoking cessation along with immunizations, targeted screening histories, and examinations represent the mainstay of any successful health-promotion and disease-prevention effort.

CLINICAL APPLICATIONS

1. Using the U.S. Preventive Services Task Force information, look up the current recommendations for Health Maintenance for your age group.
2. Explore with your classmates the arguments used by individuals who choose to not immunize their children against life-threatening diseases. Consider how you might provide patient education concerning this issue with a parent.
3. Using Prochaska's Transtheoretical Model and his readiness to change process, develop a plan on how to effect change at each stage for someone who needs to increase physical activity in daily life.

KEY POINTS

- Students must develop an appreciation of the importance of HPDP in the care of all of their patients.
- Try to address at least one health promotion topic at each patient visit.
- Strive for primary prevention of disease, but there is also great benefit to be had with implementation of secondary and tertiary prevention as well.
- Developing a comfort level with a behavior change strategy will help you to provide your patients with opportunities to make difficult lifestyle modifications.

References

1. Zuckerman S, McFeeters J. Recent growth in health expenditures. The Commonwealth Fund (website). *http://www.commonwealthfund.org/Content/Publications/Fund-Reports/2006/Mar/Recent-Growth-in-Health-Expenditures.aspx*; Accessed July 17, 2011.
2. World Health Organization. The World Health Report (2000). Health systems: improving performance. *http://www.who.int/whr/2000/en/index.html*; Accessed July 17, 2011.
3. Woolfe SH, Jonas S, Lawrence RS. Health Promotion and Disease Prevention in Clinical Practice. Baltimore: Williams & Wilkins, 1996.
4. U.S. Preventive Services Task Force. Guide to clinical preventive services. *http://www.ahrq.gov/clinic/uspstfix.htm*; Accessed July 17, 2011.
5. Frame PS. A critical review of adult health maintenance (pts. 1-4). J Fam Pract 1986; 22:341, 417, 511. J Fam Pract 1986;23:29.
6. Zimmerman G, Olsen C, Bosworth M. A 'stages of change' approach to helping patients change behavior. Am Fam Physician 2000;61:1409.

The resources for this chapter can be found at www.expertconsult.com.

CHAPTER 20

Family Medicine

Lawrence Herman

CHAPTER CONTENTS

PRIMARY CARE CONCEPTS

In defining primary care, it is first necessary to describe the nature of services provided to patients and then to identify the primary care providers. It may appear obvious that the nexus of primary care is the patient, but this description alone is inadequate. In no other specialty is the patient more centric. Although the field of primary care includes the primary care provider, definitions that focus on providers are incomplete without including a description of the primary care practice. The American Academy of Family Physicians (AAFP) enumerates five definitions relating to primary care, all of which should be taken together (*http://www.aafp.org/online/en/home/policy/policies/p/primarycare.html*; accessed April 24, 2012). These describe the care provided to the patient, the framework of providing such care, the types of providers whose role in the system is to provide primary care, and the role of others in providing such care. Throughout each definition are woven the schemata within which patients will be the focus of and have access to efficient, effective, high-quality primary care services.

Undifferentiated Patient

Primary care is care provided by those trained for and skilled in comprehensive first contact and continuing care for persons with any undiagnosed sign, symptom, or health concern (the "undifferentiated" patient) and without limitation by problem origin (biologic, behavioral, or social), organ system, or diagnosis. This includes but is not limited to health promotion, disease prevention, health maintenance, counseling, patient education, diagnosis, and treatment of acute and chronic illnesses in a variety of health care settings (e.g., office, inpatient, critical care, long-term care, home care, day care). Primary care is performed and managed by a physician, physician assistant (PA), or nurse practitioner (NP) in collaboration with other health professionals, using consultation or referral when and as appropriate. Furthermore, primary care provides patient advocacy in the health care system to accomplish cost-effective care by coordination of health care services. Primary care promotes effective communication with patients throughout the entire health care team and encourages the role of the patient as a partner in his or her own health care.

Accessible Portal of Entry

A primary care practice serves not only as the patient's first portal of entry into the health care system but also as the continuing, ongoing, and coordinated focal point for all needed health care services. Primary care practices are organized to meet the needs of patients with undifferentiated problems, with the vast majority of patient concerns and needs being cared for in the primary care practice itself, or at the least initiation of care and stabilization followed by appropriate referral and subsequent follow-up care. Primary care practices are located and oriented to the local community and facilitate ready access to providers with time-sensitive and disease-specific orientation while maintaining availability of specialty consultation when needed. As mentioned previously, primary care practices provide health promotion, disease prevention, health maintenance, counseling, patient education, diagnosis, and treatment of acute and chronic illnesses in a variety of health care settings (e.g., office, inpatient, critical care, long-term care, home care, day care).

The structure of the primary care practice commonly includes a team of physicians and nonphysician health professionals.

Approximately one in four of all office visits, or 240 million office visits each year, are made to family practitioners. This is nearly 87 million more than the next largest medical specialty. In today's increasingly complicated medical arena, family practitioners provide more care for America's underserved and rural populations than any other medical specialty. Family medicine's cornerstone is an ongoing, personal patient-practitioner relationship focused on patient-centered integrated care (*http://www.aafp.org/online/en/home/media/releases/2012/student-interest-in-family-medicine-improves.html*; accessed April 24, 2012).

Primary Care Provider

A primary care provider is a generalist physician, PA, or NP who provides definitive care to the undifferentiated patient at the point of first contact and takes continuing and ongoing responsibility for both providing and, perhaps most importantly, coordinating the patient's care. Such a provider is trained to provide primary care services. The style of primary care practice is such that the personal primary care provider serves as the entry point for and coordinates the care for substantially all of the patient's medical and health care needs—not limited by problem origin, organ system, or diagnosis. The primary care practice should also act as a single, complete, and coordinated repository of all medical records. Primary care providers are advocates for the patient in coordinat ing the use of the entire health care system to optimize the health of the patient. They may see patients in the office hospital, nursing home, or patients' homes (Table 20-1). The typical family practitioner sees nearly 100 patients weekly, but this varies widely depending on geographic location and demand.

Non–Primary Care Providers of Primary Care Services

Providers who are not trained in the primary care specialties of family medicine, general internal medicine, women's health, or general pediatrics may also provide patient care services that are typically

TABLE 20-1 **Profile of Average Weekly Family Physician Patient Visits (April 2011)**

Setting	Average per Week
Office visits	89
Hospital visits	7
Nursing home visits	2
House calls	1
Total visits	99

From American Academy of Family Physicians website, April 2011. *http://www.aafp.org/online/en/home/aboutus/specialty/facts/12.html*; accessed April 24, 2012.

delivered by primary care clinicians. These providers may provide *episodic* care focusing on specific patient care needs related to prevention, health maintenance, acute care, chronic care, or rehabilitation, but they usually do not offer these services within the context of comprehensive, ongoing, and continuing care, nor is there a focus on coordination of care. The contributions of providers who deliver some services traditionally found within the scope of primary care practice may be important to specific patient needs. Regardless, the core concept of a single point of coordination of care requires that these individuals work in close consultation with trained primary care providers.

Nonphysician Primary Care Providers

Clearly, there are increasing numbers of providers of health care other than physicians who render some primary care services. Important to our discussion here, physician assistants (PAs) provide a significant proportion of primary care in the United States. According to the American Academy of Physician Assistants (AAPA), approximately 32% of practicing PAs list primary care as their primary practice specialty (*http://www.aapa.org/the_pa_profession/quick_facts/resources/item.aspx?id=3849;* accessed April 24, 2012). This is exclusive of PAs identifying themselves as practicing internal medicine, pediatrics, and women's health, all of which can also be considered primary care specialties. As always, medicine requires a team approach. Regardless of who provides the service, if it is provided by a consultant or the patient's primary care provider, if it is ongoing or episodic, these services should be provided in collaboration in which the ultimate responsibility for the patient resides with that primary care team.

CONGRUENCE OF FAMILY PRACTICE AND INTERNAL MEDICINE

Family practitioners are trained as generalists, and family practice is the medical field in which clinicians treat a broad spectrum of medical problems. Historically this has run the gamut of patient ages from pediatrics to geriatrics and has also included gynecology and, with decreasing frequency over time, obstetrics. In contrast, general internal medicine practices include a broad spectrum of medical problems, but internal medicine does not include pediatrics, obstetrics, or gynecology, nor does it include orthopedics or minor surgical procedures that are often performed by family practitioners. In general, internal medicine tends to be a more narrowed focus, not uncommonly with a specialization varying according to the breadth of knowledge, training, and interest of the practitioner. Yet in spite of the clear differences, both family medicine and internal medicine are considered primary care disciplines.

The training of family practitioners is especially broad, whereas training in internal medicine is more focused on in-depth adult medicine, frequently with specialization. Family practitioners may also treat minor orthopedic injuries and provide wound care and suture uncomplicated lacerations; internal medicine practices rarely provide those services. Both disciplines emphasize lifetime continuity of care, with health promotion and disease prevention, and strong attention to psychosocial issues. Both primarily treat outpatients in an ambulatory care setting but also treat inpatients. According to the American Academy of Physician Assistants (AAPA), 32% of practicing PAs identify primary care as their primary practice specialty and an additional 17% identify internal medicine (and internal medicine subspecialties) as their primary practice specialty (*http://www.aapa.org/the_pa_profession/quick_facts/resources/item.aspx?id=3849;* accessed April 24, 2012).

PRIMARY CARE INCOMES

Family physician income—and as a corollary family practice, PA income—is highly dependent on region, practice setting, and the number and mix of patients seen. According to AAFP, mean and median incomes for family practice physicians in metropolitan areas are $172,200 and $156,000, respectively, and for nonmetropolitan areas are $189,700 and $178,000, respectively (*http://www.aafp.org/online/en/home/aboutus/specialty/facts/4.html;* accessed April 24, 2012). Income for primary care PAs varies on the basis of geography, specialty, and experience. Although the median annual income for a PA in 2010 practicing family practice with urgent care was $89,000, the median annual salary for a PA practicing general pediatrics was $80,000 during the same time period (Table 20-2). Similarly, in 2010 the median annual salary for a family medicine PA with less than 1 year of experience was between $64,000 and $90,000 with a median salary of $75,000, while that same PA with more than 20 years of experience earned between $70,000 and $120,000 with a median salary of $94,000 (Table 20-3). Median annual income for a family practice PA in Pennsylvania was reported as $71,000, whereas the family practice PA in Alaska reported a median annual income of $105,000. The family practitioner's adaptability and flexibility to tailor clinical services offered to patients can shape income, and there remains a large variability in terms of in-office procedures performed. Variability in services performed is considerable (Table 20-4). For example, family practitioners with more experience, those in more rural settings, those who do more sophisticated in-office procedures, those who see a higher volume of patients, and those who see patients in the hospital tend to have a higher income.

TABLE 20-2 Total Earning of PAs by Primary Care Specialty in the United States (2010)

Specialty	Median Annual Salary
Family Medicine	$84,000
Family Medicine with Urgent Care	$89,000
General Internal Medicine	$85,000
General Pediatrics	$80,000
Obstetrics/Gynecology	$82,000

From American Academy of Physician Assistants 2010 Annual Salary Survey.

EXPANDING CRISIS IN PRIMARY CARE AND FAMILY PRACTICE

Current reimbursements in primary care, and therefore family practice, make this one of the least profitable specialties. As such, salaries tend to be lower and this corresponds to an increasing difficulty in recruiting providers to primary care due to relatively depressed salaries. The AAPA reported that in 2010 the median annual salary for a primary care PA was $85,000, whereas a PA in emergency medicine had a median annual salary of $101,000 (Figure 20-1). Within what is considered traditional primary care disciplines, there is variability in median annual salaries, which in 2010 ran from a low of $80,000 in general pediatrics to a high of $89,000 in family practice with urgent care (Table 20-5). In fact, family practices across the country bear witness to this by the reality of lower salaries mandated by falling practice profitability over time. Although PA salary increases in general and specifically in family practice will likely be tempered, demand for family practice job PAs are

TABLE 20-3 Total Earning of PAs in Family Medicine by Years of Experience in the United States (2010)

Years of Experience	10th	25th	Median	75th	90th
<1	$64,000	$70,000	$75,000	$81,000	$90,000
1-4	$65,000	$71,400	$75,000	$85,200	$100,000
5-9	$67,000	$75,000	$85,000	$98,000	$110,000
10-14	$71,000	$80,000	$90,000	$105,000	$120,000
15-19	$72,000	$80,000	$90,000	$108,898	$130,000
≥20	$70,000	$80,555	$94,000	$105.000	$120,000

From American Academy of Physician Assistants 2010 Annual Salary Survey.

TABLE 20-4 Performance of Diagnostic Procedures in Family Physician Practices

Procedure	*Perform in Office*
Dermatologic procedures	87.3%
Tympanometry	39.3%
Circumcision	29.3%
Colposcopy	29.2%
Holter monitoring	23.9%
Physical therapy	13.6%
Loop electrosurgery (LEEP)	10.6%
Nasopharyngoscopy	6.7%
Laryngoscopy	6.6%
Botox	6.6%

From American Academy of Family Physicians, Practice Profile II Survey, April 2011. *http://www.aafp.org/online/en/home/aboutus/specialty/facts/12.html.* Accessed April 24, 2012.

predicted to continue to increase owing to the market forces associated with increasing cost containment, physicians electing to enter other specialties, and the dramatic increase in the number of insured Americans with the Affordable Care Act.

PARTNERSHIP BETWEEN FAMILY PHYSICIANS AND PAs

Family practice PAs work in teams with primary care physicians in a variety of settings, such as multispecialty clinics, private offices, county clinics, urgent care clinics, and hospitals. PAs may practice in a setting that is geographically removed from the physician. Currently, there are 10,022 family practice resident physicians in the 451 three-year family practice residency programs with fewer than 3300 residents entering the field annually for the foreseeable future, an inadequate number to treat our expanding

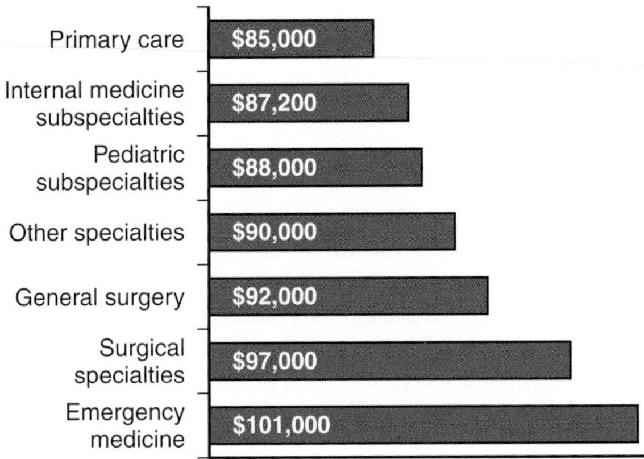

FIGURE 20-1 Total earning of PAs by selected specialty in the United States (2010). (From the American Academy of Physician Assistants website. *http:/www.aapa.org/research/data_and_statistics.aspx.* Accessed April 26, 2012.)

TABLE 20-5 Total Earning of PAs by Specialty in the United States (2010)

Specialty	Median Annual Salary
Family Medicine	$84,000
Family Medicine with Urgent Care	$89,000
General Internal Medicine	$85,000
General Pediatrics	$80,000
Obstetrics/Gynecology	$82,000

From American Academy of Physician Assistants 2010 Annual Salary Survey. *http:/www.aapa.org/research/data and statistics.aspx.* Accessed April 26, 2012.

and aging patient population (*http://www.aafp.org/online/en/home/aboutus/specialty/facts/4.html;* accessed April 24, 2012). PAs have been identified consistently as one solution to this gap between the numbers of patients needing treatment compared with those who have access to a primary care provider.

Significantly, in February 2012 the American Academy of Family Physicians (AAFP) and American Academy of Physician Assistants published a joint monograph including six specific policy statements regarding the interdependence of the two professional organizations and professions.[1] The AAFP-AAPA statement's joint policy positions follow:

1. AAFP and AAPA believe that family physicians and PAs working together in a team-oriented practice, such as the patient-centered medical home, is a proven model for delivering high-quality, cost-effective patient care. National and state legal, regulatory, and payment policies should recognize that PAs function as primary care providers in the patient-centered medical home as part of a multidisciplinary, physician-directed clinical team.
2. AAFP and AAPA encourage interprofessional education of medical students, family medicine residents, and PA students throughout their educational programs.
3. AAPA and AAFP encourage education programs of both professions to expand family medicine rotation sites for PA students, medical students, and residents.
4. AAPA and AAFP should continue to be represented on the accrediting and certifying bodies of the PA profession (ARC-PA and NCCPA, respectively).
5. AAFP and AAPA believe that national workforce policies should ensure adequate supplies of family physicians and PAs in family medicine to improve access to quality care and to avert anticipated shortages of primary care clinicians.
6. AAPA and AAFP promote flexibility in federal and state regulation so that each medical practice determines within a defined spectrum appropriate clinical roles within the medical team, physician-to-PA ratios, and supervision processes, enabling each clinician to work to the fullest extent of his or her education and expertise.

According to the statement, both organizations agree on this point: "The future of health care delivery will require inter-professional teams of health care professionals working together to provide patient-centered care. AAFP and AAPA are committed to building on the common ground that family physicians and PAs share in order to ensure an adequate, well-educated family medicine workforce to meet the health care needs of the U.S. population."

Not coincidentally, a similar joint policy monograph was published by AAPA and the American College of Physicians (ACP) at almost the same time detailing how PAs and physicians in internal medicine can and must work together in a nearly identical manner.[2]

HISTORY OF FAMILY PRACTICE

The roots of the family medicine and the family practitioner lie deep within the realm of what was previously known as the *general practitioner*, or simply GP. Until World War II, the realm of generalist medicine included general practitioners. Most of these GPs did not complete a residency, at least in part because there were relatively few graduates of what was then only a handful of general practice residency programs in existence. Regardless of whether they completed a residency, these general practitioners (physicians who took care of families) constituted the membership of the American Academy of General Practice (AAGP). Throughout the 1940s, the number of general practitioners fell steadily as the number of specialists grew, in part fueled by a technologic explosion in the United States. Supply and demand shifted, and in the late 1960s the need for well-trained generalists who could not only treat common medical problems in all age groups, including obstetrics, but also provide preventive care, led to a resurgence of generalists. In 1969, the specialty of family practice formally began with a radical restructuring of the old AAGP to form the AAFP. The AAFP implemented new standards for a 3-year residency, board certification, and recertification examinations and was the first physician specialty to do so. The end result was a fundamental redefinition of family practice to include emphasis on continuity of care, disease prevention, family dynamics, counseling, and psychology. Simultaneously, more medical schools began departments of family practice, inspiring students to enter family practice. During the 1970s, the number of family practice residency training programs in the United States exploded from 12 to more than 350. This expansion has slowed—and some say peaked—because in 2011 there were 451 family practice residencies. The 1970s were an era of social consciousness, and many students selected family practice as a way to make a contribution to society through medicine.

In the 1980s, the focus of medical training shifted and embraced specialization and the subspecialties. Driven by the powerful market force of reimbursement emphasizing payment for procedures, procedure-oriented specialists began earning many times more than family physicians. The specialists' increased earning potential lured many individuals to specialization and therefore away from primary care (family practice, general internal medicine, pediatrics, and obstetrics and gynecology) to specialties.

Family practitioners tend to be more cost-effective than subspecialists because they can treat medical problems in all age groups and in all organ systems without specialist referral and therefore remain an attractive group for hospitals, health systems, and health maintenance organizations (HMOs), who continue to use family practitioners extensively. This is, however, offset by the lower revenue that can be generated by specialists. In 2000, it was determined that approximately 25% of family practice physicians aided in routine obstetric deliveries, 28.7% managed their patients in intensive care, 48% managed patients in coronary care settings, and 36% performed minor surgery in the hospital. AAFP reports that in 2009, the most recent year for which data are available, it was determined that only 10% of family practice physicians aided in routine obstetric deliveries, 34.24% managed their patients in intensive care, only 28.7% managed patients in coronary care settings, and 34% performed minor surgery in the hospital (*http://www.aafp.org/online/en/home/aboutus/specialty/facts/17.html;* accessed April 24, 2012). The salary for family physicians in 2009, as reported in the last survey by the AAFP, indicated a mean of $173,300 annually with a range of $145,000 to $189,700 (*http://www.aafp.org/online/en/home/aboutus/specialty/facts/4.html;* accessed April 24, 2012). As is the case with most PAs, family practice PA salaries tend to parallel family practice salaries.

HISTORY OF INTERNAL MEDICINE

After the *Flexner Report* was published in 1910, medicine and its specialties evolved relatively rapidly into the system we know today. In 1932, the Commission on Medical Education advised: "A particular identification for those who profess to be specialists should be created." As a result, a number of specialty boards were incorporated between 1932 and 1940. Internal medicine became a board-certified specialty with the incorporation of the American Board of Internal Medicine (ABIM) in 1936. The move to specialize quickly found support, but not necessarily for the original reasons.[3]

Originally, internists considered virtually all of medicine (save for surgery, pediatrics, and obstetrics and gynecology) to be their domain. However, as various specialties and subspecialties formed their own boards, the focus of internal medicine narrowed considerably, and the raison d'être for board certification as a minimum standard shifted. Originally, the ABIM's purpose was to set high standards for the certification of a few internists who would be outstanding consultants ready to receive the referrals of general practice physicians. However, during and after World War II, the incentives (in terms of credentialing, finance, and prestige) for physicians to become board certified were considerable. Certification soon became the norm rather than the exception.

WHAT IS FAMILY PRACTICE?

Because family practitioners exclusively manage the lion's share of the problems they encounter, family practice demands a knowledge base that is arguably greater in breadth than any other specialty. The required broad knowledge base is focused on the most common diagnoses and management, rather than on the less common ones, the latter of which may require referral. But "jack of all trades, master of none" does disservice in describing the family practitioner, who is trained to diagnose and treat common problems thoroughly and to recognize an unusual or complex diagnosis at its undifferentiated stage.

Family practitioners perform focused and comprehensive histories and physical examinations, as well as treat chronic and acute illnesses and conditions in patients of all ages. Additionally, women are commonly seen for their general gynecologic problems, annual pelvic examinations, birth control, and prenatal care. Although some family physicians perform obstetric deliveries, malpractice costs have significantly reduced the number of family practitioners involved in obstetrics.

Going to core values of family practice, family practice treats the whole family and, as such, focuses on the patient holistically. Family practitioners may be as much concerned with patients' feelings, family lives, and jobs as they are with patients' presenting complaints or illnesses. The family practitioner is frequently perceived by the patient as a friend and confidante, and the family practitioner often counsels a patient for common problems associated with stresses of living. Some family physicians also counsel couples, perform crisis intervention, and manage acute psychiatric illnesses.

Because the family practitioners provide not simply a unique continuity of care but a continuity over the spectrum of a lifetime, the patient is able to see the *same* clinician on each visit. This unique continuum enables these practitioners to know their patients more completely and to develop a fundamental understanding of problems resulting in deeper and tightly coupled healing relationships. When a patient's problems are beyond the scope of the family practitioner, the patient may be referred to one or more subspecialists, and care is coordinated by the family practitioner.

Health care maintenance is not simply an important component of family practice; it remains essential to the core values. This includes immunizations and other preventive measures that are age and disease specific, including diet, exercise, and overall well-being. In some family practice settings, to remain financially viable, practices have moved away from the otherwise time-consuming counseling associated with handling stress that has been important to family practitioners.[4]

These core concepts, including, but not limited to, continuity of care and health care maintenance allow family practitioners to provide less costly health care to their patients. Advocating for and assisting with the implementation of healthy lifestyles and appropriate screening examinations are critical not only for preventing disease and maintaining optimal health of patients but also for discovering illness in its earliest stages, when it is both less costly to treat and likely to result in a better outcome. Continuity of care allows the practitioner to know the patient well and to follow the patient's lifestyle changes or chronic illnesses closely so that problems are less likely to develop in the first place, and if they do they tend to not spiral out of control and become more costly to manage.

WHAT DISTINGUISHES FAMILY PRACTICE FROM INTERNAL MEDICINE?

Internal medicine may best be defined by its focus of medical problems: The internal medicine practitioner's approach is similar to the approach of the family practitioner except that the focus is exclusively on adult medicine and specifically excludes surgery. Furthermore, internal medicine may not incorporate all areas of psychosocial medicine. As a result, each step along the way may allow those practicing internal medicine to be more focused and narrow. Not dissimilar to the family practitioner, the internist's method is to work with a differential diagnosis that begins with the chief complaint and enlarges to account for the various details of the history. Also, similar to family practice, the internist's physical examination narrows the differential and usually helps to stratify the differential. Diagnostic laboratory and radiology further narrow the logical choices. With the most complex problems, internal medicine may "drill down" deeper to address disease cause and treatments rather than refer out.

In large measure, the attitudes and methods of internal medicine were created by the "fathers"of medicine, such as William Osler. Many of the "pearls" (e.g., Osler's nodes) now associated with particular diseases were originally "found" in the careful observations by these physicians. Some would argue that internists are more methodical to reach a diagnosis and are more given to deliberation over the details of the case.

PAs EMPLOYED IN FAMILY PRACTICE AND INTERNAL MEDICINE

Historical Perspectives

The PA profession began in the United States in 1965, when it was perceived that most of the population had access to care save for the disenfranchised: the old, the poor, and both the rural and inner city populations. The priority for improvement in health care was for the patients who frankly lacked access to care at all levels. The number of physicians in primary care was simply inadequate to accommodate all the patients, and as a result barriers to care developed. One national strategy was to increase the number of medical students, but that addressed only part of the problem, inasmuch as many of these medical students graduated and were attracted away from primary care due to higher specialist reimbursement rates.

The PA profession was started in response to this need for access to medical care in underserved areas. All early graduates were trained in primary care, and most worked in primary care practices upon graduation. These early graduates practiced in rural clinics, public health clinics, institutions, prisons, and general and family medicine practices in small communities.[5]

Demographic Changes of Recent PA Graduates

It would be unreasonable to view characteristics of recent PA graduates in a vacuum. These characteristics can be identified, but when making workforce assessments they must be viewed within the global context of all primary care providers, including physicians and NPs, due to complex market forces that affect these characteristics as a group. Any aggregate data for PAs in general must be further scrutinized because of the disproportionate number of new graduates affecting aggregate data. It is important to note that new graduates in the past 7 years represent half of the PA profession, and as has been the case each decade since inception of the profession, the ranks of the profession are expected to continue to double in number each decade for the foreseeable future. Additionally, the profession is now 61% female and that number is increasing dramatically with each graduating class. As a result, the proportion of younger and newer PAs, as well as gender shifts, may dramatically affect the workforce dynamics associated with specialty choice.

Since 1985, practicing PAs in primary care have declined steadily. This is attributed to many forces, but the market forces of reimbursement for primary care drive both physician salaries and PA salaries and result in changes in levels of attractiveness for each of the specialties. Trends in primary care specialty selection of recent graduates loosely parallel the same downward trend for family practice and the same increase in internal medicine, but not nearly as dramatically. Nevertheless, it can be said that both experienced PAs and new graduates are choosing primary care with less and less frequency.

Challenges and Rewards in Family Practice

Like physicians in family practice, PAs in family practice often have their own panel of patients who regularly return to them each time they are seen for a medical problem. As is the case with any clinician, this affords the patient continuity of care. It also allows the PA the greatest opportunity to know the patient and understand the psychosocial impact of that patient's health. PAs also treat patients in the context of the family, often treating the children, the parents, and the grandparents in the same family. The opportunity to observe individuals and families as they develop, change, and grow is one of the greatest rewards unique to family practice. Also, identification of stressors in one family member that affect other family members provides insight into the forces contributing to health or illness of the individual. For the clinician, having such a comprehensive picture of the patient is essential in that it removes much of the mystery in discovering the cause of the individual's disease; at the same time, it is also rewarding.

Because PAs in family practice treat patients in all age groups, of both sexes, and regarding all organ systems, their care can be comprehensive. The focus on health maintenance and disease prevention has been shown to make major contributions to the patient's health.

PAs can manage 80% to 90% of the outpatients seen in a family practice, and just as a physician would seek out a consultant when presented with a particularly complicated case, PAs usually consult their physician colleague if confronted with an unfamiliar problem. PAs in family practice are intimately involved in the team approach to medicine as they work with psychologists; social workers; teachers; medical and surgical specialists; nutritionists; occupational, speech, and physical therapists; and clergy.

Some PAs are involved in the ongoing care of hospitalized patients, and many are the major communication link between patients and their families. They may make rounds, write orders on patients, and review cases on a daily basis with the physician. When the patient is ready for discharge, the PA is commonly involved in discharge planning.

The challenge of working in family practice is its breadth. Family practitioners truly need to know something about everything across the entire spectrum of medicine. Knowing the standard of care requires that the family practitioner knows the evidence and is aware of the latest guidelines in an extensive range of disease states and then incorporates those guidelines into routine care on a daily basis. Maintaining such a large database of patients and a repository of knowledge of disparate guidelines requires significant multitasking skills and constant discipline. Family practice PAs must also acknowledge their limitations and request guidance whenever appropriate.

The case histories that follow provide examples of a typical day for a PA working in family practice. The cases chosen would be treated in family practice and probably would not be treated in internal medicine. If these cases were treated by a subspecialist, health care maintenance and other age-specific patient education might not necessarily be discussed.

CASE STUDY 20-1

MP, a 35-year-old Caucasian woman, presents to your office with pain when she urinates, worsening over 3 days. She is a single mother of two children ages 3 and 9. She admits to having multiple sexual partners. She has not used any form of birth control since undergoing tubal ligation after the birth of her last child. She is not sure when her last menstrual period was because her menses have always been irregular. She believes it was 6 weeks ago. She states that she has been in good health save for a recent cold. She has no other complaints.

Upon further questioning you learn that MP does have frequency and urgency, along with nocturia last night. Although she has not taken her temperature, she says she has "felt feverish now and then" over the past week but dismisses this as part of her recent cold symptoms. She denies blood in her urine, nausea, vomiting, or chills. She admits that she has been feeling fatigued and run down lately. Her job is becomingly increasingly stressful as she takes on more responsibility. When asked about her sexual history, she states that since the divorce she has been seeing "a few guys she met in local clubs," and she volunteers that this is just a phase of "sowing her wild oats." She says she married and had children at such a young age that she missed out on a lot of the experiences other women her age have already enjoyed. She loves her children but finds them overwhelming when they "act like little devils."

Further Questioning of MP Reveals the Following

Medical History

Asthma, allergic rhinitis

Past Surgical History

Appendectomy at age 13
Tubal ligation after the birth of her last child

Medications

Albuterol inhaler as often as she can get samples from the city clinic and over-the-counter (OTC) loratadine

Social History

She works full time as a checker at the local grocery store. Only recently has she begun receiving health insurance benefits. She has not had regular annual gynecologic examinations or received any consistent health care. She drinks two to three beers per day, usually more on the weekends to help her deal with the stress of her children. She denies tobacco or illicit drug use.

Family History

Mother has type 2 diabetes and hypertension.
Father died last year of a myocardial infarction at age 60.

Vitals

Temp 99.0, Pulse 82, BP 127/84, Resp 16/min

HEENT

Head normocephalic. PERRL. EOMI. Oropharynx and TMs clear

Neck

Some nodal enlargement in the anterior cervical chain. Nontender
CV: S1, S2, RRR. No murmurs, rubs, or gallops appreciated.

Chest

Good air exchange. Slight expiratory wheezes over upper lung fields. No crackles. No CVA tenderness

Abdomen

Positive bowel sounds, soft, ND. Diffuse mild lower quadrant tenderness with some increased suprapubic tenderness to pressure. No rebound or guarding. She has no CVA tenderness.

Extremities

Peripheral pulses strong and equal bilaterally. DTRs 2+ upper and lower extremities.

Rectal

Deferred by patient

Gynecologic

Normal external genitalia without lesions. Cervix and vaginal wall appeared normal. No bacteria or fungus were seen on KOH prep and wet mount. GC and chlamydia cultures sent. Bimanual examination shows normal size uterus, no cervical motion tenderness, and no adnexal masses or tenderness.

A DIPSTICK ANALYSIS IS PERFORMED ON MP IN YOUR OFFICE. THE RESULTS ARE

2+ leukocyte esterase
1+ nitrites
pH 7.4
Negative blood, ketones, glucose, protein, bilirubin
A urine pregnancy test is negative. No further tests are performed.

CONCLUSION

Because this is MP's first urinary tract infection (UTI), you treat her empirically with TMP-SMX for 3 days and instruct her to return if her symptoms do not resolve or if she experiences fever, back pain, nausea or vomiting, or a worsening of symptoms. You choose this antibiotic specifically because this is her first UTI, the antibiotic cost is low, and historically there has been a low resistance rate in your community. You also counsel her on the importance of using condoms for STI prevention. You spend a few extra minutes counseling her for her increased stressors and then focus on her risky behaviors.

Modified from Family Medicine online, Penn State College of Medicine.

CASE STUDY 20-2

It is about 4:30 PM, and you are beginning to see the end of a long day as the acute care PA in your family medicine clinic. Just as you finish up with your last patient, you see that there is an "add on." You inquire as to the nature of the visit with the nurse who took the telephone call. She explains that the patient was a male teenager, a college freshman, known to the practice, but that the patient did not wish to disclose the reason for his appointment. As you are finishing up your electronic health record on your previous patient, the college student arrives at your clinic. You quickly gather your thoughts, knock, and then enter the room.

Upon entering the room, you find George, an 18-year-old, somewhat distressed young man wearing a soccer jersey. He is seated on the examination table with an anxious look on his face. Upon your inquiry, George states: "I have pain down there," pointing to his genitals. Further tactful questioning reveals that George's pain is in his scrotum, in particular, the right side.

Continuing the clinical interview, you obtain the following information. George began to experience pain in his right testicle approximately 3 days ago. This discomfort has gradually worsened, and he has noticed some scant redness and tenderness, along with some questionable swelling of his scrotum. He further notes the presence of a yellowish discharge from his penis in the last day or so and explains that he woke up last night and felt that he had a fever, although he did not take his temperature.

George has a burning sensation upon urination that began about a day or so before the onset of the right testicular pain. He also claims that he has been urinating more often in the past 2 days and that his urine is dark yellow and has a strong, foul smell.

In social history, George explains that he has been sexually active since the age of 16 and has had two female sexual partners since that time. He states that he has been careful about using condoms, but he readily admits that he did have one recent sexual encounter with a new girlfriend in which he did not use a condom. The encounter was over the past weekend. He adamantly denies ever having had a sexually transmitted infection (STI), homosexual contact, intravenous drug use, and smoking.

The patient has had no previous medical problems and has never required surgery. To the best of his knowledge and according to his chart, both of his testicles were normally descended at birth. He takes no medications, and although you review his family history, it is noncontributory to this current complaint. He has no known medication allergies. He denies joint pain, rash, burning eyes/conjunctivitis, or hematuria. Additionally, the patient has no history of trauma to the genital region or lower abdomen; no nausea, vomiting, or change in bowel habits; no recent viral illness or "colds"; no history of urinary tract infections or testicular symptoms; and nothing like his current problem in the past.

If the vital signs are stable, the physical examination in this patient should be directed to a thorough examination of the genitals and surrounding anatomy. However, with STIs clearly high on the differential, one should also examine the conjunctiva, oral cavity, skin (for rashes/lesions), and joints despite the negative review of systems (ROS) from the patient history.

It is important to prepare a systematic approach to the genital examination just as it is for any other region of the body. However, this is particularly important with the genital region because this examination is frequently embarrassing for the patient. It is essential that you be thorough yet expedient to minimize patient apprehensiveness. Remember, although clinicians do not "feel" but palpate instead, it is necessary to balance verbiage with patients so as to encourage understanding without being unprofessional. Typical medical terminology may be completely misunderstood, whereas colloquialisms may be inappropriate. As with any other part of the body, it is important to examine above and below the area of concern. In this patient, that would include an abdominal examination and examination of the perineum, inguinal region, and upper portion of the lower extremities. Begin by examining above and below the genital region, saving that region for last.

When treating adolescents, except for issues such as but not limited to sexual abuse and suicidal ideations, confidentiality should be maintained and discussed with the patients. Depending on state laws and ages, especially with most sexually active teens, assurance that information will be disclosed only with their permission will foster trust and enhance the chances that the patients will be honest in giving an accurate history and discussing concerns.

You perform a directed physical examination on George, with the following results:

General appearance: The patient is an athletic-appearing, apprehensive, 18-year-old male who appears to be slightly uncomfortable.

Vital signs: BP 130/85; HR 95; RR 13; Temp 100° F

Abdominal examination: Positive bowel sounds, nontender/nondistended, no masses or hepatosplenomegaly

Inguinal/upper thigh examination: no evidence of direct hernia, nontender, no redness or local skin changes, no evidence of femoral hernia

Genital examination: You observe scant erythema of the right-sided scrotal skin, the skin is warm to the touch, and the entire scrotum is slightly tender and swollen; there is no evidence of other skin changes on the scrotum or perineal skin, there is trace yellowish discharge from urethral meatus, and the testicles are normally descended, normal in size and shape, symmetric, and nontender. There are no masses palpated in the testicles, the right epididymis is tender and enlarged, and the vas deferens is normal in size and shape bilaterally and slightly tender on right side. Elevation of the right testicle reveals a reduction in pain (positive Prehn's sign), the cremasteric reflex is present bilaterally, and there is no hernia palpated through the external ring.

You order antibiotic therapy for epididymitis (presumptively caused by gonorrhea and chlamydia) according to Centers for Disease Control guidelines, perform additional testing including syphilis and HIV testing after consenting George to the tests, and also administer the first injections of the hepatitis A vaccination protocol, something he had previously refused. You discuss and George agrees to return to have his sexual partner(s) evaluated for treatment. You spend a considerable period of time discussing risky sexual behavior and risky behavior in general, including drugs and alcohol. Lastly, you further explain that it may take 2 to 4 weeks for the pain and swelling to completely resolve, and you then send the patient home with instructions to call or return to the office if his symptoms worsen or fail to improve in the next few days. You also schedule a follow-up appointment in a few days to more thoroughly address the issues encountered in this case, to gain further insight into the health risks faced by this patient, and to counsel the patient accordingly.

The urethral culture results return 2 days later and confirm your suspicion of *Neisseria gonorrhoeae.* Because gonorrhea and chlamydia are reportable diseases, this patient's infection should be reported to the state to help track the incidence and distribution of sexually transmitted infections. Although the list varies by state, the following STIs are generally considered as noteworthy: acquired immunodeficiency syndrome (AIDS); chancroid; genital infection with *Chlamydia trachomatis;* gonorrhea; hepatitis A, B, and C; human immunodeficiency virus (HIV); and syphilis.

Modified from Family Medicine online, Penn State College of Medicine.

CASE STUDY 20-3

Ms. A.J., a 30-year-old woman, presents to your office for the first time because she has recently had difficulty keeping up with her friends in her biweekly volleyball game. She had a "cold" 5 weeks ago (stuffy nose, cough, sore throat), which has gotten better except for the persistent cough. The cough is productive of green phlegm, and she gets short of breath with exertion. She tells you that she thinks she has "bronchitis" because she had bronchitis frequently as a child. She is requesting antibiotics because that is what her doctor "always" gave her for the bronchitis. She has recently tried over-the-counter inhalers but finds they offer little relief of her symptoms. She does not smoke. She coughs daily and is awakened from sleep at least one or two nights a week with cough. Her cough is worsened by cold weather, and she is noticing decreased exercise tolerance over the past several months. She volunteers, "I do *not* have asthma." Review of systems is otherwise negative. There is no personal history of asthma. She thinks her mom had asthma, and her brother has "allergies." She has never been hospitalized. She denies any allergies to medication or environmental allergens. The patient denies symptoms of gastroesophageal reflux disease.

ON EXAMINATION

General: She is a neatly dressed Caucasian woman who appears to be her stated age and in no respiratory distress.
Vitals: BP 110/70; RR 12; HR 68; Temp 97.5° F; Ht: 6′1″; Wt: 190 lb
HEENT: PERRL, EOMI, anicteric sclera, tympanic membranes visualized bilaterally, clear nasal discharge noted, nasal mucosa pink and without inflammation. No frontal or maxillary sinus tenderness. Pharynx without erythema, tonsils without exudate. Neck is supple, without adenopathy, no thyromegaly
CV: Heart rate regular without murmurs, rubs, or gallops
Lungs: Clear to auscultation in all fields bilaterally
ABD: Soft, positive bowel sounds, nontender, nondistended; no masses, guarding, or organomegaly
GU/Rectal: Deferred
Extremities: Without clubbing, cyanosis, edema
Chest radiograph: Showed no infiltrate, no mass, no cardiomegaly or increased vascular markings

The patient's peak flow is 350 (expected is 630). You discussed a possible underlying etiology of "reactive airway disease," which is dismissed by the patient, who is insistent on antibiotics. The cough cleared quickly with the regimen you prescribed, and she cancelled her 2-week follow-up visit. Although you called and counseled the patient on the telephone, she did not reschedule an appointment as you had requested in that telephone consultation.

Six months later, Ms. A.J. presented to the office reporting that she continues to have wheezing with exercise and it is taking increasingly longer to get rid of the "winded" feeling she gets. The wheezing episodes occur about two to three times a week. She also wakes occasionally from sleep short of breath. She notices that her symptoms have worsened since the weather has gotten colder. Her examination is unremarkable except for expiratory wheezes. Ms. A.J. agrees to your plan (a combination low-dose inhaled corticosteroid with a long-acting beta$_2$-agonist twice daily along with a short-acting rescue inhaler as needed). You also give her a peak flow meter and teach her how to use it and to record her daily readings. You see her in follow-up 1 month later and ask how she has been doing. She states that she feels much better and has symptoms only about once a week. Her peak flows on most days are more than 540, although on a few particularly cold days, her peak flows were only about 400. You discuss seasonal variations that may occur in her asthma and schedule a 6-month follow-up appointment with instructions to return immediately if her peak flow falls off at any time.

Modified from Family Medicine online, Penn State College of Medicine.

Challenges and Rewards in Internal Medicine

The PA in internal medicine will find the same collegial relationships that are found in other branches of medicine. The daily routine includes seeing patients, taking histories, performing examinations, ordering diagnostic aids, prescribing courses of treatment, and arranging follow-up. Additionally, the internal medicine PA may make nursing home visits or hospital rounds or may perform special procedures such as treadmill tests or flexible sigmoidoscopies. However, internal medicine PAs do not see children, do not do surgical or gynecologic procedures, and generally see fewer patients per day than do PAs in other specialties, including family practice. The patients are adult and tend to be skewed to an older population. Histories may be taken more slowly and may be augmented with history from a spouse, child, or caretaker. Examinations are thorough, with a search for subtle clues to subacute or uncommon chronic diseases. More time is taken to educate the patient about the possibilities, the workup, and the various potential outcomes. Treatment plans are often not so clear-cut. The benefits and risks of a treatment plan are discussed, and the choice is selected in partnership with the patients and their family.

Many internal medicine PAs develop areas of special knowledge or skill such as treadmill testing, diabetic education, or arthritis management. The outlook for internal medicine PAs is generally excellent. Many group practices and multispecialty clinics are finding PAs a welcome addition. Because PAs share the load of routine cases, internists are free to spend more time at the hospital or on more difficult cases.

A typical day for a PA in an internal medicine practice might include the following cases.

CASE STUDY 20-4

You are the acute care PA at the Internal Medicine Clinic, seeing Mrs. Brown for the first time. Mrs. Brown is a 67-year-old woman with a 2-day history of swelling and pain in her right lower leg. The pain worsens with walking. She remembers first noticing right calf pain when arising from bed yesterday morning. She noticed the right lower leg was swollen and red. She denies any traumatic event or recent strenuous activity. In fact, she just returned from her winter stay in Florida, and the long drive gave her legs a needed rest. The leg pain worsens with walking, especially pushing off with her toes. The pain is relieved with rest and elevation, but her calf continues to hurt. She describes the pain to be most severe "inside her calf." She has not had this leg swelling and pain previously and has never had leg edema. She denies fever or night sweats. She cannot recall any reason for her skin to be infected. She recalls no bites or scrapes to her calf area. Four months ago, Mrs. Brown had a breast mass removed that was found to be malignant. A local surgeon is following her and told her the nodes were cancer free and the tumor was completely removed.

ROS: Generally Is Negative, and Specifically the Patient

Denies fatigue
Denies headache
Denies chest pain, palpitations
Denies shortness of breath
Denies nausea, vomiting

Medical History

Hypertension (HTN): controlled; osteoarthritis; breast cancer
Menopause at age 55

Surgical History

Right breast lumpectomy, 4 months ago, negative nodes
Total knee replacement 2 years ago

Meds

Atenolol 50 mg once daily
Naprosyn OTC PRN

Allergies

Penicillin (hives)

Social History

Tobacco—1 PPD × 25 years, stopped 4 months ago
No alcohol use
Married, lives with husband. Retired school teacher with two daughters

Family History

No cancers
No peripheral vascular disease
No hypercoagulable conditions

Physical examination: On physical examination, Mrs. Brown is a pleasant woman, alert, oriented, and in no apparent distress (NAD). She has a supple neck without lymphadenopathy or jugular venous distension. Lung sounds are coarse throughout bilaterally. Her cardiac examination is normal—regular rate of 92 BPM and normal rhythm without murmurs. Abdominal examination is benign with normoactive bowel sounds, nontender, and no organomegaly. On inspection, the right lower extremity (RLE) appears edematous and mildly erythematous distal to the knee compared with the left. The right calf is 24 cm, and the left is 20 cm. There is no skin breakdown appreciated. On palpation, the right calf is warmer and firmer than the left, and the edema is nonpitting. Superficial palpation of the right calf is nontender. There is moderate tenderness to deep palpation over the calf and popliteal vein. Femoral, popliteal, posterior tibialis, and dorsalis pedis pulses are all 2+ and equal bilaterally. Homans' sign is not present. Sensation is intact bilaterally.

Mrs. Brown is sent to the nearby hospital for a diagnostic duplex ultrasound of the lower extremities and D dimer. While waiting in the emergency department waiting room, she develops sudden chest pain and shortness of breath. She is immediately taken to a room where hand-carried records from your practice are quickly reviewed while the nurse takes her vital signs: BP 150/96 mm Hg; RR 22; pulse 109.

Mrs. Brown's lab results reveal a normal CBC, lytes, PT/PTT, and cardiac profile. However, she has an elevated D-dimer—4026.

Her chest radiograph (CXR) and electrocardiogram (ECG) are as follows:

CXR: Without active disease. No definite infiltrate. Possible left atelectasis and elevation of the right hemidiaphragm

ECG: Sinus tachycardia with any ST-segment changes, normal axis, negative ectopy

With her labs in hand and the suspicion for pulmonary emboli (PE) high, she is sent to radiology for a spiral chest CT. The chest CT demonstrates multiple PE bilaterally. Small pleural effusions and atelectasis are also noted. Given her initial presentation, she is now sent for a duplex ultrasound of the lower extremities to determine if a deep vein thrombosis (DVT) was the source of her PE. The ultrasound is positive for a DVT in her right lower extremity. Mrs. Brown has a calf vein thrombi extending to the popliteal veins. No further studies are necessary in this case, but for your benefit, two venogram studies follow, exhibiting obvious calf vein clots. Unfortunately for Mrs. Brown, she has a PE and DVT. The good news is that these conditions can be effectively treated if diagnosed and acted on promptly. You anticoagulate her using enoxaparin, transition her to oral warfarin, and eventually discharge her home with a good outcome to follow up with you.

Modified from Family Medicine online, Penn State College of Medicine.

CASE STUDY 20-5

Mrs. White is a 56-year-old white woman with a 4-month history of increasing fatigue and frequent urination. She denies fever, chills, back pain, or hematuria. She denies any recent viral illnesses. Her height is 5′1″, and her weight is stable at 190 lb. Her appetite is normal. Fatigue is chronic over the past few months, which has made it difficult for her to carry out her duties as a cashier at a local grocery store.

MEDICAL HISTORY

Hypertension—controlled
Menopause age 53

SURGICAL HISTORY

Tonsillectomy age 6
Laparoscopic cholecystectomy age 51

FAMILY HISTORY

Father deceased, age 68, of myocardial infarction. History included HTN & type 2 diabetes mellitus (T2DM).
Mother deceased, age 74, of ruptured aortic aneurysm. History included osteoarthritis and HTN.
Brother alive, age 61—T2DM, HTN, BPH
Maternal grandmother deceased, age 54, of breast cancer
Maternal grandfather deceased, age 31, of industrial accident
Paternal grandmother deceased, age 70, of a stroke. History included HTN, T2DM, obesity.
Paternal grandfather deceased, age 45 of myocardial infarction

Medications

Hydrochlorothiazide 25 mg daily

Social History

Married, rare alcohol intake and has never smoked
Employed as a cashier in a local grocery store
Three grown children. Good relationship with her husband. Completed high school education

Results of Your Physical Examination Are as Follows

Height 5′1″; weight 190 lb (86.36 kg)
B/P 146/88 mm Hg; pulse 82 and regular; RR16 BPM
Ophthalmologic exam—PERRL, EOMI
Funduscopic exam—disc sharp, macula appears normal, vessels without nicking, no abnormalities noted
Cardiac exam—regular rate and rhythm, without murmurs, rubs, gallops, PMI normal (see following tables)

Laboratory results (and normal ranges for your laboratory for women) for the patient are as follows:

Plasma glucose (70-100)	160
Sodium (135-145)	141
Potassium (3.5-4.5)	3.6
Chloride (80-110)	92
Serum creatinine (0.8-1.4)	1.4
Red blood cell count (3.6-5.0)	4.3
Hgb (12-16)	13.7
Hct (37-47)	38.6
MCV (87-103)	96
MCH (26-34)	28
ALT (7-35)	25
AST (10-36)	28
Total bilirubin (0.1-1.2)	1.0
Alkaline phosphatase (40-130)	88
TSH (0.3-5.0)	3.2
Total cholesterol (<200)	212
LDL-C (<130)	151
HDL-C (>45)	38
Triglycerides (<150)	165

ALT, alanine aminotransferase; AST, aspartate transaminase HDL-C, high-density lipoprotein cholesterol; LDL-C, low-density lipoprotein cholesterol; MCH, mean corpuscular hemoglobin; MCV, mean corpuscular volume; TSH, thyroid-stimulating hormone.

U/A

pH	5.0
Specific gravity	1.020
Leukocytes	Neg
Nitrates	Neg
Protein	Neg
Glucose	Neg
Ketones	Neg
Urobiligen	Neg
Bilirubin	Neg
Blood	Neg

Pulses—femoral, popliteal, dorsalis pedis, posterior tibial normal. No bruits noted
Thyroid—smooth, not enlarged, no nodules palpated
Skin exam—multiple nevus (normal appearing), few seborrheic keratoses on back, no skin lesions or ulcers noted
Neurologic exam—grossly intact
Dental exam—edentulous, upper and lower dentures removed; no ulcers or lesions noted. Well-fitting dentures
Foot exam—skin and nails free from breaks in the skin/ulcers, 6-mm callous plantar surface of L foot, monofilament testing reveals normal sensation. Proprioception intact R & L. Gait reveals pronation of both feet during walking.

You start Mrs. White on lisinopril, 10 mg daily, for her blood pressure; atorvastatin (Lipitor), 20 mg each evening, for her hypercholesterolemia; and aspirin, 81 mg daily. You arrange for her to return to repeat her fasting glucose but presumptively diagnose her with type 2 diabetes pending that second result. You also add an HbA_{1c} to her previous blood work. You also schedule her to meet with a dietitian and diabetes educator for diet and exercise guidance, as well as to obtain a home blood glucose monitor and be instructed in its use. She will also monitor her blood pressure at home.

Mrs. White returned the following week for a repeat fasting glucose, which was 152 mg/dL and you have now diagnosed her with T2DM and prescribed metformin 500 mg once daily with breakfast for 2 weeks and escalated to two twice daily with breakfast and dinner. She returns 2 months later telling you she initially had some nausea with the metformin, but that quickly passed. She has tried to follow her diet and exercise program as outlined, and she has had a 3-lb weight loss. Her home glucose monitoring for the past 3 days is as follows (see table):

Day/Time	Monday	Tuesday	Wednesday
Fasting AM	131	145	139
PM 2 hours after dinner	201	196	211

Today her blood pressure is well controlled at 118/76 mm Hg. The remainder of her vital signs are also normal. Her hemoglobin A1C is 7.9% (normal 4% to 6%), and her repeat LFTs and kidney function testing are normal. Her cholesterol panel on atorvastatin 20 mg has changed as follows (see table):

Laboratory results (and normal ranges for your laboratory for women) for the patient are as follows:

Test	Initial	Today
Total cholesterol (<200)	212	148
Low-density lipoprotein cholesterol (<130)	151	98
High-density lipoprotein cholesterol (>45)	38	44
Triglycerides (<150)	165	132

Mrs. White has made progress with regard to both her glycemic control but is still not well-controlled, whereas most would agree that her cholesterol levels are controlled adequately. With an HbA_{1C} of 7.9 and especially with elevated postprandial glucose levels, you elect to both increase her metformin to maximal dose of 1000 mg twice daily with breakfast and dinner and add a DPP-4 inhibitor to better control postprandial glucose elevations. Statistically, you would anticipate her HbA_{1C} would likely drop about another 1% to 1.5% with this regimen and adhere to ADA and EASD guidelines for treatment to T2DM. You will see her in approximately 4 weeks for a follow-up and follow her for continued management of her diabetes and her coexisting problems, which include obesity, hypertension, and hyperlipidemia.

CONCLUSION

In 1996 Simon[6] detailed the critical requisite skills for a PA to succeed in the new job market, and these skills have become only more important. A PA needs to be as follows:

1. Technically competent, which will include functioning as a case manager and overseeing a large group of patients who may be monitored by in-home devices.
2. Oriented toward consumer satisfaction. Consumers have many choices and will leave the health plan if they are not satisfied.
3. Flexible. Generalist training is more important than ever. PAs need to be able to adapt to changing assignments throughout their careers.
4. Excellent communicators. Communication with patients will be all-important, including communication through video and electronic media.
5. Innovative. PAs need to constantly monitor their performance, working to be more time-efficient while providing quality care as judged by the consumer. The consumer, not the provider, will determine quality.
6. Multiskilled. PAs need to bring not only their generalist training but additional skills to the practice.
7. Technologically competent. PAs need to constantly adapt to new technologies.
8. Visionary. PAs need to be able to look into the future and predict what will be necessary to compete well in a few years, in 5 years, and in 10 years. The health care system is not going to be static. This is a difficult task that requires PAs to be constantly observing and staying informed.

In addition, PAs in the 21st century must be lifelong learners and must be able to critically evaluate the medical literature. Although Simon has not listed anything about being familiar with the business of medicine, successful PAs must understand how the marketplace affects the financial success of the practice and, therefore, the individual PA.

Opportunities abound for PAs in primary care disciplines. Reimbursements are driving practices to examine cost-saving options closely coupled with revenue-producing options. PAs will remain high on the list of cost-effective choices that provide quality care. No longer can we simply say that PAs are an attractive alternative when physicians cannot otherwise be attracted to rural or inner city locations. Although this is true, PAs are rapidly becoming essential to allowing practices to remain financially viable.

As a student, what should you know at the start of a primary care rotation?

Be familiar with performing focused and comprehensive history and physical examinations, ordering and interpreting basic laboratory tests for common diseases (especially dyslipidemia, diabetes, and thyroid dysfunction), and formulating a differential diagnosis of common complaints across the continuum of the lifespan. Think about the chronic care model, things such as diabetes, hypertension, and cardiovascular disease, as well as strategies to prevent these diseases in the first place, and treat them should those efforts not be successful. Be aware of health maintenance guidelines and milestones in children, adolescents, adults, and older adults. Know the top two or three drugs for each category of major drug classes including antibiotics, antihypertensives, cardiovascular, diabetic, thyroid disease, and musculoskeletal complaints. You may also be asked to provide Current Procedural Terminology (CPT) codes and International Classification of Diseases, ninth revision (ICD-9) (and soon ICD-10) codes for billing. Be familiar with these, and you will be a stand-out student!

Family practice job description: Although all family practitioners share a core of information and skills, and therefore do similar things, the dimensions of knowledge, the skill, and especially the day-to-day tasks performed vary with the individual family practitioner. Patient needs differ in various geographic areas, and the content of the family practice varies accordingly. For example, the knowledge and skills useful to a family practice PA practicing in an inner city may vary from those needed by a family practice PA with a rural practice. Furthermore, the scope of an individual family practice changes over time, evolving as competency in current skills is maintained and new knowledge and skill are obtained through continuing medical education.

As a student, what should I expect on this rotation?

Expect to spend considerable time learning every possible aspect of your patient's lives. Expect to be incredibly busy in most practices. Get to know the patients and their personal environment. Be prepared to perform many routine tests repeatedly, including things such as intramuscular injections, venipunctures, finger sticks, throat cultures, vaginal examinations, incision and drainage procedures, ECGs, ankle/brachial indices (ABIs), pulmonary function tests (PFTs), suturing, and splinting, to name only some of what most students learn and do in a busy family practice. You may round in the hospital, nursing home, or do house calls! On this clerkship you can laugh and cry with the patients.

Who are the members of the team? This typically includes a family physician and/or PA, the medical assistants and nurses, your consultants, the receptionists, perhaps the billers and coders, and depending on the office, the technologists who do things such as radiographs and sonograms. Remember that these folks are truly team members and can give you incredible insight into the patient they have known for years and you are just meeting for the first time. Do not anger these team members, or your life can be "difficult," or much worse. And remember this team taking care of the patient always includes the patient's friends and family, too!

What is the culture of the setting? Hours? Personalities? Philosophy? Clothing? Formality? Hierarchy? Stress-level? Scheduling? The culture tends to be fast-paced, friendly, and incredibly broad in terms of knowledge base and skill set. You will be in awe of a good family practice physician or PA and not ask, "Do you know … ?" but rather ask, "Is there anything you *don't* know?" Most family practice physicians (see later) are people persons, so they are friendly and like to talk. Most wear laboratory coats with open collared shirts (for men) and slacks (for women). Staff usually wears scrubs. Usually, there is a long-established senior partner (or practice manager) in charge. Stress levels can be high or low, depending on patient load, volume, and complexity, along with the level of support staff available. You can be a big help if you know what you are doing or an anchor if you do not. Be prepared ahead of time, and you will be liked. Some offices are 5 days a week, with one or two late nights, and every other Saturday. Some offices are 7 days a week, 12 hours during the week with shorter days on weekends.

Terminology, acronyms, and slang: An FP is a family practitioner. A PA is just as likely to be a "prior authorization" for an expensive medication as it is a term for a physician assistant. A "rep" is not something you do at the gym; rather, it is the pharmaceutical representative who fills the sample closet, may bring you lunch, or tell you about a job opening in a nearby hospital or practice. Be respectful!

Equipment you will encounter during the rotations: basic things including electronic prescribing, electronic health records, injections, vaccines, ECGs, throat cultures, ABIs, PFTs, vaginal exams, suturing, splinting, and perhaps interpreting radiographs. You will not be cracking chests or running codes, but you will be doing a lot of health maintenance and treatment of common diseases. The lives you save likely will be after you have counseled patients, changed their lifestyle, and gotten them to stop smoking. You may never know the impact you had, but rest assured, you will change lives for the better in family practice.

Challenges and rewards: There is rarely enough time in a day to do what you want and barely enough time to do what is absolutely essential. Try to become as efficient as possible. Good practices have efficiencies built in and you should try to emulate those. Every day is different, more so than any other field. There are continuous surprises and "Ah-ha!"moments. There is no specialty as fulfilling as primary care where you truly get to know your patients and they become the closest thing to family members imaginable.

Emerging issues in the field: The patient-centered medical home and the failing profitability of primary care all will necessitate a realignment of resources focused away from procedures and toward keeping patients healthy. Suddenly adding 40 million to the rolls of the insured through the Affordable Care Act , if it is sustained by the U.S. Supreme Court, will dramatically add an unsustainable burden on primary care unless we dramatically change our health care system to emphasize primary care services.

Common Clinical Problems in Primary Care

Health maintenance should be performed at each and every visit in primary care. This includes discussing healthy lifestyle choices, such as exercise, weight loss, and smoking cessation, as well as both vaccinations and milestones associated with specialized testing to detect illnesses and diseases. This later description includes things such as mammograms and colonoscopies. Overlooking an opportunity to perform, recommend, or refer is an opportunity lost than may never be recouped. Making recommendations on the basis of guidelines from organizations such as the USPSTF are appropriate to detect disease early, reduce morbidity and mortality, and contain health care costs.

Hypertension is perhaps one of the single most common chronic diseases that is treated in primary care. Do not treat blood pressure in a silo. Treating blood pressure to goal requires taking into consideration patient comorbidities. Fortunately, we have a plethora of effective inexpensive generic blood pressure medications. Do not be fooled by the patient who insists his or her blood pressure is only high in your office and is normal every other time it is taken. Use an ambulatory blood pressure machine to get accurate 24-hour readings. Chances are if the patient gets an elevated blood pressure because of you, the same thing happens whenever he or she argues with a co-worker or gets cut off driving to work.

Obesity is clearly epidemic in this country, and it seems like every other patient is overweight or obese. Clearly, obesity is an increasing problem. But just a few minutes at each and every visit reviewing alternatives including healthy eating and exercise choices can make significant changes in a significant proportion of patients.

Smoking cessation and tobacco addiction are health maintenance issues that frustrate many in primary care. But do not be dissuaded by the fact that patients do not necessarily stop smoking when you counsel them. Utilize motivational interviewing techniques to determine where patients are in terms of changing behavior, and make appropriate counseling decisions on the basis of their stage of change. Remember that the average person makes between six and eight attempts at stopping smoking before achieving success.

Diabetes is epidemic in this country, and the trend is only worsening. However, screening patients and telling them that they are "at risk" for diabetes may have significant impact in many of these patients. By losing between 5% and 10% of their weight when at risk, patients may have a dramatic impact on their ongoing risk for diabetes. By intervening early, you can have an impressive impact on outcomes. Diabetes, like hypertension, cannot be treated in isolation. Every risk factor must be addressed at every visit. By treating diabetics consistently and to goal at each and every visit, the downstream sequelae of diabetes can be ameliorated to a large degree.

Dyslipidemia, not unlike hypertension, is a silent killer that patients frequently only understand after a cardiac event. Fortunately, we have a number of safe, effective, inexpensive, and powerful generic drugs that can control lipid levels. Make certain you test patients, especially those with cardiovascular disease and family history risk, as well as those with diabetes, and then treat accordingly with both lifestyle changes and medications. Then continue testing twice yearly, and do not get bogged down in clinical inertia and wait. Rather, escalate therapy immediately whenever necessary.

Upper respiratory infections are one of the single most common sick visits in primary care. Most patients need antihistamines, perhaps decongestants, but rarely do they need antibiotics. Rapid strep-positive infections are the exception that first comes to mind. Even for sinus infections, data show evidence that antibiotics are not only unnecessary but potentially dangerous, especially with the increasing incidence of antibiotic-induced *Clostridium difficile* infections. Resist the urge to prescribe and explain why to your patients. They will be healthier in the long run.

Mechanical low back pain is a common sick visit, most commonly occurring after weekends and involving yard work, lifting something heavy around the house, or the result of a "weekend warrior" suddenly trying to do more than usual. These complaints rarely, if ever, need imaging studies (i.e., radiographs and magnetic resonance imaging). Check patients for red flags that alert you to potentially dangerous conditions (e.g., numbness, tingling, foot drop, bowel or bladder problems), and if they are absent, which is almost always the case, a nonsteroidal antiinflammatory (unless contraindicated) and 3 to 5 days of self-performed physical therapy involving stretching will almost always do the trick.

Vaccinations are lifesaving. Unquestionably, in both adults and children, vaccinations are a central focus of primary care and preventative medicine. Be prepared to discuss the true facts regarding vaccines with patients, including those parents and patients who are "antivaccine." We now have two cancer-preventing vaccines (hepatitis B and human papillomavirus), and we have many lifesaving vaccines, including meningitis and influenza. Post the Advisory Committee on Immunization Practices/Centers for Disease Control–recommended vaccine schedules in each examination room as a reminder and institute standardized protocols to allow nurses to consent and administer vaccines under preapproved practice guidelines.

CLINICAL APPLICATIONS

1. What is different about the chronic care model as opposed to the acute care model of health care?
2. Think of strategies to incorporate multiple issues into a single 15-minute office visit. What will you do when you simply cannot accomplish everything you would like to accomplish in this one visit?
3. Practice with a classmate who role-plays as an obese patient. Explain why and how this obese patient should lose weight and begin an exercise regimen, even when the patient is not motivated to do so.

KEY POINTS

- Primary care uses the chronic care model to treat the undifferentiated patient across the spectrum.
- Primary care is at a breaking point in many parts of the country with not enough providers and too many patients.
- Family practitioners see 240 million office visits annually, 87 million more than the next nearest specialty, and the average family practitioner sees about 100 patients weekly.
- Examples of common primary care issues a PA will see and treat on an ongoing and regular basis include hypertension, diabetes, dyslipidemia, upper respiratory infections, mechanical lower back pain, addressing health maintenance and vaccinations, and counseling patients with obesity and tobacco addiction.
- As the U.S. population ages and more patients acquire health insurance as a result of the Affordable Care Act, PAs will play an increasingly important role in providing primary care

References

1. Family Physicians and Physician Assistants. Team-Based Family Medicine. A joint policy statement of the American Academy of Family Physicians and the American Academy of Physician Assistants. Published online February 11, 2011 at *http://www.aapa.org/news_and_publications/news/item.aspx?id=454&terms=aafp*; accessed April 24, 2012.
2. Internists and Physician Assistants. Team-Based Primary Care. A joint policy statement of the American College of Physicians and the American Academy of Physician Assistants. American College of Physicians 2010; Policy Monograph.
3. Howell JD. The invention and development of American internal medicine. J Gen Intern Med 1989;4:127.
4. Siegel B. Love, Medicine and Miracles. New York: Harper & Row, 1986.
5. Schafft GE, Cawley JF. The Physician Assistant in a Changing Health Care Environment. Rockville, MD: Aspen Publishers, 1987.
6. Simon A. A glimpse of the future. Proceedings from Defining the Future Characteristics of Physician Assistant Education. Alexandria, VA: Association of Physician Assistant Programs, 1996.

The resources for this chapter can be found at www.expertconsult.com.

improved with nasal cannula O_2. An echocardiogram was unremarkable with an ejection fraction (EF) of 65% and normal pulmonary artery (PA) pressure, and it was unchanged from a previous study 3 years earlier. Because a side effect of felodipine can be peripheral edema, it was recommended that he discontinue felodipine and watch his home blood pressure carefully. In the meantime, because of the unusual pattern of MCP DJD and elevated AST, iron studies were obtained. Serum transferrin iron saturation was found to be 82%, and ferritin was 714 µg/L. Hemochromatosis DNA showed the patient was a heterozygote for the H63D allele. Because of the increased MCV, vitamin B_{12} was checked and found to be slightly low at 209 pg/mL. Subsequent serum homocysteine was slightly elevated at 15.1 µmol/L, but methyl malonate was normal at 0.31 µmol/L. Antiparietal cell antibodies were negative.

SUMMARY AT THIS POINT

1. The patient's peripheral edema appears not to be related to either heart or lung disease on the basis of the echocardiogram. He was started on home O_2 because of the exercise desaturation. Furosemide had been started, but felodipine was also discontinued to see whether the edema would improve or resolve.
2. The patient's slightly increased MCV may be due to excess alcohol intake or to low vitamin B_{12} stores, although homocysteine was barely elevated and methyl malonate was normal. Although he did not have anemia, he described a bit of ataxia on careful questioning. Therefore, oral vitamin B_{12} supplementation was started with a plan to recheck the serum level in several months.
3. The patient's abnormal liver function test, MCP arthritis, and increased iron may be related to a combination of excess ethanol intake and heterozygosity for the H63D hemochromatosis allele, although this allele is not typically associated with severe iron overload. It was recommended that he remain abstinent from ethanol for 6 months, at which time serum iron will be rechecked. If there is substantial decrease in iron stores and normalization of liver function tests (LFTs), he will be advised to remain off ethanol. If there is no improvement in iron and/or liver function deteriorates, liver biopsy will be considered.

CASE STUDY 21-2

A 79-year-old woman was admitted to the hospital with fever and upper abdominal pain of several days' duration. She had been relatively well until this acute illness. Her temperature was 38.9° C. Her conjunctivae were yellowish in color, and there was mid-epigastric and right upper quadrant (RUQ) tenderness. Admission laboratory evaluation showed leukocyte count (whole blood cell count [WBC]) of 16,800/µL with 86% polymorphonuclear neutrophils (PMNs), serum alanine transaminase (ALT)/AST 325/368 U/L, alkaline phosphatase 456 U/L, total/direct bilirubin 3.6/2.9 mg/dL, and amylase 220 U/L. Urine was positive for urobilinogen. Abdominal computed tomography (CT) showed swelling in the area of the ampulla of Vater, slight dilation of the common bile duct, mild edema of the pancreas, and several small stones in the gallbladder. Blood cultures were taken, and the patient was started on intravenous ciprofloxacin (250 mg every 12 hours). That evening she was taken to the gastrointestinal (GI) endoscopy suite, where endoscopic retrograde cholangiopancreatography (ERCP) was performed. No obvious obstructing stone could be identified, but a sphincterotomy and biopsies at the ampulla of Vater were performed without complication. By the next morning, the patient had defervesced and felt substantially better. Her laboratory tests were rapidly returning to normal. She was able to begin eating and drinking and was discharged the next morning to be followed as an outpatient.

SUMMARY AT THIS POINT

She probably had a small gallstone that impacted the common bile duct and pancreatic ducts at the ampulla of Vater, leading to cholangitis and pancreatitis. The subsequent decision will be whether to perform elective cholecystectomy to prevent recurrence. Biopsies positive for malignancy at the ampulla would alter the plan.

CASE STUDY 21-3

A 72-year-old man presented with right lower quadrant (RLQ) pain of 3 days' duration with low-grade fever and WBC 13,000/µL with left shift. History was significant for type 2 diabetes, hyperlipidemia, gout, hypertension, GERD, allergic rhinitis, and anxiety disorder. His medicines were simvastatin (40 mg every day), allopurinol (100 mg every day), losartan (50 mg every day), atenolol (50 mg every day), omeprazole (20 mg every other day), fluticasone nasal (100 µg every day), and paroxetine (20 mg every day). Chemistries were normal except for a glucose of 179 mg/dL; urinalysis was normal. The working diagnosis was diverticulitis, and he was started on ciprofloxacin and metronidazole. Abdominal CT scan with contrast confirmed the diagnosis. After 2 weeks, he continued to have mild RLQ pain and low-grade fever. WBC was 8000/µL, hematocrit (Hct) 37%, and glucose 146 mg/dL. Repeat CT scan with contrast showed a 3-cm RLQ abscess probably from perforated diverticulitis. Ciprofloxacin and metronidazole were restarted, and CT-guided percutaneous drainage was scheduled, but at the time of the procedure, 3 days after the second CT, the patient felt better and the loculated fluid had resolved, so the procedure was cancelled. Follow-up colonoscopy 1 month later showed diverticuli but no other abnormalities.

He presented again 1 month after the colonoscopy with weakness, anorexia, lightheadedness, and a 15-lb weight loss. Physical examination was nonspecific. Laboratory testing was notable for Hct 35%, glucose 144 mg/dL, blood urea nitrogen (BUN) 39 mg/dL, and creatinine 2.6 mg/dL. Additional testing showed albumin 3.3 g/dL, total bilirubin 2.2 mg/dL, AST 186 U/L, ALT 116 U/L, total cholesterol 587 mg/dL, triglycerides 2981 mg/dL, and high-density lipoprotein (HDL) cholesterol 22 mg/dL. Urinalysis showed a large amount of blood and protein. He was admitted to the hospital briefly, at which time serum myoglobin was 541 ng/mL, total creatine kinase (CK) 375 U/L, amylase normal, and lipase, 177 U/L. Simvastatin and losartan were held. He began to feel better and was discharged from the hospital. One week later, significant laboratory tests showed Hct 31%, BUN 24 mg/dL, creatinine 1.5 mg/dL, AST 76 U/dL, ALT 66 U/L, myoglobin and CK normal, lipase 84 U/L, total cholesterol 366 mg/dL, triglycerides 881 mg/dL, HDL cholesterol 31 mg/dL, and urinalysis 1+ blood, 2+ protein. Fenofibrate was started.

Two weeks later, he continued to feel better, but follow-up laboratory testing revealed triglycerides 1035 mg/dL. Other laboratory tests continued to return toward normal. Two weeks later, triglycerides were 1999 mg/dL. The patient recalled that some years earlier he had been on a combination of cholestyramine and gemfibrozil for a mixed hyperlipidemia. When statins became available, he had been switched over to simvastatin with good control. However, in the past 2 weeks he had returned to his longstanding pattern of having three alcoholic beverages per day. It was recommended that he restart simvastatin and discontinue alcohol. Two weeks later, his fasting lipid panel was total cholesterol 223 mg/dL, low-density lipoprotein (LDL) cholesterol 125 mg/dL, HDL cholesterol 58 mg/dL, and triglycerides 198 mg/dL.

One month later, he had returned to having a bit of nighttime alcohol and his lipid panel showed total cholesterol 411 mg/dL, HDL cholesterol 31 mg/dL, and triglycerides 2014 mg/dL. After another month of alcohol abstinence, his lipid panel was total cholesterol 248 mg/dL, LDL cholesterol 135 mg/dL, HDL cholesterol 55 mg/dL, and triglycerides 135 mg/dL. Ultimately, after another 6 months, he was on simvastatin and fenofibrate, having a small amount of alcohol in the evening, and had total cholesterol 182 mg/dL, LDL cholesterol 82 mg/dL, HDL cholesterol 64 mg/dL, and triglycerides 178 mg/dL.

SUMMARY AT THIS POINT

This patient has underlying metabolic syndrome manifested by central adiposity, glucose intolerance, hypertension, dyslipidemia, and gout. His diverticulitis resulted in dehydration, and the CT scans used radiocontrast material. The combination in this patient with diabetes and taking a statin likely resulted in mild renal insufficiency, rhabdomyolysis, and hepatitis. His underlying hypertriglyceridemia was exacerbated and also resulted in mild pancreatitis. In the months that followed, as his other metabolic abnormalities resolved, his hypertriglyceridemia remained sensitive to alcohol. Eventually, that stabilized as well on simvastatin and fenofibrate, and he was able to return to using small amounts of alcohol.

CASE STUDY 21-4

A 60-year-old woman with a 15-year history of hypothyroidism and hypoparathyroidism secondary to thyroid surgery and ^{131}I ablation for Graves' disease was seen with a complaint of shoulder pain, right greater than left. She noted that she was no longer taking 50,000 international units (IU) of vitamin D per day and instead was taking only 400 IU. She also noted morning stiffness and mild jaw claudication. Laboratory testing showed calcium 8.7 mg/dL, erythrocyte sedimentation rate 83 mm/hour, and C-reactive protein (CRP) 18 mg/dL. She was started on prednisone, 60 mg per day, and sent for right temporal artery biopsy, which did not show active inflammation but did show evidence of healed vasculitis. There was no evidence of other inflammatory disease. She was started on alendronate. By several weeks later, her symptoms had largely resolved, inflammatory laboratory tests had returned to normal, and her prednisone dose had been tapered to 30 mg per day. She was developing cushingoid features and self-tapered further to 10 mg per day over the next month. Over the next several months, the patient had minimal symptoms, continued to taper her prednisone, and ultimately stopped about 9 months after starting. She continued to have morning stiffness lasting from 15 to 60 minutes and was offered 2 to 3 mg prednisone per day but declined to restart the prednisone. Serum inflammatory markers remained low.

One year later she presented to the clinic 5 days after an episode of syncope that occurred while talking, standing, bending over, and then standing. There was no observed seizure activity, tongue biting, incontinence, or postictal symptoms. An electrocardiogram (ECG) showed a new left bundle branch block (LBBB). Subsequent 48-hour Holter monitor and cerebrovascular ultrasound were normal. An exercise thallium scan showed ischemia of the apical two thirds of the anteroseptal and apical walls, but there were no stress ECG abnormalities. Cardiac catheterization showed minimal atherosclerosis. The syncope was thought to be vasovagal.

Six months later, she had another episode of syncope, this time occurring in bed at night while preparing to put in eye drops, and a presyncopal episode while walking a few days later. The syncopal episode was not witnessed, but there was no tongue biting or incontinence. She was sent for electrophysiology study, where pronounced His-Purkinje conduction disease was found and a pacemaker was implanted.

Over the next year, she felt well and had no further syncope or presyncope, although her pacemaker was found to have seldom been in pacing mode when the memory was interrogated. She did develop recurrent mild left temporal discomfort and mild jaw claudication and was restarted on low-dose prednisone.

SUMMARY AT THIS POINT

The etiology of her syncopal episodes remains undetermined, although she does have demonstrable cardiac conduction dysfunction. Some episodes may indeed be vasovagal, and she has been instructed to carefully avoid dehydration, especially in warm weather. The pacemaker would cover episodes of conduction block. There is no clear evidence of association of her presumed vasculitis and His-Purkinje dysfunction.

CASE STUDY 21-5

This male patient was first seen at age 47 following a non-Q wave myocardial infarction (MI) with thrombolysis, angioplasty, and multiple left anterior descending (LAD) and right coronary artery (RCA) stents. He was readmitted to the hospital soon after with unstable angina and underwent quadruple coronary artery bypass surgery. The postoperative course was complicated by *Helicobacter pylori*–positive upper gastrointestinal (UGI) bleeding. Coronary artery disease risk factors included hyperlipidemia and hypertension. Medicines 2 months later were atorvastatin (20 mg every evening), atenolol (25 mg every day), lisinopril (10 mg every day), and aspirin (81 mg every day). He subsequently failed to return for follow-up. When he returned to the clinic 2 years later for a medication refill, his blood sugar was 250 mg/dL and HbA_{1c} was 8.3%. Metformin was started, but he was again lost to follow-up.

He next returned a year and a half later with polyuria and polydipsia. Blood sugar was 460 mg/dL, and HbA_{1c} was 10.1%. Insulin was started.

He next returned a year later with nonsteroidal antiinflammatory drug (NSAID)-induced UGI bleeding.

When he next returned, the following year, he began somewhat more regular clinic follow-up. In subsequent years, LDL cholesterol was lowered and blood pressure was brought under better control. Episodes of nighttime and early morning hypoglycemia were corrected when it was discovered that he was mistakenly taking short-acting insulin at bedtime. When last evaluated, his medicines were 70/30 insulin 25 U before breakfast and 15 U before dinner, metformin (850 mg twice daily), atorvastatin (40 mg every evening), lisinopril (20 mg twice daily), EC aspirin (81 mg every day), omeprazole (20 mg every day), amlodipine (5 mg every day), and for early symptoms of benign prostatic hypertrophy (BPH), he was started on doxazosin (2 mg every day). A recent stress ECG was normal, and laboratory evaluation showed HbA_{1c} 6.1%, creatinine 1 mg/dL, urine albumin/creatinine ratio 5.7 mg/g, total cholesterol 137 mg/dL, LDL cholesterol 88 mg/dL, HDL cholesterol 35 mg/dL, triglycerides 72 mg/dL, and LFTs normal.

SUMMARY AT THIS POINT

Despite difficulty in follow-up with this patient, he had done fairly well over the years. He had been compliant using medicines and was improving with clinic follow-up. He responded well to education regarding diabetes management, including frequent blood sugar monitoring and modification of his insulin regimen. Because of continued borderline blood pressure control, chlorthalidone was recently started and he was measuring blood pressures at home. His HDL cholesterol remained low. Niacin was discussed, recognizing that it might adversely affect his blood sugar control. However, because of side effects with previous attempts at using niacin, he was unwilling to start a trial of low-dose niacin to see if the dose could be gradually increased. Likewise, LDL cholesterol should be further lowered and he was considering the recommendation to add ezetimibe to his regimen.

CASE STUDY 21-6

A 51-year-old woman with Turner's syndrome has been followed regularly for many years. In addition to short stature and infertility, her major problems have been atopic disease (with severe asthma, allergic rhinitis, and atopic dermatitis), and multiple food and drug allergies. She has had marked arthralgias without evidence of destructive joint disease and past mild hemolytic anemia of unclear etiology. Her current medicines include gabapentin (200 mg three times daily), acetaminophen/oxycodone (325 mg/5 mg, ½ pill per day), nortriptyline (30 mg at bedtime), pantoprazole (40 mg every day), hydrochlorothiazide (25 mg every day), doxepin (100 mg every day), montelukast (10 mg every day), hydroxyzine (50 mg at bedtime), ranitidine (300 mg twice daily), potassium chloride (30 mEq twice daily), fexofenadine (180 mg twice daily), cetirizine (10 mg twice daily), sulindac (150 mg twice daily), fluticasone/salmeterol inhaled (500 μg/50 μg twice daily), budesonide inhaled (180 μg every day), tacrolimus topical (0.1% up to four times daily), alendronate (70 mg every week), fluocinolone topical solution (0.01% up to four times daily), budesonide nasal (64 μg twice daily), triamcinolone intramuscular (20 mg every week), cromolyn ophthalmic (2 drops each eye four times daily), albuterol inhaled (180 μg four times daily as needed), azelastine nasal (274 μg twice daily as needed), and pseudoephedrine (30 mg four times daily as needed). She has regular screening for sequelae of Turner's syndrome. She has a bicuspid aortic valve without aortic root dilation and mixed conductive/sensorineural primarily high-frequency hearing loss. However, she does not have evidence of metabolic syndrome (except for a recent AST of 47 U/L), renal structural abnormalities, hypothyroidism, liver function abnormalities, or inflammatory bowel disease.

SUMMARY AT THIS POINT

This patient with Turner's syndrome, severe and difficult-to-manage allergic disease, and severe arthralgias is followed jointly by general internal medicine, allergy, and rheumatology. In addition to management of her ongoing medical problems, she needs periodic surveillance for the sequelae of Turner's syndrome.

CASE STUDY 21-7

A 58-year-old woman is followed for several problems.

1. Type 2 diabetes. Blood sugars are generally in good control, but she has been sensitive to sulfonylureas with hypoglycemia in the past. She arrived by trial and error at her current regimen of metformin, 1000 mg twice daily, and glipizide, 1.25 mg at night, as long as her dinner and bedtime blood sugars are at least 150 mg/dL, and 2.5 mg if blood sugar is more than 200 mg/dL. On this regimen, fasting and predinner blood sugars are typically 100 to 130 mg/dL, and bedtime blood sugars are 135 to 145 mg/dL. Most recent HbA_{1c} was 6.7%.
2. Mixed hyperlipidemia. She has severe familial hypertriglyceridemia, with previous triglycerides as high as 7000 mg/dL resulting in pancreatitis on two occasions and necessitating partial pancreatectomy. Lipids have been stable for several years on atorvastatin (10 mg every evening) and gemfibrozil (600 mg twice daily). Most recent fasting lipid panel: total cholesterol 132 mg/dL, LDL cholesterol 58 mg/dL, HDL cholesterol 47 mg/dL, and triglycerides 132 mg/dL.
3. Hypertension. Well-controlled on enalapril (20 mg every day).
4. GERD. Well-controlled on lansoprazole (30 mg twice daily).
5. Hypothyroidism following radioiodine ablation of Graves' disease. Well-controlled on levothyroxine, 0.1 mg every day.
6. History of unexplained iron deficiency. One small colonic polyp was removed by colonoscopy; the colon was clear at 3-year follow-up. Upper GI endoscopy including biopsies was normal. She is postmenopausal.
7. Neurologic issues. Most troublesome in recent years have been several neurologic problems. She has a several-year history of migraine headaches with at least two episodes of prolonged lateralizing neurologic deficit after severe headaches but normal visualization studies. The most recent episode was in 2000, when symptoms of right arm and leg weakness and numbness, slurred speech, and blurred vision resolved only after several weeks. Nortriptyline (50 mg at bedtime) was successful in preventing further headaches.

In 2001 she had C5-6 anterior cervical diskectomy and fusion for a left C5-6 radiculopathy.

In August 2006, she was admitted to another hospital for generalized seizures including several observed in the hospital. Magnetic resonance imaging, cerebrovascular angiogram, and two electroencephalograms were unremarkable. She was started on topiramate. The nature and cause of the seizures remain unclear, although hypoglycemia is considered a possibility, presumably a less likely explanation for the seizures in the hospital. Four months later, her husband called to say she had had two more seizures while out of state visiting family. There was no associated tonic-clonic movement, tongue biting, or incontinence. One month later she was stable but somewhat ataxic on topiramate (150 mg twice daily).

SUMMARY AT THIS POINT

This patient has had a number of significant medical, metabolic, and surgical difficulties over the years. Most critical at this time is careful ongoing assessment with the patient of her metabolic parameters, especially blood sugars (looking for hypoglycemia) and lipids (checking triglycerides). Her migraines have been well-controlled for several years with nortriptyline prophylaxis, but the nature of her seizures remains unclear, and, therefore, a definitive plan of prophylaxis is as yet undeveloped.

CASE STUDY 21-8

A 74-year-old man presented for a second opinion about symptoms that were vaguely organized but included malaise, markedly decreased functional capacity, and a reported 40-pound weight loss. He had been followed at another institution and brought a list of medicines that included daily atenolol, 50 mg, and levothyroxine, 0.2 mg. As-needed medicines included dicyclomine (20 mg), acetic acid (which he put in his ears), triamcinolone cream (0.1%), colchicine (0.6 mg), ranitidine (150 mg), HCTZ (25 mg), simethicone (80 mg), psyllium wafers, and over-the-counter gestazyme, ibuprofen, glucosamine/chondroitin, multivitamins, and a calcium/magnesium/zinc pill. From the combination of his list of medical problems and his medicines, it appeared that he was treated for hypertension, hypothyroidism, irritable bowel syndrome, and lower extremity atopic dermatitis. However, most striking on physical examination were obvious changes of rheumatoid arthritis in his hands with bilateral loss of intrinsic muscle mass and synovial thickening of MCPs and wrists. When questioned, he acknowledged a 1-year history of morning stiffness, especially of shoulders and hips, and increasing muscle weakness but denied hand pain. He had severe extensive atopic dermatitis on both forearms and both lower legs with chronic scratching and lichenification. He was sent for diagnostic testing and encouraged to use the triamcinolone cream twice daily on the areas of involved skin.

Laboratory testing showed WBC 13,500/μL, glucose 182 mg/dL, rheumatoid factor 20 IU/mL, erythrocyte sedimentation rate 39 mm/hour, CRP 63.5 mg/L, anti-cyclic citrullinated peptide antibody (anti-CCP) less than 10 U/mL, and thyroid-stimulating hormone (TSH) 0.8 μU/mL. Radiographs showed multiple hand and wrist erosions consistent with rheumatoid arthritis, normal feet, and cervical osteoarthritis, especially at C4-5. He was seen by the rheumatology service, which added laboratory tests for CPK (normal) and antinuclear antibodies (ANA; negative). He was started on prednisone (15 mg every day) for a most likely diagnosis of anti-CCP–negative rheumatoid arthritis. By 1 week later, his symptoms were 80% to 90% improved. His prednisone dose was decreased to 10 mg every day, and he was started on methotrexate, 7.5 mg weekly. During the following weeks, his symptoms flared if his prednisone was decreased below 10 mg every day. Methotrexate was increased to 15 mg weekly, and the potential use of etanercept was discussed in an effort to decrease or discontinue prednisone if possible. However, the cost precluded that option. His blood sugar control worsened on prednisone, and, therefore, metformin was added.

At 7 months after initial presentation, he was pain free and had returned to regular walking and swimming. He felt well, with good strength. His blood sugars were reasonably well controlled, and episodic hyperglycemia was decreasing as his understanding of diabetes and diet improved. His most recent HbA_{1c} was 6.5%. Blood pressure was averaging 125/75 mm Hg. His extensive atopic dermatitis had entirely resolved. CBC and chemistries, including LFTs, were normal. CRP was 12.8 mg/L.

SUMMARY AT THIS POINT

Observation of the obvious physical findings of rheumatoid arthritis led to dramatic and rapid improvement in this patient's symptoms and functional quality of life. However, this was achieved with medicines that have significant toxicities—prednisone and methotrexate. It will be important to continue to monitor for these toxicities and to respond appropriately as they develop and evolve.

KEY POINTS

- Internal medicine is the specialty that deals with the nonsurgical, nongynecologic medical diseases of adults.
- There are a number of recognized subspecialties of internal medicine, each with its own training and board-certification examinations.
- Internal medicine practices range from general internal medicine primary care to highly specialized care of patients with only particular types of medical problems.
- The most complex and challenging medical problems are usually found in internal medicine practices.
- Internists typically strive for completeness and thoroughness in their medical practice from a sense of the responsibility to provide definitive care to patients, from those with straightforward medical problems to those with the most complex difficulties.

- Internists frequently serve on difficult cases as consultants for their medical colleagues.
- Many PAs work in internal medicine, from general internal medicine primary care to subspecialty practice. There are many and increasing opportunities for PAs in both outpatient and inpatient internal medicine.

References

1. Beck AH. The *Flexner Report* and the standardization of American medical education. JAMA 2004;291:2139.
2. American College of Physicians home page. *http://www.acponline.org*. Accessed March 27, 2007.
3. American Board of Internal Medicine home page. *http://www.abim.org/*. Accessed March 22, 2007.
4. Duty Hours Language. For Insertion into the Common Program Requirements for All Core and Subspecialty Programs by July 1, 2003. Chicago: Accreditation Council for Graduate Medical Education; 2003. *http://www.acgme.org/acWebsite/dutyHours/dh_Lang703.pdf*. Accessed March 22, 2007.
5. Becoming certified. American Board of Internal Medicine website. *http://www.abim.org/certification/*. Accessed March 22, 2007.
6. American College of Physicians: ACP offers new affiliate membership class for members of the American Academy of Physician Assistants. *http://www.acponline.org/college/pressroom/phys_assis.htm?hp*. Accessed March 22, 2007.
7. American Board of Medical Specialties home page. *http://www.abms.org/*. Accessed March 22, 2007.
8. Accreditation Council for Graduate Medical Education home page. *http://www.acgme.org/acWebsite/home/home.asp*. Accessed March 22, 2007.
9. 2006 AAPA Physician Assistant Census Report. Alexandria, VA: American Academy of Physician Assistants; 2006. *http://www.aapa.org/research/data_and_statistics/resources.aspx*. Accessed March 23, 2007.

The resources for this chapter can be found at www.expertconsult.com.

CHAPTER 22

EMERGENCY MEDICINE

Edward M. Sullivan

CHAPTER CONTENTS

Many people can relate a vivid story involving themselves or a family member in an emergency department (ED). From personal experience to syndicated TV programs, the stories of life and death drama that take place in a busy ED can be both exhilarating and traumatic for both patients and providers. Health care providers will experience a high level of anxiety from their personal experiences, as well as from the stories they have heard from their co-workers. Patients seeking treatment in an ED usually expect the worst, and each visit can be terrifying. Expectations are always high for both, and striving for a good outcome is always the main objective. It is the purpose of this chapter to give the ED provider some basic information that will help dissipate some of the concerns and fears and will provide some explanations for the stories that circulate through the medical ED circle.

With the formation of the American College of Emergency Physicians (ACEP) in 1968, the ED gained recognition not only as a clinical specialty but also as an academic discipline. As such, some 10 years later, the word "room" was dropped and the discipline matured into a full "academic department."

The first emergency medicine residency training program was established at the University of Cincinnati in 1970, and 12 years later, the Accreditation Council for Graduate Medical Education approved the specific requirements for emergency medicine training programs. In keeping with this philosophy, the physician assistant (PA) profession has, from its inception, required emergency medicine education as part of the curriculum. Additionally, postgraduate residency programs for those PAs who desire more training in this specialty have been developed.

The emergency department (ED) health care philosophy has changed over the past 30 years. The ED is now viewed more as the property of the community at large than as a for-profit medical facility providing a specifically designed service. Some patients view the ED as an outpatient or family practice walk-in clinic rather than a true ED. Because of this attitude, some patients may perceive their problem as urgent and feel that their presence in the ED is sufficient to categorize their complaint as an emergency. Additionally, ED personnel adhere to an unwritten law that "the patient defines the emergency," regardless of the true nature of the illness or injury. To accommodate these attitudes and to take care not to injure a patient, EDs are open 24 hours a day, 7 days a week, 365 days a year. In view of this changing attitude, ED personnel have had to adjust their treatment philosophy to handle the increased patient load. To meet this increased demand, hospital-based EDs began to employ full-time emergency medicine physicians to staff their EDs. As this practice became more prevalent, a few visionary physicians formed organizations to provide emergency services on a contract basis and began to hire physicians to support these contracts.

PRINCIPLES OF EMERGENCY MEDICINE

The emergency medicine approach to patient care is an important concept to understand because it is unique within the health care system. It is primarily a *complaint-oriented* rather than a *disease-specific* specialty. The objective is to focus on the single most important reason the patient has reported to the ED. This philosophy may, at times, seem uncaring, but it is necessary for quick, correct treatment and the smooth functioning of the ED. The provider must be able to get to the "bottom line" as quickly as possible, rule out life- or limb-threatening conditions, and complete the patient's stay in the ED in a timely fashion.

To aid in decision-making, the ACEP and the emergency medical system (EMS) established some general principles governing the practice of emergency medicine. This set of principles can be found in some form or another in all the classic emergency medicine texts.[1] Practitioners and students routinely exercise these principles in developing a foundation in emergency medicine that will aid in their approach to all patients seen in the ED.

Triage

Triage is the sorting of patients according to their specific health care needs and matching those needs with the ability of a specific ED to provide that care. Most EDs are equipped to treat any patients regardless of the complaint. However, those who cannot be treated in a given ED are stabilized and transferred, usually by ambulance or helicopter, to a medical center that can better serve their condition.

General Emergency Department Principles

Unfortunately, many of the patients seen in the ED do not conform to an established algorithm, which usually leaves the health care provider frustrated and confused. The following general principles were established to give the provider some basis to start the evaluation when a patient enters the ED. These principles should be used as *guidelines only*.

1. **Identify a life-threatening condition.** The moment the patient presents to the ED, the possibility of a life-threatening condition must be ruled out. This attitude is deliberately cultivated by health care providers in emergency medicine. The patient is considered unstable until demonstrated otherwise, usually by history, physical examination, and laboratory evaluation (e.g., electrocardiography [ECG], radiographs, blood studies). Health care providers in the ED must be able to identify those patients in need of immediate lifesaving intervention, must be able to initiate those measures, and must solicit the assistance of all ED staff in stabilizing the patient to reverse a life-threatening condition.
2. **Stabilize a life-threatening condition.** This is the mandate for prehospital care through the EMS, as well as all ED personnel. How this is done is usually as individual as the patients themselves. Stabilizing measures are the subject of courses in advanced cardiac life support (ACLS) and advanced trauma life support (ATLS), as well as of the paramedic manual and the first third of most ED textbooks. ACLS and ATLS courses are open to most midlevel practitioners and play a leading role in initial lifesaving management of an unstable patient. The role of the midlevel practitioner in this setting can vary from one ED to another and from one supervising physician to another, but the learned lifesaving measures are standard and reliable with any unstable patient. All ED health care providers should be certified in ACLS at the minimum.
3. **Find an explanation for the life-threatening condition.** Once the patient is stable, the health care provider should develop a differential diagnosis for the condition and coexistent disease that may still result in a life-threatening consequence. Once this has been initiated, the health care provider can then consider other medical needs of the patient. When this phase begins, the patient can be considered truly stable.
4. **Recognize coexistent pathology.** This may be related to the original complaint, or it may be an incidental finding during the history and physical examination. For example, the patient who has been seen in the ED on numerous occasions for alcohol abuse may have other alcohol-related disease that will need follow-up after the patient has been discharged from the ED.
5. **Determine why the patient has presented *now* rather than earlier or later.** The answer to this question may reveal a great deal about the course of the patient's pathology and may present important information about the patient's mental, physical, emotional, and social reserves for dealing with illness. Consider the following examples.

CASE STUDY 22-1

A patient with known coronary artery disease experiences daily angina and presents by ambulance to the ED. The usual questions on character of pain, location, radiation, and duration fail to reveal any difference in this episode of chest pain from the patient's usual experience of angina. Further questioning reveals that the patient has experienced three episodes of numbness and weakness of the right arm over the past 2 hours. The review of systems may have revealed these new symptoms, but direct questions such as, "What is different now?" and "What made you call the ambulance?" can give the patient an avenue for short-circuiting the usual pattern of questions.

CASE STUDY 22-2

A woman who has had a vaginal discharge for 2 weeks reports to the ED because "that's when she could get a babysitter for her children and a ride to the hospital."

CASE STUDY 22-3

Another patient reports to the ED with difficulty breathing. When questioned, he relates that he has lost his job and has run out of his seizure medication and cannot afford a refill.

In each case, the health care provider should be able to follow a clear sequence of events that logically led the patient to the ED door. If this is not clear, the provider should ask, "Why now?"

6. **Address the patient's symptoms.** Every effort should be made to relieve the patient's complaint whether by medication or by treatment (e.g., suturing a laceration or simple reassurance). If, however, the patient's symptoms cannot be relieved in the ED, the patient may need hospitalization or referral to another physician whose specialty may include the patient's findings. *Every patient leaving the ED should have the name of a physician who has been identified to follow up his or her complaint.*
7. **Consider the necessity for determining a diagnosis before the patient leaves the ED.** To the disappointment of patients and the health care provider, some patients leave the ED with no definitive diagnosis. The health care provider can make every effort to find the cause of the patient's complaint, but in some cases, it is just impossible. What the patient should receive in these cases is an explanation of the diseases and conditions that have been ruled out. Consider the patient with painless vaginal bleeding. She may leave the ED knowing that she is not pregnant, she is not anemic, she does not have a readily identifiable disease, and she has a follow-up appointment the next day with a gynecologist, but no definitive diagnosis. Each ED patient should be informed of what has been discovered about his or her condition and what remains to be investigated; he or she should be reassured that the condition is not life threatening, told what can be done for the symptoms, and be informed of where the patient should go to pursue a diagnosis if one has not been rendered.
8. **Decide on the patient's disposition.** Can hospitalization provide more of the patient's needs than an outpatient setting at this time? How will follow-up be accomplished? Does the ED have the resources for the necessary follow-up? What is the worst-case scenario of the patient's condition if the patient is lost to follow-up? These questions should have answers, and the patient or the patient's family must have a clear understanding of "where to go from here," if necessary.
9. **Discuss the ED course and the plan for follow-up with the patient and his or her family.** What are the patient's expectations? Have they been met? Patients need to know that the health care provider has understood their concerns and expectations. Each patient should be given the opportunity to ask questions and participate in his or her own health care. The patient should be told what to anticipate from the therapy prescribed, what type of adverse effects to expect, if any, and when and where to obtain needed follow-up.
10. **Record the entire visit in the patient's record.** Document *all* the information gathered during the patient's stay in the ED. Remember, the health care provider is responsible for knowing the information in the nursing record as well.

It is quickly obvious that patients' reasons for coming to the ED are many and varied. Although patients may label their medical problems as "emergencies," only a small percentage of visits to an ED fit that medical definition. Medical emergencies fall into three commonly recognized categories—*critical*, *acute*, and *urgent*.

Critical or life-threatening emergencies are those that require reversal of the pathologic state within minutes in order to prevent the patient's death—for example, cardiac arrest, airway obstruction, or severe hemorrhage.

Acute emergencies are conditions that will deteriorate into critical emergencies if therapy is not instituted within the first hour of the patient's presenting to the ED—for example, pulmonary edema, acute asthma, or ruptured ectopic pregnancy.

Urgent emergencies can be described as disease processes or injuries that have the potential to progress to life-threatening conditions, if untreated. This category includes pneumonia with hypoxia, small-bowel obstruction, testicular torsion, acetaminophen overdose, acute glaucoma, and periorbital cellulitis. The provider who is geared psychologically and educationally to take care of "emergencies" only will be at odds with the patient who comes to the ED with a nonemergent complaint.

Role of Midlevel Health Care Providers in the Emergency Department

Midlevel practitioners—PAs and NPs—work not only with a variety of patients but also with a combination of other physician-supervisors, nurses, clerks, and consultants. They must possess a great deal of tact and skill in communicating and in coordinating patients' care with these other caregivers and providers. In emergency medicine, as in medicine in general, there may be several ways to treat a given disease process. Because the patient is always referred to another physician for follow-up, the patient's care becomes the responsibility of more than one provider. The EDA must be able to balance a variety of therapeutics and referring physicians' preferences and remain an advocate for the individual patient's circumstances. Also, the PA should become familiar with each physician on the referral list so that when the patient reports for follow-up, all pertinent information (i.e., history, physical examination, laboratory tests, radiograph results plus any specific tests unique to the referred physician) is present in the patient's record.

One of the attractions of ED work for PAs is the lack of predictability. The flow of patients is variable, and the diagnoses and complaints are equally challenging. The PA is in the unique position to learn from everyone, especially the patients. The following examples illustrate this axiom. A patient who speaks only Russian may be on adequate therapy for gastritis despite the fact that the tablets are unfamiliar and the writing on the bottle is in Russian. The sickle cell patient who knows his disease and symptoms reports that morphine and not meperidine (Demerol) works better for a painful crisis. If a patient's chief complaint is chest pain, regardless of the patient's age, cardiac disease must be ruled out. Making a diagnosis may be only part of the job; discovering the patient's "agenda" is equally important.

The role of the PA in emergency medicine is evolving, and practice will continue to vary from academic, urban-based emergency medicine to rural, single-coverage sites. In 1990, the ACEP published the following position statement on the use of PAs in emergency medicine: "The PA is called on to be flexible as well in his or her role in the ED. Sometimes a leader, but always a member of the health care team, a PA needs to communicate well on all levels."[2] The PA who continues to work in emergency medicine will grow in clinical knowledge and find variations in treatment modalities for each individual patient. At each level, from student to experienced emergency clinician, the PA needs to identify resources within and outside the department to complement his or her skills.

PAs are currently providing services in a variety of positions within EDs, including those in prehospital patient care, patient triage, and patient care within the ED, as well as selective administrative functions. To further assist its members, ACEP has developed the following guidelines regarding the role of PAs in EDs that are open and staffed 24 hours a day by emergency physicians.[3] These guidelines should not be interpreted as mandatory by legislative, judicial, or regulatory bodies or by the ACEP.

1. PAs should be placed in clinical and administrative situations where they will supplement, but not replace, the medical expertise and patient care provided by emergency physicians.
2. PAs should work clinically under the supervision of an emergency physician who is physically present in the ED, who evaluates the care of each patient, and who assumes ultimate responsibility for the patient. The number of PAs whose clinical work can be simultaneously supervised by one emergency physician must be defined.
3. The PA's scope of practice must be clearly delineated. Minimally, this delineation should include the following:
   a. A description of the PA's role and responsibilities in the ED.
   b. A listing of the types of patients and conditions the PA has credentials to treat.
   c. A listing of the types of patients and conditions the PA may not treat.
   d. A listing of the types of patients and conditions that require immediate consultation with the supervising emergency physician.
   e. A listing of the procedures the PA may perform before or after consultation with the emergency physician, and those he or she may perform only under the direct supervision of the emergency physician.
4. Credentialing procedures must be specifically stated and should be similar to those required of other allied health professionals. All ED PAs should be nationally certified or should meet the requirements of the state or federal jurisdiction in which they function.
5. The medical director of the ED or a designee has the responsibility for providing the overall direction of the activities of the PA in the ED.
6. PAs working in EDs should have or acquire specific experience or specialty training in emergency medicine. They should receive a supervised orientation program, preferably by

the medical director of the ED and appropriate training and continuing education in emergency medicine. They should also acquire knowledge of specific ED policies and procedures. Additionally, PAs must be aware of and participate in the quality-assurance activities of the ED.

7. There should be a written contract that clearly addresses all of the items previously listed and other standard contractual issues.

Fast Track

To meet the increasing demands of the community and to accommodate the changing philosophies of emergency medicine, many of the busiest EDs have created an "Urgent Care Clinic" or a "Fast Track" within the physical confines of the ED. These areas are specifically designed for the treatment of minor injuries or illnesses that do not require the full services of the ED. EDs that are treating more than 2000 patients a month have discovered that setting aside one or two beds that are used solely for this designation can greatly relieve the congestion in waiting rooms where patients have had to wait sometimes 4 to 6 hours for treatment of a simple laceration.

The fast track area has traditionally been located in a region of the ED that previously was used only for overflow on busy nights or a back room or a wide hallway converted to a treatment area by adding a few beds and some curtains. In newer EDs, this area may be physically set apart from the regular ED and occasionally may even have its own entrances and waiting rooms. This fast track area has become the domain of the PA for the treatment of minor, uncomplicated diseases and injuries.

The types of patients seen and treated in a fast track vary, but some of the more common diagnoses are sprains, simple fractures, simple lacerations, uncomplicated otitis media, colds, cough, sore throat, bronchitis, ingrown toenails, foreign body in the foot or hand, low back pain, abscessed tooth, uncomplicated urinary tract infection, rashes, minor cellulitis, uncomplicated diarrhea, insect bites, minor dog bites, first- and second-degree burns, simple abscesses, poison ivy rash, motor vehicle accident with minor injuries brought to the ED for evaluation, and aches and pains from shoulders to feet.

In all of these cases, the PA in the fast track has the ability to upgrade a patient from fast track to full ED if the patient's condition warrants more complicated treatment or additional evaluation. The most valuable asset to the ED with a fast track is a good triage nurse who can spot a potentially bad situation and route that patient to the main ED for appropriate treatment.

PA Student in the Emergency Department

The emergency medicine rotation is usually one of the most enjoyable for the PA student, regardless of the intended future direction of his or her career. The student is likely to see a variety of patients and diseases. Additionally, the student learns by being available to listen to the many presentations made by other team members to the supervising physician. Typically in an academic institution, the PA student has more contact with the staff physician and the senior emergency resident than on any other inpatient service. This is a distinct advantage when performing procedures, correlating laboratory results with clinical presentation, confirming physical findings, and interpreting imaging studies. The staff physician and the senior resident provide guidance and suggestions that are unavailable in textbooks, especially during treatment, and referral options based on their accumulated clinical experience.

As a PA student gains skill in the practice of emergency medicine, it may help to identify staff members who will encourage and support the development of the PA's clinical judgment and who will also endorse the expansion of his or her responsibilities in the ED. The relationship between the emergency medicine physician and the emergency medicine PA must be based on mutual trust of each other's integrity and abilities.

It is impossible to generalize about the role of the PA student in a particular ED. However, the following suggestions may help make the experience smoother and more meaningful:

1. Identify the immediate supervisor.
2. Are there protocols restricting the type of patients PA students can or cannot see?
3. At what point in the workup should the student present the case to the supervisor?
4. What are the protocols for unstable patients?
5. What laboratory studies may the PA student order without first consulting the supervisor?
6. When do PA student orders have to be cosigned?
7. At the end of the shift, to whom does the PA student report?

The PA student should keep in mind that each rotation is not just an opportunity to learn a different branch of medicine but a chance to evaluate each field for possible employment. It is also a time to reflect on that specialty's approach to the patient, the pace and rhythm of the discipline's work, and its present and potential utilization of PAs.

Who's Who in the Emergency Department

Personnel in Table 22-1 might be found in a hospital-based ED with a level I trauma center and an associated residency training program with elaborate social services support. The ED in a small rural community will have a completely different makeup (i.e., minimal staffing of a physician or midlevel practitioner and a nurse). Most EDs fall somewhere between these two extremes. The role and functions of a PA in the ED are affected by the types and numbers of other providers. The PA may work with a single physician and split the patients according to severity, or he or she may be required to see all patients and then present the findings to a staff physician whose only function is to consult and advise.

TABLE 22-1 **Emergency Department Personnel**

Providers	**Caregivers**	
Staff physicians who supervise	Charge nurses	
Residents	Primary RN supervisor	
Midlevels	Nursing assistants	
Medical and PA students	Nursing students	
Consultants		
Private primary care providers		
Physician specialists		
Nonphysician therapists		
Ancillary Personnel		
PREHOSPITAL	IN-HOSPITAL	POSTHOSPITAL
EMS personnel	Unit clerks	Chemical dependency units
Security	Social services	Shelters
Poison control	Translators	
Chaplains		

EMS, emergency medical service; PA, physician assistant; RN, registered nurse.

Residents

The presence of physician residents adds another dimension to an ED practice. A full-time emergency department PA can provide consistency and stability in a department that is in constant change with rotating interns and residents. The PA who has been employed in an academic ED for any length of time must now take on the additional task of teacher.

Primary Care Providers. Community primary care providers and specialists play a significant role in the smooth functioning of all EDs. Ideally, each patient should have a primary care physician or clinic where they usually seek their first medical treatment. Additionally, every primary care physician expects to see his or her patients after an ED visit. Specialists, on the other hand, depend on consults from the ED staff. All of this requires a tremendous amount of communication. Regardless of the care given in the ED, it is important that the ED professional staff stresses the continuing role of the primary care physician and encourages the patient to return to his or her primary care physician as soon as possible after an ED visit.

Specialists. The determination of when to consult a specialist and who presents the patient to the specialist is not clearly delineated in most EDs. Some specialists want to talk only to the ED physician; others want to talk to the provider who has done the workup on the patient. There are many unwritten protocols that the emergency care provider must be made aware of as he or she learns the resources and habits of physicians in the practice community, most of which will be learned on the job.

Nursing Staff. The ED does not run without its nursing staff. Nurses are vital to the smooth functioning of the department. They usually spend more time with the patient than anyone else, including the provider. They are one of the few constants in a department in which provider turnover is the rule. ED nurses have a wealth of knowledge and experience that can be useful to all providers. Occasionally, the technical functions of the PA and a nurse overlap. This is probably truer in small EDs. Because of this, communication within the team is essential. The PA who works closely with the nursing staff in providing patient care will maintain a good productive relationship that contributes to the smooth running of the ED.

PROBLEM-ORIENTED HISTORY AND PHYSICAL EXAMINATION

The ED history and physical examination are reviewed and refined to support the overall concept of the ED. Because of this, most ED charts have a small space reserved for the admitting problem and physical findings associated with that problem. Brevity, without compromise of important facts and findings, is the rule.

History

There is nothing intrinsically difficult or different about obtaining a history from a patient in the ED. It is important to discern early what the determining factor was that required the patient to seek treatment in the ED. The importance of the chief complaint (CC) takes on a new meaning because that is the problem that will be addressed by the ED staff. Those patients with multiple problems or chronic diseases who have acute exacerbation of their symptoms (e.g., sickle cell crises) are usually referred to their primary care physician once it has been determined that the ED has addressed and treated any immediate complication to their chronic existing problems.

The initial interview concerning the patient's CC should take place as soon as possible after the patient reports to the ED. It must be determined early in the patient's workup whether the complaint is a new problem or an exacerbation of an old illness. If this is an old complaint, the previous history regarding any prior diagnosis, treatment, and its effectiveness must be documented. The importance of this information should be emphasized to avoid the possibility of additional blood tests, radiographs, or a hospital admission. Too often, a patient waits until discharge and announces, "That's what the last doctor did and it didn't help."

There are some significant differences between the history of an injury and the history of a medical complaint. The cause of an injury may be as significant as the injury itself. Consider the following: A patient presenting with a broken wrist from a fall on the ice is treated differently from a patient who fainted, fell on the ice, and broke his or her wrist. In the second case, the injury to the wrist becomes secondary until the cause of the syncope episode is investigated. Patients who cannot give a history of an injury because of intoxication or decreased level of consciousness must be suspected of having occult serious pathology.

The time elapsed after an injury is another important factor, especially in cases of lacerations or fractures. Some wounds are left to heal secondarily if too much time has elapsed between the injury and the patient's reporting to the ED.

The mechanism of injury and a description of the instrument causing the injury should be recorded whenever possible. This information may help in selection of initial treatment by revealing the amount of tissue damage and the potential for infection at a later date.

Additional pertinent information that is dependent on the chief complaint is equally important to ascertain (e.g., Which is the dominant extremity of a patient with an injury to an arm or hand? Does the patient with bronchitis smoke? In the case of a dog bite, how was the dog acting at the time the patient was bitten? Has the dog bitten more than one person? Where is the dog now?) The patient also needs a tetanus immunization. Other crucial information includes a history of allergies, chronic diseases such as diabetes, chronic renal failure, hypertension, or peptic ulcer disease; anything that may have an implication or that might cloud the issue of the patient's chief complaint should be recorded.

The ED PA must often rely on sources of information other than the patient to obtain an entire history. Non–English-speaking patients need a translator. The patient with altered mental status needs additional sources for information on the family—primary care provider, an old chart, or any other hospitals or medical agencies where the patient may have been treated. In some instances, ED personnel may know the patient and can provide valuable input regarding their condition. Occasionally, simultaneous treatment and obtaining a history may take place. For example, a patient with an acute exacerbation of asthma may feel more comfortable answering questions while receiving a breathing treatment.

Physical Examination

The first data recorded in the physical examination are the patient's vital signs. The supervising physician in the ED should be made aware of all patients with significantly abnormal vital signs as soon as they are obtained. What constitutes significantly abnormal vital signs occupies chapters in emergency medicine textbooks and encompasses 90% of the course of study of emergency medical technicians (EMTs) and paramedics. Serial vital signs, those taken every 5 to 10 minutes, are an important indicator of the patient's response to treatment. These, plus the patient's general appearance, may provide an overall picture of the patient's medical condition.

The next statement should include the patient's level of awareness and orientation. "Alert and oriented times three" means patients are aware of the following:

1. Who they are
2. Where they are
3. What has happened to them

Additionally, a general psychological statement using well-defined phrases such as *cooperative*, *anxious*, or *hostile* may set the tone for the patient's examination. The speech pattern or content, the manner of dress, and the patient's personal hygiene should all be documented.

The following two examples illustrate what may appear in the patient's chart during workup.

CASE STUDY 22-4

Mrs. Jones is a 42-year-old woman appearing older than her stated age who smells unwashed, looks disheveled, and is wearing multiple layers of filthy clothing, including a parka in the month of August. She stated she was homeless and living on the street. After initial observation, the health care provider assesses the patient's mental, physical, and emotional capacity and how well she is dealing with her environment. Her chief complaint is observed as a mild cellulitis of the left foot. Determining that she is not diabetic and that her tetanus is up to date, the health care provider prescribes the appropriate treatment for her cellulitis and advises her to elevate her foot for 3 days. The health care provider then addresses the circumstance that put the patient at risk for this illness and determines that it may be impossible for her to comply with the treatment because she is homeless.

For children, the provider must substitute interactions, verbalizations, and spontaneous activities for the mental status and psychiatric examinations normally obtained in an adult.

CASE STUDY 22-5

A 3-year-old girl enters the ED with her mother and baby sister. The patient smells unwashed, looks disheveled, and is dressed in dirty shorts, T-shirt, and no shoes. It is August, and the ED is located in a small town. The mother reports that the child has a fever and is complaining of ear pain. The mother is neatly and appropriately dressed for the weather. The second child, a baby, is clean, dressed in diapers, and asleep on the mother's shoulder. Meanwhile, the 3-year-old spends time alternating between whining and resting her head on the mother's knee or actively tearing up the waiting room. The health care provider should not have the same concerns with the appearance of this patient as he or she would have for the patient in Case Study 22-4. Unkempt and dirty can be considered the natural state of a 3-year-old during the summer months. The presence of the mother and the other sibling, as well as the patient's interaction with the mother, gives invaluable clues on the coping mechanisms and relationships of this patient to the family.

Another area of pertinent information about patients in the ED is their comfort or pain level. Some phrases that are commonly used to describe this include the following: no distress, no pain with normal gait and stance, moderate respiratory distress, uncomfortable with movement, writhing during examination.

Finally, the hydration and nutrition status of the patient should be assessed. This is especially important in geriatric and pediatric populations. Neither elderly nor very young patients tolerate dehydration well; prompt intervention with intravenous (IV) fluids may be needed before a full assessment can take place. IV fluids may be initiated in the early phase of any ED visit while other causes for the patient's condition are being considered.

The remainder of the physical examination is based on the differential diagnosis generated during the history. A thorough examination of the system within which the chief complaint originated must be performed; "abdominal pain," for instance, demands an examination of all contiguous areas, including the chest, the pelvis, and the back. There are many causes for abdominal pain, and if the answer is not forthcoming in the routine examination, the diagnosis may be found in remote areas (e.g., the thyroid gland or a spider bite on an extremity). A chief complaint of dizziness requires examination of the cardiovascular system, the neurologic system, the visual system, and the vestibular system.

Once the history and physical examination have been completed, a differential diagnosis or working diagnosis is established. Constant reassessment and reexamination may change the working diagnosis or may confirm the original diagnosis; studies usually aid in this determination.

Laboratory Tests

The health care provider must remain cognizant of the need for a diagnosis when ordering laboratory tests and medical imaging studies. A minimum amount of testing combined with the history and physical examination may offer the diagnosis. However, some questions need to be considered before any laboratory testing is ordered.

- **Will the test results provide additional information for determining the patient's diagnosis and treatment?** For example, an otherwise healthy 4-year-old child is brought to the ED with a temperature of 101.8°F (38.8°C) and is pulling at his ear. Physical examination reveals a bulging, red tympanic membrane. The diagnosis is made by history and physical examination. A complete blood count (CBC) shows a mildly elevated white blood cell count (WBC), which does not alter the diagnosis or the treatment.
- **Will laboratory test results alter the workup or treatment of the patient?** The same patient

with a minimally elevated WBC count may not need antibiotics, and the patient with a markedly higher WBC count may need to be admitted to the hospital for IV antibiotic therapy.

- **Will the results of the tests be back before the patient leaves the ED?** Consider the following:

CASE STUDY 22-6

A 21-year-old man reports to the ED with a simple, uncomplicated laceration to his forearm. During the history, the patient reveals that he has had a 15-lb weight loss over the past 6 months and occasionally some bloody diarrhea. He requests an HIV test. Should this be considered part of the treatment for his laceration? It seems clinically indicated by his history. The facility has the ability to do an HIV test, but the results will not be back before the patient is discharged. Is it the ED's responsibility to act on the results? Is there a mechanism within the ED for follow-up of a patient with serious pathologic laboratory test results? In this case, the patient could be better served in an outpatient setting by a primary care provider.

- **Do the laboratory test results need interpretation that the ED cannot provide?** The ED physician is responsible for the initial interpretation of radiographs. However, the overall interpretation of the entire radiographic study for liability issues should be performed by a licensed radiologist. Most ED physicians will overread a radiograph and treat the patient conservatively rather than wait for an interpretation by the radiologist the next day.
- **Will the laboratory test results aid in the patient's follow-up care?** ED health care providers make it a priority to know each individual consultant and the specific laboratory tests they may favor. Additionally, the ED provider often orders these tests and will have the results before the consultant sees the patient. Community practices vary widely in mechanisms and protocol for obtaining outpatient imaging studies from the ED. However, acting in the patient's best interest and efficiently with the local system may dictate that the laboratory test should be initiated in the ED.

The ED record is a chronologic summary of the patient from the occurrence of the injury or start of the illness to the patient's discharge or release from the ED. It should contain a complete history of the activity of the patient while in the ED. A good format to follow is the subjective, objective, assessment, and plan (SOAP) note. Many laboratory tests are available to most hospital-based EDs. However, only a few of these tests are commonly performed in EDs. The following list indicates those tests that have proved to be the most cost-effective in revealing the broadest range of relevant information in the shortest amount of time.

Diagnostic Tests Commonly Ordered in the Emergency Department

1. CBC with differential and indices.
2. Electrolytes, including blood urea nitrogen, creatinine, and Ca^{2+}.
3. Arterial blood gas with O_2 saturation.
4. Carbon monoxide level.
5. Urinalysis.
6. Pregnancy test (urine or serum).
7. Lipase and amylase.
8. Wet prep and potassium chloride (KOH) level of vaginal secretions.
9. Serum levels of drugs (e.g., acetaminophen, theophylline, phenytoin).
10. Gram's stain and cell count of various body fluids (e.g., cerebrospinal fluid, joint fluid).

THE COMMUNITY

It is extremely useful for the health care provider in the ED to know the community in which the ED is located and the specific population it serves. Occasionally, the ED provider may be unable to address some of the patient's complaints because of a lack of understanding concerning the culture and background in which the patient resides. A knowledge of the community allows the health care provider to appreciate disease patterns and predilections with regard to race, geography, and socioeconomic status. This type of preparation expands the differential diagnosis of patients to include those diseases that are more prevalent in each distinct community.

Another significant factor affecting both the types of diseases and the volume of patients using the ED for their primary health care is the fluctuation of the local economy. Health insurance plays a major role for these patients. Any loss of benefits may result in an increased number of patients who cannot afford to visit a family physician. Even worse, such a loss may cause the patient to delay seeking medical treatment until illness is much more advanced, placing an even greater stress on the health care system. A number of studies have been done to attempt to correlate various economic factors with ED use. Brunette and coworkers[4] investigated the timing of the volume of 911 calls to the distribution of the welfare checks in Hennepin County, Minnesota. They also looked at the numbers of patients served in the Hennepin County Medical Center ED, the numbers of patients admitted to the county alcohol receiving center (ARC), and the admissions to the Hennepin County jail around the time of the check dispersal. This study revealed a significant drop in these volumes of patients as the number of days elapsed after the checks were distributed. The authors noted that the largest volume recorded was an increase in ARC admissions. ED volume and the number of Hennepin County ambulance runs were also significantly increased at check dispersal and tapered off as time elapsed. The authors were careful to point out, however, that a cause-and-effect relationship had not been established with these data, and they could only speculate on the possible relationship of increased cash flow with an increased consumption of alcohol. Some of the major factors affecting a health care provider's understanding of the cultural attitudes toward health, disease, and therapeutics follow:

- Economic status
- Religious beliefs
- Ethnic and racial background
- Social differences

An appreciation of what sickness is and how it relates to these factors in each different group can aid the ED provider in prescribing those therapies that will result in the successful treatment of each individual patient.

ROLE OF THE EMERGENCY DEPARTMENT WITHIN THE HEALTH CARE SYSTEM

Regardless of the size of the ED or the type of hospital it serves, the ED usually functions as an independent clinic where patients are admitted and discharged by ED personnel alone. Other departments of the hospital depend on the ED to properly triage sick and injured patients and stabilize those patients who may require further hospitalization. Each department usually has an agreement or a protocol for the joint management of the patient in the ED. These protocols are as individual as the hospital, and the provider must make every effort to stabilize the patient according to established protocols before transferring the patient to the hospital ward. Certain types of patients, such as major trauma victims, unstable pediatric patients, or pregnant women with other medical conditions, may be best handled by those specific departments, and communication with that department is the most important factor in the initial management of those patients.

The ED operates under both internally and externally imposed mandates. ED providers can serve as gatekeepers to admittance of patients to the rest of the hospital. They are expected to handle an ever-changing set of circumstances and a random stream of patients exhibiting a random set of medical illnesses that may or may not result in specific diagnosis and treatment. They protect vulnerable patients, act as the medical witness in matters of litigious personal injury, and assume leadership in disaster management. The ED is responsible for maintaining acceptable standards of quality assurance in patient care. If the hospital participates in training programs, the ED may also be required to provide an education for physicians, PAs, nurses, EMTs, and paramedics.

Most hospitals that support the ED have plans for dealing with unstable medical or major trauma patients. Often hospitals use a "code team" to respond to cardiac arrests within the institution; this may mean that physicians from the ED participate in those codes. Specified members of this team are alerted when patients requiring stabilization or resuscitation are identified.

Ideally, the PA is part of a code team. In a busy ED where more than one resuscitation may be conducted at a time, the PA may be called on to "run" the code. All PAs working in emergency medicine should be ACLS certified and must be able to direct a code according to those protocols. Most PAs, however, will find themselves working in a department with experienced physicians, nurses, and paramedics. They will have the opportunity to participate in numerous resuscitations and learn the variations on the ACLS theme before they are asked to run a code.

The principles taught in advanced trauma life support (ATLS) are invaluable in the organized approach to a critically injured patient. Certification in ATLS is not available to PAs; however, all PAs working in an emergency setting are strongly encouraged to take advantage of this course. ATLS principles and skills are an invaluable tool for recognizing physical findings and initiating proper treatment to help stabilize the patient.

It has been the experience of many PAs working in the ED that their skills in managing minor trauma (e.g., simple lacerations) are extremely valuable. If there is a niche for PAs in the ED, this seems to be it. Here, PAs tend to shine clinically. They provide a high degree of quality care with speed and accuracy. This ability is extremely desirable in many health care settings, from busy metropolitan EDs with multiple-provider coverage to rural health care clinics where the PA may work alone. Consequently, this allows the physician the latitude to concentrate on other tasks.

Disaster management from earthquake preparedness to toxic decontamination control is an important aspect of today's industrialized world. Disaster management is already a structured entity within most towns and urban centers. In place are designated disaster offices and volunteer teams and protocols that involve many different community service organizations such as fire, civil defense, hazardous waste management, and search and rescue teams. It is inevitable that the ED, including the prehospital team, will be an intrinsic part of a disaster response separate from the emergency management of individual patients. The PA may well have a place on the team, especially if he or she is willing to play a different role than in the ED. If the PA develops an interest in these areas, he or she might be in a position to provide a unique service to the community in conjunction with the disaster relief team. A member of such a team can expect instruction in disaster management principles and an orientation to the highly choreographed response to various possible disaster scenarios.

The ED that hosts an emergency medicine residency program is ripe with opportunities for the experienced PA in teaching and conducting and participating in clinical research. Students, interns, and emergency medicine residents enter the department with widely varying experience in ED procedures. An experienced PA working in an emergency setting is in an ideal position to teach procedures such as suturing, IV access techniques, immobilization and casting techniques, orthopedic procedures, abscess and wound care management, and use of specialized equipment. The PA has the opportunity to acquaint new residents and students with the accepted standards of practice regarding the techniques and supervision of ED procedures. More importantly, the PA has the obligation to educate these new health care providers to the PA concept, PA practice, and the role of the PA in emergency medicine.

Patient follow-up is traditionally a weak link in emergency medicine. Once the patient leaves the ED, the emergency clinician usually hears from or about the patient again only if there is a complication. Because EDs were originally conceived of for a one-time visit for an unstable patient, follow-up was an unaccustomed bonus for a physician wishing to see the final result of his or her treatment. Today, many patients depend on the ED for their primary health care, and follow-up has become a legal and practical dilemma for all EDs. The use of PAs for patient follow-up and call-back is widening. Occasionally, PAs are employed in EDs strictly for follow-up of abnormal laboratory values or radiograph-reading discrepancies. Some departments use midlevel providers to review charts for completeness and adherence to predetermined protocols. Different EDs have different follow-up needs, but again, because of their temporal stability and familiarity with department protocols, procedures, and resources, PAs are excellent candidates for organizing and staffing a follow-up program.

In 1990, Beth Israel Medical Center published an overview of its 8-year experience with PAs in the ED.[5] One of the unique features of the Beth Israel ED was the emphasis on patient follow-up. All the PAs employed in the ED participated in quality assurance chart reviews and in recontacting a statistically select group of patients for a follow-up phone call and revisit if indicated.

Ideally, the ED should function as the patient's health care source for only a short period of time. That often means that the ED provider may not know what happens to the patient when he or she leaves the department. Even with the best intentions and best follow-up instructions, the ED loses track of patients. Because the ED staff does not establish an ongoing relationship with the patients they treat, they must be able to tolerate a lack of closure both intellectually and emotionally.

The next section of this chapter is designed to give a new provider in the ED some practical information and "how-to" tools for evaluating some of the more common complaints that are seen in most busy EDs today. These are meant as guidelines only. For treatment of wounds and specifics on laceration repair, please refer to Chapter 11.

GENERAL APPROACH TO THE EVALUATION OF ABDOMINAL PAIN

The approach to the patient with abdominal pain involves a directed history, a complete physical examination, selected laboratory tests, and selected radiographic procedures.

History. The history should include the following:

- Description of the pain—onset, duration, quality, radiation, exacerbating and relieving factors
- Prior similar pain
- Gastrointestinal symptoms, including vomiting, diarrhea, last normal bowel movement, appetite, food intolerance
- Urinary tract symptoms—dysuria, frequency, hematuria
- Gynecologic review—last normal menstrual period, gravida and para status, number of abortions and miscarriages, discharge, dyspareunia

- Prior abdominal surgery
- Prior diagnostic evaluations—upper gastrointestinal series, barium enema, intravenous pyelogram (IVP), ultrasound, computed tomography (CT)

Physical Examination. The physical examination should be head to toe and should include a rectal examination with a stool guaiac and a pelvic examination for women with lower abdominal pain.

Laboratory Studies. The laboratory evaluation involves selection from a menu of laboratory and radiograph studies depending on clinical impressions from the history and physical examination. The laboratory menu includes CBC, urinalysis (UA), SMA-7, aspartate transaminase (AST), alanine aminotransferase (ALT), bilirubin (total, direct, indirect), alkaline phosphatase (AP), amylase, and lipase. The x-ray menu includes flat plate abdomen, upright film abdomen, upright posteroanterior (PA) chest film for free air, ultrasound of the gallbladder and pelvis, and IVP and CT scan with double contrast (IVP dye and oral contrast).

Acute Cholecystitis

History. The patient presents with pain in the right upper quadrant that is of rapid onset and variable in character. The pain may be described as sharp, aching, or cramplike. It often radiates to the back and is usually accompanied by nausea with or without vomiting. Patients may have a history of similar episodes for some time in the past that lasted minutes to hours and often left them tender to touch for a few days. The pain may be brought on by eating fatty or greasy food.

Physical Examination. The hallmark is the physical examination, which reveals tenderness to palpation in the right upper quadrant of the abdomen. The tenderness may increase when the PA has the patient take a deep breath while palpating the right upper quadrant (Murphy's sign). The patient may also have epigastric tenderness, particularly if there is concomitant pancreatitis. The patient may be febrile.

Laboratory Studies. Laboratory evaluation should include CBC, UA, amylase and lipase, AP, bilirubin, AST, and ALT. Gallbladder disease is a leading cause of pancreatitis, the other common cause being alcohol. Eighty percent of gallstones are radiolucent, so a flat plate of the abdomen will show gallstones only 20% of the time. Ultrasound identifies gallstones reliably and is noninvasive. The definitive test for cholecystitis is the nuclear hepatoiminodiacetic acid (HIDA) scan. If the common bile duct becomes visible and the gallbladder does not, there is a functional obstruction in the cystic duct. Although ultrasound can detect gallstones, it does not detect obstruction of the cystic duct. The HIDA scan is particularly useful in differentiating appendicitis from cholecystitis.

Treatment. Patients with fever, complicating pancreatitis, or unremitting pain require admission to the hospital for IV fluids and parenteral antibiotics and analgesics. Patients who have normal laboratory studies, no fever, and bearable pain can be sent home with oral pain medication, next-day follow-up with a surgeon, and instructions to return immediately if the pain intensifies or fever occurs.

Ureteral Colic

History. Patients with ureteral colic present with a spectrum of pain. At one end is the patient who presents with severe pain in the right lower quadrant that is sharp and constant and may radiate to the costovertebral angle (CVA) area or the testicle on the same side. At the other end of the spectrum, the patient exhibits mild pain somewhere in the area stretching from the kidney down to the lower abdomen and into the testicle or vagina on the affected side.

Physical Examination. The patient is in marked distress—pale, diaphoretic, nauseated, and writhing on the examination table with pain. The hallmark of a stone is that in spite of the severe pain, tenderness is usually minimal. It may require careful questioning to establish that palpation really is not increasing the severity of the pain the patient is experiencing.

Laboratory Studies. Laboratory evaluation usually consists of a CBC, SMA-7, and routine UA with culture and sensitivity, if indicated. UA usually shows microscopic hematuria, unless the stone is completely blocking the ureter. An IVP is obtained to definitively diagnose the problem and guide management. All urine should be strained while the patient is undergoing evaluation in the ED, and any stone passed should be sent to the pathology laboratory for analysis.

Treatment. When the provider is confident from the patient's history and physical examination that he or she has a stone, an IV infusion with Ringer's lactate should be started. The patient may be given morphine sulfate IV in increments of 5 mg every 3 to 5 minutes or until the pain can be tolerated. The patient should also be given an IV antiemetic such as prochlorperazine (Compazine), 5 mg, or promethazine (Phenergan), 25 mg. IV ketorolac tromethamine (Toradol), 30 mg, is also effective in pain relief.

Indications for Admission. The indications for admission include the following:

1. Stone greater than 5 mm in size
2. Accompanying urinary tract infection requiring emergency urologic consultation for decompressive procedure
3. High-grade obstruction on IVP
4. Intractable pain (often accompanies high-grade obstruction)

The patient with a stone less than 5 mm in size without high-grade obstruction or accompanying infection, and without intractable pain, may go home. The patient should be given a urine strainer and should be instructed to strain all urine and save for analysis any stone passed regardless of size. The patient should also be given a potent oral analgesic (Lorcet 10 [hydrocodone 10 mg plus 650 mg of acetaminophen]) and should be told to return immediately if severe pain or fever develops. The patient should also be instructed to force fluids and to follow up with a urologist in 2 to 3 days with radiographs, laboratory results, and a copy of the ED record.

Appendicitis

History. Patients with appendicitis can be easy or difficult to diagnose. The patient who is easy to diagnose presents with a history of pain that was initially periumbilical and crampy, but within 12 to 24 hours, the pain localized in the right lower quadrant. The pain is worse with movement and is accompanied by nausea and anorexia. Unfortunately, many patients with appendicitis have atypical histories and their laboratory and radiograph findings do not fit the classic picture. The hallmark in these difficult cases is the consistent presence of tenderness in the right lower quadrant. Temperature can be normal, the patient can be hungry, and WBC counts can be normal. If the patient has consistent right lower quadrant tenderness and if a ureteral stone, as well as gynecologic pathology, have been ruled out, a surgical consult is warranted.

In many cases, the patient will have nonspecific abdominal pain with no clues for the diagnosis of appendicitis in the workup and still may turn out to have this problem. In any patient with abdominal pain of unknown cause whom the provider is electing to send home without a baseline examination by a surgeon, a follow-up examination in 6 to 12 hours is mandated. The patient should be instructed to return to the ED immediately if the pain worsens or localizes to the right lower quadrant.

Physical Examination. On physical examination, the patient has a mild fever and localized tenderness in the right lower quadrant at McBurney's point. Pressing deeply on the left side of the abdomen, which causes the patient to experience pain in the right lower quadrant, is a positive Rovsing's sign. Coughing intensifies right lower quadrant pain. A tap on the patient's heel also intensifies the pain, and the patient has tenderness on the right side on rectal examination.

Laboratory Studies. The patient's WBC count is usually more than 10,000/mm^3 but less than 15,000/mm^3 with a left shift. The abdominal film reveals a fecalith in the right lower quadrant, and a few air-fluid levels in the small bowel in the right lower quadrant may be visible.

Treatment. The treatment for suspected appendicitis is surgery.

Diverticulitis

History. The patient presents to the ED with pain in the left lower quadrant. However, the diagnosis of diverticulitis in the ED is a clinical one.

Physical Examination. The hallmark of the physical examination is localized tenderness in the area of the inflamed diverticulum. Patients exhibit rebound tenderness and fever.

Laboratory Studies. Leukocytosis is found on the CBC.

Treatment. These patients should be admitted for IV fluids, parenteral antibiotics, analgesics, and frequent reexamination. In cases in which there is no rebound tenderness and no significant fever, and the patient is able to keep fluids down, the patient may be discharged from the ED. If this is the case, an oral antibiotic should be prescribed, as well as bed rest, a low-residue diet, and next-day follow-up examination.

Cystitis

History. The diagnosis of cystitis is usually straightforward. The patient complains of frequency and dysuria.

Physical Examination. The physical examination is usually unremarkable with only mild suprapubic tenderness. In cases that are not clear-cut, there is the possibility that the bladder-irritating symptoms are coming from an adjacent inflammatory condition, such as pelvic inflammatory disease (PID), diverticulitis, or appendicitis. However, the tenderness on palpation is much more prominent in these other conditions than would be expected for cystitis. Sometimes a stone lodged at the ureterovesical junction will cause irritative bladder symptoms, but the pain from a stone is usually much more intense and the urine has no WBCs unless there is a complicating infection.

Laboratory Studies. Urinalysis shows variable numbers of WBCs and red blood cells (RBCs). The patient may have a positive nitrite and leukocyte esterase on urine dipstick test. A urine culture and sensitivity should be sent in all patients with impaired defenses, history of recurrent infections, or past surgery of the urinary tract.

Treatment. Treatment regimens seem to change frequently. One of the best sources for antibiotic therapy is *Sanford's Guide to Antimicrobial Therapy*.[6] This booklet is updated yearly and currently suggests 3-day therapy with a number of different antibiotics, depending on the specific needs of the patient.

Pyelonephritis

History. Pyelonephritis is usually a straightforward diagnosis. The patient may complain of a few days of urinary frequency and dysuria followed by fever, chills, myalgia, nausea, and back pain. The patient may also complain of nonspecific abdominal pain and have nonspecific abdominal tenderness on examination.

Physical Examination. The hallmark is CVA tenderness, especially reliable if it is unilateral. This can be demonstrated most reliably by sliding the hand under the supine patient and pressing upward into the CVA area. Occasionally, pyelonephritis can be extremely difficult to diagnose. Consider it in young children, usually girls, who present to the ED with fever and no identifiable source evident after history and physical examination. Also consider pyelonephritis in adults with nonspecific abdominal pain, low-grade fever, and mild unilateral CVA tenderness.

Males with pyelonephritis usually fit into one of the following groups:

1. Very young with a congenital malformation of the urinary system
2. Older patients with obstruction due to prostatic hypertrophy
3. Any patient with an indwelling catheter

Laboratory Studies. A urine culture and sensitivity should always be ordered on all patients suspected of having this problem. Blood cultures at two sites are indicated in all febrile patients. These patients should be admitted unless they exhibit a mild case without significant fever or vomiting.

Treatment. If the patient is admitted, IV antibiotics should be given. If the patient is discharged, oral antibiotics should be given with 24-hour follow-up instructions.

FEMALE WITH LOWER ABDOMINAL PAIN AND VAGINAL BLEEDING

General

History. The history should include the pertinent information (either positive or negative) about any of the following:

- Pain—onset, duration, character, radiation, exacerbating, and relieving factors
- Prior similar episodes
- Last normal menstrual period, gravida and para status, number of abortions and miscarriages
- Gastrointestinal symptoms—vomiting, diarrhea, last normal bowel movement
- Urinary tract symptoms—dysuria, frequency, hematuria
- Gynecologic symptoms—vaginal discharge, dyspareunia
- Prior gynecologic problems—pelvic infection, ovarian cyst, endometriosis
- Prior abdominal surgery

Physical Examination. A complete physical examination should be done to record tenderness or masses on the abdominal examination, discharge, the appearance of the cervix on pelvic examination, and tenderness on rectal examination. A tilt test should be done routinely on all female patients who have vaginal bleeding and lower abdominal pain.

Laboratory Studies. A CBC, UA, and urine pregnancy test should be done on all women of childbearing age. In addition, during the pelvic examination, cultures for *Gonorrhoeae* and *Chlamydia* should be collected. A blood type and Rh factor should be done in all women who are diagnosed with an abortion or an ectopic pregnancy. If the Rh factor is negative, the patient should receive a RhoGAM [Rh_0(D) immune globulin] injection.

Pelvic Ultrasonography. A patient with abdominal pain, tenderness on pelvic examination, and a positive pregnancy test will need a pelvic sonogram. To definitively diagnose an ectopic pregnancy, the fetal heartbeat must be visualized in an adnexal mass. However, the unusual report shows the uterus to be empty, some free fluid in the cul-de-sac, and a suggestion of an adnexal mass. An elevated quantitative beta–human chorionic gonadotropin (β-hCG) will correlate with a lower abdominal mass noted on sonography for the diagnosis of an ectopic pregnancy. By the fifth week of gestation, a gestational sac should be detectable in the uterus. By 6 weeks, a fetal pole can be seen, and by 7 weeks a fetal heartbeat can be observed. The quantitative β-hCG level is around 1500 IU/L at 5 weeks. A β-hCG level greater than 1500 IU/L with an empty uterus on sonography should arouse suspicions for an ectopic pregnancy. Pelvic sonography is also helpful in the pregnant patient with vaginal bleeding in whom the viability of the fetus is of concern. In this situation, the lack of significant pain is not indicative of an ectopic pregnancy, and a sonogram should not be considered as part of an ED workup. However, a sonogram should be obtained as soon as possible during normal working hours.

Pelvic Inflammatory Disease

History. Patients with pelvic inflammatory disease (PID) present with a spectrum of pain ranging from a mild-to-moderate constant aching pain to severe, constant pain with fever. The latter patient often walks into the ED with a slow shuffling gait, bent over, and clutching her lower abdomen with both hands. This presentation is characteristic and common enough to be dubbed "the PID shuffle." Patients with PID are frequently menstruating or have recently finished a period.

Physical Examination. The hallmark of PID is pain with cervical motion tenderness and diffuse pelvic tenderness on bimanual examination. Fever may or may not be present.

Laboratory Studies. The patient's WBC count may or may not be elevated. Ectopic pregnancy must be ruled out by a urine pregnancy test. It is cost-effective to add a screening test for syphilis in any patient with a clinical diagnosis of PID.

Treatment. With the information gained in the evaluation, patients can be sorted into three categories using the following criteria:

1. Patients who need admission: Temperature of 101° F (38.3° C) or higher, WBC count of 15,000/mm^3 or higher, and rebound tenderness on examination of the abdomen. These patients should be treated with cefoxitin, 2 g IV every 6 hours, coupled with doxycycline, 100 mg IV every 12 hours, until the patient has responded clinically and the WBC count returns to normal. Patients treated as outpatients should get a ceftriaxone (Rocephin, 250 mg) injection intramuscularly followed by a 10-day course of doxycycline, 100 mg twice daily.
2. Patients who can be treated with antibiotics as outpatients: Temperature less than 101° F (38.3° C), WBC count less than 15,000/mm^3, and no rebound tenderness.
3. Patients who can be treated symptomatically pending the results of cervical cultures: Reliable patients who are afebrile with minimal tenderness.

Tubal Pregnancy

A female of childbearing age who has lower abdominal pain is considered to have an ectopic pregnancy until proven otherwise.

History. A patient with tubal pregnancy usually presents 6 to 8 weeks past her last menstrual period with fairly sudden onset of unilateral sharp pain that becomes constant and is exacerbated with motion. If bleeding is massive, she may have fainted or may complain of dizziness on standing. Pain may radiate to the shoulder if blood is irritating the diaphragm. There may be a history of prior PID or a previous ectopic pregnancy.

Physical Examination. Physical examination demonstrates a spectrum of findings based on the underlying pathophysiology. At one end of the spectrum, the patient exhibits severe pain, shock, and an abdomen distended with blood. At the other end, the patient complains of mild aggravating unilateral pain and mild-to-moderate tenderness on examination.

Laboratory Studies. These patients require a urine pregnancy test. Patients with pain and a positive pregnancy test need an emergency pelvic sonogram and an immediate obstetric-gynecologic (OB-GYN) consultation. As has been mentioned previously, the quantitative β-hCG is useful to correlate with sonographic findings in arriving at a presumptive diagnosis.

Treatment. The treatment for a tubal pregnancy is emergency surgery. The patient can rapidly develop life-threatening complications, mainly internal hemorrhage.

Threatened Abortion

History. It is useful to consider vaginal bleeding a complication of a pregnancy until it can be ruled out by a urine pregnancy test. In patients who are pregnant and bleeding, it must be determined whether they are in danger of having a miscarriage, are in the process of having a miscarriage, or have completed having a miscarriage.

Physical Examination. Usually the assessment of the cervical os enables the PA to differentiate these possibilities. The patient who presents with slight bleeding, mild or no cramps, a closed os, and no significant tenderness on pelvic examination can be diagnosed as having a threatened abortion. The patient with significant bleeding and cramps in which the os admits a ring forceps is in the process of miscarrying. It is more difficult to diagnose threatened abortion in multiparous patients because the os is often stretched from previous childbirth and may appear open on casual visualization.

Laboratory Studies. A quantitative β-hCG is helpful as a baseline test in these patients because in normal pregnancies, the quantitative β-hCG doubles every 2 days during the first trimester. Sonography is an extremely helpful adjunct in cases that are questionable. It is wise to do an emergent pelvic sonogram to make the differentiation.

Treatment. Occasionally, the patient is bleeding profusely and tissue may be noted protruding from the cervical os. Removing the tissue with a ring forceps should be done immediately and often results in a marked decrease in bleeding. If the patient is having a miscarriage, an immediate OB-GYN consultation should be obtained. If the patient has a closed os and a normal hematocrit and is not bleeding massively, she may be discharged from the ED with instructions to go home and rest. She should return to the ED if the bleeding increases or if she has any tissue loss. Refer the patient for follow-up the next day to her regular OB-GYN physician.

Vaginitis

The patient who complains of a vaginal discharge requires a pelvic examination, a cervical culture for *Gonorrhoeae* and *Chlamydia*, and a wet prep for yeast and *Trichomonas*. The diagnosis is often straightforward from the history and physical examination.

Yeast Vaginitis. Yeast vaginitis usually causes intense itching, and the patient complains of the characteristic white "cottage cheese" discharge. The vulva may be inflamed.

Treatment of yeast vaginitis is accomplished by any number of antiyeast regimens.

***Trichomonas* Vaginitis.** *Trichomonas* vaginitis causes a copious, malodorous discharge that is yellow-green in color and often frothy. Itching may be present but is much less prominent than in yeast infections.

Treatment of *Trichomonas* vaginitis is metronidazole (Flagyl) in a single 2-g dose administered to the patient and her sexual partner. If the patient is in the first trimester of pregnancy, a 20% saline douche or clotrimazole may be used.

Bacterial Vaginosis

Bacterial vaginosis usually presents with a grayish white discharge that is malodorous but not frothy, and itching is not prominent. The wet prep may show "clue cells," which are desquamated epithelial cells with clusters of bacilli clinging to their surfaces, giving them a stippled appearance. *Gardnerella vaginalis*, *Peptococcus*, and non-*fragilis Bacteroides* have all been implicated as etiologic. Bacterial vaginosis is treated with metronidazole, 500 mg twice daily for 7 days, with no treatment of the sexual partner. Because treatments change from year to year, the reader should consult *Sanford's Guide to Antimicrobial Therapy* for the latest recommendations.[8]

MANAGEMENT OF THE FEBRILE CHILD YOUNGER THAN 2 YEARS

Child Younger Than 3 Months

The child younger than 3 months of age with a temperature greater than or equal to 100.4° F (38° C) should undergo a full septic workup, be placed on parenteral antibiotics, and be admitted to the hospital. A full septic workup includes a CBC, SMA-7, blood cultures at two sites, routine UA and culture (preferably obtained by suprapubic aspiration), stool for fecal leukocytes and culture (if diarrhea is present), lumbar puncture, and chest radiograph. Refer to the current issue of *Sanford's Guide to Antimicrobial Therapy* for the latest antibiotic recommendations.[8]

Child 3 Months to 4 Years of Age

Regardless of the level of temperature, if the child appears acutely ill, he or she must be admitted for treatment. If the child does not appear acutely ill and has a focus of infection on examination that most likely is the source of the fever, the infection should be treated and the parents asked to contact their pediatrician within the next 24 hours. For example, the child who has bilateral otitis media with a temperature of 102° F (38.8° C) but is taking fluids well and does not appear toxic can be treated and discharged from the ED.

If the child is not toxic in appearance, has a temperature of 102° F (38.8° C) or higher, and has no focus of infection on examination, the child is at risk for bacteremia. A WBC and differential should be obtained. If the WBC is greater than 15,000/mm^3, blood culture should be done along with a UA and chest radiograph. The child should be treated with a parenteral antibiotic, and instructions should be given to the parents to contact their pediatrician in 12 to 24 hours.

If the child is not toxic in appearance and has a temperature of 102° F (38.8° C) or higher, no focus of infection on examination, and a WBC less than 15,0000/mm^3, he or she should be treated symptomatically with reexamination in 12 to 24 hours.

EYE EMERGENCIES

Initial Evaluation

All persons with eye complaints should have a *visual acuity* recorded on their chart as the first step in evaluation. This should be done with the patient wearing his or her glasses or contacts if possible. If glasses or contacts are not available, use a piece of cardboard with a pinhole to correct refractive errors. The Snellen eye chart is a satisfactory method for assessing visual acuity in most cases.

In many cases, the patient will be having so much discomfort that a *topical anesthetic* will need to be instilled in the eye before the visual acuity testing can be done. The skin should be gently pinched under the lower lid and the lid pulled outward to form a small pouch. Warn the patient that the medication will sting, and place a drop or two of the anesthetic into the pouch; have the patient gently close his or her eye for a few seconds. This pouch technique is much more comfortable to the patient than is dropping eye drops directly onto the surface of the cornea.

Direct inspection with a light source directed onto the eye from the side will show obvious abnormalities and is a good way to evaluate the depth of the anterior chamber. Usually, the entire anterior chamber will be illuminated, but in the case of a shallow anterior chamber, only the lateral half illuminates and the medial half remains in a shadow. Eyes with shallow anterior chambers should not be dilated because glaucoma can be precipitated.

If there is any suggestion in the patient's history of a problem that might involve a disrupted corneal epithelium (e.g., foreign body sensation, eye pain, or chemicals in the eye), it is helpful to add *fluorescein dye* to the eye before the slit lamp or Wood's lamp examination. Fluorescein-impregnated paper strips are moistened with ophthalmic irrigating solution and are touched lightly to the lower palpebral conjunctival surface to instill the dye. Excess dye is rinsed away with the ophthalmic irrigating solution if necessary, and the eye is viewed under a black light. Areas of disrupted corneal epithelium fluoresce brightly.

Slit lamp examination should be learned by direct demonstration and hands-on instruction.

Lid eversion is necessary to evaluate foreign body sensations in the eye or when corneal examination reveals vertical linear abrasions. The patient is asked to look down, and the upper lid eyebrows are grasped gently between the thumb and index finger and pulled outward. A cotton-tipped swab is used as a fulcrum behind the tarsal plate over which the lid is everted. The swab is then removed and the lid held everted with the thumb. It is helpful to keep the patient looking down during this maneuver because if the patient looks up, the lid spontaneously reverts to its normal position. This maneuver can be done at the slit lamp and allows the provider to scan the undersurface of the lid with the slit lamp, searching for any foreign body.

Funduscopic examination with the direct ophthalmoscope is part of every standard eye examination. This can usually be accomplished without dilating the pupil.

Tonometry with the Shiøtz tonometer should be done on any eye in which the history and eye examination suggest glaucoma. With the patient supine, the eye is anesthetized topically, the lids are gently retracted with caution not to touch the globe, and the tonometer is placed on the cornea. It is helpful to have an assistant place a finger 3 feet over the patient's face so that the patient can fixate on it to help hold the eye still. The scale reading on the tonometer is converted to millimeters of mercury (mm Hg) by a chart that accompanies the tonometer. Normal intraocular pressure is 16.1 ± 2.8 mm Hg. In acute glaucoma, intraocular pressure is usually markedly elevated (40 to 50 mm Hg), and in iritis, the intraocular pressure may decrease. Application tonometry using the slit lamp and the new Tono-Pen (Automated Ophthalmics, Columbia, Md.) are more advanced ways to measure intraocular pressure.

If the history suggests possible penetrating ocular injury, radiographs of the orbit for foreign body should be obtained. A Waters view of the orbits is helpful in the evaluation of possible fractures associated with blunt trauma to the eye. Tomograms of the orbital floor or a CT scan may be necessary to diagnose a blowout fracture of the orbital floor, if clinical suspicion is high and routine radiographs fail to show the fracture.

Common Eye Infections

Stye. A stye (external hordeolum) is a staphylococcal infection of small glands along the external lid margin. A red swelling appears in the lash line of the lid margin, accompanied by pain, tenderness, and often considerable edema of the lid. Eventually, a yellow summit appears, indicating suppuration. Treatment consists of hot compresses to hasten suppuration and a local antibiotic instilled into the eye. Incision is usually not indicated, and systemic antibiotics should be withheld unless the infection is spreading into the eyelid with poor localization. A stye may also occur on the inside of the lid (internal hordeolum), and the treatment is identical.

Conjunctivitis. Conjunctivitis is inflammation of the conjunctival surfaces of the eye. Conjunctivitis has diverse causes, including bacterial infection, viral infection, allergy, ultraviolet light exposure, and trauma. In most cases, the patient presents with eye discharge, redness, and mild pain. In simple cases, it is standard practice to treat with a local antibiotic and refer to an ophthalmologist if the patient fails to respond to treatment. Conjunctivitis in newborns and infants requires special considerations that are beyond the scope of this discussion.

Acute purulent conjunctivitis is characterized by a profuse purulent eye discharge. Causative bacteria include pneumococci, streptococci, *Haemophilus influenzae* (Koch-Weeks bacillus), *H. conjunctivitis*, staphylococci, and *Neisseria catarrhalis*. Mixed infections are common. Treatment is started empirically with an antibiotic eye drop or ointment, and Gram stain and cultures are reserved for resistant cases.

Viral conjunctivitis is also characterized by an eye discharge. It differs from bacterial conjunctivitis in that the discharge is less profuse, and preauricular lymph node enlargement is often present. Gram stain shows a preponderance of lymphocytes and mononuclear cells without bacteria. However, because routine Gram stains are not recommended, treat with an antibiotic eye drop or ointment, and reserve Gram stain and cultures for resistant cases.

Allergic conjunctivitis is distinguished by itching, watering, redness, and mucoid discharge. Edematous swelling is noted in which the bulbar conjunctival surface may protrude out of the eye or overlap the cornea in ballooning folds. The clinical picture is distinct, and treatment is with an antihistamine vasoconstrictor eye drop (Vasocon-A).

Traumatic conjunctivitis is an acute purulent conjunctivitis induced by traumatic contamination.

Ultraviolet keratoconjunctivitis is caused by exposure to ultraviolet radiation. Common sources include welders' electric arcs, sunlamps, or sunlight reflected by snow. Around 12 hours after exposure, the patient develops severe bilateral eye pain, watering, and photophobia. The pain is usually so intense that the eyes cannot be opened until a drop of topical anesthetic is instilled. Slit lamp examination with fluorescein stain reveals a diffuse stippled uptake of dye over the surface of the cornea, and the conjunctival surfaces are diffusely injected. Treatment is an antibiotic eye drop, a cycloplegic, and patching of both eyes. Systemic analgesia is usually required.

Orbital Cellulitis. Orbital cellulitis is a serious infection of bacterial origin. The patient has high fever, eye pain, redness and swelling of orbital tissues, and ophthalmoplegia in severe cases. Infection may extend from an infected sinus or tooth, or there may be a primary site of infection. In children, orbital cellulitis is usually a primary infection. In either case, treatment is immediate referral for hospitalization and IV antibiotics.

Corneal Infections. Corneal infections may be primary or may arise after trauma has broken the corneal epithelium. Bacterial ulcers are frequently associated with purulent conjunctivitis and have a grayish appearance. Immediate ophthalmologic consult should be obtained. Any corneal abrasion may become secondarily infected with bacteria, fungi, or herpes virus. When the fluorescein-stained cornea is examined under the slit lamp, a characteristic dendritic pattern is often seen with herpes virus infection. An ophthalmologic consult should be obtained immediately, and antiviral eye drops should be prescribed.

Placing topical steroids in an eye with a herpes virus infection has resulted in rapid progression of the infection with corneal destruction. This danger is one of the main reasons for the dictum that under no circumstances should a nonophthalmologist ever prescribe topical steroids for eye problems.

Ocular Foreign Bodies

Conjunctival Foreign Bodies. Conjunctival foreign bodies cause pain and a sensation that something is in the eye. Those in the lower conjunctival sac are easily removed with a moistened cotton-tipped applicator after topical anesthesia. Foreign bodies under the upper lid are exposed by everting the lid, as discussed earlier. They are usually found 2 to 3 mm from the lid margin and are also easily removed with a moistened cotton-tipped applicator. The cornea must be examined carefully under the slit lamp with fluorescein staining to search for multiple vertical corneal abrasions. These scratches are caused by the motion of the foreign body back and forth across the cornea each time the patient blinks. If abrasions are present, instill a topical antibiotic, a cycloplegic, and double-patch the eye for 24 hours. If no abrasion is present, prescribe a topical antibiotic eye drop to instill four times daily for 2 to 3 days to prevent traumatic conjunctivitis. If the eye is patched, it should be reexamined in 24 hours. Patching is for comfort only and is optional.

Corneal Foreign Bodies. Corneal foreign bodies also cause pain and a sensation that something is in the eye. The foreign body is usually easily seen by direct vision or slit lamp examination after topical anesthesia. Removal is accomplished with an eye spud, a 25-gauge needle attached to a cotton-tipped applicator, or the special ophthalmologic corneal burr attached to a battery-operated drill. The latter technique is especially efficient if there is a metallic corneal foreign body because a *rust ring* usually remains in the cornea after removal of the metal. It is important to use the drill to remove these rust rings as completely as possible. Any residual rust increases the healing time of the abrasion and the inflammatory response of the eye. After removal of the foreign body and any residual rust, instill an antibiotic eye drop, a cycloplegic, and double-patch the eye. Patching is for comfort only and is optional. Reexamination is necessary in 24 hours. Avoid placing steroids in the eye because these reduce the resistance of the cornea to infection. Do not use an antibiotic ointment unless the abrasion is very superficial (there have been instances in which a drop of ointment has been epithelialized in the abrasion, with formation of an ointment "cyst" that later requires operative removal).

Intraocular Foreign Bodies. Intraocular foreign bodies are easily overlooked if the index of suspicion is not high. Obtain orbital films any time the patient gives a history of striking a hammer on a piece of metal, or similar activity in which a small foreign body could be projected into the eye with enough force to penetrate the eye. If the radiograph is positive for a foreign body, immediate ophthalmology consultation is required.

Eye Injuries Arising from Direct Trauma

Hyphema. A hyphema may result from blunt trauma to the eye that causes bleeding into the anterior chamber. The bleeding may completely fill the anterior chamber, resulting in an "eight-ball" appearance. More commonly, the anterior chamber is partially filled with blood layering out inferiorly. Immediate ophthalmology consultation is required.

Iritis. Iritis may follow trauma to the eye. The patient complains of pain and photophobia. The bulbar conjunctivae are diffusely injected, especially in the perilimbal region. The pupil is miotic, and visual acuity is decreased. On slit lamp examination, WBCs are seen in the anterior chamber. Ophthalmology consultation should be obtained.

Traumatic Mydriasis. Traumatic mydriasis may occur occasionally following blunt trauma to the eye. Usually, the dilated, fixed pupil reverts to normal in a few days without specific treatment. Rarely, the dilatation may be permanent.

Retinal Detachment. Retinal detachment is heralded by a decrease in vision, often described as light flashes followed by a "curtain" type of field defect. The fundus appears gray and rippled or undulating, and the retinal vessels are elevated and abnormally tortuous. If the retina is detached only peripherally, it may not be visible on direct ophthalmoscopy, and vision may be normal. For this reason, it is prudent to refer patients with significant blunt trauma for ophthalmologic examination if any suspicious history is present (i.e., light flashes, black spots, film or cloud over vision, curtain coming down).

Orbital Blowout Fracture. Orbital blowout fracture may occur when an object larger than the orbital rim strikes the eye, compressing the orbital contents. The increased intraorbital pressure "blows out" the thin and weak orbital floor. The inferior rectus and inferior oblique muscles may prolapse into the defect, causing diplopia on upward gaze. Plain radiographs may not reveal the fracture. A CT scan or tomograms of the orbital floor may be necessary to demonstrate the fracture.

Differential Diagnosis of the Red Eye

Conjunctivitis. In conjunctivitis, the eye is diffusely injected. There is no change in visual acuity, intraocular pressure, or pupillary size and reaction.

Iritis. In iritis, the injection is concentrated in the perilimbal area. The visual acuity and intraocular pressure are decreased. The pupil is miotic, and cells are present in the anterior chamber.

Acute Glaucoma. In acute glaucoma, the eye is diffusely injected. The visual acuity is decreased, and the intraocular pressure is markedly elevated. The pupil is dilated and frequently reacts sluggishly or not at all. The cornea often has a hazy appearance.

Chemicals in the Eye. The first thing that should be done is to immediately instill a topical anesthetic and irrigate the eye profusely. Hang a 1000-mL bag of normal saline, and run the entire amount over the surface of the eye. Any particles of material should be removed with a moistened cotton-tipped applicator. Assessment of the eye is then done in standard fashion. Superficial corneal injuries are treated in the same way as abrasions from other causes with a topical antibiotic, a short-acting cycloplegic, and patching, with reevaluation in 24 hours. The patch is for comfort only and is optional. Severe corneal burns or alkali burns require ophthalmologic consultation.

EAR, NOSE, AND THROAT EMERGENCIES

Epistaxis

The first step in the treatment of epistaxis is to have the patient squeeze the nose firmly between the thumb and index finger and not let go for at least 10 minutes. However, if the patient is in shock or has uncontrolled hypertension, immediately give the usual treatment for those entities while the patient holds his or her nose.

History. In the vast majority of cases, patients are stable. The history is taken while focusing on the common causes of epistaxis—trauma, respiratory infection, hypertension, or underlying hemostatic defect.

Physical Examination. Examination of the nose is accomplished with an ear, nose, and throat (ENT) headlight, a nasal spectrum, a metal tip attached to suction, a pair of bayonet forceps, a small medicine cup, cotton balls, and 4% cocaine solution.

Laboratory Studies. Consider laboratory studies in patients who have unstable vital signs or a history of hemostatic defect. A CBC, platelet count, prothrombin time, partial thromboplastin time, SMA-7, and type and cross-match are the tests selected according to the clinical picture. Again, most patients do not require laboratory work.

Treatment. The provider should place a gown over his or her clothes and give the patient an emesis basin to catch any bleeding. An attempt should be made to visualize the site of bleeding. First, remove clots from the patient's nose with the forceps or by having the patient blow the clots into the emesis basin. If active bleeding is occurring, have the patient lean forward and let the blood run into the basin. The goal is to differentiate anterior from posterior epistaxis and to visually identify the bleeding site if it is anterior.

Anterior Epistaxis. The most common site for epistaxis is anterior. A small, pumping blood vessel can be located on the anterior inferior portion of the nasal septum. It often appears to be a tiny worm sticking out of the ground and waving in the breeze.

Once the site has been identified, take the bayonet forceps and wrap part of a cotton ball around the forceps, making a pledget of cotton. Soak the pledget in cocaine, squeeze out the excess, and insert it into the nose. Leave it in place for 10 minutes, remove it, and cauterize the bleeder with a silver nitrate stick. Hold the silver nitrate stick in place for 10 seconds, and then observe for cessation of bleeding. Once the bleeding has been controlled, place a small anterior petroleum jelly gauze pack and a Band-Aid with a space for the nostril cut out on the side that does not have the packing. Instruct the patient not to do any physical exertion and to keep the head elevated above heart level for 48 hours. Give the patient a referral for removal of the packing in 48 hours and instructions to return immediately if bleeding recurs.

Posterior Epistaxis. Patients with posterior epistaxis need a nasal pack and may need admission to the hospital. Insertion of a nasal pack is extremely uncomfortable. Anesthetize the whole nasal passageway using cocaine-soaked cotton pledgets inserted deeply into the nose and layered to fill the cavity. Consider premedicating the patient with an injectable analgesic. A useful first step is to insert a Merocel foam (Uline, Waukegan, Ill.) nasal pack after coating it with antibiotic ointment. Drip saline from a 10-mL syringe on the packing, and it will expand into a spongelike pack that fills the nasal cavity. It should be removed in 48 hours and must be remoistened before removal.

The Nasostat (Sparta, Pleasanton, Calif.) is a commercially available device that can be inserted into the nose and inflated carefully by following the directions that come with the device. It has an anterior and a posterior balloon that can be filled with saline.

In a patient whose hemorrhage cannot be controlled with the measures mentioned earlier, a No. 10 or a No. 12 Foley catheter with a 30-mL balloon can be inserted into the nose until it can be seen in the posterior pharynx. Inflate the balloon with water and pull it snugly against the posterior aspect of the nares. Take petroleum jelly gauze and pack it in with bayonet forceps, starting along the bottom of the nasal passageway and layering it upward to fill the nose. An assistant is needed to hold traction on the Foley catheter as the pack is placed in the nose against the balloon. A small square of sponge cast padding with a slit in it is used as a pad between the nose and a small C-clamp. If this fails to control the hemorrhage, get an ENT specialist to help. These patients all need admission to the hospital.

Removal of Intranasal Foreign Body

The usual patient is a child who has put some small object up his or her nose and comes into the ED with the mother. These patients rarely present with a unilateral purulent nasal drainage. Phenylephrine nasal spray often works in trying to coax the child to blow the foreign body out of the nose.

The easiest way to remove most foreign bodies from the nose is with an ear curette. The child should be restrained in a papoose board with an assistant positioned to control the patient's head. Gently slide the curette over the top of the foreign body and then drag it out. This succeeds in nearly all cases. If the object is suitable for grabbing, remove it with a small pair of alligator forceps. No special treatment is needed after removal.

Septal Hematoma

It is important in any case that involves trauma to the nose to look for a septal hematoma and to document on the chart its presence or absence. Failure to diagnose a septal hematoma can be disastrous for the patient. The septal hematoma may become infected, leading to destruction of the cartilage of the nasal septum and subsequent collapse of the nose with saddle deformity. Immediate ENT consult is indicated for drainage of the hematoma and packing of the nose.

Ruptured Eardrum

History. Usually, the patient presents complaining of ear pain following trauma. Most commonly, the patient may have been slapped on the ear or may have fallen while water-skiing and slapped the ear on the water. Rarely, the trauma is due to an object introduced into the ear in an attempt to remove earwax.

Physical Examination. The physical examination reveals a defect in the eardrum that is clearly evident.

Treatment. Treatment consists of keeping the ear dry and administering an oral analgesic and a systemic antibiotic appropriate for otitis media. Patients seem to feel better if they place a small, dry cotton ball in the ear. These small perforations heal in nearly all instances, and the patient can simply be reassured. It should be recommended that the patient follow up with an ENT specialist or the family doctor in 2 weeks or immediately if increased pain, fever, or purulent ear drainage occurs.

NECK PAIN AND LOW BACK PAIN

When dealing with a patient who is complaining of neck or low back pain in the ED, the following questions should be answered:

- Is there a fracture or other abnormality of the bones?
- Is there a radiculopathy (diseased condition of roots of spinal nerves)?
- Is there a muscle or ligament abnormality?

History. An accurate history includes every episode of this pain both past and present.

Physical Examination. The physical examination is the key to detecting signs of radiculopathy.

Neck

1. Palpate areas of tenderness.
2. Check and record the *range of motion.* Have the patient turn the neck to the right as far as he or she can until the pain begins, and record the rotation in degrees. Then have the patient turn to the left.
3. Perform a nerve root–directed *motor and sensory examination* (Table 22-2).

Radiculopathy can usually be detected with the motor and sensory examination. Reflexes are not as helpful because multiple nerve roots are reflected by reflexes in the arms.

TABLE 22-2 **Motor and Sensory Examination of Nerve Roots—Neck**

Nerve Root	Motor	Sensory	Reflex
C5	Deltoid	Lateral shoulder	—
C6	Biceps	Thumb	Biceps
C7	Wrist extensors	Long finger	—
C8	Finger flexors	Little finger	—
T1	Finger abductors	Inner upper arm	—

Laboratory Studies. Obtain radiographs, which show bony abnormalities. Disk space narrowing, spur formation, congenital abnormalities, and postsurgical changes (prior fusions) are most common. There may be a straightening of the normal C-shaped curve of the cervical (C) spine. This is due to spasm of the surrounding muscles. Of course, if the patient is presenting with neck pain following recent trauma, the first step is to get a full C-spine series to rule out fracture before performing the physical examination. Using the previously described format, an example of the patient's chart would be as follows.

CASE STUDY 22-7

History

A 40-year-old man with a 3-week history of increasing pain in the posterior neck that radiates into the right arm and has a burning quality. No prior similar pain, no history of injury.

Physical Examination

Pain to palpation of right paraspinous muscles
Right rotation, 30 degrees; left rotation, 60 degrees
Motor, C5-T1: Weakness in right biceps; otherwise normal
Sensory, C5-T1: Decreased sensation to touch and pinprick in right thumb; otherwise normal
Triceps reflex normal; biceps reflex decreased

Laboratory Studies

Radiographs reveal disk space narrowing with large hypertrophic spurs at the C5-6 level.

Diagnosis

C6 radiculopathy (herniated disk vs. pressure from spur).

Treatment

In this case, treatment can be selected from muscle relaxants, analgesics, antiinflammatory drugs, and physical therapy. Patients who do not respond to conservative therapy need orthopedic or neurosurgical referral for consideration of surgery.

Lower Back

- Palpate areas of tenderness.
- Check and record the range of motion. Have the patient bend forward as far as he or she comfortably can, as if doing a "toe touch," and record where the fingertips rest (e.g., floor, knees, mid-thigh).
- Do a nerve root–directed motor and sensory examination (Table 22-3).

Straight Leg Raising

Straight leg raising (SLR) should be tested and recorded. Raise the patient's straightened leg slowly from the table until a point is reached that intensifies the pain in the back. Record it as, for example, "SLR positive at 30 degrees" or "SLR negative to 90 degrees." If the patient experiences pain in the opposite side of the back and the opposite leg, this is uggestive of a ruptured disk. This phenomenon is called *crossed straight leg raise,* and in some studies, it is 90% correlated with a ruptured disk.

The patient's chart may read as follows.

CASE STUDY 22-8

History

A 35-year-old man with a history of sudden onset of pain in the left lower back 2 weeks ago while lifting a 50-lb box at work. The pain now radiates into the left leg, and he occasionally feels numbness in his foot. Several milder episodes of pain have occurred over the past 3 years, none severe enough for a physician visit.

Examination

Pain to palpation of left paraspinous muscles, left sacroiliac joint, and left buttock over the sciatic nerve.
Forward flexion: Fingertips to knees.
Motor, L4-S1: Subjective weakness in left calf with toe raises; otherwise normal.
Sensory, L4-S1: Decreased sensation over the lateral foot; otherwise normal.
Knee jerk: Normal.
Ankle jerk: Normal, right; absent, left.
SLR L to 30 degrees; crossed SLR R to L to 60 degrees.

Laboratory Studies

Radiographs reveal disk space narrowing of L5-S1.

Diagnosis

Acute low back pain with herniated disk and S1 radiculopathy.

Treatment

In this case, treatment can be again selected from muscle relaxants, analgesics, and antiinflammatory drugs. Recent studies have shown that patients with low back pain do better with "activity within the limits of pain" than with bed rest or physical therapy. Patients who do not respond to conservative treatment need orthopedic or neurosurgical referral for consideration of surgery.

TABLE 22-3 **Motor and Sensory Examination of Nerve Roots—Lower Back**

Nerve Root	Motor	Sensory	Reflex
L4	Quadriceps	Above knee	Knee jerk
L5	Great toe extensor	Medial foot	—
S1	Calf	Lateral foot	Ankle jerk

SPRAINS

Differentiating Sprains

A ligament is a tough fibrous structure that runs from bone to bone. Sprains are ligamentous injuries, and it is essential to divide them into three categories for treatment purposes.

First-Degree (Mild). Some fibers of the ligament have been torn, but there is no loss of function and no loss in the strength of the ligament.

History. Historically, one finds only mild disability. Indeed, the disability may be so mild that the patient does not even seek the advice of a physician.

Physical Examination. Physical examination reveals mild tenderness and swelling over the injured ligament, with no instability.

Treatment. The treatment is *RICE* (rest, ice, compression, and elevation). In this case, the ligament is not weakened and a cast or a brace is not necessary.

Second-Degree (Moderate). A larger portion of the ligament is torn, enough to weaken it functionally. It is difficult to determine clinically the extent of the damage and just how much of the ligament is torn.

History. Historically, there is some degree of immediate disability. The patient is unable to continue to use the joint normally.

Physical Examination. The physical examination reveals a moderate amount of local tenderness and swelling over the injured ligament, but no instability.

Treatment. Treatment consists of immobilizing and protecting the injured ligament while it heals. In this case, the ligament is only partially torn, and wide retraction of the ends of the torn ligament is not part of the injury process. Therefore, satisfactory healing should occur provided the joint is adequately immobilized and protected. The specific method of immobilization depends on the joint involved and is discussed later.

Third-Degree (Severe). The entire ligament is torn with complete functional loss.

History. Historically, there is immediate and complete loss of function of the affected joint. Severe second- and third-degree sprains cannot be separated on the basis of the history alone because loss of function occurs in both.

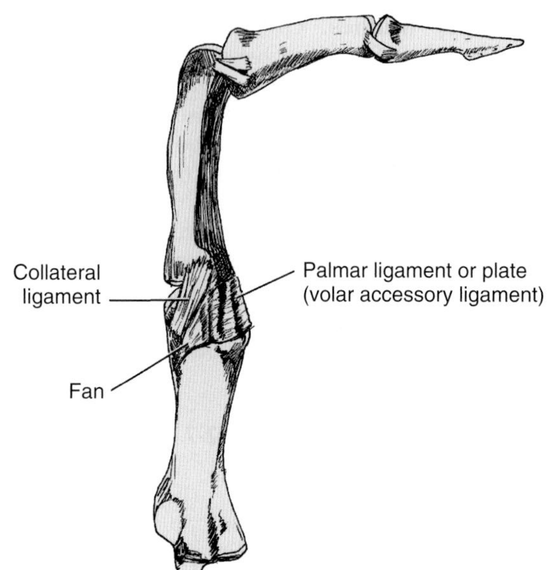

FIGURE 22-1 The metacarpophalangeal joint of the thumb has collateral ligaments and a strong palmar ligament (volar plate).

Physical Examination. The physical examination reveals marked tenderness and swelling over the torn ligament.

Laboratory Studies. The diagnosis depends on demonstrating abnormal motion of the involved joint by radiograph, with stress on the joint, or both.

Treatment. Treatment is usually surgical. Efficient repair is dependent on the apposition of the torn ends of the ligament, which may be widely separated. A less satisfactory alternative is to treat third-degree sprains with immobilization, with the hope that the ends are close enough together to heal. A secondary surgical procedure is then done if subsequent instability occurs.

Specific Sprains

Metacarpophalangeal Joint of the Thumb. The metacarpophalangeal joint of the thumb (Figure 22-1) has collateral ligaments and a strong palmar ligament (volar plate).

History. The history reveals that the patient's thumb has been subjected to a hyperabduction stress. This occurs most commonly from the steering wheel in deceleration accidents, from the ski pole in falls while snow-skiing (ski-pole thumb), and from other injuries in which the thumb is hyperabducted.

Physical Examination. The physical examination reveals swelling and tenderness at the

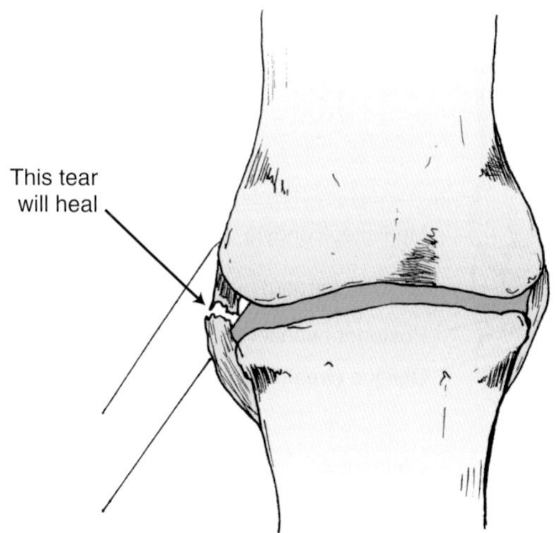

FIGURE 22-2 Grade III rupture of the ulnar collateral ligament with the ligament ends in apposition.

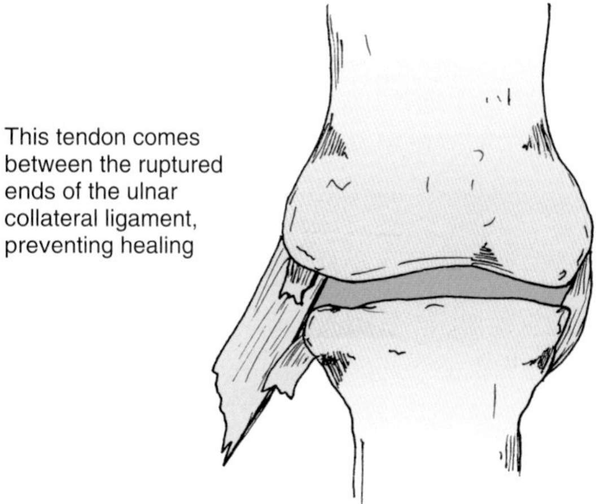

FIGURE 22-3 Grade III rupture of the ulnar collateral ligament with interposition of the adductor aponeurosis and turnback of the proximal end of the ligament.

metacarpophalangeal joint. Gentle hyperabduction stress reveals instability if a complete tear of the ulnar collateral ligament is present.

Laboratory Studies. Radiographs are normal.

Treatment. An immediate orthopedic consultation is necessary. There is controversy about the best way to treat this injury. If the ligament ends are in apposition, a satisfactory result can be obtained by immobilization in a thumb spica cast. A grade III rupture of the ulnar collateral ligament is exhibited by an interposition of the adductor aponeurosis and a "turning back" of the proximal end of the ligament (Figure 22-2). A second-degree sprain would be treated with a thumb spica splint for 3 weeks. A first-degree sprain would be treated symptomatically. Occasionally, the adductor pollicis brevis aponeurosis interposes itself between the torn ends of the ligament. In this situation, surgical intervention is mandated to repair the instability and avoid a rapidly progressive degenerative arthritis in the joint (Figure 22-3).

Metacarpophalangeal Joint of the Fifth Finger

History. The history reveals an injury that puts a hyperabduction stress on the radial collateral ligament of the metacarpophalangeal joint of the fifth finger.

Physical Examination. The physical examination reveals tenderness and swelling in the joint. If the ligament is completely ruptured, it will be unstable with stress, and sometimes the short abductor pulls the finger into ulnar deviation.

Treatment. Treatment for first-degree sprains is symptomatic. Second-degree sprains can be treated by taping the fourth finger to the fifth finger; immediate orthopedic referral is provided for complete ruptures. Ruptures of the collateral ligaments of other metacarpophalangeal joints are rare and do not need operative repair, owing to the stability provided by surrounding structures.

Proximal Interphalangeal Joint. The proximal interphalangeal joint has collateral ligaments and a thick volar plate, as does the metacarpophalangeal joint. These ligaments may rupture with or without an associated dislocation.

History. The history reveals an injury to the finger. Sometimes the patient describes a dislocation that was self-reduced or was reduced by a friend before arrival in the ED.

Physical Examination. The physical examination reveals tenderness and swelling, and radiography is negative for fractures. Gentle stress of the collateral ligaments reveals instability if a complete rupture is present. The volar plate is tested by gently hyperextending the joint.

Treatment. Treatment is immediate orthopedic referral if collateral ligament instability is found. Some orthopedists treat with surgical repair, whereas others treat conservatively with splinting. Second-degree sprains can be immobilized for 3 weeks by buddy-taping the injured finger to the adjacent finger and encouraging active range of motion. First-degree sprains are treated symptomatically.

Wrist Sprains. Wrist sprains are uncommon. Most wrist sprains are actually strains of tendon attachments or bony injuries. Navicular fractures in the wrist are notorious for not appearing on radiographs initially. Additionally, they have a high incidence of avascular necrosis of the proximal fragment. When this occurs,

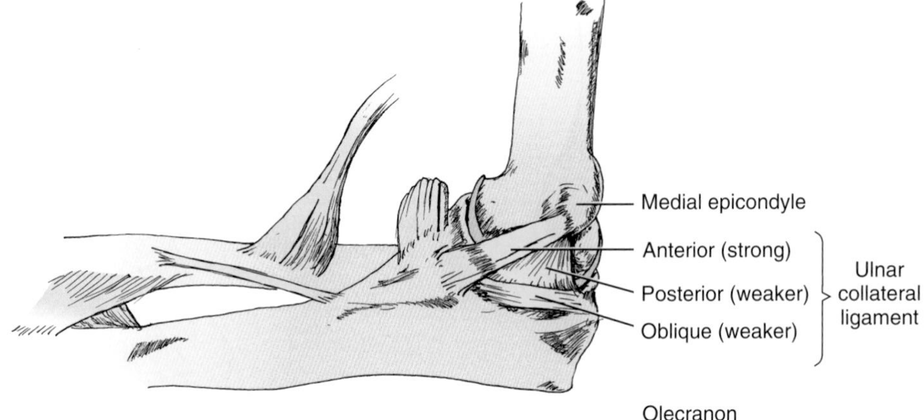

FIGURE 22-4 Ulnar collateral ligament of the elbow.

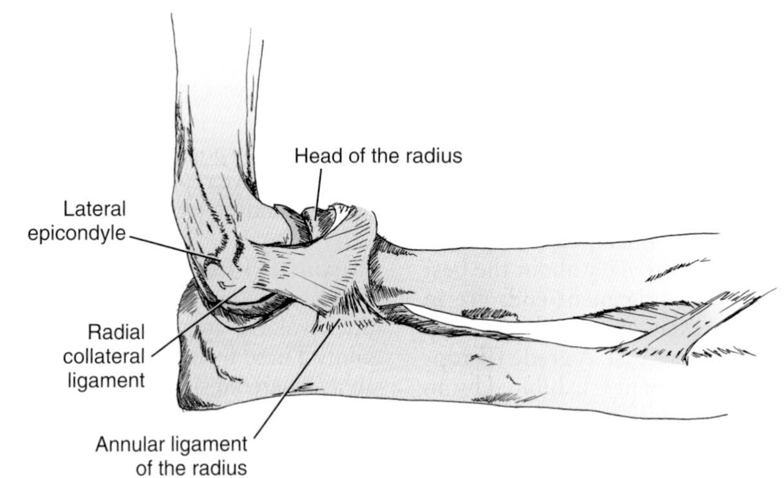

FIGURE 22-5 Radial collateral ligament of the elbow.

the patient requires surgery to remove the devascularized portion of the bone. It is good practice to splint any significant wrist injury and have the patient follow up with an orthopedist. A thumb spica splint should be used if a navicular fracture is suspected.

Elbow Sprains. The ulnar collateral ligament of the elbow is attached to the humerus superiorly and the ulna inferiorly on the medial aspect of the joint (Figure 22-4). The elbow also has a lateral ligament known as the *radial collateral ligament*, which extends over the radial head as the annular ligament of the radius (Figure 22-5). A ligamentous injury here is relatively uncommon. The ligaments may be torn by hyperextension or lateral motion (forced abduction of the extended arm). If radiographic studies are negative, it is not necessary to stress-test for instability. The elbow joint has inherent bony stability and is a non–weight-bearing joint. A good result is obtained regardless of the degree of sprain by using a protective sling and gradually increasing the motion within the limits of pain until the joint is pain free.

Ankle Sprains. The lateral side of the ankle is supported by the anterior talofibular, calcaneofibular, and posterior talofibular ligaments. Anterior and posterior tibiofibular ligaments bind the fibula to the tibia (Figure 22-6). The medial side of the ankle is supported by the multiple components of the thick deltoid ligament (Figure 22-7).

Eighty-five percent of all ankle sprains are inversion injuries. This force is usually an internal rotation and plantar flexion of the foot in relation to the leg. The anterior talofibular ligament is always injured first, followed by the calcaneofibular ligament, and in severe cases with dislocation, the posterior talofibular

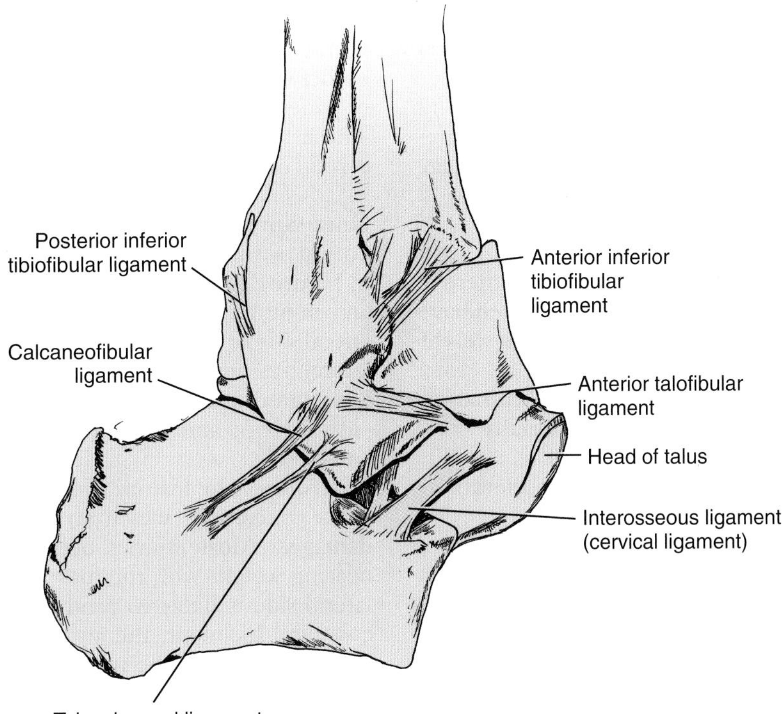

FIGURE 22-6 Lateral view of the ligaments of the ankle.

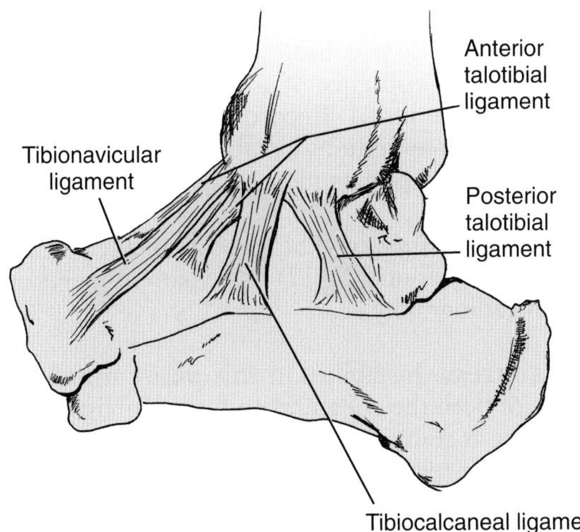

FIGURE 22-7 Medial view of the ligaments of the ankle.

ligament. It is difficult to clinically differentiate a severe second-degree sprain from a third-degree sprain of the ankle.

Some physicians recommend local or IV regional anesthesia followed by stress radiography to demonstrate instability and also recommend surgical repair of complete ligament ruptures, especially in competitive athletes. Other physicians recommend treating both second- and third-degree sprains by cast or brace immobilization and reserve surgery for patients who demonstrate an unstable joint after the conservative treatment has been completed and the ankle has healed. The following treatment, from the *Manual of Acute Orthopaedic Therapeutics* by Iversen and Swiontkowski,[7] is a useful approach for the nonorthopedist for this type of injury.

History. The history should focus on the mechanism of injury and the amount of functional disability for grading the sprain. Information on previous injuries to the ankle and their treatment should be obtained.

Physical Examination. Inspection will reveal ecchymosis and swelling of the ankle. Palpate carefully over the posterior talofibular ligament, calcaneofibular ligament, anterior talofibular ligament, deltoid ligament, and the anterior capsule to define the areas of injury. In addition, check for instability by performing the anterior drawer test. This is performed by holding the leg with one hand and grasping the heel with the other. Gently pull forward on the heel, and subluxate the talus anteriorly within the ankle mortise. A positive anterior drawer test indicates complete rupture of the anterior talofibular ligament. In addition, significant tenderness and swelling over the deltoid ligament or anterior capsule indicate that a severe sprain has occurred.

Laboratory Studies. Radiographs should be obtained, provided that the patient meets the criteria outlined in the ED.

Treatment. Treatment consists of synthesizing information from the history and physical examination to determine the severity of the sprain and diagnosing it as first, second, or third degree.

First-Degree Sprain

History. The patient sustains an injury, but there is little functional disability. The patient may even have been able to finish the activity and can bear weight without much discomfort.

Physical Examination. Physical examination reveals mild tenderness and swelling, usually confined to the anterior talofibular ligament.

Treatment. RICE (rest, ice, compression, elevation)

Second-Degree Sprain

History. The patient usually has functional disability immediately after the injury and is unable to continue activity. The patient bears weight poorly or not at all.

Physical Examination. Physical examination reveals moderate-to-severe swelling and tenderness over both the anterior talofibular and the calcaneofibular ligaments. There is usually no significant tenderness over the deltoid ligament or the anterior capsule, and the anterior drawer test is negative.

Treatment. Treatment consists of immobilizing the ankle, placing the patient on crutches, and referring the patient to an orthopedist in 24 to 48 hours for reevaluation. Immobilize by cast or splint. The ankle can be wrapped in two 4-inch rolls of cast padding followed by an Ace bandage or by using a plaster stirrup splint.

Third-Degree Sprain

History. The patient experiences immediate loss of function of the injured ankle and may relate that the ankle "feels" unstable with any attempt at weight bearing.

Physical Examination. Physical examination reveals severe swelling and tenderness over the anterior talofibular ligament, the calcaneofibular ligament, and, occasionally, the posterior talofibular ligament. There is also tenderness over the deltoid ligament and the anterior capsule, and the anterior drawer test is positive.

Treatment. The orthopedist should be contacted immediately. This allows the orthopedist the option of obtaining stress films and treating the injury surgically. It also gives the orthopedist the option of conservative treatment (i.e., soft roll, Ace bandage, ice, elevation, non–weight-bearing with crutches for a few days, followed by a short leg walking cast or ankle fracture splint for 6 weeks). If long-term lateral instability results from non-operative treatment, surgical repair will be necessary.

Ankle sprains have a high risk for morbidity. The average duration of disability has been reported to be between 4 and 26 weeks, and only 25% to 60% of patients are symptom free 1 to 4 years after injury. These so-called minor injuries, therefore, deserve careful diagnosis and treatment.

Knee Sprains. The medial side of the knee is supported by the tibial collateral ligament. The diagrams in Figure 22-8 illustrate the tibial collateral ligament and bony attachments to the femur and tibia. The lateral side of the knee is supported by the fibular collateral ligament and the iliotibial band (Figure 22-9). The anterior and posterior cruciate ligaments provide anterior and posterior stability (Figures 22-10, and 22-11).

History. The history of injury provides important clues concerning which structures may have been damaged. Most injuries occur while the patient is bearing weight with the foot fixed. A blow from the lateral side is likely to produce a tear of the medial collateral ligament, the anterior or posterior cruciate ligament, and the medial meniscus. Blows from the medial side, although rare, produce tears of the lateral collateral ligament, the iliotibial band, and the lateral meniscus. A hyperextension injury either forward or backward may produce tears of the cruciate ligaments.

Physical Examination. The physical examination begins with gentle palpation for areas of tenderness. The presence or absence of an effusion (fluid in the joint) should be noted. Record the range of motion and check for ligamentous instability. Lay the patient down with the knee extended, and gently apply varus and valgus stress.

Laboratory Studies. The knee is imaged to rule out a fracture (Figure 22-12) if the patient meets criteria for radiography.

Valgus Stress. Instability in this position indicates rupture of both the collateral and cruciate ligaments. If the knee is stable in extension, flex the knee 25 to 30 degrees to relax the cruciate ligaments and repeat the examination. Instability in this position indicates medial or collateral ligament tears (Figure 22-13A).

Anterior Drawer Sign. Have the patient flex the injured knee to 60 to 90 degrees and place the foot firmly on the table. It is easy to fix the foot in this position simply by sitting on it, which leaves both hands free to examine the knee (Figure 22-13B).

Pull the lower leg forward and backward, looking for any movement or instability in the joint. Any movement forward is positive for a tear of the anterior cruciate ligament, and any movement backward is positive for a tear of the posterior cruciate ligament.

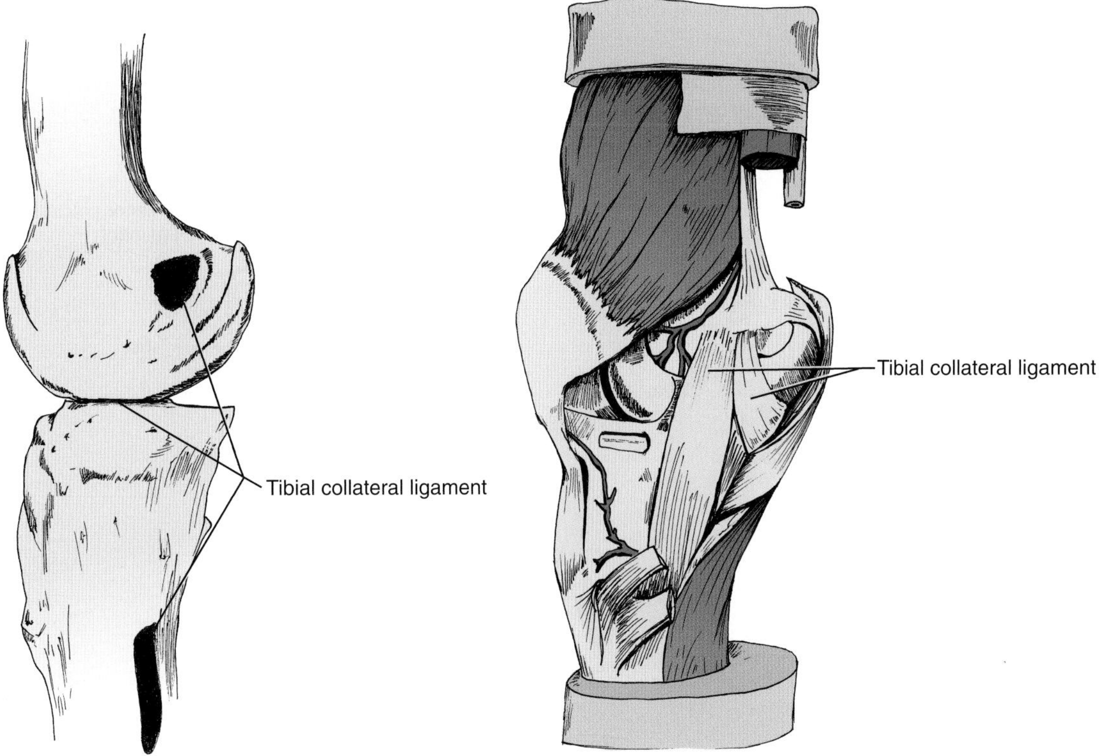

FIGURE 22-8 Tibial collateral ligament of the knee.

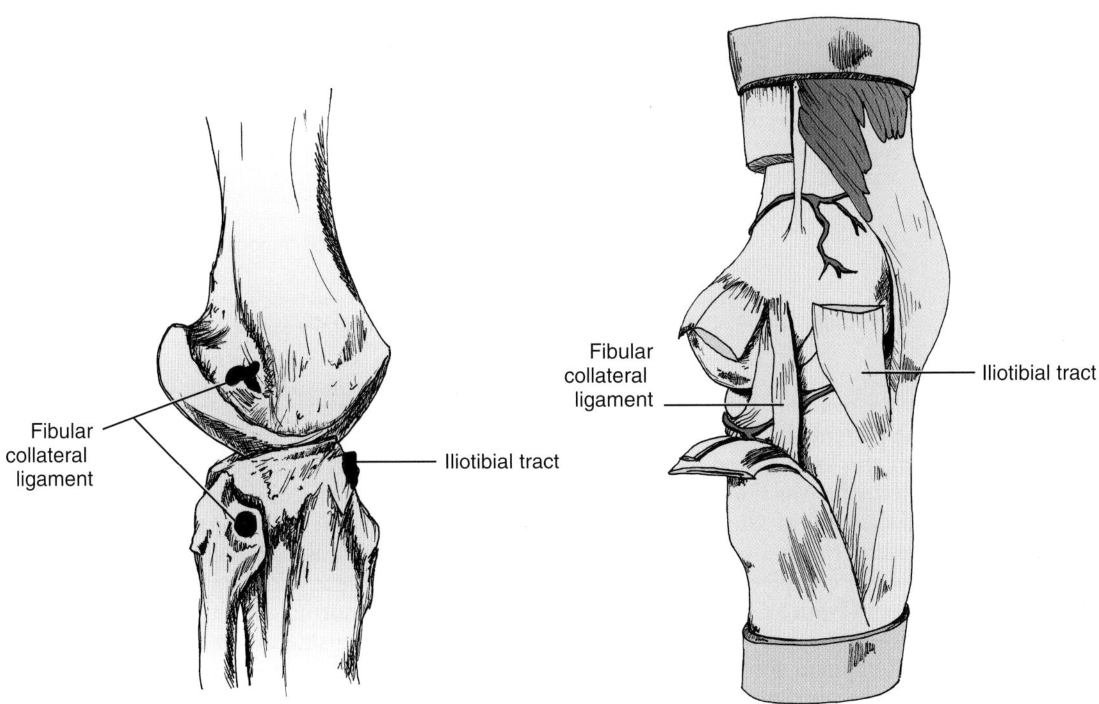

FIGURE 22-9 Fibular collateral ligament and iliotibial band.

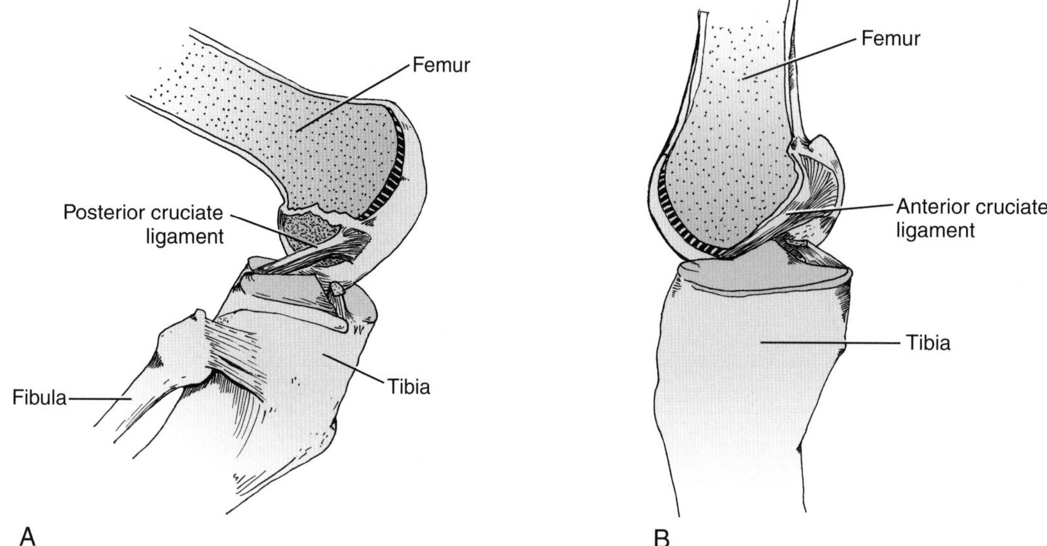

FIGURE 22-10 The posterior **(A)** and anterior **(B)** cruciate ligaments of the knee.

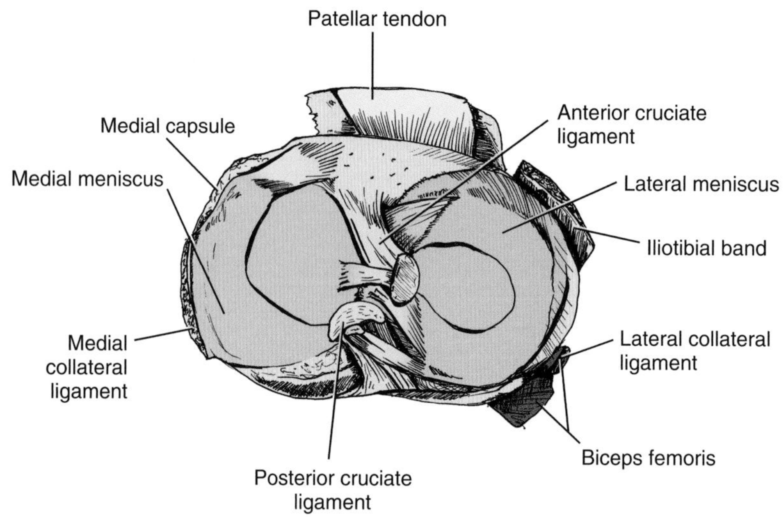

FIGURE 22-11 Cross-section showing the ligaments of the knee.

An alternative way to test the anterior cruciate ligament is to have the patient sit on the side of the examination table with the knee flexed 90 degrees. Gently pull forward on the proximal lower leg, looking for forward displacement of the tibia on the femur. If motion is present, this is a positive anterior drawer sign and indicates a complete rupture of the anterior cruciate ligament (Figure 22-14A and B).

Lachman Test. The Lachman test is also helpful for demonstrating anterior cruciate ligament instability. With the knee flexed 30 degrees, gently pull the lower leg forward on the femur, again looking for abnormal anterior motion. Assessment of the stability of the ligaments is difficult if the examiner is rough. Pain will cause the patient to contract the powerful thigh muscles, which may mask significant instability. Additionally, it is extremely important to examine both of the patient's knees, comparing the injured knee with the normal knee. This should be done because of the considerable variation from patient to patient in normal ligamentous laxity. Knee sprains are divided into first-, second-, and third-degree for treatment purposes.

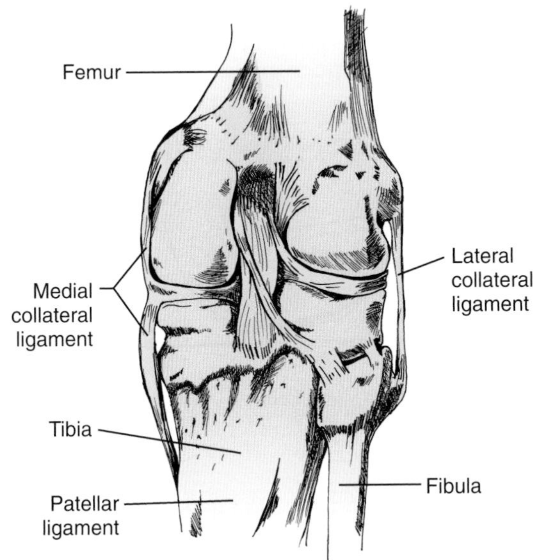

FIGURE 22-12 The knee from the front with the superficial structures removed.

First-Degree Knee Sprain

History. The patient experiences mild or no immediate loss of function.

Physical Examination. Physical examination reveals tenderness and mild swelling over the involved ligament. An effusion is not present. Gentle passive movement of the joint reveals a normal or near-normal range of motion. Stressing the ligaments may cause pain, but no instability is evident.

Treatment. Treatment is RICE: rest with activity within the limits of pain, ice, compression with an Ace bandage, and elevation.

Second-Degree Knee Sprain

History. The patient usually has some immediate loss of function.

Physical Examination. Physical examination reveals more swelling and tenderness over the involved ligament, and an effusion is often present. Range of motion is decreased. Stress testing reveals mild or no instability.

Treatment. In this case, the treatment is protection and referral. A useful approach follows.

- Aspirate the joint if a large effusion is present and is causing severe pain.
- Wrap the knee with an Ace bandage, starting at the foot and wrapping to above the knee to avoid a tourniquet effect.
- Apply a prefabricated posterior knee splint.
- Place the patient on crutches.
- Instruct the patient to apply ice for 20 minutes every 2 hours while awake.
- Prescribe a non-steroidal antiinflammatory drug as an analgesic.
- Have the patient perform ten 7- to 10-second isometric quadriceps contractions every hour while awake.
- Refer the patient to an orthopedist for follow-up in 24 to 48 hours.

Third-Degree Knee Sprain

History. The patient has immediate loss of function and may report that the knee feels unstable with attempted weight bearing.

Physical Examination. Severe tenderness and swelling are usually present over the involved ligaments. An effusion is usually present, although, if the joint capsule is torn, the blood may leak out into the surrounding tissues. Range of motion is severely decreased, and stress testing reveals instability, which is the hallmark of a third-degree sprain.

Treatment. Immediate orthopedic consultation is indicated if instability is demonstrated. It is important not to diagnose a second-degree sprain if a third-degree sprain is really present because the treatment for a third-degree sprain is usually surgical. Therefore, if the examination is inadequate because the patient is experiencing too much pain to relax the knee, consult an orthopedist immediately. The orthopedist may want to examine the patient under anesthesia.

Approximately 85% of patients who sustain a hyperextension injury of the knee and have a bloody effusion on examination have an anterior cruciate ligament tear. In light of this fact, it is prudent to obtain a next-day orthopedic consultation, even if instability could not be demonstrated on examination. The classic example of this type of injury in football is the punter whose down leg is hyperextended by a defender attempting to block the kick. It is difficult to diagnose a cartilage injury in an acutely injured knee unless the knee is "locked." This occurs when the torn cartilage blocks full extension of the knee and the patient reports that something is preventing him or her from straightening the knee. The knee is usually locked in 20 to 30 degrees of flexion. Consult the orthopedist immediately and follow the treatment regimen for second-degree knee sprains.

Patellar Dislocation. A common injury easily confused with a sprain is a patellar dislocation.

History. The patient relates that the knee went out of joint or dislocated. Complete loss of function is present if spontaneous reduction has not occurred.

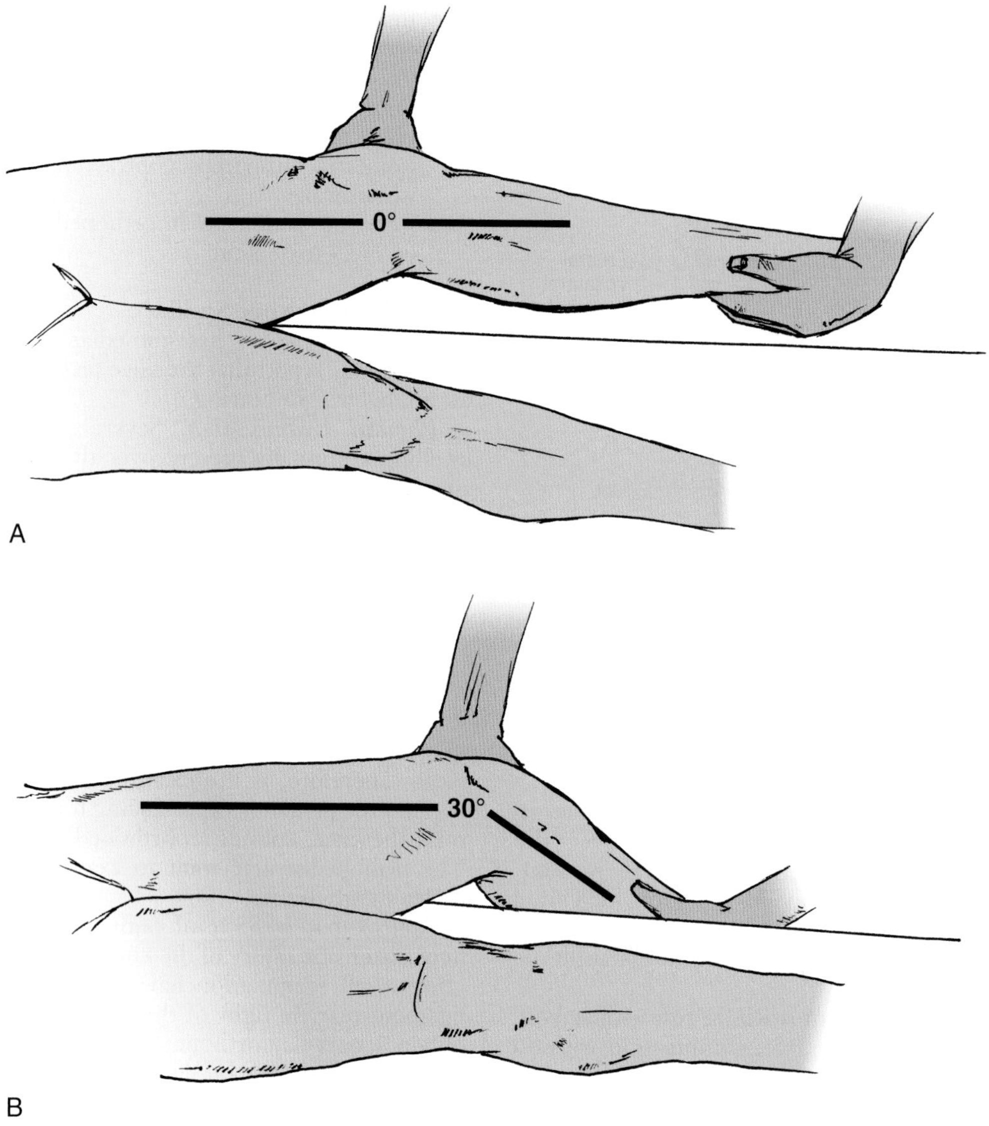

0°

A

30°

B

FIGURE 22-13 ■ Negative movement **(A)** and instability **(B)** of the knee under valgus stress.

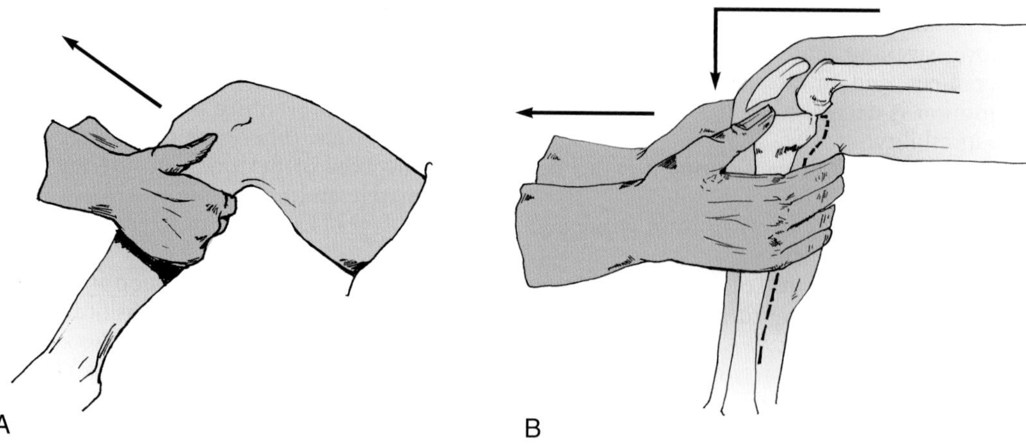

FIGURE 22-14 ■ Anterior **(A)** and alternative **(B)** drawer signs.

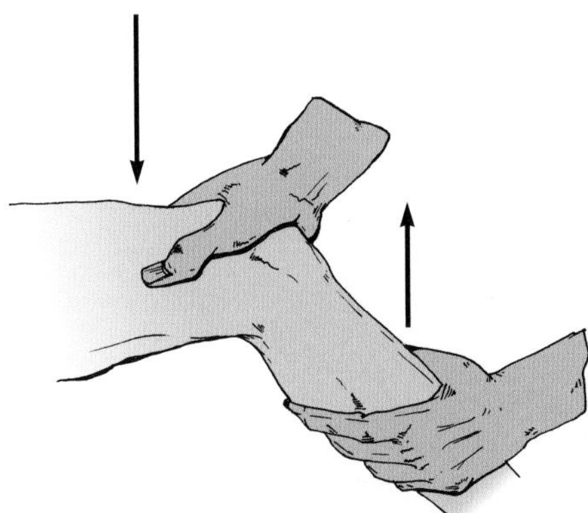

FIGURE 22-15 Lachman test.

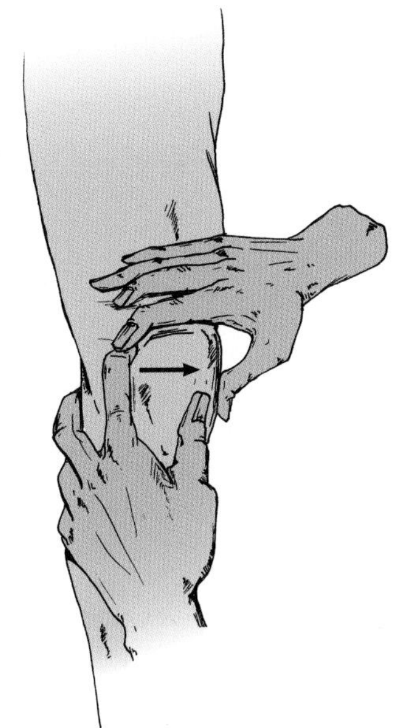

FIGURE 22-16 Patellar apprehension test.

Physical Examination. Physical examination reveals that the patella dislocated laterally and the patient is holding the knee at around 30 degrees of flexion. If the patella has spontaneously reduced, an effusion is usually present and tenderness is marked along the medial aspect of the patella, where supporting tissues were torn when it dislocated. Bending the knee slightly and applying a gentle force to the medial aspect of the patella with the fingers may demonstrate the instability of the tendon and redislocate the patella. Usually the patient apprehensively stops the examination at this point.

Treatment. If the dislocation is still present, it can easily be reduced by straightening the knee and pulling the patella toward the midline. Often, the dislocation has spontaneously reduced before examination. Although radiographic results are usually negative, occasionally a thin sliver of patella may appear medially to the patella. This sliver was avulsed as the kneecap dislocated laterally out of the femoral groove. A sunrise view of the patella is helpful in ruling out this fracture (Figures 22-15 and 22-16).

Shoulder Sprains and Strains. Patients reporting to the ED with shoulder pain frequently have negative results on standard radiography; however, many have significant injuries that require specialized care. Always helpful are a good understanding of the anatomy of the shoulder and an awareness of the clinical presentations of dislocations, acromioclavicular sprains, rotator cuff tears, and ruptures of the long head of the biceps tendon.

A fibrous capsule holds the humeral head in the glenoid cavity. Any sprain of the shoulder injures this capsule. The tendons of the muscles of the shoulder, which make up the rotator cuff, blend with this capsule, making it difficult to differentiate sprains from strains, but it is not important from the standpoint of treatment.

Figure 22-17 shows the posterior portion of the rotator cuff, which is made up of the infraspinatus and teres minor tendons. The infraspinatus has been cut and lifted to show the fibrous capsule underneath. The axillary nerve, which supplies motor power to the deltoid muscle and sensation to the lateral upper arm, is also visible. The tendons of the supraspinatus and subscapularis muscles form the superior and anterior portions of the rotator cuff. The long head of the biceps tendon enters the shoulder joint and is attached to the superior rim of the glenoid (Figure 22-18).

Anterior Dislocation of the Shoulder

History. The patient reports experiencing a force that caused a combination of abduction, extension, and external rotation of the shoulder. The capsule of the shoulder joint is torn from the glenoid, and the humeral head rests inferiorly and anteriorly in a subcoracoid position.

Physical Examination. The physical examination finds the patient holding the arm in slight abduction. The acromion will be prominent, and the deltoid will be flattened. Exclude neurovascular injury by feeling pulses, checking the function of the axillary nerve (most commonly injured), and checking the function of the musculocutaneous nerve. The axillary nerve provides sensation to the lateral upper arm and motor power to the deltoid, which abducts the shoulder.

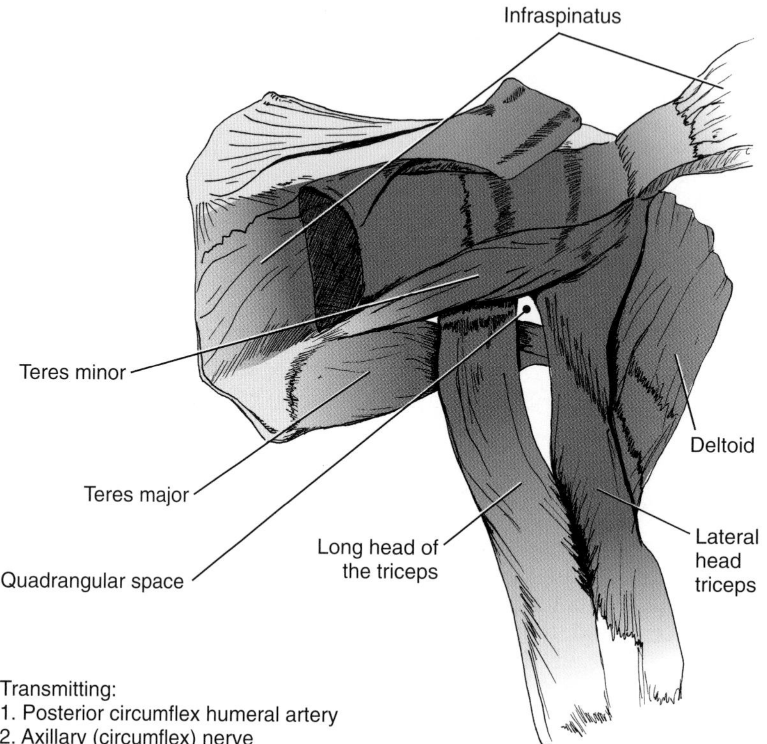

FIGURE 22-17 ■ Posterior portion of the rotator cuff of the shoulder.

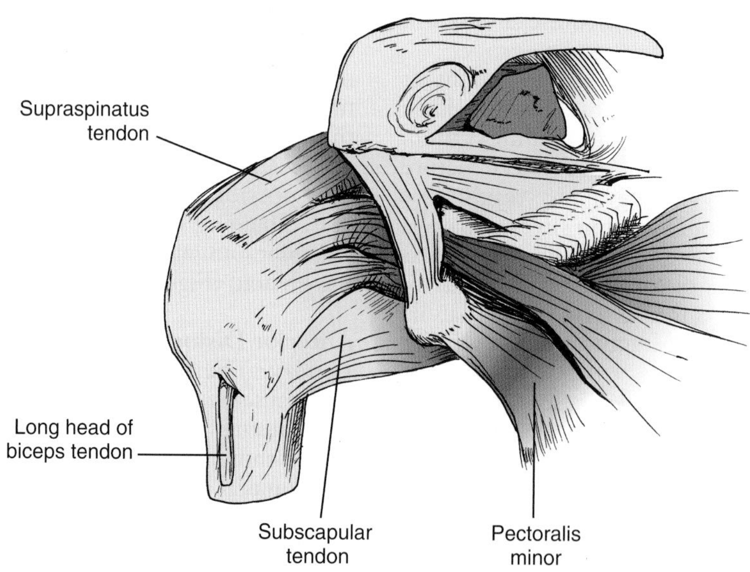

FIGURE 22-18 ■ Anterior portion of the shoulder.

The musculocutaneous nerve provides sensation to the volar radial side of the forearm and motor power to the biceps muscle. Loss of function is usually due to a contusion of one of these nerves and usually resolves spontaneously in a few weeks to 3 to 4 months.

Before examination, an analgesic should be administered parenterally and radiographs should be obtained. If a fracture is revealed, especially one involving the greater tuberosity or humeral head, immediate orthopedic consultation should be sought.

Treatment. If no fracture is present, the shoulder reduction can be accomplished in several ways; however, only the countertraction method is discussed here. With the patient supine, an assistant should position himself at the head of the bed on the side opposite the dislocated shoulder. A sheet should be looped over the patient's chest through the axilla, on the injured side, returning the sheet under the patient's back to exit near the assistant. The assistant stabilizes the patient and applies countertraction as the shoulder is reduced. The operator, using both hands to grasp the wrist on the arm with the injured shoulder, applies gentle traction, straightening the arm to 20 to 40 degrees of abduction. The operator can then lean back slowly, allowing his or her own body weight to apply even and steady traction and encouraging the patient to let the shoulder muscles relax and "turn into jelly." It is helpful to coach the patient in letting the muscles relax more and more with each exhalation. If reduction is not achieved in 2 to 3 minutes, midazolam (Versed) should be administered through an IV line at 1 mg every 30 to 60 seconds until relocation occurs or a maximum dose of 10 mg is reached. Follow the conscious sedation protocol for the ED when using IV midazolam. After reduction, the arm is placed in a shoulder immobilizer and the patient is referred to an orthopedist within the next 7 days.

Posterior Dislocation of the Shoulder. Posterior dislocations of the shoulder are rare and may be easily missed.

History. The mechanism of injury is usually a direct driving force against the lower end of the humerus while the arm is flexed forward. These injuries usually occur during a seizure with convulsions or from severe trauma. The force is transmitted up the arm, driving the humeral head posteriorly behind the glenoid. The patient experiences intense pain and is unable to move the arm, while the outward appearance of the shoulder is deceivingly normal. The patient holds the arm fixed to his or her side, usually with the forearm across the abdomen.

Physical Examination. The patient resists any attempt to examine or externally rotate the arm or shoulder.

Laboratory Studies. The AP radiograph appears normal because the head of the humerus moves almost straight backward and is not displaced inferiorly to any significant extent. An oblique radiograph must be taken with the patient erect and facing the cassette. This allows the central beam of the radiograph to correspond to the plane of the body of the scapula. In difficult cases, a transaxillary view taken while the arm is abducted with the patient under general anesthesia is diagnostic.

Treatment. Orthopedic referral is indicated immediately.

Rotator Cuff Tears

History. Rotator cuff tears may accompany shoulder dislocations and severe shoulder strains. They are difficult to diagnose unless massive.

Physical Examination. On physical examination, the patient is unable to initiate abduction and the arm falls to the patient's side when passively abducted to 30 degrees and dropped (drop arm test). If the patient can actively abduct the arm as little as 15 to 20 degrees, a complete rotator cuff tear can be ruled out.

Laboratory Studies. The tear can be confirmed with an arthrogram, and surgical repair is necessary, especially in athletes.

Treatment. Orthopedic consultation should be obtained if this complication is diagnosed.

Acromioclavicular Joint Sprains. The clavicle is connected to the acromion process of the scapula by the acromioclavicular (AC) ligament (AC joint). The AC ligament is weak and is easily ruptured with mild trauma. The clavicle is anchored to the coracoid process of the scapula by the strong coracoclavicular ligament.

History. The mechanism of injury is a downward force over the superior acromion process, resulting in varying degrees of sprain to the AC joint. The most common example of this is a fall on the point of the shoulder, as from a horse or a motorcycle. It is critical to diagnose the degree of sprain in a shoulder injury. A first-degree sprain exhibits an incomplete tear of the AC ligament without subluxation of the joint. A second-degree sprain is more severe and demonstrates a disruption of the AC ligament that allows partial separation of the AC joint, while the coracoclavicular ligaments remain intact. A third-degree AC sprain (complete shoulder separation) is a complete tear of the AC and coracoclavicular ligaments with a complete dislocation of the AC joint (Figures 22-19 through 22-21).

Physical Examination. In a first- or second-degree sprain, the patient has point tenderness and swelling over the AC joint. Deformity is not present or is negligible.

Laboratory Studies. If standard shoulder radiographs are negative, stress radiographs should be taken. A single view of both AC joints is made with a 5- to 10-lb weight attached to the wrists of a standing patient. The patient must be educated

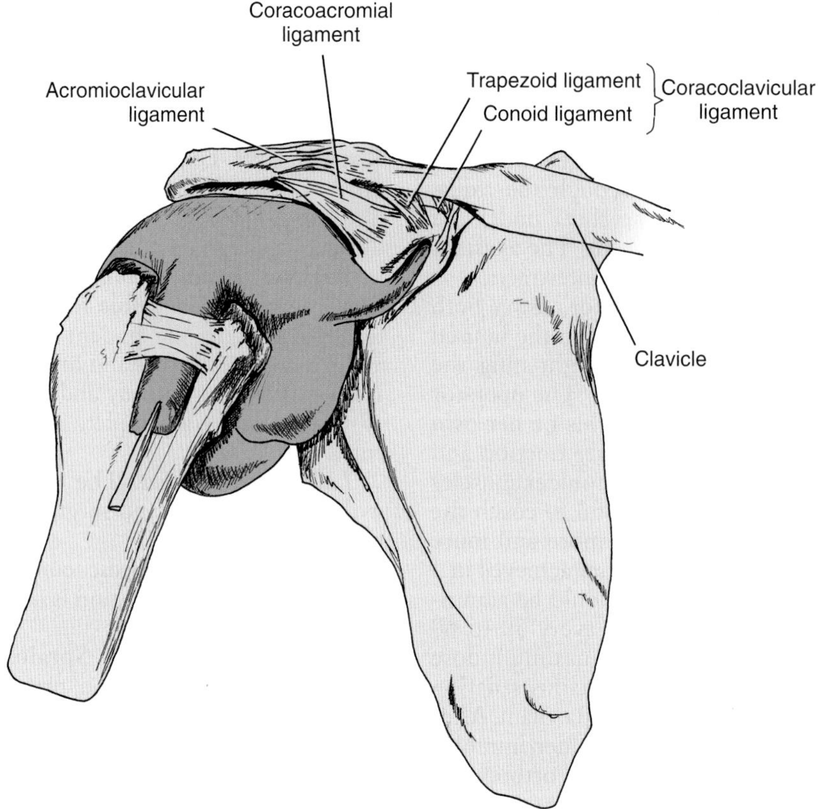

FIGURE 22-19 ■ Ligaments of the shoulder.

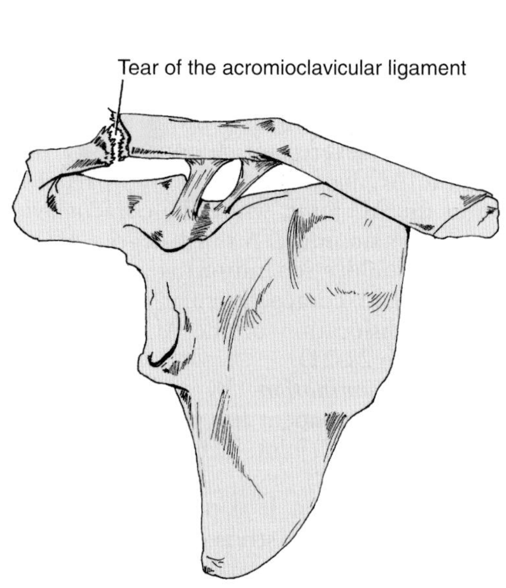

FIGURE 22-20 ■ Second-degree sprain of the shoulder, with tear of the acromioclavicular ligament.

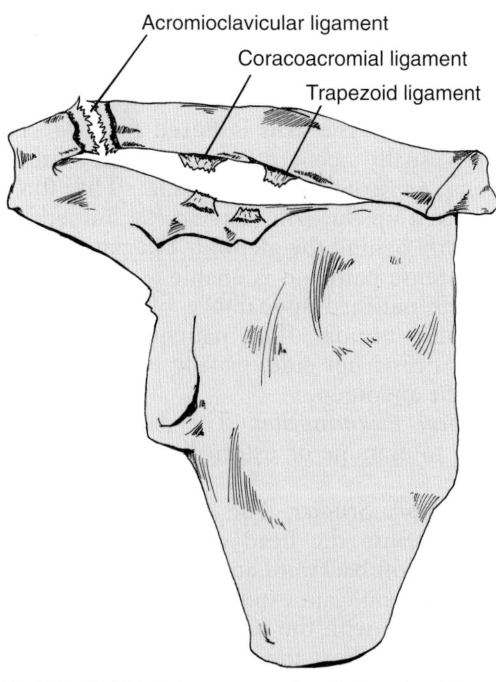

FIGURE 22-21 ■ Third-degree sprain of the shoulder, with complete shoulder separation.

not to take the strain off the AC joint by contracting the biceps muscles, or a false-negative result may occur. A *first-degree* sprain has a normal stress film. A *second-degree* sprain shows widening of the AC joint but no increased distance between the coracoid and the clavicle. The upward displacement of the distal clavicle should not be more than the full diameter of the clavicle. These injuries may be treated symptomatically with pain relievers and immobilization with a sling for 10 days to 3 weeks, followed by a rehabilitative exercise program.

The patient with a *third-degree* sprain has an obvious deformity with the skin tented by the distal end of the clavicle and the shoulder dropped down. Routine views of the shoulder usually show the clavicle to be riding high, completely out of the AC joint, with a widened space between the clavicle and the coracoid. Third-degree sprains require orthopedic referral. Currently, most orthopedic surgeons advocate surgical repair, especially in athletes (see Figure 22-21).

Rupture of the Long Head of the Biceps Tendon
The biceps tendon runs in the intertubercular groove of the humerus through the shoulder joint to attach to the posterior superior aspect of the glenoid.

History. This injury is most commonly found in the elderly, usually as a result of attrition due to chronic bicipital tenosynovitis. Under these circumstances, it acquires a secondary attachment to the intertubercular groove and is discovered at autopsy. Clinically, this would be an elderly patient with a chronically painful shoulder that suddenly quits hurting when the rupture is complete. The muscle belly bunches up and appears prominent in the distal arm; however, surgical repair is generally not indicated in this group of patients.

Acute rupture in a younger person occurs as a result of forceful contraction of the biceps muscle or forceful downward movement of the arm with the biceps contracted. The diagnosis is readily apparent when the patient contracts his or her biceps with the arm abducted 90 degrees and externally rotated.

Treatment. Treatment is always surgical, whereby the long head of the biceps tendon is fastened into the intertubercular groove of the humerus.

MISCELLANEOUS CONDITIONS

Baseball Finger

Also known as *mallet finger*, the pathology is pictured in Figure 22-22.

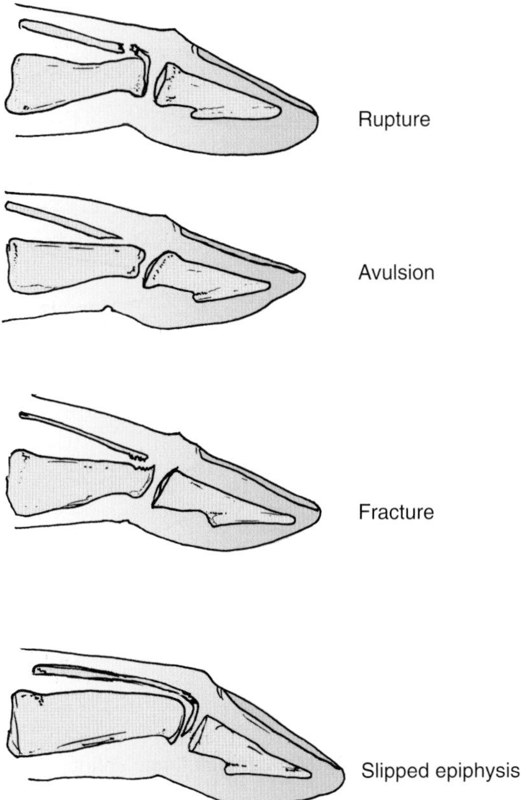

FIGURE 22-22 Baseball finger (mallet finger).

History. The patient presents with a history of blunt trauma to the end of the finger.

Physical Examination. Physical examination reveals tenderness, swelling, and inability to extend the distal interphalangeal (DIP) joint. The DIP joint is pulled into flexion by the unopposed flexor digitorum longus tendon.

Laboratory Studies. Radiographic results range from normal to an avulsion fracture or may reveal an epiphyseal fracture.

Treatment. If the extensor tendon is avulsed from its attachment to the distal phalanx with no fracture or a small avulsion fracture, treatment consists of immobilizing the distal phalanx in hyperextension. A commercially available Stack finger splint (Bird & Cronin, Eagan, Minn.) is excellent (Figure 22-23).

If the Stack splint is not available, peel the foam off a piece of padded aluminum splint material and construct a small metal dorsal mallet finger splint (Figure 22-24).

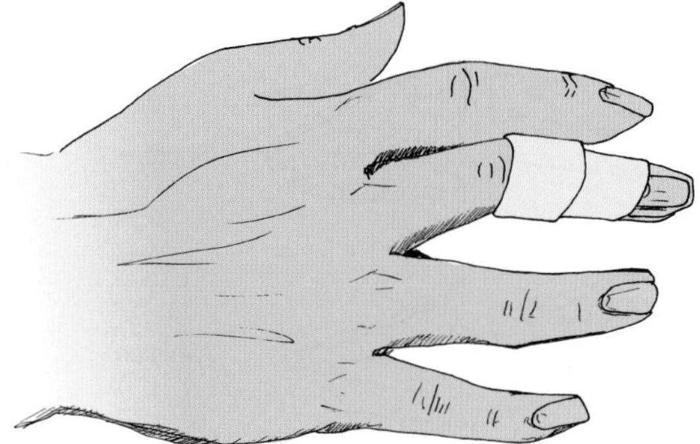

FIGURE 22-23 ■ Stack finger splint.

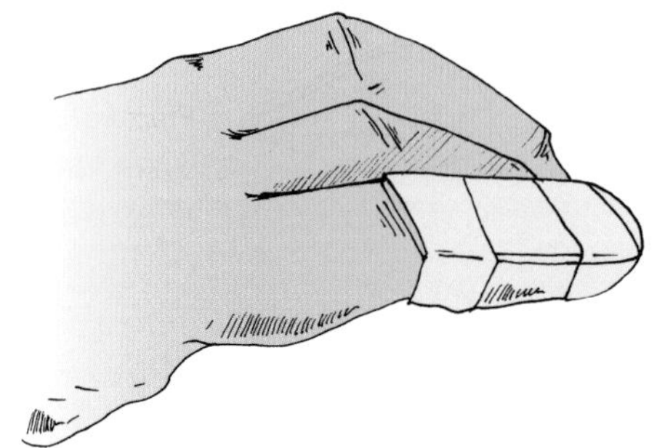

FIGURE 22-24 ■ Metal mallet finger splint.

If the avulsed fragment involves one third or more of the articular surface, immediate orthopedic consultation is indicated for surgical repair.

Ruptured Central Slip of the Extensor Tendon

The central slip of the extensor tendon attaches to the base of the middle phalanx. The lateral bands converge and attach to the base of the distal phalanx (Figure 22-25).

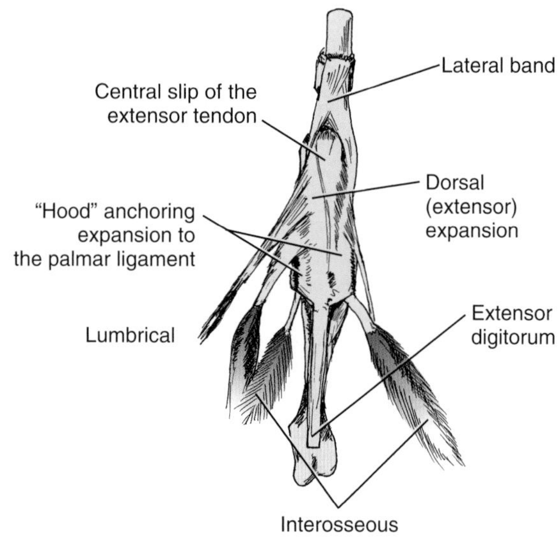

FIGURE 22-25 ■ Dorsal view of the middle phalanx, showing the central slip of the extensor tendon.

History. The patient who ruptures the central slip presents with a jamming injury to the finger.

Physical Examination. Physical examination reveals tenderness and swelling over the dorsum of the proximal interphalangeal (PIP) joint. The patient is unable to extend the PIP joint or extends it weakly. Careful testing of extensor function must be done with every PIP joint sprain, or this injury is easily missed.

If it is missed, over time the lateral bands will slip below the axis of motion of the PIP joint and pull the PIP joint into flexion and the DIP joint into hyperextension. This is called the *boutonnière deformity*, and the patient ends up with a serious problem requiring surgical correction (Figure 22-26).

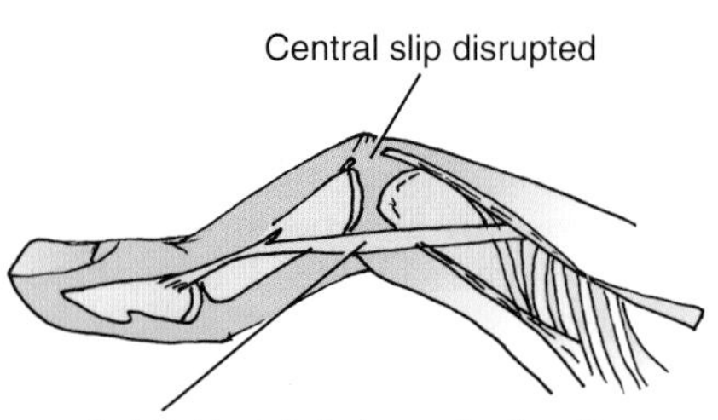

FIGURE 22-26 ■ Central slip disrupted.

Laboratory Studies. Radiography results are negative.

Treatment. If injury is detected early, splinting in extension for 3 weeks usually results in adequate healing.

Rupture of the Extensor Pollicis Longus

The extensor pollicis longus tendon is the sole extender of the interphalangeal (IP) joint of the thumb (Figure 22-27).

History. The patient presents with a history of blunt trauma to the thumb or with a spontaneous inability to extend the distal phalanx of the thumb sometime after a fracture of the distal radius. It also occurs occasionally in people who have occupations that require continuous motion with the wrist in dorsal flexion and radial deviation (drummers). The tendon runs obliquely across the dorsum of the radius and is gradually destroyed from friction.

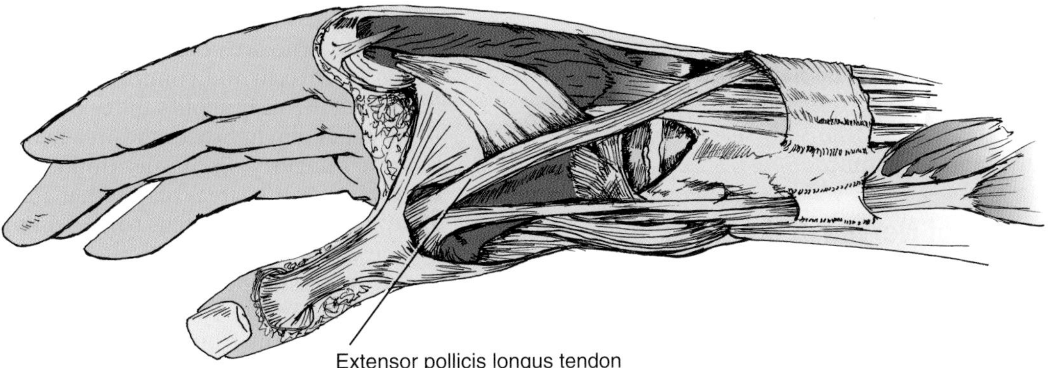

FIGURE 22-27 ■ Extensor pollicis longus tendon.

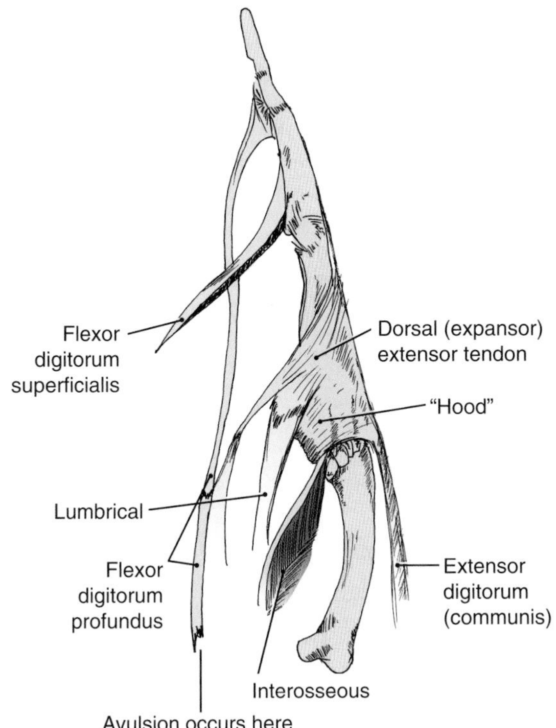

FIGURE 22-28 ■ Flexor digitorum profundus tendon.

Dislocation of the Extensor Tendon at the Metacarpophalangeal Joint

History. Here the radial aspect of the joint capsule of the metacarpophalangeal (MP) joint will rupture, usually following a blunt trauma.

Physical Examination. When the patient tries to extend the finger actively, the tendon will slip off to the ulnar side at the MP joint. Passive extension of the finger "pops" it back into place.

Treatment. An orthopedic consultation for surgical repair is indicated.

Rupture of the Flexor Digitorum Profundus

The flexor digitorum profundus tendon attaches to the base of the distal phalanx and flexes the DIP (Figure 22-28).

History. The patient sustains some blunt trauma, which results in disinsertion of the profundus tendon from its attachment on the volar aspect of the base of the distal phalanx.

Physical Examination. Physical examination reveals inability to flex the distal phalanx.

Laboratory Studies. This may occur with or without a tiny bone chip being evident on radiograph.

Treatment. Referral for surgery is indicated.

NEUROLOGIC AND TENDON EVALUATION OF THE FOREARM, WRIST, AND HAND

Median Nerve

Motor function is tested by having the patient touch the tip of the thumb to the tip of the fifth finger. Sensory function is tested on the volar aspect of the distal phalanx of the index finger.

Ulnar Nerve

Motor function of the ulnar nerve is tested by having the patient pinch the thumb against the index finger while the examiner palpates the dorsal interosseous muscle for contraction. An alternative method is to have the patient lay his or her hand palm-down flat on the table and adduct and abduct all the fingers. Sensory function is tested on the volar aspect of the distal phalanx of the fifth finger.

Radial Nerve

Motor function is tested by having the patient dorsiflex the wrist. Sensory function is checked on the dorsum of the hand in the web space between the index finger and the thumb.

Distribution of Nerves of the Hand

The standard distribution of the cutaneous nerves to the palm and dorsum of the hand is shown in Figure 22-29. There are many variations in this pattern, and it is helpful to know the areas of the hand that are supplied by this nerve. These areas are called the autonomous zones and are represented by the *dark shading* within each dermatome.

Testing for sensation can be done in several ways.

- *Sharp-dull:* A sterile, 18-gauge needle can be used to touch the patient in various places over a specific dermatome, using both the point and the hub of the needle to determine whether the patient can differentiate between the two.
- *Light touch:* The examiner touches the area to be examined lightly with his or her finger, comparing the sensation with the uninjured extremity.
- *Two-point discrimination:* Using a straightened paper clip bent into a U shape, the patient is asked to determine whether two points are felt or just one. The examiner positions himself or herself in such a way that the patient cannot observe the area being tested. The patient should be relaxed and comfortable. The examiner simultaneously applies the two blunted ends of the paper clip lightly to the area being tested. A normal finger pulp can discriminate points 2 to 4 mm apart. On areas of skin that are callused and tough, this area widens to 4 to 6 mm apart. On the dorsum of the hand, the patient should be able to determine a normal distance of about 8 to 10 mm. Another useful point is that sweating will be absent from the skin when sensory innervation has been interrupted.

Tendon Laceration Injuries

A laceration on the dorsum of the distal forearm, wrist, and hand can cause tendon injuries that are difficult to diagnose if one does not have a thorough knowledge of the anatomy. Evaluating these types of injuries involves testing the function of the tendon both actively and actively against resistance while directly visualizing the wound, with bleeding controlled by a tourniquet.

This is important because if the common extensor to the middle finger is lacerated proximal to the intercommunicating slips from the other extensor tendons, the patient will still be able to actively extend the middle finger. Also, a laceration of the

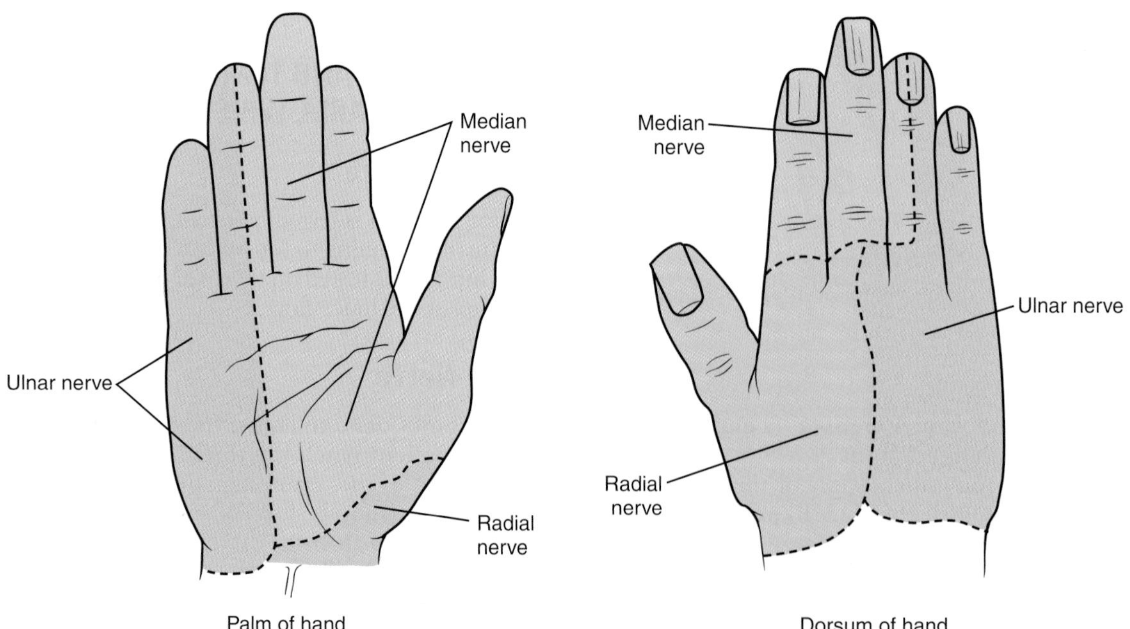

FIGURE 22-29 Sensory nerve distribution of the hand.

extensor pollicis brevis is easily missed because the extensor pollicis longus is capable of extending both the MP joint and the IP joint. The extensor carpi radialis longus can be bisected, and the patient could still be able to extend the wrist with the extensor carpi radialis brevis and vice versa. For these reasons, it is critical to evaluate the tendons not only functionally but also under tourniquet control to directly visualize any tendon injury. This is the only way to reliably diagnose complete and partial tendon ruptures.

Testing Tendon Function. To test *extensor digitorum communis* tendon function, have the patient actively extend each finger and hold it extended against resistance. Significant pain or weakness may indicate a partial laceration of the tendon. Have the patient extend the thumb against resistance while the *extensor pollicis longus* and the *extensor pollicis brevis* tendons are palpated. These tendons will be tense if they are intact. Test wrist extension against resistance using the other hand to palpate over the *extensor carpi radialis longus*, *extensor carpi radialis brevis*, and *extensor carpi ulnaris* tendons. Intact tendons should feel tense and be strong.

The volar aspect of the forearm, wrist, and hand is equally treacherous. Knowledge of the anatomy and how to test each tendon is required to avoid morbidity.

The *flexor digitorum superficialis* functions to flex the PIP joint of the fingers. Because the flexor digitorum profundus can also flex the PIP joint, its influence must be eliminated during the examination. This can be accomplished by holding all the fingers in extension except the finger to be tested. Have the patient rest his or her hand on a flat surface palm-up and stabilize all the fingers in extension, except the finger to be tested. The patient should then flex the remaining finger at the PIP joint actively and actively against resistance. Pain and weakness may indicate a partial laceration. If the tendon is completely transected, there will be no flexion.

The *flexor digitorum profundus* is tested by holding the PIP joint in extension and checking for flexion of the DIP joint actively and actively against resistance.

The *flexor pollicis longus* flexes the IP joint of the thumb and can be tested in like manner.

The *flexor carpi radialis* and *flexor carpi ulnaris* flex the wrist and are tested by having the patient flex the wrist against resistance while palpating each of the tendons in turn.

The *palmaris longus* tendon has no essential function and may be left alone or repaired at the physician's and the patient's discretion. Any laceration of this tendon can be diagnosed only by direct visualization under tourniquet control.

Tourniquet control of bleeding can be achieved by inflating a blood pressure cuff on the upper arm. With the patient in a supine position, have him or her point the injured extremity toward the ceiling while straightening the arm and holding it there for a couple of minutes, to allow as much venous blood to drain as possible. With the arm still elevated, the blood pressure cuff should be inflated to 250 mm Hg and held there during the examination. This procedure provides the examiner a bloodless field, and, although it is uncomfortable for patients, most can tolerate it for up to 15 minutes.

WILDERNESS MEDICINE

Since the early 1950s, when Outward Bound *(www.outwardbound.org)* moved from England to the United States, outdoor pursuits have become the fastest growing segment of recreational life in this country. Sixty years ago, a person could hike all day in the Catskills or backpack for a week in the Rocky Mountains without seeing another person. However, in 1964 the U.S. Congress passed the Wilderness Act. The original bill established 9.1 million acres of federally protected wilderness in America's national forests. This simple publicity popularized the notion that the average American could venture into the wilderness. Americans began turning more attention to the outdoors and the environment. Unprecedented numbers of people now enter into environments previously reserved for the most stout-hearted adventurers.

In 1965, Paul Petzolt founded the National Outdoor Leadership School (NOLS: *www.nols.edu*). His goals were to have people learn to care about and protect the wilderness. Both the Outward Bound and NOLS organizations had within their curriculum first aid and survival courses; however, if someone became injured or lost in the wilderness, he or she was left to his or her own ingenuity, physical stamina, and wilderness savvy to survive. In many cases, victims were rescued by their companions or by Good Samaritans. Search and Rescue (SAR) was conducted by the local police or sheriff's office, and the actual treatment of injuries and illnesses was left to the emergency physician after the injured party reached the hospital.

In 1971, the Yosemite Institute *(www.yni.org)* began sponsoring outdoor educational programs at Yosemite National Park. Four years later, they held the first yearly symposium and other conferences focused on mountain and wilderness medicine. Health care workers from all aspects of medicine attended these meetings in droves. Attendees included a few visionary emergency physicians who recognized the need for health care providers to obtain the necessary skills to diagnose and treat wilderness medical emergencies. In 1983, the first edition of the textbook that became *Wilderness Medicine*, currently in its fifth edition and edited by Paul Auerbach, was published with 27 chapters. The book now has 97 chapters and 157 contributing authors, truly "the bible" on wilderness medicine for health care providers.

At approximately the same time as publication of the first edition of the textbook, three California physicians—Paul Auerbach, Ed Geehr, and Ken Kizer—incorporated the Wilderness Medical Society (WMS: www.wms.org) as a nonprofit organization designed "to encourage, foster, support, and conduct activities or programs concerned with the life sciences, which may improve the scientific knowledge of the membership and the general public in matters related to wilderness environments and human activities in these environments." Its mission remains "to advance healthcare, research, and education related to wilderness medicine." The pillars of the program include hazards of environmental exposure such as heat and cold injury, altitude illness, hyperbaric medicine, and trauma in the wilderness; hazardous marine life; mammalian bites; venomous bites and stings; survival techniques; search and rescue; resuscitation; infectious disease associated with travel; medical fitness and nutrition for wilderness activities; and expedition medical planning. They explore health risks and safety issues in extreme locations such as mountains, jungles, deserts, caves, marine environments, and space. The WMS was first accredited by the Council for Continuing Medical Education in 1990 and has maintained its accreditation every 4 years since then. Excellence in programming is the key feature of the society's educational efforts.

The society holds its annual meetings in spectacular locations noted for their outdoor lure and wilderness activities. These locations include Yosemite National Park, where the first meeting was held in November 1984. Other noted locations are the Grand Tetons, Wy.; Big Sky, Mont.; Keystone, Colo.; Snowmass, Colo.; Stratton Mountain, Vt.; Park City, Utah; Snowbird, Utah; Lake Placid, N.Y.; and Kananaskis, Canada.

Topic-specific meetings began in 1991 with "Winter Wilderness Medicine" in Crested Butte, Colo. Since then, specialty meetings have developed in travel medicine, desert medicine, and dive medicine. In 1991, the first World Congress on Wilderness and Mountain Medicine was held in Whistler, British Columbia, Canada, setting the stage for cooperation among other related organizations from around the world, such as the International Society of Mountain Medicine, the International Society of Travel Medicine, and the International Commission for Alpine Rescue.

"Wilderness Medicine," the official newsletter of the Wilderness Medical Society, made its debut in January 1984 and has been published quarterly since. It is currently in magazine format. In 1987, the *Journal of Wilderness Medicine* began publication. In 2000, the name was changed to *Journal of Wilderness and Environmental Medicine* to more accurately portray its contents. In 1990, an educational lecture slide series was inaugurated; it covers a variety of wilderness medicine topics, "written by doctors for doctors, medical students, and other health care providers." This series was revised in 2001 and is currently undergoing further revision. The WMS also supports an extensive bibliography of more than 160 pages divided into 29 sections, with more than 350 listings covering all aspects of medicine for the outdoors.

Wilderness medicine is for people who love the outdoors, have a deep respect for the environment and our precious natural resources, and want to combine these with their chosen field of medical expertise. With about 272 million visitors to America's national parks in 2006 and 2007, there were 15,846 incidents requiring emergency medical response. That figure had increased from 13,898 in the previous year, 2005. The more adventure travelers extend themselves into the wilderness, the greater the risk for injuries and survival situations. Because of the foresight of a few individuals who loved the outdoors and combined this love with their profession, wilderness medicine has now been added to many of the nation's medical school curricula and has become a medical specialty.

The Coalition of Outdoor Medicine Physician Assistants (COMPAS) is an interest group of the WMS. The group has two goals. First, health care providers have the mission to further promote their profession within wilderness and travel medicine; second, these providers should pursue their passion for the outdoors.

MISCELLANEOUS CONDITIONS

Insect in the Ear

The patient presents to the ED in distress with a history of awakening from sleep with pain and motion in the ear. The usual culprit is a roach that has crawled into the ear canal while the patient was asleep. Occasionally, and less commonly, the patient relates that something flew into his or her ear. To kill the insect, fill the ear canal with Auralgan ear drops, alcohol, or 2% lidocaine. After the insect is dead, it can be removed by flushing the ear with a Water-Pik or a

22-mL syringe with a 14-gauge angiocath attached. Only lukewarm water should be used. If this method fails, the insect will have to be removed piece by piece with a small pair of alligator forceps, using an otoscope for direct visualization.

Fishhook Removal

The most common and effective way to remove a fishhook is first to anesthetize the entire area surrounding the hook. Push the hook barb through the skin. Cut off the barb with a small pair of wire cutters. Withdraw the hook by reversing it through the original puncture site. Note: While cutting off the barb, catch it before it flies away by placing a 4 × 4 gauze over the hook barb before clipping it with the wire cutters.

Ingrown Toenail

Patients often present to the ED with an infected ingrown toenail, usually on the big toe. The standard treatment is to remove the ingrown portion of the nail, thereby releasing pressure on the surrounding tissue. This is best accomplished by a digital block with 0.5% bupivacaine (Marcaine) and removal of the lateral one fourth of the nail on the affected side. Once adequate anesthesia has been achieved, slide one half of an opened hemostat under the edge of the nail from the top to the cuticle margin. Close it and roll the edge of the nail toward the center, pulling it from beneath the inflamed nail fold. The hemostat can then be removed and the freed edge of the nail cut off with a pair of scissors. Dressing the toe should include antibiotic salve, nonadhering dressing pads, and a small roller gauze. Systemic antibiotic and analgesic should be prescribed, and the patient should be instructed to follow up with the regular family physician for a wound check in 48 hours.

DRUG AND ALCOHOL POISONING IN THE EMERGENCY DEPARTMENT

Alcohol and drugs are estimated to be involved in more than 50% of all visits to the ED. This is true from small suburban EDs to large county trauma centers. Recognizing the physical and physiologic patterns of intoxication will help the ED provider with the early management of these patients and may predict other concurrent pathology, any possible sequelae, and their eventual disposition. Several factors work against the health care provider when he or she is attempting to treat a patient in the ED who is under the influence of alcohol or drugs. These patients are often unwilling or unable to give a clear history of the events that led to the ED visit. There are considerable consequences involved both legally and socially with substance abuse, and patients often consider it in their best interest to prevaricate. Despite this, the ED provider is asked to distinguish the differences between the patient with an acute intoxication and a patient with preexistent pathology. Additionally, the ED provider may be confronted by a patient with both a preexistent illness and an acute intoxication. In this case, the medical history will help to determine specific management.

Alcohol creates a myriad of pathologies. It leaves no system untouched and remains a difficult addiction to treat. A complete discussion on alcohol and its associated complications is beyond the scope of this chapter; however, a brief explanation of the additional history needed for the completeness of the treatment of an intoxicated patient admitted to the ED is warranted.

Considering that what looks, smells, and tastes like alcohol is not always alcohol and, conversely, that ethanol is an ingredient in many substances, it is imperative that the cause of the patient's condition be identified before any medical intervention is initiated. Additionally, its presence is not always readily appreciated by the history. A Breathalyzer is a quick, cheap method for confirming the presence of alcohol in a patient, but it is not sufficient to rule out other ingestions. If the patient arrives by ambulance, EMS personnel who were first to treat the patient may provide valuable information about the circumstances and condition. Questions should be asked, such as: Who called the ambulance? Where was the patient picked up? What containers or paraphernalia were apparent at the scene? Were there any witnesses, and what did they report? Was there any trauma? Do the paramedics know this patient from previous runs? At this point, it is extremely important to know this patient's drinking habits. The patient's drinking pattern may predict withdrawal complications, and the health care provider has the ability to plan for the patient's recovery in a safe environment.

Alcoholism is a physiologically global addiction that affects all the major organ systems. A comprehensive physical examination must be part of the treatment. The vital signs and a complete visual examination of the skin are two of the most important steps that can be accomplished when evaluating the patient. Completely undress the patient and take care to look for obvious trauma. This information should correlate directly with the history. Keep in mind that intoxication can historically and physically mask signs and symptoms of trauma. Laboratory tests should be judiciously guided by the history and physical examination.

A few simple laboratory tests should be considered for all intoxicated patients. These patients are frequently hypoglycemic, and a blood glucose level should be determined as soon as the patient is stable. Alcoholics are prone to metabolic and electrolyte imbalances, as well as dehydration. Pulse oximeters should be initiated soon after the patient reports to the ED for determination of the patient's oxygen saturation level; cardiac monitors will provide reassurance during the treatment of the patient.

The provider should know what resources within the hospital and community are available to patients with alcohol-related problems. Before the patient leaves the ED, two questions should be answered: Is this an opportunity to offer the patient and family assistance with alcoholism? Does this patient have medical follow-up?

Alcohol is not the only recreational drug with medical complications. Cocaine is probably the most often used and most commonly encountered recreational drug nationwide. Narcotics, hallucinogens, benzodiazepines, and the ever-changing designer drugs are popular and all carry health risks. These classes of drugs can often be recognized by their characteristic physical signs, and it is imperative that the PA knows the pattern, complications, and treatment for these drugs.

The distinction between a drug of abuse and a medication is largely a legal definition rather than a medical one. Any patient with an overdose is considered to be the responsibility of the ED to evaluate and manage. Fortunately, there is an extensive network of poison control centers around the nation to assist in identifying and isolating the toxic substance and recommending appropriate therapy.

Following are some general principles for treating the patient with an acute overdose:

1. Identify the patient and get an accurate history about the ingestion as soon as possible. Details may tend to blur or be forgotten altogether as time elapses after an ingestion. Inquire about the amount of the drug ingested, its strength, and over what period of time the drug was taken. Was the drug combined with any other medications? Is this a regularly prescribed medication or an over-the-counter medication? Has the patient eaten, or is there any alcohol involved? Did the patient vomit? If so, when and how many times, and what was in the vomitus? What was the maximum number of milligrams that the patient could have taken, on the basis of the historical evidence and the scene? What did the patient say about the ingestion during transport? Does the patient have any medical problems? Again, the family and the prehospital personnel are good sources of information. Question the EMT about the condition of the scene. The unintentional overdose is most often by its nature a single-agent ingestion. The suicide attempt, however, must always be suspected to be a multidrug ingestion. Commonly available and potentially lethal substances such as aspirin and acetaminophen may complicate the picture of an overdosed patient. Additionally, these medications are clinically undetectable.
2. Monitor the patient while gathering information about the overdose and while considering the treatment options. In addition to monitoring of vital signs, a stable patient should be placed on a cardiac monitor and a pulse oximeter. An IV line will allow quick intervention in the patient who is unstable. Monitoring for expected signs and symptoms of the drug's toxicity is inexpensive and offers immediate intervention as soon as the drug or drugs are identified. There are relatively few specific antidotes to most of the available drugs; however, oxygen, glucose, and naloxone (Narcan) are commonly used and are standard drugs for paramedics to administer to patients in the field. These three medications should not be neglected in the ED. Other antidotes require specific clinical or laboratory evidence of ingestion and toxicity before their use, and the descriptions are found in most standard ED texts. In most overdoses, patients who are clinically stable receive activated charcoal to absorb any drug remaining in the gastrointestinal tract.

The patient admitted to the ED with a deliberate overdose activates a special and unique set of guidelines. The health care provider is obliged to treat this patient, regardless of the circumstances and occasionally with full knowledge that the patient may make another attempt as soon as he or she leaves the facility. It may be impossible to sort patients with a deliberate overdose from those experiencing an accidental overdose. Initially, the health care provider must assume all overdoses are intentional and that all patients need to be protected from themselves. The precautions taken to ensure the patient's safety while in the ED vary from community to community, and most EDs are aware of the ramifications of holding a patient against his or her will. Patients cannot be restrained or detained without cause, and usually this is delineated in a document called a "hold." Each state has specific guidelines that must be met when providers are attempting to hold a patient, and in most cases, PAs are not authorized to sign and initiate the hold. A hold initiates a cascade of events that should include informing the patient and family that a hold has been signed, why it was thought necessary, what restrictions will be placed on the patient's movements, and how and when the patient will be released from the hold. Holds, although necessary, should not be initiated thoughtlessly and should be frequently re-evaluated for their continued necessity.

Some key questions in evaluating the intoxicated patient include the following:

1. How did the patient come to the attention of the ED?
2. Is trauma involved? Can the patient protect his or her own airway?
3. Is alcohol intoxication confirmed? How?
4. Is ethanol alone responsible for the patient's clinical state?
5. Is the patient progressing as expected in his or her detoxification? If not, have other pathologies been considered?
6. Has the patient's disposition been planned, and how will he or she be kept safe until then?

LEGAL AND ETHICAL DECISIONS IN EMERGENCY MEDICINE

The emergency arena presents some unique ethical and legal choices to the medical practitioner. The issues of treatment of minors, resuscitation of the terminally ill, elder abuse, attempted suicide, mental illness, and determination of incompetence are just a few examples. Providers in some branches of medicine may work with one or more of these issues on a regular basis. In this case, the patient is known and the clinician has access to the medical chart for completeness. The ED clinician is at a considerable disadvantage in attempting to treat a patient because of this lack of knowledge; therefore, the physician or PA must proceed with the belief that the treatment given to the patient in the ED is desired. In retrospect, the treatment may be resented, contraindicated, unnecessary, or controversial. Some of these cases have been litigated so extensively that formal guidelines covering the permutations and combinations of a situation have been established. Decisions to act or not act, to investigate or not investigate, and to uphold the rights of one party over the wishes of another are less clearly defined. The outcome depends on the practitioner's willingness to accept responsibility for these moral questions as part of the job. Few clinicians relish this kind of unhappy controversy and may use the situation as an opportunity to educate a patient and family about the options and consequences of each procedure and to empower them to participate in the decision-making process. Allowing the patient and family this freedom creates a jointly shared responsibility and is more likely to result in a more favorable outcome for all involved.

One of the least acknowledged but most frequently encountered ethical decisions in emergency medicine is the decision to treat the sickest patient first. The long-cherished belief in "first come, first served" is frequently disregarded from the time the patient enters the ED and remains throughout the stay. Although the concept is not new to most patients, it still causes protests at the triage desk.

Privacy, both physical and informational, is a concern of all branches of medicine. Because of the physical layout of most EDs, privacy is a difficult commodity to ensure. Patients and families themselves often forget that their conversations can be overheard by the patient in the next cubicle. PAs should avoid contributing to this unrestrained exchange of information by presenting their patients quietly when on rounds; refraining from discussing a conscious, competent patient's condition with family or friends without the expressed consent of the patient; and ensuring the privacy of the physical examination. When in doubt about how the patient wants the examination conducted or his or her test results discussed, it is prudent to discuss everything with the patient first. Questions from a patient about other patients in the ED often reflect the inquirer's anxiety about his or her own medical problem. Reasonable curiosity and human concern can be met with reasonable replies. The PA should deflect with tact and compassion the questions that pry into another patient's private business.

Information regarding the patient's visits to other hospitals is protected under the right to privacy act. The patient must sign a consent form authorizing the release of these records to another facility. All states have exceptions to the privacy of information act and require reporting of cases in one or more of the following areas: communicable diseases; victims of violence, including child and elder abuse; animal bites; venereal diseases; poisonings; and unexplained death. The patient must be informed that this information will be reported to the public health services, social services, or the appropriate law enforcement agency.

The medical system's obligation in treating minors (those younger than age 18) has always been a gray area. The law provides the following guidelines:

1. If an emergency exists, treat.
2. If the patient is a minor who presents for evaluation of pregnancy-related problems, venereal disease, or substance abuse problems, most states provide for treatment of the condition without prior consent or reporting to the parent or guardian.

3. If the patient presents for a nonurgent condition, obtain consent of the legal guardian before the patient is treated.
4. If a legal guardian is unavailable, a court may appoint a guardian.

Regardless of the law involved, remember that these children are still entitled to participate in their own care and to be informed of their diagnoses and possible treatments.

ED personnel are often in the position of evaluating patients whose mental competence is in doubt. Indeed, people are sometimes brought in from the community solely for the purpose of having the ED physician determine their mental competence. The elements of competence should be reviewed in advance. People are judged to be competent if they:

1. Have the ability to understand options.
2. Can understand the consequences of choosing each of those options.
3. Can evaluate the relative merits of those options with regard to their value system.
4. Can communicate with their wishes.

Occasionally, patients are admitted to the ED from nursing homes or a psychiatric facility with their mental competence and legally appointed guardian previously determined. This is usually documented in the forms that accompany patients from their residences. Frequently, these patients have a terminal condition. The legal guardians appointed to make decisions will have been consulted and will have signed forms attesting to how they believe the patient would wish to be treated or not treated as they approach death. Do-not-resuscitate (DNR) means that in the event of cardiac arrest, cardiopulmonary resuscitation and ACLS measures to restart the heart should not be used. Do-not-intubate (DNI) would seem to be a fairly self-explanatory order but actually has some important and common exceptions that need to be considered before the patient has respiratory compromise. The intent of the DNI order is to prevent a terminally ill patient from being intubated and becoming ventilator dependent with no hope for regaining independent respiratory function. On the other hand, elderly patients or patients with eventually terminal diseases can suffer temporary respiratory complications, such as pneumonia, from which they could fully recover if they were temporarily assisted by intubation and ventilation. When this circumstance is explained to the patient or family, they can appreciate the distinction between the two anticipated outcomes and may well suspend the DNI order.

DNR and DNI do not mean that patients cannot be treated. The patient who is admitted to the ED with these standing orders should still be treated for reversible conditions. This treatment may include IV fluids, antibiotics, diuretics, antiarrhythmics, oxygen, Foley catheter, or whatever is clinically indicated to relieve the presenting complaint. In addition to the DNR or DNI order, the patient may have written orders further limiting care (e.g., no IV antibiotics or no hyperalimentation). Laws vary from state to state concerning advance directives and decision-making for incompetent patients. In the absence of clear, written documentation of the patient's wishes, the department is obliged to proceed with resuscitation.

SPECIAL CONSIDERATIONS

The ED is also the repository for a heterogeneous group of patients with a chief complaint of "bizarre behavior." During the initial evaluation of these patients, it is imperative that the cause of their behavior be considered organic and correctable. Unlike most of the other patients in the ED, these patients usually do not author their own chief complaint and are often denying it vigorously. These patients generally have a difficult time understanding why they have been detained in the ED to begin with. "Bizarre behavior" or "altered mental status" encompasses a wide range of disease processes. The diagnosis of a psychiatric disorder may precede the true cause and relationship of an intracranial bleed. Patients who appear "high" act bizarre, as do patients who are hypoxic. Delusional patients may view the health care provider as a threat and strike out. They may have a violent psychotic personality or they may be hypoglycemic. Patients who will not answer questions may be stubborn and angry, or they may be recent stroke victims. The ability to triage these patients appropriately takes a special appreciation of all the possibilities.

Occasionally, some of these patients may exhibit violent behavior. The first rule for the provider in attempting to treat these patients is to protect himself or herself. The second rule is to protect the other patients in the ED, and the third rule is to protect the patient in question. The patient who is restrained and is in police custody is usually the accompanying officer's responsibility. However, if the patient is not under arrest, it is up to the ED personnel to appropriately restrain and/or isolate the patient. The ED provider is now in the delicate position of making a judgment about the potential for a patient to become violent solely on the basis of the history provided by others relating to the patient's behavior before arrival in the ED.

When patients are considered to be at risk for harming themselves or others, the ED is obliged by law to ensure that this does not happen. If the ED provider elects to use physical restraints, he or she must ensure the patient's safety by frequent and periodic reassessments. The evolution of these events may be a relatively rare occurrence in certain EDs and may be a daily routine in others.

There are many legal and ethical questions involved in restraining patients against their will. The law provides for medical "holds" on patients if:

- The patient is considered to be a danger to himself or herself.
- The patient is considered to be a danger to others.
- The patient is considered to be unable to care for or make decisions for himself or herself.

Although the PA may initiate a hold on a patient by virtue of being the first to evaluate the patient, the physician of record is responsible for signing the hold. There is no correct answer, only a weighing of the risks and benefits of restraining patients and placing them on hold and the importance of an accurate history and physical examination as soon as a patient reports to the ED.

When a provider is confronted by a patient who is acting strangely and cannot give a history regarding the illness, the physical and mental assessment may be inadequate. In most EDs, four quick diagnostic screens that may identify a life-threatening condition in these types of patients are available:

- Oxygen saturation
- Serum glucose level
- Electrocardiogram
- Blood alcohol level

Other valuable diagnostic tests that may be considered but for which the results will take longer to obtain are:

- Serum electrolyte levels
- Blood urea nitrogen level
- Arterial blood studies
- Urinalysis

Drug or medication overdose should always be a consideration in evaluation of the patient with an altered mental status or abnormal behavior pattern. Medications prescribed and taken in overdoses may be the problem, and any indication of a specific substance that may be found in the patient's blood should be relayed to the laboratory. This information can often direct the laboratory in deciding which test should be conducted. However, the laboratory should not be solely depended on for providing a diagnosis. The history and physical examination along with the laboratory findings will reveal the most appropriate treatment for the patient. It is imperative that each health care provider in the ED is familiar with the categories of chemicals that laboratories may screen for, what type of specimen that laboratory may need, and the time it takes to report the results. Additionally, the PA must be aware of what prescriptive and nonprescriptive drugs commonly cause behavioral changes, as well as how to counteract them. Considering these questions may save valuable time when one is confronted with an uncooperative patient with an inadequate history.

Patients with psychological illness are sometimes identifiable by their typical patterns of behavior; however, organic pathology in a patient with a known psychological illness must be considered. This is especially true for the patient presenting to the ED with a significant change in behavioral routine. In this case, the old chart may be a most helpful clue to the patient's illness and may reveal an identifiable profile or characteristic that the patient is not exhibiting at the time of examination.

Most ED providers are not well versed in the evaluation of patients with psychological illness, and the activity in a typical ED is not an ideal environment for a comprehensive psychological workup. First, all medications and their prescribed dosages must be reviewed. The patient may be in the ER because of a medication change or a dosage change, or because of an interaction of a medication with another drug, or the patient for some reason has been unable to take a scheduled medication. Psychotropic medications are well known for side effects, abnormal interactions with other drugs, and individually narrow therapeutic windows. If the evaluation of a patient with a known psychiatric illness fails to reveal any physical cause of this ED visit, reevaluation by a psychiatrist or other specialists in mental health must be initiated.

More than in any other medical setting, the ED personnel are confronted with patients and families in crisis. Providers here experience firsthand how families with different cultural and religious beliefs deal with unexpected medical emergencies. Managing the reactions of patients with minor illnesses and their families may demand more flexibility on the part of the ED personnel than the responsibility incurred at the time of another patient's death within the department.

The ED is one of the few socially acceptable public places where people tend to "let their hair down," and the emotions expressed may reflect a reaction to much more than the patient's medical emergency. Individual patients vary in their reactions to the loss of control, to pain, or to the uncertainty of a medical illness, as do their families. Sometimes the behavior of the patient and his or her family seems totally inappropriate and disproportionate to the patient's situation. This may be a culturally comfortable way for the patient and the family to react, but it may not be comfortable for the ED staff. It is important for each provider to recognize this and allow the patient some latitude, thus giving back to the patient some of the control lost when his or her life was interrupted by the event that necessitated the ED visit.

However, when one patient's method of coping is total decompensation, it is time for the ED staff to step in. If the department is big enough and empty enough, this may simply be a matter of moving the patient to a more secluded area. When this is not possible, the ED provider must impress on the patient that moderating his or her behavior is mandatory, to the extent of threatening to expel the patient from the ED if the behavior does not change. It is preferable to give the options and allow the patient to suggest a resolution, but most importantly, the patient, family, friends, and anyone else in the ED must realize that the ED provider is in command and that he or she has the authority to maintain control by whatever means necessary within the law.

ED personnel are confronted with patients in pain, fearful of a serious diagnosis, hostile, distrustful, worried, anxious, humiliated at the loss of privacy, and angry at their incapacity. These predominantly negative emotions inevitably surface in some patients and occasionally may be directed at a provider. The provider experiences similar emotions when confronted by a hostile, angry patient. Pain may arouse fear. Fear can create anxiety. Anxiety begets anger and hostility. *The alleviation of pain may be the single most important act a provider can perform in the ED.* In addition, this simple understanding may short-circuit the cascade from pain to hostility and avoid serious confrontations.

CLINICAL PEARLS IN EMERGENCY MEDICINE

The following is a list of selected clinical pearls gathered by the authors of the textbook *Emergency Medicine: An Approach to Clinical Problem-Solving*, Hamilton and co-workers,[1] reprinted here with permission from W.B. Saunders Company. Many of these pearls apply to everyday care in the ED. Many will stand the test of time; others will be forgotten as research proves them obsolete. Currently, they offer an insight into the hazards and rewards of the specialty. Reviewing them before each tour of duty is a worthwhile exercise. Although many others are worth learning, these are some of the best.

A. The New Job

1. Respect is earned.
2. Befriend, through a show of respect, the nursing staff.

B. Maximizing Patient Satisfaction with Your Care

1. Avoid medical jargon.
2. Learn how to tell a patient you do not know what is wrong.
3. Let the patient know he or she is always welcome to return.

C. Minimizing Patient Dissatisfaction

1. One hour feels like three behind a curtain.
2. A companion makes the wait less unbearable.
3. Give the patient an estimate of the time needed to complete the evaluation. Significant delays require an honest accounting.

D. You Are the Patient's Advocate

1. If you must, err on the side of helping the patient.
2. Respect the patient's need for privacy.
3. Always consider the "costs" of your interventions.
4. Do not negotiate any medically important decision with a patient with an altered sensorium, particularly if it is due to alcohol or other substance abuse.
5. If a patient is a source of potential harm to himself or herself or others, or cannot take care of himself or herself, he or she must stay for observation or admission.
6. Physical restraint may be necessary and appropriate to protect the patient or ED staff.
7. Do not discharge a now "sobered" patient who has recovered from acute alcoholism without performing a repeat history and physical examination.
8. Anxiety and hysteria are diagnoses of exclusion.

E. Clinical Judgment

1. When the clinical impression does not fit with the history, physical examination results, or laboratory evaluation, STOP! Rethink and expand the differential diagnosis.
2. If the patient cannot walk, he cannot go home.
3. If the ancillary data do not fit the clinical picture, reconfirm the accuracy of the data before making treatment and disposition decisions.
4. If you seriously consider a specific diagnosis when working through a differential diagnosis, you should rule it out with the appropriate tests.
5. "If you don't know what to do, do nothing." Observe the patient closely for the evolution

of the disease process instead of gambling on a marginally indicated therapeutic intervention.
6. Always assume that females of childbearing age might be pregnant and act accordingly.
7. The patient who returns to the ED on an unscheduled basis is first assumed to be at high risk for a serious illness.
8. Abnormal vital signs must be repeated and explained.
9. A patient who will not look at you during the history and physical examination is usually either depressed or manipulative. Almost never is such a person shy.
10. Patients usually have one major medical problem for each decade of life after the age of 60.
11. Never completely trust a younger child, a geriatric patient, an alcoholic, or a drug abuser. That is, corroborate the history and carefully interpret the physical findings in each of these patients.
12. Listen closely to the suggestions of patients and their families about what is wrong and how they should be treated.

F. Specific Clinical Situations

During the winter months, if the whole family has "the flu," be sure to consider carbon monoxide poisoning.

Ask what caused the trauma in the patient you are treating. Trauma is often considered the only problem and not potentially the result of another problem.

1. Consider the diagnosis of ruptured (or expanding) abdominal aortic aneurysm in all patients older than 60 years who appear to have renal colic.
2. Because the eye is to see, record its acuity.
3. Always confirm a field or bedside glucose oxidase strip reading in the ED with a blood glucose level.
4. Multiple drug allergies often correlate highly with functional or psychogenic complaints.
5. Chest pain radiating below the umbilicus or above the maxilla is seldom cardiac in origin.

G. Pediatric Encounter

1. Speak to children in language they can understand.
2. Allow parents to stay in the room. Observing the child's interaction with his or her parents is an important part of the evaluation.
3. Children are rarely hypochondriacs.
4. Examine neurovascular and motor integrity before focusing on the injured area.

H. Communicating with the Attending or Consulting Physician

1. Confirm admission or discharge with the primary physician before committing yourself to the patient.
2. When in doubt, a second opinion to confirm a clinical impression is always appropriate.

I. Avoid Supporting the Legal Profession

1. Do not think you are going to win just because you are "right."
2. Protect yourself by protecting the patient.
3. A printed form never saved anyone.
4. One of the most hazardous moments in emergency medicine is "signing out" patients to a colleague at the end of one's shift. A complete and accurate exchange of information and impression is necessary.

J. Destroying Your Credibility

1. Subvert the call schedule or be chronically late.
2. Yell at someone.
3. Give an opinion before looking at the patient.
4. Treat a number, not the patient.

K. Your Mental Health

1. Every physician/PA/student has moments of self-doubt.
2. There is always a disposition.
3. When you find yourself becoming angry with a patient ("positive personal hypertension sign") during history taking, you must step away momentarily. The patient may be malingering and withholding or providing misleading information, or you may be fatigued or have lost your perspective in your role. In any case, the emotion and its origin must not be allowed to influence or impair your judgment.

L. Do's

1. Meet every patient turned over to you at the change of shift.
2. Order soft tissue radiographs to rule out suspected soft tissue foreign bodies.
3. Respond to complaints by private attendings immediately to avoid irreparable damage.
4. Always see and interpret the diagnostic studies you have ordered.

M. Don'ts

1. Never say: "There is nothing wrong with you."
2. Do not expect patients to remember verbal information.
3. Do not try to weasel out of accepting responsibility when you blew it. Admit the error, apologize, and get on with life.

CLINICAL APPLICATIONS

1. Describe how the perceptions of emergency medicine by patients and clinicians have changed over the past 30 years.
2. Identify 10 general principles that guide the practice of emergency medicine.
3. Define the following categories of medical emergencies—critical, acute, and urgent.
4. Describe the typical role of a PA in an ED.
5. If you accepted a position in an ED, how would you update your knowledge base and clinical skills for this practice specialty? What might you expect to be the challenges and satisfactions that you would experience as a PA in emergency medicine?

KEY POINTS

- Emergency medicine has experienced some drastic changes over the past 20 years.
- Triage is still the most important initial tool for the clinician in an ED setting.
- The problem-oriented history and physical examination is the staple of all the providers.
- The development of a separate Fast Track section in an ED is becoming commonplace, taking the true non–life-threating patients out of the mix and treating them from a walk-in clinic setting.
- More and more EDs are staffing their Fast Tracks with PAs.

References

1. Hamilton G, Sanders A, Strange G, et al. Emergency Medicine: An Approach to Clinical Problem-Solving. Philadelphia: WB Saunders; 1991.
2. American College of Emergency Physicians Position Statement on PAs in Emergency Medicine. Irving, TX: ACEP, 1990.
3. American College of Emergency Physicians Position Statement on PAs in Emergency Medicine. Irving, TX: ACEP, 1990.
4. Brunette DD, Kominsky J, Ruiz E. Correlation of emergency health care use, 911 volume, and jail activity with welfare check distribution. Ann Emerg Med 1991;20:739.
5. Beth Israel Medical Center, 1990.
6. Gilbert D, Moellering R, Sande M, (eds). The Sanford Guide to Antimicrobial Therapy. Sperryville, VA: Antimicrobial Therapy Inc., 1998.
7. Iversen LD, Swiontkowski MF. Manual of Acute Orthopaedic Therapeutics. 4th ed. Philadelphia: Lippincott Raven, 1994.
8. Mengert T, Eisenberg M, Copass M. Emergency Medical Therapy. 4th ed. Philadelphia: WB Saunders, 1996.

The resources for this chapter can be found at www.expertconsult.com.

CHAPTER 23

PEDIATRICS

Linda M. Dale • Lois C. Thetford • Linda J. Vorvick

CHAPTER CONTENTS

The skills of the physician assistant (PA) involve both the art and science of medicine. The role of the PA in pediatrics is to be a resource and guardian for the physical, emotional, and mental health of infants, children, and adolescents as they evolve along a continuum of growth and development. Helping parents with the anxieties of the responsibility of a new life, seeing the tangible effects of using healing skills on behalf of a child, working with special needs children to grant them the dignified life they are entitled to, and getting to know families and watching their children mature are just a few of the rewards. As in the practice of medicine in any other realm, there are also tragedies and losses that require commitment and compassion if the PA is to be of true service to children and families. The privilege of working with young people as they grow and mature cannot be underestimated.

In this chapter, the history of the practice of pediatrics in the United States, the role of PAs in pediatrics, issues in pediatric medicine as they help define pediatric practice, settings and areas of specialization in which PAs work within pediatrics, and challenges for the future are reviewed.

HISTORICAL PERSPECTIVE

In the United States, pediatrics did not emerge as a distinct area of medicine until the late 1800s. The first infant mortality studies were done in Philadelphia in 1871. The Society for the Prevention of Cruelty to Children was founded in 1876. Public health efforts on behalf of children began in 1897, when the New York state legislature mandated that New York City hire doctors and nurses to work with families in an attempt to alleviate the suffering of infants dying of "summer diarrhea." White House Conferences on Children began in 1910 during the administration of Theodore Roosevelt. Subsequent conferences have been held every decade since then. The Child Labor Law was passed in 1916. In 1930, the American Academy of Pediatrics was founded. The Shepard-Towner Act, passed in 1921, authorized health care funds for mothers during childbearing years and for infants. This act served as the foundation for Title V programs that mandated health services for indigent mothers and children, to be administered by health agencies in states and territories. Services for crippled children were also provided. In the 1960s, services for children were expanded with the Maternal and Child Health, Crippled Children, Head Start, Job Corps, and Medicaid programs.[1,2] There have been numerous advances and losses in the provision of health care on behalf of children. Experience has proved that in periods of economic uncertainty, programs for children are among the most vulnerable to governmental cutbacks.

The contributions of PAs to pediatric health care began in 1969, with Henry K. Silver, MD, and the innovative Child Health Associate Program at the University of Colorado School of Medicine. The 3-year Master of Science program was designed to create new professionals who were able to provide comprehensive health services to children in an era when it was anticipated that resources for children would continue to be strained. As envisioned by Silver, child health associates are trained to work with physicians as colleagues and associates. They provide a wide range of diagnostic, preventive, and therapeutic services for children, as well as parent and patient education, support, and counseling.[3]

Although the Child Health Associate Program was designed to offer specialized training in pediatrics, all current PA training programs that emphasize primary care provide pediatric training. Graduates of many programs may choose pediatrics as an area of focus. PAs identifying pediatrics or pediatric subspecialties as their areas of practice represent 4.1% of the members of the American Academy of Physician Assistants (AAPA).[4]

TABLE 23-1 **Percentage of Infant Deaths, United States, 2007***

RANK	CAUSE OF DEATH	PERCENTAGE
1	Congenital anomalies	19.9
2	Disorders relating to short gestation and unspecified low birth weight	16.7
3	Sudden infant death syndrome	8.4
4	Newborn affected by maternal complications of pregnancy	6.1
5	Accidents (unintended injuries)	4.4
6	Newborn affected by complications of placenta, cord, and membranes	3.9
7	Bacterial sepsis of newborn	2.8
8	Respiratory distress	2.7
9	Diseases of the circulatory system	2.1
10	Neonatal hemorrhage	2.0
	All other causes	31.0
Total		100.0

From Xu J, Kochanek KD, Murphy SL, Tejada-Vera B. Deaths: final data for 2007. Natl Vital Stat Rep 2010;58:1. *http://www.cdc.gov/nchs/deaths.htm*. Accessed August 2, 2011.
*The 10 leading causes of death before age 1 year, per 100,000 live births.

ISSUES IN PEDIATRICS

Pediatric practice encompasses the care of patients from birth through adolescence. One way to define the scope of pediatric practice is to look at the risks to health and development that affect children and adolescents. Health supervision and attention to both acute and chronic illness should be provided to all children as they mature.

Table 23-1 ranks the causes of infant (<1 year of age) mortality in the United States.[5] The U.S. infant mortality rate is 6.75 infant deaths per 1000 live births with a range of 13.25 for African Americans to 4.59 for Cuban Americans.[5] The infant mortality rate is higher in the United States than in many other developed countries. In 2005, the United States ranked 30th in infant mortality among European countries.[6] Many of the deaths in this age group could be prevented by provision of adequate health services to pregnant women. Preterm delivery is more than twice as likely in the United States compared with European countries.[6] If the rate of preterm delivery was consistent with other European countries, the infant mortality rate in the United States would decrease by 33%.[6] The risk for prematurity, low birth weight, and perinatal infection can in many cases be minimized by appropriate intervention. The death rate for African American infants during the first year of life is 2.3 times greater than for white infants.[6] The higher number of deaths among African American infants reflects the higher percentages of infants born in low- and very-low-birth-weight categories.[6] Access to health care and socioeconomic status partially explain this discrepancy, but efforts at prevention continue to challenge health care providers.

Table 23-2 reviews the major causes of death among children in the United States who are older than age 1 year.[7,8] Unintentional injuries rank first for all age groups. Suicide and homicide are prominent in the teen years.

When assessing risks to children's health, one should note that many of the conditions affecting children are

TABLE 23-2 **Leading Causes of Death in Percentage by Age, United States, Ages 1–24, 2007, and 12–19, 2006***

	AGE (YR)	
CAUSES OF DEATH (%)	**1–24**	**12–19**
Accidents (unintentional injuries)	43	48
Assault (homicide)	13	13
Intentional self-harm (suicide)	9	11
Malignant neoplasms	7	6
Diseases of the heart	3	3
Congenital anomalies	0	2
All other causes	25	17
Total	100	100

Modified from National Vital Statistics, National Center for Health Statistics, Centers for Disease Control.[7,8]
*Percentage of all deaths.

avoidable. A major component of pediatric care focuses on health promotion and disease prevention. The goals of the American Academy of Pediatrics's Bright Futures initiative for child health include the following:

1. Work with states to make the Bright Futures approach the standard of care for infants, children, and adolescents;
2. Help health care providers shift their thinking to a prevention-based, family-focused, and developmentally oriented direction;
3. Foster partnerships between families, providers, and communities; and
4. Empower families with the skills and knowledge to be active participants in their children's healthy development.[9]

The status of children in the United States today illustrates some of the problems encountered in the provision of health care. National crises such as inadequate health care services, poverty, and homelessness take their toll on children. Eight million children are among those Americans who lack health insurance. Millions more are underinsured. Uninsured children are 10 times more likely to have untreated medical issues, such as asthma, diabetes, or obesity. They have not had a medical visit in more than 2 years (16.5% uninsured vs. 2.6% insured) unless they have had an emergency visit (6% uninsured vs. 7.3% insured).[10] Families with health insurance may find the cost of preventive care (i.e., immunizations) or outpatient care for acute illnesses prohibitive. These services may not be covered or may not be sought because of high deductibles. The State-Sponsored Children's Health Insurance Program (SCHIP) has improved this situation in many states, but barriers persist, especially for immigrant children. Among the populations most threatened by the free-market insurance approach are children, particularly those with special needs.[10]

The result of the medical neglect of children is readily apparent when one examines the problems facing youth today. Threats to children's health are exacerbated by lack of access to health care and by poverty. Poor children are much more susceptible to the effects of prematurity, perinatal infections, infectious diseases of early childhood, child abuse, accidents, homicide, suicide, teen pregnancy, and school failure. Poor, homeless, and inner city children are much less likely to receive required immunizations by age 2.[10]

Some of these issues may not have easy solutions. It is tempting to be overwhelmed by the magnitude of problems facing our youth. Individual contributions by committed health professionals, however, often make an enormous difference in the lives of specific children and their families. Resourceful, innovative approaches allow individual PAs to make a difference both with families facing multiple problems and families blessed with stability and healthy children. Giving advice about topics as mundane as teething, pacifiers, sleep habits, and picky eating is one of the ways that a PA may help break a family deadlock and enable a child and parents to focus more on positive issues than on the inevitable struggles involved in child-rearing.

WHAT IS THE PRACTICE OF PEDIATRICS?

CASE STUDY 23-1

Parents of healthy 6-month-old twins bring the babies in for a routine checkup. The mother has several questions about the boy, Thomas, who still wants to eat every hour, is irritable, and cries for hours in the evening. The girl, Theresa, is an "easy baby," who smiles readily, eats every 3 to 4 hours during the day, and settles down to sleep without difficulty.

1. What additional information would help you problem-solve this difference?
2. How would you change the framing of this question from good/bad?
3. What is the "normal" feeding interval at this age?

The realm of pediatric care includes monitoring the health and normal progression of children's growth and development. Care provided to children encompasses visits for periodic health supervision, acute illness, and chronic illness, as well as case management for children with special needs. The psychosocial arena in which children function has an impact on their ability to meet and adapt to challenges to optimal growth. All of these areas offer the PA the opportunity to contribute in a meaningful way to children and families. Figure 23-1 provides a format for the content and tasks of periodic child health supervision visits.[11]

Pediatric Interview

The first part of any medical encounter focuses on the medical history. For many encounters in pediatrics, the history is related by a third party (caregiver), not the patient. The level of concern expressed by the parent or caregiver should never be underestimated. A parent's concerns and suspicions are often the most accurate. It is important to keep in mind that parents might not implement a treatment plan if they feel that their concerns were not heard. The practitioner needs to hone observation skills about normal child development and behavior to augment and interpret the information given by the parent.

Appropriate methods of inquiry are always open-ended, allowing the people with the concerns to delineate their worries in their own words and to elaborate on their own observations. Frequently, it is important for the PA to clarify these concerns by following up with questions such as these: "What worried you most about her?" "Why did that worry you?" and "What were you hoping we could do for her today?" These questions often are useful in sorting out underlying fears and concerns that parents have about their children.[12] Examples of questions that parents might not be able to ask directly include the following: "Will allowing my baby to sleep on her stomach cause sudden infant death syndrome?" "Will this cold turn into asthma?" "Will flying on a plane with this ear infection burst my child's eardrum?"

When the clinician is assessing developmental milestones, it is often the quality of the child's interaction that gives clues about the capacity of the child to develop skills necessary to interact with, manipulate, and master tasks for learning, language, and movement. Gentle but thorough inquiry gives the clinician a complete database, which is critical toward reaching the appropriate diagnosis and treatment plan.

The interview with an adolescent can be more complex and challenging for some practitioners. However, it can be immensely rewarding to observe and participate as teens define themselves as separate and distinct from their family. Parents of teens also want to talk with the PA and to have their concerns heard. It is essential that the adolescent be allowed the opportunity to be interviewed independently, providing the possibility of discussing issues of a confidential nature. This practice encourages teens to take responsibility for their health behaviors. Often a young person may have an apparently superficial concern that serves as a means of asking about bigger worries, such as the possibility of an unwanted pregnancy or a sexually transmitted disease, or the means of obtaining a safe, effective, birth control method. These types of concerns illustrate the need for the adolescent to feel assured that confidentiality will be preserved and that the practitioner can be trusted. The PA, the teen, and the parent(s) should meet at the end of the visit in a joint conference to review the health status of the adolescent and to go over the information shared with the teen that is not of a confidential nature.

Most states offer specific legal protection to health care providers who provide services that are confidential to a teen. Examples of confidential visits include counseling about birth control, sexually transmitted disease, drug and alcohol use or abuse, and mental health issues. It is also important for the provider to be honest about the limits of confidentiality. In general, when the PA judges that the topics discussed by the teen arouse apprehension about the safety of that teen or others, for instance remarks that seem suicidal or homicidal, confidentiality should not be protected. Being up front and honest with the teen about these concerns will often protect the professional relationship between the provider and the teen.[13]

Physical Examination

The physical examination in pediatrics requires a thorough and comprehensive approach. Many findings on physical examination need to be tied to age-specific norms. For example, vital signs demonstrate wide variation from infancy through adolescence. The appropriate approach to the patient requires techniques that are age related.

When the patient is an infant, it is reassuring to a parent to observe that the PA handles the baby with confidence and with sensitivity. A particularly irritable infant may be exquisitely sensitive to touch and handling. Sometimes it is helpful to parents to validate their observations by demonstrating specifically how an infant responds to the stimulation of the physical examination. The spectrum of temperamental style is often readily apparent during the newborn period, and coping strategies might be discussed during the first visit.

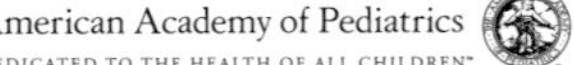

American Academy of Pediatrics
DEDICATED TO THE HEALTH OF ALL CHILDREN™

Recommendations for Preventive Pediatric Health Care

Bright Futures/American Academy of Pediatrics

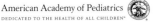

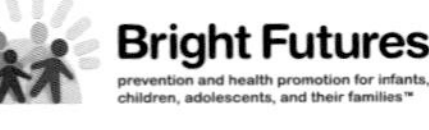

Bright Futures. prevention and health promotion for infants, children, adolescents, and their families™

Each child and family is unique; therefore, these **Recommendations for Preventive Pediatric Health Care** are designed for the care of children who are receiving competent parenting, have no manifestations of any important health problems, and are growing and developing in satisfactory fashion. **Additional visits may become necessary** if circumstances suggest variations from normal.

Developmental, psychosocial, and chronic disease issues for children and adolescents may require frequent counseling and treatment visits separate from preventive care visits.

These guidelines represent a consensus by the American Academy of Pediatrics (AAP) and Bright Futures. The AAP continues to emphasize the great importance of **continuity of care** in comprehensive health supervision and the need to avoid **fragmentation of care.**

The recommendations in this statement do not indicate an exclusive course of treatment or standard of medical care. Variations, taking into account individual circumstances, may be appropriate.

	INFANCY								EARLY CHILDHOOD							MIDDLE CHILDHOOD						ADOLESCENCE										
AGE[1]	PRENATAL[2]	NEWBORN[3]	3–5 d[4]	By 1 mo	2 mo	4 mo	6 mo	9 mo	12 m	15 mo	18 mo	24 mo	30 mo	3 y	4 y	5 y	6 y	7 y	8 y	9 y	10 y	11 y	12 y	13 y	14 y	15 y	16 y	17 y	18 y	19 y	20 y	21 y
HISTORY																																
Initial/Interval	●	●	●	●	●	●	●	●	●	●	●	●	●	●	●	●	●	●	●	●	●	●	●	●	●	●	●	●	●	●	●	●
MEASUREMENTS																																
Length/Height and Weight		●	●	●	●	●	●	●	●	●	●	●	●	●	●	●	●	●	●	●	●	●	●	●	●	●	●	●	●	●	●	●
Head Circumference		●	●	●	●	●	●	●	●	●	●	●																				
Weight for Length		●	●	●	●	●	●	●	●	●	●																					
Body Mass Index												●	●	●	●	●	●	●	●	●	●	●	●	●	●	●	●	●	●	●	●	●
Blood Pressure[5]		★	★	★	★	★	★	★	★	★	★	★	★	●	●	●	●	●	●	●	●	●	●	●	●	●	●	●	●	●	●	●
SENSORY SCREENING																																
Vision		★	★	★	★	★	★	★	★	★	★	★	★	●[6]	●	●	●	★	●	★	●	★	●	★	★	●	★	★	●	★	★	★
Hearing		●[7]	★	★	★	★	★	★	★	★	★	★	★	★	●	●	●	★	●	★	●	★	★	★	★	★	★	★	★	★	★	★
DEVELOPMENTAL/BEHAVIORAL ASSESSMENT																																
Developmental Screening[8]								●			●		●																			
Autism Screening[9]											●	●																				
Developmental Surveillance[8]		●	●	●	●	●	●		●	●		●		●	●	●	●	●	●	●	●	●	●	●	●	●	●	●	●	●	●	●
Psychosocial/Behavioral Assessment		●	●	●	●	●	●	●	●	●	●	●	●	●	●	●	●	●	●	●	●	●	●	●	●	●	●	●	●	●	●	●
Alcohol and Drug Use Assessment																						★	★	★	★	★	★	★	★	★	★	★
PHYSICAL EXAMINATION[10]		●	●	●	●	●	●	●	●	●	●	●	●	●	●	●	●	●	●	●	●	●	●	●	●	●	●	●	●	●	●	●
PROCEDURES[11]																																
Newborn Metabolic/Hemoglobin Screening[12]		←	●		→																											
Immunization[13]		●	●	●	●	●	●	●	●	●	●	●	●	●	●	●	●	●	●	●	●	●	●	●	●	●	●	●	●	●	●	●
Hematocrit or Hemoglobin[14]						★			●		★	★		★	★	★	★	★	★	★	★	★	★	★	★	★	★	★	★	★	★	★
Lead Screening[15]							★	★	●or★[16]		★	●or★[16]		★	★	★	★															
Tuberculin Test[17]				★			★		★		★	★		★	★	★	★	★	★	★	★	★	★	★	★	★	★	★	★	★	★	★
Dyslipidemia Screening[18]												★			★		★		★		★	★	★	★	★	★	★	★	←		●	→
STI Screening[19]																						★	★	★	★	★	★	★	★	★	★	★
Cervical Dysplasia Screening[20]																						★	★	★	★	★	★	★	★	★	★	★
ORAL HEALTH[21]							★	★	●or★[21]		●or★[21]	●or★[21]	●or★[21]	●[22]			●[22]															
ANTICIPATORY GUIDANCE[23]	●	●	●	●	●	●	●	●	●	●	●	●	●	●	●	●	●	●	●	●	●	●	●	●	●	●	●	●	●	●	●	●

1. If a child comes under care for the first time at any point on the schedule, or if any items are not accomplished at the suggested age, the schedule should be brought up to date at the earliest possible time.
2. A prenatal visit is recommended for parents who are at high risk, for first-time parents, and for those who request a conference. The prenatal visit should include anticipatory guidance, pertinent medical history, and a discussion of benefits of breastfeeding and planned method of feeding per AAP statement "The Prenatal Visit" (2001) [URL: http://aappolicy.aappublications.org/cgi/content/full/pediatrics;107/6/1456].
3. Every infant should have a newborn evaluation after birth, breastfeeding encouraged, and instruction and support offered.
4. Every infant should have an evaluation within 3 to 5 days of birth and within 48 to 72 hours after discharge from the hospital, to include evaluation for feeding and jaundice. Breastfeeding infants should receive formal breastfeeding evaluation, encouragement, and instruction as recommended in AAP statement "Breastfeeding and the Use of Human Milk" (2005) [URL: http://aappolicy.aappublications.org/cgi/content/full/pediatrics;115/2/496]. For newborns discharged in less than 48 hours after delivery, the infant must be examined within 48 hours of discharge per AAP statement "Hospital Stay for Healthy Term Newborns" (2004) [URL: http://aappolicy.aappublications.org/cgi/content/full/pediatrics;113/5/1434].
5. Blood pressure measurement in infants and children with specific risk conditions should be performed at visits before age 3 years.
6. If the patient is uncooperative, rescreen within 6 months per the AAP statement "Eye Examination in Infants, Children, and Young Adults by Pediatricians" (2007) [URL: http://aappolicy.aappublications.org/cgi/content/full/pediatrics;111/4/902].
7. All newborns should be screened per AAP statement "Year 2000 Position Statement: Principles and Guidelines for Early Hearing Detection and Intervention Programs" (2000) [URL: http://aappolicy.aappublications.org/cgi/content/full/pediatrics;106/4/798]. Joint Committee on Infant Hearing. Year 2007 position statement: principles and guidelines for early hearing detection and intervention programs. *Pediatrics.* 2007;120:898–921.
8. AAP Council on Children With Disabilities, AAP Section on Developmental Behavioral Pediatrics, AAP Bright Futures Steering Committee, AAP Medical Home Initiatives for Children With Special Needs Project Advisory Committee. Identifying infants and young children with developmental disorders in the medical home: an algorithm for developmental surveillance and screening. *Pediatrics.* 2006;118:405–420 [URL: http://aappolicy.aappublications.org/cgi/content/full/pediatrics;118/1/405].
9. Gupta VB, Hyman SL, Johnson CP, et al. Identifying children with autism early? *Pediatrics.* 2007;119:152–153 [URL: http://pediatrics.aappublications.org/cgi/content/full/119/1/152].
10. At each visit, age-appropriate physical examination is essential, with infant totally unclothed, older child undressed and suitably draped.
11. These may be modified, depending on entry point into schedule and individual need.
12. Newborn metabolic and hemoglobinopathy screening should be done according to state law. Results should be reviewed at visits and appropriate retesting or referral done as needed.
13. Schedules per the Committee on Infectious Diseases, published annually in the January issue of *Pediatrics.* Every visit should be an opportunity to update and complete a child's immunizations.
14. See AAP *Pediatric Nutrition Handbook*, 5th Edition (2003) for a discussion of universal and selective screening options. See also Recommendations to prevent and control iron deficiency in the United States. *MMWR.* 1998;47(RR-3):1–36.
15. For children at risk of lead exposure, consult the AAP statement "Lead Exposure in Children: Prevention, Detection, and Management" (2005) [URL: http://aappolicy.aappublications.org/cgi/content/full/pediatrics;116/4/1036]. Additionally, screening should be done in accordance with state law where applicable.
16. Perform risk assessments or screens as appropriate, based on universal screening requirements for patients with Medicaid or high prevalence areas.
17. Tuberculosis testing per recommendations of the Committee on Infectious Diseases, published in the current edition of *Red Book: Report of the Committee on Infectious Diseases.* Testing should be done on recognition of high-risk factors.
18. "Third Report of the National Cholesterol Education Program (NCEP) Expert Panel on Detection, Evaluation, and Treatment of High Blood Cholesterol in Adults (Adult Treatment Panel III) Final Report" (2002) [URL: http://circ.ahajournals.org/cgi/content/full/106/25/3143] and "The Expert Committee Recommendations on the Assessment, Prevention, and Treatment of Child and Adolescent Overweight and Obesity." Supplement to *Pediatrics.* In press.
19. All sexually active patients should be screened for sexually transmitted infections (STIs).
20. All sexually active girls should have screening for cervical dysplasia as part of a pelvic examination beginning within 3 years of onset of sexual activity or age 21 (whichever comes first).
21. Referral to dental home, if available. Otherwise, administer oral health risk assessment. If the primary water source is deficient in fluoride, consider oral fluoride supplementation.
22. At the visits for 3 years and 6 years of age, it should be determined whether the patient has a dental home. If the patient does not have a dental home, a referral should be made to one. If the primary water source is deficient in fluoride, consider oral fluoride supplementation.
23. Refer to the specific guidance by age as listed in Bright Futures Guidelines. (Hagan JF, Shaw JS, Duncan PM, eds. *Bright Futures: Guidelines for Health Supervision of Infants, Children, and Adolescents.* 3rd ed. Elk Grove Village, IL: American Academy of Pediatrics; 2008.)

KEY

● = to be performed ★ = risk assessment to be performed, with appropriate action to follow, if positive ←—●—→ = range during which a service may be provided, with the symbol indicating the preferred age

FIGURE 23-1 Committee on Practice and Ambulatory Medicine and Bright Futures Steering Committee. Recommendations for preventive pediatric health care. (From Pediatrics 2007;120:1376. *http://pediatrics.aappublications.org/content/120/6/1376.full.html.* Accessed August 2, 2011.)

As a baby grows and develops, stranger anxiety may make a physical examination more difficult because the infant reacts to the unfamiliar health care provider. An active, curious infant often will want to inspect and handle diagnostic equipment. At this age, it is wise to have toys in one's "bag of tricks" with which to distract the infant. A toddler approaching independence may perceive the physical examination as both invasive and limiting. From the age of 9 months to about 3 years, it is often helpful to do much of the examination with the child in the parent's lap. This may reassure the anxious child, and the parent may provide a helpful extra set of hands as the examiner interacts with the child. It is wise to set up the examination to proceed from least invasive (i.e., inspecting fingers and toes, testing extraocular movements with a finger puppet) to most invasive procedures (i.e., pneumatic otoscopy, looking at the back of the throat) to maximize the cooperation of the child.

At about 3 to 5 years of age, children are usually delightful, cooperative, eager to please, and genuinely interested in what the examiner is doing. If, at this age, a child is still extremely anxious about getting a physical examination, further investigation is warranted. Perhaps the child has been ill and has undergone some traumatizing procedures. Sometimes messages from elsewhere intimidate the child with threats about "shots." It is always important for the PA to be alert to extreme anxiety or indifference because these symptoms are potential manifestations of reactions to child abuse. For a child who is temperamentally more anxious without specific cause, playing with a "doctor kit" or reading books about going to the doctor can help the child feel some mastery of the experience of a medical visit.

As a child approaches the early school-age years, his or her need for modesty becomes more evident during the physical examination. Appropriate gowns and drapes may help alleviate the child's discomfort. During the course of the physical examination, the PA may take the opportunity to focus exclusively on the child and engage him or her independently in conversation.

In a child who is approaching the end of the latency period, the clinician must be attuned to signs of the development of secondary sexual characteristics. Again, concerns about modesty and normality can be paramount for the patient. It is not uncommon for clinicians to feel some discomfort in working with teens as they go through the physical process of sexual maturation. Frequently, working with patients in this age group provides a stimulus for health care providers to consider feelings and issues about their own adolescent experience. Potentially, this stimulus may enable the clinician to be more genuinely attuned to the teen's experience, serving to enhance the overall rapport.

Care of Patients

Growth. Assessment of growth is one of the most important indicators of overall health in childhood. Measurements of morphologic growth give evidence of underlying biochemical, organic, and developmental competencies.[14] There are noticeable differences in the rates of growth and maturation of organ systems. In neural, lymphoid, general, and genital development, various age-specific phases of accelerated development can be noted.

From infancy through age 3 years, height, weight, and head circumference are measured at every health supervision visit. After age 3 and through adolescence, weight and stature measurements are obtained. These parameters are plotted on growth charts (Figure 23-2) recommended by the Centers for Disease Control and Prevention (CDC). The recommended growth charts for 0 to 2 years old are now produced by the World Health Organization (WHO). The WHO charts provide norms of growth from children who are primarily breast-fed to 4 months old and continue breast-feeding to 1 year old. After 2 years old, the CDC growth charts are developed from actual growth in a cross-section of children from the United States representing various ethnic and economic groups. As norms, the growth curves provide a background against which to assess the growth of an individual child. It is important to realize that once a child has established a pattern and velocity of growth, evidence of continuation of that pattern indicates the integrity and ability of the child to attain overall growth potential. Variations in normal patterns may reflect nutrition problems, physical illness, and psychosocial disruptions. Concerns arise with disproportionate acceleration or deceleration in growth.[15,16]

Text continued on p. 337

CASE STUDY 23-2

Ericka is 15. She is petite and will be competing in gymnastics again this year. She needs a physical examination to participate in her sport. In taking the history, the PA learns that Ericka has not started menstruating yet. Her mother started her periods when she was 12, and her older sister started in "seventh grade." Ericka's parents are both small: Mom is 5 feet, 3 inches, and Dad is 5 feet, 7 inches.

1. Is this delayed puberty?
2. What factors do you consider in evaluating her lack of menarche?
3. How do you counsel her on nutrition and growth?

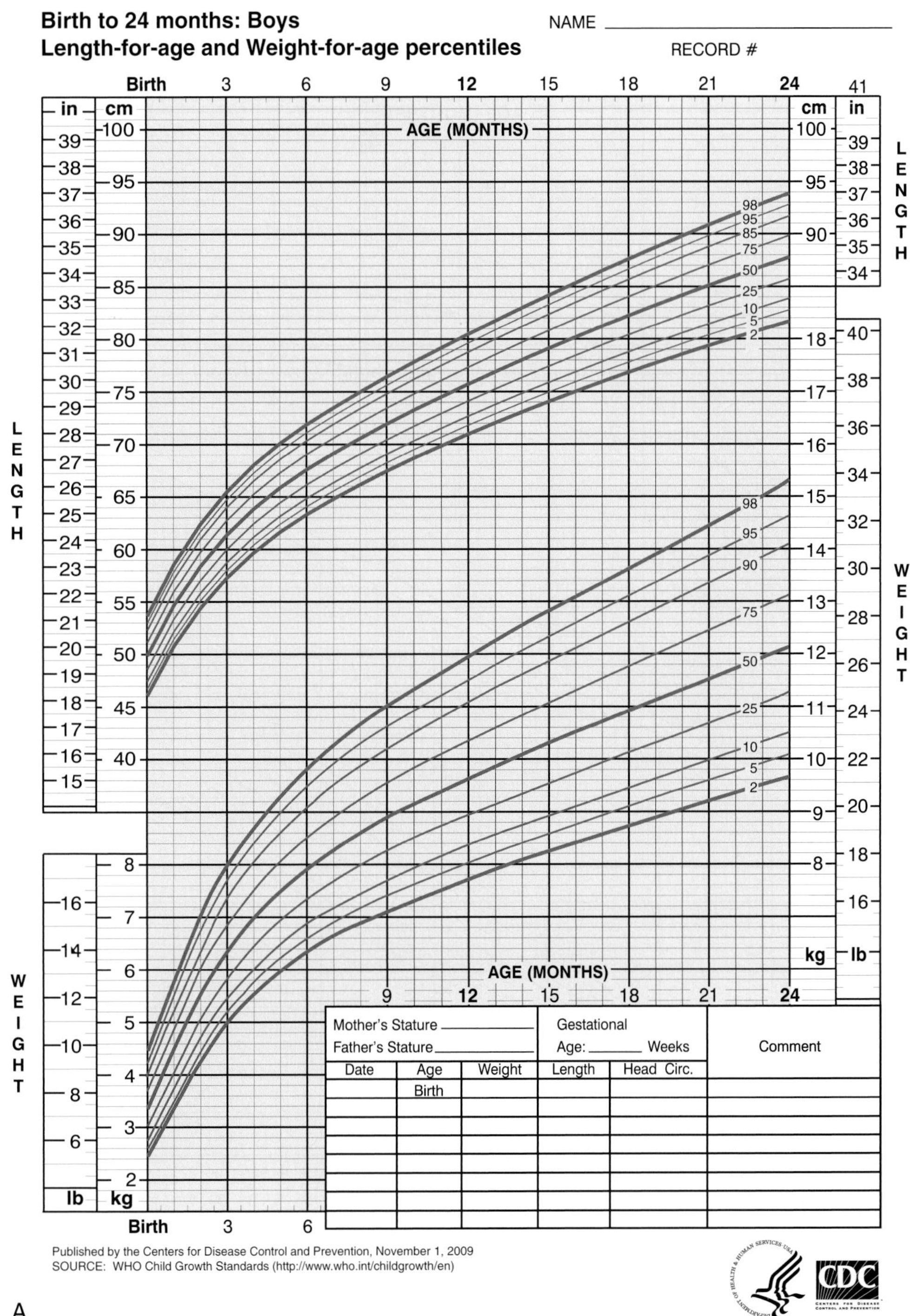

FIGURE 23-2 Physical growth charts from the World Health Organization. **A,** Birth to 24 months: boys' length-for-age percentiles and weight-for-age percentiles. (From *http://www.cdc.gov/growthcharts/who_charts.htm.*)

Continued

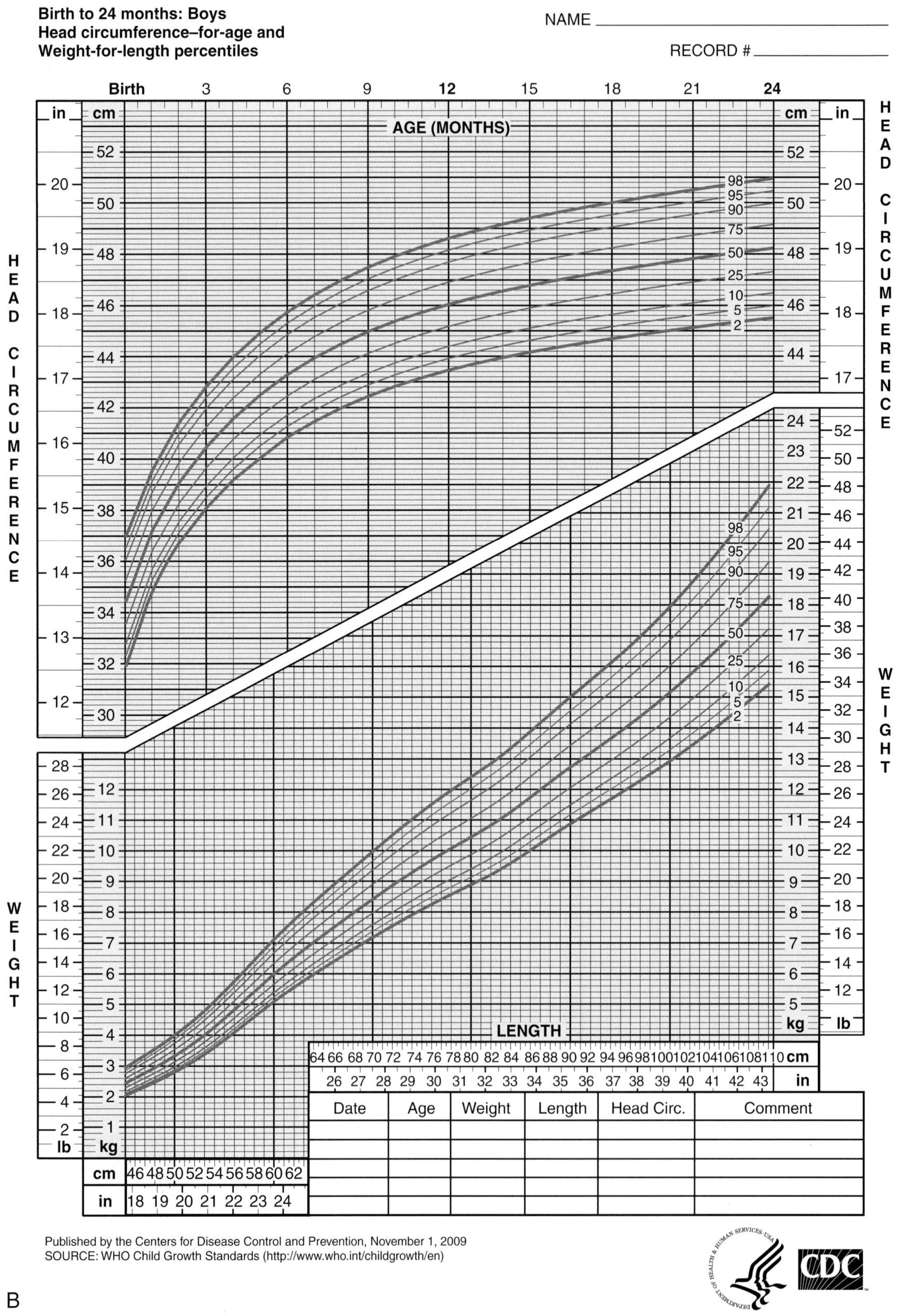

Birth to 24 months: Boys
Head circumference–for-age and
Weight-for-length percentiles

NAME ________________________________

RECORD # ______________

Birth 3 6 9 12 15 18 21 24

AGE (MONTHS)

HEAD CIRCUMFERENCE

in: 12 13 14 15 16 17 18 19 20

cm: 30 32 34 36 38 40 42 44 46 48 50 52

98 95 90 75 50 25 10 5 2

WEIGHT

lb: 2 4 6 8 10 12 14 16 18 20 22 24 26 28 30 32 34 36 38 40 42 44 46 48 50 52

kg: 1 2 3 4 5 6 7 8 9 10 11 12 13 14 15 16 17 18 19 20 21 22 23 24

98 95 90 75 50 25 10 5 2

LENGTH

cm: 46 48 50 52 54 56 58 60 62 64 66 68 70 72 74 76 78 80 82 84 86 88 90 92 94 96 98 100 102 104 106 108 110

in: 18 19 20 21 22 23 24 25 26 27 28 29 30 31 32 33 34 35 36 37 38 39 40 41 42 43

Date	Age	Weight	Length	Head Circ.	Comment

Published by the Centers for Disease Control and Prevention, November 1, 2009
SOURCE: WHO Child Growth Standards (http://www.who.int/childgrowth/en)

B

FIGURE 23-2, cont'd B, Birth to 24 months: boys' weight-for-length percentiles and head circumference–for-age percentiles. (From *http://www.cdc.gov/growthcharts/who_charts.htm.*)

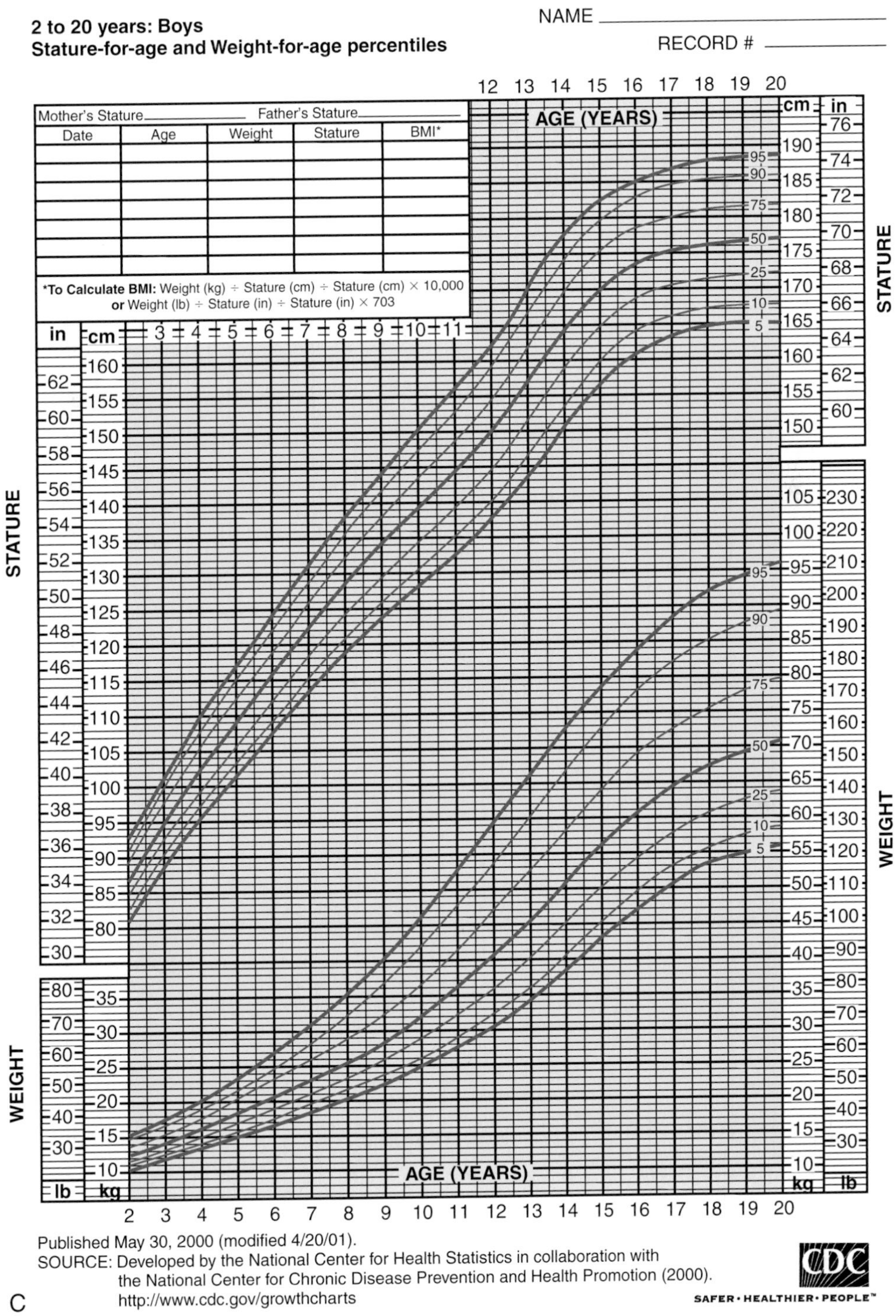

C

FIGURE 23-2, cont'd C, 2 to 20 years: boys' stature-for-age and weight-for-age percentiles. (Developed by the National Center for Health Statistics in collaboration with the National Center for Chronic Disease Prevention and Health Promotion [2000]. From *http://www.cdc.gov/growthcharts/clinical_charts.htm.)*

Continued

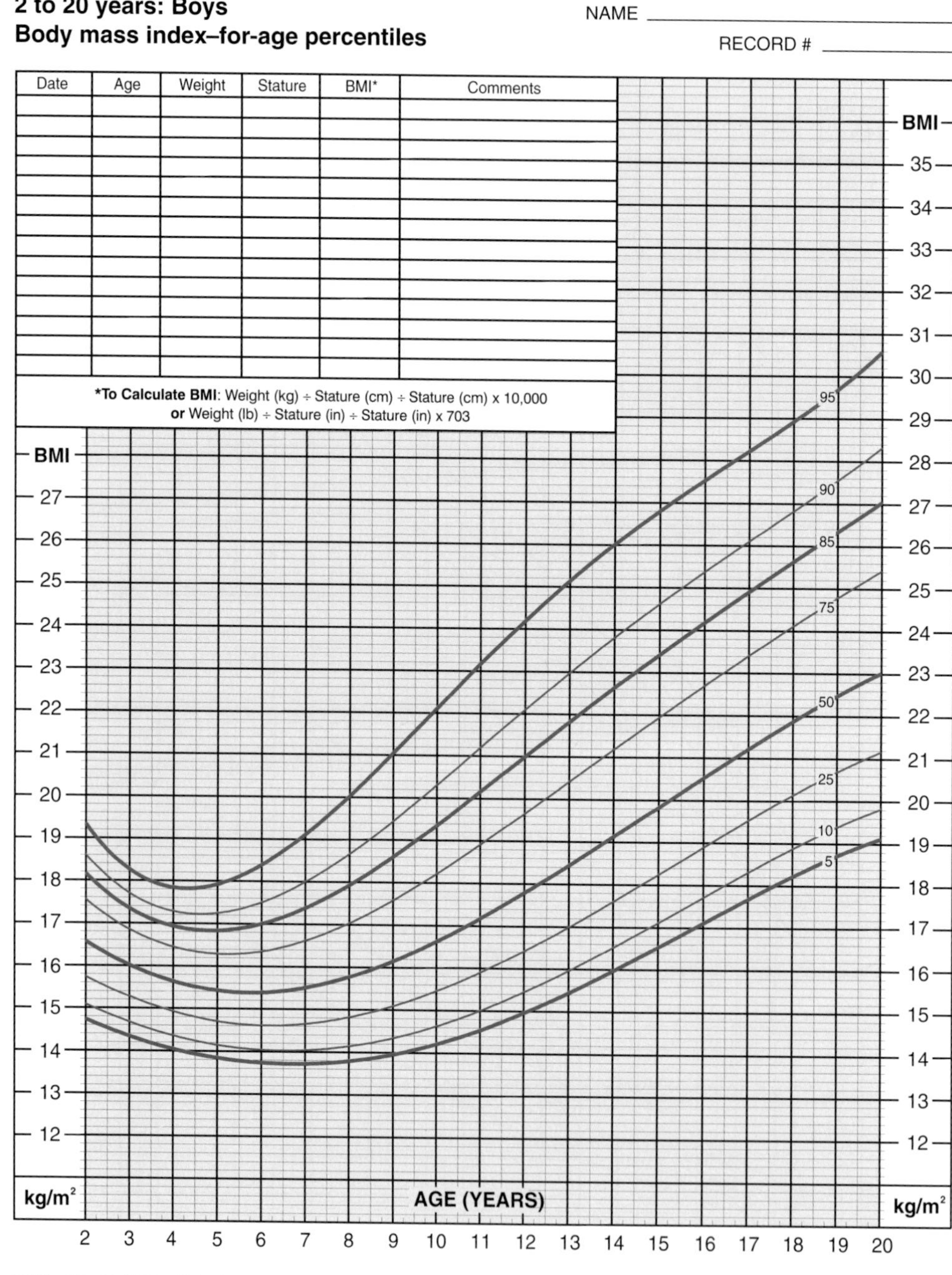

FIGURE 23-2, cont'd D, 2 to 20 years: boys' body mass index–for-age percentiles. (Developed by the National Center for Health Statistics in collaboration with the National Center for Chronic Disease Prevention and Health Promotion [2000]. From *http://www.cdc.gov/growthcharts/clinical_charts.htm.*)

In adolescence, an estimate of sexual maturity rating (SMR) is added. This is helpful in determining how a teen is progressing through the period of rapid growth and in assessing the rate and pattern of sexual development.

The Tanner (SMR) scale presents ranges of normal development with descriptions for each stage of growth for penis, testes, and pubic hair development in males and pubic hair and breast development in females. This is useful clinically in helping the clinician to predict height spurt for both sexes and menarche for females. These norms also alert the clinician to precocious or delayed puberty.

Nutrition. Concerns about feeding are common in pediatrics. Adequacy of the diet influences overall health status and growth of the child. Nutrition habits from childhood carry over to adulthood and therefore potentially have consequences for health risks throughout life.

Questions about feeding are initiated when parents make choices about breast-feeding or bottle-feeding. Although breast-feeding is recognized as preferable, PAs in primary care pediatrics should be able to discuss the advantages and disadvantages of both breast-feeding and bottle-feeding and should be sensitive to the parents' feelings as they make the decision for the child. The ideal is to promote a feeding style that provides the optimal nutrition status and feeding relationship for the child and family.

After early infancy, parents may seek advice about the initiation of solid food and about the quality and balance of the child's diet. The clinician needs to have a working knowledge of food sources that supply adequate calories, protein, vitamins, and minerals to assess the nutritive value of the child's diet. It is also necessary to be attuned to normal fluctuations in the child's appetite. Feeding problems include difficulties with the feeding interaction, overfeeding, and underfeeding. The complications of failure to thrive, obesity, attitudes toward food, and unusual eating behaviors, such as anorexia or bingeing and purging, may have lifelong repercussions.

Laboratory Screening. Routine laboratory screening is also a part of the pediatric health supervision examination. All children should be screened in the newborn period for metabolic diseases and hemoglobinopathies. Vision, hearing, and blood pressure determinations are also performed routinely. Utilization of tuberculosis, cholesterol, anemia, urine, and lead screens is subject to an assessment of prevalence and risk factors for individual patients and communities.

Immunizations. In the years just before 1900, 20% of children died before 1 year of age from infectious diseases.[17] The treatment of infectious diseases has dramatically improved, as many serious or fatal infectious diseases of childhood are preventable through vaccination. Immunization remains a cornerstone of pediatrics. The most updated immunization recommendations for the United States are available at *http://www.cdc.gov/vaccines/recs/acip/default.htm* (approved by the Advisory Committee on Immunization Practices). Current vaccine guidelines include immunization against diphtheria, acellular pertussis, and tetanus (DTaP); poliovirus (IPV); measles, mumps, and rubella (MMR); hepatitis B virus (HBV); pneumococcus (PCV or PPV); varicella-zoster virus (VZB); and *Haemophilus influenzae* type B conjugate vaccine (Hib). In recent years, vaccine recommendations have been revised. These revisions have been prompted by the development of new vaccines for rotavirus, hepatitis A, and H1N1. The resurgence of measles and the rising rates of hepatitis B and pneumococcal infection have also influenced these changes.[18]

CASE STUDY 23-3

Three-year-old Katie's father brings her to the emergency department for evaluation of fever and irritability. She has been ill for 2 days with a cold and has not been eating well. In talking with the father and by reviewing the medical records, the PA ascertains that Katie has not had a routine checkup since she was 6 months old. The family has no consistent source of health care. The father does not think Katie has had shots since she was 6 months old.

1. Which immunization series are reduced or eliminated because she is now 3?
2. Which series are the most important to bring up to date as soon as possible?
3. How do you counsel parents regarding fever and immunization?

Because access to and utilization of health care greatly influence the chance that a child will be fully immunized, the PA should take advantage of every opportunity to bring a child up to date on immunization by reviewing the record of immunization at each encounter. It is imperative that the expected and more serious adverse reactions to immunizations be discussed with parents as a part of the informed consent process. Significant adverse reactions should be reported. The National Childhood Vaccine Injury Act allows compensation to families for significant events following vaccination.[19]

Interruption of the routine immunization schedule can cause some confusion about how to bring a child's immunization status up to date. If a child comes in with lapses in DaPT, HbCV, IPV, and HBV schedules, the next doses should be given as if the interval were usual. Missed immunizations do not require that the entire series be reinstituted.[19]

Sometimes clinicians are hesitant to immunize a child because of concerns about contraindications or reactions. This reluctance contributes to the unacceptable number of children in the United States who are not fully immunized. Afebrile minor illnesses, such as colds and diarrheal illnesses, in a child who is otherwise in good health are not contraindications to immunization. Vaccination should be deferred if an adverse effect or an adverse reaction to the vaccine could potentially exacerbate an illness.[19]

Special consideration is given to immunization of immunocompromised patients and of preterm infants. Alterations in immune function can result from immunosuppressive therapy such as corticosteroids, chemotherapeutic agents, and transplant-recipient regimens. Patients with congenital disorders of immune function are also more susceptible to adverse outcomes from immunizations, especially with live viral vaccines. Live bacterial and viral vaccines (MMR, and varicella) and bacillus Calmette-Guérin (BCG) are contraindicated for patients with congenital disorders of immune function.[19] The inactivated polio vaccine (IPV) can be used safely. Patients on immunosuppressive therapy require a thorough evaluation of the underlying disease and the type of therapy, as well as its schedule and dose, previous infectious disease, and immunization history. Patients with symptomatic human immunodeficiency virus (HIV) infection should not receive live viral vaccines. Because of the risk for complications from measles, however, it is recommended that MMR be given regardless of symptoms.[19]

Preterm infants can be immunized safely at the usual chronologic age. For example, if a baby is still in the nursery at 2 months old, all recommended 2-month-old vaccinations can be given.[19]

Development and Behavior

CASE STUDY 23-4

Four-month-old Angela is brought in by her mother for shots. During the visit, the mother tells the PA that she is worried about the baby because the grandmother thinks that the baby is not "acting right." Grandma has noticed that the baby does not look around and watch when people walk into the room and talk to her. Further review of the family history reveals that the mother has two other children who have been removed from the home because of suspicion of child abuse.

1. What other family history is relevant about this behavior?
2. Why is this behavior significant?
3. What parenting questions would you ask?

A cornerstone of pediatrics is an appreciation of how children progress through normal development. Components of this process include the cognitive, affective, motor, and language skills that a child attains throughout normal maturation. Because none of these processes happens in a vacuum, an understanding of the circumstances of the home and community in which the child functions is important.

Freud, Erikson, Piaget, and Mahler have influenced the assessment of childhood development. The observations and theories established by these and other analysts of human behavior have allowed the formulation of general principles, many of which are included in developmental screening tests. The following basic principles apply to human development:

- Development is a continuous and dynamic process.
- The sequence of development is generally the same for all individuals.
- The pace or rate of development is variable for each child.
- Development is affected by the overall health of the child. Acute and chronic illness may adversely affect the performance of a child on a screening test.
- Major events in the child's milieu may also alter the performance of the child on developmental screening. Examples of potentially stressful events are deaths, separations, moves, and the illness of a family member.[14]

For PAs working with families, attention to development during infancy and early childhood is a necessity. The timing and frequency of health supervision visits enable the PA to take on the roles of family advisor and advocate for the child. Periodic screening with developmental tests such as the Denver II and Bayley Infant Development Scales allows measurement against norms for age. Marked deviation from norms mandates a more intensive and specific developmental evaluation. Many readily available checklists of developmental milestones may facilitate developmental screening.

CASE STUDY 23-5

Seven-year-old Brett is brought in by his parents. They have recently attended a school conference, at which the teachers reported noticing that Brett has a lot of difficulty staying "on task." He is up and out of his seat, frequently disturbing other children. He is about 6 months behind the other children in reading. At home, he is "creative" and loves Nintendo but "forgets" and loses things, talks loudly, and interrupts at meals. He needs frequent reminders to do simple things, such as getting ready for school in the morning. Any chores he does require constant supervision.

1. Why is the onset of this behavior important?
2. What diagnoses does this behavior indicate?
3. Why is the parents' educational background important?

Although early childhood is a period of rapid acquisition of new skills, developmental issues continue to be evaluated in patients through adolescence. During the school years, it is important to be cognizant of the child's capacity for learning, social interaction, and motor skills. With teenagers, topics address how a patient is managing in school, at work, with peers, and with family. It is reassuring to both patients and families to know that the issues that arise in the process of maturation are normal and expected. Discerning when patterns and progression through development are not consistent, either for the patient or in comparison with norms, is critical.

The individuality of each child manifests itself throughout the child's life. These stylistic characteristics are often apparent in infancy. Temperamental styles influence how the child reacts to stimuli and how he or she is perceived by the family, as well as by teachers, peers, and co-workers. Qualities such as shyness, adaptability, and creativity are among the many traits to which others in the child's environment respond. The perception of and value placed on these traits play a role in the child's integration of self and development of self-esteem. Coping skills and stylistic traits influence the child's adaptation to stressful events such as changes in schools, moves, losses, and divorce. Because no child is protected completely from difficulties while growing up, it may be helpful to the family for the clinician to recognize how the child responds to these events.

Health care providers are in a unique position to observe a child and family throughout the child's growth to maturity and are frequently solicited for advice about behaviors. Sometimes this advice focuses on suggestions about setting limits and applying discipline as the family strives to live harmoniously. When conflicts arise, interactions may reflect the inability of family members to recognize temperamental patterns and to develop mutually acceptable alternative behaviors that are complementary. PAs can be helpful by communicating their observations to the family and offering alternatives for management of these issues. Many of the issues come under the heading of "parenting." Some of the problems for children, however, are a predictable part of developmental and maturation processes and should be addressed routinely through anticipatory guidance during health supervision visits.

PAs must also be attuned to deviations from expected behavior. Children are not immune to serious psychiatric disturbances. Although it is important for the PA to appreciate normal behavior, it is equally important that he or she be aware of symptoms of underlying psychopathology. Appropriate referral for therapeutic intervention may be essential in helping the child and family.

Anticipatory Guidance

CASE STUDY 23-6

Eleven-year-old Jason is in for a routine camp physical. In reviewing his general health and activities, the PA finds that Jason enjoys riding his bike, rollerblading, and skateboarding. He has had two trips to the emergency department this year—one for stitches and one for a possible concussion. He does not wear a bicycle helmet or use pads when rollerblading or skateboarding. He does not use seat belts while riding in the car, and neither do his parents.

1. How do you broach safety issues with this family?
2. How important are statistics in your pitch?
3. Is there a bike helmet coupon provided by your hospital or insurance network?

Preparing parents for expected milestones in a child's health and development is an integral part of the practice of pediatrics. Information about growth, development, behavior, day care, nutrition, family functioning, television use, injury prevention, and management of illnesses is a part of every visit. Discussion of these topics by PAs builds alliances with parents by offering support and acknowledging the parents' competency to provide for the child. Anticipatory guidance should be timed for age-appropriate tasks and skills.

As a child approaches adolescence, the health care visit includes topics about which the young person will have to make decisions. Discussions about risk-taking behavior, peer pressure, smoking, alcohol, drugs, sexuality, and safe sex are all relevant.

Because accidents are the leading cause of death in childhood after infancy, a discussion of safety and injury prevention should be a component of every health maintenance visit. The list of topics should be adapted to the risks associated with the child's age. The American Academy of Pediatrics' Injury Prevention Program (TIPP) provides a questionnaire that assesses hazards and offers information to parents. Subjects for discussion range from use of car seats to avoidance of burns, falls, head injuries, drowning, choking, and poisoning. Home safety topics must include the availability of a working smoke alarm. As the child grows, possible further topics include bicycle safety, use of helmets and seat belts, and firearms in the home.[20]

Acute Illnesses

CASE STUDY 23-7

His mother brings in 2-year-old Matthew with concerns about persistent diarrhea. The diarrhea started 10 days ago, maybe with a "low-grade" fever. Although the stools were initially quite frequent (8 to 10 per day), the diarrhea has now tapered off to about four "really mushy," foul-smelling stools each day. Matthew was almost potty-trained but is now back in diapers. The mother thinks Matthew is beginning to look like he has lost weight. Workers at his day care center are also concerned.

1. What is your biggest concern with diarrhea in a toddler?
2. What questions would you have for the daycare center?
3. What immunization questions would you ask?

While caring for their ill child, parents interpret symptoms and make judgments about their severity. With a preverbal infant, it is sometimes difficult for parents to decide how ill the child is. Sometimes, the first provider contact with the family will occur over the telephone, helping the family determine whether the child needs to be seen by the provider. In the outpatient setting, the PA will evaluate information from the history, perform a thorough physical examination, decide on diagnostic studies, make the diagnosis, offer appropriate therapy, and discuss with the family the nature and course of the illness and the means of making the child comfortable. The PA's supervising physician is always available for consultation on difficult cases.

Elements of appropriate patient management include telephone and office triage skills and decisions about home management versus hospitalization. It is essential to keep access to care and transportation in mind when planning for follow-up. During the physical examination, subtle clues such as whether the child is playful and smiling often help the PA ascertain important features about the severity of illness.[21]

Anticipatory guidance also occurs during an illness visit. It is important to discuss with the parent the signs of worsening illness and when to call or bring the child in for reevaluation. Parents frequently have questions about contagion, return to day care or school, and timing and adverse effects of medications. Addressing all of these issues facilitates satisfying the family's needs and helps ensure compliance with therapy. It also helps build the parents' confidence and ultimately enables the PA to feel at ease with the reliability of the family.

Chronic Disease Visits

CASE STUDY 23-8

Three-year-old Felicia, who has spina bifida, is brought to the clinic for her biannual evaluation. She is an only child, and her parents do not want to have any other children. She is still in diapers. Both parents work, and although an aunt has been able to provide day care until now, the aunt is moving away. Felicia's last hospitalization was 3 months ago for foot surgery. She had a bad bladder infection a month ago and is still on antibiotics. Felicia's parents want to know when she will be potty-trained and also think she has outgrown her leg braces.

1. What disabled services does this family need?
2. How do you coordinate care for this child?
3. How do you counsel this family?

The spectrum of afflictions that affect children chronically is broad and includes entities such as recurrent otitis media, asthma, abdominal pain, congenital anomalies, sequelae of prematurity, developmental delays, and mental retardation. Current estimates are that approximately 9% of pediatric patients are affected by chronic illness that limits the child's activities. Some of these conditions are limited to one organ system and respond well to interventions. Others are multifocal and include mental health issues that impact the child's life throughout many areas of functioning.[22]

PAs are increasingly assuming the important role of case manager. Because patients with chronic illnesses need ongoing follow-up and evaluation, a multidisciplinary team approach is commonly used in providing their care. The team includes various medical and surgical specialists, a nutritionist, a physical or occupational therapist, a speech and language therapist, a social worker or psychologist, and a teacher. The case manager facilitates a coordinated approach to address the child's needs. Ideally, all those involved in the child's care meet on a regular basis to assess the child's progress, establish goals, and work with the parents to implement a realistic treatment plan. The child's and family's processes of adjustment to the illness or disability are ongoing. With each developmental stage, new issues arise. The ultimate goal is to maximize the child's potential through early intervention and to support family members as they work with the child's special needs.[22]

Care of the Hospitalized Patient

PAs are also increasingly involved in the management of hospitalized patients. In some settings, the PA will have primary responsibility for ongoing patient care and will review cases with an attending physician on a daily basis. PAs make daily rounds on patients, write progress notes, evaluate laboratory data, and write orders for patient care. The type and severity of illnesses the PA follows vary among settings.

Skills for appropriate patient management ultimately are the same as for office practice. They include the ability to take a complete history that comprises essential elements to reveal the correct diagnosis; in addition, a thorough physical examination must be performed, laboratory or diagnostic studies must be used judiciously, and the information obtained must be critically analyzed. The utilization of observational skills in evaluating and reevaluating the patient as the illness takes its course, arranging discharge, and formulating follow-up plans are also components of comprehensive hospital care. The PA is involved in helping the family understand the illness and is often aware of the psychosocial aspects of case management. It is in this interface with the family that the PA provides the "care" for the patient that is most highly valued.

CHOICES FOR PRACTICE

The opportunities available to a PA who wants to practice in pediatrics are ample. PAs are used as a vital part of health care teams providing services to children. Physical settings include ambulatory clinics for children and adolescents in both private and public sectors. Sites include health maintenance organizations (HMOs), private offices, public health facilities, migrant and inner city clinics, and emergency departments. PAs also provide inpatient health care services in hospitals and facilities for the chronically ill and disabled.

Specialization within the field of pediatrics is also increasingly available. PAs work as specialists or subspecialists in neonatology, pediatric asthma and allergy, endocrinology, hematology and oncology, orthopedics, child abuse and neglect, and adolescent medicine, to name just a few. The opportunity and availability of other settings continue to grow because of the interest and ability of well-trained PAs to bridge gaps in pediatric care.

Challenges in Pediatrics

The image of childhood is accompanied by the promise of hope and opportunity. That image, coupled with the dictum of medicine that in order to care *for* a patient one begins by caring *about* the patient, presents the pediatric PA with many challenges.

Provision of comprehensive and compassionate health care to children sometimes leads one to question expectations of what life should be like in childhood. Some children are not blessed with a carefree and safe existence. It may be difficult to deal with a child and family who are forced to relinquish expectations and to grieve when a child is diagnosed with a debilitating birth defect, chronic disease, or terminal illness. Some children are victimized by gruesome acts of maltreatment at the hands of adults through either neglect or outright abuse. Abject poverty does not seem fair in a country with so many resources.

Despite these injustices, every child is in need of care and advocacy by committed professionals. Putting aside strong feelings to move through a difficult situation requires dedication, reflection, a supportive team, and the ability to see that growth occurs even in the midst of sadness. The patient needs the PA's talents. Difficult as these occasions are, they are ultimately opportunities for true service and often yield meaningful professional and personal lessons.

Rewards and Satisfactions

The practice of pediatrics offers numerous professional opportunities for pleasure and affirmation. Children are frequently delightful and charming. They are always spontaneous and guileless. It is from opportunities to interact with children in a helpful and productive way that many rewards come. As a PA, one has the chance to observe growth and evolution, not just as children mature physically, but also as they develop personality and character.

The intellectual challenge of understanding the disease processes of childhood and providing appropriate diagnoses is also rewarding. For the most part, children are readily healed. Medical care given to children is affirming because, in most instances, their physical resilience is exceptional.

The provision of empathetic listening and appropriate reassurance from an individual removed from the immediacy of problems is highly valued by parents as the pace of society becomes more frenetic and mobility interrupts important connections to the extended family. Parents want to do the best they can for their children, even in the most difficult circumstances. It is a genuine privilege for the PA to be able to provide guidance to families and young children. The role offers the opportunity to help families build on inherent strengths and maximize their confidence in their ability to provide appropriate support and nurturing.

Pediatrics, like other primary care subspecialties, is filled with variety. A day in a pediatric office can be filled with many "routine" visits for which the intervention is relatively simple. There are many times, however, when diagnostic acumen and the ability to appreciate subtleties make a difference in the life of a particular child and family. The niche of a pediatric PA requires a knowledgeable and experienced view of what to expect from normal processes in childhood, as well as expertise in pathologic processes in children.

CONCLUSION

There is no doubt that PAs will continue to be in demand for their ability to provide high-quality health care to pediatric patients. Traditionally, PAs have augmented and amplified the availability and quality of health care for children. Crises in provision of health care services for children will, unfortunately, continue to expand the areas for contribution. In the United States, as a result of chemoprophylaxis of HIV-infected pregnant women, transmission of the AIDS virus is estimated to occur in less than 2% of newborns. However, pediatric AIDS is a leading cause of death in children throughout the world, and it was estimated at the end of 2009 that there were 2.5 million children living with HIV/AIDS.[23] Infants are also subject to the ravages of intrauterine exposure to drugs and alcohol. Lack of prenatal care directly influences the number of infants born prematurely and with congenital problems. Poor access to health care exacerbates complications from illnesses and disabilities. Children who are homeless face a multitude of health and psychosocial problems. Domestic violence affects children from the perinatal period through adolescence. Teen pregnancy remains an ongoing problem in the United States.

Although this litany may seem like a cry of despair, *all* children in the United States are in need of care. PAs are uniquely able to provide this care and meet children's health care needs. As Osler[24] wrote, "Useful your lives must be, as you will care for those who cannot care for themselves, and who need about them, in the day of tribulation, gentle hands and tender hearts."

CLINICAL APPLICATIONS

CASE STUDY 1

It is February. The McCarthys have brought 9-month-old Robert in because of a cough. He is in the third day of this illness and has not run a fever. They state that this is "really weird" because he seems fine during the day—coughs occasionally and is hoarse but is eating great and playful. He was up most of last night with a dry, barky ("almost honking") cough. The McCarthys live in a small rural community in the mountains, 45 minutes away when the roads are not snowy.

1. What would be your differential diagnosis for this illness?
2. How would the family's access to care affect your treatment decisions?
3. How would the child's age affect your treatment decisions?

CASE STUDY 2

Ms. Tannenbaum is here with 16-month-old Rebecca for an ear check. It is her fourth ear infection since she started day care 6 months ago. Ms. Tannenbaum is almost in tears because she cannot take any more time off from her job and wants to know what to do to prevent Rebecca from getting any more infections.

1. What questions would you ask to help her think through Rebecca's risk for ear infections?
2. Would you advise her to take her child out of day care? Why or why not?
3. What about the day care center's contribution to Rebecca getting ear infections? Are there other options for child care? What would you recommend?

CASE STUDY 3

Mr. Fletcher brings in 10-year-old Jeff to the HMO where you work. The family is on their way out of town to Disneyland for a long-awaited family vacation. Jeff announced last night that he had a sore throat, and he seems to have the sniffles this morning. Mr. Fletcher seems rushed and lets you know that their old family doctor treated any sore throat with antibiotics. They really want to start him on penicillin today before their 4:00 PM flight.

Jeff has a 3-year-old sister, and his grandmother is joining them on this trip. Mr. Fletcher is concerned that the whole family will end up sick if Jeff does not start on antibiotics.

1. What additional history would you take about Jeff's symptoms?
2. What are the risks and benefits of starting Jeff on antibiotics?
3. What are your options for laboratory diagnosis, and how reliable are they for predicting whether this is an infection that requires antibiotics?

General Clinical Application Questions

1. If you accepted a position as a PA in pediatrics, how would you update your knowledge base and clinical skills?
2. What do you think you would find personally challenging and rewarding about working in pediatrics?

KEY POINTS

- The role of the PA in pediatrics is to be a resource for the physical, emotional, and mental health of infants, children, and adolescents.
- During periods of economic uncertainty, programs for children are among the most vulnerable to governmental cutbacks.
- PAs identifying pediatrics as their areas of practice represent 4% of the members of AAPA.
- Threats to children's health care are exacerbated by lack of access to health care and by poverty. Poor children are much more susceptible to the effects of prematurity, perinatal infections, infectious diseases of early childhood, child abuse, accidents, homicide, suicide, teen pregnancy, and school failure.
- Poor, inner city children are much less likely to receive required immunizations by age 2.
- The PA practitioner needs to hone observation skills about normal child development and behavior to augment and interpret the information given by the parent.
- Most states offer specific legal protection to health care providers who provide confidential services to teens. Examples of confidential visits include counseling about birth control, sexually transmitted disease, drug and alcohol use or abuse, and mental health issues.
- The pediatric physical examination requires a thorough and comprehensive approach and needs to be tied to age-specific norms.
- Assessment of growth is one of the most important indicators of overall health in childhood. Measurements of morphologic growth give evidence of underlying biochemical, organic, and developmental competencies.
- A cornerstone of pediatrics is an appreciation of how children progress through normal development.
- PAs must be attuned to deviations from expected behavior.
- In the role of case manager, the PA's ultimate goal is to maximize the child's potential through early intervention and to support family members as they work with the child's special needs.

References

1. Rudolph A. The health care system. In: Rudolph R, Oglesby A (eds). Pediatrics. New York: Appleton-Century-Crofts, 1977.
2. Rudolph A. Pediatric health supervision. In: Overby K (ed). Rudolph's Pediatrics. Norwalk, CT: Appleton Lange, 1991.
3. Silver H, Ott J. The child health associate: a new health care professional to provide comprehensive health care to children. Pediatrics 1973;51:1.
4. American Academy of Physician Assistants. 2009 AAPA Physician Assistant Census National Report. *http://www.aapa.org/research/data_and_statistics/resources/item.aspx?id=600*; Accessed August 3, 2011.
5. Xu J, Kochanek KD, Murphy SL, Tejada-Vera B. Deaths: final data for 2007. Natl Vital Stat Rep 2010;58:1. *http://www.cdc.gov/nchs/deaths.htm*; Accessed August 2, 2011.

6. MacDorman MF, Mathews TJ. Behind international rankings of infant mortality: how the United States compares with Europe. NCHS Data Brief 2009;23. *http://www.cdc.gov/nchs/data/databriefs/db23.htm#citation*; Accessed August 2, 2011.
7. Miniño AM, Xu J, Kochanek K, Tejada-Vera B. Death in the United States, 2007. National Center for Health Statistics Data Brief 2009;26:26. *http://www.cdc.gov/nchs/fastats/deaths.htm*; Accessed August 3, 2011.
8. Miniño AM. Mortality among teenagers aged 12-19 years: United States, 1999-2006. U.S. Department of Health and Human Services, Centers for Disease Control and Prevention, National Center for Health Statistics, *http://www.cdc.gov/nchs/fastats/deaths.htm*; Accessed August 3, 2011.
9. American Academy of Pediatrics, Bright Futures. Bright futures goals. *http://brightfutures.aap.org/goals.html*; Accessed August 2, 2011.
10. Children's Defense Fund. The state of America's children. 2010. *http://www.childrensdefense.org/child-research-data-publications/data/state-of-americas-children-2010-report.html*; Accessed August 2, 2011.
11. Committee on Practice and Ambulatory Medicine and Bright Futures Steering Committee. Recommendations for preventive pediatric health care. Pediatrics 2007;120:1376. *http://pediatrics.aappublications.org/content/120/6/1376.full.html*; Accessed August 2, 2011.
12. Korsch B, Freemon B, Negrete V. Practical implications of doctor-patient interaction analysis for pediatric practice. Am J Dis Child 1971;121:110.
13. Society for Adolescent Medicine. Confidential health care for adolescents: position paper of the Society for Adolescent Medicine. J Adolesc Health 2004;35:160.
14. Keane V. Assessment of growth. In: Kliegman RM, Stanton BF, St. Geme III JW, et al (eds). Nelson Textbook of Pediatrics. Philadelphia: Elsevier Saunders; 2011.
15. Centers for Disease Control and Prevention. WHO growth standards are recommended for use in the U.S. for infants and children 0 to 2 years of age. *http://www.cdc.gov/growthcharts/who_charts.htm*; Accessed August 2, 2011.
16. Centers for Disease Control and Prevention. Clinical growth charts. *http://www.cdc.gov/growthcharts/clinical_charts.htm#Set1*; Accessed August 4, 2011.
17. Stanton BF, Behrman RE. Overview of pediatrics. In: Kliegman RM, Stanton BF, St. Geme III JW, et al (eds). Nelson Textbook of Pediatrics. Philadelphia: Elsevier Saunders, 2011.
18. Centers for Disease Control and Prevention. Recommended immunization schedules for persons aged 0-18 years—United States, 2012. MMWR 2012;61(05):1–4. *http://www.cdc.gov/vaccines/recs/schedules/child-schedule.htm#hcp*; Accessed August 1, 2012.
19. Centers for Disease Control and Prevention. General recommendations on immunization. MMWR Recomm Rep 2011;60(2):1–64. *http://www.cdc.gov/vaccines/pubs/ACIP-list.htm*; Accessed August 2, 2011.
20. American Academy of Pediatrics. The Injury Prevention Program (TIPP). Age-related safety sheets: a guide to safety counseling in office practice. *http://www.aap.org/family/tippmain.htm*; Accessed August 2, 2011.
21. Saunders M, Gorelick MH. Evaluation of the sick child in the office and clinic. In: Kliegman RM, Stanton BF, St. Geme III JW, et al (eds). Nelson Textbook of Pediatrics. Philadelphia: Elsevier Saunderss, 2011.
22. Chamberlain LJ, Wise PH. Chronic illness in childhood. In: Kliegman RM, Stanton BF, St. Geme III JW, et al (eds). Nelson Textbook of Pediatrics. Philadelphia: Elsevier Saunders; 2011.
23. Yogev R, Chadwick EG. Acquired immunodeficiency syndrome (human immunodeficiency virus). In: Kliegman RM, Stanton BF, St. Geme III JW, et al (eds). Nelson Textbook of Pediatrics. Philadelphia: Elsevier Saunders, 2011.
24. Osler W. Doctor and nurse. In: Osler W (ed). Aequanimatas, with Other Addresses to Medical Students, Nurses and Practitioners of Medicine. Philadelphia: The Blakiston Company, 1932.

The resources for this chapter can be found at www.expertconsult.com.

CHAPTER 24

Obstetrics and Gynecology

J. Kirkland Grant • Edward M. Sullivan

CHAPTER CONTENTS

Midlevel providers have long been involved in the practice of obstetrics and gynecology (OB-GYN), dating back to early midwifery. Certified nurse midwives (CNMs) play a large role in some OB-GYN practices, performing all uncomplicated vaginal deliveries, with the doctor called in for complicated vaginal deliveries or cesarean sections. Most OB-GYN physicians, however, do not have much experience with any sort of midlevel provider, particularly physician assistants (PAs). The practice of medicine has changed considerably over the past few years, with OB-GYN physicians taking on increasing primary care roles and reimbursement steadily declining with the growth of managed care and discounted fees. This offers an ideal opportunity for the growth of PAs in the field of obstetrics and gynecology. The broad primary care training of PAs allows them to fit into this niche and make a substantial contribution. The PA can pick up abnormal findings on physical examination and has a broad understanding of other disease processes as they relate to obstetrics and gynecology and to primary care. The fact that PAs are trained by physicians gives PAs a point of view parallel to that of their OB-GYN supervisors.

Most midlevel clinicians working in obstetrics and gynecology are women and have been easily accepted by both physicians and patients. Some women feel more comfortable being examined by a woman clinician and actively seek out an OB-GYN practice where female clinicians are available. If the clinician is a caring individual with a willingness to listen and can put the patient at ease quickly, that woman will become a long-term patient regardless of the sex of the clinician.

One attribute of obstetrics is a uniquely hectic schedule. In large practices, one physician may be scheduled out of the office all day to cover deliveries. Smaller practices do not have this luxury, and often a physician is called away from a busy office to deliver a baby or attend other surgical emergencies. PAs can provide an ideal solution to such problems. Through planning of enough flexibility into the office schedule, the PA can cover many of these absences and minimize patient rescheduling. Although some patients may still choose to reschedule for a physician's appointment, most would prefer to be seen in a timely fashion. Utilization of a PA to provide backup and allow flexibility in scheduling also gives peace of mind to the physician, who can be assured that patients will be seen in his or her absence and that rescheduling or lengthy waiting room stays can be avoided.

Additionally, a PA is ideally suited to assist a physician in surgery. In most hospitals, PAs can first-assist on all surgical cases. Familiarity with the physician's technique in the OR allows the PA to anticipate the physician's needs. This can help the procedure go more smoothly. Too often the scrub technicians are different for each case and may not be accustomed to working with a particular physician.

COUNSELING

The daily routine of an OB-GYN clinician includes extensive and intensive opportunities for counseling of patients. Although it would be generally inappropriate for the OB-GYN physician to delegate all counseling tasks to the PA, it is equally true that the PA can provide these services cost-effectively, particularly for patients with extensive and complicated concerns. Although many patient education videos are available, these sometimes raise more questions and a PA can help put in perspective and individualize these videos for each patient. A patient who is about to undergo a surgical procedure will benefit from multiple counseling visits to ensure that she understands the scope of the procedure and its benefits, as well as its potential limitations.

By seeing a PA, the patient can be counseled thoroughly regarding her goals and expectations. Any specific concerns can be referred to the physician for further consultation if necessary. Preventive care is one of the most important services health care providers can offer their patients and is most effectively achieved through patient education, counseling, and consistent follow-up. PAs working in obstetrics and gynecology are particularly proud of the relationships they develop with their patients throughout pregnancies and other transitions in their lives.

The differential diagnosis of a medical problem, as well as appropriate education and counseling, may be influenced by the patient's sexual orientation. PAs must take care not to assume that their female patients are heterosexual. During the initial history, asking patients whether their sex partners are male, female, or both can elicit valuable information with a nonjudgmental approach. For example, right lower quadrant pain in a lesbian patient is less likely to be caused by pelvic inflammatory disease than in the heterosexual population. PAs who acknowledge the sexual orientation of lesbian, bisexual, and heterosexual women will be better able to develop positive relationships with their patients.

Patient Concerns

The PA has the opportunity to provide in-depth **counseling** and information about female anatomy and physiology, contraception, the menstrual cycle, sexually transmitted diseases (STDs), sexual problems and concerns, infertility, premenstrual syndrome, conception, prenatal care, breast-feeding, sterilization, breast self-examinations and mammograms, menopausal symptoms, hormone replacement, and a multitude of other reproductive and general health concerns. Despite the increasing availability of women's health information, women have many questions about the reproductive **process.** They often turn to the Internet for guidance, but some of the information posted on the Internet **can be** false or misleading. It is important that the PA reviews this information carefully with the patient and puts it in proper perspective for the individual that he or she is **counseling**. Similarly, the press often releases information **via news outlets** before it is available for review by health care providers. A thorough understanding of these issues can help the clinician put the information in perspective for the patient.

Counseling can take many different paths. Women may not know when they ovulate and are therefore subject to becoming pregnant unintentionally. Some women think that the birth control pill can also protect against STDs. Although it is true that the hormone effect causes thickening of the cervical mucus and may help retard the upward spread of chlamydia or gonorrhea into the fallopian tubes, this offers no protection against herpes, acquired immunodeficiency syndrome, *Trichomonas*, or *Condyloma*. Many women are also misinformed about their anatomy. A common question, especially among teenage girls, is whether a tampon or diaphragm can "get lost." Patient education and counseling are essential parts of the role of PAs in obstetrics and gynecology.

First Pelvic Examination

CASE STUDY 24-1

A 16-year-old high school student comes to the office for her first pelvic examination and Papanicolaou (Pap) smear. Her mother accompanies her. The patient appears apprehensive, showing little eye contact with the PA. After a focused history and physical examination, the PA performs the pelvic examination using the techniques described in the box on p. 347. The PA offers the patient a mirror to view her cervix. After seeing her cervix, the patient becomes more animated and asks several questions about the examination, providing the PA an opportunity to educate the patient about normal female anatomy and physiology.

The first pelvic examination illustrates the importance of taking time for patient education and discussion. A woman coming in for her first examination may be apprehensive and afraid. Unfortunately, many of her friends and relatives may have shared with her detailed descriptions of painful and humiliating pelvic examination experiences. Some women are still virgins and are concerned that they cannot be examined without tearing of their hymen. These situations require a sensitive, caring clinician who will take the time to explain clearly what a pelvic examination involves and thereby alleviate the patient's anxiety. This explanation should be presented by a clinician who has performed many pelvic examinations and has developed techniques to make the examination more comfortable. The procedure described in the box below can be applied to a first pelvic examination or any pelvic examination when appropriate.

PELVIC EXAMINATION PROCEDURE

- Show the patient the speculum and how it works.
- If the patient is a virgin, smaller speculums should be available. Make sure they are ready before the patient is placed in a lithotomy position (in stirrups). Assure the patient that the hymen will remain intact.
- Describe the process for obtaining a Pap smear, reassuring the patient that it generally takes more time to describe the process than to perform it.
- Describe the bimanual examination and tell her how to relax. Instruct the patient to keep her bottom on the table and allow her knees to fall apart. If her knees are together, this tightens the introitus and makes the speculum examination and bimanual examination more difficult. She should try to keep her face and neck relaxed, focusing on a relaxing poster placed on the ceiling above the examination table. Remind her not to hold her breath but to continue slow, deep breathing in through her nose and out through her mouth. An experienced nursing assistant in the room can help the PA and talk with the patient.
- Elevate the head of the examination table to give her a sense of greater participation and control.
- Have a mirror available to let her see her cervix.
- When the patient has her legs in stirrups, drape a sheet discreetly over her knees. Gently touch the inner part of her thigh, then slowly slide your gloved hand down to the vulva, so as not to startle the patient.
- Explain that you will first examine the external glands and urethra. Then gently insert a finger into the vagina and gauge the opening for selection of a speculum of proper size.

After the pelvic examination has been performed, the clinician may spend additional time talking with the patient about anatomy, the menstrual cycle, STDs, contraception, and other issues that the patient may have concerns about.

A teenager may be accompanied to her examination by a parent, usually her mother. Although this can be beneficial to the patient, sometimes the parent's presence can cause the patient to be inhibited and she may not want to talk about some of her concerns. The clinician must be sensitive to this and must know when to discreetly remove the parent from the examination room and ask the patient whether there are any issues she would like to discuss in private. Any issues of confidentiality she may have should be met with reassurance that information from her medical record, including topics of discussion, is not available to other individuals, including her parents, without her permission.

Often, a teenager may have scheduled the appointment to obtain birth control. It is important that the clinician discusses all the available methods, along with their risks, benefits, and possible adverse effects, to help the patient make an informed decision. Once she has selected a method of birth control, she needs further careful instruction on how to use the method correctly. It is especially important that a clinician is available to a teen for questions and to deal with any potential problems that could cause her to stop using her chosen method. The patient should understand that the clinician is available by telephone and that makers of oral contraceptive pills (OCPs) have toll-free lines that offer answers to many questions about the OCP. The patient should be advised to call before discontinuing the use of any method because of a problem or uncertainty. Minor adverse effects often resolve within the first 2 or 3 months of use. Any major adverse effects should be reported immediately.

Teens are also often unaware of the types of STDs to which they can be exposed and the possible consequences of these diseases. Every patient encounter should include review and reinforcement of this information. It is important for the clinician to emphasize that although the birth control pill may prevent pregnancy, it will not provide protection from STDs.

Sexual Issues

Many women have questions and concerns about sexuality but are uncertain and embarrassed about expressing them to the clinician. PAs in OB-GYN need to be knowledgeable and comfortable with discussing any of the patient's sexual concerns and problems. Skill in taking a detailed history of a sexual encounter is a required competency for the OB-GYN clinician, as is knowledge of appropriate treatment interventions and resources. Most patients will not volunteer any information about sexual problems. If they perceive that the clinician is hurried or uncaring, they will not mention the problem even if they are asked.

Open-ended questions are usually helpful in drawing out the patient. It is essential that the clinician maintain a nonjudgmental attitude. Often the patient simply needs to be reassured that what she is experiencing is normal or common among women. Documentation of items discussed is important to refresh the PA's memory when the patient returns for future visits but need not be extremely detailed unless such detail is pertinent to the patient's problem.

Premenstrual Syndrome

Many women experience premenstrual syndrome (PMS) with its many physical and psychological symptoms. Unfortunately, the exact cause of PMS remains unknown, which hampers clinicians' ability to counsel and treat their patients. Sometimes PMS is blamed for symptoms that are actually the result of other problems. The PA should be familiar with PMS, including its signs and symptoms and their timing in the cycle; he or she must also be attuned to other possible causes of a patient's symptoms. Having the patient keep a detailed monthly chart or diary of her periods, noting the timing and severity of her symptoms, can help the clinician determine if the condition is truly PMS and can help in identification of the primary symptoms. Recently, severe PMS has been categorized as PMDD (premenstrual dysphoric disorder). A plethora of information is available on the Internet, which can be a good resource for patients if they take the time to make sure that they are viewing reputable sites.

Many treatment modalities have been recommended for PMS. Because no single treatment or combination of treatments is effective for all women, it is best that the treatment plan be tailored to fit the individual patient. All women benefit from exercise, diet modification, and vitamin and mineral supplementation. Extra vitamins C, E, and B complex, as well as calcium and magnesium, may help diminish the symptoms of PMS. Hormone supplementation, diuretics, antidepressants, anxiolytics, and antiprostaglandin agents (nonsteroidal antiinflammatory drugs [NSAIDs]) all have roles in the treatment of specific complaints. In some cases, biofeedback or professional counseling may be necessary. In every case, thorough discussion of the treatment plan and close follow-up contribute to successful treatment.

The most effective treatment in studies to date has been the selective serotonin reuptake inhibitors (SSRIs) and related drugs. Some studies have shown up to a 70% response. Fluoxetine hydrochloride (Prozac) has been marketed under the label Sarafem for the targeting of PMDD. Some women have responded to the medication after taking it for only 7 to 10 days before their expected menses, although peak effects of the drug are not usually noted until after 6 weeks of continuous use. For those with more severe PMDD or for those who do not respond to the premenstrual regimen, daily doses through the month should be offered.

Conception

Unfortunately, many women do not seek medical advice when they are planning to get pregnant. Too often the emphasis is placed on preventing unplanned pregnancies rather than preconception planning for those ready. Studies now indicate that taking vitamins (particularly folic acid) before conception can reduce the incidence of certain birth defects, such as spina bifida and anencephaly, and may lower the incidence of spontaneous abortion. It is important for a couple to verify immunity to rubella before planning a pregnancy; those patients who are not immune should be immunized. Rubella vaccine (or measles, mumps, rubella [MMR]) should not be given to a pregnant woman, and pregnancy should be delayed 3 months after immunization. If the woman is diabetic, strict control of her blood sugar before conception can reduce the incidence of birth defects. Certain medications that women may be taking, such as antihypertensive, antiepileptic, or anti–acne medications, are contraindicated during pregnancy and should be changed before pregnancy is attempted, or immediately on discovery of a pregnancy. Overweight women should be instructed about eating a healthy diet. The effects of tobacco, alcohol, drug, and caffeine use before and during pregnancy should be reviewed.

Information about the normal menstrual cycle and ovulation and the optimal timing and frequency of intercourse can be of help. If patients are taking the OCP, they should be advised to wait at least two cycles after discontinuing the pill before attempting to conceive. If they do conceive before that time, they can be reassured that the pregnancy will most likely proceed without complication. Patients using medroxyprogesterone acetate (Depo-Provera) should know that it may take up to a year for their menstrual cycle to return to normal and for ovulation to resume. Any other health issues should be addressed before conception if possible.

Infertility

Infertility often requires extensive counseling by the clinician. Couples who have problems conceiving are often anxious and frustrated. They usually have friends who have conceived easily or who have had rapid success with infertility workups, and they cannot understand why they are having problems. Many feel pressured by family members and colleagues to produce offspring, and this compounds the anxiety. Although most causes of infertility fall into three major categories (anovulation, tubal blockage, and low sperm count), there are hundreds of other potential causes and only a systematic investigation may uncover them. Some women would like a single test to see if they can get pregnant. Unfortunately, the only such test is a positive serum or urine HCG test. Other patients come in seeking a "fertility pill," thinking that it will help them get pregnant no matter what the cause of their infertility may be. Education and explanation of various tests, their results and meaning, and the implications of those results for future pregnancy need to be provided in great detail to this type of patient. They need to understand that there is only one chance a month to get pregnant, and even if everything is in working order, the chances of getting pregnant during any one cycle may be only 20%. As a result, some infertility workups can last for years. Both the patient and her spouse should be encouraged to come to office appointments whenever possible so that they can be updated on the status of the workup. It is often difficult for patients to adequately understand detailed and complicated physical and laboratory findings. Special laboratory tests must be done on specific days of the menstrual cycle, and, therefore, detailed instructions must be given and followed. Some OB-GYN practices are hiring PAs to work exclusively in the area of infertility because it is such a labor-intensive aspect of practice.

Pregnancy

A pregnant woman experiences many hormonal and physical changes and sometimes is uncertain whether these changes are normal. Previous pregnancies are of no help because each pregnancy is different and may bring new questions and concerns not previously addressed. Adequate counseling and education can help prevent a plethora of concerns that will usually alleviate most anxiety. Couples want to know about the growth and development of the fetus, changes in the mother's body throughout the pregnancy, and when quickening (first time fetal movement is felt) occurs. The fetal heartbeat can first be detected usually at 5 to 6 weeks by sonogram (depending on the machine), at 10 weeks by Doppler, at 15 weeks by fetoscope, and at 20 to 22 weeks by regular stethoscope. Numerous good reference books are geared toward pregnant women, and prenatal classes should be encouraged, but these sometimes raise other questions that the clinician should be prepared to answer.

Pregnant women should be counseled about which over-the-counter (OTC) preparations are safe. If they have questions about any medications that they are currently taking or that have been prescribed by other physicians during their pregnancy, they should call before initiating the medicine. The *Physicians' Desk Reference (PDR)* and other drug-prescribing handbooks list the pregnancy category of each drug. In general, category A and B drugs can be used safely during pregnancy, although some are contraindicated in the first trimester and others in the third trimester. Category C drugs can be used if the benefits outweigh the risks. Drugs such as phenytoin (Dilantin), which is known to cause an increased incidence of birth defects, may need to be continued despite the risks. Consultation with appropriate specialists will help the patient decide if the medication should be discontinued or changed.

Warning signs to be discussed with the pregnant patient differ with each trimester. Bleeding in the first trimester may be indicative of a threatened abortion, an ectopic pregnancy, or just cervical irritation. Severe vaginitis may at times cause bleeding, as well as cervical polyps or vaginal lacerations. In the third trimester, placenta previa or abruptio placentae need to be ruled out. This can usually be accomplished by a sonogram. Discharge in the third trimester might occur with premature rupture of the membranes (PROM), but infections that could precipitate PROM should be identified and treated. Braxton Hicks contractions begin at the start of the third trimester, but if they are strong and regular, premature labor must be ruled out. Cystitis may be the cause of uterine irritability; if untreated, it may progress to premature labor. A patient should be instructed to call if contractions are more frequent than 10 minutes apart and she is less than 37 weeks, but to wait until the contractions are strong and regular if 37 weeks or over.

When diabetes or another high-risk factor is identified, patients need extensive education to help prevent possible complications. Counseling and education of the pregnant woman constitute a major part of good prenatal care. Special considerations for teen pregnancies, single mothers-to-be, elderly gravidas, and other conditions should be incorporated into the patient education. Consultation with other specialists such as a perinatologist should be done in a timely fashion. Depending on the scope of the physician's practice, these patients may be referred to a high-risk center and they may be followed in conjunction with the specialist.

Prenatal Care

Pregnant women are seen in the office numerous times during their pregnancy, which offers a unique opportunity for PAs to develop close rapport with their patients. Every prenatal visit should include assessment of weight and blood pressure, urine checks for glucose and protein, measurement of fundal height, auscultation of fetal heart tones after 10 weeks, evaluation of any new signs and symptoms, discussion about patient concerns, and education appropriate to the stage of pregnancy. Initial laboratory work during pregnancy includes a complete blood count (CBC); a blood type Rh and antibody screen; screening for rapid plasma reagin, hepatitis B antigen, human immunodeficiency virus, and rubella; and a Pap smear. Abnormal findings should be reviewed with the patient, and tests should be repeated as needed.

After 14 weeks, a maternal serum alpha-fetoprotein level should be obtained. When this result is abnormal, the patient is understandably fearful because it may indicate birth defects in the fetus and the clinician must appropriately counsel the patient. The patient should be reassured that there are often false-positive results, but the possibility of a serious problem cannot be totally discounted. An ultrasound or sometimes an amniocentesis may be necessary to determine the cause of an abnormal value. All pregnant women have a disruption of their glucose metabolism, and hypoglycemia is a frequent cause of dizziness and fainting that patients usually do not recognize as such. Implementation of a proper diet will usually relieve these symptoms.

When entering the third trimester, the patient may develop hyperglycemia and screening should be done on all patients. This usually consists of a blood glucose test on blood drawn 60 minutes following a 50-g glucose load. If elevated, further studies should be done to confirm gestational diabetes. If gestational diabetes is diagnosed, the patient needs to understand the need for tight glucose control to prevent macrosomia and to reduce the incidence of stillbirth, birth trauma, and neonatal metabolic problems. Fetal well-being tests should be instituted, such as nonstress tests, which in some cases can be performed in the office under supervision by a PA.

Some OB-GYN practices alternate a patient's prenatal visits between the physician and the PA. Others may designate specific visits to specific providers. Some physicians prefer to have the PA complete the initial history and physical examination. Others prefer to use this longer visit as an opportunity to bond with the patient. In some clinics, PAs provide prenatal care for low-risk patients and physician services are reserved for high-risk cases. At any visit, if the PA detects potential problems or complications, he or she is able to refer the patient to the physician for immediate evaluation.

Postpartum Concerns

Once a woman has delivered, she often has questions and concerns about the postpartum period and breast-feeding. Postpartum depression is common and must be evaluated so that the clinician can judge whether medication or counseling may be necessary. Couples will have questions about when they can resume sexual intercourse, how soon after delivery they might get pregnant again, and how contraceptives should be used in the postpartum period. Progestogen-only contraceptive pills have been used in breast-feeding women, but they are not as reliable and usually are not used in other situations.

A woman must make many adjustments to her life with a newborn baby. The lack of sleep and emphasis on the baby may leave her tired and disinterested in sex, while her partner may begin to feel unloved or left out. She must be encouraged to take some time out for herself, and her partner should be educated about normal postpartum conditions. If the partner is supportive and helps with the care of the baby, their relationship will be strengthened.

Menopause

Women have questions from their mid-30s on about the onset of menopause. This is an area of misinformation and often unfounded concerns. Many women believe that the current cultural preoccupation with youth devalues women as they leave their childbearing years. Women in the perimenopausal period may experience mood swings, hot flashes, sleep disturbance, and changes in their body habitus. Postmenopausal women can have vaginal dryness, breast atrophy, and other physical changes. The challenge to the clinician is to provide information on menopause as a normal developmental phase rather than an illness. Prevention of osteoporosis and cardiovascular disease and consideration of hormone replacement must be discussed. Reports of a possible association between breast cancer and estrogen replacement must be put into perspective. The long-term benefits of preventive care must be emphasized, especially for women who are already postmenopausal and may not be experiencing any menopausal symptoms.

CASE STUDY 24-2

A 49-year-old paralegal visits her OB-GYN office after 6 months of amenorrhea. During the preceding year, she experienced irregular menstrual periods with slightly lighter flow, sometimes skipping a month. She complains of fatigue, night sweats, and hot flashes. She has also noticed a decreased interest in intercourse with her long-term partner and complains of decrease in lubrication when having intercourse. The physical examination and pelvic examination are normal except for atrophic-appearing vaginal mucosa.

The PA discusses the risks and benefits of hormone replacement therapy with the patient. Because she has no medical history that would contraindicate hormone replacement and because she is at risk for osteoporosis, the patient decides to start replacement therapy. A combination of estrogen and progesterone is initiated with good results. The patient's symptoms abate, and her sexual activity and enjoyment increase. The patient is educated about the importance of breast self-examination and regular follow-up with the PA for breast and pelvic examinations and Pap smears.

The continued need for annual pelvic examinations and regular Pap smears must be explained because women often feel they no longer need this care after they have completed their childbearing years. After age 50, annual mammograms are recommended. Although they may be uncomfortable, newer mammogram units and experienced technicians can minimize discomfort. New bone density measurements can be obtained to gauge the degree of osteoporosis when appropriate. The need for continued exercise, diet modifications, and increased calcium intake must be explained. The clinician must be sure to obtain a sexual history in menopausal women and must not assume that they are no longer sexually active. If the patient complains of dyspareunia (painful intercourse), a careful history and examination can determine whether this is due to atrophic vaginitis, inadequate lubrication, infection, or possible anatomic changes.

TASKS AND PROCEDURES

Annual Examinations

The most routine activity for OB-GYN clinicians is the performance of annual examinations. Every woman coming in for her yearly examination needs a history update or a complete history if she is a new patient, a complete physical examination, a Pap smear, and appropriate laboratory studies for routine screening. This is also the time to teach or reinforce proper technique and timing of the breast self-examination and the indications and timing for mammography. It is not uncommon for an astute clinician to pick up previously unnoticed problems, such as an enlarged thyroid, a heart murmur, or a pelvic mass in a patient who presents for a yearly examination without any problems or complaints.

Patients often will not volunteer information about problems, either out of embarrassment or because they think a symptom is normal. Women with endometriosis may have severe dysmenorrhea but may think that all women have severe cramps during their menses. Patients may not know that NSAIDs are generally superior to acetaminophen in helping to alleviate menstrual cramps. In some cases, laparoscopy may be warranted to diagnose the problem and treat the symptoms.

Questions about incontinence should always be asked during history-taking because many women are reluctant to volunteer information about bladder control problems. Even young women may lose urine with coughing, sneezing, or jumping up and down. It can also be helpful to put a poster in the restroom that may prompt reticent women to ask about treatment options. A routine examination is also the time to provide counseling about anatomy, physiology, the normal menstrual cycle, nutrition, contraception, STDs, sexual problems and concerns, and normal developmental changes.

Contraception

Most women of childbearing age come to an OB-GYN practice for a prescribed method of birth control. It is important for the clinician to review all options to help the patient select the optimal method for her use. It is also important to take a detailed history, including a sexual history, to help determine which method to recommend. The OCP is still the favorite choice for most women. Its safety record, effectiveness, and relatively low incidence of adverse effects cannot be overlooked. Studies have also shown that the OCP lowers the incidence of endometrial cancer and ovarian cancer. Most women have some relief of dysmenorrhea, and there is even an OCP with a Food and Drug Administration (FDA) indication for the treatment of acne. Teenagers often have trouble remembering to take the pill at the same time each day. Although there are ways to help them remember, such as placing the pill pack next to a toothbrush, this still remains a challenge. Women smokers older than age 35 or women with a history of thrombosis, hypertension, or other medical problems are not candidates for the OCP.

Careful instruction on when to begin and how to take the OCP is essential. If a woman forgets to take a pill, she should be instructed to take the missed pill as soon as possible or to take two the next day. If she forgets for 2 days, she should take two pills each day for the next 2 days. If she forgets for longer than 2 days, she should discontinue that pack and begin a new pack the following week. Patients must be reminded that the OCP may not be effective if pills are missed and that they may experience breakthrough bleeding.

Depo-Provera has been approved for contraceptive use in the United States after decades of use in other countries. Depo-Provera is a slow-release, long-acting progestin that is given as an injection every 3 months. This works very well for women who have trouble remembering to take a pill every day. Depo-Provera is even more effective than the OCP in preventing pregnancy. The drawbacks include a greater number of adverse side effects than are experienced with the OCP, including weight gain, hair loss, and menstrual disruption. After long-term use, most patients experience amenorrhea, and it may take up to 1 year before they can conceive after discontinuing the use of Depo-Provera. It can offer an alternative for the smoker who is older than 35 years of age and desires to use a hormonal contraceptive method.

Intrauterine devices (IUDs) are undergoing resurgence after litigation troubles in the mid-1980s. Currently, three IUDs are available in the United States—the Progestasert, the ParaGard, and a newer IUD, which is like a marriage of the other two. The Progestasert is filled with progesterone hormone, which is supposed to decrease vaginal bleeding. The hormone is gradually consumed, and the IUD must be replaced every year. It offers a good choice for women who want relatively short-term contraception. The ParaGard consists of a T-shaped, copper-wrapped device that has now been approved for 10 years. The Mirena is a copper-wrapped IUD that also contains a progestogen, which has been used extensively in contraceptive pills. It can be left in place for 5 years and has the advantage of decreasing menstrual flow. Many women will become amenorrheic while using this device. This property has led to an indication for its use for treatment of menorrhagia, outside of its contraceptive benefits. IUDs are contraindicated in women with a history of pelvic inflammatory disease (PID) and are a poor choice for women who have multiple sex partners and are likely to be exposed to STDs, such as gonorrhea and chlamydia. Effectiveness is similar to that of the OCP, although in the clinical trials for Mirena in the United States, there were zero pregnancies. The IUD also may offer a good alternative for the smoker or for the woman who is not ready for permanent sterilization but desires long-term contraception. Insertion of an IUD is a simple office procedure—taking less than 5 minutes—that any PA can learn to perform (see following box).

DR. GRANT'S PARAGARD INTRAUTERINE DEVICE INSERTION TECHNIQUE

- Before insertion, the patient should have been counseled about the IUD and the technique for insertion and given the brochure for review. Because of past litigation problems with the IUD, the information can be frightening and must be put in its proper perspective.
- An NSAID taken 30 minutes before insertion can reduce the discomfort.
- Lay out the instruments you will need for insertion—the proper IUD, a tenaculum, a sound, scissors, and sterile gloves—and pour an antiseptic (Betadine, if the patient is not allergic) into a medicine cup. A nonsterile speculum and large swabs should be available.
- With the patient in lithotomy position, perform a pelvic examination with disposable gloves to ascertain the size and position of the uterus (e.g., midposition, anteverted, retroverted).
- Change gloves, insert the speculum, and swab off the cervix with the antiseptic solution.
- Carefully open the sterile IUD package, apply the sterile gloves, and prepare the IUD for insertion by folding the arms of the T and inserting them into the introducer. Insert the plunger into the opposite end.
- I have found that unless the uterus is sharply anteflexed or retroflexed, or the cervical os is very narrow, a tenaculum is often not necessary, and thus the procedure is much less uncomfortable.
- Gently insert the IUD with a slight curve, matching the uterine position, until resistance is met. If the IUD has been inserted 7 to 8 cm, you have reached the fundus. While keeping pressure on the plunger, withdraw the introducer, which will allow the arms of the T to re-extend.
- If the IUD does not go past the internal os, have an assistant open the sterile tenaculum, grasp the anterior lip of the cervix, and place gentle traction on the uterus, which will straighten the uterus and usually allow the IUD to be inserted. If you still have difficulty, obtain an ultrasound examination of the uterus to identify the canal. Trim the two strings with scissors. Have the

patient feel the strings so that she knows what they feel like.

- Give the patient a prescription for an antibiotic and stress that it is important she fills it right away. One or two doses are usually sufficient for prophylaxis. (Give samples if available.)
- Instruct the patient to check periodically that the strings are in place. If she cannot feel them, she should re-check after her next menses. If she still cannot find the strings, she should come in to be checked to see if the IUD is still in its proper place. Sometimes the strings can curl up in the os and can easily be removed with a cotton-tipped swab.
- Have the patient follow up in 6 weeks to ensure that the IUD is in place.

The technique for the newer Mirena is somewhat different, and I recommend that you attend one of the training sessions to gain proficiency in its insertion. The Progestasert insertion is essentially the same as the ParaGard.

A diaphragm fitting must include teaching the patient how to insert and remove the diaphragm, as well as how to use and care for it. The patient should be allowed time to insert and remove the diaphragm herself under supervision. Omission of this important step is linked to noncompliance. The patient who is uncertain about her ability to correctly place her diaphragm is unlikely to use it consistently. A major advantage of the diaphragm is its lack of any hormonal adverse effects. Studies of certain cohorts of women using the diaphragm for contraception have shown respectable success rates. One complaint about the diaphragm is the lack of spontaneity involved in having to insert it just before intercourse. Patients should be counseled that they can insert the diaphragm several hours in advance, and if longer than 2 hours has elapsed, an applicator for spermicide can be inserted into the vagina without the need to replace the diaphragm. It should not be removed before 6 hours after intercourse.

Rhythm and withdrawal are relatively ineffective methods that some couples practice. Spermicides alone offer slightly better protection. Although a condom is not as effective as the other methods detailed here, it does offer the benefit of protection from many STDs. Women who are not in a long-term, mutually monogamous relationship should be counseled to use a condom even if they are using one of the other methods for contraception.

Over the past several years a full array of new contraceptive techniques has been developed. Some of these have been immensely popular, and in others, the popularity has waned. The Implanon is one of these. It consists of one polymeric silicone (Silastic) implant containing a progestogen that is inserted into the upper arm. Training and practice are required to make insertion smooth and correct. The manufacturer of the Implanon provides training materials and workshops to teach the technique, which involves making a small incision in the upper arm and using a trocar to insert the capsule. Its 3-year life span makes it attractive to patients who want long-term contraception. Adverse effects are relatively common, including menstrual disruption, bloating, weight gain, and hair thinning. Counseling is particularly important for determining whether Implanon is a good choice for the patient and for providing education about its adverse effects.

The contraceptive patch is popular. This is essentially the birth control pill that can be taken (applied) once a week, 3 weeks on, 1 week off. Patch technology has matured to yield a patch that is well tolerated and associated with minimal loss, although a replacement patch is available at the pharmacy should a patch fall off prematurely.

Lunelle is a once-a-month injection that is similar to taking a pill-pack at a time. The patient will continue to have regular menses, unlike with Depo-Provera, and generally has fewer adverse effects than with Depo-Provera.

Also available is a self-inserted contraceptive ring that is left in place for a week.

Regardless of the type of birth control method chosen by the patient, the clinician's role is to recognize any problems associated with the selected method of birth control and to manage those problems appropriately. Because many OB-GYN physicians think that their time can be most effectively spent performing deliveries and surgery or dealing with complicated patients, the PA can assume an essential role in addressing the patient's common contraceptive needs.

Common Problems and Complaints

Frequently, patients come to an OB-GYN practice for evaluation of specific problems and complaints. The PA should be able to initiate evaluation of these common problems and should know when to refer the patient to the physician. Common problems include vaginitis, urinary tract infection (UTI), symptoms of STD, pelvic pain, pelvic infection, abnormal bleeding, abnormal menses, infertility, and abnormal Pap smear.

The PA should be able to diagnose and appropriately treat the simpler problems without physician consultation. When the patient complains of vaginal itching or discharge, diagnosis can often be made via a wet prep. *Trichomonas* is easily diagnosed, and yeast can be seen under the microscope. The presence of clue cells indicates bacterial vaginosis. Vaginal pH can also be helpful, and newer DNA probes are now available to diagnose the more common pathogens. Less commonly, beta streptococcus, *Escherichia coli*, or other bacteria may be causing the symptoms and can be detected by culture.

A purulent cervical discharge may be seen with chlamydia, gonorrhea, or other less common pathogens, some sexually transmitted and others not. Cultures and DNA probes are available to make the diagnosis. If an STD is suspected, appropriate tests should be obtained. Because a definitive diagnosis cannot be made without the culture results, the clinician should inform the patient that cultures are being taken.

A urinalysis can easily be performed in the office with the aid of simple dipsticks and a centrifuge to spin down the urine. The presence of leukocytes or bacteria in the urine alerts the clinician to the possibility of a UTI. Red blood cells may be seen with a severe, acute UTI but may also be seen with urolithiasis or other kidney disease. With a more involved problem, the PA can assist the physician by taking a careful history of the problem, performing a careful and thorough physical examination, and ordering appropriate laboratory work before referring the patient to the physician. Thus, the physician is saved the time and effort of the initial work and can use the information gathered by the PA to make a diagnosis and recommend an appropriate treatment plan more quickly.

Obstetric and Gynecologic Emergencies

A clinician must always be alert to the possibility of overlooking a serious problem. The signs and symptoms that a patient presents with do not always mirror those described in the textbook. A perfect example of this is a woman presenting with an ectopic pregnancy. The classic symptoms are unilateral pelvic pain, spotting, and a pelvic mass. The pain may be intermittent at first, becoming severe only when the ectopic begins to rupture. The patient may have had what she describes as a normal menstrual period only 2 weeks before the time she presents to the office. A positive pregnancy test may be the only thing that alerts the clinician to the lurking danger. Ectopic pregnancy is still one of the leading causes of pregnancy-related death. If diagnosed early, an unruptured tube can often be salvaged. Appendicitis in pregnancy can be difficult to diagnose because of the physiologic changes of pregnancy and the upward displacement of the appendix by the enlarged uterus. A strong index of suspicion is the key to timely diagnosis of these and other potentially life-threatening conditions.

PRACTICE CHOICES IN OBSTETRICS AND GYNECOLOGY

Practice settings for PAs in OB-GYN range from strictly outpatient to strictly inpatient settings. Some PAs move back and forth between the hospital and the clinic as part of their daily routine. Some practices are based on the assumption that the PA is best used in providing continuity in the office during the frequent and unplanned absences of the physician for deliveries and surgeries. Other practices with a large proportion of hospitalized patients may choose to assign the PA exclusively to the performance of hospital tasks, including managing patients in labor, assisting at surgery, and providing preoperative and postoperative care. It is common for OB-GYN PAs in an outpatient clinic to have their own schedules of patients to see each day. Because physician schedules may be full for weeks in advance, the PA's schedule may include a number of patients with complicated problems that cannot wait (e.g., bleeding problems, possible infections, pelvic pain). Additionally, the PA's daily schedule might include several routine annual examinations, follow-up visits with previously treated patients, and overflow patients from physicians called away from the office.

Many OB-GYN PAs report that the variety of patients they see on a daily basis is one of the most rewarding aspects of their practices. This variety also gives the PA the opportunity to perform a wide range of procedures in evaluating problems. PAs routinely perform cervical biopsies, vulvar biopsies, endometrial biopsies, and destruction of genital warts using chemicals or cryosurgery. Some PAs are actively involved in the evaluation and treatment of breast disease. Although some clinicians may choose to restrict their practice to routine visits, PAs working in any specialty over time generally expand their clinical and procedural expertise. A professional development plan for any clinical job should ideally include active planning for the acquisition of further skills and expanded responsibilities.

CONCLUSION

Growing concerns for women's health issues and health care reform plans that increase access to OB-GYN services are resulting in greater utilization of PAs. Many clinics are making the decision to expand the mix of providers (PAs, nurse practitioners [NPs], and CNMs) rather than adding physicians to OB-GYN practices. Some primary care clinics are hiring PAs with OB-GYN backgrounds specifically to provide family planning and prenatal services to their patients. Health maintenance organizations (HMOs) increase access to all OB-GYN services through the utilization of PAs and NPs. Research projects investigating women's health issues actively seek PAs and NPs to conduct the clinical components. Clinics serving HIV-positive women utilize PAs and NPs to provide evaluation and treatment services. OB-GYN clinics in small communities are choosing PAs to expand services when they are unable to economically support additional physicians. In all of these situations, PAs are filling important niches in the health care system and are increasing patient access to OB-GYN services.

CLINICAL APPLICATIONS

1. Identify the steps in performing a pelvic examination.
2. Describe common symptoms of premenstrual syndrome and appropriate treatment approaches.
3. Discuss an approach to screening and preventive measures for the best outcomes of pregnancy for mother and child.
4. Identify typical symptoms of perimenopause and the risks and benefits of hormone replacement therapy.
5. Discuss typical roles of PAs working in OB-GYN. What would you find challenging and rewarding about practicing in OB-GYN?

KEY POINTS

- The majority of OB/GYN providers are female, and this adds legitimacy to this type of practice.
- Contraception needs to be tailored to the individual patient's needs.
- Pregnancy routines should also be tailored to the individual patient with the focus placed on protecting both mother and baby.
- Sexually transmitted infections have been increasing at an alarming rate among all females regardless of age.

The resources for this chapter can be found at www.expertconsult.com.

CHAPTER 25

SURGERY

Edward M. Sullivan

"Experience is best borrowed and not learned."
—ANONYMOUS

CHAPTER CONTENTS

The advent of the physician assistant (PA) profession in 1965 created a uniquely skilled clinician who bridged the gap between the medical and the nursing professions. Initially, a majority of PAs chose to practice in general and family medicine, with a few migrating to the surgical theater and the care of the surgical patient. PAs in general surgery and the surgical subspecialties are well represented in the profession today. Most PAs, by virtue of their broad clinical training and on-the-job experience, exhibit significant versatility and work in surgery without additional formal training beyond PA school. However, a handful of PA surgery residency programs offer advanced training for graduate PAs, illustrating a continued demand for surgically trained PAs. These residencies allow PAs to learn and perform surgical house staff functions.

Surgical PAs work both in inpatient and outpatient settings, often augmenting resident staff or substituting for resident coverage in hospitals not using resident staff. Working within a team model with the surgeon as "captain of the ship," they are employed by university-based academic hospitals, community hospitals, individual and group surgical practices, and health maintenance organizations (HMOs), as well as preferred provider organizations (PPOs) and institutions representing all areas of surgery and surgical subspecialties, including general and vascular, orthopedic, transplantation, pediatric, cardiothoracic and thoracic, neurosurgical, plastic and reconstructive, otolaryngologic, urologic, trauma, obstetrics-gynecology, and surgical critical care. The roles assumed by surgical PAs reflect the flexibility and high quality of training demonstrated by performance of surgical house staff functions traditionally delegated to the surgeon in training. The PA provides a reliable standard of care for the teaching surgical staff; becomes a liaison with the surgeons, medical staff, and allied health professionals; and, most important, provides continuity of care for the team as the surgery resident staff rotates through the various surgical services. Both patient and family benefit from increased contact with a surgical staff member who can provide advocacy and prompt evaluation and education when required.

The American College of Surgeons recognizes PAs as valuable members of the first-assistant team, even though the tasks performed by PAs on a surgical service encompass the entire spectrum of care. PA surgical duties also involve initial patient evaluations (history and physical), admission orders, and preoperative preparation; first- and second-assisting in the operating room (OR), including independent procedures (e.g., harvesting of saphenous vein, insertion of invasive monitoring lines and assist devices, incision closure); providing postoperative care through discharge from the hospital; and evaluating and treating patients during postoperative visits in an outpatient setting. Thoracentesis and chest tube insertion, lumbar puncture, central venous catheter placement, paracentesis, and advanced cardiac and trauma life support are within the expertise of, and are common practice for, most surgical PAs. Many surgical PAs provide formal instruction to residents, medical students, other PAs, and team members. PAs may also be involved in clinical research and publication. Most third-party payers cover PA services in surgery, and payment is provided to the PA's employer. Law mandates Medicare coverage with a PA first-assistant at surgery at a reimbursement rate of 85% of that allowed for a physician providing the same services. Detailed information on third-party reimbursement for PAs may be obtained from the American Academy of Physician Assistants in Alexandria, Virginia.[1]

> *"We should always let our judgments and recommendations be guided by the fact that we operate on patients, not on diseases."*
>
> STANLEY O. HOERR
> *AMERICAN JOURNAL OF SURGERY* (1962)

All PA students are required to participate in a minimum of one surgical rotation as part of their training program. This chapter is constructed to serve as a practical primer of surgical principles and routine tasks, in the hope that it will alleviate some of the anxiety a PA student may feel when introduced to a busy surgical service. The spectrum of surgical practice is exceedingly broad, and no single chapter can present a comprehensive guide for each student's educational requirements. Therefore, a general surgery perspective is used to illustrate this overview and to emphasize the basic skills that are universally used in surgical practice. The "Clinical Procedure" sections are highlighted to emphasize key elements of performance. Other areas offer only brief overviews, with the hope that the student will pursue a detailed study of these areas as he or she continues training.

Much of this chapter concentrates on the specific actions required of the PA in the OR, where technical demands allow few mistakes. The remainder of the chapter discusses the appropriate preoperative evaluation of the patient in preparation for surgery, routines and requirements important to bringing the patient safely through surgery to discharge, and a few of the more common postoperative problems and complications.

GENERAL OVERVIEW

Practice and repetition are the essential elements of successful surgery, particularly when one is developing and refining manual dexterity; thus, one can comprehend the lengthy period required to train a surgeon. The PA should focus on this simple understanding when approaching surgical rotations or a new postgraduate position: Sustained effort brings maximum reward.

Surgical PAs must remember that they are part of a team and that the patient is the ultimate benefactor of the team's efforts. To form a cohesive unit, each member should understand the others' roles, and personality conflicts should be identified early and resolved in a manner that optimizes patient care. Surgery requires stamina and emotional stability. Many long hours are spent at the operating table during lengthy procedures, and a strong constitution is needed to meet the demands experienced by the tense situations that may be encountered by the team. A good sense of humor, solid interpersonal skills, and a steady sense of self are necessary assets for keeping the team working toward a common goal with élan and efficiency, resulting in effective patient care.

To be an effective team member in this milieu, one must learn self-control and self-discipline. These strengths are often learned by observing senior, experienced team members and should be consciously cultivated, for they are equally as important as knot-tying and suturing. PAs are often called on in critical situations to perform highly technical tasks with little margin for error and to make decisions that may directly and quickly affect the health of a patient. Self-control and disciplined behavior are major assets enabling the PA to provide quality surgical care.

LEARNING THE ROPES

The practice of surgery comprises an enormous scope of patient physiology and care conditions. It can be as uncomplicated as suturing a clean superficial finger laceration in the emergency department or as complex as caring for a neutropenic cancer patient who must undergo major chest surgery that requires an extended ventilator-dependent period and postoperative total parenteral nutrition. Therefore, the practice of surgery requires an intimate and detailed understanding of anatomy and pathophysiology.

Most PAs learn anatomy in the context of what is joined to what, as well as where structures are located. The surgeon, on the other hand, is concerned with how each structure interrelates with the adjacent and adjoining structures in its vicinity, as well as how altering the anatomy and function of each structure affects the individual patient. Three-dimensional, spatial understanding of this concept is critical to the safe and effective performance of any surgical or invasive procedure. This concept can be illustrated by considering the insertion of a subclavian central venous catheter, a common surgical task. An iatrogenic disaster can occur if one does not understand the position of the subclavian vein and artery beneath the clavicle relative to that of the lung. A pneumothorax or an undetected subclavian artery cannulation may occur as a result of deep probing beneath the clavicle during this procedure.

Sound knowledge of the methods of accurate diagnosis, through the history and physical examination (PE), understanding of normal body physiology and adaptation to stressors, and a detailed comprehension of the pathogenesis and natural history of surgically treatable diseases allow the preservation and manipulation of the patient's physiologic processes during surgical care. This concept is aptly demonstrated during cardiac surgery, during which an artificial physiologic state is created when the native circulation is manually bypassed and the heart is stopped with a cardioplegic solution. Oxygenation, electrolyte and acid-base balance, and vascular volume are all controlled extracorporeally by the perfusionist. Postoperatively, the patient's cardiac preload, afterload, and inotropic efficiency are manipulated pharmacologically to optimize tissue perfusion and adequate cardiac output, and the heart rate is controlled by an external, computer-controlled pacemaker. Pulmonary function is controlled by ventilator respiration.

Many textbooks are available for learning techniques of surgical diagnosis, indications for surgery, specific treatment regimens, surgical procedures, and complications. They are elemental to acquiring essential surgical knowledge and serve as invaluable guides for the novice and the experienced surgical PA alike. The surgical resident should be able to suggest one or two textbooks recognized as standards for the care, treatment, and evaluation of diseases germane to their particular surgical specialty. Many texts are available that present guidelines for the routine care of the surgical patient. These provide capsulated, practical information on writing orders, treating common problems, and so forth.

Surgical anatomy texts and operative atlases are available for each of the commonly performed surgical procedures. Atlases detail each important step of a procedure, emphasizing anatomic landmarks, routine surgical maneuvers, and the use of important specialty instruments and techniques. Anatomic plates feature detailed dissections of pertinent tissues.

Surgical intensive care manuals and surgery physiology texts, coupled with physician guidance and practical experience, are useful means of mastering the preoperative and postoperative aspects of patient care. This approach is especially fitting for patients requiring complex physiologic support.

ASSISTANT IN SURGERY

Historically, the roles of first- and second-assistant in surgery have been filled by experienced surgeons, nurses, and certified surgical technicians. The proliferation of qualified PAs trained in surgical assisting now brings the skills of another practitioner, trained in the medical model, to the operating suite.

The *first-assistant* is the person directly opposite the surgeon at the OR table, who actively participates in conducting the procedure. Most PA surgical rotations are dominated by members of the surgical residency and by fellows, who seek practical hands-on experience in the OR. The educational opportunity available within a group of surgical patients for first-assisting is limited, and often the roles of second- and even third-assistant are relegated to PAs and medical students. This may displace the student from the operative field, thereby diminishing his or her ability to adequately practice the harmonized and educated movements of an experienced surgical team. In these instances, however, the student has a unique opportunity to learn many of the subtleties and nuances that will serve well when the opportunity to actively first-assist arises. Although tugging at the end of a retractor may seem like an interminable task, it enables one to observe and appreciate the practiced movements and coordinated efforts of the surgeon and first-assistant without peril of poor performance from lack of experience. The basic techniques of incision creation, appropriate tissue retraction, gentle tissue handling, hemostasis, knot-tying, and wound closure can all be gleaned from keen observation at the table.

JUDGMENT, HANDS, TOOLS, AND DEVICES

Surgical procedures are composed of a series of physical motions centering on tissue dissection and manipulation, with experienced judgment directing the action. All operations are memorized step by step, including common intraoperative alternatives, in order to achieve the optimum result. The proper use of surgical instruments must be mastered, but more important, the PA must learn to use each one efficiently, effectively, and safely. Maneuvers such as the use of the scalpel, suturing, knot-tying, tissue retraction, and intravenous (IV) and chest tube insertion require learned manual dexterity and hand-eye spatial coordination that are mastered with study and practice. An assistant's hands are the most valuable tools he or she brings to the table, next to sound surgical decision-making skills.

Surgical judgment is the ability to recognize what should or should not be done during an operation or during the care of a surgical patient. This judgment can be acquired only through active immersion in the surgical environment. The frequently touted axiom "See one, do one, teach one" does not embody the value of experience to the surgical PA. The appropriate "whens" and "hows" for manipulating a nerve, holding the large bowel, using electrocautery, or adjusting a ventilator's settings come with time and demonstration, not with trial and error. This is why the chapter's opening quote is so poignant.

Academicians often refer to the concept of the "practice" of surgery. This state of constant renewal and relearning must occur as new techniques and modifications, materials, and devices are applied to care for the surgical patient. The OR and intensive care unit (ICU) are replete with devices requiring electrical input and computer control; all essential personnel are required to be skilled in their use and maintenance, and many require attention and oversight from PAs. It is extremely important for the clinician to know completely each device's operation and to be able to troubleshoot that device if an emergency arises from its malfunction. Intraoperatively, such malfunctions may account for an inordinate rise in total anesthetic time and an increase in morbidity.

Each instrument, retractor, and needle has inherent properties of action that, in the hands of an experienced user, become direct extensions of the hands and fingers. Spending time in the instrument cleansing and sterilization area is an excellent opportunity for the PA to handle instruments and practice their use without the pressure of timed performance in the OR. The staff can aid in instrument identification, and the novice PA can handle each of the commonly used instruments of the specialty and practice proper hand position and control of the instrument with the goal of understanding its actions and precise use. A short time spent practicing outside the OR can prevent fumbling and uncoordinated movements during the actual operation.

WHO'S WHO IN THE OPERATING ROOM

Surgical Team

The surgical team may consist of all or a combination of the following people: attending surgeon, fellow, fifth-year resident, junior resident, intern, and student(s).

Attending Surgeon. In most academic centers, the attending surgeon is an experienced staff member who has the ultimate responsibility for the surgical team's patients. He or she is responsible for the training of the fellows and fifth-year surgical residents and frequently teaches the more difficult and complex surgical techniques and decision making to this group. Attending surgeons often have particular areas of clinical interest (e.g., oncology, intensive care, trauma, burns, gastrointestinal disorders) and are commonly involved in research. The attending surgeon participates in the training of students on the surgical rotation as well and is called on to personally operate on the more difficult surgical cases that require experienced judgment.

Fellow. A graduate of a surgical residency, a fellow has elected to continue studies in a specific subspecialty (e.g., vascular, trauma, cardiac, neurosurgery). Each fellowship lasts between 1 and 3 years, during which an intense training regimen prepares the fellow to practice in the chosen specialty. Much of this training is spent in the OR, learning and performing specific specialty procedures. Many fellowships include a specified opportunity to conduct research activities.

Fifth-Year Resident. The fifth is the last year of residency for most general surgery programs, although some extend to 7 years. The fifth-year resident is responsible for the overall day-to-day patient care provided by the team. He or she performs the most complicated operations with the attending surgeon, instructs junior residents in the OR, and provides consultation on the care of newly admitted patients and complicated cases.

Junior Resident. The junior resident is the workhorse of the residency staff. This person is responsible for the minute-to-minute care of the patient as provided by the surgical team. The junior resident does a large volume of the service's operating and is responsible for the training of the second-year resident and intern. A resident in the second year of training along with the intern does much of the admitting and discharging of the service's patients. Additionally, the second-year resident usually serves extended rotations in the emergency department and ICU to hone emergency care, triage, and surgical intensive care unit (SICU) skills.

Intern. The first-year resident, or intern, is a recently graduated medical student and a new arrival on the surgical service. He or she is responsible for the brunt of the everyday tasks required for patient care/routine orders, admissions, discharges, consults, night call, IV lines, tubes, laboratory tests, and radiologic studies. Interns are engaged in learning the basic surgical skills and techniques required for general patient care. They are excellent sources of information for PA students, and because of the great burden of tasks thrust on them, interns commonly allow PA students to learn by doing.

Student. Medical and PA students are a valuable part of the surgical team in that students provide the additional staff required to efficiently operate a large-volume service. While constantly observing, students help manage the day-to-day needs of their assigned patients—history and PE, beginning IV lines, drawing blood specimens, inserting chest tubes, casting, wound care, emergency department duties, patient assessment, patient transport, dressing changes and wound care, and monitoring response to treatment. In addition, PA and medical students learn basic surgical techniques such as suturing and knot-tying, inserting monitoring lines, and first-, second-, and third-assisting in surgery. After adequate observation and performance of techniques monitored by senior team members, the student's motto should be, "I will do that for you."

Anesthesia Team

The anesthesiologist is responsible for evaluating the patient for anesthesia and, in coordination with the operating team, for providing safe conduct of the patient through the chosen anesthetic technique. Anesthesiologists care for the patient throughout the recovery room period and into the SICU if required. Many have particular expertise in pain management.

Certified registered nurse anesthetists (CRNAs) train in nurse residency programs to perform many of the same tasks as a physician or a doctor of osteopathy (DO) anesthesiologist. Deeply versed in anesthetic practice, CRNAs provide quality care, often without the direct supervision of an anesthesiologist, and are used by many surgeons for uncomplicated surgical procedures. Limitations on CRNA practice are dictated by hospital and state regulations and vary from institution to institution and from state to state.

Anesthesiology assistants (AAs) are individuals who attend a training program to conduct anesthesia but who are not physicians or CRNAs. Several training programs are available in the United States, although only a handful of states have regulations or laws that allow administration of anesthesia by AAs. AAs perform anesthesia practice under the supervision of a licensed anesthesiologist and are valued members of the anesthesia team, on which they are used.

Operating Room and Recovery Team

Postanesthesia Recovery Unit (PARU)/Recovery Room Nurse. The PARU nurse is trained in assessing and treating the patient in the immediate postoperative period, including maintenance of hemodynamic and cardiopulmonary stability, pain management, and crisis intervention when necessary. Such professionals are invaluable sources of guidance and information on postanesthesia patient care.

OR Director. Usually a veteran registered nurse (RN), the director controls the overall activity of the OR and is responsible to the chief of surgery (a surgeon) and the hospital's director of nursing. The OR director represents the OR to other hospital departments, manages the department's fiscal requirements, and oversees the management of OR personnel. He or she can set the tone for a favorable climate for PAs in the OR.

OR Supervisor. Also usually an RN, the OR supervisor manages the day-to-day activities in the OR and makes important policy decisions in conjunction with the OR director. The supervisor is responsible for problem-solving, overall procedure and OR staff scheduling, instrument purchases, and staff training.

Control Room Supervisor. As the title implies, the control room supervisor controls the scheduling of surgery and personnel assignments on a daily basis. He or she checks for the proper availability of equipment for each case and acts as a traffic coordinator for busy surgery departments.

Head Nurse. There is usually one head nurse per shift. He or she helps micromanage the OR environment for smooth and efficient daily operations. Often, the head nurse is an experienced nurse with good problem-solving abilities and adaptability. He or she is a liaison between the OR staff and the surgeon.

Staff Nurse. Staff nurses are usually RNs and licensed practical nurses (LPNs). They have two overlapping roles—circulating nurse and scrub technician or scrub nurse.

Circulating Nurse (Circulator). The circulator supervises the general activity of each individual in the OR, including assessing the patient in the holding area before bringing him or her into the OR and transporting the patient to the recovery area after surgery. Patient safety, also the responsibility of the circulator, centers on appropriate positioning of the patient on the OR table and preparation of the patient by scrub preparation of the skin before the incision. The circulator assists the scrub nurse in assembling the supplies and instruments required for the operation and in accounting for all sponges, needles, and instruments before and after each operation. Circulators provide additional supplies for the operative field when required. They receive and connect the various tubes and wires coming from the sterile field (e.g., suction tubes, laparoscopic equipment, and electrocautery wires) to the appropriate devices. They operate and troubleshoot non-sterile equipment and prepare tissue specimens received from the surgeon for transport to the pathologist for analysis.

Scrub Nurse. Scrub nurses assist the surgeon by providing all instruments, sutures, and supplies required for the smooth execution of each procedure. Scrub nurses anticipate the needs of the surgeon and first-assistant by understanding each step of a procedure and by monitoring the progress of the operation, often handing the appropriate instrument to the surgeon without prior request. In addition, the scrub nurse occasionally assists in retracting tissues, cutting sutures, sponging blood from the field, and operating the suction. A well-trained and experienced scrub nurse often performs certain portions of the procedure without direct supervision by the surgeon. One of the scrub nurse's primary responsibilities is knowing the location and count of all items in the sterile operative field before, during, and after surgery, ensuring that nothing has been left in the wound. The scrub nurse is an invaluable source of information on the conduct expected of the PA or medical student in the OR and the skills required at the OR table. Also, a scrub nurse who has worked frequently with a given surgeon may have invaluable information regarding that surgeon's preferences and dislikes in the OR.

Certified Surgical Technologist (CST). Although not an RN or LPN, the CST is trained by an American Medical Association (AMA)-approved center and meets rigid certification examination criteria to perform a wide variety of functions in the OR. Many of these responsibilities parallel those of the scrub nurse, although many large institutions do not allow CSTs to circulate during surgery. CSTs often assist the surgeon while scrubbed and fill an important position in the operating suite.

PREOPERATIVE PATIENT EVALUATION

"For us, an operation is an incident in the day's work, but for our patients, it may be and no doubt it often is the sternest and most dreadful of all trials, for the mysteries of life and death surround it, and it must be faced alone."

SIR BERKELEY MOYNIHAN (1865-1936)

The most important portion of the evaluation of surgical patients (after stabilization in emergencies) is assessing their ability to safely undergo the proposed surgical procedure. This assessment concentrates on the patient's replies to questions derived from the past medical history and systems review. Information gained from past medical records and family members is equally as important as PE findings, diagnostic laboratory results, and radiology reports.

SAMPLE ADMISSION ORDERS

- Admit to
- Diagnosis
- Condition
- Vital signs
- Allergies
- Nursing (tubes, wound care, respiratory care, oxygen, etc.)
- Diet
- IV fluids
- I/O (fluids into and out of patient), daily weights
- Medications
- Studies (chest radiograph, electrocardiogram, pulmonary function tests, etc.)
- Laboratory tests
- Call house officer for (limits of temperature, vital signs, urine output, drain output, etc.)

THE FIVE Ps OF MEDICATIONS

Pain: Oral or parenteral pain meds (scheduled or as needed [prn]). Consider patient-initiated pain pump.
Pillow: Sleeping pill (prn).
Poop: Stool softener or cathartic (scheduled or prn).
Pus: Antibiotics; topical agents for skin or wound care.
Previous: Long-term medications the patient has been using; may need to be changed postoperatively.

Obtaining a comprehensive history is critical Most surgeons do not assess all physiologic systems before surgery, often relegating this task to the PA. This is a prime opportunity for the PA to establish a trusting relationship with the patient and family. It is during this initial contact that the PA can explain the usual preoperative preparations, the planned surgical procedure, its risks and benefits, and the expected postoperative course.

History

Each type of surgery demands different information about the history of present illness. In acute, life-threatening emergencies, a paucity of information may be available. In acute surgical cases (allowing several hours before surgical intervention), the history of present illness should detail the type, severity, and duration of symptoms; associated symptoms (e.g., pain, nausea, vomiting, syncope); previous similar episodes; previous evaluation, if any; previous treatments; family history of similar problems or anesthesia complications; and last oral intake. A detailed history should center on past operations, particularly those that may have a bearing on the present illness. Electively scheduled surgery allows a more leisurely but thorough patient evaluation.

Detecting "comorbidity" by eliciting information on coexisting diseases that could lead to complications before, during, or after surgery is a prime focus in taking the history of a surgical patient. Comorbid disease can increase the risk of complications, which could be ameliorated or prevented with preoperative medication or treatment. Early identification allows appropriate consultation with other services and preemptive treatment of expected postoperative problems. Table 25-1 lists diseases and conditions that must be detected and evaluated before surgery.

In general, the information required during the preoperative evaluation is as follows:

- An assessment of the general state of health, including exercise tolerance, recent weight gains or losses, usual state of emotional health, and frequency of routine medical care.
- A review of the patient's current drug use, which should alert the PA to underlying pathophysiologic diseases that may affect the course of surgery (e.g., digitalis as a clue to heart disease). Obtain a history of drug use, both prescribed and over-the-counter, including tobacco, aspirin, nonsteroidal anti-inflammatory drugs, street drugs, and herbs or other alternative or complementary medications used. The quantity and duration of use of tobacco products should be identified and chronicled in the chart and discussed with the surgical team.
- An identification of all medication and food allergies, including type and severity of reaction (e.g., pruritus, respiratory distress).
- A thorough menstrual and obstetric history from female patients, including any anesthetic complications that occurred during childbirth. Menstrual history is especially important for patients who may not suspect that they are pregnant or for patients who could be anemic from heavy menstrual blood loss.
- Previous hospital charts, when possible, to review the patient's past surgical performance (e.g., type of surgery and anesthesia, complications, anesthetic problems, blood transfusions, extended ICU admissions).

TABLE 25-1 **Major Diseases or Conditions Requiring Evaluation before Surgery**

- Diabetes mellitus and other endocrine diseases
- Cardiac disease
  - Rheumatic heart disease
  - Valvular disease
  - Arrhythmias
  - Prior myocardial infarction
  - Angina
  - Severe hypertension
  - Congestive heart failure
- Pulmonary disorders
  - Moderate to heavy smoking
  - COPD
  - Asthma
  - Obesity
- Hematologic diseases
  - Bleeding disorders
  - Thrombocytopenia and hemophilia
  - Moderate to severe anemia (sickle cell, iron deficiency, etc.)
  - Thromboembolic disease (deep vein thrombosis, pulmonary embolism)
- Thyroid disease
  - Hyperthyroidism
  - Hypothyroidism
- Adrenal dysfunction
- Liver disease
  - Hepatitis (drug-induced, viral, cholestasis)
  - Cirrhosis
- Electrolyte disorders
  - Calcium, potassium, phosphorus, sodium, magnesium
- Acute or chronic renal failure
- Neurologic diseases
  - Seizures
  - History of stroke or transient ischemic attacks
  - Myasthenia gravis
  - Multiple sclerosis
- Pregnancy
- Peripheral vascular disease
- Rheumatologic diseases
  - Rheumatoid arthritis
  - Systemic lupus erythematosus
  - Gout
  - Sarcoidosis
- Psychiatric disease
  - Heavy alcohol use, schizophrenia, bipolar disorder
- Risk factors for HIV and hepatitis
- IV or other street drug use/abuse

COPD, Chronic obstructive pulmonary disease; HIV, human immunodeficiency virus.

The review of systems (ROS) is especially useful in determining the patient's overall health status. Regardless of the schedule of the patient's usual health care, important problems may have developed in the interim that need evaluation before surgery. Attention should be given to detecting risk factors for communicable viral diseases such as hepatitis and the human immunodeficiency virus (HIV).

In the ROS, questions should be directed toward problems involving the cardiopulmonary and endocrine systems because these systems account for a majority of postoperative deaths and morbidity.

SAMPLE ROS QUESTIONS FOR PREOPERATIVE EVALUATION

These sample pertinent questions are not a comprehensive guide to ROS questioning but are useful as a basis for review of each system during the preoperative evaluation.

GENERAL

How is your general health?
If emergent surgery required—When was your last meal?
Have you been sick lately, or are you under the care of a doctor for any problems?
What are the names of any other physicians providing care for you?
Any history of cancer?
Tell me about your weight and appetite.
How is your energy level?
When was your last tetanus immunization?
Have you had a Pneumovax immunization? (splenectomy or older than age 65)

DRUGS

Ask the patient to bring all home medications to the hospital or office for evaluation.
Do you take any prescription medications? Which ones? Do you take them on a regular basis?
Have you taken, or are you now taking, oral or injected steroids?
Do you take any over-the-counter medications, including vitamins and cold medicines (antihistamines and ephedrine-like medications)? Have you used any aspirin, ibuprofen (Advil, Motrin), or other antiinflammatory medications over the past 10 to 14 days?
Do you take any herbs or home remedies?
Do you use marijuana, heroin, cocaine or crack, methamphetamines, opioids, or barbiturates? Any other street drugs?
Do you drink alcohol? How much per day or week and for how many years? Have you ever been admitted or evaluated for alcohol problems?
Use the answers to these questions to investigate specific systems affected by the medications cited (e.g., ask diabetes/endocrine questions if patient is taking oral antihyperglycemic agents).

RESPIRATORY

When was your last chest radiograph?
Do you smoke? If yes, how many packs a day and for how long?
Have you been diagnosed with asthma, bronchitis, emphysema?
Have you ever been hospitalized for pneumonia, bronchitis, or asthma?
Have you ever been on a ventilator after surgery or for any other reason?
Do you cough every morning or on some mornings? Do you ever cough up anything? Describe it. Have you had a recent cough or cold?
Have you ever been exposed to or had tuberculosis? If so, which treatment did you receive and for how long?
Are you prone to sinus infections?
What medications do you take for your respiratory problems?
Do you need oxygen at home to breathe?

CARDIAC

What heart medications are you taking?
Do you have high blood pressure? How long have you had it?
What was your last measured blood pressure?
Do you have high cholesterol or triglycerides?
When was your last electrocardiogram?
Have you ever had a stress test or a cardiac echo or catheterization?
Have you ever been told you have a heart murmur?
Have you ever had a heart attack or rheumatic fever? When was your heart attack?
Do you have an irregular heart rhythm? Do you have an implanted pacemaker?
Have you ever had heart surgery?
Do you ever get chest pain? How often? Related to what activity?
Are you ever short of breath, or do you ever wake up at night short of breath?
How many pillows do you need to sleep on? If you have climbed any stairs recently or walked around the block, how far did you go before becoming short of breath?
What is the hardest work you have done in the past couple of weeks and how did you tolerate that?
Do you have pain in your legs when you walk? Does it subside with rest?
Do you have any swelling in your feet or your hands?

ENDOCRINE

Do you have diabetes or thyroid disease? For how long? Which medications do you use?

SAMPLE ROS QUESTIONS FOR PREOPERATIVE EVALUATION—CONT'D

Have you had any complications/problems related to your diabetes/thyroid disease?
Have you ever had any problems with your adrenal glands?
Have you taken any steroids in the past year? Do you have heat or cold intolerance?
Do you get up at night to urinate? If so, how many times?
Do you urinate frequently?
How well do you sleep?
Are you nervous?
Have you had any weight gain or weight loss lately?
Are you frequently thirsty?

Hematologic

Do you bleed easily?
When you cut yourself, do you quickly stop bleeding?
Do you have frequent nosebleeds?
Does anybody in your family bleed easily?
Has anyone in your family been told they have von Willebrand disease or hemophilia?
Do you bleed when you brush your teeth?
Have you ever been told that you are anemic?
Have you been told you have too much blood (polycythemia)?
Do you have any history of thrombophlebitis or blood clots in the lungs or legs?
Have you had any blood transfusions in the past? If yes, how many units or what kind? Any problems associated with them?

Gastrointestinal/Nutrition

How is your appetite?
Have you had any weight gain or loss?
Are you nauseated or do you have vomiting? Have you had any abdominal or pelvic operations?
Have you ever vomited up blood?
Have you ever had bloody or tarry stools?
Have you ever had an ulcer?
Do you have abdominal pain (type, location, relation to foods, treatment)?
What are your bowel habits like?
Have you ever been jaundiced?
Have you had hepatitis in the past?
Are there any foods that you cannot eat?
If diabetes or neurologic disease, have you ever been told that you have trouble with emptying your stomach (delayed gastric emptying)?
Have you ever had an upper or lower endoscopy?

Genitourinary

Have you ever had any kidney or renal diseases?
Are you prone to bladder infection or prostate infection?
Do you have a history of kidney stones or blood in your urine?
Do you have any problems with urinary incontinence?
Do you have any problems with urinary incontinence?
Do you have difficulty with urination?
Do you get up at night to urinate?

Neurologic and Psychiatric

Have you ever had a seizure or a convulsion? Do you take any medications for this? Which ones and for how long?
Do you have history of a stroke or transient ischemic attacks?
Have you ever had an arm or leg go dead, or have you ever been paralyzed or had a numb limb?
Have you ever had trouble with your vision, either loss in one eye or seeing double?
Do you have frequent headaches?
Do you have any impairment of your memory or speech?
Do you have any difficulty with your motor coordination?
Do you have any problems with vertigo (dizziness)?
Have you seen a psychiatrist or psychologist?
Do you have any anxiety or nervous disorders?
Do you have a history of depression?

Gynecologic/Obstetric

Have you been pregnant? How many times? What were the results of those pregnancies?
Did you have any complications?
Do you think you could be pregnant now? When was your last menstrual period?
Are you using birth control pills or another type of birth control?
What is your usual menstrual flow?
Do you have any trouble with your menstrual period, especially significant bleeding?

Anesthesia

Have you or has anyone in your family had problems with anesthesia?
Have you or has anyone taken a long time to wake up from anesthesia (antipseudocholinesterase deficiency)?
Have you or has anyone in your family had a high temperature as a result of anesthesia (malignant hyperthermia)?
Have you ever had to stay on the ventilator after surgery? (Important question for chronic obstructive pulmonary disease [COPD] patients.)

Musculoskeletal

Do you have arthritis of any kind?
Are any of your joints frozen or hard to move?
Do you have any back problems?
Do you have any muscle diseases?
Do you have any artificial joints?

Physical Examination

A complete physical examination (PE) should be performed on each patient if time permits. The value of a complete PE in identifying possible sources of complications that can be managed expectantly cannot be overestimated. Preoperative physical findings are often used in the postoperative period to explain new signs and symptoms, as evidenced by the following example.

CASE STUDY 25-1

A 45-year-old man admitted with acute gastrointestinal bleeding from a perforated duodenal ulcer undergoes a successful 2-hour operation through a midline incision under general anesthesia. He is transferred to the PARU extubated and in good condition. The PARU nurse notes that the patient is unable to move the fourth and fifth fingers of his right hand and is too groggy to appropriately answer questions relating to this alarming finding. The anesthesia staff is concerned that the patient was improperly positioned on the OR table and may have experienced pressure on the ulnar nerve at the elbow or from inordinate traction on the brachial plexus at the shoulder during the surgical procedure.

If a thorough history and PE had been performed on admission, the patient's previous trauma-related ulnar nerve injury would have been detected, eliminating needless panic among the staff.

Although a complete PE should be performed, its focus should be on the state of the patient's cardiopulmonary and vascular systems, where many surgical complications may arise. Full vital signs, with the blood pressure measured in both lying and standing positions, may reveal orthostatic changes. Thorough examination of the vascular system, including the carotid, aortic, and femoral arteries for bruits, may indicate vascular or cerebrovascular disease. A peripheral vascular examination is useful in assessing edema, signs of superficial or deep phlebitis, varicose veins, or distal limb perfusion problems. Shiny atrophic skin, thick ridged nails, and ulcers on the foot may be signs of chronic arterial insufficiency. Edema may be a sign of congestive heart failure or serum protein insufficiency of liver disease or malnutrition. The limbs and neck should be examined for adequacy of IV or arterial vascular access and evidence of IV drug abuse. The remainder of the examination should focus on the detection of physical signs of comorbid diseases or factors that may affect postoperative recovery such as ambulatory difficulties; visual, hearing, or coordination impairment; diminished pulmonary reserve; and easy fatigability due to congestive heart failure or chronic obstructive pulmonary disease.

Laboratory and Radiologic Evaluations

The approach to the preoperative laboratory examination has undergone revision over the past 10 years and is reduced to a minimum for most patients. The underlying methodology for ordering laboratory tests should be based on a thorough history and PE and not on a routine testing template. A significant amount of a patient's hospital bill is accumulated by laboratory and diagnostic testing. The PA can play an important role in cost containment. Most hospitals require all patients to have a complete blood count (CBC) with differential and a chemistry panel, including electrolytes, glucose, blood urea nitrogen, and serum creatinine before surgery. Chest radiography is performed only when an abnormality is suspected on the basis of history or physical findings, or when preexisting cardiopulmonary disease is present. A history of tobacco use should be elicited in all patients. Electrocardiograms are recommended for patients older than 40 years if review of the cardiac system reveals any positive findings or if the patient is known to have cardiac disease.

The history and physical findings should provide justification for other laboratory studies that may be indicated before surgery. Prothrombin time (PT) and partial thromboplastin time (PTT) tests are ordered for patients who give a specific personal or family history of coagulopathies or who are taking warfarin or heparin. A bleeding time may also be ordered for patients taking platelet aggregation inhibitors (e.g., aspirin, ibuprofen, dipyridamole [Persantine], other nonsteroidal antiinflammatory drugs, coagulation inhibitors). Patients with known risk factors for liver disease should undergo liver function testing, and a history of genitourinary disease or symptoms should prompt urinalysis or 24-hour urine collections for creatinine clearance. Patients taking medications such as digoxin, quinidine, theophylline, or antiepileptics may require evaluation of serum drug levels before surgery.

A history of significant pulmonary disease or suspected pulmonary dysfunction (e.g., in heavy smokers) requires pulmonary function testing and arterial blood gas sampling before surgery. Echocardiograms and exercise stress testing are usually indicated for patients with a history of untreated angina, previous myocardial infarction, or significant hypertension.

A rational approach to identifying those patients with infectious viral diseases, notably HIV and hepatitis, should involve asking questions about risk factors associated with acquiring these diseases, even though all patients should be treated with the use of universal precautions.

Guidelines for mandatory testing of such patients vary by state and are controlled by hospital policies.

Check with the hospital's infection control committee to obtain this information.

A final note on preoperative evaluation: The examiner should use PA and physician medical and surgical consultations to further evaluate patients when he or she is unsure of the severity or importance of a particular disease process. Consultants can often suggest methods by which the patient's ability to tolerate surgery can be assisted with an emphasis on postoperative care in difficult cases.

Preoperative Evaluation of Elderly Patients

As the U.S. population of patients 65 years and older increases, PAs should expect to be an integral part of their care. The elderly are at higher risk of morbidity and mortality in the perioperative or postoperative period because of their age-altered physiology. The American Society of Anesthesiologists categorizes individuals as high operative risks solely because of an age greater than 75 years, acknowledging the problems related to the care of the elderly surgical patient.

The overall effect of aging is a decrease in the physiologic reserve of the elderly individual as a consequence of normal changes in various organ systems. Cardiovascular system changes are related to decreases in cardiac output and are a response to exogenous stressors. The heart undergoes ventricular hypertrophy, often with calcification of the mitral and aortic annuli. Vascular tree resilience decreases, and peripheral vascular resistance increases. The final result is a higher risk of developing additional problems such as fluid overload, septic shock, and renal failure, all of which can be iatrogenically induced.

The renal system undergoes a marked reduction in number of nephrons, and the glomerular filtration rate slows with age. Importantly, these changes are not often reflected in the serum creatinine level because of the dependence of this measurement on muscle mass. Because muscle mass is decreased in elderly patients, reliance on serum creatinine level as a predictor is inaccurate.

In the nervous system, there is a decrease in cerebral blood flow in coordination with variable age-related changes in problem-solving skills and short-term memory. Elderly patients may have significant declines in vision and hearing. In the postoperative period, these losses, coupled with sensory deprivation in the foreign environment of the hospital room, recovery area, or ICU, can cause confusion and agitation. Delirium is a more common finding in postoperative elderly patients, secondary to the altered pharmacodynamic and pharmacokinetic processing of anesthetic and analgesic agents. This alteration is primarily a result of the changes in volume, distribution, and reservoir for deposition of such drugs.

The pulmonary system undergoes significant changes secondary to age, with smaller thoracic cage volume and greater thoracic rigidity. Respiratory muscle strength and endurance both decline. Measurements of pulmonary function may show larger functional residual capacity and dead space, as well as a decrease in the forced expiratory volume and peak expiratory flow rate. These changes contribute to the elderly patient's sensitivity to the effects of general anesthetics and increase the risk of postoperative pneumonia and atelectasis.

The geriatric patient population may present with a broad spectrum of disease processes inherent to their advancing age. Myocardial infarctions, hypertension and hyperlipidemia, cancers, neurologic disorders such as Parkinson's disease or dementia, diabetes mellitus, and rheumatic disorders occur more often among the elderly.

For patients with evidence of malnutrition, a nutritional analysis will be helpful in evaluating total protein, albumin, prealbumin, transferrin, calcium, phosphorus, magnesium, vitamin B_{12}, and folic acid levels. Pulmonary function testing with the addition of arterial blood gas values may be ordered for patients undergoing thoracic or upper abdominal procedures, to furnish baseline values in the event of postoperative pulmonary problems. Pulmonary artery catheterization and echocardiography may be indicated in patients with significant murmurs, congestive heart failure, or significant preexisting pulmonary disease.

The most common postoperative and perioperative complications for elderly patients are myocardial infarction, heart failure, fluid overload, pneumonia, and pulmonary embolus. Other complications include urinary tract infection (UTI), septic complications, renal failure, and metabolic problems. Common diseases, such as pneumonia and dehydration, do not manifest in the typical manner; the patient who has a UTI, pneumonia, or a myocardial infarction may become confused rather than present with the typical manifestations of these conditions.

Postoperative rehabilitation is important for all patients, but greater emphasis is required for the older patient. Patients who spend extended periods in bed are at increased risk for thrombophlebitis, pulmonary embolus, and atelectasis proceeding to pneumonia.

A final area of preoperative importance for the geriatric surgical patient regards provision of prophylaxis against common postoperative complications. These include encouraging smoking cessation, ordering preoperative and postoperative use of bronchodilators in patients with bronchospastic pulmonary disease, and providing preoperative and postoperative chest physiotherapy, including incentive spirometry, coughing, and deep breathing. Prophylaxis also involves preoperative treatment of pulmonary infection and infected sputum, as well as early postoperative ambulation.

Discharge Planning. Planning for home care and discharge should begin when the patient is first admitted to the hospital. It is critical that elderly patients' current level of physical, mental, and emotional functioning be assessed, along with their ability to care for themselves after discharge. Interviews with the family, nursing home workers, and the patient will provide a baseline assessment of the patient's ability to manage activities of daily living (ADLs). Questions should be directed toward assessing the patient's level of independence and needs for assistance with feeding, bathing, and self-cleansing, as well as his or her ability to ambulate, sit, stand, and walk. It is useful in this instance to enlist the aid of a medical social worker, a discharge planner, or a geriatric clinician to obtain an in-depth analysis of the patient's and family's ability to provide care and resume ADLs.

BLOOD AND BLOOD PRODUCTS

Few deaths per year occur among the 4 million transfusions received each year in the United States, but the recognition and identification of the acquired immunodeficiency syndrome (AIDS) and hepatitis C as blood-borne diseases have led to a national effort to rethink transfusion requirements for surgical patients. Historically, patients undergoing surgery were thought to require transfusion if their hemoglobin fell below 10 mg/dL. Currently, patients with healthy cardiovascular, neurologic, and pulmonary systems are often closely evaluated for hemodynamic instability during and after surgery before the ordering of blood transfusions. Hemoglobin values of 7 to 8 mg/dL are now thought to be acceptable for a healthy group of select patients.

Often the PA must explain to the patient and family the potential need for blood and blood product transfusion during surgery. Reports of HIV, hepatitis C, and other blood-borne infections linked to blood transfusions have elevated public fears. Legally, every patient should be informed of the possible need for blood transfusion before surgery, when applicable. Many institutions ask all surgical patients to sign consent for transfusion. The fundamentals of informed consent for homologous transfusion (of community-acquired banked blood) include the following:

1. Explaining the risks, benefits, and alternatives.
2. Allowing an opportunity for the patient to ask questions.
3. Obtaining a signed consent.

The patient undergoing an operation in which blood transfusion may be needed should understand that the American Association of Blood Banks (AABB) has instituted regulations that exclude high-risk individuals from the donor pool for blood and blood products. Self-exclusion is promoted to potential donors, and lengthy questioning of all potential donors screens other high-risk individuals from donation. Assays for the HIV antibody and hepatitis C are used to screen for seropositive blood products; very few donors who are infected with these diseases, and who are not seropositive, are missed by these methods. Patients found to be seropositive for hepatitis and HIV are permanently excluded from donating blood or blood products in the future.

The viral agent most commonly transmitted by transfusion is cytomegalovirus (CMV). Harbored in leukocytes, CMV is not a significant problem for nonimmunocompromised patients. However, blood specifically screened for CMV is required for immunocompromised patients (including bone marrow and solid organ transplant recipients), CMV-seronegative pregnant women who require blood, premature infants, and HIV-positive patients who are CMV-negative.

Less life-threatening complications related to homologous blood transfusion include febrile reactions and urticaria. Fever is the most common problem occurring in transfusion. It appears in approximately 5% of all transfusions and manifests as a transient elevation in basal body temperature of 1° to 2° C, although serious cardiopulmonary compromise can occur on rare occasions. Antipyretics or antihistamines frequently are given prophylactically to blood recipient patients. Urticaria is easily managed with antihistamines and antipyretics. More serious symptoms associated with transfusion are rare (<1%). They include pulmonary edema, renal failure, anaphylaxis, bacterial contamination, and death.

Alternatives to Blood Transfusion

The following techniques have gained increased utilization as alternatives to homologous banked blood. These can be considered when religious beliefs (e.g., some Jehovah's Witnesses) or fears regarding blood-borne contagious diseases lead patients to refuse banked blood transfusion.

Autologous Blood Donation. The patient's own blood is preoperatively collected for storage and eventual transfusion. This gives the patient the comfort of knowing that his or her own blood will be used to replace the amount lost during surgery. Preoperatively, donation is scheduled as frequently as 1 unit of blood every 72 hours, provided that the hematocrit remains greater than or equal to 33%. Patients are routinely given iron supplementation to spur erythropoiesis; the number of units obtained depends on the patient's erythropoietin response and increase in blood cell production. This blood can be stored a maximum of 30 to 42 days. Planning and foresight are required to enroll the patient in an autologous deposit program.

Designated Blood Transfusion. Patients often ask whether donors known to them can deposit blood for use in homologous blood transfusion. There have been blood supply shortages in the United States, and encouraging individuals to donate blood products benefits all patients. However, there is no evidence to date indicating that this type of blood transfusion is safer than the homologous blood from the general population. In addition, family members who are at high risk for HIV or hepatitis may be forced to reveal this status when they must decline to participate in designated donation. A patient who makes such a request should be made to understand that there are no guarantees for an exact match between donor and recipient, even if they have the same blood type. Educating the patient and family about the safety of the blood supply in general and informing them of other alternatives should be part of all presurgical counseling.

Autologous Blood Salvage (Autotransfusion) Intraoperative blood salvage from the sterile surgical field entails passing the recovered blood through a cell saver via washing and centrifugation. This procedure removes the active products of coagulation and the heparin anticoagulant used in the collection system. Of great benefit during orthopedic and cardiac operations, autologous cell salvage has reduced homologous blood transfusions significantly over the past several years for selected procedures. This concentrated collection is primarily composed of red blood cells with a hematocrit of approximately 55%. Total recovery of cells is approximately one half to two thirds of the initially collected volume, possibly eliminating the need for transfusion.

Transfusion Adjuncts

Several pharmacologic agents provide alternatives for the patient who requires autologous blood transfusion. Recombinant erythropoietin is used in patients with renal failure to increase red blood cell (RBC) mass. Another agent is desmopressin, a synthetic analog of vasopressin (antidiuretic hormone). It has no important vasomotor effects and has been shown to increase levels of factor VIII and von Willebrand factor.

Hemodilution. Preoperative hemodilution consists of a one-for-one exchange of whole blood with a crystalloid or colloid IV solution after anesthesia induction but before skin incision. Patients can be hemodiluted to a hematocrit of 22% to 25%. As blood loss commences and the hematocrit drops below 20% to 22%, it is replaced with the collected blood.

Hemoglobin Substitutes (Artificial Blood). Intensive research efforts continue to search for a safe but inexpensive solution containing synthetic hemoglobin molecules for use in humans. Several models exist for this technology, but their applicability outside research institutions has not been established.

Ordering and Administering Blood and Blood Products

Type and Crossmatch (T&C). The patient's blood is matched for A, B, O, and Rh type against specific donor units. When a T&C is ordered, the number of units that may be required should be specified on the request form. These units will be held in reserve for approximately 24 hours. If it is anticipated that the blood will not be required during or after surgery, the T&C order should be canceled, freeing the blood for other patients.

Type and Hold (Type and Screen). The patient's A, B, O, and Rh type are established and screened for antibodies. *No blood is available for this patient until further ordered by crossmatch!*

Blood Bank Products.

Whole Blood. All blood elements are available in this blood. One unit equals approximately 450 mL. This form is not often used.

Packed Red Blood Cells (PRBCs). Almost all plasma is removed. One unit equals approximately 250 to 300 mL. This is the most commonly used red blood cell replacement product.

Platelets. Platelets are supplied in packs equal to 1 unit of whole blood. They may be collected from a single donor but are usually pooled from many donors. One pack is approximately 50 mL. Platelets are usually given in multiples of 6 to 10 packs per patient.

Cryoprecipitate (Cryo). This pack contains factors VIII and XIII, von Willebrand factor, and fibrinogen. Cryoprecipitate is used in patients with bleeding disorders, particularly secondary to von Willebrand's disease and fibrinogen deficiency.

Fresh Frozen Plasma (FFP). FFP contains coagulation cascade factors II, IV, VII, IX, X, XI, XII, and XIV. It is used primarily for patients with an undiagnosed bleeding condition or when large quantities of packed RBCs (usually >10 units of blood) may be required. FFP comes in packs of approximately 150 to 250 mL per unit.

Washed RBCs. Almost all white blood cells (WBCs) are removed from blood products given to decrease the antigenicity of this fluid. Washed RBCs are used in patients who are to undergo renal or other transplantation, who are severely immunocompromised, and who have a history of previous transfusion reactions.

Leukocyte-Poor Blood Cells. Most of the WBCs are removed to make the compound less antigenic. Leukocyte-poor blood cells are less pure than washed RBCs, and one unit equals 200 to 250 mL.

Transfusion Procedures. A large-bore needle of 18 gauge or larger must be used for blood transfusion. Any patient receiving blood is first identified with a wrist bracelet containing specific information about blood type and Rh compatibility. It is mandatory that the patient's identification information from the ID bracelet be verified by comparison with the identification information contained on the label on the matched donor blood unit. Typically, two individuals cross-check each other before blood is administered to the patient.

Blood products are transfused only with isotonic saline. Mixing of blood products with other IV solutions may cause cell agglutination or lysis. Blood is frequently given quickly through pressure IV bags that accelerate administration. Additionally, cold blood is infused through a blood warmer to prevent cooling of the patient's core temperature.

After transfusion, all of the empty blood packs are banded together and sent back to the laboratory. In the event of a febrile transfusion reaction, small quantities of the blood left in the bags are used to determine antigenic status and to investigate possible pathogenic contamination of the blood administered to the patient.

DOCUMENTATION

"If it was not written down, it has not been done."

Specific entries are placed into every patient's chart for tracking and documenting care. Absence of these entries may delay or even cause the cancellation of a surgical procedure.

Consent

This includes explaining the proposed procedure to the patient and family or legal guardian, including the benefits and risks, and available alternatives. This explanation must always include the possibility of bleeding complications, infections, allergic reactions to medications or anesthesia, the possibilities of blood clot, possible damage to adjacent organs, lung or heart problems, and even death. Other risks specific to the proposed procedure should be disclosed. Consents for photography and observers in the OR may be appropriate as well. A witness who is not directly part of the surgical team (e.g., a staff nurse) should witness the explanation and sign the consent along with the patient and the PA. A skilled translator must be used to obtain consent from a patient whose native language is not English. A physician member of the team obtains most surgical consents.

Implied consent is used for patients with life- or limb-threatening emergencies who are incapable of understanding the implications of the proposed operation. Patients who are in shock or who are unconscious are often treated under this category. Attempts should always be made to locate a family member or guardian, and any efforts to do so should be documented.

Preoperative Note

The preoperative note is documented on the patient's chart in paragraph or list form before surgery to reiterate and substantiate important issues about the patient's preparation for surgery. It contains a statement regarding the patient's need for surgery, a basic review of the patient's preoperative condition, and the type of procedure proposed. Results of a brief PE are also included. This note reviews only the pertinent laboratory values and important radiographic findings. The consent status is documented, noting whether the patient, family, or other decision maker (e.g., legal guardian) has signed the consent or if implied consent is in effect. Risks and possible complications are listed for medical legal documentation, particularly if the patient is undergoing a difficult surgical procedure (e.g., possible loss of finger function for repair of a crushed hand injury, risk of cerebrovascular accident after carotid endarterectomy).

The expected disposition of the patient (e.g., admission to ICU or rehabilitation unit after surgery) is included to notify and prepare other services for future patient arrivals.

PREOPERATIVE NOTE

- To be written the afternoon before the planned procedure; serves as checklist and to document that someone actually checked laboratory reports, studies, and availability of blood products.
- Date
- Preoperative diagnosis
- Procedure planned
- Laboratory results
- Chest radiograph
- Electrocardiogram
- Other preoperative diagnostic studies (angiography results, CT/MRI findings, etc.)
- Risks and possible complications
- Consent signed
- Expected patient disposition

Postoperative Note

The operative note, handwritten into the chart directly after surgery, records the intraoperative findings and conduct of the patient's surgery. This note is particularly valuable to other practitioners who are following the patient postoperatively, especially in light of the fact that the typed operative note, which is a complete description of all events that occurred during the course of surgery and is dictated by the surgeon after surgery, may not be transcribed and available on the chart for 2 or 3 days postoperatively.

The postoperative note contains the following information in list form:

- Preoperative diagnosis(es).
- Postoperative diagnosis(es). May be different from the preoperative diagnosis (e.g., suspected malignant mass found benign by intraoperative pathology analysis).
- Name of the procedure. If multiple procedures were performed, they are named either sequentially or in decreasing order of "severity."
- Surgeon's name. Occasionally, a cosurgeon is also listed.
- Name(s) of assistant(s). All those assisting in surgery, including students, are listed here.
- Anesthesiologist's and/or anesthetist's name.
- Type of anesthesia administered (e.g., regional, general, spinal, local).
- Important intraoperative findings. Describes what was anatomically and clinically discovered during the procedure; may include the results of frozen section specimens sent to the pathologist, intraoperative radiologic examinations, foreign objects found, and organs affected.
- Estimated amount of blood loss (EBL). This is an estimation of the amount of blood measured in the suction reservoirs combined with an approximation of the amount of blood soaked into the sponges used and an estimation of the loss of blood intraoperatively onto the drapes. Blood loss is usually established by consensus between the anesthesiologist and the surgeon.
- Urine output during the operation, usually measured by an indwelling urinary catheter.
- Intraoperative IV fluids. Types and amounts of fluids given to the patient during surgery. IV fluid replacement often necessitates the use of multiple agents, including crystalloid and colloid solutions, blood and blood products, and, in some cases, medications that require large amounts of IV fluids as a vehicle for delivery (e.g., mannitol, sodium bicarbonate).
- Specimens sent to pathology. Can be a useful paper trail if specimens are misplaced.
- Drains. Each drain is listed by type, location, and type of collection reservoir.
- Tubes and lines. Lists all tubes and IV lines, including those inserted preoperatively and during the course of the procedure. Chest tubes, arterial lines, bladder catheters, nasogastric (NG) tubes, or pulmonary artery lines may be inserted. The author must be sure to include the size and location of each one (e.g., "18-gauge right radial arterial line").
- Implants. Lists any artificial materials implanted into the patient, such as joints, penile or breast prostheses, mesh materials, heart valves, and dialysis conduits. This should include the manufacturer's name, type of prosthesis, and registration

POSTOPERATIVE NOTE

- Preop Dx
- Postop Dx
- Procedure(s)
- Surgeon(s)
- Assistant(s)
- Anesthesiologist/CRNA/AA
- Intraoperative findings
- Type of anesthesia
- EBL (estimated blood loss)
- Urine output
- IV fluids
- Specimens
- Drains
- Tubes and lines
- Implants
- Complications
- Disposition

number for each. Any registration stickers or cards should be stamped with the patient's identification information and mailed to the registration agency of the manufacturer, after copies have been placed in the chart.

- Complications. Accurately describes what occurred, with specifics as to what was done to correct the problem, as well as the status of the patient on delivery to the recovery room.
- Disposition of patient. Should note how and for what destination the patient left the operating suite (e.g., to the PARU, extubated and in satisfactory condition, or to the ICU intubated and in poor condition).

PREPARATION FOR SURGERY

A significant portion of the surgical PA's responsibility outside the OR involves preparing the patient, the patient's family, and the hospital staff for surgery. This includes identifying the patient's diagnosis and need for surgery but also requires establishing the patient's ability to tolerate the proposed surgical procedure, while fully educating the patient and family and orchestrating the many details required to safely lead the patient through the upcoming ordeal. The PA may act as the team coordinator before surgery, a role that is invaluable to most surgeons.

Patient and Family Education

The patient should be well versed about what is about to take place. The patient and family should understand the need for surgery, the routines required for preoperative evaluation and preparation, and the usual preoperative and postoperative courses of events. This education also includes a complete explanation of the risks and benefits of the proposed procedure. All consents should be signed and witnessed, including consents for the specific type of procedure(s) and for the administration of blood and blood products. The patient's apprehension should be expected because of anticipated future pain, possible loss of function, the question of ability to continue working, and the general environment of the hospital. The PA has the ability and the time to sit down with the patient and family to explain upcoming events from the admission process through the postoperative course and must allow time for the patient and his or her family to vocalize their concerns and fears. Patients who have received education regarding the expected level of pain and the activities they will be required to perform after surgery have been shown to require fewer analgesics, cooperate more willingly after surgery, and have less protracted recoveries. By providing preoperative instruction on the value of deep breathing and early ambulation after the procedure, along with an explanation of the probable tubes and lines remaining after surgery, of where the patient may be for a short period (i.e., ICU), and of the known efficacy of prescribed analgesics, the PA can ensure better patient compliance and cooperation during postoperative convalescence.

Many patients have concerns and fears because of previous difficulties with surgery and anesthesia. Older anesthesia practices may have caused prolonged nausea and vomiting or severe headaches from spinal anesthesia. In addition, patients recall "horror stories" from family and friends about their surgical experiences, which are usually embellished by time. Each patient should be prompted to voice these concerns so that they may be discussed and alleviated as much as possible before surgery.

Excluding the family from the education process eliminates an informed source of support for the patient in times of crisis and may propagate unwarranted tension between the staff and family. An explanation of the facilities and services available for the family's support should include access to the medical social worker and chaplain, sleeping accommodations, meals, and visiting hours. Hospitals often have staff members responsible for such education, but supplying it during the early phases of care encourages trust and exhibits compassion.

The PA should be readily available when the family needs information and can serve as a liaison between the family, hospital staff, and surgeon. This role includes interpreting medical jargon, explaining the ramifications of laboratory or radiologic results, personally performing routine procedures if the family asks, and sending progress reports to the family from the OR during long procedures.

Preparing Hospital Staff

The OR staff should be informed about the type and anticipated length of the procedure and should be promptly notified of unanticipated changes or special requirements. If the patient requires preoperative antibiotics for a procedure that has a high risk of infection (e.g., gastrointestinal, genitourinary, or gynecologic procedure; infected wound; endocarditis prophylaxis), these should be administered 30 minutes before skin incision to ensure adequate tissue drug levels. The PA should review all laboratory, radiologic, electrocardiographic, and other preoperative test results before the operation and should immediately investigate and report any abnormalities. If a frozen section examination of tissue is required, the pathology department should be informed of the approximate time the specimen will be available to ensure the presence of a pathologist to process the specimen. The PA should also inform Radiology if any intraoperative radiographs are anticipated (e.g., arteriograms, cholangiograms, bone fixation, post–joint replacement films).

Other preparations include ascertaining the availability of special items specifically required for the planned procedure. When a special tissue or device is needed, the matter should be brought to the attention of the OR staff as soon as possible before surgery to facilitate the ordering and arrival of these materials.

Pertinent radiographs, computed tomography (CT) scans, and magnetic resonance imaging (MRI) scans should always be available in the room for intraoperative reference and surgical planning.

Before the procedure begins, the PA should work with the team to make certain the patient is correctly and safely positioned on the OR table, with all bony prominences cushioned, and that the security straps are in place. Invasive monitoring lines and tubes should be inserted after the patient has been sedated or anesthetized, if prudent, to avoid undue patient discomfort and anxiety.

Note on Deep Vein Thrombosis and Pulmonary Embolism

The severe morbidity and mortality of postoperative deep vein thrombosis (DVT) and pulmonary embolism require routine prophylaxis for all high-risk surgical patients. DVT and pulmonary embolism may occur because of the venous stasis created by various patient positions on the OR table (e.g., lithotomy with pressure on the calves) or by low-flow states occurring during hypotension. Risk factors for these postoperative complications include age older than 40 years, obesity, history of malignancy, previous history of DVT or pulmonary embolism, and long or complicated surgical procedures.

Two methods may be used, in addition to early postoperative ambulation, to prevent DVT and pulmonary embolism. Either low-dose heparin or a heparin analog may be used as pharmacologic prevention. Externally applied pneumatic compression and pressure gradient elastic stockings are effective mechanical means of preventing DVT (Figure 25-1). These can be applied at the time of surgery and can remain in place until the patient is ambulatory.

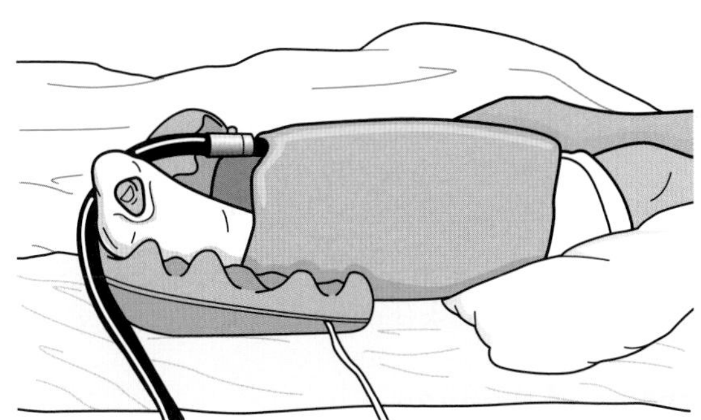

FIGURE 25-1 External pneumatic gradient antiembolism stocking.

ASEPSIS AND INFECTION CONTROL IN THE OPERATING ROOM

By advocating a controlled OR environment with sterile OR attire and precision housekeeping methods, surgeons can safely perform deeply invasive procedures and care for traumatic and dirty wounds with confidence to avoid surgical infection. Methods of controlling iatrogenic contamination, in conjunction with the development of heat and chemical sterilization processes to effectively kill microorganisms, ensure that modern surgery is now practiced in an environment that is maintained in as clean and sterile a state as possible.

The concept of aseptic technique is simple. Sources of contamination should be isolated from the area where surgery is being performed. All procedures should be done in a field devoid of living microorganisms, including patient skin flora, to decrease the morbidity and mortality associated with wound infections. Asepsis also involves recognizing and alleviating conditions advantageous to the growth of bacteria (e.g., removal of dead tissue, serum, and blood from the wound or incision) and avoiding gaps or "dead space" between wound tissues, which might result in hematoma formation. It also comprises the use of preoperative antibiotics.

Operating Suite Geography

To protect the actual OR from contamination by outside microorganisms, the surgery department is divided into several geographic zones to promote isolation. Entry into the *periphery* of the operating suite, where patients are delivered and received in preparation for surgery, is unrestricted. Family members may be allowed in this area with staff permission, and hospital personnel are not required to wear specific clothing here. The *intermediate zone*, clearly marked by signs and closed doors, is restricted to persons appropriately dressed in hospital scrub clothes; street clothes are forbidden in this area. Finally, the *sterile OR* itself, including the scrub rooms and the areas immediately adjacent to the actual operating suite, is limited to those personnel prepared to work in an aseptic or sterile environment. Personnel in the OR suites must have clean scrubs, shoe covers, a hat or a cap, and a facial mask (Figure 25-2).

Dress and Hygiene

To promote good aseptic technique, OR staff must adhere to strict personnel hygiene regimens to reduce iatrogenic contamination of the OR. Major areas of microbial burden are the head, neck, axilla, hands, groin, perineum, legs, and feet. Hair is an excellent place for bacteria to reside, and hair proteins can cause significant foreign body reactions during the healing process. Personnel must cover all head hair with a hat or a hair bonnet. Those with beards should wear a hood that covers the sides of the face and chin.

Anyone entering the intermediate zone of the suite must wear appropriately laundered scrub attire as provided by the hospital. Scrubs laundered at home should not be worn in surgery. Shoes worn in the OR are not worn outside the OR unless they are covered by "clean" shoe covers to remove the risk of trailing blood and body fluids through the hospital. Any scrub attire worn outside the OR suite should be covered with a long, buttoned laboratory coat.

Universal Precautions and Surgery

Proper OR attire also gives personnel protection from inadvertent exposure to infectious agents. Although asepsis protects the patient from iatrogenic infection, sterile clothing also insulates the health care provider from diseases transmitted by the patient. Both the Centers for Disease Control (CDC) and the Occupational Safety and Health Administration (OSHA) have established standards for the prevention of transmission of infectious diseases, including HIV, in health care settings. Universal precautions mandate that all human body fluids, blood, and tissues be considered potentially contaminated and containing viral pathogens. PA students are required to receive hepatitis B immunization several months before exposure to direct patient care.

Surgical Garments

Surgical garments are considered barriers against patient-borne diseases, as well as iatrogenic transmission of infection to patients.

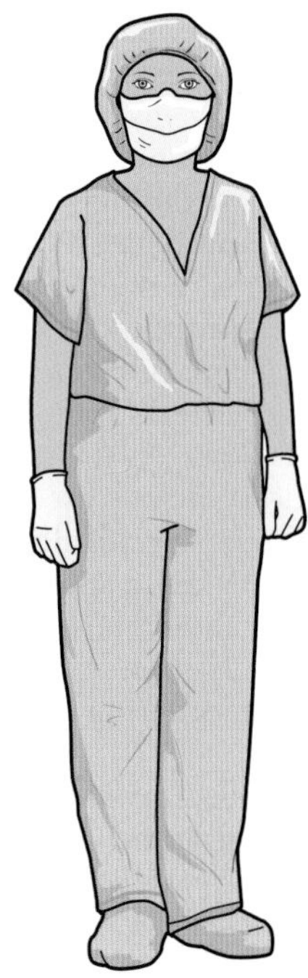

FIGURE 25-2 Typical surgical garment. Note cap, mask, and shoe covers. The shirt is tucked into the pants, and no jewelry is worn.

Masks and Goggles. Respiratory droplet infection from the oral and nasal pharynx has been identified as a major source of contamination. Therefore, an impermeable mask must be worn in the OR to cover the nose and mouth. The least effective mask is the molded, preshaped mask with an elastic string because of its poor conformance to most facial contours. Its preformed dimensions allow escape of excess droplets from the mask's sides.

To be efficacious, a surgical mask must be worn over both nose and mouth so that air passes only through the filtering system. It should be firmly molded around the nose, with the upper strings tied at the back of the head and the lower strings tied behind the neck. Crossing the strings across the back of the head distorts the compliance of the mask along the cheek, resulting in leakage of expired air. This is problematic for health care providers who wear glasses because when the expired warm air mixes with cold OR air, lenses are fogged. Some masks contain adhesive strips across the nose to prevent this problem. A strip of surgical tape may also be used to seal the top of the mask. Additionally, it may be necessary to apply a defogger to glasses before entering the OR to prevent this nuisance.

Masks also protect the wearer from patient-borne pathogens. Gerberding and colleagues[2] found that a high percentage of OR personnel were exposed to blood through facial mucocutaneous splashes and identified several variables associated with increased risk of blood exposure—loss of more than 300 mL of blood, procedure lasting longer than 3 hours, emergency procedures, major surgical procedures, procedures required for trauma or fracture, laparotomies, intraabdominal gynecologic procedures, vascular procedures, otolaryngologic procedures, and cutaneous abscess drainage.

All personnel at the operating table, including anesthesia staff, must wear goggles, glasses with specifically designed splash guards attached to the sides, or masks with splash guards attached to decrease the transmission of communicable diseases. These precautions prevent contamination from splashes on odd trajectories from the operative field. Glasses alone are not adequate to prevent splashes from the side or between the glasses and the cheek.

Some masks are designed to filter microorganisms transmissible to the wearer. These are effective for procedures during which voluminous smoke plumes containing viral agents (as small as 0.3 μm) are generated, such as laser ablation of lesions containing human papillomavirus from genital or rectal lesions. High-filtration masks should be used for these procedures.

Masks should be changed between cases and whenever saturated by moisture from respiration.

Gloves. Sterile gloves are designed to provide maximum sensitivity for the user while providing a sterile barrier to disease transmission. A discussion of the appropriate choice of glove size and type is not within the scope of this chapter. Glove allergies, caused by the talc used to lubricate the hand for entry into the glove or by the latex materials used in manufacturing, can cause severe dermatitis in a small number of wearers. For such persons, some gloves are designed to be hypoallergenic. In severe cases, a dermatologist may prescribe a topical steroid cream until the irritation subsides.

Double Gloving. Wright and associates[3] showed that 27% of the glove tears from sharp instrumentation occurred on hands that were retracting tissues during surgery. Of that group, 67% were caused by needles, 10% by scalpels, and 23% by other instruments, such as cautery tips, wire, skin staples, bone cutters, and bone chisels. An additional 15% of glove tears occurred on hands holding instruments, and a small subset occurred during hand-typing of sutures ("suture cuts"). Other mechanisms of glove tears occurred during the passing of sharp instruments between individuals at the table and contact with sharps (e.g., needles, scalpels) laid on the table during activities such as suture-tying. Bleeding occurred in more than 80% of sharps injuries in this study. A majority of glove tears occurred on the fingertips. Quebbeman and co-workers[4] demonstrated the inadequacy of single-gloving practices among surgical personnel, documenting a glove failure rate of approximately 51%, glove failure being defined as tears in the glove after surgery, or when there is blood on the hand after glove removal without known trauma or penetration of the gloved hand by a sharp instrument.

Both studies advocated the use of double gloves by OR personnel to reduce risks of blood-borne contamination. Additionally, these reports demonstrate a significant decrease in finger contamination rate, from 51% to 7%, for those who wore double gloves. Of 130 participants in the Quebbeman study,[4] 7% found that two gloves were too tight and caused numbness and 1% found them too baggy. Almost 88% were in favor of wearing two gloves, however. Finally, 82% of the participants indicated that they would wear double gloves routinely, and an additional 2% said that they would wear double gloves when operating on high-risk patients. Eighty-eight percent of these participants remarked that tactile sensation and comfort were satisfactory with double gloves.

Gowns and Shoe Covers. The surgical gown is a principal barrier against disease transmission. High-risk procedures, as previously noted, should probably mandate the addition of a sterile sleeve over the gown's arms to prevent strike-through (i.e., penetration of moisture through protection, resulting in possible microbial transmission).

The shoe cover is an overlooked place of potential disease transmission. Most personnel in surgery wear lightweight shoes with cloth or synthetic material shoe covers. Particularly during urologic and arthroscopic irrigation procedures or trauma resuscitation, large quantities of fluid may accumulate on the floor, saturating the wearer's shoes. All OR personnel should be aware of this mechanism of blood exposure and should don lightweight, knee-high disposable boots in situations with potential for exposure to this problem. These procedures may also require that personnel wear a plastic "cook's apron," which slips over the head and ties behind the back, protecting the front of the wearer from seepage through the front of the gown.

The following precautions should be taken by persons performing surgical procedures:

1. Goggles, glasses with side guards, face masks, knee-high shoe covers, waterproof aprons, and additional sleeves should be worn, depending on the type of surgery expected.

2. Double gloving reduces blood-borne contamination.
3. Extreme care should be exercised when sharps are present on the table. Instruments should be passed via an intermediary table or tray, if possible. *The assistant's immobile, retracting hand should be safeguarded while sharps are in use.*
4. During suturing, the needle should not be kept in the hand while knots are being tied. Optimally, the needle should be cut from the suture as soon as the suture is in place. If this is not possible, the point of the needle should be clamped within the needle holder and placed on the sterile field away from the hands. The needle should always be grasped with forceps immediately after it pierces the tissue and should be transferred back to the needle holder without direct touching of the needle with the gloved hand.
5. All scalpel blades should be placed onto and removed from the knife handle by a hemostat. Hypodermic needles should not be recapped.
6. Some glove tears and finger cuts result from hand-tying of sutures. The distal or proximal interphalangeal crease should not be used as a fulcrum for tying knots. The pads of the fingers should be used to tighten knots to prevent "suture cuts."
7. Gloves should always be worn when there is a risk of contracting a patient's body fluids. Even the seemingly innocuous tasks of phlebotomy, cleansing of the patient after surgery, dressing changes, and insertion of NG tubes can result in inadvertent pathogenic exposure of the health care provider.
8. All accidental mucocutaneous inoculation, needlesticks, cuts, and so forth should be reported to the surgical team and OR staff to ensure proper serologic evaluation of the patient in the postoperative period.
9. Operative personnel with open lesions, weeping dermatitis, and so forth should refrain from close contact with patients. This precaution can be a problem for operative personnel who experience "washing trauma" from frequent hand washings, which may cause cuts, abrasions, and minor lesions. Keeping the skin of the hands well moistened helps prevent such trauma.

SKIN PREPARATION

Remember: Handwashing between patient PEs eliminates the leading cause of nosocomial infection.

Appropriate attire, preparation of the hands at the scrub sink, shaving and preparing the patient's skin for incision, erecting barriers against microbial contamination, meticulous tissue handling, and an expeditious work ethic during surgery contribute to maintaining low patient morbidity and mortality. Complete elimination of all skin flora and of all microorganisms from the operative field is preferable, although an altogether aseptic operative field is not possible. However, appropriate skin preparation can reduce the numbers of microorganisms to an absolute minimum.

Resident flora is removed from the skin on and around the operative site with a combination of mechanical scrubbing with an antibacterial soap and application of an antibacterial solution after the scrub. Although some operative areas, such as the eye, ear, nose, throat, mouth, and perineal and perianal regions, cannot be adequately sterilized, aseptic techniques are used to prevent further contamination of the surrounding field.

The operative area is shaved to remove only the hair that may interfere with the incision and surrounding region. Wet shaving with a safety razor is preferred to dry shaving, which can cause razor drag, leaving abrasions, tiny lacerations, and greater postoperative discomfort.

Agents Commonly Used for Operative Site Skin Preparation and Surgical Hand Washing

Povidone-iodine or iodophor products are supplied in two distinct liquid versions. For the operative site preparation, a detergent *scrub* is first applied with sponges to mechanically remove gross dirt and oils from the skin. After the skin has been blotted with a sterile towel, a nondetergent *solution* is "painted" onto the area. This thin film of povidone-iodine continues to have bactericidal action for up to 8 hours after application. The solution's brown color also effectively outlines the borders of the surgical scrub, allowing accurate placement of the towels and drapes before incision. Patients and OR staff who have a history of sensitivity or allergic reaction to iodine should refrain from the use of either of these preparations for surgical scrubs.

Chlorhexidine gluconate, when used in a 4% concentration, is bactericidal and has persistent antimicrobial activity after application. Repeated scrubbing throughout the day enhances its activity. Because this agent is nonirritating for a majority of the patient population, it is commonly used for hand washing and preparation of the operative site. Chlorhexidine gluconate scrub soap adequately prepares the skin, and no solution is required after the scrub.

Parachlorometaxylenol (PCMX) is a useful skin preparation agent, particularly for those allergic to iodine-containing preparations. This agent is often combined with an emollient to reduce skin drying.

Hexachlorophene, although used infrequently, is an effective skin preparation solution for those patients and staff allergic to povidone-iodine and chlorhexidine gluconate. It accumulates on the skin after several days of use, causing an overall decrease in skin flora.

CLINICAL PROCEDURE

During skin preparation of the operative site, personnel must make sure that the solution does not pool beneath the patient. Such a pool might serve as an electrical ground to the table during the use of electrocautery or, if unnoticed during postoperative skin cleansing, may lead to chemical skin burns. In addition, the PA should always check the safety profile for use of these agents in sensitive areas such as the eye, ear, vagina, and rectum.

SURGICAL HAND SCRUB

Agents commonly used for hand scrubbing often come in sterile prepackaged brush and sponge units. Alternatively, brushes are packaged separately, and the scrub soap is kept at the scrub sink in containers with foot-operated dispensing controls.

CLINICAL PROCEDURE

Povidone-iodine solutions tend to be drying, and multiple scrubs throughout the day can produce drying and cracking of the cuticles and hands. Personnel who frequently scrub for surgery should take care to apply emollients and non–oil-based lotions to their hands several times during the day, if possible, to prevent the occurrence of these potential conduits for bacteria. Chlorhexidine gluconate, PCMX, and hexachlorophene are often combined with emollient lathering agents and may be less drying than the povidone-iodine solutions for those who scrub frequently.

GENERAL PREPARATIONS

The PA should inform the scrub nurse before scrubbing, so a gown and appropriate gloves will be ready. The skin should be kept clean and in good condition. *Anyone with open wounds or weeping dermatitis evident on the hands or arms should not scrub for surgery.* Fingernails should not reach beyond the fingertips, to reduce trauma to the patient and inadvertent glove punctures. All hand and wrist jewelry should be removed. A cap and mask should be in place, glasses or goggles should be adjusted, and all neck jewelry should be covered or removed before scrubbing. Shoe covers should be worn at all times within the OR, and the ties from surgical scrubs and shoelaces should be tucked inside the waistband or shoe cover.

Five-Minute Scrub

1. A scrub brush impregnated with the choice of antiseptic agent is chosen. The package is opened and saturated with solution from the foot-controlled dispenser.
2. The water temperature is adjusted to a comfortable level.
3. The hands are passed beneath the running water with one or two motions, allowing the water to flow from fingertips to elbow and wetting to 3 inches above the elbow. The hands are kept above the waist.
4. The soap solution is used to wash the hands and arms and to remove the gross dirt and dead skin.
5. The hands and brush are rinsed.
6. The brush is again saturated with soap.
7. Under running water, the fingernails of one hand are cleaned with a sterile pick to remove subungual debris (the brush is kept in the hand holding the nail pick) and rinsed.
8. The process is repeated for the other hand.
9. The time should be noted. The fingers are scrubbed with a circular motion for one minute, including the nails, knuckles, and web spaces. The fingers and hand are regarded as having four sides for the purpose of the scrub.
10. Circular scrubbing is continued for 1 minute on the arm, roughly dividing it into thirds and scrubbing to 3 inches above the elbow (Figure 25-3).
11. The brush is transferred to the scrubbed hand, and the process is repeated on the unscrubbed arm and hand.
12. When 5 minutes have elapsed, the brush is discarded and the hands and arms are rinsed of lather by passing them through the water stream, allowing the water to cascade from fingertips to elbow—never in the reverse direction. One or two passes should be sufficient to remove the lather.
13. The water is turned off with the knee.
14. The arms are held above the waist so that any residual water drips from the fingers to the elbows.

All subsequent scrubs of the day should last 5 minutes.

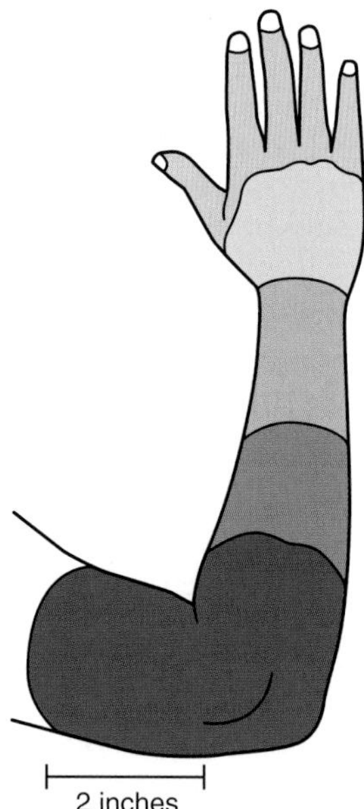

FIGURE 25-3 ■ Divide your hands and arms into sections for the surgical scrub.

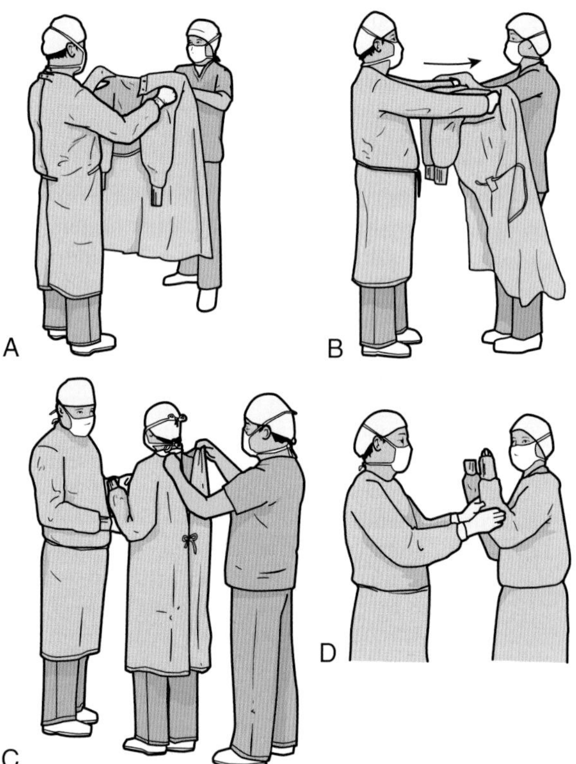

FIGURE 25-4 ■ Being gowned. Place your outstretched arms into the armholes **(A)**. The circulator will pull the gown onto your shoulders **(B)** and fasten the ties **(C)**. The scrub nurse will adjust the sleeves before gloving **(D)**.

GOWNING AND GLOVING

Drying Hands and Arms

Hands and arms must be dried thoroughly before gowning and gloving. The towel is passed from the sterile table by the scrub nurse, or it is taken from the sterile instrument table, with care taken not to drip any water onto the table. The towel is opened to its fullest length and is kept well away from the scrub clothes. Only one end of the towel is used to dry the first hand and arm. A blotting and twisting motion is used as the fingers and arms are rotated. Each finger is dried individually; then the process is completed, working from wrist to elbow. Once the first arm has been dried, *the opposite end of the same side of the towel is used to dry the other hand and arm in a similar manner*. The towel is then discarded by being given to a waiting circulating nurse or dropped into a soiled cloth receptacle.

Donning Gown and Gloves

Donning the sterile gown depends on the method used to place gloves on the hands. When the gloves are donned without assistance (closed-glove technique), the hands and fingers are kept within the gown sleeve. Partial finger extrusion is needed when someone else (i.e., the scrub nurse) applies the gloves (Figure 25-4).

For the *closed-glove method*, the gown is carefully removed from the sterile field (without dripping water onto the field) and is gently shaken, well above the floor, to loosen the folds and fully extend the gown. The hands are placed into the armholes, and the circulating nurse, who is unsterile, pulls the gown onto the wearer's shoulders and fastens the gown from behind. The hands are not placed through the wrist cuffs but remain within the sleeve of the gown itself. The gown's cuffs may be used like mittens to manipulate the fingers and hands into the first glove, without touching the glove with the bare hand (Figure 25-5).

The *open-glove method* requires assistance from a sterile team member. The gown may be donned as previously described or may be placed by the scrub nurse. The arms are extended at a 90-degree angle in front of the body, and the gown is placed over the shoulders by the scrub nurse. The fingers are partially extruded through the wrist cuffs so that the cuff end rests just below the thumb.

The right glove is placed first. The fingers are slightly abducted, and the hand is gently inserted into the glove as the scrub nurse circumferentially expands the wrist cuff. The scrub nurse then expands the left glove's wrist cuff. With the right hand, the wearer

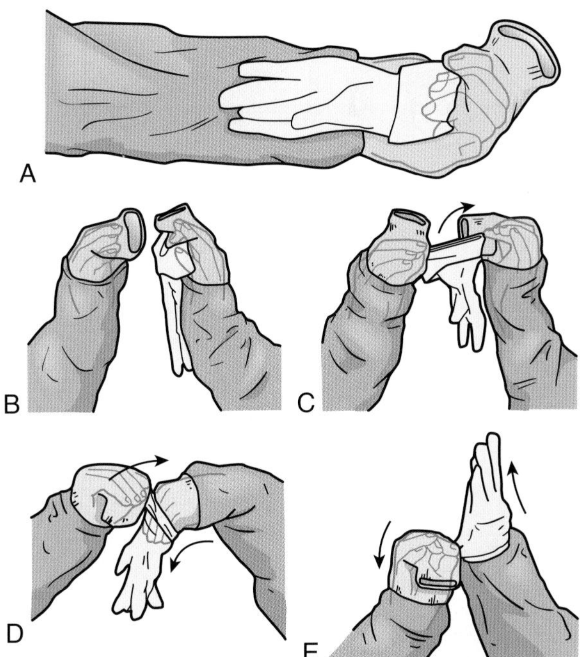

FIGURE 25-5 Gloving yourself. **A,** Keep the fingers within the gown's cuff, and use the cuff as a mitten to manipulate the fingers into the glove. **B,** Place the glove's thumb-side down onto your hand and wrist, with the fingers pointing toward your elbow. **C** and **D,** After grasping the edge of the cuff between your thumb and index finger, flip the glove over while using your other hand to pull the glove onto your hand. **E,** Adjust the gown cuff for comfort. Repeat for the other hand.

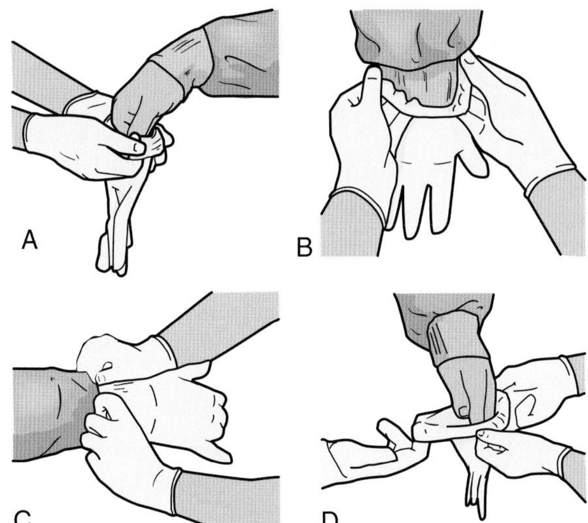

FIGURE 25-6 Being gloved by another. Insert your right hand into the opened glove held by the scrub nurse (**A** and **B**), pushing deeply into the glove to seat your fingertips (**C**). Grasp the left cuff's edge with your right hand and insert fingers (**D**). Adjust cuffs for comfort.

gently pulls the edge of the cuff toward the body and places the left hand into the glove (Figure 25-6).

Even appropriately sized gloves can cause distal hand paresthesias if the gown's cuff is bunched over the median nerve at the volar wrist. The midarm section of the gown is held stationary with the opposite hand during the open-glove method, and the cuff is adjusted after the closed-glove method.

Occasionally, a glove becomes contaminated or sustains a puncture or tear during surgery and must be changed. If this occurs, step back from the sterile field and extend the wrist of the contaminated hand up to the circulating nurse, who will pull the glove from the contaminated hand. The scrub nurse assists with a new glove placement by the open-glove method. Care must be taken to keep the exposed hand away from any portion of the sterile field.

All surgical gowns have a wraparound tie at the waist that prevents the back of the gown from becoming unfastened. On disposable gowns, the paper "handle" is carefully handed to the circulating nurse while the person donning the gown turns in a circle or pirouette. The tie is gently pulled from the paper handle, with no touching of the contaminated handle, and is secured to the front tie of the gown. For nondisposable gowns, the wraparound tie must be given to a sterile person. Alternatively, the tie may be wrapped in an empty sterile glove wrapper, which is handed to a nonsterile person as the turn is made. If the tie is dropped, an unsterile team member may fasten the back of the gown with a hemostat or other instrument. The wearer must remember not to discard the instrument into the trash or soiled cloth receptacle at the end of the procedure.

Removing Gown and Gloves

The gown is always removed before the gloves by pulling it forward across the shoulders and down onto the arms after the rear ties have been released. The gloved hands are then removed from the gown cuffs. The gown is rolled into a ball, with all contaminated surfaces kept in the interior of the ball, and is discarded into the appropriate receptacle. The gloves are removed by grasping the outside of one glove near the wrist with the other hand and turning the glove inside out as it is removed. This glove is held in the palm of the remaining gloved hand. The ungloved hand then reaches inside the cuff of the remaining glove and pulls it from the hand, inside out, encompassing the glove previously removed. The gloves are discarded into the appropriate receptacle. This method internalizes all fluid-contaminated portions

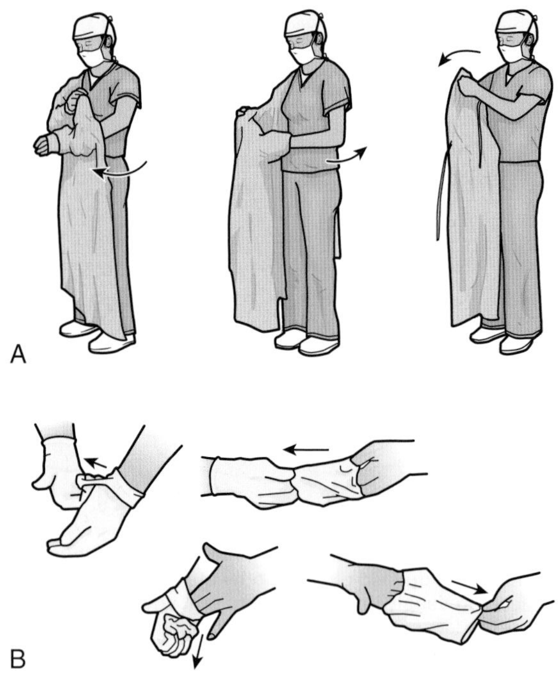

FIGURE 25-7 Removing gown and gloves. **A,** With gloves on, and after the front and back ties are loosened, pull the gown from your shoulders, rolling the soiled exterior into a ball. **B,** Grasp the outside of the first glove's cuff and pull from your hand. Hold the removed glove in the remaining glove. Grasp the inside of the remaining glove, removing it inside out while enveloping the previously removed glove.

of the gown and gloves and prevents accidental contamination of the skin (Figure 25-7).

MAINTAINING A STERILE FIELD

The area immediately surrounding the operative site, the sterile instrument tables, and any open sterile instrument packs is designated as the "sterile field" (Figure 25-8). There are no intermediates between sterile areas in the operating suite and the unsterile areas.

All personnel in the operating suite are responsible for the maintenance of the sterile environment. The cardinal rule is to replace any item *suspected* of contamination, even if contamination was not directly observed.

In most institutions, students are encouraged to approach the sterile field to observe the conduct of surgery. The student should do the following:

1. Use a short step platform to see over the operating staff's shoulders.
2. Ask anesthesia personnel for a position near the head of the table to observe over the drapes.

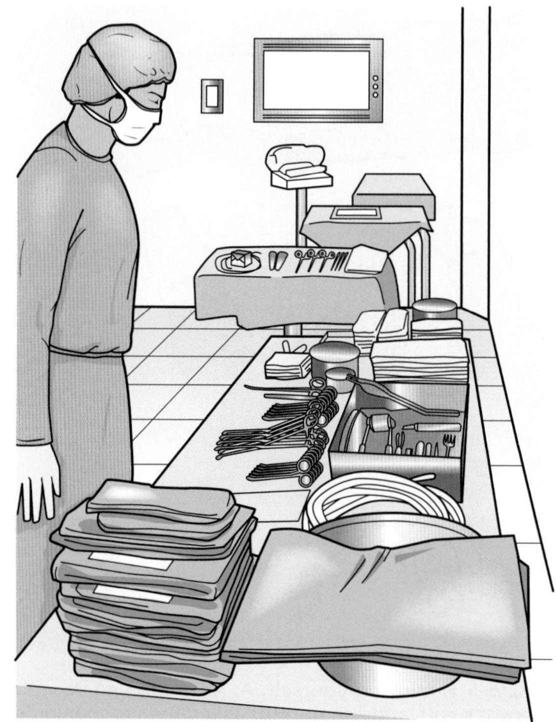

FIGURE 25-8 A typical sterile field. See text for explanation.

CLINICAL PROCEDURE

Although it seems redundant to say that only sterile items are used within sterile fields, this axiom is of paramount importance. Use the following "rules" for maintaining the sterile field in the OR:

- Only the front of the gown is considered sterile in the areas from the axilla to the waist and from the fingertips to approximately 3 inches above the sleeves.
- Hands should be kept in front, in sight, and above waist level at all times. They should never touch the face or be folded beneath the axilla.
- If some portion of the arm or elbow becomes contaminated, a sterile "sleeve" can be placed by the scrub nurse or CST to cover that area and eliminate the need for a complete gown change.

Nonsterile persons reaching across a sterile field contaminate the entire area. A wide margin of safety should be maintained by those working around a sterile area. Nonsterile persons should always pass behind those who are scrubbed and in sterile attire for surgery.

All those involved in draping the patient should stand an arm's length from the OR table to prevent gown contamination. Sterile persons should pass each other back to back so that their unsterile areas are facing each other. A sterile person should face a sterile area to pass it. In addition, sterile persons should stay within the sterile field and should not walk around the OR suite or go outside the room unless absolutely necessary. Those considered sterile should keep contact with the sterile area to a minimum by not leaning on the instrument tables or the draped patient. Sitting or leaning on a nonsterile surface is considered a break in technique unless the operating team must be seated to perform a specific procedure.

Tables are sterile only at tabletop level; any part of the sterile drape that falls over the edge is considered contaminated. The table height should be appropriately adjusted to maintain a maximally sterile field. Any items that drop below waist level are considered contaminated and should be discarded from the field.

Disease transmission may occur as a result of strike-through, or penetration of moisture in whatever form, through the protection of gown or drapes. This can occur when sterile packages are laid onto wet areas or when the drying cycle of heat sterilizers does not completely dry the enveloping package wrapping. It may also result when blood or other fluids penetrate the gown of the assistant or surgeon. Choosing gowns with waterproof front panels, wearing oversleeves, and using waterproof coverings on instrument tables can prevent iatrogenic transmission of infectious agents via strike-through.

CLINICAL PROCEDURE

Drape placement usually requires monitoring by the circulating nurse and/or anesthesia staff, who ensure adherence to sterile technique. The following guidelines should be used:

- Drapes should be held high enough above the table to prevent contamination from the unsterile area of the table and the patient.
- Walk around the table to complete the draping procedure when necessary, and never reach across the table.
- When a drape is placed near a nonsterile area or is handed to the anesthesia team to create the sterile barrier between them and the operating team, the drape should form a cuff over the gloved hand of the sterile person, who offers it to the unsterile area in that manner. This technique prevents drape contamination as the anesthesiologist or other nonsterile person pulls a portion of the drape into position.
- Sterile personnel should touch no part of the draping material that falls into a nonsterile area. If a portion of the draping material becomes contaminated and needs replacement, the circulating nurse will grab its edge and slowly pull it off the table. It then can be replaced with a new drape.

Handling Tubes and Lines

After the patient has been draped, the tubes, wires, and cords required for the procedure will be passed from the sterile field to a waiting non-sterile person. These may include electrocautery pencil wires, suction tubing of various sorts, cardiopulmonary bypass tubing, cell-saving equipment, laparoscopy cords, and ultrasound transducers. They are usually contained on the scrub nurse's back table until needed. The ends are handed to the circulating nurse or anesthesia staff.

CLINICAL PROCEDURE

The equipment tubes are tightly clipped to a fold of drape with a nonpenetrating towel clip or Allis clamp, to prevent the weight of the tubing from pulling them off the sterile field. A fold of the drape is gathered to encompass the tube and wire and is tightly clamped shut with the Allis clamp or towel clip.

PATIENT POSITIONING

Patients receiving anesthesia, whether general or regional, are at great risk for injury caused by improper physical movement or improper placement on the OR table. Abnormal pressure on nerves for extended periods may result in palsy or irreversible paralysis of muscle innervation or sensory distribution of that nerve. Stretching the brachial plexus by abducting the arms more than 90 degrees during a breast or chest procedure can result in hand dysfunction, as can pressure on the ulnar nerve by the hard table surface (Figure 25-9). Pressure on the proximal calf and the peroneal nerve in the lithotomy position can cause footdrop or venous stasis in the calf deep veins, with subsequent deep vein thrombosis and pulmonary embolus.

The surgeon and/or assistant guides the positioning with the anesthesia team. Other members of the operative team assist the process. Proper patient positioning facilitates access to the operative site and provides maximum patient safety. The chosen position is decided by the patient's age, height, weight, cardiopulmonary status, and preexisting diseases, such as rheumatic disorders. For example, the extremely

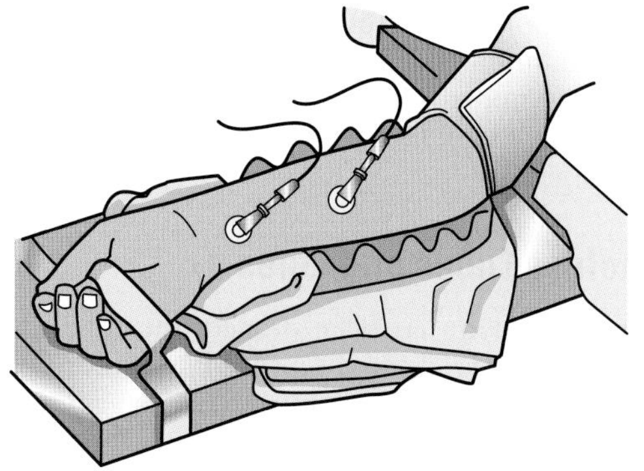

FIGURE 25-9 Safety padding for the patient's wrist and elbow to prevent nerve or vessel injury. Note the proper anatomic alignment of the wrist.

obese patient is positioned with a slightly elevated head and thorax to facilitate mechanical ventilation during surgery.

Most OR tables are manually or electrically controlled through hydraulic lifts and gears that allow a table to be manipulated into various positions, including lateral inclines and Trendelenburg or reverse Trendelenburg tilts. The head and feet can be independently controlled or removed from the main table, and a middle portion of the table (the "kidney rest") allows elevation of the central portion of the body. Parallel side rails allow the attachment of retractor devices and arm supports. The PA should become familiar with all these functions and should be able to manipulate a table into all of its positions. Additionally, the PA should understand how to remove the various table segments as required to position the patient for surgery and should be competent in attaching devices such as retraction systems and arm boards to the table.

Common Patient Positions (Figure 25-10)

Supine. The patient is placed flat on the back with arms either outstretched at less than 90 degrees or placed at the sides. This position is used for access to any anterior body part, particularly the chest, abdomen, pelvis, and extremities.

Prone. The patient is placed face down. If general anesthesia with endotracheal intubation is planned, the patient is first placed in the supine position. Anesthesia is induced, the endotracheal tube is placed, and the patient is turned over. This position is useful for access to the posterior portions of the body.

Jackknife. The torso and legs are lowered slightly after the patient is placed in the prone position. This position is useful for lower spine and rectal procedures.

Lithotomy. The legs are positioned slightly flexed above the table and are supported in slings or stirrups with the patient lying supine. The table portion beneath the legs is then removed from the upper table or is lowered to hang perpendicularly. The patient's buttocks can then be positioned at the edge of the table, allowing access to the genitals, perineum, and anorectal anatomy. This position is used primarily for obstetric, gynecologic, urologic, and anorectal operations.

CLINICAL PROCEDURE

Several important considerations for proper patient positioning are given here. The PA should assist the anesthesia team and the circulating nurse in safely positioning the patient on the table and during the induction of anesthesia. All staff should keep in mind that inadvertent injury may occur beneath the drapes as a result of poor positioning and may remain unnoticed until the end of the operation. Such an injury may not respond to therapeutic treatment and may result in permanent paralysis or dysfunction.

- Wheels on both the table and the transport stretcher should be locked before transfer of the patient to or from the OR table.
- Anatomic alignment of the patient on the OR table should be maintained as close to normal as possible. This prevents overstretching of, or pressure on, nerves and blood vessels. Proper anatomic alignment can be facilitated by inserting pillows between the legs of a patient in the lateral position or behind the knees of a patient in the supine position.
- Pad all bony prominences to prevent nerve or vessel injury. The thorax of a prone patient should be supported with foam pillows to facilitate chest wall excursion and adequate ventilation.
- Never cross the patient's legs in the supine position.
- Give careful consideration to the patient's joints during transfer or positioning so that they are not moved past their normal range of motion. This is especially important for positioning the legs and hips in the lithotomy position. Older patients with osteoarthritis or rheumatologic diseases require careful padding and positioning to avoid iatrogenic injury.
- All fixed appliances or instrumentation that come into contact with the patient's skin must

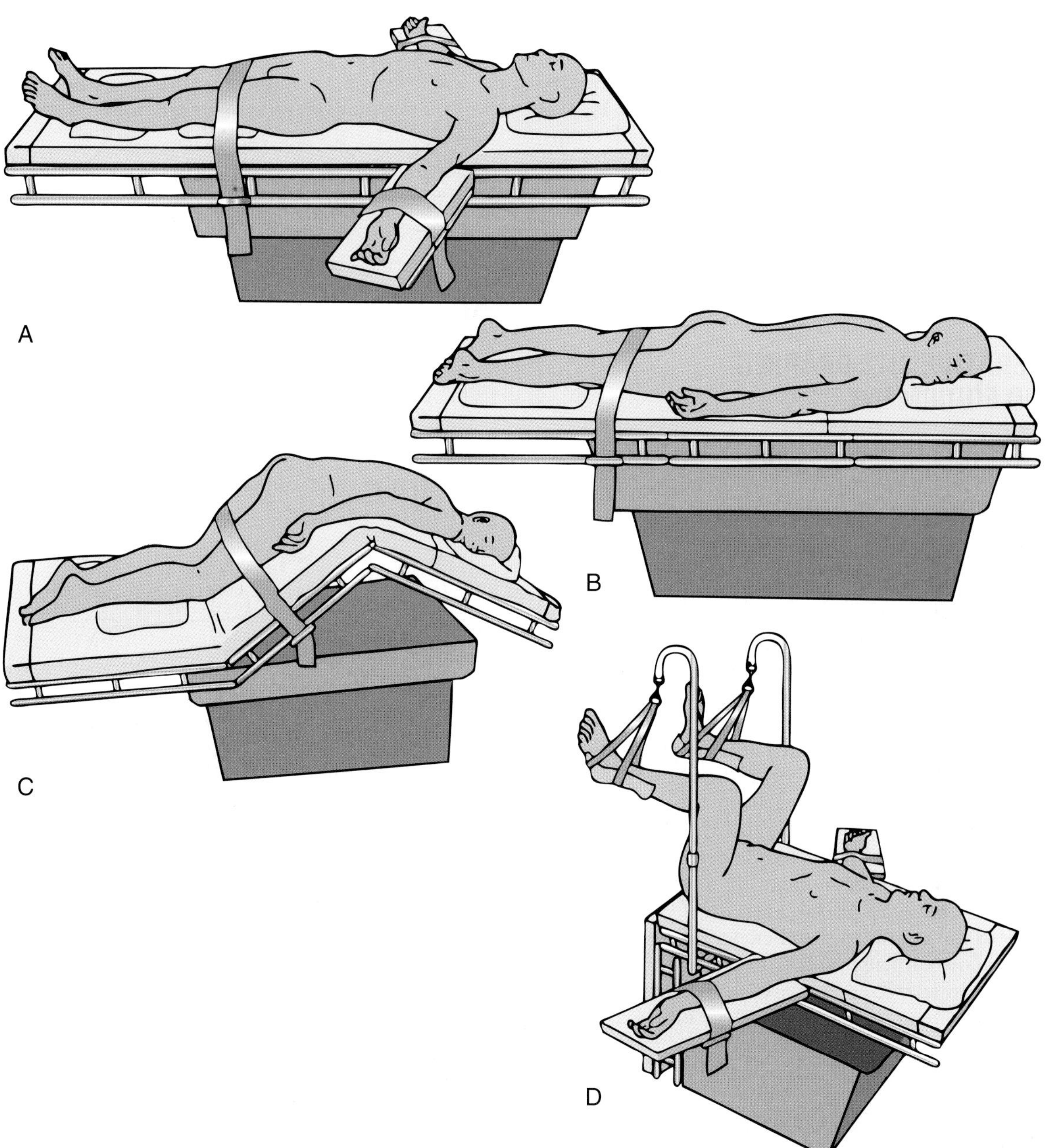

FIGURE 25-10 ■ **A,** Supine position. Patient is placed on back with arms at sides or extended to 90 degrees and head in alignment with body. Legs are uncrossed, with a safety strap placed above knees. **B,** Prone position. Patient is usually anesthetized while supine and then turned. Arms are placed at sides, with rolls beneath axilla to facilitate respiration. **C,** Jackknife position. Patient is usually anesthetized while supine and then turned. Knees are flexed slightly to reduce lumbosacral stress. **D,** Lithotomy position. Patient is on back, and foot section of operating table is removed or lowered to 90-degree angle. Buttocks are moved to table's edge. Feet are suspended in straps to flex knees. Legs are placed into or removed from the stirrups simultaneously to avoid hip injuries.

be adequately padded (e.g., leg slings or stirrups for lithotomy, sleighs or sheets to keep arms tucked at the patient's side, foam pads on wrists or elbows on arm boards, foam heel pads).

- Every patient is secured to the table with straps or tape to prevent accidents. Patients under the influence of sedative, narcotic, and anesthetic agents are prone to confusion and agitation, especially when awakening from general anesthesia, and often attempt to sit up or get off the table before they are fully awake and competent.

OPERATIVE SITE DRAPING AND EQUIPMENT

One of the most important steps in preparing the operative site is appropriate draping of the patient to create a sterile area around the incision. Several layers of materials are used for this purpose, and each surgical specialty has special draping procedures and drape material specifically designed for each procedure.

After aseptic preparation of the skin by application of the appropriate agent, as was previously discussed, the operative site should be rectangularly draped with folded cotton towels held in place with towel clips. Because these towel clips pass through the towels into a nonsterile area, they are always considered contaminated after placement. If the clips need to be removed, they are discarded from the sterile field, and the area where they penetrated the drapes should be overlaid with additional sterile draping material.

A large sterile sheet containing a fenestration, or central opening, is placed over the field, allowing access to the operative site. Fenestration size is chosen to allow sufficient access to the area of incision and to allow a large enough area for use of the appropriate equipment (e.g., retractors) for limb manipulation and so forth.

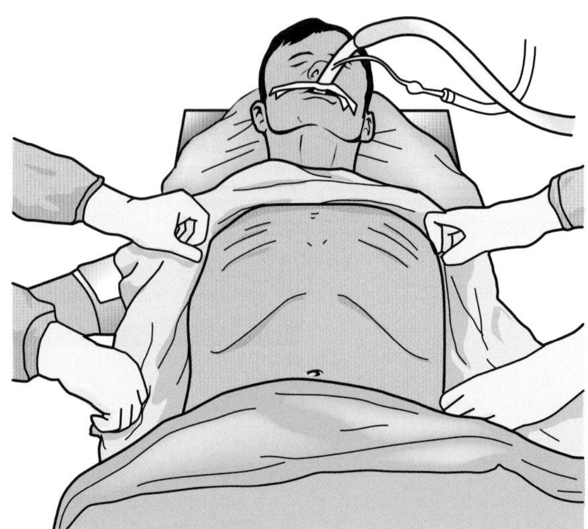

FIGURE 25-11 Widely draping the abdomen for incision.

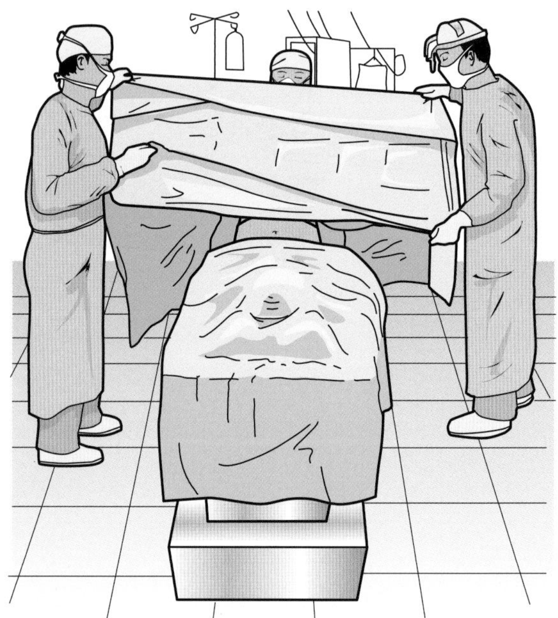

FIGURE 25-12 Placing the drapes between the anesthesia area and the surgical team.

CLINICAL PROCEDURE

Personnel should always drape with cotton towels an area wider and longer than the planned incision. Incisions may need to be lengthened during the course of the procedure (Figure 25-11). After placement of the towels, nonwoven fabric or disposable paper drapes are used to completely isolate the remainder of the exposed patient from the incision site. These drapes are called quarter-, half-, or three-quarter sheets according to their size. They are placed over the patient's feet, torso, limbs, and head as required for each procedure (Figure 25-12). Occasionally, a limb will be draped in a sterile plastic tunnel with one closed end if that limb requires manipulation by the surgeon or assistant.

SURGICAL ASSISTING AND INSTRUMENTATION

The principal means of preparing to assist at an operation is to study the proposed operation before the procedure. All assistants should be prepared to answer questions

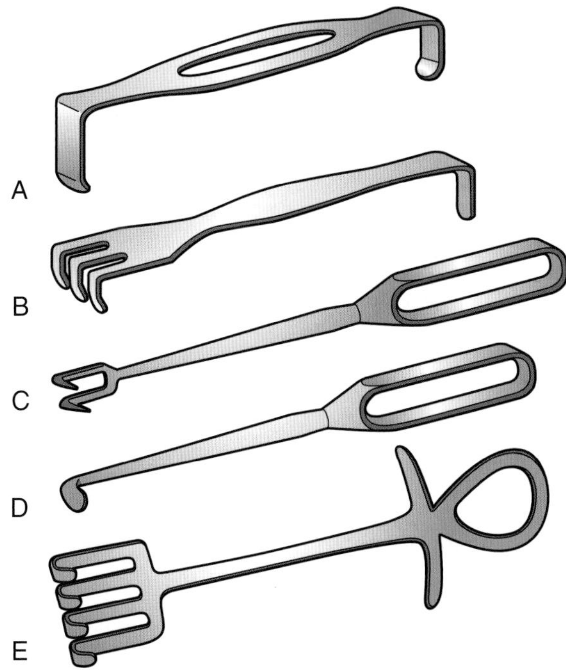

FIGURE 25-13 Handheld retractors. **A,** Army-Navy retractor. **B,** Senn retractor. **C,** Skin hook. **D,** Vein retractor. **E,** Rake.

regarding the current indications for the planned procedure, its attendant complications and expected results, and possible alternative procedures. Review of the pertinent regional anatomy and the steps of the operation is required so that a minimum of instruction is required from the surgeon during the operation, excluding those instructions needed to direct the assistant's hands or for discussion of intraoperative decisions.

Surgical assistants must be intimately familiar with the instrumentation used to extend the functions of their hands. After mastering the use of basic surgical equipment and instrumentation, the surgical PA can progress to understanding the nuances of the surgical procedure itself. Many eponyms are used to describe similar instruments; therefore, descriptive names are used here to avoid confusion.

Retraction Devices

Many kinds of retractors are used to provide exposure. Some are manually controlled extensions of the assistant's hands, as in the Senn, Army-Navy, Richardson, Deaver, and Harrington retractors. Others are self-retaining locking devices, such as the Weitlaner, Balfour, Bookwalter, and Iron Intern retractors. Only a handful are used with any frequency, despite the many types available for each surgical specialty.

Handheld Retractors

Army-Navy and Senn Retractors Of the smaller retractors, the Army-Navy and Senn are used to retract small amounts of superficial tissue. The Army-Navy retractor (Figure 25-13A) has two flat blades of different lengths. The Senn retractor (Figure 25-13B) has a rake on one end and a flat blade on the other.

Richardson Retractor. The Richardson retractor (Figure 25-14A) is manufactured with blade widths from small to large and often has two different blade widths on opposite ends for quick size changes. It is used primarily for retracting tissues within cavities (abdomen and pelvis) and for deep incisions.

Deaver and Harrington Retractors. The Deaver retractor (Figure 25-14B) is a curved instrument with a narrow to wide, flat blade. It is used for viscera and abdominal wall retraction. The Harrington or "sweetheart" retractor (Figure 25-14C), so named because of its characteristic heart-shaped shovel, provides deep retraction within a cavity without disturbance of more superficial structures. This instrument is also used for delicate organs such as the lobes of the liver.

Ribbon or Malleable Retractor. Another commonly used retractor is the ribbon or malleable retractor (Figure 25-14D). It has a flat blade and can easily be formed into different useful shapes where preformed retractors prove inadequate. The ribbon retractor is also used to keep the viscera within the confines of the abdomen during closure of an abdominal incision.

CLINICAL PROCEDURE

A retractor used on delicate tissues or that will be held in one place for an extended period should be padded with a wet saline gauze pad to prevent tissue desiccation or trauma. Because students frequently find themselves attached to a retractor, learning some simple tips can aid the process.

- Flat-bladed instruments without rounded handles should be padded with a sponge pad to ease the holder's hand pain.
- Retraction can be a tedious affair, resulting in fatigue and fidgeting. The student should use retraction time to observe how the surgeons work as a team and how tissues are handled. The best method of becoming a good first-assistant is to observe and copy accomplished assistants.
- The retractor holder must be especially aware of the tissues against which he or she is pulling. Care should be taken with delicate tissues, such as the liver, nerves, lungs, or blood vessels, which

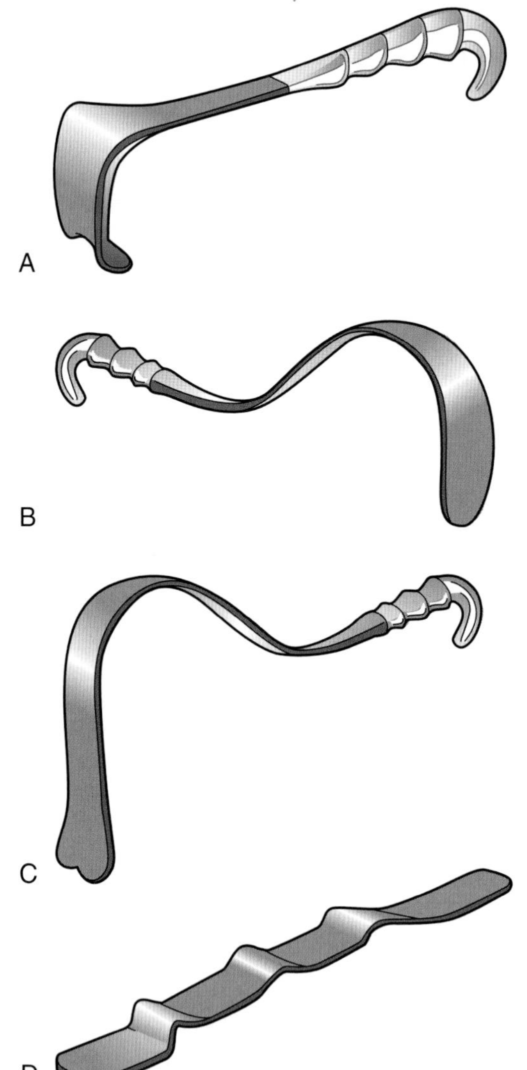

FIGURE 25-14 Handheld retractors. The blades of these retractors should be padded with moistened gauze pads to prevent injury to the viscera. **A,** Richardson. **B,** Deaver. **C,** Harrington. **D,** Ribbon or malleable.

could be permanently damaged by overaggressive retraction. Usually, the surgeon positions the retractor and adjusts the amount of tension required from the assistant to facilitate tissue exposure. The student should constantly monitor the retraction instrument and strive to maintain the appropriate amount of exposure required. If asked to reapproximate the retractor, ask for specific instructions. Some instructions may entail "towing in," which means to lift up on the handle of the retractor while pulling downward with the tip of the retractor, or "towing out," which means precisely the opposite actions.

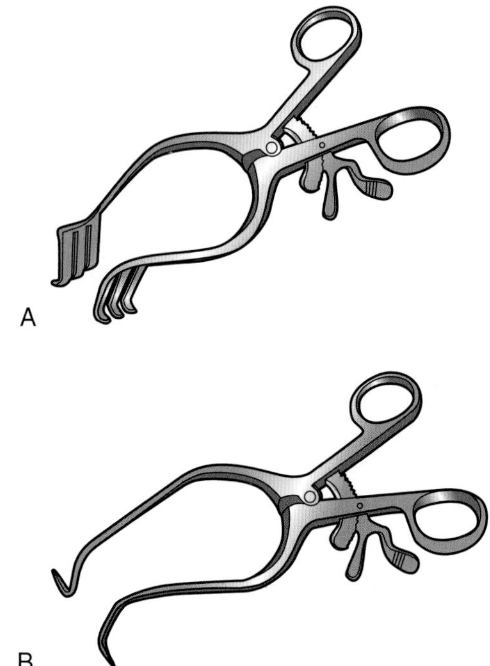

FIGURE 25-15 Self-retaining retractors. **A,** Weitlaner. **B,** Gelpi.

Self-Retaining Retractors. Self-retaining retractors have locking mechanisms that keep the blades apart and in place while spreading the edges of the incision and holding other tissue in place, thus freeing the surgeon's and assistant's hands for other tasks.

Weitlaner and Gelpi Retractors. Two of the most commonly used self-retaining retractors are the Weitlaner and Gelpi retractors (Figure 25-15). These are used to retract skin edges for superficial procedures. Care must be taken not to puncture vital tissues or oneself with the sharp points of these retractors.

Balfour and Bookwalter Retractors. The Balfour and the Bookwalter are self-retaining abdominal wall retractors with various deep and shallow blades that can be attached and removed as needed. The Balfour retractor is placed within the incision, spread apart as needed, and locked in place by tightening of a wing nut (Figure 25-16). The Bookwalter retractor has a single post that attaches to the table's side rail. This attachment takes some practice to master. A crossbar mounted on the post holds an oval or round ring to which various sizes of Richardson, malleable, and Deaver-like blades may be attached with adjustable, ratcheted "clips."

Goligher Retractor and Iron Intern. The Goligher retractor (Figure 25-17A) is used for abdominal operations in the superior regions of the peritoneal

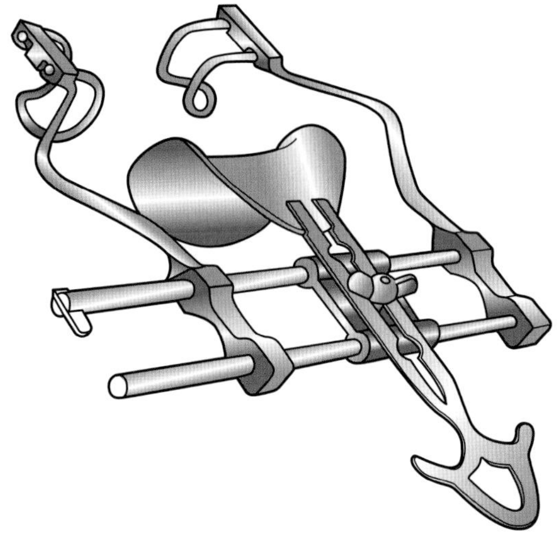

FIGURE 25-16 ■ The Balfour self-retaining retractor uses deep and shallow blades to separate the abdominal incision. The perpendicularly placed bladder blade can keep the bladder out of the operative field. Place a hand between the viscera and the abdominal wall to prevent inadvertent trapping of viscera while opening this retractor.

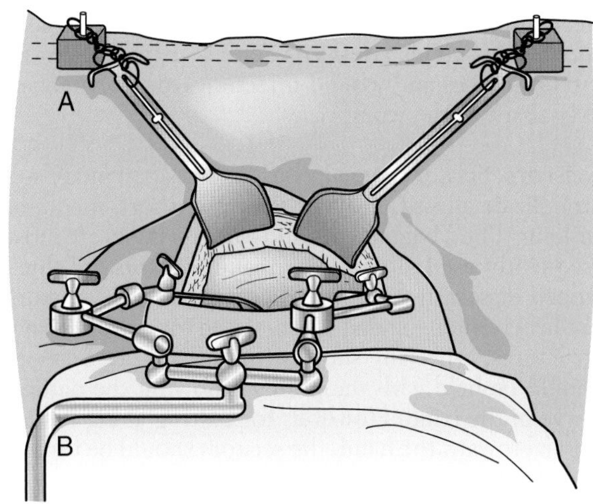

FIGURE 25-17 ■ **A,** The Goligher retractor (shown elevating the upper abdomen) is attached to a bar crossing the head of the table. It is useful for liver, biliary, stomach, diaphragm, and lower esophageal surgeries. **B,** The Iron Intern (shown retracting the lower abdomen) has multiple arms and can be adjusted to hold a variety of differently shaped retractor blades.

cavity, particularly for gallbladder, liver, and stomach procedures. It is easily attached to a crossbar placed onto the head of the OR table. The Iron Intern (Figure 25-17B) uses a series of locking arms and joints to position retractors within the abdomen or pelvis.

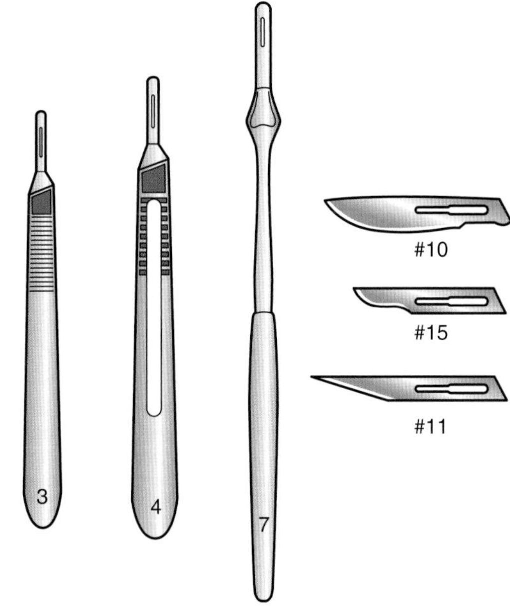

FIGURE 25-18 ■ Scalpels and scalpel blades. Note the shapes of the No. 10, No. 11, and No. 15 blades. They are frequently used with the No. 3 or medium handle. A No. 7 or small handle can be used for precise blade control. The No. 4 handle, slightly larger than the No. 3, may be used by individuals with large hands or for indelicate incisions.

Learning to Use Retractors. It should be noted that each specialty has its own specifically designed retraction devices that must be mastered as the student rotates to each surgical service. The student should not experiment with these instruments directly before or during the surgical procedure because of the risk of accidental instrument contamination; however, when the patient has been successfully delivered to the recovery area and the instruments have been transferred to the instrument washing room, there is an excellent opportunity for hands-on experience and for learning how to use these devices.

Cutting Instruments

Scalpels. The single most common cutting instrument in the OR is the scalpel (occasionally called a knife). The four most-used scalpel blades are the No. 10, No. 11, No. 15, and No. 20. A medium No. 3 scalpel handle is used with all blades except the No. 20 blade, which requires a larger (No. 4) handle. The No. 10 and No. 20 blades are general-purpose blades used to create most large incisions. For safe practice, the scalpel should be engaged and removed from the handle with a ratcheted, locking hemostat to prevent injury (Figures 25-18 and 25-19).

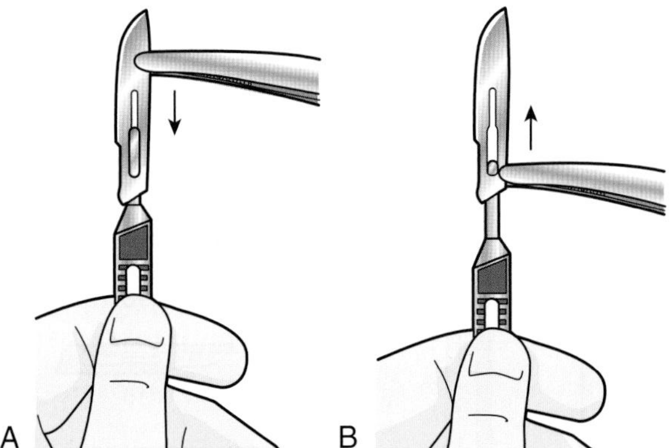

FIGURE 25-19 ■ **A,** The scalpel blade is placed by use of a hemostat. The key-shaped groove is inserted into the side grooves of the handle and slowly snapped into place. **B,** The heel of the blade is lifted with a hemostat and is slid away from the assistant to remove it.

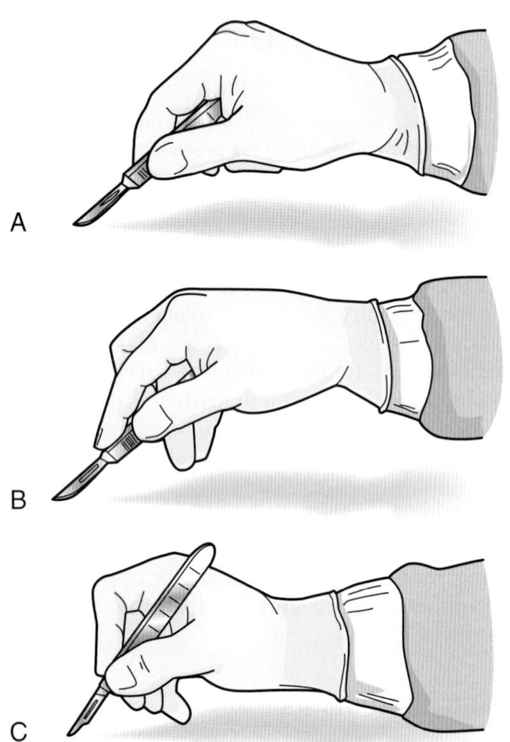

FIGURE 25-20 ■ **A,** The balance grip. The scalpel is allowed to pivot against the middle finger while the lateral movements are controlled with a gentle pinch between the index finger and the thumb. The end of the handle rests within the palm. Only a slight downward pressure is needed to cut through the dermis. **B,** The index finger can be placed on top of the knife handle to further control unwanted lateral blade movement. **C,** Holding the scalpel in the pencil or precision grip exercises maximum control on the blade's movement. The hand is usually rested on the tissue for further stability. This grip should be used only for short incisions.

For large incisions, the scalpel is held in the palm of the hand so that the belly of the blade is used to make the incision (Figure 25-20A and B). Scalpels require minimal downward pressure from the operator to incise the skin. The skin should be held firmly under retraction with the other hand to provide a smooth surface upon which to cut. The entire arm of the operator is moved from the shoulder as the scalpel is held perpendicular to the skin and pulled toward the operator.

Finer, more intricate incisions are created with the No. 15 blade with the scalpel handle held like a pencil. This allows maximum accuracy, especially when incisions other than straight lines are made. Placing the middle, fourth, and fifth fingers of the hand on the patient's skin provides a point of stability for more accurate control of the point of the scalpel (Figure 25-20C).

The pointed No. 11 blade has several uses. It is often used for incising abscesses; the sharp edge of the blade tip is thrust up into the abscess and pulled outward with a sawing movement to incise the skin.

Most scalpel incisions are made precisely perpendicular to the skin. An angled or beveled cut undermines the dermis and epidermis, possibly resulting in necrosis of the skin secondary to circulatory impairment. This yields a less cosmetic scar in the best of circumstances and wound infection from devitalized skin tissue in the worst cases.

Scissors. Scissors come in various sizes and models—straight or curved, heavy or delicate; short, medium, or long. The Metzenbaum and Mayo scissors are most frequently used. The Metzenbaum scissors are thin-tipped dissecting scissors, whereas the Mayo scissors are heavy, blunt-bladed scissors used for cutting heavy structures, especially sutures (Figure 25-21). Scissors should be held with the points following the natural curve of the hand. However, for cutting along tissues curved toward the hand, the scissors should be turned over for proper usage.

Assistants are frequently asked to cut sutures; although this in itself is a simple maneuver, a few words of advice are warranted. Use heavy scissors to cut sutures; delicate scissors are more expensive and can be dulled if they are used to cut suture material. A steady hand held palm-down against your other arm or hand, or against the patient, gives excellent control of the tips of the scissors, which is the only portion that should be used for cutting sutures. The slightly open blades of the scissors should be placed on the upheld suture and slid down the sutures until the knot is felt against the blades of the scissors. The blades of the scissors should be rotated 45 degrees and closed to cut the suture. Care must be taken

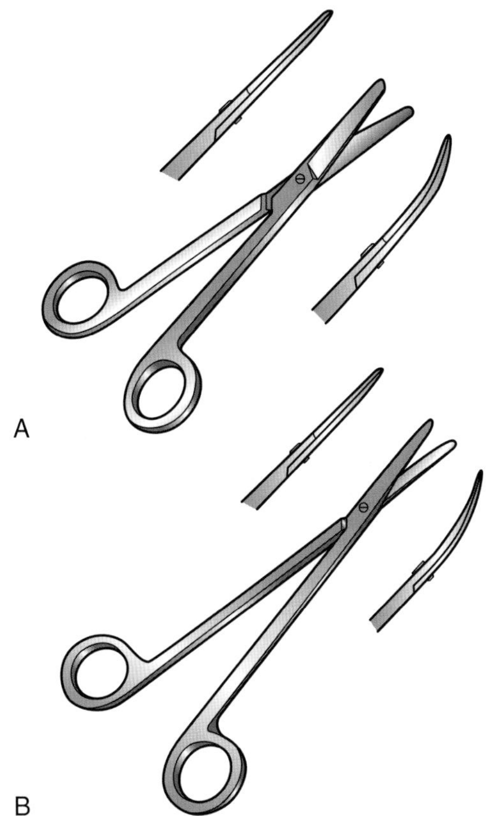

FIGURE 25-21 ■ **A,** Mayo scissors are used for cutting thick structures and sutures. **B,** Metzenbaum scissors are used for dissecting, transecting vessels, and opening viscera.

to ensure that the scissors do not cut anything but the suture and that the suture does not get caught within the blades. Otherwise, the scissors may pull the suture from the tied tissue, causing bleeding or other adverse effects.

When absorbable sutures such as chromic and plain gut are cut, a tag of 3 to 4 mm is left to prevent the knot from unwinding. Synthetic nonabsorbable sutures, such as nylon and Prolene, have a springlike memory and require a tag of 7 to 10 mm to prevent unwinding. Nonabsorbable sutures such as silk and surgical cotton usually do not require a tag and may be cut on the knot. The tails of a closely placed series of sutures can be easily controlled and cut using the maneuver illustrated in Figure 25-22.

CLINICAL PROCEDURE

"Pass pointing" occurs when the tips of the scissors extend past the structure or suture chosen for cutting and accidentally sever an unintended structure on the other side. Keep the tips of the scissors in your direct line of vision to avoid this complication. If there is any question, another team member should be asked to make the cut.

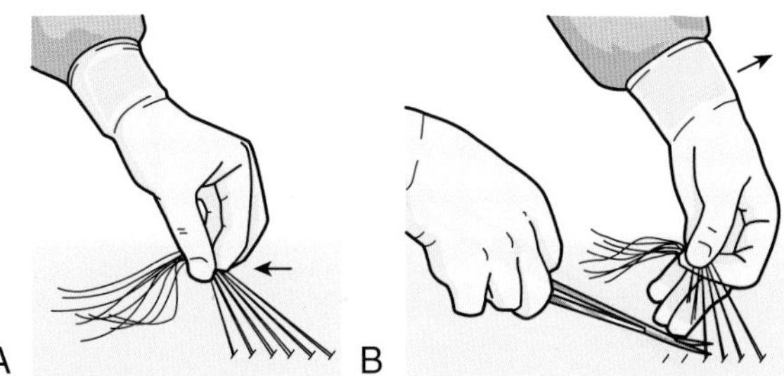

FIGURE 25-22 ■ **A,** Rows of tied sutures can easily be cut by gathering all the suture ends into one hand and pulling the ends toward you, graduating the suture tail lengths. **B,** Apply upward tension while cutting the suture closest to you, to keep previously cut tails out of the scissors' blades.

Surgical Sponges and Pads

Removing blood from the wound allows exposure and examination of the anatomy. Dabbing the wound with absorbent gauze pads or sponges of various sizes is usually sufficient, but with copious bleeding, suction devices are important for clearing the operative field of fluids. Sponges are designated with various eponyms: 4- × 8-inch coarse-weave sponges ("4 × 4s," "Raytecs") are used for minimal bleeding in smaller areas. Larger, tightly woven laparotomy sponges ("laps," "lap pads") are used to absorb many times their weight in blood and fluids.

CLINICAL PROCEDURE

All surgical gauze pads have a blue radiopaque thread either woven into their substance or attached as a loop. These blue threads are readily located on radiography if a sponge has been inadvertently left within a body cavity after surgery. All sponges used during surgery must be accounted for by OR personnel and therefore should not be used for bandages or wound dressings.

Suction Devices

The *Yankauer tip (tonsil tip)* is one of the most commonly used suction tips. It allows for aspiration of large volumes of fluid, although it has the disadvantage of easily clogging or occluding when the tip is brought into close approximation with tissues or large blood clots. Placing a gauze sponge over the tip and suctioning fluid through the gauze may

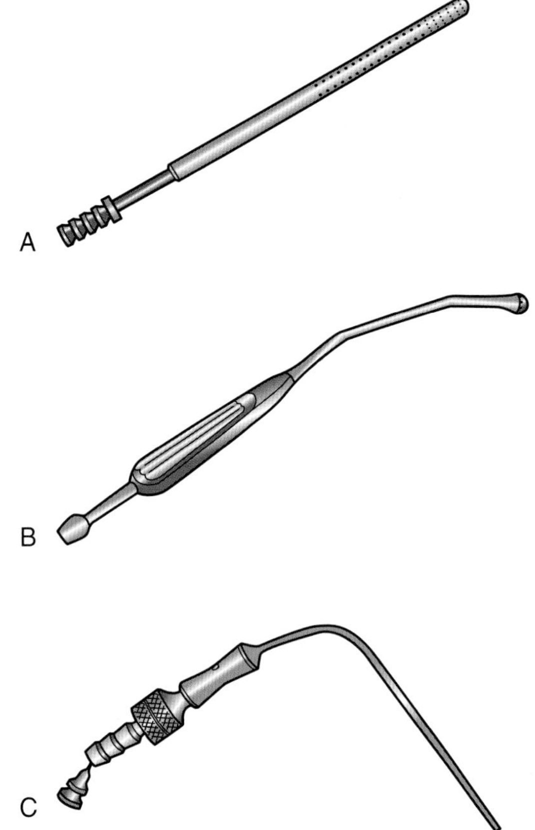

FIGURE 25-23 ■ Suction tips. **A,** Poole tip. **B,** Yankauer or tonsil tip. **C,** Frazier or neuro tip.

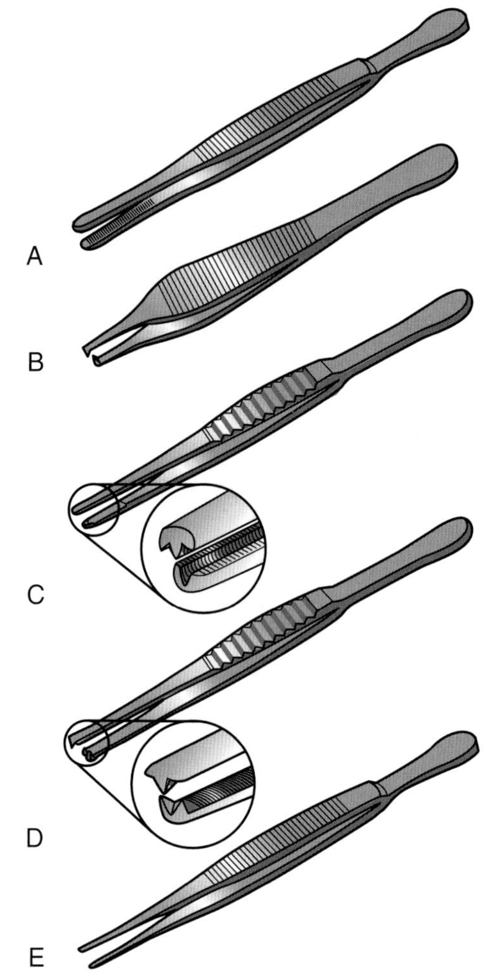

FIGURE 25-24 ■ Thumb forceps. **A,** Plain. **B,** Adson with teeth. **C,** DeBakey. **D,** Toothed. **E,** Cushing.

prevent clogging. The Poole tip has an inner canal surrounded by a fenestrated outer sleeve containing smaller holes that prevent inadvertent occlusion. For use in delicate procedures, a *neuro* or *Frazier* suction device uses a 3- to 5-mm cannula opening with a vented side port on the handle to control the suction force applied at the tip (Figure 25-23).

CLINICAL PROCEDURE

Use a pencil grip to hold suction tips. This allows defined, precision control of the instrument, which is especially important for delicate vascular and microsurgical procedures.

Forceps, Clamps, and Needle Holders

Forceps are divided into two categories: those with teeth and those without teeth. Thumb forceps require finger apposition in the form of a pencil grip to handle tissues. Ratcheted forceps (clamps) can be locked onto tissues and left in place, freeing the hands for other efforts.

Thumb Forceps. Toothed thumb forceps (Figure 25-24D) are used on tissues that require a firm grip, such as fascia, or for abdominal wall closure. *Bonney* and *rat-tooth* forceps are good examples of heavy-toothed thumb forceps. Small *Adson* forceps (Figure 25-24B) are ideal for everting the skin edges when staples are placed for incision closure. One should never use toothed forceps on nerves, blood vessels, bowel, or other viscera.

Smooth forceps are used for handling delicate structures. *DeBakey* forceps (Figure 25-24C), a useful variant of the smooth forceps, were originally designed for vascular surgery. Their unique, interpolating, smooth tooth design causes minimal tissue crushing by distributing the grasping forces equally throughout the tips. *Cushing* (Figure 25-24E) and *Potts* forceps are smooth, finely tipped forceps used for similar purposes.

Smooth forceps should not be used to handle fascia or skin because the excessive force required will damage these instruments.

CLINICAL PROCEDURE

Knowing how much tension to apply to each type of tissue is a key element of tissue preservation. Grasping the tissue closest to the site of action imparts the greatest control over the tissue's movement. Only a minimal amount of pressure is then required to move the tissue. For nerves and blood vessels, the enveloping adventitia should be grasped to prevent vessel-crushing injuries. Manipulate the skin by grasping the dermis located beneath the epidermis or by using a skin hook (see Figure 25-13C).

Locking (Ratcheted) Forceps. Ratcheted or locking forceps ("clamps") are instruments known by many eponyms (Figure 25-25). The *hemostat* clamp (Figure 25-25A) may be straight or curved and may have serration on all or part of the blade length. Smaller hemostats, called *mosquito* clamps, have fine tips. *Crile* and *Kelly* clamps are larger versions of the hemostat. Even larger are the *Peán* and *Carmalt* clamps, which are used to clamp large blood vessels before transection and tying. *Right-angle* clamps (Figure 25-25C) can be used to dissect around veins or arteries or to pass suture material around tubular structures.

The *Kocher* clamp (Figure 25-25G) is a traumatic toothed clamp applied to hold structures that will be removed or will not undergo harm from severe crushing, such as the rectus sheath fascia. *Allis* clamps (Figure 25-25I) have perpendicular teeth along their edges but by design are less traumatic than Kocher clamps and can be used on structures for retraction or for apposition of tissue edges. A *Babcock* clamp (Figure 25-25H) is used to gently hold delicate viscera or to encircle tubular structures for gentle retraction.

Needle Holders. Needle holders ("needle drivers") are designed with fine, medium, and heavy tips with a variety of handle lengths (Figure 25-25F). The driver's tip size is determined by the delicacy of the needle used for suturing. The depth at which the suturing occurs determines the length of the handles. Generally, the shorter lengths are easier to guide and are used for suturing with precise control. Using a delicate needle holder for a heavy needle destroys the integrity and locking ability of the instrument.

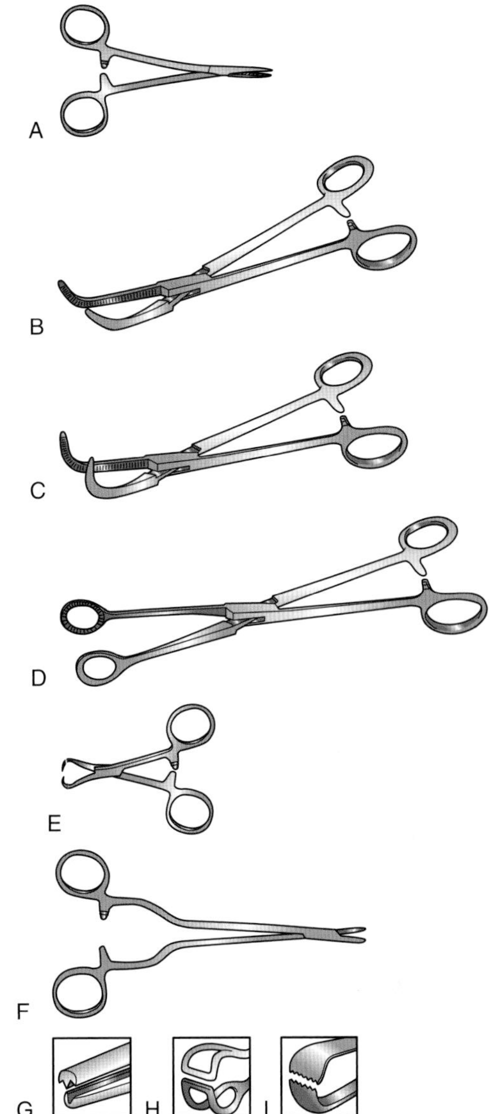

FIGURE 25-25 Ratcheted locking forceps (clamps). **A,** Straight hemostat. **B,** Large clamp. **C,** Right-angle clamp. **D,** Ring (sponge). **E,** Towel clip. **F,** Needle holder. **G,** Kocher. **H,** Babcock. **I,** Allis.

CLINICAL PROCEDURES

Unfortunately, ringed instruments (such as clamps, needle holders, and scissors) are designed for right-handed individuals. All surgeons and assistants should be proficient in the use of these tools with either hand because frequently, the instrument will be used in the nondominant hand. The left-handed assistant may have to practice using these instruments more than the right-handed person. It takes precisely the opposite motions and movements to control these instruments with the left hand, particularly for opening ratcheted clamps or cutting with scissors. Perfection requires concerted effort and practice. Several guidelines follow.

Do not allow your fingers to protrude through the rings past the distal interphalangeal joint. Placing the proximal interphalangeal joint through the rings severely restricts the ability to quickly disengage the instrument from the hand. The thumb ring should be controlled with the thumb's pad only. Occasionally, it is useful to place the ring and little finger into the other ring for control. The index finger can be placed onto the shaft or middle of the instrument, to provide better control, in the "tripod grip" (Figure 25-26). At best, lack of proficiency with these instruments may cause delay; at worst, finger fumbling with an instrument may avulse a vessel, causing unnecessary bleeding.

The clamp's locking ratchets allow a mechanism to release the instrument from the hand while continuing to grip the tissue. To disengage a ratcheted clamp in the right hand, the thumb pushes outward and the remaining fingers pull inward to release the locking mechanism. The opposite movements are needed for the left hand (Figure 25-27A and B). Practice using these instruments with both hands, with the curved tip pointing up and then with the tip pointing down. Similar finger motions are required for proper cutting action with scissors (Figure 25-27C and D).

As with thumb forceps, ratcheted forceps should encase only enough tissue in the tips of the instrument to enable a firm grip. For instance, blood vessels should be grasped without trapping surrounding structures. Finally, although blunt by design, the forceps' ratchets can tear gloves or accidentally entrap other tissues or sutures. Caution should always be used when applying and disengaging these instruments.

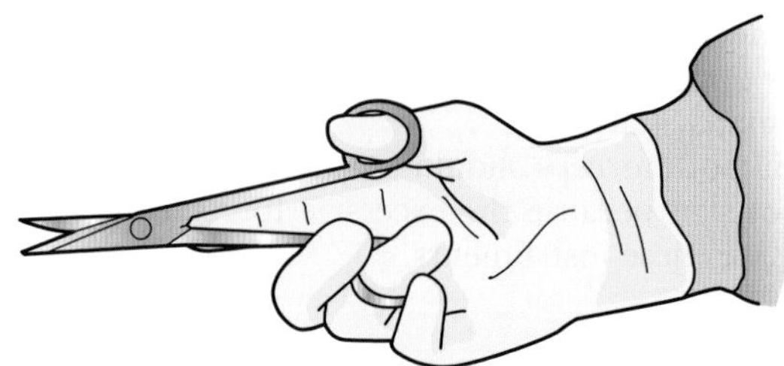

FIGURE 25-26 ■ The tripod grip can be used with a ringed forceps to optimize control of the instrument's tips. The index finger helps guide and stabilize the instrument, thereby reducing hand tremor. Rotate the hand palm-down for the best hand muscle control and strength.

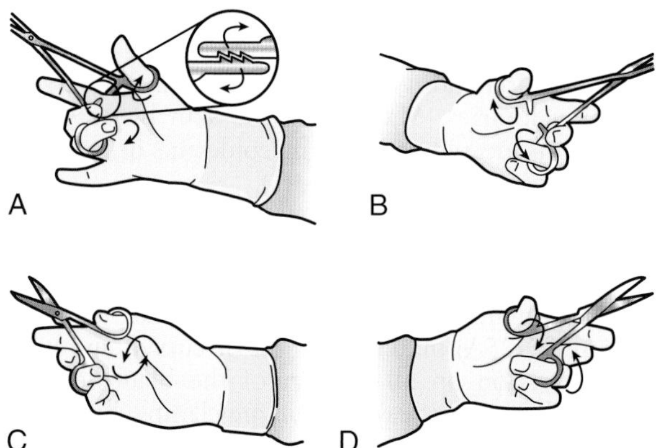

FIGURE 25-27 ■ Control of ratcheted instruments takes practice, particularly with the nondominant hand. **A,** To open locking ratcheted forceps with the right hand, the thumb is pushed toward the body and upward while the other fingers are pulled toward the palm. **B,** The reverse relationship holds for the left hand. **C,** Creating close contact of the blades during closure allows scissors to cut rather than tear tissues. In the right hand, the thumb moves away from the palm and body as the other fingers pull toward the palm. **D,** Again, the opposite holds for the left hand.

Drains and Tubes

Drains are placed *prophylactically*, to prevent accumulation of fluids and to encourage the obliteration of dead space, or *therapeutically*, to promote escape of fluids that have already accumulated.

General Precautions. Drains act as two-way conduits. The benefits of a drain must be weighed against the risk of introducing infection.

- Because a drain permits bacterial ingress and prevents full closure of a wound, it should never be brought out through the operative incision.
- A drain should always be fixed to the skin with sutures.
- A drain that is too hard or stiff may cause pressure necrosis of surrounding tissues, especially if placed near a large blood vessel, tendon, nerve, or solid organ.

Types of Drains and Tubes. Drains may be classified into four basic categories: sump drains, self-suction drains, straight drains, and chest tubes.

Sump Drains. Sump drains have two parallel lumina leading to a multiholed distal tip. One lumen is used to aspirate fluid, and the second lumen allows air to enter the cavity being aspirated, thus preventing undue suction from pulling of tissues into the aspiration ports and clogging of the holes. Salem sump NG tubes are characteristic of this drain type.

Self-Suction Drains. A self-suction or closed-suction drain is attached to a vacuum device, bulb, or wall suction to provide continuous drainage of a wound site or cavity. Bulbs are usually hand-charged (squeezed) to initiate suction. Hemovac, Jackson-Pratt

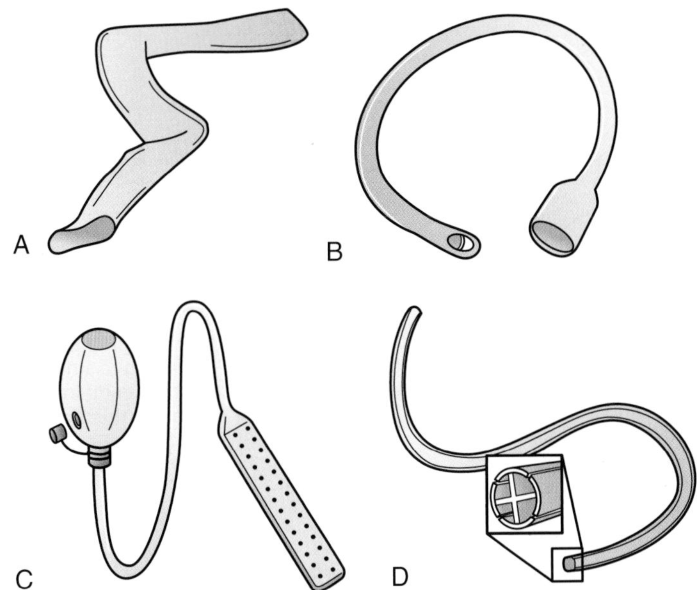

FIGURE 25-28 ■ Four frequently used drains. **A,** Penrose. **B,** Red rubber catheter. **C,** Jackson-Pratt. **D,** Blake. **Inset,** Cross section of Blake drain, showing channels that run its entire length.

(see Figure 25-28C), and Blake (see Figure 25-28D) drains are self-suction drains.

Straight Drains. Straight drains do not use suction; rather, gravity is used to facilitate fluid movement. The Penrose drain (Figure 25-28A), a flat latex tube, is a good example of a straight drain. This category also includes gastric and jejunal tubes (tubes placed directly through the skin into the stomach or jejunum), which may be used to drain the gastrointestinal tract or to provide infusion of enteral nutrition.

Chest Tubes. Chest tubes inserted through the chest wall into the thorax are suction drains designed to help maintain lung inflation and drain fluids or blood from the pleural space. They are connected to a water seal and then to a suction source. The water pressure prevents an accidental lung collapse if the suction source is intentionally or accidentally discontinued. A seal is maintained at the chest wall to prevent air leaks by wrapping a petroleum jelly-impregnated gauze strip around the skin entrance of the tube.

CLINICAL PROCEDURE

A Penrose drain is secured to the skin with a simple suture or a large safety pin designed to keep the drain from slipping out of the exit site or back into the body. A Salem sump tube is taped to the nose or face to secure its position. Chest tubes and self-suctioning drains are secured with a suture tied to the tube and sewn to the skin. Figure 25-29 illustrates how to sew a drain to the skin.

Removal of Drains. Drains should be removed as soon as drainage has subsided.

1. Warn the patient that there will be some pain; consider premedication for anxious patients.
2. Remove surrounding bandages and cut attaching skin suture.
3. *Always release suction before pulling.*
4. Be prepared for leaks and drips.

MINIMALLY INVASIVE SURGERY

In the late 1980s, Eddie Jo Reddick, MD, brought advanced technology into general surgery when he published several reports regarding the first laparoscopic cholecystectomies performed in the United States. Endoscopy and laparoscopy techniques date back to the early 1800s, but Reddick and surgeons in France working at the same time can be credited with introducing surgeons from all disciplines to the concept of performing surgery with minimal incisions and decreased recovery times (minimally invasive surgery [MIS]). For many diseases requiring surgical evaluation, intervention, or treatment, a laparoscopic or endoscopic procedure may be considered the first-line approach (Figure 25-30A-C).

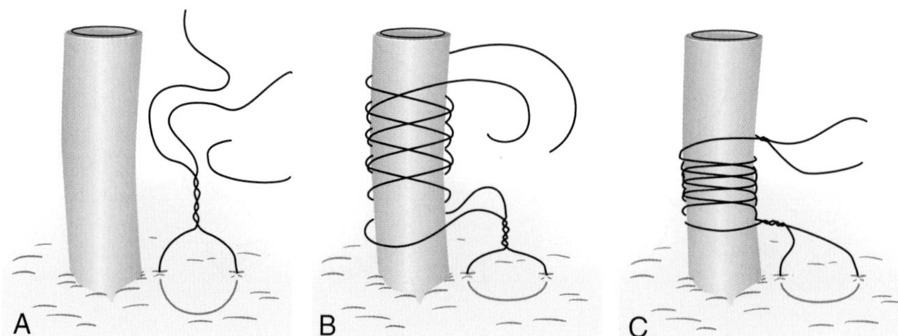

FIGURE 25-29 Sewing a drain to the skin. **A,** Create a loop by driving the needle through the skin. Pull the two suture ends to equal lengths, cut off the needle, and tie four or five half-knots above the skin, leaving room for postoperative tissue edema and to prevent the suture from cutting through the skin. **B,** Sandal-lace the suture ends loosely around the tube three or four times. **C,** Gently push the sandal lacing together while tightening the loops. Do this firmly but not too tightly to avoid strangulating the flow of fluid within the tube.

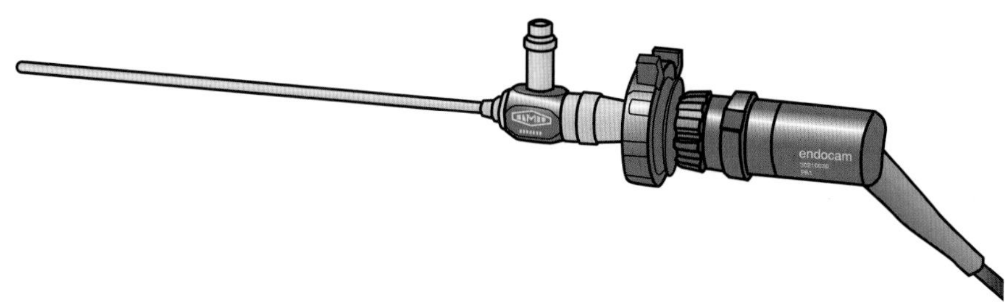

FIGURE 25-30 Laparoscope and camera head.

MIS includes the realm of arthroscopy employed by orthopedists worldwide. A large number of procedures are performed intraluminally via endoscopes through bronchoscopy, colonoscopy, and esophagogastroduodenoscopy. This section concentrates on general MIS in the abdomen and thorax (Figure 25-31A-C).

An entire culture blossomed around MIS in which much of the equipment is disposable. Equipment manufacturers developed MIS forceps, needle holders, suturing devices and ligatures, irrigation and suction, biopsy devices, retractors, and hemorrhage control methods (Figure 25-32A-E). One of the major advances allowing safe performance of laparoscopic cholecystectomy was the development of a preloaded device to apply titanium clips to close the cystic duct and control blood vessels via the laparoscope. It is safe to say all American hospitals performing surgery have MIS equipment. Approximately 85% of cholecystectomies and a majority of kidneys removed from living donors for transplant in the United States are performed with the use of MIS.[5]

Minimally invasive surgical techniques reduce cosmetic deformity and essentially minimize damage to the patient during surgery. Laparoscopy can be defined as insufflation of the abdomen, leading to MIS. Thoracoscopy (or video-assisted thoracic surgery [VATS]) entails deflating the lung and introducing the camera through the chest wall. Other MIS procedures are performed beneath the skin, as seen in endoscopic saphenous vein harvesting for coronary artery bypass grafting. A thoracotomy may be replaced by VATS through several small punctures in the intercostal spaces, and the 8-inch incision from a traditional cholecystectomy is replaced with four, 1- to 2-cm punctures in the anterior abdomen from a laparoscopic approach, with patient recovery measured in days and not weeks. The list of procedures performed via minimally invasive techniques has grown significantly since the late 1980s (Table 25-2) and will continue to expand as techniques are perfected and data analysis demonstrates which procedures offer the best outcomes for the patient. The complete value of MIS has not been proved in all cases, and some procedures are best left to classical open surgical approaches.

MIS typically involves replacement of human binocular three-dimensional vision by the use of a small video camera that projects two-dimensional images onto monitors posted around the OR table. Some advanced systems use dual cameras to mimic a three-dimensional surgical field, but these are not in common use. The surgeon makes a 1-cm incision to blindly introduce a needle used to introduce

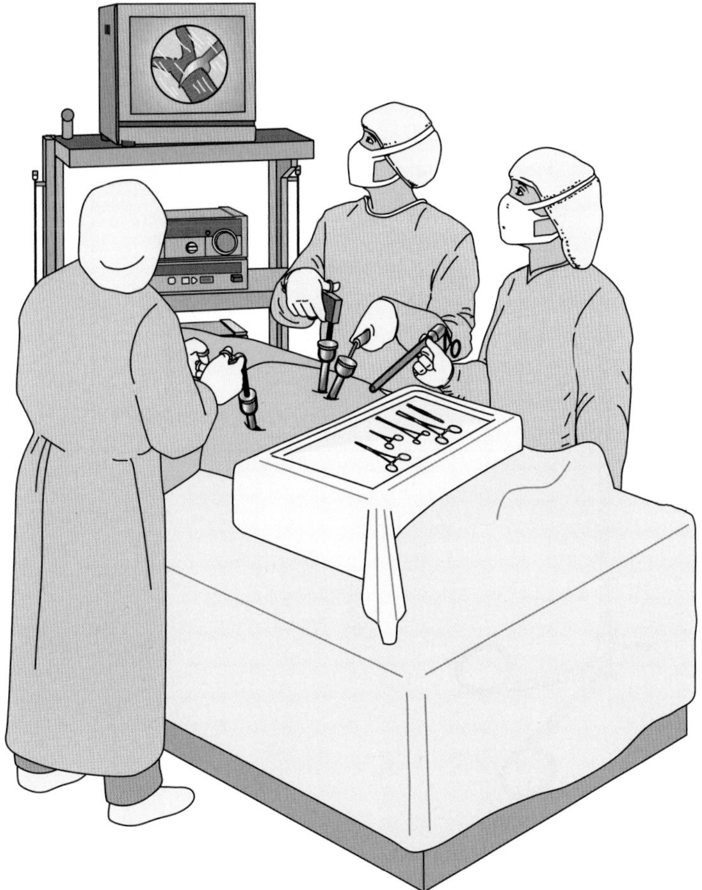

FIGURE 25-31 ■ Typical operating room layout for cholecystectomy.

CO_2 into the abdomen to raise the anterior abdominal wall away from underlying viscera (Figure 25-33A-C). The surgeon pushes a sharp trocar through another small incision and slides the camera down the hollow sleeve or "port" left after the inner trocar obturator is removed. Ports have valves that trap gas within the abdomen while allowing instrument passage down the inner lumen. Side valves allow attachment of tubing for gas insufflation (Figure 25-34A and B). Twelve- to 15-inch-long instruments are then used to perform the surgery (see Figure 25-32B). Electrocautery may be used for dissection and hemorrhage control. An ultrasonic dissecting device, the Harmonic Scalpel, can be used to avoid inadvertent burns from cautery use.

Laparoscopic video images are confined to the immediate field of vision directly in front of the camera, and the loss of the three-dimensional spatial relationships ordinarily seen with binocular vision requires careful instrument use, judicious use of electrocautery, and meticulous control of bleeding. MIS eliminates the familiar tactile sensations associated with open surgery tissue handling, and suturing can be extremely frustrating in a two-dimensional environment. American College of Surgery data show that the learning curve for MIS procedures is steep, and an average of 25 to 30 procedures is required before a surgeon is considered skilled in that particular procedure.

Surgical PAs are often asked to assist with MIS procedures. Most MIS requires at least a camera holder, while many such procedures require active participation by the first-assistant. The best method of acquiring the skills necessary for MIS proficiency is to spend time in an MIS laboratory within your training institution or hospital. There, trocar insertion, camera manipulation, and acquiring an understanding of the operating characteristics of the various instruments and devices can be practiced without risk of patient morbidity.

The references that follow this chapter contain several excellent sources of information on MIS procedures and instruments that are not mentioned or

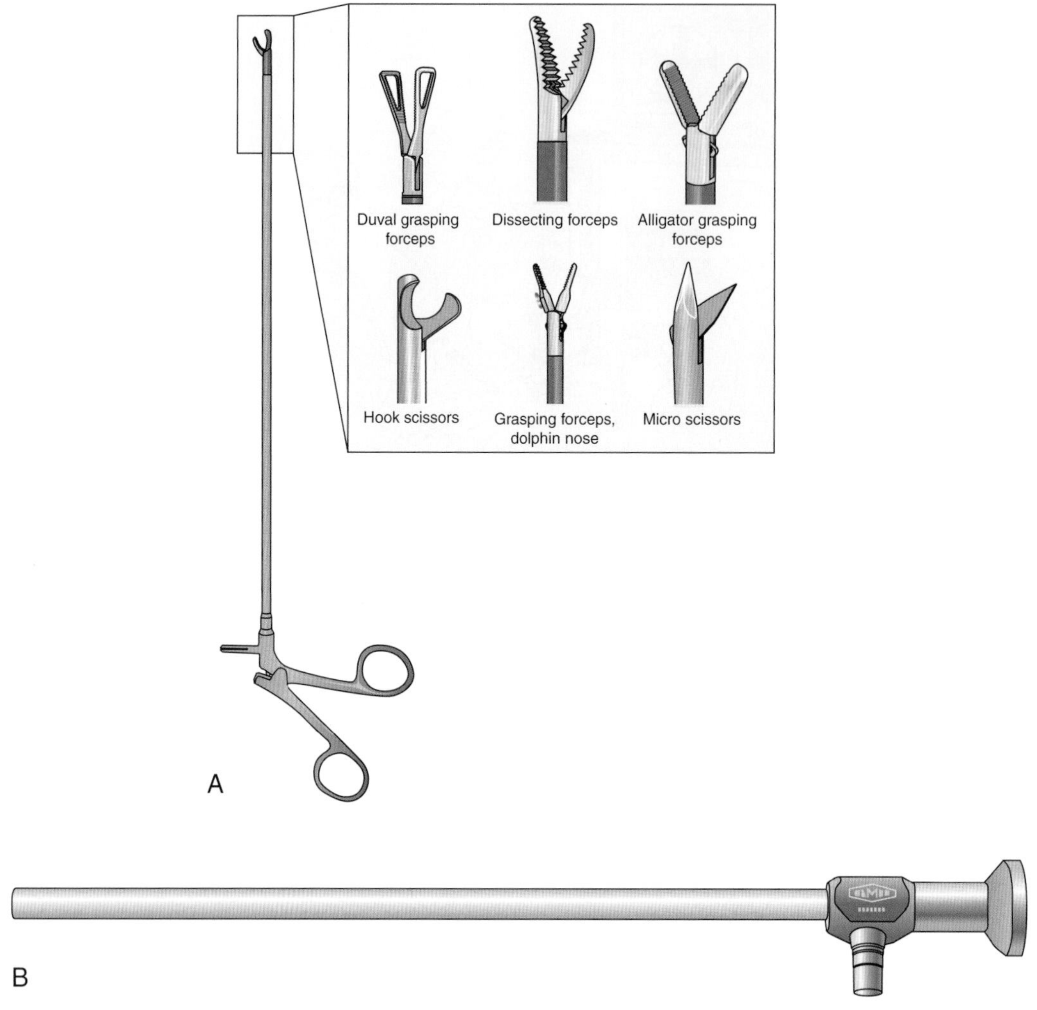

FIGURE 25-32 ■ **A,** Laparoscopic instruments with a variety of heads. **B,** Laparoscope.

adequately detailed in this section. We advise students to spend time with the laparoscope, CO_2 gas insufflator, videoscope light source, and associated instruments to gain understanding of their use at the operating table and to learn techniques for troubleshooting this high-tech equipment during surgery.

CLINICAL PROCEDURE

The field of view is often reversed on the video monitor from what you do with your hands for instrument manipulation. For example, the port acts as a fulcrum through the abdominal wall. Pushing down on the handle of the instrument outside the body causes the tip of the instrument to move up within the abdominal cavity. Rightward movements of the handle cause leftward movement of the instrument tip.

Depth perception on the video monitor comes with practice. Watching your hands outside the abdomen and estimating how deeply the instrument is inserted within the patient can assist with acquiring an understanding of how to safely move instruments within the abdomen or chest. Observe for shadows, the position of other instruments, and the relationship of your instruments to the anatomy to gain confidence with tissue and instrument control.

The camera operator becomes the surgeon's eyes. The only important field of view is where the surgeon is working; therefore keep the camera focused on the surgeon's working instruments and the anatomy under scrutiny. Try to avoid tissue spray during dissection and irrigation splashes onto the camera lens. Lens fogging can be problematic and is best addressed before surgery by wiping a commercial antifogging agent onto the lens and warming the

TABLE 25-2 **Minimally Invasive Surgery Procedures**

Laparoscopic cholecystectomy
Laparoscopic appendectomy
Laparoscopic colon resection or colostomy formation
Laparoscopic inguinal and umbilical herniorrhaphy
Laparoscopic Nissen fundoplication
Laparoscopic kidney harvesting for donation
Laparoscopic adhesiolysis
Laparoscopic Heller myotomy
Laparoscopic nephrectomy
Laparoscopic gastrostomy and jejunostomy feeding tube insertion
Laparoscopic adrenalectomy
Laparoscopic bladder and gynecologic procedures
Hysterectomy
Bladder suspension
Thoracoscopic bleb resection, lung and pleural biopsy
Thoracoscopic sympathectomy
Thoracoscopic lung volume reduction
Thoracoscopic esophagectomy
MIS harvesting of the internal mammary artery
MIS harvesting of the saphenous vein

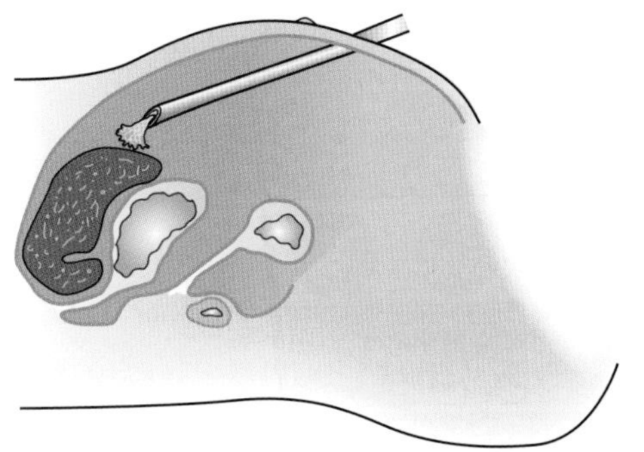

FIGURE 25-33 Abdominal wall separated from viscera by CO_2 gas.

scope before introducing it into warm humid tissue. Dabbing the lens onto the liver or other relatively fat-free tissue can also wipe the lens clean. A well-directed stream from an irrigation device is also helpful.

Electrocautery energy can arc within a body cavity or ground to an adjoining metal instrument, thereby transferring energy to a distant site and causing a serious injury or an occult burn that is not obvious until 1 or 2 days postoperatively. Use extreme care when using electrocautery and examine surrounding tissues at the end of the procedure to look for signs of electrothermal injury.

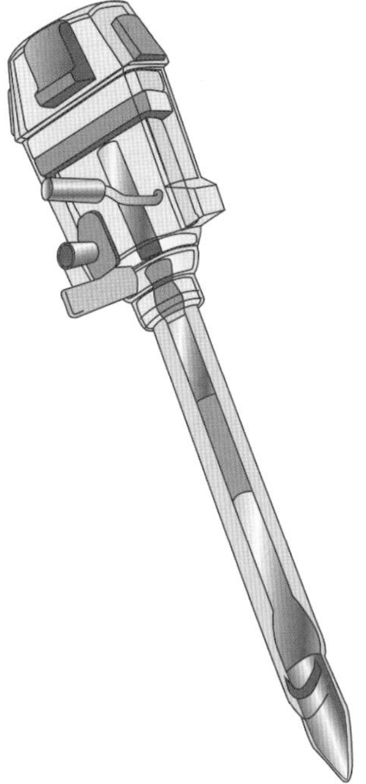

FIGURE 25-34 Trocar.

Anatomy identification is critical to success with MIS. The most common intraabdominal injuries for MIS include visceral perforation (bladder, bowel, intestine) and damage to tubular structures such as the ureter, common bile and cystic ducts, and blood vessels.

All MIS procedures carry risks. Each procedure should be treated as if it could be converted into a traditional open operation if difficult anatomy, uncontrollable bleeding, or a complication warrants improved access to the surgical field. A good assistant must know the surgical conduct required for both MIS and open approaches and must expect that some procedures will be converted. The OR staff should have full traditional instrumentation immediately available in the OR for such unanticipated events.

SURGICAL BLEEDING

The secret of controlling intraoperative hemorrhage lies in its prevention. There are several reliable methods to control surgical bleeding. Some take advantage of the body's intrinsic clotting mechanisms (e.g., direct pressure), and some are artificially applied (e.g., topical thrombin). Bleeding compounded by coagulation defects is a broad topic beyond the scope of this chapter.

Direct Pressure

The easiest way to stop bleeding from small vessels is to apply gentle manual pressure. The systolic pressure in small vessels (between 5 and 10 mm Hg) is easily controlled in this manner. Direct pressure can be achieved by gently pushing the vessel against the underlying tissue with a finger or with the tip of a hemostat, sponge, scalpel, suction unit, or sponge attached to a long-handled clamp (ring forceps). Squeezing the vessel with forceps or between the fingers is also effective. Normal clotting for small vessels takes place within 15 to 30 seconds and may be all that is required for control. Direct pressure also gives the surgeon time to control bleeding in larger, high-pressure vessels with a hemostatic clamp or ligature if needed (see later).

During some procedures, diffuse bleeding may require pressure for extended periods; for example, a large sponge may be packed against the bleeding surface and held in place by the assistant's hand or with a retractor while some other portion of the procedure is completed. This is especially efficient for areas that have innumerable small or pinpoint "bleeders" that would be time-consuming to control individually.

CLINICAL PROCEDURE

When sponging blood from an area, do not aggressively drag or scrape the sponge across the tissue. This action removes coagulated blood products from the ends of blood vessels and allows bleeding to resume. Blotting is the safest method. Large amounts of clot can be removed by irrigating the area with saline and using suction or by scooping them by hand into a basin.

Electrocautery

The electrocautery unit (Bovie, cautery, or electrosurgical unit) (Figure 25-35A) uses high-frequency electrical energy to cut tissue or coagulate bleeding. The preferential conduction of electrical energy by blood

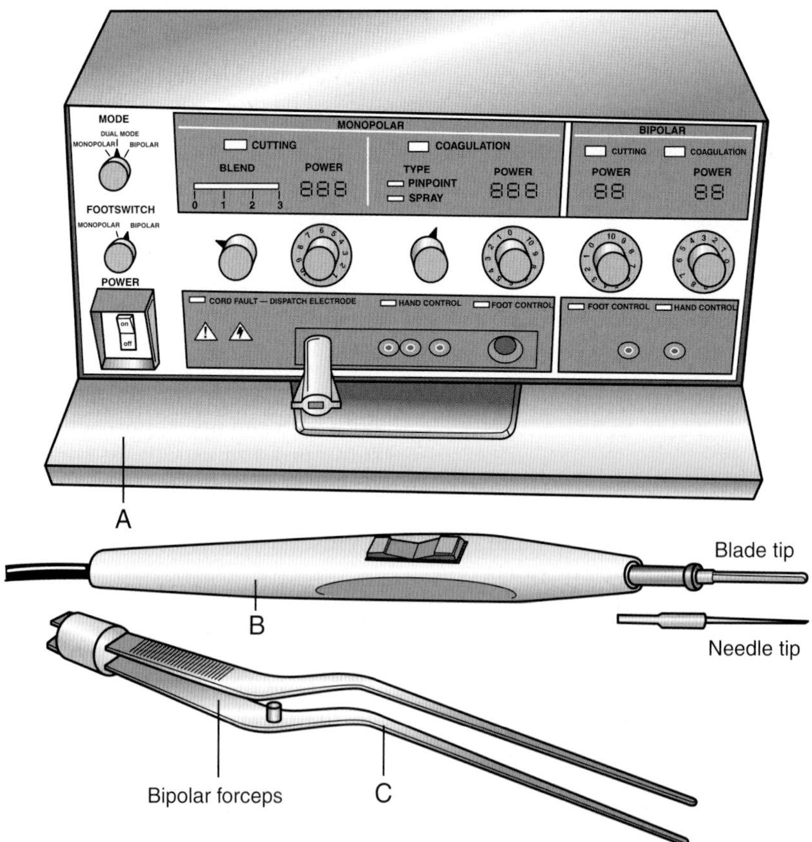

FIGURE 25-35 ■ **A,** Typical electrocautery unit. **B,** The monopolar electrosurgical "pencil" can cut or provide hemostasis through activation of the handle switch. **C,** Bipolar tips provide precise application of energy to the tissues.

vessels facilitates coagulation. It is crucial to remove pooled blood and irrigation fluids from the operative field that may act as an insulator or disperse the cautery's energy, thereby diminishing its effectiveness.

Electrocautery may be used in two different ways. In the bipolar mode, a tweezers-tip instrument is used to control bleeding vessels when the two tips complete the electrical circuit at the point of application (Figure 25-35C). The advantage of bipolar cautery is its precise application of energy to small and delicate areas. This is particularly efficacious for microvascular surgery, microneurosurgery, and plastic surgery procedures. Most bipolar units are operated by the surgeon through a foot-controlled switch.

In the monopolar mode, a grounding pad is attached to the patient from the electrocautery unit and an electrosurgical "pencil" is used to complete a circuit through the patient when it touches bleeding tissues (Figure 25-35B). This "pencil" has a rocker switch or two buttons on its shaft that activate either a continuous application of electrical energy for cutting through tissue or pulses that can coagulate specific sources of bleeding. Most units can produce a blend of cut and coagulation waveforms to combine the desired features of each.

The cut mode easily cleaves most tissue and does not penetrate deeply into the surrounding tissue. It is not effective for coagulating bleeding.

In the coagulation mode, the metal blade or needle tip can be directly applied to the tissue or to an intermediary instrument, such as a clamp or forceps, that has been placed onto a bleeding vessel. It can also be used to coagulate a small blood vessel along its visible length before the vessel is transected. The coagulation mode penetrates deeply into the surrounding tissues and can cause thermal damage to unseen arteries, nerves, and other delicate tissues surrounding the cautery tip and vessel surface.

CLINICAL PROCEDURE

Judgment involving the practical use of this instrument comes only with experience, through which one learns which vessels will respond to electrocautery coagulation. Great care must be taken when touching an intermediary instrument such as a clamp or forceps for coagulation because it will burn all tissues it comes in contact with. Before engaging the coagulation mode, be sure the grasping instrument is not touching the skin or other important tissues in the vicinity of the vessel being coagulated.

Although there is little risk from this technology, holes in gloves can allow burns through electrical conduction to the hands or fingers and loose grounding pads can cause severe electrical burns to the patient. The grounding pad should be in full contact with the chosen skin site and should not be placed on a bony prominence or over an implanted metal prosthesis (e.g., hip prosthesis). This is just one aspect of OR safety, and PAs should become familiar with the correct and safe use of this device. The manufacturer of the specific electrocautery machine in use in the OR can provide in-service instruction to OR staff and students.

Clamps, Clips, Ligatures, and Sutures

Larger hemorrhaging blood vessels are not safely controlled by direct pressure, packing, or electrocautery, and a wide variety of clamps, ligatures, sutures, and clips are available for this purpose.

Clamps. Bleeding from larger blood vessels may be controlled by the application of a clamp or ratcheted forceps appropriate to the size of the vessel's diameter. If the vessel is already cut and bleeding, grasp it with smooth thumb forceps to temporarily control the flow and then apply the ratcheted forceps. A vessel to be clamped before cutting should be held in place with thumb forceps and carefully isolated from the surrounding tissues with blunt dissection with a small hemostat. To accomplish this maneuver, gently advance the clamp parallel to the vessel while opening and closing the jaws to create a tunnel under and around the vessel (Figure 25-36). Both sides require dissection. Place two hemostats, tips facing each other, on opposite ends of the vessel. A small overhang of each tip around which to wrap the suture should extend past the vessel. Close the clamps and transect the vessel with Metzenbaum scissors. Only the vessel itself should be included in the jaws of the clamp. Frequently, the surgeon or assistant will tie a suture beneath these clamps to achieve hemostasis. Very small vessels may be coagulated with electrocautery.

Often, the student or new assistant will be asked to control the clamp when the surgeon ties a suture around the vessel. Give the surgeon a clear view of the vessel. Provide adequate exposure by keeping your hands out of the surgeon's line of sight and by retracting surrounding tissue away from the vessel being tied. "Rock" the clamp away from the underlying tissue as the tie passes around the back of the clamp. Then gently rock the clamp in the opposite direction, elevating the tip so that the suture may be passed completely around the vessel (Figure 25-37). The vessel end with the highest pressure should be tied first. Do not pull the clamped vessel up during this maneuver; pulling might avulse vessels, resulting in the retraction of the open bleeding vessel deep into the surrounding tissue with resultant hemorrhage that is difficult to control.

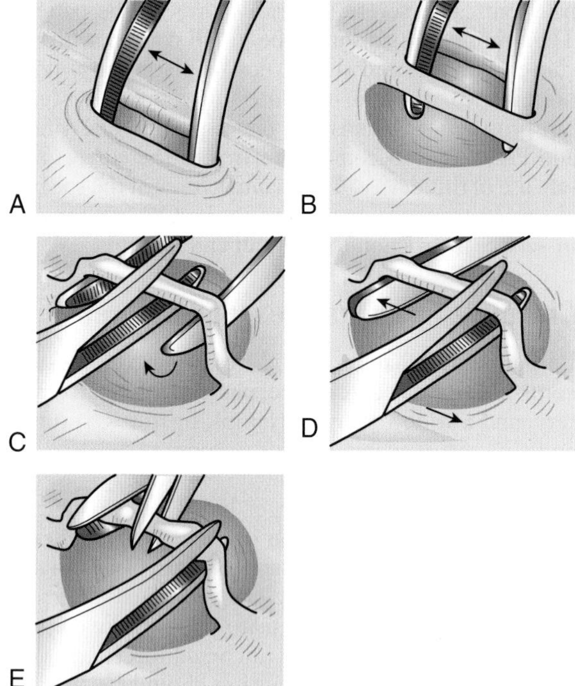

FIGURE 25-36 **A** and **B,** Clamps can be used to dissect the loose areolar tissues surrounding blood vessels. Small movements of the tips during spreading prevent tearing of unseen adjacent blood vessels. **C** and **D,** After a clear tunnel is developed, hemostats are placed on both ends of the vessel, which is then divided with scissors **(E)**. The end closer to the main circulation is tied first to prevent hemorrhage if the vessel slips from the clamp.

CLINICAL PROCEDURE

After the surgeon has tightened the first throw of the knot, slowly open the clamp and withdraw it from the wound. Occasionally, the surgeon asks the assistant to "flash" the clamp during tightening of the first throw of the knot. To do this, slowly release the clamp *while keeping tension on the tissue within its jaws. Do not let go of the vessel.* As the surgeon tightens the first throw, firmly reapply the clamp and hold steady while the remainder of the knot is completed. "Flashing" is especially useful for controlling vessels that have the potential to retract deeply into the surrounding tissue, where they would be inaccessible for further hemostasis. Flashing is also useful when a large-diameter vessel must be "bunched up" to allow more tissue to be encompassed within the knot and when another tie, clip, or ligature is required for complete control of the vessel.

When sutures are tied to replace a series of clamps, the clamp closest to the person tying the sutures should be tied first. This prevents snagging of the suture on adjacent clamps.

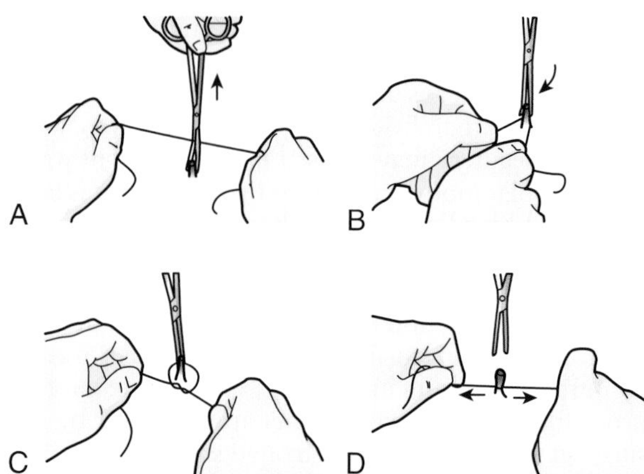

FIGURE 25-37 Tying a vessel held within a clamp. **A,** The heel of the instrument is raised to allow passage of the suture behind the clamp. **B,** The clamp nose is then slightly lifted to allow circumferential wrapping of the suture. **C** and **D,** The clamp is released when instructed, or when the first half-knot is securely tightened. Note the position of the tying fingers parallel to the vessel during knot-tightening to prevent accidental avulsion from shearing forces. Withdraw the clamp parallel from the vessel to avoid entangling the suture ends. This maneuver takes coordination and communication with the person tying the suture.

Clips. Titanium clips are used to control bleeding and occasionally serve as radiopaque markers in cancer patients who are expected to have postoperative radiation therapy. Clips are easy to apply and take less time than tying sutures, a characteristic advantage in many situations. Long-handled applicators are used to place clips in narrow or deep spaces where suture-tying is difficult. Clips are significantly more expensive than sutures, however, and can obscure the surrounding anatomy through signal scatter during computed tomography.

Clips are placed on bleeding vessels in the same manner as sutures. A clamp or forceps is used to occlude the end of the vessel, and the vessel is clipped before division. Clips are applied by firm squeezing of the handles of the applicator.

CLINICAL PROCEDURE

Clips must completely encompass the vessel to provide reliable hemostasis. If this is not possible, a suture tie or ligature must be used. Clips loaded onto nondisposable applicators are tricky to use. If the clip handle is slightly squeezed and released before the clip is applied, the clip will fall from the applicator tip and another will need to be reloaded, wasting valuable time. This is not the case with preloaded, multiclip, disposable instruments.

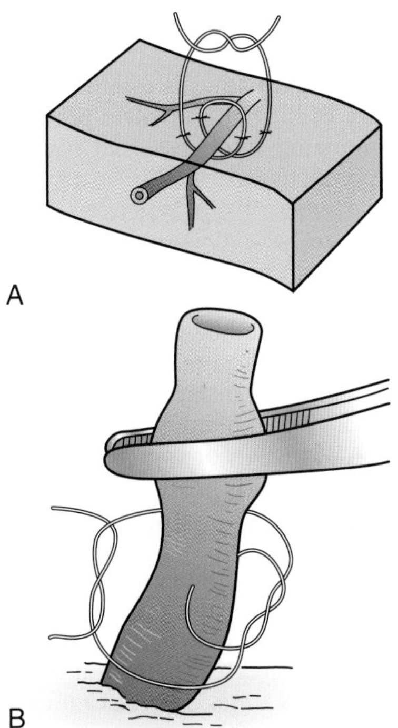

FIGURE 25-38 ■ **A,** Vessels hidden beneath enveloping tissues that cannot be readily located or are diffusely bleeding may be controlled with the figure-eight suture shown here. Care must be taken not to ligate important surrounding structures. **B,** The suture ligature prevents suture slippage on large or high-pressure vessels.

Suture Ligatures. Suture ligatures are used to attain hemostasis of larger veins and arteries when simple suture ties or clips are deemed inadequate or inappropriate. They are particularly useful on vessels of larger caliber and close to the higher systolic pressure of the central circulation, which have the potential to dislodge a simple suture tie or a clip over time.

A figure-eight suture ligature can be used to control vessels that retract deep into the surrounding tissues, cannot be located for clamping, and do not respond to the application of electrocautery. This ligature encompasses surrounding tissues and directly compresses the bleeding vessel (Figure 25-38A). Care must be demonstrated to avoid inclusion of valuable structures in the suture ligature and to avoid narrowing the lumen of adjacent tubular structures.

Another variation of the suture ligature enables hemostasis of large vessels. The suture is passed *through the middle* of the vessel being held within the jaws of a hemostat; then the ends are brought around the clamp from opposite directions before being tied (Figure 25-38B).

Absorbable Hemostatic Agents

Several agents are used to control bleeding by promoting the formation of an artificial clot or by providing a matrix framework for a clot to form. They are designed to control oozing in instances of hemorrhage from multiple tiny vessels. Hemorrhaging from solid organs with enveloping capsule damage (e.g., small spleen or liver tears) can be controlled in this manner. Occasionally, such agents can be applied to a vascular anastomosis to control needle-hole bleeding.

Thrombin. Thrombin applied topically as a powder or solution is particularly useful for capillary oozing. In its liquid form, it can be used in conjunction with an absorbable gelatin sponge to form a bulky hemostatic plug for highly vascular regions such as the liver or spleen.

Absorbable Gelatin Sponge (Gelfoam). Gelfoam helps form a bulky artificial clot in vascular areas, as mentioned previously. It is usually wetted with thrombin or isotonic saline to allow pliability (saline) or greater clot formation (thrombin). It can be left in the surgical site and will be absorbed in 4 to 6 weeks. The diffuse but copious bleeding frequently encountered in liver surgery, including biopsies, can often be controlled with this agent.

Oxidized Cellulose (Surgicel). A treated surgical gauze, oxidized cellulose acts as a physical matrix for clot formation and does not actively cause any alteration of the clotting cascade. It is produced in several forms, including strips, gauze pads, and pledgets. Pledgets can be sewn into place with sutures to seal needle punctures created during vascular or cardiac procedures. Oxidized cellulose can be left in the surgical site, but it is commonly removed after coagulation has taken place.

Microfibrillar Collagen Hemostat (Avitene, Angiostat). This agent is packaged as a friable, flat pad that works through adhesion to the bleeding site by platelet aggregation. This agent is efficacious for spleen or liver tears and for diffuse bleeding from multiple small vessels.

CONCEPTS FOR SURGICAL ASSISTING

Suturing, Knot-Tying, and Staples

Understanding suture and needle construction, their handling characteristics, the differences between absorbable and nonabsorbable sutures, the probable rate of absorption for each type of suture, and surgical knot-tying is a key element of surgical practice. When an improperly tied suture fails, serious hemorrhage, wound dehiscence, or incisional hernias may occur. It is beyond the scope of this chapter and it would be unreasonable to duplicate the excellent efforts of preexisting instruction manuals to adequately address this topic, with the exception of several pieces of advice.

Students should obtain a manual for knot-tying techniques and a knot-tying board. These items can be obtained through the PA training program or from one of the major suture manufacturers (USS/Davis and Geck or Ethicon; see Resources). The student should begin practicing *before* the first surgical rotation. Like playing a musical instrument with accomplishment, knot-tying requires dedicated practice. The speed at which knots are tied is not as important as accurate placement of a reliable series of knots ("throws") with the suture material. Creating a tight knot without *strangulating* the tissue takes practice and avoids unnecessary ischemia that may impede tissue healing. Wearing a pair of gloves and wetting the suture can approximate the in vivo environment. Use the pads of the fingers when tightening knots to prevent cuts in gloves and fingers. Stainless steel staples can be used to close the skin incision in lieu of sutures. They are less likely than sutures to leave scars tied across the skin, which may leave "railroad tracks" perpendicular to the incision (Figure 25-39). Staples are usually not used on the face or on very thin skin.

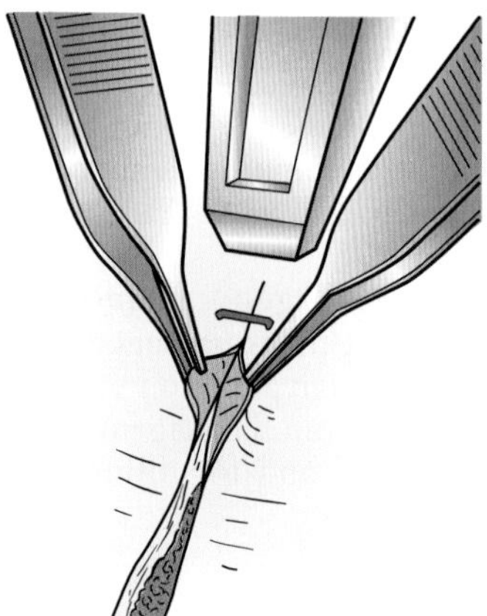

FIGURE 25-39 Use Adson forceps with teeth to evert the skin edges when placing skin staples. Center the stapler head on the incision, and gently push downward before pulling the stapler handle. Pull backward after setting the staple to disengage the skin. Occasionally, keeping the handle squeezed after firing the staple stabilizes the skin, allowing easier relocation of Adson forceps for the placement of the next staple.

Tissue Preservation

Preserving exposed tissues is essential to promoting postoperative healing and involves preventing desiccation, minimizing fluid loss, and handling tissues gently. Exposed tissues should be kept moist with saline-soaked gauze or repeated irrigation when possible. The gauze-padded blades of locking retractors should also be kept moist. Gentle handling of tissues with forceps and hands is paramount, and a minimum amount of force should be used to accomplish tissue movement. For instance, tearing of the spleen's capsule during retraction or laceration of the short gastric vessels has caused many bleeding injuries during manipulation of the left or transverse colon.

Facilitating the Procedure

Anticipation of the surgeon's movement through thorough knowledge of the procedure allows a system of teamwork to develop between the surgeon and assistant. It also decreases the length of both operative and anesthesia time. The assistant can become intimately familiar with the nuances and preferences of each surgeon, further facilitating the team approach. The alert assistant should be one step ahead of the surgeon in anticipating the next phase of the procedure and should know what instruments and maneuvers are required to accomplish that step. For example, as the surgeon makes an abdominal incision, the assistant should place proper countertraction opposite the surgeon's hand to facilitate the scalpel's penetration of tissue planes. Additionally, when a blood vessel is to be ligated, it is dissected free of the surrounding tissue and clamped with two hemostats—usually one placed by the surgeon and the other by the assistant.

Providing adequate exposure and visibility is a mainstay task of assisting. An old surgery axiom holds: "If the surgeon is struggling, then the exposure is inadequate." If the first-assistant adjusts the overhead surgical lights to illuminate the central operative field and controls the retraction devices, including directing the hands of the second-assistant, the surgeon can concentrate on the operation without distraction. Understanding what the surgeon needs to see comes with experience and knowledge of the steps involved in the procedure. Use instruments that are long enough to keep fingers out of the line of the surgeon's sight. Once good exposure is achieved, hand movements and retractors should remain in place unless a more refined move will benefit the surgeon. For routine operations, the team eventually uses fewer moves and needs little discussion to complete the procedure.

CLINICAL PROCEDURE

Surgery is a two-handed act. Each hand should be doing something, whether retracting, suctioning, or sponging. Good combinations include the suction tip or sponge and a retractor; forceps and suction tip; or forceps and needle holder. Some instruments, such as the thumb and ratcheted forceps, can be "palmed" in the hand to free the fingers for other tasks (Figure 25-40). This maneuver eliminates the need to frequently regrasp the same instrument if a task such as suctioning blood from the field requires attention for a brief moment.

Traction

Surgical exposure requires the judicious use of tissue traction. Not to be confused with retraction, tissue traction allows continuous exposure of underlying structures during the cleavage of tissues with scissors, scalpel, forceps, or electrocautery by gentle pulling of joined tissues in opposite directions. The initial use of traction occurs during the skin incision, as the surgeon or assistant uses the scalpel to divide the skin. Both the surgeon and the assistant pull on opposite sides of a line created by the scalpel to spread the tissue as it is cleaved (Figure 25-41A). Alternatively, a finger can be placed on either side of the incision to be made by the scalpel, if the incision is being accomplished without assistance (Figure 25-41B). Forceful traction, however, can cause immense harm by injuring delicate nerves, tearing arteries and veins, and causing uncontrolled hemorrhage, or by tearing organs, particularly the liver and spleen.

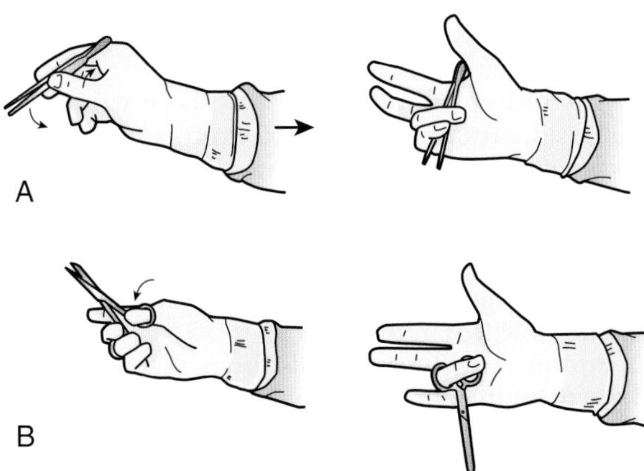

FIGURE 25-40 **A,** Hold the thumb forceps in a balanced grip similar to the precision grip described earlier, and "palm" it into the hand, leaving the thumb and index and middle fingers free for other tasks. **B,** Ringed instruments can also be palmed to free the fingers for other tasks. One ring is held on the second interphalangeal segment of the ring finger and is supported in place by the fifth finger. The instrument is flipped into position, and the thumb is inserted into the ring for use.

Dissection

Tissue dissection should always follow anatomic planes when possible, many of which are defined by the surrounding loose areolar tissues. Gentle traction helps separate and expose structures, so less force may be needed during *sharp* dissection with the scissors or scalpel. In addition to opening and closing scissor blades to cut tissues, long cuts can be accomplished by enclosing fascial tissues into the crotch of the partially open blades of a pair of scissors and pushing the scissors along the intended cut without further moving of the blades. This is particularly helpful when dissecting adventitia away from arteries and veins. The closed blades can also be pushed gently into tissue planes, gently spread, and then removed to dissect with minimal trauma. The closed blades can be gently used to elevate structures before dividing them. A cardinal rule for surgeons and assistants alike is this: *Never dissect or cut tissue that cannot be seen.* Experienced surgeons understand that this maneuver is dangerous and that use of knowledge, judgment, and extreme caution is needed.

Blunt dissection, less refined and controlled, is accomplished with instruments that are not considered sharp. It can be useful for separating sheets of loose areolar tissue but should be confined to places where vessel, nerve, or organ tearing is unlikely. Dissection is truly learned through experience, which has no substitute.

POSTOPERATIVE CARE

With normal postoperative recovery, the patient should demonstrate each day objective evidence of improvement, and postoperative care is directed toward promoting healing and resuming the normal ADLs. The

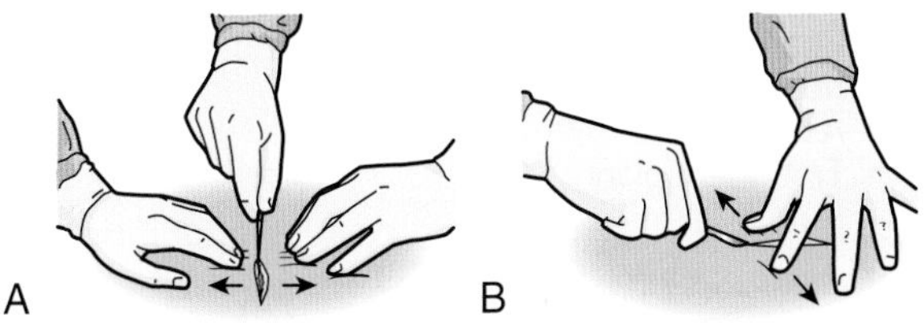

FIGURE 25-41 Traction placed onto both sides of the incision and during dissection allows visualization of underlying structures and the application of less force to cleave through tissue. **A,** Two-handed traction during abdominal incision. **B,** One-handed traction.

goals of postoperative care are to anticipate and avoid common problems and to discover problems early so that prompt intervention can prevent serious complications. Because the realm of postoperative complications is broad, a cursory overview is provided here to guide the student toward further learning.

Postoperative Notes

All postoperative patients should be evaluated soon after surgery. These checks are an excellent opportunity for a student to learn how a postoperative patient should look and are the times at which many acute postoperative problems are detected.

The first postoperative note documents how well the patient has done since leaving the OR. Subsequent notes document the patient's recovery process and response to treatment. The first note includes the patient's subjective comments, mental status, vital signs, hemodynamic stability, IV fluid volume infused since surgery, oral intake if any, urinary and drain outputs per hour or per 8-hour shift, current medications, and ventilator settings. It should also include results of a relevant problem-oriented PE. The assessment of the patient's status is noted in the chart, as are therapeutic plans until the next evaluation.

POSTOPERATIVE CHECK

To be made after the patient leaves the recovery room and before the PA leaves for the day.

- Time and date
- Vital signs
- Verbalized complaints, if any
- Physical findings
  - Neurologic (alertness, any gross deficits)
  - Lungs
  - Heart
  - Abdomen (be extremely gentle after abdominal operation)
  - Incision/dressing (do not remove dressings unless severe bleeding is noted)
  - Extremities (lesions, swelling)
- I/O (urine output, emesis, NG, and drain output)
- Postoperative laboratory findings or other diagnostic studies
- Assessment
- Treatment plan

Morning Rounds

A PA surgical assistant's day begins early, with evaluation of assigned patients *before* the surgical team meets for formal morning rounds. The nursing staff that follows the patient through the night should be consulted often and should be encouraged to discuss their assessment of the patient's progress. A clipboard, personal digital assistant (PDA), or index card system can help maintain an updated log on each patient's serial laboratory findings and serum drug levels, radiologic and diagnostic evaluations, vital signs and daily weights, and intake and output records. A reliable system will help alert the team to any abnormal trends. The team should know the medications and dosages of each patient, including the number of days the patient has been taking critical medications such as antibiotics.

Formal rounds involve seeing the patients with the rest of the team. The previous day's notes should be reread, and the PA or PA student should anticipate questions from the attending residents or interns, which could range from, "What were the patient's intake and output?" to "What are the most common etiologies of this patient's disease process?" A textbook is a good source for gaining understanding of the patient's disease and should be read as soon as the patient is assigned to the team and a free moment occurs in the PA student's schedule.

Present the patient to the team with the following information: name, number of days after operation, procedure performed, important comorbid diseases, the overnight course, vital signs, input and output (I&O), pertinent laboratory and x-ray data, and weight (noting any change up or down). A list of the pertinent positive findings on PE, any problems noted, and what should be done for the patient that day, such as advancing the diet, removing tubes, ordering laboratory or radiological studies, discharge, and preoperative preparation, should be compiled. The presentation should be concise.

The orders and notes may have been written or will need writing after rounds. Postoperative chart documentation is an important part of the medical legal record (Table 25-3). Surgeons are prone to writing abbreviated notes to save time. Brevity may be efficient for charting in surgery, but remember that all patient complaints need to be fully evaluated and documented in the chart.

Postoperative notes (aside from the brief note written for the first postoperative check) or daily progress notes always contain two important accounting dates at the top of each note: the number of days since surgery (postoperative day [POD]; day 1 is the day *after* surgery) and the number of days of antibiotic therapy and the names of antibiotics. Patient status after whichever procedure (status post or "S/P") follows. The postoperative note follows the typical SOAP format described in other chapters and is briefly reviewed here. Emphasis should be given to the patient's pain control, diet, nausea or vomiting, bowel function, ambulatory status, and vital signs, which can all be used as indicators of the patient's progress.

SOAP Format for Postoperative Notes

Subjective. Patient comments may be passing flatus, eating well/ready to eat, nauseated, pain medications insufficient, feel good, feel bad, and so forth. The note should always include patient complaints. The examiner should also include any subjective observations of the patient; for instance, "Looks better."

Observation. The vital signs, total I&O (which includes an accurate accounting of oral intake), IV fluids, medications, drains, urine and stool, and daily weight should be recorded.

Record a general description of the patient (e.g., awake and alert, intubated, in bed, sedated).

The PE consists of auscultation of the heart and lungs and palpation of the abdomen. The extremities should also be checked for signs of DVT. The operative site and wound should be observed under aseptic or sterile conditions. The appearance of the wound (erythematous, dry, presence of bleeding or exudate, intactness of staples or sutures) should be recorded. All IV lines, tubes, and drains should be examined for signs of infection. The patient's mental status should also be noted (e.g., awake, confused, easily aroused).

Laboratory and other *diagnostic test results* are also reported here.

Assessment. A number of terms and phrases can be used to describe the patient's progress through recovery—stable, improved, worse, nauseated, pain well managed, diet progressing adequately; IV fluid volume and urine output are sufficient. All the patient's

CONTENTS OF POSTOPERATIVE (DAILY PROGRESS) NOTE

POSTOPERATIVE DAY (POD) # X; TYPE OF ANTIBIOTIC(S) AND NUMBER OF DAYS PATIENT HAS RECEIVED THEM

S(ubjective)

- Patient comments (include all complaints)
- Family and allied health observations
- General observations (e.g., "Looks better")

O(bservation)

- Vital signs
- Daily weight
- General
- I&Os
- Oral
  Drains
  IVF (intravenous fluids)
  NG tube
  Urine (since surgery if immediately postoperative; otherwise, per 24 hours)
- Important medications
- Laboratory test results
- X-ray findings
- Other (ventilation/pacemaker settings, etc., as applicable)
- Physical findings (mental status, surgical site, heart, lungs, abdomen, extremities, other as needed)

A(ssessment)

- How is the patient progressing? Any complications? Recommendations from consultants?

P(lan)

- What should be done for the patient (stop IV, increase dietary level, increase ambulation, dressing change, etc.)?

TABLE 25-3 **Charting Tips**

Purpose of chart notes	Daily checklist for writer Communication with other members of team Communication with other health care teams Documentation for historical reference Legal document
Important items to include	Give laboratory, x-ray, and other results in objective section, and use the assessment section to say whether values are normal, abnormal, etc. Date and time of EVERY note and order Signature; printed last name; title of writer; pager number may be useful to nursing staff Cosignature for student notes and orders
Important items to exclude	1. Editorial comments a. Would you want the patient to read what you have written? b. Would you want it read out loud in court? 2. Use of "VSS" (vital signs stable) or "stable" is not good documentation of patient status 3. Any mention of exact discharge date. Instead say, "Discharge when ..." or "Discharge if ..."

complaints should be addressed here as well, and conclusions should be drawn as to what may be the cause of each complaint. Evidence must be provided for any conclusions.

Plan. Actions or investigations needed to address any patient complaints are recorded here. Questions and suggestions for plans should be part of the verbal presentation to the team. However, no changes should be made until a senior team member has cleared the new orders.

Daily Considerations in Patient Care

Basic questions that need to be answered each day concerning the patient are as follows:

- Can the dietary level be advanced? Most patients proceed from nothing by mouth (NPO) to clear liquids to regular diet. Feeding usually resumes once the patient has bowel sounds, is passing flatus or has bowel movements, and mentions being hungry.
- Can the patient ambulate? Get up to sit in a chair? Use the bathroom or shower?
- Can any of the IV medications be given by mouth or stopped entirely?
- Can oxygen therapy be cut back or discontinued?
- Can any tubes be removed? NG tubes should be removed before feeding resumes. Urinary catheters are usually removed when accurate measurement of I&O is no longer necessary and the patient can take care of this function without assistance.
- Can the sutures or staples be removed?
- Can the drain(s) be removed? Wound drains are usually removed when the output is less than 30 mL per day.
- Are any laboratory, radiologic, or other diagnostic studies needed?
- Does the patient need respiratory, physical, or occupational therapy?
- Does the patient need a social worker or discharge planner to help arrange home care after discharge?

Notes on Wound Care

The initial operative dressing or bandage should stay in place for 2 to 4 days. If blood continues to soak through a dressing, fever appears, or wound pain increases, the wound should be examined promptly. Circling the shape of blood soaking through the bandage and observing further spread can indicate how brisk the bleeding is. Wounds that are left to heal by secondary intention should be packed with moist, isotonic saline-soaked gauze pads that are replaced every 8 hours. This process mechanically débrides the wound, allowing the removal of necrotic tissue and providing a clean bed for healing.

Common Postoperative Problems

There is no substitute for experience, but preparation and suspicion can assist in early detection of postoperative problems. PA students interested in surgery should find time during their surgical rotation, or should request a separate elective rotation, to care for patients in the surgical ICU. Encountering the spectrum and severity of SICU problems is an excellent means of learning about complex IV fluid infusion therapy, acid-base imbalance, electrolyte abnormalities, and physiologic monitoring systems. It also provides an opportunity to better understand and practice the techniques and theory of pulmonary ventilation, polypharmacy, and insertion and monitoring of invasive lines and devices.

Postoperative complications can be divided into two categories—those occurring as a result of altered physiology and preexisting disease and those created by the staff (iatrogenic). Complications can range from simple postoperative fever to bleeding and shock requiring resuscitation and reoperation.

Postoperative Fever. Fever is probably the most common postoperative dilemma the student will encounter on the surgical service. Fever is not normal in the postoperative patient, and any significantly elevated temperature must be evaluated. Febrile patients should receive a thorough PE, a chest radiograph, a urinalysis with culture and sensitivity, and a CBC with differential. Fever secondary to an infection or inflammation that is subsequently resolved by surgery (e.g., cholecystitis) should defervesce within several days after surgery. The patient with an oral temperature of 99.5° F probably can be watched for several hours in lieu of initiating a full diagnostic battery. However, high fever (>101.5° F [38.6° C]), tachycardia, decreased blood pressure, or diminished urinary output should be evaluated emergently by the senior staff and will require a full workup comprising the previously listed diagnostic tests with blood cultures to rule out sepsis.

Most postoperative fevers fall into the following etiologic categories (the "Four Ws"): wind, wound, water, and walk.

Wind. Temperature elevations during the first 48 hours are usually of pulmonary origin. Thus, the value of the cough, deep breathing, and incentive spirometry exercises should be taught preoperatively to all patients undergoing major surgery. The lungs are predisposed to be a source of fever because of the following:

1. Hypoventilation from general endotracheal anesthesia or the effects of narcotics.
2. The tendency to avoid coughing, secondary to pain (of note with abdominal and chest incisions).
3. Simply sedation.

A chest radiograph is obtained to evaluate for pneumonia and atelectasis due to alveolar collapse. Purulent sputum should be sent to the laboratory for Gram's stain and culture and sensitivity testing, including anaerobe identification.

Atelectasis is treated by encouraging the patient to cough and take deep breaths and by the use of incentive spirometry. Early patient mobilization and ambulation with assistance from physical therapy also helps prevent postoperative fever from a pulmonary source. Pneumonia can occur at any time during the postoperative course and should always be a part of the differential diagnosis for fever.

Wound. Wound infections, including intra-abdominal abscesses, usually declare themselves on the fourth through seventh postoperative days. In general, the sooner an infection manifests, the more virulent the pathogen and the more serious the sequelae. The dressing should be removed and the wound examined for purulent drainage, expanding erythema or induration, and, most important, increasing pain and tenderness at the operative site. The first indication of wound infection is increasing pain. Dark discoloration, blisters, and foul-smelling exudates are grim signs and should be evaluated by a senior team member. Removal of a single stitch or staple may allow the escape of trapped pus and introduction of a sterile swab into the wound to gently search for pockets of infection. Aerobic organisms cause most wound infections, but all exudates should be sent to the laboratory for aerobic and anaerobic microbial culture and sensitivity testing. Fungal infections occur, albeit rarely, and immunocompromised patients are at highest risk. Grossly infected wounds must be reopened and drained. Superficial infections may be managed with oral antibiotics after drainage, but most nosocomial infections demand parenteral antibiotics.

If no other source for a fever can be located, a CT scan or MRI may reveal the source. An intra-abdominal abscess may be difficult to diagnose. Abdominal trauma, undergoing a contaminated abdominal procedure (e.g., ruptured diverticulitis or appendix), a history of peritonitis, and the creation of an intestinal suture line (e.g., bowel resection with reanastomosis) are all potential sources of intra-abdominal abscess. CT-guided drainage or reoperation may be necessary.

Water. Indwelling urinary catheters cause most UTIs. They rarely cause sepsis unless the upper tract is involved. Upper UTI can manifest as fever, chills, and flank pain. A urine sample should be sent for a urinalysis along with aerobic and anaerobic culture and for sensitivity testing. Patients may complain of dysuria or frequency after an indwelling catheter has been removed; however, the results of the urinalysis should guide treatment. Elderly patients may have had a UTI before admission; this is more prevalent in men with bladder outlet obstruction and urostasis secondary to prostatic hypertrophy. Such patients may benefit from the insertion of a urinary catheter to drain the infected region.

Walk. DVT usually occurs around the 5th to 14th postoperative days. The best method of treating DVT and the subsequent catastrophic possibility of pulmonary embolism is prophylactic therapy through the use of intermittent external compression devices, gradient pressure leg stockings (see Figure 25-1), or pharmacologic agents such as subcutaneous heparin or heparin analogs. The index of suspicion should always be high for this disease because the physical findings may be unreliable. The patient's leg may be tender, hot, edematous, or indurated, but more commonly, no abnormalities are noted. Homans sign (pain in the calf when the foot is dorsiflexed) is rarely present.

The gold standard for diagnosis is the injection of radiopaque contrast material into a foot vein after application of a tourniquet on the proximal leg, which forces contrast material into the deep venous system. Complete blockage or irregularities of the normally smooth vein wall are diagnostic of DVT. Duplex scanning combines both Doppler and B-mode ultrasound imaging and is the quickest method by which to diagnose DVT. A positive duplex scan is grounds for instituting anticoagulation with heparin. Phlebography can be used to diagnose cases in which patients' results of duplex scans are equivocal. Patients with DVT should be considered for admission to the SICU for observation. All patients will require heparinization.

Other Causes of Fever. Abrupt, high, spiking fevers should lead to the evaluation of existing indwelling devices. All intravascular devices can cause fever if they become infected. Heart valves, IV catheters, central venous catheters, arterial lines, pulmonary artery catheters, and NG tubes (which may cause sinusitis) can be sources of infection. The physical findings may be subtle (mild erythema or cellulitis at the catheter entry site) or completely nonexistent. Heart valves can be evaluated by echocardiography and blood culture; a cardiology consultation should be requested if an infected valve is possible. *The possibility that the fever is caused by one of these devices should be strongly considered when the blood culture yields* Staphylococcus aureus.

Treatment dictates that the device be removed and 7 to 10 days of antistaphylococcal antibiotic coverage be initiated. An infectious disease consult may be warranted. Fevers from gram-negative infections usually defervesce quickly after removal of the foreign device, unless florid gram-negative sepsis has developed.

Avoiding Iatrogenic Problems. *A final word on a practical topic.* Many postoperative problems occur as a result of forgetting of the organized routine in the rush of managing a busy surgical service. Iatrogenic complications are almost always preventable with forethought and the development of a system for approaching every patient and his or her management. It is beyond this discussion to consider all iatrogenic omissions in the detailed context they deserve. The student is encouraged to address the evaluation and treatment of common postoperative problems through reading one of the texts listed in the Resources list and by gaining experience under the guidance of a senior surgical mentor.

These are a few pearls of wisdom for avoiding the common pitfalls of routine postoperative care:

- Know the I&O status of each patient and the IV solution's base composition, additives, and rate. *Vascular volume overload from inappropriate or overaggressive IV therapy is preventable.*
- Potassium is easily lost through the urine, NG tube, diarrhea, or vomitus, and intravascular potassium can be diluted by IV fluid replacement. IV fluids should include potassium to account for those losses. Even mild hypokalemia can cause prolonged bowel immotility (ileus) or cardiac arrhythmias in patients receiving digitalis.
- Tubes should be removed promptly when no longer needed. UTIs often result from urinary catheters left in place too long.
- All intravascular devices, incisions, and wounds should be inspected daily.
- Early ambulation and mobilization should be encouraged.
- Medication dosages for elderly patients and patients with renal or liver failure should be titrated. Drug levels for aminoglycosides, vancomycin, or cardiopulmonary medications (e.g., digitalis, theophylline) should be monitored when appropriate.
- A thorough PE should be performed each day and with each call to evaluate a sick patient. Every attempt should be made to discover problems early in their evolution (e.g., congestive heart failure, sepsis, respiratory distress). Pulmonary embolism, myocardial infarction, or cerebrovascular accident should always be considered in patients with shortness of breath, chest pain, or unexplained hypotension.

CONCLUSION

The future of PAs in the health care arena is not only secure but also expanding within all aspects of medicine, including new and existing roles in the surgical theater. The ingenuity and resourcefulness of individual PAs will shape and expand the existing roles for the surgical PA. This responsibility lies not only in the hands of the PA but also in the hands of the supervising physician and the institutions that employ surgical PAs. As teaching hospitals cut back on the numbers of residency slots in surgery and try to meet restrictions on the number of hours worked by residents each week, it is conceivable that PAs will be expected to fill these vacant positions.

RESPONSIBILITIES OF THE PA STUDENT ON SURGICAL ROTATION

I. Give total care to each patient.
  A. Preoperative.
    1. Admission history and PE.
    2. Admission orders.
    3. Preoperative orders.
    4. Preoperative note.
    5. Insert IV lines, tubes, or catheters, if asked.
  B. Perioperative.
    1. Accompany patient to OR; first-assist or second-assist at procedure.
    2. Operative note.
    3. Postoperative orders.
    4. Postoperative check.
  C. Postoperative.
    1. Daily patient care.
      a. Early morning evaluation, assessment, plans for day, orders.
      b. Morning rounds with patient progress reports.
      c. Accompany patient to diagnostic procedures when feasible.
      d. Perform diagnostic and therapeutic procedures when feasible (NG intubation, arterial blood gases, venipuncture for laboratory studies, venous catheterization, spinal tap, thoracentesis, etc.).
      e. Write daily progress notes.

f. Quick afternoon assessment.
g. Evening rounds with report of daily activities, laboratory results, diagnostic study results, etc.
h. Check final pathology results (24-48 hours postoperatively).
i. Speak with the patient's family.

2. Assist with writing of discharge orders, prescriptions, and other discharge paperwork.
3. Date and time on all notes and orders.

II. Read about the patient's specific disease processes and planned procedure before surgery.
III. Attend all rounds, conferences, and lectures pertaining to the surgical service and surgical rotation.
IV. Be the patients' and families' advocate. Find answers to their questions; do not be afraid to say, "I don't know, but I'll find out."
V. Ask questions.

PAs are well suited for these tasks, and with proper supervision and direction from the surgical house staff and faculty, the PA can make the transition from physician resident to PA house staff smooth and uncomplicated for both the institution and the surgical teams involved. The cost-effectiveness and excellence in patient care exhibited by PAs in all aspects of medicine have been repeatedly verified and are emphasized by the dramatic increase in applications to, and the number of, PA programs across the nation. PA education must meet this challenge by incorporating into the curriculum options for PA students in surgical education and allowing students some aspect of freedom in choosing their clinical experiences. There is a demonstrated need for PAs in surgical health care today, and the program curriculum that meets this need will stand at the forefront of PA education and provide a strong and viable future that is versatile enough to meet changing health care environment demands.

CLINICAL APPLICATIONS

1. Identify the members of a typical surgical team and describe their functions.
2. Identify the members of a typical OR and recovery team and describe their functions.
3. Discuss the key elements of an admitting history and PE for a surgical patient.
4. Identify the elements and format of a preoperative and an operative note.
5. List three "rules" for maintaining the sterile field in the OR.
6. Identify the elements and format of a postoperative check and a postoperative daily progress note.
7. What do you think you would find personally challenging and rewarding about practice as a PA in surgery?

KEY POINTS

- PAs in a surgery setting are well respected and accepted.
- A PA student is part of the surgical team working alongside the interns and residents both in the operating theater and on the surgical wards.
- A solid understanding and knowledge of anatomy is essential to any surgical procedure.
- A PA student, as well as a seasoned surgical PA, must have an intricate knowledge of the instruments that are unique to the operating room.

References

1. American College of Surgeons. Statements on Principles. Qualification of the first assistant in the operating room. *www.facs.org/fellows_info/statements/stonprin.html#2b*.
2. Gerberding JL, Littell C, Tarkington A, et al. Risk of exposure of surgical personnel to patients' blood during surgery at San Francisco Hospital. N Engl J Med 1990;322:1788.
3. Wright JG, McGeer AJ, Chyatte D, Ransohoff DF. Mechanisms of glove tears and sharp injuries among surgical personnel. JAMA 1991;266:1668.
4. Quebbeman EJ, Telford GL, Hubbard S, et al. Risk of blood contamination and injury to operating room personnel. Ann Surg 1991;214:614.
5. Comaro A. Tiny holes, big surgery. Minimal surgery hurts less and scars less—but is it right for you? U.S. News and World Report 2002;133(3); Section: America's Best Hospitals, Special Report.

The resources for this chapter can be found at www.expertconsult.com.

CHAPTER 26

GERIATRIC MEDICINE

Freddi Segal-Gidan • Gwen Yeo

CHAPTER CONTENTS

This chapter provides an overview of geriatric medicine oriented to the beginning clinician, including basic information and clinical perspectives that are useful to the health care provider in approaching the social and medical complexities associated with care of the older person. The health care of elders in the United States presents the clinician with numerous challenges. In addition to the complex medical conditions, many older patients present with social, spiritual, economic, and political challenges. When these challenges are successfully met, however, physician assistants (PAs) in a geriatric practice can experience enormous satisfaction and provide an important contribution to the well-being of both patients and society.

Our society is growing older just as our medical care has become more sophisticated at an ever-increasing cost. By the year 2030, projections are that one in five Americans will be 65 years of age or older, and there will be twice as many people 65 and older as there were in 2000. This huge increase began in 2011 when the first cohort of baby boomers reached age 65.[1] These older Americans will also be increasingly diverse with one third of them belonging to one of the minority populations by mid-century. Medical practices are experiencing the effects of this increase in the older population just as many also experience fewer resources and more uncertainty about the structure of medical care in the future. PAs are providing an increasingly important role in general geriatric care, specialty care, and long-term care. The challenge to all PAs is to provide competent, cost-effective, functionally oriented, ethnically competent health care to each older person in their practice.

GERIATRIC CARE

Chronic Conditions

There are some significant differences in providing appropriate geriatric care that likely require PAs to make a clear shift in the goals they usually have in patient care. Because most of the health conditions older adults present with are likely to be chronic rather than acute, it requires the provider to concentrate on *management* in most cases rather than *treatment* in the expectation that the condition will be cured. Because the chronic conditions are not time limited, additional chronic diseases are frequently added, so geriatric clinicians are most often faced with trying to manage a patient's multiple conditions, which usually entail multiple medications as well. Figure 26-1 illustrates the most common chronic diseases experienced by older adults in the United States. The goal is to help elders maintain the highest possible function to maximize their quality of life in the context of their chronic conditions.

Functional Status

This emphasis on functional status is a critical component of good geriatric care and requires the clinician to use the measure of function as a constant tool. The two principal methods of functional assessment are determining the level of independence or dependence in performing activities of daily living (ADLs) and instrumental activities of daily living (IADLs). See Table 26-1 for a list of ADLs and IADLs and Figure 26-2 for the profile of Medicare enrollees who have limitations in either measure.

Dependence on ADLs is commonly used as a measure for eligibility for services such as nursing homes, adult day health care, or in-home support services. There are several different versions of the lists of ADLs and IADLs, but they all contain the basic activities. Scoring schemes vary from yes/no answers to questions such as, "Do you need help performing the following activities?" to five categories of dependence for each activity.[2]

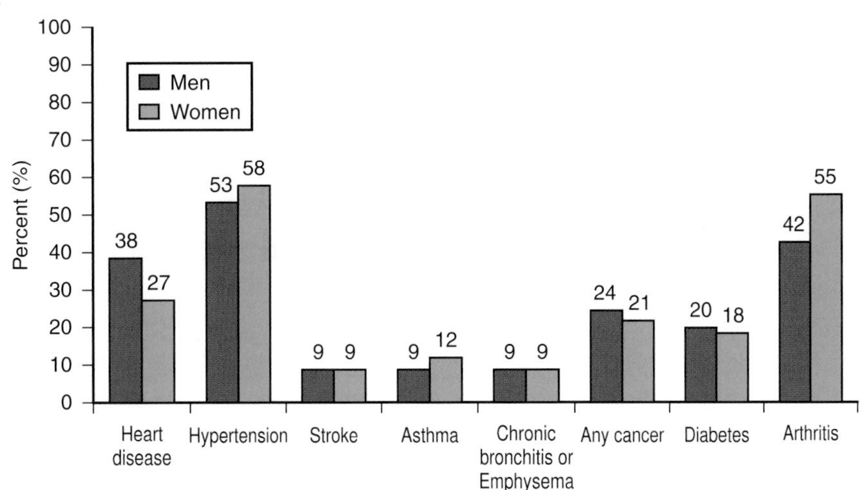

FIGURE 26-1 Chronic health conditions among the population, age 65 and older, by sex, 2007-2008. (From Centers for Disease Control and Prevention, National Center for Health Statistics, National Health Interview Survey.)

TABLE 26-1 Activities of Daily Living (ADLs) and Instrumental Activities of Daily Living (IADLs)

ADLs
Feeding
Dressing
Ambulation
Toileting/Continence
Bathing
Transfer (bed, chair, toilet)
IADLs
Cooking/Food preparation
Shopping
Laundry
Housekeeping
Using telephone
Managing medications
Ability to handle finances/money management
Transportation

In the routine clinical encounter, function needs to be a constant concern. Can a diabetic patient see well enough to be able to self-administer insulin? Can a patient easily swallow antibiotic tablets for bronchitis, or would a liquid be easier and promote compliance? Can a patient limited by arthritis remove the cap from the medication bottle or easily remove the tablets from the office samples given him or her? The question that should always underlie any change of condition or new diagnosis is, "How does this affect the person's ability to manage the activities of daily living?"

Time and Perspective

Geriatric practice often differs in time and perspective in that PAs working with geriatric patients frequently need to spend more time learning and understanding their patient's medical status. In many cases, care of older adults includes working with family members or other caregivers, which involves additional time

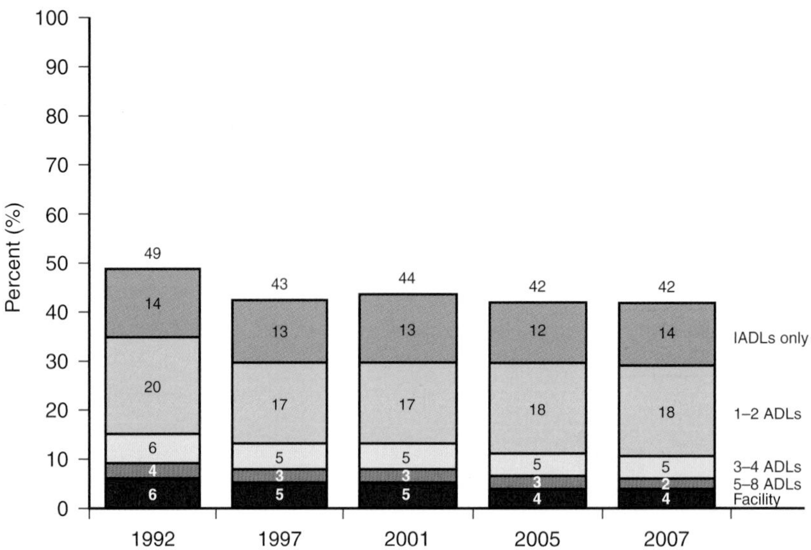

Note: The Medicare Current Beneficiary Survey replaced the national Long Term Care Survey as the data source for this indicator. Consequently, the measurement of functional limitations (previously called disability) has changed from previous editions of *Older Americans*. A residence (or unit) is considered a long-term care facility if it is certified by Medicare or Medicaid, has 3 or more beds, and is licensed as a nursing home or other long-term care facility and provides at least one personal care service or provides 24-hour, 7-day-a-week supervision by a nonfamily, paid caregiver. ADL limitations refer to difficulty performing (or inability to perform for a health reason) one or more of the following tasks: bathing, dressing, eating, getting in/out of chairs, walking, or using the toilet. IADL limitations refer to difficulty performing (or inability to perform for a health reason) one or more of the following tasks; using the telephone, light housework, heavy housework, meal preparation, shopping, or managing money. Rates are age adjusted using the 2000 standard population. Data for 1992 and 2001 do not sum to the totals because of rounding. Reference: These data refer to Medicare enrollees.

FIGURE 26-2 Percentage of Medicare enrollees age 65 and older who have limitations in activities of daily living or instrumental activities of daily living (IADL) or who were in a facility from 1992-2007. (From Centers for Medicare and Medicaid Services.)

and a unique set of skills. Time is often the critical factor in eliciting a thoughtful and comprehensive history, especially in cases with multiple chronic conditions. Many older patients need more time to disrobe and dress again. The PA may have to work into his or her schedule driving time to a patient in a nursing home whose condition has changed or for a routine continuity-of-care visit. When an older patient who is chronically ill develops an acute condition, a prior therapeutic relationship with the patient and a clear sense of the patient's baseline are extremely important because these enable the provider to identify the subtle signs (e.g., confusion, decreased appetite, listlessness) that may often be the only clues for a new underlying disease process. Although initially the PA may need to spend more time getting to know an elderly patient, he or she will find it easier to spot acute or chronic change and be able to preempt the problem. Once such a meaningful therapeutic patient/PA relationship has been established, the PA will be of enormous help to the physicians in that he or she will be able to establish the contextual framework for the patient's illness, thereby significantly increasing the overall efficacy of the practice (Table 26-2).

AGE-RELATED CHANGES

Aging is commonly viewed as the gradual loss of function and independence with increasing years. Successful aging is remaining active and functional in the physical, cognitive, and emotional realms until death.[3] The aging process depends on the complex interaction of genetics, disease, health habits (e.g., smoking and alcohol consumption), diet, and exercise. In differentiating disease from aging, it is important for PAs to have an understanding of important age-related changes that tend to occur even in those who have an active and healthy lifestyle. Common age-related changes are summarized by system in the sections that follow.

Sensory Changes

With older age, there is an increased incidence of cataracts and a consequent decrease in visual acuity resulting in, among other risks, an increased incidence of falls. There is an age-related reduction in the ability to hear higher frequencies (presbycusis), resulting in communication difficulties. When one is communicating with an older person who is known to have sensory impairment, it is important to speak slowly and clearly, sit close to the person, and make sure one's face is in the light. These simple measures can reduce confusion and anxiety and make for a more successful clinical encounter.

There also appears to be a decrease in acuity of taste with increasing age, so food tends to be perceived as bland. The clinical consequences can be a decreased appreciation for food and a loss of appetite, which can lead to significant weight loss and nutrition deficiency, and increased use of seasoning to enhance taste, such as salt or sugar, which can exacerbate underlying medical conditions and their treatment (e.g., hypertension, heart failure, diabetes). The aging skin is more porous, and therefore there is an increase in loss of body. The result is increased risk with ambient temperature changes for hypothermia and hyperthermia among the elderly and a propensity for dry skin (xerosis), skin breakdown, and ulcerations.

Cardiovascular Changes

The resting cardiac output does not change with age. However, there is a slight decrease in the heart rate and a compensatory increase in stroke volume. Heart rate response to exercise is decreased in the elderly secondary to a decrease in the beta-adrenergic response. Also, diastolic dysfunction may be seen during both rest and exercise in older adults. Systolic blood pressure tends to rise with age more than diastolic, and sustained elevations (hypertension) in either one or both increase the risk for stroke and heart disease.

Coronary artery disease is the most common cause of death among those 65 years and older. A well-balanced healthy diet and regular exercise have a tremendous positive impact on the cardiovascular changes associated with aging. A *reasonable* diet and exercise program should be strongly encouraged for persons in advanced years. They can increase their stamina and aerobic fitness level if they exercise regularly.[4]

Endocrine Changes

Aging is associated with deteriorating glucose tolerance changes, and peripheral glucose utilization is thought to be the major factor in this phenomenon.[3] Thyroid function is generally normal in physiologic aging, although older patients tend to have low triiodothyronine (T_3) levels. There is an increase of 2% to 5% in the prevalence of hypothyroidism in those older than age 65, and the prevalence continues to rise with age. The clinician should consider hypothyroidism when confronted with complaints of fatigue, depression, loss of initiative, confusion, dry skin, and constipation in an older patient. Serum parathyroid

TABLE 26-2 **10-Minute Screener for Geriatric Conditions**

Problem	Screening Measure	Positive Screen
Vision	Two parts: 1. Ask: "Do you have difficulty driving or watching television or reading or doing any of your daily activities because of your eyesight?" 2. If yes, then: Test each eye with the Snellen chart while the patient wears corrective lenses (if applicable)	Yes to question and inability to read >20/40 on Snellen chart
Hearing	Use audioscope set at 40 dB; test hearing using 1000 and 2000 Hz	Inability to hear 1000 and 2000 Hz in both ears, or inability to hear frequencies in either ear
Leg mobility	Time the patient after asking: "Rise from the chair. Walk 10 feet, turn, walk back to the chair, and sit down."	Unable to complete task in 10 sec
Urinary Incontinence	Two parts: Ask: "In the past year, have you ever lost your urine and gotten wet?" If yes, then ask: "Have you lost your urine on at least 7 separate days?"	Yes to both questions
Nutrition, weight loss	Two parts: Ask: "Have you lost 10 lb over the past 6 months without trying to do so?" Weigh the patient.	Yes to the question or weight < 100 lb
Memory	Three-item recall	Unable to recall all items after 1 minute
Depression	Ask: "Do you often feel sad or depressed?"	Yes to the question
Physical disability	Six questions "Are you able to do strenuous activities like fast walking or bicycling?" "... do heavy work around the house, like washing windows, walls, or floors?" "... go shopping for groceries or clothes?" "... get to places out of walking distance?" "... bathe, either a sponge bath, a tub bath, or a shower?" "... dress, including putting on a shirt, buttoning and zipping, and putting on shoes?"	No to any of the questions

From Moore AA, Siu AL. Screening for common problems in ambulatory elderly: clinical confirmation of a screening instrument. Am J Med 1996;100:438.
Modified from Kane RW, Ouslander JG, Abrass IB. Essentials of Clinical Geriatrics, 3rd ed. New York: McGraw-Hill, 1994.

hormone (PTH) increases in the elderly, and this increase correlates with a decline in vitamin D levels; treatment with 1,25-$(OH)_2$-D_3 results in a decrease in PTH levels. Age-related increases in PTH are thought to be a major factor accounting for age-related bone loss.

Immunologic Changes

There is an overall decrease in immunity with age, resulting in a greater prevalence of infections (e.g., pneumonia and urinary tract infections), shingles, gram-negative bacteremia, and severe episodes of influenza. Aging is accompanied by changes in both cellular and humoral immunity. The function of lymphocytes is altered with decreased proliferative capacity of T lymphocytes. Macrophage function is altered, and delayed-type skin hypersensitivity (DTH) declines. Elders will often present an atypical clinical picture, with absence of fevers, presence of hypothermia, altered eating patterns, delirium, and agitation in response to infection. They may also fail to mount a leukocytosis in response to an infection but will frequently have a left-shift in the face of a normal leukocyte count. The clinical implication is that even simple illnesses in the elderly need to be monitored closely and treated aggressively as indicated.

Renal Function

There is an overall decrease in kidney mass and loss of parenchymal mass over time. The total number of glomeruli decreases with age, and the renal vasculature undergoes sclerotic changes. All of these changes result in a progressively decreasing glomerular filtration rate (GFR). Concomitantly, with increasing age, there is a reduction in lean body mass, which results in decreased creatinine production. Therefore, the creatinine can continue to remain falsely low or "normal," even in the face of decreasing GFR and compromised renal function. Even the commonly used Cockcroft and Gault equation can lead to a mean underestimation of the measured creatinine clearance of 12.1 mL/minute in a group of healthy patients.[5] Therefore, calculated creatinine clearances should be avoided in the elderly in favor of short-duration, timed urine collections to measure the actual creatinine clearance. To avoid overmedication, any medicine excreted by the kidneys must be carefully considered for dosing and closely monitored.

$$\text{Creatinine clearance} = [140 - \text{age}] \times \text{Body weight in kilograms}/[72 \times \text{Serum creatinine}]$$

GERIATRIC SYNDROMES

Dementia

Dementia is the most common cause of mental decline with increasing age. Dementia is defined as an acquired syndrome of decline in memory (impaired ability to learn new information or recall previously learned information) and one or more other areas of cognitive function in the following list sufficient to affect daily life in an alert patient[6]:

- Aphasia (language disturbance)
- Apraxia (inability to perform complex movements)
- Agnosia (failure to recognize or identify objects)
- Executive function (judgment and reasoning, problem-solving)
- Visuospatial ability
- Calculation

Dementia affects the physical, psychosocial, and economic well-being of patients and their families, as well as society at large.

Alzheimer' disease (AD) accounts for approximately two thirds of all dementia cases, and vascular dementia (multiple infarcts in the cortical and subcortical gray matter and the internal capsule, or white matter demyelination in the cerebral cortex) causes an estimated 15% to 25% of dementia cases in the United States. In recent years, dementia associated with Lewy bodies (DLB—dementia plus parkinsonian signs, detailed visual hallucinations leading to secondary delusions and alterations of alertness or attention) and frontotemporal dementia (FTD) have received increased attention. As people age, they may experience such cognitive changes as slowing in information processing, where it takes longer or more repetitions to learn new information, but these kinds of changes are benign. In contrast, dementia is a progressive and disabling pathologic condition that is not considered part of normal aging.

Alzheimer disease is the most common and well-known form of dementia. It is estimated to affect 5.4 million people in the United States.[7] It is also expected that an estimated 14 million Americans will suffer from AD by the year 2040. The prevalence of AD increases with age with an estimated 6% to 8% occurring in patients 65 years of age or older and an estimated 30% noted among those age 85 or older.

Caregivers and patients often misinterpret initial symptoms of AD (e.g., memory loss) as normal age-related changes. The two greatest risk factors for AD are age and family history. Genetic mutations on chromosomes 1, 14, and 21 are responsible for the rare forms of familial AD that begin before age 60 (presenile or early-onset AD). The apolipoprotein E gene *(APOE)* on chromosome 19 is the only identified genetic risk factor presently for the more commonly occurring late-onset AD.

Gradual onset and progressive decline in cognitive functioning characterize AD. Motor and sensory functions are usually spared until late stages. Memory impairment, for new material, is a core symptom of any dementia, and this is seen even in the earliest stages of AD. Typical cognitive symptoms of AD include the following:

- Difficulty learning and retaining new information
- Disorientation, first to time and then to include place
- Language ability, particularly word finding
- Visuospatial dysfunction (getting lost)
- Impaired judgment and reasoning

The cognitive loss with dementia initially affects the patient's IADLs and then later their ADLs so that eventually the patient becomes completely dependent on others. Recognition of dementia may be further complicated by the presence of depression and the need for the PA to be aware of treatable conditions that can mimic dementia by their clinical presentation (Table 26-3). Patients with primary dementia commonly experience symptoms of depression, and depressed patients present with cognitive complaints that exceed objectively measured deficits.

TABLE 26-3 **Mnemonic for the Treatable Causes of Dementia**

D	Drugs
E	Emotional disorders
M	Metabolic or endocrine disorders
E	Eye and ear dysfunctions
N	Nutrition deficiencies
T	Tumor and trauma
I	Infection
A	Arteriosclerotic complications (myocardial infarction, congestive heart failure) and use of alcohol

Modified from Kane RW, Ouslander JG, Abrass IB. Essentials of Clinical Geriatrics, 3rd ed. New York: McGraw-Hill, 1994.

Dementia Workup. Patient and family member interviews and office-based clinical assessment are the most important diagnostic tools for dementia. This should include the following:

- A comprehensive history with special attention to the onset and rate of cognitive and functional change
- Use of validated screening tests of cognitive function (Table 26-4)
- Physical examination, with special attention to cardiovascular and neurologic function
- Laboratory evaluations (complete blood cell count [CBC], thyroid-stimulating hormone [TSH], Venereal Disease Research Laboratory [VDRL]) and vitamin B_{12} are recommended.[8] Brain imaging studies should be considered in patients if the following conditions apply:
  - Dementia onset occurs at an age younger than 65 years.
  - The condition is post acute (symptoms have occurred < 2 years).
  - Focal neurologic deficits are present.
  - The clinical picture suggests normal-pressure hydrocephalus (triad of onset within 1 year, gait disorder, and unexplained incontinence).

Management of Dementia. Primary treatment goals for patients with dementia are to enhance and preserve quality of life and to optimize functional performance by improving cognition, mood, and behavior.[9] Working closely with the patient and caregivers to establish a trusting relationship and a therapeutic alliance facilitates management. Current recommendations are for pharmacologic therapy to be started early in the disease process, beginning with an acetylcholinesterase inhibitor and then adding an *N*-methyl-d-aspartate (NMDA) agonist:

- Acetylcholinesterase inhibitors NMDA glutamate agonist

TABLE 26-4 **Mental Status Screening Tools**

Instrument
Folstein Mini Mental State Examination (MMSE)
Modified Mini-Mental State Examination (3MS)
Montreal Cognitive Assessment (MOCA)
Mini-Cog Screening
St. Louis University Mental Status (SLUMS)

- Donepezil (Aricept) memantine (Namenda)
- Rivastigmine (Exelon)
- Galantamine (Reminyl)

Nonpharmacologic treatments, such as physical and cognitive stimulation and reminiscence therapy, are also important components. It is of critical importance that clinicians initiate discussion about long-term health and financial care plans while the patient is still in the early stages of dementia when he or she can participate in these crucial decisions. Caregivers are often subject to enormous stresses and should be referred to caregiver support groups which have been shown to be effective in alleviating stress and preserving caregiver health. Respite care and other community resources like dementia adult day care offer caregivers relief and help postpone patient institutionalization. Familiarity with community resources and referral to social work care management or organizations such as the Alzheimer's Association is an essential component of care for patients with dementia and their families.

Delirium

Delirium or an "acute confusional state" is a common geriatric syndrome that is often overlooked and underdiagnosed. Up to one third of all hospitalized elderly patients exhibit some level of delirium.[10] Delirium is an independent risk factor for poor medical outcomes in the elderly. An advanced age, history of dementia, poor functional status, and sensory impairment are known predisposing factors for delirium. The Confusion Assessment Method (Table 26-5) is a practice and useful tool for detecting delirium, particularly among institutionalized elderly.[11] Acute infection, postoperative state, acute myocardial infarction, and alcohol withdrawal are common precipitating factors. Iatrogenic delirium is extremely common among the elderly, and drugs with anticholinergic effects are some of the most common culprits. Other causative drugs include antihistamines, antiparkinsonism drugs, benzodiazepines, and

TABLE 26-5 Confusion Assessment Method

For a diagnosis of delirium, a patient must have:
1. Presence of an acute and fluctuating course
   and
2. Inattention
   and either
3. Disorganized thinking OR
4. Altered level of consciousness

Source: Inouye SK, van Dyk CH, Alessi C, et al. Clarifying confusion: the confusion assessment method. A new method for the detection of delirium. Ann Intern Med 1990;113:941.

H_2-blockers. Management of delirium includes the following:
- High index of suspicion and early identification
- Withdrawal of suspected offending drug/drugs (if any)
- Treatment of the underlying cause
- Supportive care, including a well-lit, safe, and familiar environment
- Reassurance for both the patient and the family

CASE STUDY 26-1

Mr. S is an 88-year-old white male veteran with a medical history that includes AD, mild hypertension, and gallbladder disease status post cholecystectomy (35 years ago). The Veterans Affairs (VA) geriatric clinic interdisciplinary team was familiar with Mr. S, having cared for him for the past 3 years. His AD had been diagnosed 5 to 6 years ago. He had initially lived by himself, but as his AD progressed, his daughter Sandy, who is his surrogate decision-maker, moved him to a residential care facility. Over the past year, Mr. S seemed to be deteriorating, with increased memory problems and difficulty recognizing acquaintances, as well as needing some help with ADLs. His recent Mini-Mental State Examination (MMSE) was 17/30 (his education level was high with a master's in aeronautic engineering).

Sandy brought Mr. S to clinic and requested to see only the geropsychologist, saying, "Today, Daddy's issues are not medical problems; it is purely psychiatric." The residential facility staff had noted that the patient had become confused and agitated over the past week. His confused mood was noted to wax and wane over the course of the day. The agitation had not been related to any particular events, nor had there been any new employees or any other changes in residential care routines. On two notable occasions, Mr. S was heard screaming out, "Fire! Fire!" and one night, he actually dialed 911 and reported a fire in the facility, which had led to a police investigation of the premises. Further history revealed that the residential facility staff had in fact noticed that he had been eating poorly. He was afebrile and otherwise asymptomatic.

Patient's medications:
Lisinopril, 10 mg per day
Multivitamin, 1 tablet per day
Tylenol, 500 mg, three times daily, for arthritis
No history of other over-the-counter medications or herbal medications
Allergies: No known drug allergies
Physical examination: Mr. S was able to recognize his primary care physician (PCP) but seemed listless. When asked about the fire episode, he became agitated and repeatedly said, "Fire! Fire," and was clutching his groin region while saying this. His daughter Sandy was embarrassed at this and admonished her father for this behavior.
Vitals: Temperature of 97.6° F, BP 134/82, RR 12, and HR 76
Head, eyes, ear, nose, throat: Normocephalic, atraumatic. Pupils reacting equally to light and accommodation
Neck: Supple with trachea in the midline
Chest: Clear to auscultation bilaterally
Heart: Regular rate and rhythm with no murmur, rub, or gallop
Abdomen: Soft, positive for bowel sounds, mild diffuse tenderness to percussion, especially in the suprapubic region with voluntary guarding to palpation
Extremities: No cyanosis, clubbing, or edema
Rectal examination: Significantly enlarged hard, nodular prostate with guaiac-negative stool

DISCUSSION

At this point, the physician believed that Mr. S's enlarged prostate had probably caused urine retention with a secondary urine infection confirmed by the suprapubic tenderness. His delirium was thought to have been secondary to urinary tract infection. A bladder scan determined that Mr. S's postvoidal residue was 280 mL. The result of the stat urinalysis was consistent with a urinary tract infection, and Mr. S was started on a course of antibiotics, tamsulosin and phenazopyridine hydrochloride (Pyridium).

Of bigger concern was the newly diagnosed prostate enlargement. A prostate-specific antigen was ordered, and a follow-up appointment was scheduled for 2 weeks. Over the next several days, Mr. S's confusion lessened, but he continued to remain weak and listless. His prostate-specific antigen (PSA) came back as significantly elevated at 125 units. A clinical diagnosis of prostate cancer was made, and the geriatrician offered to refer Mr. S to a urologist for further workup. Because the patient was deemed incompetent to make any medical decisions, further discussions were held with his daughter, who was his durable power of health care attorney. After several discussions with Sandy, a bone scan was performed and showed extensive bony metastasis. Sandy refused further workup of the presumed prostate cancer because her father had previously specifically expressed the wish not to have any invasive medical procedures. A prostate biopsy was therefore not an option. Mr. S continued to deteriorate rapidly and was admitted to the VA Inpatient Hospice Unit for comfort care. He died peacefully 2 weeks later, and an autopsy confirmed the diagnosis of metastatic prostate cancer.

Urinary Incontinence

Unfortunately, incontinence is frequently not mentioned by patients and is not often asked about by providers. It is all too often mistakenly assumed by patients to be a normal function of aging. In reality, it is not inevitable and is usually treatable. Urinary incontinence of one or more episodes in the past month affects about 20% of people older than age 60, 50% of those in institutions, and twice as many women than men.[12] One third to half of affected patients have never sought medical attention for incontinence.

The adverse effects of incontinence can be extremely troubling, resulting in skin breakdown, frequent urinary tract infection, and falls from an unsteady gait rushing to the toilet or slipping on some urine. The psychological impact of incontinence can lead to social isolation and depression. There can be tremendous stress on the caregivers, and the resulting dependency can result in institutionalization.[13] The economic costs can be considerable when supplies, laundry, labor, and the medical cost of managing complications are totaled. The total direct costs alone have been estimated at more than $14 billion per year in the United States alone.[14,15]

Incontinence can be classified as acute or chronic. Acute incontinence in an otherwise healthy person is usually secondary to infection or inflammation (e.g., atrophic vaginitis, urethritis). It is important to note that the differential diagnosis for acute incontinence covers a wide range of possibilities, including restricted mobility.

The principal types of chronic urinary incontinence can be categorized as stress, urge, overflow, functional, or mixed, involving more than one type.

Stress Incontinence. Involuntary loss of urine, usually a small amount, secondary to increased intra-abdominal pressure from a cough or laugh. Common causes are weakness and laxity of the pelvic floor musculature and weakness of the bladder outlet or urethral sphincter

Urge Incontinence/Overactive Bladder (OAB). Leakage of urine, usually a large amount, due to the inability to delay voiding after the sensation of bladder fullness is perceived. Common causes are detrusor muscle instability, alone or associated with a local genitourinary condition (urinary tract infection, urethritis, tumor, stones) and central nervous system disorder (parkinsonism, cerebrovascular accident, dementia).

Overflow Incontinence. Leakage of urine results from mechanical forces in an overdistended bladder. Common causes are anatomic obstruction (urethral stricture secondary to benign prostatic hypertrophy or cystocele), acontractile bladder (associated with diabetes or spinal cord injury), and neurogenic bladder (result of detrusor-sphincter dyssynergia associated with multiple sclerosis and other suprasacral cord lesions).

Functional Incontinence. The inability to toilet due to impaired cognitive or physical function, environmental barriers, or psychological unwillingness (depression, anger, or hostility).

The PA's approach to incontinence should include the following measures:

- A thorough history to quantify the amount of urine lost and circumstances of the incontinent episodes sufficient to affect daily life in an alert patient.
- A physical examination, including abdomen, genital, rectal, and neurologic screening and mobility/joint examination.
- Laboratory assessment of urine with culture and sensitivity testing.
- Other laboratory tests or referral to a specialist (gynecologist, urologist, neurologist) depending on history and physical findings.

Management of urinary incontinence is usually based on the classification or type. For the most common types affecting older women—stress and urge—the nonpharmacologic, noninvasive behavioral intervention known as *pelvic floor muscle training* or *Kegel exercises* has been found in a majority of cases to substantially reduce or eliminate incontinence problems.[16] PAs can improve the quality of life of many of their older patients who have lost control of their urination by giving them the instructions described in Box 26-1, and then scheduling regular follow-up visits to monitor and reinforce their progress. Pharmacologic intervention with anticholinergic,

BOX 26-1 INSTRUCTIONS FOR PELVIC MUSCLE (KEGEL) EXERCISES

Identifying and Contracting (Tightening) Your Pelvic Muscle

The pelvic muscle is the muscle you tighten to stop your urine flow and to keep from passing gas or, if you are a woman, to "pull up" your vagina. Women can easily feel if they are tightening this muscle by placing one or two fingers in their vagina and contracting around their fingers.

It is important to be able to contract your pelvic muscle without contracting your abdominal muscles, which could cause you to leak urine. To determine if you are tightening your abdominal muscles, place a hand on your abdomen while you tighten your pelvic muscles. If you feel your abdomen tighten, you need to practice relaxing your abdomen while continuing to contract your pelvic muscles.

Practicing Pelvic Muscle Exercises

First, empty your bladder. Sit or lie in a comfortable place and relax for a minute. Then, tighten your pelvic muscle (without tightening your abdomen). Keep it tight for 10 seconds. Relax for 10 seconds. Repeat for a total of 15 contractions. Do these 15 contractions three times each day. If you are not able to hold the muscle tight for 10 seconds or are unable to repeat 15 times, just do it as many times as you can. Your ability to perform the exercise will improve with time.

What to Expect

The benefit increases the longer you practice the exercises. Most women notice a decrease in their frequency of incontinence within 4 to 6 weeks. Studies have shown that this exercise program is effective in reducing incontinence by an average of 70% and completely eliminates incontinence in about one third of women after 6 incomplete weeks. As the exercises become familiar, you can practice them anytime, such as when you are watching television, driving, or in bed.

If Incontinence Persists

If incontinence persists, there are additional treatment options of medication or surgery that you may want to discuss with your doctor.

antimuscarinic medications such as oxybutynin, tolterodine, solifenacin, darifenacin, tropsium, and fesoterodine are commonly used for urge incontinence if the behavioral interventions are unsuccessful. The side effects that profile these agents (dry mouth, constipation, dry eyes, blurred vision) limit their tolerability in the elderly.

Instability and Falls

Falls account for a significant number of cases of injury and death among the elderly. Accidents are the sixth leading cause of death among the elderly, and falls account for two thirds of accidental deaths.[17] Besides the acute trauma noted in patients who present in the emergency department or office, a significant number of falls with resulting soft tissue injury and psychological stress occur and are unreported. This leads to decreased independence, a reduced sense of autonomy, and for some, a fear of falling again that can be disabling.

Falls are a multifactorial problem in the elderly.

The intrinsic factors affecting stability and predisposing an older person to falls include the following:

1. Changes in vision, including depth perception and acuity
2. Decreased proprioception
3. Decreased lower-extremity muscle strength
4. Increased postural sway
5. Changes in gait, both speed and height of step
6. Almost any disease process that exacerbates the expected aging changes, especially dementia, depression, cardiovascular disease, arthritis, podiatric problems, diabetes, peripheral neuropathy, and stroke

The extrinsic factors play an important role in falls and include the following:

1. Poor lighting
2. Irregular surfaces (cracks in the sidewalk, short or irregular steps)
3. Slick surfaces (throw rugs)
4. Furniture too high or too low
5. Bathroom fixtures without support bars or at an inappropriate height

Patients who have fallen require a careful and complete medical evaluation, including assessment of orthostatic blood pressure changes, cardiovascular status, neurologic deficits including mental status, musculoskeletal conditions, foot disorders, and sensory deficits (especially visual). A careful review of medications, particularly psychotropic agents, and nonprescription/over-the-counter, along with prescription medication, is especially important for those elderly patients who report a history of falls.

Fall prevention strategy requires attention to those factors that can be medically or surgically corrected (e.g., cataract surgery, medication adjustment). Observation of the patient arising from a chair and walking ("Get Up and Go Test") is an essential component of fall prevention and evaluation. Physical disabilities can be addressed with physical therapy and, if appropriate, assistive devices such as walkers and canes. A home health nursing evaluation or a home visit by the PA may help identify and address the extrinsic factors. Community resources like the senior center and Area Agency on Aging (AAA) often provide information on low-cost installation of bathroom and hallway bars.

Eight key factors found to influence falls in the elderly have been identified[18]:

1. Postural hypotension
2. Use of sedative/hypnotic medication
3. Use of more than four medications
4. Toilet and bathtub safety
5. Environmental hazards
6. Abnormal gait, transfers, and balance
7. Lower- and upper-extremity strength and range of motion
8. Foot problems

Exercise plays an important role in the prevention of falls. Studies demonstrate that even the very old (80+) can benefit from exercise and weight training. Even the practice of Tai Chi has been shown to improve balance, leading to reduced incidence of falls.[19]

COMMON PROBLEMS IN GERIATRIC CARE

Screening and Health Promotion

Preventive health practices are an important, and often overlooked, part of caring for older adults. Cancer is the second major cause of death in people older than 65 years of age, following cardiovascular disease.[20] Leukemia, as well as cancer of the digestive tract, breast, prostate, skin, and urinary tract, increases in incidence up to the age of 84. PAs should take every opportunity when caring for an older patient to incorporate primary and secondary disease prevention strategies into both routine and episodic care. These include screening for common age-related diseases (hypertension, diabetes, osteoporosis, hyperlipidemia) and updating immunizations (tetanus, pneumonia, herpes zoster). Table 26-6 lists comprehensive recommendations for screening and health promotion strategies for older adults.

Complications of Pharmacotherapy

CASE STUDY 26-2

Mrs. S is a 72-year-old widow who lives alone in an apartment complex. Her two sons live nearby. In her early 20s she was diagnosed as having schizophrenia and has had several hospitalizations over the years, but overall she has been well managed with medications and ongoing psychiatric care. Currently she has been experiencing increased paranoia and agitation. During the past 10 years, Mrs. S has also been diagnosed as having congestive heart failure, hyperparathyroidism, hypertension, and chronic obstructive pulmonary disease.

One day, she is brought into the office by her older son, who reports that her landlady found Mrs. S wandering in the snow, talking incessantly, disoriented, tearful, and apparently hallucinating. She had fallen several times on the ice. Her face is flushed and she is lightly clad, even though it is cold outside. Her temperature is 102° F, pulse and respirations are rapid, and pupils are dilated. She is apparently agitated but cannot speak above a whisper. She appears frightened but recognizes and embraces the doctor. Her lips and mucous membranes are bone-dry. Examination reveals the following: bruises over the arms and legs and on the forehead; lung fields clear, heart-sinus tachycardia, no murmur, moderate cardiomegaly; abdomen—no organomegaly, no tenderness or decreased bowel sounds, and a hard stool in the rectum.

Mrs. S's son has brought all her current medications as he was instructed to do when he phoned for the same-day appointment. The following medication bottles are pulled from the bag: digoxin, 0.125 mg daily; potassium (Slow-K); furosemide (Lasix), 20 mg twice daily; Fleet Phospho-Soda, 1 tsp three times daily; oxybutynin (Ditropan XL) 10 mg, once daily; olanzapine (Zyprexa) 7.5 mg twice daily; one propantheline bromide (Pro-Banthine), 15 mg before meals; thioridazine (Mellaril), 50 mg three times daily; amitriptyline (Elavil), 75 mg before bed; ibuprofen (Motrin), 400 mg three times daily; flurazepam (Dalmane), 15 mg before bed, as needed; and benztropine mesylate (Cogentin), 2 mg twice daily.

TABLE 26-6 **Summary of Preventive Medicine and Screening Recommendations for Older Adults***

Maneuver	Evidence†	Recommendation (Source)	Grade†
Screening‡			
Blood pressure	I	Every examination at least every 1-2 yr (USPSTF)	A
Physician breast examination	I	Annually after age 40 (ACS, USPSTF)	A
Mammogram	I	Annually after age 50 (ACS) or every 1-2 yr, ages 50-69 (USPSTF, ACP); continue every 1-3 yr, ages 70-85 based on life expectancy (AGS, USPSTF)	A;C > age 69
Pelvic examination/Pap smear	II	Every 2-3 yr after 3 negative annual examinations; can be discontinued after age 65-69 (ACS, USPSTF, CTF, AGS)	A;C > age 65
Cholesterol	I-III	Adults every 5 yr (NCEP); less certain for elderly	B; C > age 65
Rectal examination	II	Annually after age 40 (ACS)	C
Fecal occult blood test	II	Annually after age 50 (ACS)	B
Colonoscopy	II	Every 10 yr age 50-75 (ACS)	B
Visual acuity test	III	Periodically in older adults (various)	B
Test/inquire for hearing impaired	III	Periodically in older adults (various)	B
Mouth, nodes, testes, skin, heart, lung examinations	III	Annually (ACS, AHA)	C
Glucose	III	Periodic in high-risk groups (USPSTF)	C
Thyroid function	III	Clinically prudent for elderly, especially women (USPSTF)	C
Electrocardiogram	III	Periodically after age 40-50 (AHA)	C
Glaucoma screening	III	Periodically by eye specialist after age 65 (USPSTF)	C
Mental/functional status	III	As needed; be alert for decline (USPSTF)	C
Bone mineral density (women)	III	Once after age 65, then as needed (USPSTF)	C
Prostate examination/ prostate-specific antigen	III	NR; Symptomatic after age 50. Not after age 75 (USPSTF)	C-D
Chest radiograph	III	If needed for treatment decision (USPSTF)	D
Prophylaxis/Counseling			
Exercise	I-II	Encourage aerobic and resistance exercise as tolerated (USPSTF, AHA)	A
Tetanus-diphtheria vaccine	I-II	1 series, then booster every 10 yr (ACP, USPSTF)	A
Influenza vaccine	I-II	Annually after age 65 or chronically ill (ACP, USPSTF)	B
Pneumovax	II	23-valent at least once after age 65 (ACP, USPSTF)	B
Herpes zoster			
Calcium	II	800-1500 mg/day (various)	B
Aspirin	I-II	Men after age 50, 80-325 mg every day, every other day (various) (USPSTF)	C

From American College of Physicians (ACP), American Cancer Society (ACS), American Geriatrics Society (AGS), American Heart Association (AHA), Canadian Task Force (CTF) of the Periodic Health Examination, National Cholesterol Education Program (NCEP), U.S. Preventive Services Task Force (USPSTF), and authors' interpretation of the literature.

Modified from Goldberg TH, Chavin SI. Preventive medicine and screening in older adults. J Am Geriatr Soc 1997;45:351.

*Recommendations on prevention and screening in older adults, summarized from this paper and other literature.

†Grades of evidence and recommendations adapted primarily from U.S. Preventive Services Task Force. Grades are those given by the Task Force except when none are available and grades are assigned by authors.

‡Screening recommendations apply only to asymptomatic individuals; specific clinical circumstances may necessitate different testing and treatment schedules. Where no upper age limits are listed, screening should continue until approximately age 85 or when the patient is not a treatment candidate because of limited active life expectancy/quality.

NR, Not recommended for routine screening in asymptomatic individuals, although it may be useful when clinically indicated.

Mrs. S is hospitalized, and all medications are stopped. Infection, injury, and thyroid, diabetic, and metabolic/electrolyte imbalances are ruled out. Over the course of a week, she returns to normal. The diagnosis of anticholinergic psychosis is confirmed.

In later discussions with Mrs. S and with the psychiatrists and other physicians who treated her, the PA pieces the following history together. Different doctors had seen her at different times, and each had given her medications for the current complaint without looking at the entire set of medications. When she began showing symptoms that could have been adverse effects of previous medications, such as depression or agitation, new drugs were added for those symptoms. Primary care providers had been hesitant to change her psychiatric medications, and psychiatrists left adjusting her somatic drugs to her other providers.

How could this happen? Unfortunately, this is not uncommon. Some examples of these causes include elderly patients taking a large number of over-the-counter medications in addition to those prescribed by different providers. Confusion is a common reaction to toxic medication levels and drug interactions in the elderly. Family members and others often attribute confusion to "just getting old" or "senility" and are unaware of the various medications prescribed for their loved ones. For appropriate prescription practices and avoidance of polypharmacy, the following recommendations have been made to health care providers by the American Geriatrics Society[2]:

Obtain a Complete Drug History. Be sure to ask about previous treatments and responses, as well as about other prescribers. Ask about allergies, over-the-counter (OTC) drugs, nutrition supplements, alternative medications, alcohol, tobacco, caffeine, and recreational drugs.

Avoid Prescribing before a Diagnosis Is Made Consider nondrug therapy. Eliminate drugs for which no diagnosis can be identified.

1. *Review medications regularly and before prescribing a new medication.* Discontinue medications that have not had the intended response or are no longer needed. Monitor the use of as-needed and OTC drugs. Know the actions, adverse effects, and toxicity profiles of the medications you prescribe. Consider how these might interact with or complement existing drug therapy.
2. Start long-term drug therapy at a low dose, and titrate dose on the basis of tolerability and response. Use drug blood levels when available.
3. *Attempt to maximize dose before switching or adding another drug.* Use combination medications cautiously. Encourage compliance with therapy. *Educate patients and/or caregivers about each medication*, the regimen, the therapeutic goal, its cost, and potential adverse effects or drug interactions. Provide written instructions.
4. Avoid using one drug to treat the adverse effects of another.
5. Attempt to use one drug to treat two or more conditions.
6. *Communicate with other prescribers.* Do not assume that patients will—they assume you do!
7. Avoid using drugs from the same class or with similar actions (e.g., alprazolam, solpidem).

Dizziness and Syncope

Dizziness can be classified as follows:

- Vertigo (rotational sensation)
- Presyncope (impending faint)
- Disequilibrium (loss of balance without head sensation)
- Lightheadedness

Benign positional vertigo (BPV) is a common cause of dizziness among the elderly and manifests as episodic dizzy spells that are usually precipitated by changes in position, such as turning, rolling over, getting into and out of bed, or bending over. These are often brief (5 to 15 seconds), usually relatively mild and self-limited. Presyncope is the sensation of near-fainting caused by diminished cerebral perfusion; it occurs secondary to cardiac causes (arrhythmias), vascular causes (orthostatic hypotension), or vagal stimulation, which in some cases can result in syncope (micturition syncope). Syncope is defined as a sudden, transient loss of postural tone and consciousness not due to trauma and with spontaneous full recovery. Like presyncope, syncope is generally caused by a reduction in cerebral perfusion. The clinical history, physical examination, and electrocardiogram have been found to be the most useful steps in evaluating syncope,[21] and they should be used in most patients to determine whether further testing is necessary.

Sleep Problems

Difficulty falling asleep, nighttime awakening, early morning awakening, and daytime sleepiness are common sleep disorders experienced by the elderly. Risk factors for sleep disturbance include chronic illness, mood disturbance, lack of physical activity, and increased physical disability. Older people report an earlier bedtime and an early awakening. They also report decreased total sleep time with fragmented sleep patterns characterized by frequent arousals during the night and diminished deep sleep (stages III and IV of sleep). Consequently, older patients may report dissatisfaction with the quantity and quality of their sleep and often attribute their low energy, easy fatigability, and excessive daytime sleepiness to poor nighttime sleep.

Screening Older Patients for Sleep Problems
The National Institutes of Health Consensus Statement on the Treatment of Sleep Disorders of Older People[22] recommends that the following three questions be asked:

1. Is the person satisfied with his or her sleep?
2. Does sleep or fatigue interfere with daytime activities?
3. Do the bed partner or others complain of unusual behavior during sleep, such as snoring, interrupted breathing, or leg movements?

Although a detailed account of the diagnosis and management of sleep problems is beyond the scope of this chapter, at minimum a thorough review of medications and medical conditions, with attention to impact on sleep, should be conducted. Long-term usage of sedative/hypnotics in older patients should be avoided because these are associated with many adverse effects, including secondary depression and increased incidence of falls with injury, especially hip fractures.

DEPRESSION

Depression is underdiagnosed and undertreated in the elderly.[23] Late-life depression has been found to be associated with higher than expected mortality rates and persistent impairment.[24] Older patients tend to be more preoccupied with somatic symptoms (e.g., constipation, insomnia, pain) and report depressed mood and guilty preoccupations less frequently, so depression may often be masked. The primary symptoms of depression, including persistent feelings of a sad mood (in the absence of normal causes like recent bereavement) and anhedonia or loss of pleasure, are hallmarks of depression and are helpful in the identification of depression in most medically ill patients.

The diagnosis of major depression in older persons is complicated by the overlap of symptoms of major depression with those of physical illness (e.g., weight loss, insomnia, loss of libido, changes in bowel habits). Debilitated patients and those with serious illness may be preoccupied by thoughts of death or worthlessness. The elderly are also often taking numerous medications (e.g., beta-blockers, steroids, H_2-blockers), which can complicate the picture even further. Certain medical conditions (e.g., hypothyroidism) that commonly occur in the older adult also predispose to depression. As individuals grow older, they often experience a loss of friends, family, personal function, economic resources, and social position. Any such loss (especially the loss of a spouse) can precipitate a reactive depression that should be addressed by the health care provider. To simply regard depression as a natural component of aging and to thereby dismiss it disregards the possible serious consequences.

Clearly, the identification of depression in the elderly is a diagnostic challenge. Untreated depression can significantly reduce the patient's quality of life and can cause immense suffering. Depression can result in increased morbidity and mortality in patients who have coexistent medical illnesses. Development of depression in patients following a myocardial infarction, congestive heart failure, or cardiac bypass surgery has been shown to increase mortality from cardiovascular events. Depression can impair judgment, leading to risks not usually taken and ultimately to an accident or fall. Lack of appetite and loss of sleep can seriously affect the frail elderly and exacerbate underlying disease. The withdrawal and apathy that may be the first signs of depression can result in severe social isolation and lack of self-care. Depression can precipitate a downward spiral of biologic and social events, ultimately leading to morbidity and death.

Depressed older patients with comorbid physical illness, who live alone, who are male, and/or who are alcoholic are at high risk for suicide. Persons aged 65 and older represent less than 13% of the population but account for 25% of suicides. The older depressed patient is more likely to attempt suicide, more likely to commit suicide violently (firearms and hanging), and more likely to succeed compared with younger counterparts. "Psychological autopsy" studies have shown that older adults who commit suicide were often suffering from a major depression. The vast majority had seen a primary care physician within 1 month of the act. Therefore, the need for frequent screening of the elderly patient for depression cannot be overemphasized. The short form of the Geriatric Depression Scale is a rapid and effective tool for screening the elderly patient for depression.

Steps in the diagnosis of depression in the older adult include the following:

1. A quick review of medications for possible depressive adverse effects (e.g., steroids, beta-blockers, benzodiazepines)

2. A social history focusing on recent changes in finances, living circumstance, new diagnosis of disease, and loss of friends or family
3. Screening with the short form of the Geriatric Depression Scale (GDS) (see Figure 26-2)
4. Focused history and physical examination for the early manifestations of disease or a change in existing disease
5. Screening of TSH to rule out hypothyroidism as appropriate

It is important to note that elderly who immigrate to the United States from other countries are at increased risk for depression. This is especially true if they come to live with younger family members and find themselves isolated at home most of the time while the others in their household are at work or if they come as refugees after having experienced traumatic events in their homeland. The availability of the GDS in multiple languages *(www.stanford.edu/~yesavage/GDS.html)* provides a tool that can help the PA when there is a lack of a common language for communication. One common difficulty in diagnosing depression among older immigrants is that the symptom complex may not be the same as those described in American psychiatric literature. Depressed Asian elders, for example, especially those from China or Southeast Asia, and Hispanics, have been found to be much more likely to present with somatic symptoms such as loss of appetite, sleep disturbances, and even headaches or stomachaches and to not reveal feelings of sadness or dysphoria.

Once depression has been diagnosed, appropriate treatment should be pursued. If necessary, referral to a psychiatrist or other therapist who specializes in the treatment of older adults should be considered. Depression is usually a treatable disease and should not be regarded as a hopeless circumstance to be endured and hidden. Antidepressant medication and psychotherapy have both been found to benefit older depressed patients.[25]

Older Women's Health

Currently, U.S. women can expect to live into their 80s and beyond. Many of the health risks that characterize these later years of life for women can be attributed to postmenopausal changes. Physiologic aging of the woman accelerates after menopause, especially in the genital tract. The ovarian follicular estrogen (estradiol) diminishes dramatically in the postmenopausal woman, and estrone—a low-potency estrogen derived from androstenedione—takes over as the major estrogen. Progesterone, derived mainly from the adrenals, also diminishes. The genital organs undergo atrophy, resulting in sclerotic ovaries, a smaller atrophied uterus, a pale foreshortened narrow vaginal canal (sometimes causing dyspareunia), and the loss of acidic vaginal pH, causing increased vulnerability to infection. Hormone replacement therapy (HRT), estrogen alone or combination of estrogen and progesterone, has been shown to be associated with a slightly increased risk of thromboembolic disease (blood clots and stroke) and breast cancer, as well as reduction in colon cancer and bone loss.[26] HRT is currently recommended for a limited time for the treatment of troubling postmenopausal symptoms (hot flashes, vaginal dryness).

Hormonal changes caused by menopause also result in accelerated osteoporosis, so by age 70 years, 50% of bone mass is lost in women, compared with men, who lose 25% of bone mass by age 80 years.[16] Recommendations include regular monitoring of bone density and use of estrogen agonists (Evista) or bisphosphonates. Increased levels of cholesterol, triglycerides, and low-density lipoprotein (LDL) and decreased levels of high-density lipoprotein (HDL) secondary to ovarian failure increase the older women's predisposition to heart disease.

SEXUALITY AND AGING

CASE STUDY 26-3

Mrs. C is 75 years of age and has been happily married for 15 years, after being widowed for 8 years. Her husband, who is in the end stages of Parkinson disease, is living in an assisted living facility because Mrs. C could no longer care for him by herself. Mr. C has become quite fond of one of the female assistants at the facility. In reviewing her circumstances with the PA, Mrs. C relates a history of physical closeness that she has cherished. When she and her husband retired to bed each night they would hold each other, kiss, and touch. They would talk and share the day's activities, as well as their hopes, dreams, and troubles. Now that her husband is unable to participate in that closeness, she says with sorrow, "When you grow old, you become withered and ugly. No one wants to touch you anymore."

As life expectancy increases, it is important to recognize that continued sexual activity is an essential component of old age in promoting satisfactory relationships and good quality of life. Many older patients maintain sexual interest and capacity as long as they have their health, a healthy partner, and a good relationship with that partner. Normal

change in sexual function in men is manifested in the following ways:
1. The need for more time for arousal
2. The need for more time for reaching orgasm
3. Less-rigid erections
4. Orgasms that last for a shorter time than when they were younger
5. Less force of ejaculation and less volume of ejaculate

Older women are often more concerned about their appearance and their desirability. Although women's multiorgasmic capacity remains throughout life, postmenopausal hormonal changes result in physical and psychological changes. In addition, older women are often primary caregivers for their aging partners and are often greatly burdened by caregiver stress syndrome. Because women tend to outlive their male counterparts, they may have difficulty finding good partners and meaningful relationships.

Often, there is a generational difference between the health care provider and the elderly patient that may cause some discomfort for both parties. The provider should approach the issue with an open-ended question that allows the patient to choose to participate and voice concerns or questions. For example, during the review of systems, the PA could ask, "Are there any sexual or relationship issues or questions you would like to discuss this visit?" A sensitively elicited sexual history; a focused physical examination as directed by the history; diagnosis and treatment of sexually transmitted diseases when present; and offering overall guidance and support continue to remain important components of care of the aging patient.

PROSTATE DISEASE

Benign prostatic hypertrophy (BPH) is one of the most common conditions among aging men, accounting for more than 1.5 million office visits and about 250,000 surgical procedures annually in the United States. A nonmalignant enlargement of the epithelial and fibromuscular components of the prostate gland that may result in irritative (frequency, urgency, nocturia) and/or obstructive (hesitancy, intermittency, weak stream, incomplete emptying) urinary symptoms is almost universal among older men. If left untreated, it can result in significantly diminished quality of life in the older man. Treatment options include lifestyle modification (avoidance of caffeine, decrease in late evening fluid intake); avoidance of problematic medications (e.g., anticholinergic drugs); and treatment with appropriate medications like alpha-adrenergic antagonists (e.g., doxazosin, terazosin, tamsulosin) and 5α-reductase inhibitors (finasteride). Surgery is reserved for patients who have severe symptoms that are refractory to medical treatment or for patients who are unable to tolerate the adverse effects of medication.

Prostate cancer is a cancer of old age. Its incidence increases with age and is rare in men younger than 40 years of age. Autopsy studies in which the entire prostate was examined have revealed histologic evidence of prostate cancer in 30% of men older than age 50 and 80% of men older than age 80. Prostate cancer usually arises in the peripheral zone of the prostate and remains asymptomatic in most patients, especially in the early stages. Currently, there is no direct evidence that early detection decreases mortality rates due to prostate cancer. Most men with prostate cancer die with the disease, not from it. Serum PSA is a nonspecific test, with elevations in PSA occurring in BPH and prostatitis and transiently in response to conditions such as ejaculation and prostatic massage, or even a digital rectal examination. The U.S. Preventive Services Task Force, the American College of Physicians, and the Canadian Task Force on the Periodic Health Examination have recommended *against* routine PSA screening for prostate cancer.

Acute bacterial prostatitis is characterized by fever, chills, dysuria, and a tense or tender prostate as seen in older men with indwelling urinary catheters; an infectious agent is not identified in 80% of cases. Treatment includes antibiotics, and hospitalization may be required in severe cases.

Chronic bacterial prostatitis presents classically as recurrent bacteriuria, and continuous low-dose antibiotic suppressive therapy can be considered for patients with frequent symptomatic relapse.

UNIQUE ISSUES IN GERIATRIC CARE

Elder Abuse

Evaluation of the geriatric patient cannot be considered complete unless the issue of elder abuse/mistreatment has been addressed. The term *elder mistreatment* denotes acts of omission or commission that result in harm or threatened harm to the health or welfare of an older adult. Abuse can be physical abuse (including sexual abuse), emotional abuse, intentional or unintentional neglect (including self-neglect), financial exploitation, abandonment, or a combination of these. Neglect is the most common type of mistreatment. It is estimated that between 2%

and 10% of elders experience abuse, and it appears to be increasing.[27] It can occur in homes of the older adult or their relatives or in institutional settings and is found among all socioeconomic strata and ethnic populations. Poverty, dependency of the elderly person for caregiving needs, functional disability, frailty, and cognitive impairment are some of the risk factors for elder abuse, along with family stress and conflict.

All states have some type of mandatory reporting requirements in which health and social service providers are required to report suspected cases of elder mistreatment to adult protective services. Primary care providers are in a unique position to detect elder abuse. Clues include patients who look ill-dressed with poor personal hygiene; are malnourished, listless, or apathetic; are brought to the clinic or the emergency department by someone other than the caregiver; present with fractures or bruises in various stages of healing, unexplained bruises, or unusual bruises (e.g., bruises in inner arms or thighs); have cigarette, rope, or chemical burns; or have facial lacerations and abrasions or marks occurring only in areas of the body usually covered by clothes. Evidence that material goods are being taken in exchange for care or that personal belongings (house, jewelry, car) are being taken over without consent or approval, as well as reports of being left in unsafe situations or of inability to get needed medication, can be indicators of underlying abuse. Astute PAs who maintain a heightened suspicion for potential elder abuse can identify cases by a careful history and a discerning physical examination, as well as by watching for subtle changes in the physical and psychosocial status of the patient over time.

Medicare and Medicaid

Medicare is the federal health insurance program for Americans aged 65 years and older and people younger than 65 with certain disabilities; 95% of older Americans have Medicare coverage. As such, it influences much of geriatric care (e.g., how long and in what circumstances Medicare pays for certain services, such as physical therapy or home health care). All of the authorization for Medicare coverage must be made by physicians. Unless the older adult is enrolled in a Medicare Advantage Plan, such as a health maintenance organization or preferred provider organization, their coverage is organized by the following parts of the original Medicare:

- Part A of Medicare helps pay for inpatient care in the hospital, medically necessary care in a skilled nursing home after a minimum 3-day inpatient hospital stay, hospice care, and medically necessary home health care for homebound patients.
- Part B helps cover 80% of many medically necessary outpatient care costs after a deductible is met. Beginning in 2011, it also covered most preventive services given by providers who accept assignment, meaning that the provider agrees to charge only what Medicare allows.
- Part D helps pay for prescription medications if the Medicare enrollee joins one of many drug plans offered by different companies, with varying deductibles and copayment options.

In general, Medicare is complicated and often confusing to both the provider and patient alike. It does not cover many of the costs of health care older adults use, such as vision care by non-physicians and glasses, hearing aids, care in assisted living homes, and long-term custodial care in nursing homes. Many older Americans also have supplementary insurance (called MediGap insurance) to help pay for the copayments and deductibles not covered by Medicare for outpatient care, and some also have long-term care insurance to help cover the costs of nursing homes and long-term in-home care.

PAs may be reimbursed for health care provided in outpatient offices or clinics without the requirement of "direct physician supervision" (interpreted as the supervising physician being onsite). PAs are also reimbursed in the hospital, surgical, and skilled nursing home settings. The rate of reimbursement in outpatient settings, first-assist in surgery, hospital care, and skilled nursing care is 85% of the rate of reimbursement for a physician. An excellent resource for the details of the latest legislation is the American Academy of Physician Assistants, Department of Government and Professional Affairs, 950 North Washington Street, Alexandria, VA, 22314-1552; phone: 703-836-2272.

Medicaid is a federal and state health insurance program for low-income people aged 65 and over, as well as those who are blind or with certain disabilities. People who have both Medicare and Medicaid coverage are called Dual Eligibles. Medicaid covers many of the costs not covered by Medicare, such as long-term custodial care in nursing homes. Reimbursement rates are generally lower for Medicaid than Medicare and vary considerably from state to state. Different states call their Medicaid programs by various names (e.g., MediCal in California).

Ethnogeriatrics

Just as the United States as a whole is becoming more diverse, the cultural heterogeneity among older Americans is growing rapidly. As mentioned earlier, the numbers of elders in the four major ethnic minority categories (American Indian/Alaska

Native, African American, Asian/Pacific Islander, and Hispanic) are growing even more rapidly than the rapidly exploding numbers of older adults in general. Within and between each of the minority populations, as well as among those considered the majority, are vast differences in characteristics that affect the health care encounter. These include acculturation level and age at immigration, religion, culturally related beliefs about causes and treatments of medical conditions, expectations and trust of health care providers based on historical experiences, and who has the authority/responsibility to make decisions about an elder's health care. Rates and risk factors for specific diseases also vary considerably by ethnic and racial population.[28] Although it is beyond the scope of this chapter to provide a detailed discussion of ethnogeriatric topics PAs are likely to face, it is important to remember some basic principles:

- Each older patient from a background other than non-Hispanic white may or may not fit the profile of the population that one might expect.
- Trained interpreters in person or by phone or video are needed for every encounter with an older patient who is limited English proficient (LEP); ad hoc interpreters (family members, friends, or untrained staff) increase the likelihood of medical errors and reduce the effectiveness of crucial communication; children should never be used as interpreters in a medical setting; documents such as consent forms should be translated into the patient's native language if they do not read English.
- Showing culturally appropriate respect to elders is extremely important in building a therapeutic relationship, especially because in many cultures elders are held in high esteem.
- It is always important to try to understand older patients' perspectives (sometimes called "explanatory model") on their own illnesses and integrate these perspectives into the management plan to increase the likelihood of their adherence to the plan.
- Family caregivers are major members of the health care team, especially in cultures in which there is a strong expectation that adult children should care for their parents; in some cases the decisions and preferences of the children may not be the same as the parents, so the parents' choices should be obtained.

For more information and resources on ethnogeriatrics, see the Stanford Geriatric Education Center website at *http://sgec.stanford.edu* and *http://geriatrics.stanford.edu/*.

Social Support and Caregiver Support

A supportive social network has been found to be a major factor in maintaining the health of older adults. For those without available family nearby or who are otherwise isolated, social support may mean having important connections with friends, neighbors, or through faith communities or other community resources, such as senior centers. PAs can help to foster those connections by encouraging their older patients to interact with others or by facilitating social work interventions to connect them with important community resources. If social work services are not available, PAs can encourage the connections themselves.

In some cases of dependent elders, the family caregiver is the major source of social support, as well as physical and instrumental support. Support of the caregiver, then, is a major part of geriatric care, especially when elders have dementia or other debilitating conditions. It is not unusual for the cause of institutionalization of an older patient to be the illness of the caregiver after long periods of extreme stress from caregiving. PAs need to monitor the stress level and health condition of primary caregivers as part of the care of their geriatric patients and help them get the health, respite, or support services they need in order to continue providing the support to the geriatric patient.

Some communities have specific programs for support of caregivers who are caring for dependent elders. They may include respite programs for someone else to care for the elder while the caregiver has some time to take care of their own needs, sometimes subsidized by public funds; support groups; or instructional programs on caring for dependent older adults. The Family Caregiver Alliance of the National Center on Caregiving has a wealth of information and materials available for caregivers (*www.caregiver.org*).

End of Life

Death and dying are a part of caring for aging adults. The majority of deaths occur in persons older than age 65, most in hospitals, but increasingly more in nursing homes and at home.[29] Discussions with patients about their wishes for care at the end of life and designation of a surrogate decision-maker should they be unable to make their wishes known are encouraged. Patients should be routinely questioned about completion of advanced directives (power of attorney for health care [POAHC] and physician orders for life-sustaining treatment [POLST]), and copies should be placed in their medical records. When appropriate, discussion of, and referral for, palliative care and hospice should occur.

COMMUNITY RESOURCES AND SERVICES

A major part of geriatric primary care is knowing the important health-related support services available for older adults in the community, knowing when they are indicated to support the maintenance of older patients' functional status and quality of life, and then helping elders access the services they need. Because a truism in geriatrics is that it is by nature a multidisciplinary enterprise, to be a successful provider is to be a team player. Unfortunately, in many medical settings, the other members of the geriatric team (e.g., social worker, psychologist, chaplain, home care nurse, therapists) are employed by other organizations and are less accessible for coordination of care than the medical provider might prefer.

This section describes some of the major types of services primary care providers should be familiar with in their local communities. Keeping current phone numbers of such resources in the office directory can be a useful means of dealing with common geriatric situations, such as the need for post-hospitalization care for an older widow who lives alone, the mild depression and growing isolation of a retiree, or the increasing stress and fatigue of an older woman trying to care for her mildly demented husband. In addition to the resources discussed here, there are hundreds of others that would be valuable in helping older patients improve or maintain their health and quality of life.

Information and Referral Services

A logical place to start for most community resources is one of the agencies organized (1) to maintain current listings of services older adults need and (2) to provide the appropriate information to elders or their advocates. To find the local equivalents of the services listed in this section, the PA could consult an Information and Assistance (I&A) service in one of two agencies.

Area Agencies on Aging (AAAs) are available to plan and coordinate services for older adults in every corner of the United States. One of the requirements imposed by the Older Americans Act, which created the AAAs, is that they maintain I&A services for the region they cover, usually including one or more counties. Unfortunately, AAAs frequently have some other official designation, such as "Department on Aging" or "Senior Services Council," and they may be associated with a governmental or private nonprofit agency, but one can usually find the phone number for the local AAA or its I&A through the listings in the front of the telephone directory under "Senior" or "Aging" services. They can also be located on the Internet by various search engines, such as Google.

Another excellent source of I&A services is the local *multipurpose senior center*, which is available in almost every town or suburb of any size. Most senior centers offer among their services a comprehensive I&A department that has up-to-date information on services elders need, such as housing, home health care, transportation, home-delivered meals, and nursing homes, for the particular area they serve.

If those resources are difficult to locate, there is a national Elder Care Locator, which has information on services in all communities by calling 1-800-677-1116.

Case Management or Care Coordination

An important role within the geriatric team is coordinating the myriad of fragmented health and social services and agencies a frail elder with multiple problems might need. A *case manager* or care coordinator not only deals with medical services but also assesses need and helps to arrange for transportation, in-home assistance (such as home-delivered meals and homemaker services), assistance with business affairs, and, if needed, more supportive housing such as assisted living. They also follow up to see that the services are delivered and are satisfactory. Unfortunately, case managers are not yet available in all communities and to all older residents, but they are increasingly part of community-based long-term care services designed to provide alternatives to institutional care for frail elders. Private case management programs are also growing in many areas.

Multipurpose Senior Centers

It is safe to say that the lives of millions of elders across the nation are enhanced by participation in their local senior centers, which typically offer a wide range of programs at no or low cost for healthy independent elders. Programs provided in a center for older adults who live in the community enable elders to do the following:

- Take classes in subjects such as fitness (frequently ranging from armchair exercises to yoga to aerobics), music of various types, languages, financial management, and self-management for chronic disease.
- Eat a nutritious, low-cost lunch subsidized with Older Americans Act funds.

- Learn about and take advantage of special services or programs for senior citizens, such as travel and tours, hypertension screening, and assistance with tax forms.
- Visit with friends in an attractive, upbeat environment that encourages older adults to be active and stay involved with the world.

PAs would do well to become acquainted with the staff and activities in the local senior center so that patients can be referred there for a wide range of health-related support services, including nutrition, fitness, health screenings, health education, health insurance assistance and counseling, and antidotes to depression for elders who are isolated and lonely.

Day Care/Day Health Care Programs

Just as multipurpose senior centers are important health centers for generally healthy, independent elders, day care (sometimes called "social day care") and day health care programs serve a similar function for frail elders. Both usually offer programs for movement-impaired or cognitively impaired older adults who need assistance, and the programs are typically offered 5 days a week. Both are designed to provide respite for the family caregivers of frail elders, frequently enabling adult children to keep frail elders in their homes when both children and spouse work outside the home. Some day centers also accept elders who are incontinent. Both models typically offer transportation, and the cost is usually figured on a sliding scale. Programs commonly include music, arts and crafts, current events, and a nutritious lunch. In addition, the day health care programs provide nursing, social work, and physical and occupational therapy services on the basis of assessed need. For the elder at risk of institutionalization, these centers are extremely important resources that can help maintain the elder at home for much longer than would otherwise be the case, because the staff can monitor changes in the patient's health and functional status on a daily or weekly basis and can keep the PA informed about problems, such as reactions to medications or acute confusion that might signal an infection.

CASE 26-4

Mr. B, an 82-year-old married African American male who had a stroke 6 weeks ago. Before his stroke he was still active in the plumbing store a few days/week that he owns with his son. Mr, B has hypertension and type 2 diabetes. He has had two transient ischemic attacks (TIAs) in the past year, one with a fall and fractured wrist. He was hospitalized for several days and then transferred to a skilled nursing facility for rehabilitation from which he was discharged 2 weeks ago. He has left-sided weakness and is walking with a pronged cane but reports that he continues to improve. His wife concurs that he is doing well and says she provides some assistance with dressing, showering, and toileting. She is worried about the possibility of another stroke and further disability. Mr. B expresses frustration with his wife "treating me like I can't do anything" and wants to resume driving and going to his shop. You review his medications: hydrochlorothiazide 25 mg once daily, lisinopril 40 mg once daily, metformin 500 mg twice daily, glipizide 5 mg 1 am and 1/2 pm, clopidogrel 7 mg once daily, calcium with vitamin D once daily, check vital signs (Wt 186#/Ht 69.6"; BP 138/84, P 86, reg), and do a brief cardiovascular and neurologic examination. You spend some time discussing with the patient and his wife what to expect in stroke recovery, some continued improvement but some increased risk for another stroke. You encourage activity and socialization for both of them and suggest they investigate a local day care program for Mr. B and activities at the local senior center. On follow-up 2 months later they report Mr. B has been attending the day care health program twice weekly, where he has continued to receive physical therapy, and Mrs. B is participating in a walking group at the senior center. They want to discuss what to do if Mr. B has another stroke and end-of-life care, topics they heard about at a stroke support group at the senior center recently attended.

In-Home Care

Many patients prefer to remain at home as long as possible, and because that desire often represents the option that both supports the patient's highest quality of life and is the most cost-effective, the goal of geriatric care is often to keep a patient at home. There is great comfort in being in familiar surroundings and, if possible, being cared for by family and friends. To that end, the PA should know about a variety of resources available to assist patients who prefer to be at home but need professional and other types of support that cannot be provided by the informal support system.

The *home health care* industry has become extremely sophisticated and offers a wide range of services to the homebound elderly person. In-home care through home health agencies should be considered as a possible resource to prevent nonacute hospitalization or placement in a skilled nursing facility. The services provided vary, depending on the agency, and can include physical therapy; occupational therapy; social work to evaluate and coordinate assistance with financial, social support, and mental health resources; hospice care for dying patients and their family members; and skilled nursing support. Skilled nursing care can include intravenous (IV) hydration, IV antibiotics, wound care, management of medication, follow-up of office assessment, fecal disimpaction, placement of urinary catheters, drawing of blood for laboratory assessment, pain control, and a nursing assessment of the patient's condition. The skilled nursing care and affiliated services provided by home health agencies can be extremely important in maintaining continuity of posthospitalization care for older patients.

The role of the PA in home health care includes the following:

- Evaluating the patient medically and recommending a course of treatment
- Documenting the need for the services provided by the home care agency
- Acting as a liaison for the agency to monitor care and outcomes and provide support for the staff if medical questions arise
- Understanding the resources and financial constraints involved in recommending home care and ensuring that all parties understand the scope of needed services and the cost

Although most PAs in practice know and work with home health agencies, older patients can often profit from less skilled and more varied support at home. In many cases, the prevention of institutionalization depends on the availability of someone to assist the elder with ADLs and IADLs at home. This assistance, referred to as *personal care* or *homemaker or chore services*, can often be provided by the same home health agencies that furnish skilled professional care. The advantages of going through the agency are that workers are screened and bonded for security, workers may have some training, and substitutes can be provided if a worker is absent. The disadvantage is that the services obtained through a home health care agency may be more expensive than those arranged privately. Some communities maintain registries of names of possible assistants.

Home-delivered meals are provided in most communities on a sliding fee scale for elders medically certified as homebound through Older Americans Act funds, but there may be a waiting list to receive such services. Other in-home services, such as *home repairs and renovations* for wheelchairs, are frequently also available; the best source of information is a case manager or an I&A service.

An especially important service for frail or at-risk elders who are living alone is an *alert system*. These are electronic monitors that can be attached to clothing or worn around the neck so that an elder who has fallen or otherwise has an emergency can easily contact a central switchboard, which then summons assistance as needed. The private systems that are widely advertised on TV tend to be much more expensive than those run in many communities through a local hospital or other health care agency. Communities also frequently have volunteer programs to provide *friendly visiting or telephone reassurance* on a regular basis for homebound elders at risk for isolation.

Senior Housing

Many choices of housing are especially designed for older adults and provide all degrees of support needed. When PAs are included in the process of recommending or deciding on residential options, it is imperative that they know the differences between levels of care so that the support available in the living environment can be matched to the level of care needed. The most important principle to use in those decisions is that of *the least restrictive environment*, meaning that elders need to be given the option of living in the type of environment that allows them the most freedom possible while giving them the support they need. The major options available in most communities are described as follows.

CONCLUSION

Caring for the elderly can be both challenging and extremely rewarding. Geriatrics, based on team care, is ideally suited to PAs with broad-based clinical medicine skills and knowledge. There is tremendous value in learning to differentiate what is "normal" and "expected" and comparing that with the physical manifestation of disease and its varied presentations with age. The geriatric population often offers the student and clinician the opportunity to observe findings associated with aging and disease processes that challenge stereotypes and sharpen the clinical learning process.

Students may struggle with the fundamentals of the history, physical examination, and diagnosis, as well as the options for treatment. However, medical care is more than ascertaining the correct diagnosis and treatment. Working with older adults enables the PA student to struggle with the social, emotional, and cultural challenges inherent in working with the medically complex person. Also, patients benefit tremendously by being in the care of a provider who takes the time to get to know the person behind the disease and to provide care that takes into account the physical, psychological, social, functional, and spiritual components of need. For the student to avoid the challenge of treating older patients because they are too complex, too hard to talk with, or simply too difficult is to lose an essential learning experience that cuts across all medical disciplines to the core of the health care experience, which is to make a difference and help patients find meaning in their lives amid the challenges generated by their illnesses.

CLINICAL APPLICATIONS

1. Summarize age-related changes for each body system that are common in elderly patients.
2. Identify four steps in assessing the medication status of elderly patients.
3. List eight common causes of reversible dementia in the elderly. Which cause is the most common?
4. Describe how you would teach pelvic muscle exercises to a patient with incontinence.
5. List eight components of a safety assessment of the home environment of an elderly patient.
6. Identify community resources commonly used by the elderly.

KEY POINTS

- Geriatrics emphasizes function, preventing functional decline, and maintenance of optimal function as goals.
- Aging is not a disease. Differentiating normal/expected changes of age from disease is often not easy.
- Polypharmacy requires frequent review of all medications (prescribed and over-the-counter) with attempt to reduce the number of medications and dosages in order to minimize risk of adverse drug reactions and interactions.
- Cognitive decline is not normal but increasingly common with age, requiring a high index of suspicion and assessment for reversible causes.
- Good geriatric care requires familiarity with the presentation and management of geriatric syndromes and common chronic conditions by health care providers.
- Knowledge about community resources and services available for older patents is an essential part of geriatric medicine.

References

1. Federal Interagency Forum on Aging-Related Statistics. Older Americans 2010: Key Indicators of Well-Being. Federal Interagency Forum on Aging-Related Statistics. Washington, DC: U.S. Government Printing Office, July 2010.
2. Reuben DB, Herr KA, Pacala JT, et al. Geriatrics at Your Fingertips: 2011. 13th ed. New York: The American Geriatrics Society, 2011.
3. Banks WA, Willoughby LM, Thomas DR, et al. Insulin resistance syndrome in the elderly: assessment of functional, biochemical, metabolic, and inflammatory status. Diabetes Care 2007;30:2369.
4. Buchner DM. Physical activity and prevention of cardiovascular disease in older adults. Clin Geriatr Med 2009:25661.
5. Malmrose LC, Gray SL, Pieper CF, et al. Measured versus estimated creatinine clearance in a high functioning elderly sample: MacArthur Foundation study of successful aging. J Am Geriatr Soc 1993;41:715.
6. American Psychiatric Association. Diagnostic and Statistical Manual IV, 2011.
7. Alzheimer's Association. 2011 Alzheimer's Disease Facts and Figures. Chicago: AA, 2011.
8. Knopman DS, DeKosky ST, Cummings JL, et al. Practice parameter: diagnosis of dementia (an evidence-based review). Report of the Quality Standards Subcommittee of the American Academy of Neurology. Neurology 2001;56:1143-1153.
9. Segal-Gidan F, Cherry D, Jones R, et al. Alzheimer's disease management guideline: Update 2008. Alzheimers Dement 2011;7:e51.
10. American College of Physicians. Delirium. Philadelphia: American College of Physicians, 2007.
11. Inouye SK. Current concepts: delirium in older persons. N Engl J Med 2006;354:1157.
12. Tennstedt SL, Link CL, Steers WD, et al. Prevalence or and risk factors for urinary leakage in a racially and ethnically diverse population of adults. Am J Epidemiol 2008;167:390.
13. Thom DH, Haan MN, Van Den Eeden SK, et al. Medically recognized urinary incontinence and risks of hospitalization, nursing home admission and mortality. Age Ageing 1997;26:367.
14. Stothers L, Thom D, Calhoun E. Urologic diseases in America project: urinary incontinence in males: demographics and economic burden. J Urol 2005;173:1302.
15. Thom DH, Nygaard IE, Calhoun EA. Urologic diseases in America project: urinary incontinence in women—national trends in hospitalizations, office visits, treatment and economic impact. J Urol 2005;173:1295.

16. Kegel AH. Physiologic therapy for urinary incontinence. JAMA 1951;146:915.
17. Centers for Disease Control. *http://www.cdc.gov/nchs/fastats/deaths.htm*. Accessed July 30, 2011.
18. Tinetti ME, Baker DI, McAvay G, et al. A multifactorial interfventin to reduce the risk of falling among elderly people living in the community. N Engl J Med 1994;331:821.
19. Liu H, Frank A. Tai chi as a balance improvement exercise for older adults: a systematic review. J Geriatr Phys Ther 2010;33:103.
20. Sahyoun NR, Lentzner H, Hoyert D, Robinson KN. Trends in Causes of Death Among the Elderly. Aging Trends; No.1 Hyattsville, MD: National Center for Health Statistics, 2001.
21. Linzer MD, Yang EH, Estes M, et al. Diagnosing syncope, Part 1: value of history, physical examination and electrocardiography. Ann Intern Med 1997;126:989.
22. Consensus Statements [Internet] NIH. National Institutes of Health (US). Office for Medical Applications of Research. Bethesda, MD: National Institutes of Health, 1977-2002.
23. NIH Consensus Conference. Diagnosis and treatment of depression in late life. JAMA 1992;268:1018.
24. Denihan A, Kirby M, Bruce I, et al. Three-year prognosis of depression in the community-dwelling elderly. Br J Psychiatry 2000;176:453.
25. Zeiss AM, Breckenridge JS. Treatment of late life depression: a response to the NIH consensus conference. Behav Ther 1997;28:3.
26. Rossouw JE, Anderson GL, Prentice RL, et al. Writing Group for the Women's Health Initiative Investigators. Risks and benefits of estrogen plus progestin in healthy postmenopausal women. Principal results from the Women's Health Initiative randomized control trial. JAMA 2002;288:321.
27. O'Brien JG. The mistreatment of older adults. In: Arenson C, Busby-Whitehead J, Brummel-Smith K (eds). Reichel's Care of the Elderly: Clinical Aspects of Aging. 6th ed. New York: Cambridge University Press, 2009.
28. Yeo G. How will the U.S. health care system meet the challenge of the ethnogeriatric imperative? J Am Geriatr Soc 2009;57:1278.
29. Miniño AM. Death in the United States, 2009. NCHS data brief, no 64, Hyattsville, MD: National Center for Health Statistics, 2011.

The resources for this chapter can be found at www.expertconsult.com.

CHAPTER 27

Behavioral Science and Medicine: Essentials in Practice

F.J. (Gino) Gianola • Ky Haverkamp • H. James Lurie • Timothy Quigley

CHAPTER CONTENTS

The physician assistant (PA) is one of the frontline providers who identifies and addresses the mental health needs of patients in the majority of clinical practices. Observations over the years indicate that this is the case regardless of practice location (inner city, suburban, or rural) or type (family practice, internal medicine, women's health, pediatrics, surgery, or transplant medicine). PAs also continue to be frontline providers in managing chronic illnesses, a task that often requires PAs to use behavioral medicine skills. In this chapter, we describe common psychiatric problems confronting the practicing PA. We then provide some basic building blocks and resources for treatment of those problems. We also review the knowledge, skills, and attitudes PAs need to guide their patients through making and sustaining lifestyle changes.

As PAs, we work each day with the sick and the worried well; we work to improve the mental and physical health of our patients. Before attempting to evaluate the mental health of a patient, clinicians should review their personal coping mechanisms to avoid projecting their own value systems onto the patient. Our task as PAs considering a psychiatric diagnosis is to gather data, evaluate, reflect, formulate, and implement therapies in contexts that are directed toward the needs of specific individuals.

We have included the American Psychiatric Association's *Diagnostic and Statistical Manual of Mental Disorders*, 4th edition (DSM-IV-TR), criteria to familiarize the student with the classification system used for mental disorders.[1] This is also a valuable resource for practicing PAs, who must use this system when completing insurance billing forms. The *Resources* section at the end of the chapter provides suggestions for further reading that can offer additional background on mental health.

MENTAL HEALTH

Improving mental health in the United States has been seen as a desirable goal. However, in recent years, restrictive guidelines for reimbursement by managed care systems and both public and private insurance providers have imposed serious limitations on the ability of clinicians to assess and treat emotional problems that present in a clinical setting. Often, it is difficult for a PA to offer the in-depth services needed. At the same time, the patient who has been referred to a mental health practitioner or behavioral medicine clinic is usually limited to a set number of reimbursed outpatient visits per year. Compounding the problem are medically underserved populations who often have little access to mental health professionals. For better or worse, in remote and rural areas, the major source of mental health services is the primary care practitioner.[2] The American Academy of Family Practice (AAFP), in its mental health position paper, "Provision of Mental Health Care Services by Family Physicians," addressed the necessity of including basic mental health care services in a uniform benefits package. This position paper estimates that depression, anxiety disorders, and somatization occur in 20% to 30% of the primary care population.[3]

It has long been recognized that depression, anxiety, and somatization are disorders that commonly present in primary care settings. At the same time, the stigma attached to seeking help for emotional problems (including acknowledging the problem to oneself) often delays recognition and treatment of these disorders, sometimes for decades. Patient attitudes may be apparent in statements such as: "If I'm a little blue or nervous, I have to deal with it myself." "If I tell my doctor I'm depressed or nervous and receive treatment, do I have to mark it on my job application or insurance forms that ask, 'Have you ever been treated for a mental illness?' Will this jeopardize my job or my insurance coverage?" These stoic feelings and apprehensions may hinder a person from seeking mental health care. An additional complication is that mental health issues are seen differently in the context of distinct racial and ethnic cultures. A problem that might be referred for psychiatric evaluation in one culture may be referred to a priest in another and a family elder in a third. It seems clear, however, that PAs should be able to make accurate assessments of the most common emotional problems that present in primary care settings, establish at least a tentative diagnosis, have definite ideas about treatment (frequently in consultation with their preceptor physicians or with a mental health professional), and be aware of community resources for referral, patient education, support, and additional treatment options.

Emotional problems that greatly impact the lives of patients have always been a major part of medicine. Research suggests that between 20% and 80% of patients who present in an outpatient primary care setting have a primary emotional problem either as a major reason for their visit or as a comorbid condition accompanying a physical complaint.[4] With the recent information explosion in neuroscience, as well as the increasing availability of pharmacologic agents to treat specific psychiatric syndromes, the armamentarium of both psychiatric specialists and primary care practitioners has been increased enormously. Despite this hopeful state, many psychiatric disorders in primary care are underdiagnosed or misdiagnosed.[5] Unless the correct questions are asked, anxiety disorders and depressive disorders—two of the most common conditions seen in primary care settings—are often missed. Often the patient then returns with a myriad of puzzling somatic complaints.

Over the past 20 years, increasing emphasis has been placed on accurate classification of mental disorders for purposes of improving treatment, research, and reimbursement. The major classification system used in the United States is published in the previously mentioned *DSM*.[1] Wherever possible in this chapter, reference to the *DSM* is made because as PAs we are expected to use this classification system when completing patient reimbursement forms for both private and public insurance providers (e.g., managed care, health maintenance organization, Medicare, Medicaid, and Social Security reimbursement forms).

The purpose of this chapter is to describe, with case examples, many of the major psychiatric syndromes likely to be seen by PAs, especially in primary care settings. We also provide some suggestions for brief psychotherapy (counseling). Because mental health issues pervade all aspects of medicine, this chapter obviously cannot be complete. However, the authors' hope is that it may serve as an introduction to psychiatric conditions, which are inseparable from those of "physical medicine," even if their descriptions appear to polarize the differences between "mind and body." This chapter also includes a description of the basic elements of an effective patient encounter.

STRUCTURE OF THE PHYSICIAN ASSISTANT–PATIENT ENCOUNTER

There are five basic components to each patient encounter: previsit preparation, medical interview, physical examination, treatment plan, and follow-up care.

Previsit Preparation

Preparing for the interview is the first step to creating a positive encounter. Take steps to provide a quiet environment, and arrange the examination room to ensure privacy and comfort. Set up the seating arrangements so that eye level is equal for the PA and patient. Do not forget to provide easy access to the examination room for those with disabilities. Consider hanging art that is accepting of cultural diversity.

As PAs we should work to eliminate personal distractions to maintain focus on the patient's problem.[6,7] This can be accomplished in many ways. Some PAs meditate or use relaxation techniques to help maintain focus.[6] Reviewing the patient's medical chart to learn about his or her previous clinic encounters provides some contextual framework. Knowledge of the patient's chronic medical conditions and/or information that may be related to the current chief complaint is particularly useful.[6]

Medical Interview

Attention to the beginning of the visit is critical to creating professional clinical encounters.[8] The first step is to greet the patient in a respectful and professional manner. This greeting should incorporate the use of the patient's formal name. It is helpful at this time to correct mispronunciations of the name and to document the phonetic pronunciation of challenging names. The PA should introduce himself or herself, using a full name and title.

Once introductions are complete, agenda setting is the next priority. Initially the PA should ask the patient to list all of his or her concerns and help in their prioritization.[7-9] Once the list is established, the PA should describe to the patient the steps that will be used in addressing the list of concerns: obtaining a history, performing a focused physical examination, developing a treatment plan, and establishing a follow-up care plan. Agenda setting and defining expectations create a transparent process for the patient.

While obtaining the history, exploring patient beliefs about the presenting problems will acknowledge the perspective of the patient's concerns. Avoid prematurely barraging patients with diagnostic questions. Be mentally present in the moment; do not get distracted by previous encounters or future concerns. Eliciting, acknowledging, and recognizing the value of the patient's perspective on his or her illness can help reduce barriers to wellness and improve the sense of partnership that can increase patient adherence to medical therapies.[8] Responding to your patient's specific concerns and questions using empathetic statements aids in establishing rapport and the trust needed for a therapeutic partnership.

Physical Examination

As with the interview, the key to success is to put the patient at ease. Many patients are curious about their own physical examination findings. Maintaining a dialogue with the patient throughout the physical examination is one more tool to establish rapport and trust. PAs can discuss with patients the presence or absence of physical findings related to the chief complaint. Some PAs combine performing the physical examination with a comprehensive review of systems to provide an opportunity for the patient to tell a more complete story of the current concern.

Treatment Planning

After obtaining the history and performing the physical examination and any ancillary tests, the PA summarizes and synthesizes the information with the patient. In a patient-centered encounter, the PA and patient together create the treatment plan. Included in this conversation is the social context of the patient's concerns and acceptable therapies.[10,11] A written summary of the treatment plans and follow-up information may increase personal investment in and compliance with the therapy.[11]

Follow-up Care

Whether patients present with a short-term illness or a chronic medical problem, the long-term relationship with patients is aided by appropriate follow-up care. Follow-up care can be delivered in many ways. For example, telephone calls, return visits to the clinic, or even secure e-mail messages can be reassuring to patients. In any mode of follow-up care, it is essential to review the course of the symptoms, inquire about new symptoms, and review the treatment plan in detail. With each method, the PA can address any potential barriers to adherence to the treatment plan.

PSYCHOTHERAPY

People come to a primary care provider because they are anxious and worried. They miss work because they are experiencing a new or chronic pain. Often, they are concerned about issues that are more vague—not feeling "right" or wondering about a new pain or physical symptom. They may be having trouble sleeping, or they may be feeling anxious about some ill-defined sense of malaise. The "conventional" separation of mind and body simply does not apply to most patients. People develop symptoms after experiencing stress, and any physical symptom in turn induces stress and worry. The internal dialogue may sound something like this: "Is this the first symptom of a fatal disease? Am I developing heart trouble like my father had when he was my age? Does this lump mean I have breast cancer? Is my PA going to suggest that my breast needs to be removed?" The PA's role is to give information, identify issues, and educate, but most of all, it is to give comfort to the suffering patient, who often has no other place to raise fears and worries with a concerned yet objective provider *and* receive assurance and comfort.

For the PA who is willing, psychotherapy in a medical context is a natural, helpful intervention, and it often takes much less time than expected. Psychotherapy in a medical context does not mean psychoanalysis. It does not mean an hour of counseling provided on a weekly basis. It does mean a focused intervention relevant to the specific patient and his or her concerns, often associated with a medical diagnosis. Following are seven suggestions about how to provide brief psychotherapy in the context of a medical encounter.

1. Listen for and inquire about the patient's concerns, both medical and psychological. Prioritize your patient's appointment time to listen, clarify, and identify the concerns of the patient. The first 5 minutes of every scheduled encounter should be spent in assisting the patient to articulate his or her genuine concerns and listening to the narrative.

   "So, since you developed that pain, you wonder if you have the same heart disease that your dad had at your age."

   Part of clarifying the patient's concerns involves finding out whether an event (e.g., a change at home or at work, an anniversary, a birthday) might be a contributing factor. Clarifying a patient's statement often means repeating it in your own words, asking, "Do you mean … ?" and restating the concerns (which may be multiple) in as simple and straightforward a manner as possible.
2. Empathize with the patient's apprehension and anxiety. Empathy is a response to the patient's feelings and is not critical or judgmental. It may be verbal or nonverbal.

   "It must be very wearing on you to have that pain and not know whether it's serious."
3. Help the patient identify how the medical or psychological concern is affecting how he or she feels. "I'm always keyed up, worrying, about what might happen to my family. I can't sleep at night, and I'm having trouble concentrating at my job. My wife noticed I'm keyed up, but I haven't wanted to worry her, too. And sometimes, I've been feeling really down."

   "So, you've been feeling anxious, fearful, and sometimes really down, too."
4. In a sensitive and empathetic manner, develop a plan with the patient to help clarify the reality of the patient's concerns.

   "What I think we should do first is to get a more detailed history of all your symptoms—anything leading up to them, any stress contributing to them. We should then do a good physical examination and get some laboratory work and an electrocardiogram (ECG), and maybe a stress test (depending on what the ECG reveals). We need to make some time to go over the results. It is also crucial that we talk about how we can deal with your anxiety, which is making you so uneasy."
5. Educate the patient in an empathetic manner about heart disease and anxiety. Affirm that feeling anxious is normal and is not a sign of weakness. Reassure the patient that depression often follows anxiety about a real or feared loss. Although this is "normal," both depression and anxiety must be monitored so that they do not turn into serious, disabling conditions. Normalizing the patient's situation can decrease anxiety.

"Many of my patients have reacted in a similar way; it's a normal response."

6. Offer your opinion about what would be helpful, but remember that the patient is the one who ultimately decides what is to be done. Arguing with or confronting the patient is rarely productive. Patients will "talk with their feet" and take neither your advice nor your medication. They are unlikely to return for the next appointment. Ultimately, by supporting the patient's choice, you can maintain an open dialogue, educate, and be available to the patient even if you disagree with his or her current choice.
7. When you meet with a patient who has a severe mental illness or who appears to be disregarding your opinions and "medical facts," it is important to explore his or her attitudes about having a particular diagnosis, taking medications, and having to change behavior for treatment to be beneficial. Try questions such as these.

   "Do you feel that taking medication for depression is a sign of weakness?"

   "Does it seem that cutting down on fats and sugars is just too much of a sacrifice?"

   A regular appointment schedule for follow-up is important in many cases. You and the patient will be able to evaluate how the patient's various concerns are resolving or whether the patient may need a referral to a mental health specialist.

SUPPORTING BEHAVIORAL CHANGE

One crucial role we PAs play in all clinical settings is to help patients construct and sustain new behaviors to improve their health. On a daily basis, we ask patients to make difficult lifestyle changes. Prochaska and colleagues[12] propose the "Stages of Change Model," which outlines six stages people commonly cycle through in their efforts to make changes. This model allows PAs to match the therapies to the patient's stage of change. When the intervention matches the stage of change, it strengthens the PA-patient relationship; greater trust is established as incremental successes follow along with change.[12,13] The six stages are listed as follows with suggested intervention strategies.

Precontemplation

In this stage patients are in denial about the problem behavior and have little awareness about the problem or its solution. The main pitfall in challenging patients in this stage is that they may become defensive. Diffuse this natural tendency by asking permission to provide information about the problem behavior. Confronting the patient in this stage means expressing concern about the problem behavior and its effects.

Example: Richard is a 55-year-old lawyer who works 60 to 70 hours per week and has a wife and three children. He is in the clinic today regarding elevated liver enzymes. During the history, the PA inquires about alcohol intake. Richard drinks four to five whiskey sours each evening but is not concerned about his level of drinking because he does not get drunk and has never been arrested for drinking and driving. After asking permission to discuss the effects of alcohol in Richard's life, the PA expresses concern that this level of drinking could cause the elevation in his enzymes. Richard is not worried about the drinking and would like to investigate other causes for his elevated enzymes. However, the PA suggests that Richard should think more about the alcohol issues and return for follow-up to discuss a comprehensive plan to investigate possible causes for the elevated enzymes.

Contemplation

This stage is marked by ambivalence to change, but the issues are defined. The patient is weighing the pros and cons of his or her behavior and is willing to discuss the behavior. Patients often have experimented with incremental changes related to the problem behavior. These attempts at change can be explored and supported, keeping in mind that it is often more effective to elicit the patient's perspective than for the PA to discuss his or her own perspective. In this stage, we as PAs can explore what patients like and dislike about the problem behavior. One should avoid pushing for a commitment to change and should encourage "change talk." Change talk is promoted when the PA elicits the patient's description of the reasons for making positive changes. Motivation to make changes comes from the combination of how important the change is to the patient and how confident he or she is that success in making and sustaining change can be achieved. Therapeutically, it is vital to ask about the concepts of importance and confidence in the context of a medical interview. Additionally, it may be helpful for the patient to try new behaviors and then report back to the PA about the trial.

Example continued: Richard returns for a follow-up appointment regarding his elevated liver enzymes. Other causes for his transaminitis have been eliminated. The PA elicits Richard's perspective first and learns that his alcohol consumption has been a source of contention in his marriage. Richard explains that things have been strained in the marriage for some time, but not just because of his drinking. He is not ready to stop drinking but thinks that if he modified his drinking, things would improve at home. The PA asks Richard about the pros and cons of his continued drinking and learns that Richard likes drinking to "take the edge off a stressful day at the office" and also that he really enjoys drinking with his friends. The cons, Richard states, are problems at home, but he does not elaborate. The PA suggests a trial of abstinence, and Richard agrees to consider a short period without drinking.

Preparation

This stage is marked by a commitment and planning to changing the problem behavior. The significance of the problem is acknowledged, and confidence in change is typically high, but patients may procrastinate and delay setting a start date. PAs should help negotiate a start date, encourage patients to declare their intent publicly (verbally), and plan for close follow-up. It is also helpful to summarize the patient's reasons for making the change.

Example continued: Richard returns to discuss his experimentation with abstinence. Since the last visit, his wife has told him she would seek a divorce if his drinking continues. Richard wants to stay married. He had a hard time stopping his drinking and asks about a detoxification program and what that would mean for him. He has heard about Alcoholics Anonymous (AA) but does not think it is for him. After summarizing Richard's reasons for stopping his drinking, the PA encourages him to announce his desire to stop drinking to those who care for him and to set a stop date. Additionally, the PA discusses various inpatient and outpatient options. Richard is opposed to inpatient options because he does not want to miss work. Richard and the PA agree on an outpatient treatment plan that includes counseling, medications, a follow-up appointment in 1 week, and a trial of AA.

Action

This stage is marked by active efforts to change the problem behavior. The patient is under maximum stress and may spontaneously abandon change efforts. It is helpful for PAs to follow patients closely in the action phase and validate the stress of trying new behaviors. PAs can help by anticipating and predicting potential problems that the patient may encounter and aid in problem-solving. If particular aspects of the plan are not working well, work to modify the plan. If patients experience setbacks, it is important to normalize these and to support sustained efforts to change.

Example continued: Richard returns for follow-up and is discouraged. He has not been drinking, but tensions with his wife are heightened. The PA validates his frustrations, reviews the treatment plan, and learns that he is tolerating his medications well and taking them as prescribed. Richard has not been to an AA meeting because work demands got in the way. Additionally he has not set up the counseling appointment yet, and his wife is upset at the delay. The PA reviews and supports the reasons for change and demonstrates an interest in Richard's plan for sobriety. The PA also works to improve the plan by discussing barriers and common pitfalls and reviews specific ways to implement the plan for change.

Maintenance

This stage is marked by a sense of accomplishment that needs to be supported and acknowledged. Patients may inadvertently be reverting to old, maladaptive behaviors. Patients will certainly have stories about how the new behaviors are impacting their lives. Their commitment to the change can be firm, or some patients may show signs of wavering. PAs should continue to elicit the patient's perspective on the situation, acknowledge the work the patient has done, reflect on the long-term nature of the changes, support the patient's active conscious efforts to maintain the new behaviors, and discuss what to do in the event of relapse. In this stage, patients may realize that having made positive strides in improving a problem behavior did not dramatically improve other areas of their lives.

Example continued: Three years later, Richard returns for an appointment with a complaint of cold symptoms. The PA asks about his drinking and learns that Richard and his wife are still happily married, he has been sober without a drink for more than 2 years, and he has changed his mind about AA (he attends one meeting per week and has a sponsor). The PA demonstrates admiration for the difficult changes Richard has made, inquires about his future expectations regarding alcohol, and asks about any relapses in the past 3 years and what Richard learned from them.

Relapse

This stage is marked by the regular recurrence of the problem behavior. It is also marked by the return to any earlier stage of change. It is important for the PA to assess the new stage of change and to target the approach accordingly. The relapse itself can be framed as a learning tool and a common experience for patients making difficult changes in their lives. Efforts should be made to reinstitute the new behaviors by reviewing and revising the action plan as needed.

Example continued: Richard returns to see the PA after a relapse. He started drinking again while on a stressful business trip. He has not told his wife or his AA sponsor, and he has stopped attending his weekly AA meetings. Since the relapse, he has been obsessed with alcohol and has been sneaking drinks on his way home from work. The PA attempts to normalize the relapse experience and to move the discussion toward talk about when Richard is going to stop drinking again. The PA also reminds Richard of all the hard work he has done and of his reasons for change. After talking about what Richard learned from the relapse, the PA and Richard decide together that telling his wife and his sponsor is the first step to getting back on track. Richard also decides to reconnect with his AA group. The PA plans to follow Richard closely again for a while and has him schedule a return appointment in 1 week.

Asking patients about both the positive and negative roles a behavior plays in their lives helps them develop a broader understanding of their problem behaviors. For example, a patient who smokes usually can think of many reasons to quit but may need a provider to discuss the enjoyable aspects of smoking. Defining the enjoyable aspects of problem behavior helps PAs and patients predict obstacles to change. Once obstacles are identified, problem-solving can address pitfalls specific to each patient.

Making lifestyle changes often takes a long time, and patients can make many cycles through the stages of change.[13] This is partly because making and sustaining the changes takes concerted effort and planning. Taking this into consideration, it is also helpful for a PA to assess a patient's readiness to change by inquiring about how important making the change is to the patient and about the level of confidence a patient has in his or her ability to change. A simple 0-10 scale to assess importance and confidence can be useful. For those who rate change as important, assessing confidence by using this simple scale can also illuminate obstacles to change. For example, a person who rates his or her confidence in the ability to quit smoking as a 4 on this scale can be asked, "Why didn't you respond with a 5?" When this question is answered, patients will describe barriers to making the change. The follow-up question is then to explore why the patient did not rate the confidence level as a 3. The response to this question gives the PA an insight into the patient's strengths and supports the patient's confidence.

REFERRAL: HOW AND WHEN

When we make a referral to a specialist for liver disease, the reason is that the issues of the disorder are beyond our scope of practice, knowledge, and skill. The referral seems straightforward, and both the PA and the patient tend to accept the need for more "expert" opinion for management and treatment.

PAs and patients tend to be much more ambivalent about referral to a counselor, a psychiatrist (a doctor of medicine trained in psychological issues and also able to prescribe medications), or a psychologist (a person with expert training in the diagnosis and treatment of psychological problems with the use of behavioral and other therapies). Patients often do not understand that a referral to someone accustomed to dealing with complex psychological situations is like any other medical referral. Rather than being an admission of failure or weakness, this referral is simply a procedure to help the patient resolve symptoms as expeditiously as possible. We need to remain positive about the referral, negotiating with the patient about keeping in touch and continuing to care for the patient's other medical problems.

> "Gordon, you have what's called technically a 'major depression,' which is a biochemical disorder of the nervous system. Although it was set off by your divorce, we've talked about how it runs in your family and you've mentioned that in the past you had a bad setback when you were in college. We've tried a couple of medications, but you're still feeling pretty teary and sad. I'm worried about you. I'd like you to see a colleague whom I've worked with, who is much more familiar with a wide variety of other treatments and medications that might be helpful for you. I want to keep seeing you here in the office and, with the help of my colleague, I'm sure this situation will improve. I need your agreement before I make the referral."

MENTAL STATUS EXAMINATION

As with other types of referrals, before you refer your patient to a mental health specialist, it is imperative that you gather data. Information on the mental status examination (MSE) can be found in Table 27-1. This formal mental status examination is used when needed, especially in cases in which you are concerned about a psychotic disorder.

The mini-mental status examination (MMSE) (Table 27-2) is most often used for determination of dementia or delirium. This test takes about 10 minutes. It includes fewer categories than the complete MSE, and the MMSE is scored. The problem with using the MMSE is that it is insensitive to patients with a low educational level, poor language skills, or impaired vision. Scores for these patients tend to be lower. The primary care provider should be aware of the cultural insensitivity of the MMSE when incorporating the tool into an examination. The clinician should also be careful not to misinterpret the cultural insensitivity of the test by presuming that the results reflect a lower educational level.

TABLE 27-1 Mental Status Examination (MSE)

Appearance	Level of consciousness: alert, hypervigilant, drowsy, stuporous Dress, grooming, idiosyncrasies
Behavior	Cooperative, aggressive, ambiguous, hostile
Speech	Rate: rapid, forced, slowed Volume: loud, soft monotone, dramatic Quality: flowing, peculiar
Affect/mood	Silly, anxious, labile, controlled, unreserved, blunted, flat
Thought process	Tangential, disorganized, loose associations, flight of ideas
Thought content	Delusions, grandiose, paranoid, bizarre Document precisely what the patient appears to believe Thought broadcasting, thought insertion Suicidal or homicidal ideations, including plan and intent
Perception	Hallucinations, illusions (auditory, visual, somatic, tactile) Belief in hallucinations that originate inside or outside, how many voices
Cognition	Level of awareness: aware of situation
Level of alertness	Orientation to person, place, and time
Memory	Immediate, short-term, and long-term
Attention	Digital span serial 7s; spell *world* backward
Calculation	Ability to calculate change from a transaction, addition, subtraction
Fund of knowledge	
Abstractions	Proverb interpretation, similarities
Insight	Knows something is wrong, understands illness is present, and considers causes
Judgment	Does the behavior match stated goals; response to standard questions (What would you do if you smelled smoke in a crowded theater?) Is the patient behaving appropriately for the situation?

DEPRESSIVE DISORDERS

CASE STUDY 27-1

A 70-year-old widower whose wife died 2 years ago presents to a primary care office because of weight loss, fatigue, a persistent cough, and "feeling run down." At one time a heavy smoker, the patient now smokes only half a pack of cigarettes a day. The patient has always prided himself on his independence and athletic stamina but began to lose interest in his usual daily walks about a year after his wife died. Clinically, the patient is alert, but he looks slightly sad and anxious. He states that he does not enjoy much of anything anymore, except for watching sports on TV. His sleep is restless. His speech is slightly slowed. His memory and concentration are slightly decreased. Physical examination reveals some bilateral rhonchi. An extensive workup was done for medical problems that might explain his symptoms. All laboratory tests, including chest radiograph, are relatively normal. On the second visit for these complaints, he begins to discuss his sorrow after his wife's death and the fact that he sometimes wishes he were dead so that he could "join her." In response to specific questions about suicidal ideation, he says he has considered suicide and has a loaded gun but "wouldn't have the guts to use it." After intensive treatment for a depressive disorder, most of the patient's symptoms disappear. Within 2 months, he says that, although he still greatly misses his wife, he now feels "more like his old self" (see Clinical Applications, question 4, at the end of the chapter).

DISCUSSION

Depression is one of the most common conditions seen in medicine, affecting 10% to 20% of the population at any given time, with 4% to 8% of the population having full-blown clinical depression. Women have twice the incidence of depression as men.[14] (In depression, as in several other disorders such as schizophrenia, Alzheimer's disease, anxiety disorders, and alcoholism, neuroendocrine differences between men and women produce different incidence ratios and different clinical courses.)[15] For unclear reasons, the incidence of depression has gradually increased throughout the past century. More people are becoming depressed and at an earlier age.[14,16] According to experts, only one quarter of depressed individuals receive treatment.[17] As was mentioned previously, some of this occurs because many people with depression feel that seeking help is a sign of moral weakness. In other cases, health practitioners either minimize depressive symptoms as "normal" or do not ask the right questions to establish a diagnosis.

Although everyone has depressed feelings or a depressed mood from time to time in a situational response to disappointment or loss, such feelings usually go away after a short time and respond to reassurance and affection. Depression as a disorder is more pervasive and disabling and does not remit rapidly. Current clinical research suggests that signs and symptoms of a depressive disorder are related to biochemical changes in the brain. Once established, such symptoms, left untreated, usually do not disappear in less than a year. Depression is also associated with a worse outcome when it occurs with physical illness, such as coronary artery disease.[17,18] It has been the authors' experience and observation that primary care providers tend to treat depressed patients for too brief a time and at too low a dose of medication.

MAJOR DEPRESSION (DSM-IV 296.2)

Signs and Symptoms

Five or more of the following symptoms during the same 2-week period are necessary for this diagnosis. At least one of the symptoms is either a depressed mood or a loss of interest or pleasure in usual activities. These (single-episode) symptoms cause significant distress, are not due to substance use, and are not caused primarily by bereavement. The PA should look for the following:

- Depressed mood most of the day, nearly every day
- Diminished interest or pleasure in most activities
- Significant weight loss (>5% body weight loss in a month) or decrease or increase in appetite
- Insomnia or hypersomnia nearly every day
- Motor agitation or retardation nearly every day
- Fatigue or loss of energy
- Feelings of worthlessness or excessive guilt
- Decreased ability to think or concentrate
- Recurrent thoughts of death, suicidal ideation, or a suicide attempt or specific plan

In Case Study 27-1, although it was possibly triggered by the death of his spouse, this man's depression fit the criteria for a major depression and required medication, supportive individual counseling, referral to a support group, and mobilization of his support network to achieve remission of his symptoms. The sleep disturbance and depressed mood responded fairly rapidly. His energy level and appetite took a longer time to readjust.

Differential Diagnosis

A number of common illnesses, nonprescription drugs, and prescribed medications can produce depression. Illnesses include cancer, viral disease, endocrine abnormalities, anemia, stroke, and liver disease. Medications, including oral contraceptives, steroids, some beta-blockers, L-dopa, and methyldopa, can cause depression. Drugs that can trigger depression include alcohol and narcotics; withdrawal from amphetamines or cocaine can do the same. Depressive symptoms can also exist in schizophrenia, dementia, and anxiety disorders. Depression is found in manic-depressive illness in which an individual has elevated mood, increased energy, decreased need for sleep, and poor judgment alternating with the more classic symptoms of major depression.

TABLE 27-2 **Mini-Mental Status Examination**

Orientation (10 points)	What is the date? (year, season, date, day, month)—5 points Where are we? (state, country, town, hospital, floor)—5 points
Registration (3 points)	Name three objects: Each one spoken distinctly with a brief pause. Patient repeats all three with one point for each. Score is determined by first repetition. Record number of trials needed to learn all three objects.
Attention and calculation (5 points)	Either serial 7s counting backward from 100, or spell *world* backward. Points are awarded for each correct answer up to the first miscalculation or misspelled letter.
Recall (3 points)	Recite the three objects memorized in the Registration Section.
Language (9 points)	Patient names two objects that he or she is shown (watch, pencil). (1 point each) Repeat a sentence: "No ifs, ands, or buts." (1 point) Follow a three-stage command: Take a piece of paper in your right hand, fold it in half, and put in on the floor. (3 points) Read and obey the following: Write on a blank piece of paper, "Close your eyes." Ask the patient to read and do what it says. (1 point) Ask the patient to copy a design (intersecting pentagons). All 10 angles must be present, and 2 must intersect. (1 point)

Total maximum score is 30 points. Commonly, a score of less than 24 is indicative of dementia or delirium.

Treatment

Treatment measures include medications, focused psychotherapy, and emotional support. Many medications are available and effective in treating depression. However, in primary care settings, patients often do not receive medications long enough and in adequate dosages for them to be effective. Prescribing a "mild" (subtherapeutic) dose of an antidepressant is often useless. If a patient's depression requires medication, the patient requires a full, therapeutic dose.

Support can come from family, friends, and primary care providers. Support represents the mainstay of treatment for depression. Experts in the treatment of depressive disorders also advise clinicians who treat depressed patients to do the following.[19]

- Establish a supportive and positive relationship.
- Have regular appointments with the patient.
- Maintain a hopeful attitude with the patient.
- Set realistic goals.
- Explore and confront negative thinking through diaries and discussion with the primary care clinician.
- Involve the family and/or other supportive individuals.

Focused counseling usually requires referral to a mental health professional and is often useful if depression persists despite adequate medication and support or if the patient has more than two episodes of major depression.

ANXIETY DISORDERS

CASE STUDY 27-2

A 16-year-old girl with spina bifida dropped out of high school after she had several panic attacks at school. These were triggered initially by the fact that she was being teased by other students for occasional episodes of urinary incontinence at school. She became increasingly fearful of leaving her house, and over several months she became fearful of being alone at home in the absence of family members. She became anxious and tremulous at the thought of going outside. During her occasional episodes of panic, she experienced rapid heartbeat, a sense of doom, a feeling that she might be choking to death, trouble catching her breath, sweating, and numbness of her hands. On several occasions, her worried parents brought her to an emergency department because she thought from her symptoms that she was having a heart attack.

Eventually, she consented to come to a primary care clinic to rule out medical causes for her condition. She had told her parents after her last panic attack (which lasted 3 hours) that she would rather be dead than continue to experience "these terrible episodes." After treatment was begun with both medication from her PA and behavioral techniques administered by a psychologist, her symptoms of both panic attacks and generalized anxiety were sufficiently alleviated that she could gradually return to school on a limited basis. Stabilization of her symptoms took a number of months and involved a number of different medication trials but eventually was moderately successful (see Clinical Applications at the end of the chapter).

DISCUSSION

Anxiety disorders are common in the general population and in primary care practice. About a third of otherwise normal individuals have sporadic panic attacks, and about 1% to 2% of the population has severe enough symptoms to be diagnosed as having a panic disorder. Severe fearfulness of leaving the home environment and severe specific phobias occur in 2% to 5% of the general population, and about one fifth of people have milder phobias. About 5% of the general population have symptoms of generalized anxiety. Anxiety symptoms are often misdiagnosed and undertreated.[17,18]

In many cases, anxiety is accompanied by depression. Although the primary care provider often treats the symptoms of anxiety adequately, the depression is frequently not treated appropriately. If medication is prescribed, it may be at too low a dose or for too short a time.

Several different conditions are included under the general heading "anxiety disorders." These include posttraumatic stress disorder (PTSD), obsessive-compulsive disorder (OCD), panic disorder with or without agoraphobia, social phobia (social anxiety disorder), and other specific phobias.

Generalized Anxiety Disorder (DSM-IV 300.02)

In this disorder, there is excessive anxiety and worry more days than not about a number of events or activities. The person finds it difficult to control the worry, and anxiety and worry are associated with three or more of the following symptoms:

- Restlessness
- Being easily fatigued
- Difficulty concentrating
- Irritability

- Muscle tension
- Sleep disturbance (difficulty falling or staying asleep or restless, unsatisfying sleep)
- Anxiety, worry, or physical symptoms cause significant distress or impairment in social, occupational, or other important areas of functioning

Pharmacologic Treatment of Anxiety Disorders

It is well beyond the scope of this chapter to describe in detail the specific treatments available for the different forms of anxiety disorder. However, pharmacologic treatments are generally used to treat each type of anxiety disorder. The difficulty in generalizing about treatment in large part results from research that increasingly indicates that different areas of the brain are involved in the different disorders, and that different neurochemical mechanisms mediate their clinical expression. In general, however, antianxiety agents, such as buspirone and the benzodiazepines, are used for generalized anxiety disorders, whereas disorders involving panic often respond to the newer antidepressants, especially the selective serotonin reuptake inhibitors (SSRIs). Older antidepressants such as the monoamine oxidase inhibitors (MAOIs) are effective but tricky to use because of their dangerous interactions with certain foods and medications.

Phobias and social avoidance problems are treated with a combination of antianxiety medications, along with behavioral treatments such as relaxation training and desensitization to the feared stimulus.[14] Certain kinds of social anxiety, such as performance anxiety, respond to beta-blockers, a type of antihypertensive agent.

Obsessive-compulsive disorder requires both treatment with SSRIs (often in high doses) and training that enables the patient to stop and interrupt obsessive thinking or compulsive rituals. "Cognitive restructuring" is often useful for this disorder. The patient learns to "correct" his or her obsessive thinking (e.g., "I know that even if I feel I must wash my hands, nothing bad will happen if I stop myself from doing it").[19]

The treatment of PTSD is highly complex and often involves specialized group and individual therapy, as well as antidepressants and antianxiety medications.

In patients with each of these conditions, the PA who is interested can often play a major role in identifying the disorder; in less complex cases, the PA can also be instrumental in providing treatment. The PA can serve as a "case manager" and triage patients with those disorders that often fluctuate in intensity throughout the life span.

Situation-Specific Anxiety in Medically Ill Patients

According to Benedek and Engel,[5] certain types of anxiety arise in response to specific situations, especially in the medically ill. These include the following general categories.

1. *Separation anxiety.* Anxiety occurs when the patient is separated from an important caregiver. This may express itself in fearfulness, disruptive behavior, physical complaints, or increased demands for attention.
2. *Stranger anxiety.* Although normal in childhood, this is manifested by distress or increased complaints when the patient is confronted by unfamiliar health care providers.
3. *Anxiety about dependency.* These individuals are threatened by any situation that makes them feel dependent. They may devalue those who offer help or may refuse to comply with treatment.
4. *Anxiety about loss of control.* This type of anxiety occurs when important decisions are taken out of the hands of patients, such as when they require hospitalization. These patients argue about diagnosis, are noncompliant, may fail to keep appointments, and may remain oppositional to regain a sense of control.
5. *Anxiety about the meaning of an illness.* Such patients may, for example, engage in inappropriately seductive behavior if they are worried about no longer being attractive.
6. *Signal anxiety.* Patients may overreact to medical situations if such situations evoke "bad" thoughts or emotions that the patient has previously tried to suppress.

Differential Diagnosis

A variety of medical conditions can produce symptoms that mimic anxiety disorders. These include cardiovascular disease such as paroxysmal tachycardia; endocrine or metabolic disorders, such as hypoglycemia or thyroid disease; multiple sclerosis; acute organic brain syndromes of any cause; tumors, such as pheochromocytoma or carcinoid; pulmonary disorders, including hypoxia and pulmonary embolism; and infectious agents such as tuberculosis. Medications and nonprescription drugs that may cause anxiety include central nervous system stimulants such as amphetamines, cocaine, caffeine, monosodium glutamate, theophylline, and neuroleptics (which produce akathisia, a kind of motor restlessness).

Nonpharmacologic Treatment Approaches

In addition to medication, a variety of other treatments are often effective for these disorders. These include reassurance, explanations, and patient education about treatments (especially if the patient has specific concerns about the treatment), systematic exposure to feared situations, and relaxation and visualization techniques to assist in immediate reduction of anxiety. To treat phobias, systematic desensitization is often used together with medication. In the office, the patient initially uses a relaxation technique and then progressively visualizes scenes of increasing anxiety, signaling the clinician as the anxiety appears, and relaxing again until the anxiety disappears. Outside of the office, the patient actually enters the scenes that were visualized, transferring the habit of relaxation to the phobic setting. Other techniques include providing support, encouraging the patient to use mechanisms such as exercise that have previously been helpful in stressful situations, and encouraging denial for those patients who tend to dwell too much on the danger they are in. Family counseling is sometimes useful to help individuals maintain progress so that the family does not inadvertently encourage dependence or regression.

Panic Disorder with Agoraphobia (DSM-IV 300.2)

Panic disorder is recognized by recurrent, unexpected panic attacks. A discrete period of intense fear or discomfort occurs, in which four or more of the following symptoms develop abruptly and reach a peak within 10 minutes:

- Palpitations, pounding, or accelerated heart rate
- Sweating, trembling, or shaking
- Sensation of shortness of breath or smothering
- Feeling of choking, chest pain, or discomfort
- Nausea or abdominal distress
- Feeling of dizziness or lightheadedness, fainting
- Feeling of unreality or of being detached from oneself
- Fear of losing control or going crazy
- Fear of dying

At least one of the attacks must have been followed by fear of having additional attacks, worry about the consequences of the attack (e.g., going crazy), or a significant change in behavior related to the attacks.

Agoraphobia is diagnosed when the following two symptoms occur.

- The patient may experience anxiety about being in places or situations from which escape might be difficult or embarrassing, or where help may not be available in case of another panic attack. (Agoraphobia often involves being outside the home alone, being in a crowd, standing in a line, being on a bridge, or traveling by car, train, or bus.)
- Situations are avoided or are endured with marked distress.

Panic Disorder without Agoraphobia (DSM-IV 300.01)

Although panic attacks occur in this situation accompanied by concern about additional attacks, the patient is not immobilized to the point of avoiding such situations.

Agoraphobia without History of Panic Disorder (DSM-IV 300.22)

The patient has a fear of developing paniclike symptoms without having experienced the symptoms that meet the criteria for panic disorder.

Specific Phobia (DSM-IV 300.29)

This is marked by an excessive or unreasonable fear in the presence or in anticipation of a specific situation or object (e.g., insects, flying, heights). Exposure to the phobic stimulus almost invariably provokes an immediate anxiety response.

Social Phobia (DSM-IV 300.23A)

This is a marked and persistent fear of one or more social or performance situations in which the person is exposed to unfamiliar people or to possible scrutiny by others. The individual fears that he or she will act in a way that will be humiliating or embarrassing. Exposure to the feared situation almost invariably provokes anxiety or a panic attack. Individuals avoid such situations or endure them with intense anxiety; this avoidance interferes with their normal routine, occupational functioning, or social activities or relationships.

Obsessive-Compulsive Disorder (DSM-IV 300.3)

The person has either obsessions or compulsions. Obsessions are recurrent, intrusive, and inappropriate thoughts, impulses, or images that cause marked anxiety or distress that the individual attempts to ignore or suppress. Compulsions are repetitive behaviors (e.g., hand washing, checking) or mental acts (e.g., praying, counting, repeating words) that the person feels driven to perform in response to an obsession. With both obsessions and compulsions, the individual recognizes that the obsessions or compulsions are excessive or unreasonable.

Posttraumatic Stress Disorder (DSM-IV 309.81)

The individual has experienced, witnessed, or been confronted by events that involved threatened death or serious injury, or a threat to the physical integrity of self or others. The person's response involved intense fear, helplessness, or horror. The traumatic event is persistently reexperienced in one or more of the following ways:

- Recurrent and distressing recollections of the event, including images, thoughts, or perceptions (e.g., "flashbacks")
- Recurrent distressing dreams of the events
- Acting or feeling that the event is recurring

This includes a sense of reliving the experience, illusions, hallucinations, or dissociative flashback episodes, including those that occur on awakening or when intoxicated. Symptoms are accompanied by intense psychological distress, including persistent symptoms of increased arousal (e.g., difficulty falling asleep, irritability, difficulty concentrating, hypervigilance, exaggerated startle response). There is persistent avoidance of stimuli associated with the trauma, as well as numbing of general responsiveness by reactions such as avoiding thoughts or conversations associated with the trauma and avoiding activities that arouse recollection of the trauma, inability to recall aspects of the trauma, diminished interest in significant activities, feelings of detachment or estrangement from others, restricted range of affect (e.g., unable to have loving feelings), and the sense of a foreshortened future (does not expect to have a career or a normal life span).

PSYCHOTIC DISORDERS

Beginning in the 1960s, motivated by the success of new antipsychotic medications, a humanitarian effort was undertaken to discharge patients from mental hospitals and place them back into their communities. For financial reasons, many individuals with chronic psychosis who previously had lived for years inside a protected hospital setting were released precipitously into the community. Although some of these efforts were successful, many patients were unable to cope with the demands of community living. They ended up homeless, in prison, or rehospitalized. In recent years, younger patients who develop severe mental illness, especially schizophrenia, may never be hospitalized but may still have great difficulty coping in the community. They run afoul of the law because of poor judgment and often use alcohol and drugs as a way of coping with their psychotic symptoms. Although many of these individuals have their mental illness supervised by mental health professionals, such individuals usually have their health care needs met by primary care providers, including PAs. It is important, therefore, for PAs to be aware of signs and symptoms of psychotic disorders and to work collaboratively with mental health professionals in identifying early symptoms of decompensation.

Schizophrenia (DSM-IV 295.xx)

Signs and Symptoms

Schizophrenia usually arises during the late teens and early 20s. It is often preceded by a "prodromal phase" in which a person whose previous functioning was reasonably good becomes disorganized, withdrawn, and suspicious. The person shows increasingly impaired reality testing. To meet DSM-IV criteria for schizophrenia, an individual must show, during the "active" phase of the disorder, continuous signs of a disturbance for at least 6 months. Two or more of the following symptoms must be present during a 1-month period.

1. *Delusions.* The patient exhibits fixed, false ideas that are inconsistent with his or her culture or religion and cannot be corrected by rational argument. They may be poorly organized or complex and somaticized. They may be bizarre and sometimes are associated with a depressed or elevated mood.
2. *Hallucinations.* These are perceptual experiences that occur in the absence of an actual stimulus. Auditory and visual hallucinations are most common. Olfactory, tactile, and complex visual hallucinations are more common with other organic mental syndromes, such as intoxication, seizure disorders, and tumors.
3. *Disorganized speech.* This symptom is often a reflection of both the individual's difficulty in concentration and the bizarre content of the individual's thoughts. It may also show the unusual form of the individual's thinking (e.g., a patient's conversation is "derailed"

when he says a word that reminds him of a word with a similar sound, even though there is no other connection between the words). A patient may also have "loose associations" in which he or she interprets abstract sayings in a highly idiosyncratic fashion (e.g., "a table and a chair are alike because they sit together to pray").

4. *Gross disorganization or catatonic behavior.* In this situation, the patient may become severely withdrawn, mute, and unresponsive to questions or requests and may even be incontinent.
5. *Negative symptoms.* The patient shows affective flattening (no emotional expression), may display limited or absent speech, and reveals the absence of interest in any activities or participation.

The person with schizophrenia also shows a marked deterioration in areas of work, interpersonal relations, and self-care compared with previous levels of functioning.

Antipsychotic medications have become increasingly refined so that newer medications produce fewer adverse effects than do the older medications used for the treatment of psychosis. Many individuals who had some remission of hallucinations and delusions were troubled by motor stiffness, involuntary motor restlessness, and at times, acute motor spasms. In addition, negative symptoms were usually not helped by the older medications. Now, many patients using the newer antipsychotic medications can live independently, can be employed, and have a much brighter affect and a higher energy level. Despite these improvements, many individuals with residual schizophrenia continue to display poor judgment, exhibit intermittent drug or alcohol abuse or dependence, have difficulty managing money, and receive marginal health care. This is often so because of poor compliance, confusion about the need for medical follow-up, poor coping and problem-solving skills, and problems in trusting authority figures. During assessment of an individual with schizophrenia who presents to a primary care setting, the following questions are crucial.

- Is the patient currently taking antipsychotic medications regularly; does he or she know how much and how often?
- What is the patient's source of financial security? Can he or she buy and take medications that the PA might prescribe?
- How impaired is the patient currently? Is the patient oriented? How intact are memory and judgment? Is the need to continue on medication and to have follow-up acknowledged by the patient? Does the patient understand the medical conditions you are assessing and treating? Can the patient be relied on to take medications? Does the patient need supervision for medication compliance?
- Is the patient currently using/abusing recreational drugs or alcohol? Are these a major impediment to compliance with the medical regimen?
- Who else in the patient's support system can be contacted for assistance to help with compliance (e.g., a case manager, mental health personnel, family members)?

Differential Diagnosis

Psychotic thinking may sometimes be associated with other disorders besides schizophrenia. These include delirium, dementia, toxic states, and mood disorders. Also included is psychosis associated with severe depressive illness or with manic-depressive illness, especially during the manic phase when grandiose delusions are common.

Treatment

Although mental health professionals usually undertake the treatment of schizophrenia, a treatment team is often necessary for an individual with schizophrenia to remain stable. This team often includes a case manager (to track the afflicted individual and often manage his or her money), family members (who need education about the disorder to help provide appropriate support and structure), a primary care team to keep track of the medical aspects of the patient's condition, and, whenever possible, a community advocacy component (such as the National Alliance for the Mentally Ill) to keep track of resources in the community, educate health and mental health providers, and serve as a source of legal and financial advocacy if necessary.

DELIRIUM AND DEMENTIA

Because the population of the United States is growing older and living longer, an important component of primary care practices involves (and will increasingly involve) assessment and management of individuals who, as they become older, develop increasing memory problems. Major diagnostic categories of particular concern are delirium and dementia.

Delirium (DSM-IV 293.0)

Delirium is a syndrome that involves a disturbance in consciousness, which shows the following characteristics:

- Disturbance of consciousness, with reduced clarity of awareness of the environment and with reduced ability to focus, sustain, or shift attention.
- A change in cognitive abilities, such as memory deficit, disorientation, language disturbance, or the development of a perceptual disturbance.
- The disturbance develops over a short period and tends to fluctuate over the course of the day.

Delirium can be secondary to medication or drug intoxication (e.g., minor tranquilizers), metabolic conditions (e.g., diabetic ketoacidosis), medication or substance withdrawal (e.g., abrupt withdrawal of benzodiazepines), or acute physical illness (e.g., a febrile illness or urinary tract infection). Because in an elderly person delirium often occurs in tandem with a more fixed and permanent memory problem (i.e., dementia), it is crucial that a primary care provider take a careful history and do a thorough mental status and physical examination to differentiate how much the memory problem is related to an irreversible process and how much is related to an acute medical problem.

Dementia (DSM-IV 290.1)

Dementia is a chronic disturbance of memory, judgment, and intellectual functioning, without prominent clouding of consciousness. Onset is often insidious. Two of the most common forms of dementia are dementia of the Alzheimer's type and vascular dementia (related to cerebral anoxia or small brain infarcts).

Dementia of Alzheimer's Type (DSM-IV 294.1x)

Criteria for dementia of the Alzheimer's type include multiple cognitive deficits manifested by the following.[1]

- Memory impairment will be noted (impaired ability to learn new information or to recall previously learned information).
- One or more of the following cognitive disturbances will be present:
  - Aphasia (language disturbance)
  - Apraxia (impaired ability to carry out motor activities despite intact motor function)
  - Agnosia (failure to recognize or identify objects despite intact sensory function)
  - Disturbance in executive functioning (i.e., planning, organizing, sequencing, abstracting)
- Cognitive deficits that cause significant impairment in social or occupational functioning and that represent a significant decline from a previous level of functioning will develop.
- The course is characterized by gradual onset and continuing cognitive decline.

Vascular Dementia (DSM-IV 290.4)

Vascular dementia has similar criteria, except that focal neurologic signs and symptoms or laboratory evidence of cerebrovascular disease is present, and the clinical course usually shows episodic rather than gradual decline (as in Alzheimer's-type dementia).[1]

A number of diagnostic tests, such as the MMSE, are useful for documenting the degree and type of impairment, especially when a patient is followed over an extended time.[20] Because elderly patients are especially sensitive and embarrassed about memory or other cognitive losses, an evaluation for dementia and delirium must be carried out with great tact, sensitivity, and reassurance.

SUMMARY

As PAs, we should be familiar with common emotional problems that present in clinical settings, be able to make an assessment (sometimes with consultation from a mental health specialist), and have sufficient knowledge, compassion, empathy, and skills to be able to develop a subsequent effective course of action, ranging from pharmacologic intervention to referral for counseling, support, additional education, or, if necessary, hospitalization. The outcome of medical treatment in primary care settings (for instance, with diabetes or hypertension) depends a great deal on awareness of the interaction or comorbidity between medical and psychological factors or conditions. The mind and body have never been separate domains; research is increasingly documenting their interdependence for homeostasis and health.[21] However, as Faber has observed, "In the final analysis, the goal of neuropsychiatric assessment is to understand the patient and explain his or her predicament, leading to maximally effective treatment. Mainly through empathy and pertinent observation, clinicians can understand psychologically the patient's pain, distress, and dysphoria."[22]

CLINICAL APPLICATIONS

1. What is the most common mental health coverage provided by Medicare, Medicaid, and private insurers? For your patients, are inpatient or outpatient therapies reimbursed better? What is the average number of outpatient visits covered? What is the ceiling coverage for inpatient care, and is there a limit to the number of times a patient can be admitted for inpatient treatment? For the clinician, does inpatient or outpatient care lead to better reimbursement?
2. What type of training do religious leaders (e.g., ministers, priests, rabbis) receive for counseling their members? Would you access members of the religious community for counseling patients in your practice who are members of their congregations? If yes, how would you access them? What about patient confidentiality?
3. What are some of the economic effects of untreated depression and anxiety? What is the effect on the patient, on the local community, nationally?
4. In Case Study 27-1 with the 70-year-old widower, what are your specific treatment options, and what specific medications would you use and why? What are your follow-up strategies? This patient states that he feels like his "old self" after 2 months of receiving your therapies. What are your major concerns? What are your follow-up plans at this point?
5. What is the estimated number of cases of depression in your community? Why? What are the percentages by age?
6. In Case Study 27-2, the 16-year-old has returned to school on a limited basis. In your community, what types of social service and school support exist for children reentering school after mental health treatment, including medications? Is there a systematic way of teaching children without disabilities about their classmate with physical and mental challenges, especially for children who are preteens and teens?
7. This teenager is currently stabilized. What is your follow-up plan for her at this point in her therapy? What is your major concern? Why? Specifically, how do you involve the family in her continued therapy?
8. Let us assume this teenager is now visiting colleges to make a choice of where to go. She and her family ask what they should look for to ensure her continued successful therapy. How would you approach this question? What would you do now?

KEY POINTS

- PAs are frontline providers who identify and address the mental health needs of patients in a majority of clinical settings, both primary and specialty care.
- Mental health concerns include anxiety, depression, and somatization, which occur in 20% to 30% of the primary care population. Employers and insurers continue to attach stigmas to mental health diagnoses.
- PAs should be familiar with common classifications in the DSM-IV, which is used for diagnosis and billing for both private and public insurance providers.
- PAs engage in psychotherapy focused on interventions associated with illness and disease and need to have an appreciation of each patient's narrative and concerns.
- The structure of the PA-patient encounter creates the basis for a trusting therapeutic relationship.
- In their therapeutic role, PAs must have an understanding of how to help patients make and sustain behavioral changes.
- Knowledge of the community that is the mental health referral system is essential for PAs. Providers to refer to may include psychologists, psychiatrists, family counselors, or clergy trained in therapeutic modalities. This includes normalizing the referral for patients who are unfamiliar with mental health providers.
- The PA should be familiar with psychotropic medications and proper dosages for common diagnoses, such as depression and anxiety.

ACKNOWLEDGMENT

The authors would like to thank Dr. Keren H. Wick for coordinating the revisions to this chapter and for her careful editorial review.

References

1. American Psychiatric Association. Diagnostic and Statistical Manual of Mental Disorders (DSM-IV-TR). 4th ed. Arlington, VA: American Psychiatric Publishing, 2000.
2. Smalley KB, Yancey CT, Warren JC, et al. Rural mental health and psychological treatment: a review for practitioners. J Clin Psychol 2010;66:479.
3. American Academy of Family Physicians. Mental Health Care Services by Family Physicians (position paper). Leawood KS: AAFP; 2001, *http://www.aafp.org/online/en/home/policy/policies/m/mentalhealthcareservices.html*; Accessed December 21, 2011.
4. Office of the Surgeon General. Report of a Surgeon General's Working Meeting on the Integration of Mental Health Services and Primary Health Care. Rockville MD: United States Department of Health and Human Services, 2001, *http://www.surgeongeneral.gov/library/mentalhealthservices/mentalhealthservices.html*; Accessed August 15, 2007.
5. Byers AL, Yaffe K, et al. High occurrence of mood and anxiety disorders among older adults—the national comorbidity survey replication. Arch Gen Psychiatry 2010;67:489.
6. Sibinga E, Wu AW. Clinician mindfulness and patient safety. JAMA 2010;304:2532.
7. Cegala DJ, Post DM. The impact of patients' participation on physicians' patient-centered communication. Patient Educ Counsel 2009;77:202.
8. Lee Yin-Yang, Julia L. Lin. Do patient autonomy preferences matter? Linking patient-centered care to patient-physician relationships and health outcomes. Soc SciMed 2010;71:1811.
9. Cegala DJ, Post DM. The impact of patients' participation on physicians' patient-centered communication. Patient Educ Counsel 2009;77:202.
10. Muma RD. An approach to patient education. In: Muma RD, Lyons BR (eds). Patient Education: A Practical Approach. 2nd ed. Boston: Jones and Bartlett, 2012.
11. Lee Y-Y, Lin JL. Do patient autonomy preferences matter? Linking patient-centered care to patient-physician relationships and health outcomes. Social Sci Med 2010;71:1811.
12. Norcross JC, Krebs PM, Prochaska JO. Stages of change. J Clin Psychol 2011;67:143.
13. Prochaska JO, Redding CA, Evers KE. The transtheoretical model and stages of change. In: Glanz K, Rimer BK, Viswanath K, (eds). Health Behavior and Health Education: Theory, Research, and Practice. San Francisco: Jossey-Bass, 2008.
14. Kessler RC, Chiu WT, Demler O, Walters EE. Prevalence, severity, and comorbidity of twelve-month DSM-IV disorders in the National Comorbidity Survey Replication (NCS-R). Arch Gen Psychiatry 2005;62:617.
15. Seeman MV. Psychopathology in women and men: focus on female hormones. Am J Psychiatry 1997;154:1641.
16. Merikangas KR, He J, Burstein M. Lifetime prevalence of mental disorders in U.S. adolescents: results from the National Comorbidity Survey Replication–Adolescent Supplement (NCS-A). J Am Acad Child Adolesc Psychiatry 2010;49:980.
17. Kocsis JH, Gelenberg AJ, Rothbaum B, et al. Chronic forms of major depression are still undertreated in the 21st century: Systematic assessment of 801 patients presenting for treatment. J Affect Disord 2008;110:55.
18. Frasure-Smith N, Lespérance F. Depression and cardiac risk: present status and future directions. Postgrad Med J 2010;86:193.
19. Polen MR. Understanding how clinician-patient relationships and relational continuity of care affect recovery from serious mental illness: STARS Study Results. Psychiatr Rehabil J 2008;32:9.
20. Folstein M, Folstein S, McHugh P. Mini-mental state: a practical method for grading the cognitive state of patients for the clinician. J Psychiatr Res 1975;12:189.
21. Andreasen NC. What shape are we in? Gender, psychopathology, and the brain. Am J Psychiatry 1997;154:1637.
22. Faber, Raymond A. The neuropsychiatric mental status examination. Semin Neurol 2009;29:185.

The resources for this chapter can be found at www.expertconsult.com.

CHAPTER 28

PHYSICIAN ASSISTANTS IN HOSPITAL MEDICINE

H. William Mahaffy

CHAPTER CONTENTS

It comes as no surprise that physician assistants (PAs) have continued to follow their physician colleagues into emerging arenas of health care practice. One of the fastest growing examples of this paradigm is the hospitalist PA. With hospitalist programs expanding at a prodigious rate, PAs are viewed as a known resource to help improve care and safety in the inpatient setting. The flexibility provided to health care systems through the integration of PAs into hospitalist teams has shown the same benefits seen in other inpatient settings. Hospital medicine (HM) has undergone explosive growth over the past decade and is now considered an integral part of the management model for inpatient care. According to a *New England Journal of Medicine* article: "The Society of Hospital Medicine (SHM) estimated a 20% increase in the number of hospitalists between 2005 and 2006. A 2005 survey by the American Hospital Association showed that 40% of community hospitals had hospitalist programs, and a 2006–2007 survey showed that at least 59% of all hospitals in California had hospitalist programs."[1]

HISTORY AND CURRENT STATUS

The hospitalist designation was coined in 1996 by Robert M. Wachter, MD.[2] HM has emerged more as a specialty of process and efficiency versus one of organ-system expertise. HM practitioners come from a variety of clinical backgrounds. Although initially most hospitalists were internists, the hospitalist of today comes from a variety of medical specialties including internal medicine, family practice, pediatrics, cardiology, and critical care. Hospitalists are extremely adept at orchestrating the diagnostic and therapeutic options needed to treat the patient effectively and in a timely manner. Some HM models incorporate staff with a range of subspecialty expertise (e.g., critical care, geriatrics, palliative care). This brings an added quality of focus and understanding to the overall patient management environment. Initially, the end points for measuring effectiveness of the HM model were recognized as improvement in outcomes and a reduction in length of stay (LOS). Although these are still important metrics to track, additional focus has been placed on patient safety, inpatient quality initiatives, and improving the critical transition between the inpatient and outpatient setting. Project BOOST (**B**etter **O**utcomes for **O**lder adults through **S**afe **T**ransitions) is a national initiative conceived and sponsored by the SHM to address this significant interval in the overall patient management scheme.[3]

The rise in hospitalist programs was not universally welcomed in the early years. There was a perceived threat to the autonomy of primary care practitioners (PCPs) as they relinquished the "control" of their patients to the inpatient care team. However, hospitalists have remained responsive to these concerns and focus on methods to make the transition of care from the acute setting back to the outpatient realm as safe and stress free as possible. Discussions with the PCP on the day of discharge followed by a detailed discharge summary are the main tools used by the hospitalist to maintain a seamless transition for the patient and PCP. Numerous surveys have shown high satisfaction ratings from both patients and PCPs when the process is structured to provide early, focused follow-up after discharge.

Specialists have also voiced concern that hospitalists would be less inclined to seek consultation and the patient would not receive the benefit of their specialty training. This concern has not been consistently borne out in actual practice. Specialist consultations have remained prominent components of many admissions. Hospitalists are not tasked with performing upper and lower endoscopies, nonemergent cardioversion, electroencephalogram interpretation, echocardiography, lymph node biopsy, and other procedure-based specialty services. In fact, specialists are finding the hospitalist-generated consults are more problem specific and actually use their expertise in a more focused manner.

The hospitalist practice structure has evolved out of the economic considerations found in today's health care environment. Many PCPs find they can increase their office availability and, therefore, productivity by eliminating the "hospital rounds" component of their practice. Coupled with decreasing reimbursement for inpatient services, this model works well for both patient and practitioner. Some PCPs strive to make daily "continuity rounds"—a brief visit with their admitted patients and an equally brief discussion with the hospitalist team to keep abreast of the patient's progress. This activity takes far less time than the standard rounding requirement and provides additional benefit at the time of outpatient follow-up. Although this practice can occasionally lead to patient confusion about "who their doctor is," the majority find it comforting to know that their family doctor remains interested and involved in their overall care plan.

SCOPE OF PRACTICE

In a traditional patient management model, the patient's PCP would be called on to admit the patient to the hospital, round on them daily, and consult specialists for specific problems. The hospitalist model provides the efficiencies of a dedicated team functioning exclusively in-house and focuses on the coordination of care during the patient's hospital stay. This becomes increasingly important if more than one specialty becomes involved in the case. This patient care strategy is well known in larger medical centers that have used a "house staff" to provide the daily (and nightly) medical coverage on the floors. However, smaller hospitals without residency program resources have not had the advantages of 24/7 in-house coverage. Other factors have also conspired to make the hospitalist model attractive to hospital administrators. Even with residents available to handle the daily patient care duties, work-hour restrictions have significantly impacted a hospital's ability to provide consistent in-house coverage. In many areas, hospitalist services have stepped in to fill this gap.

The setup of a hospitalist service is also uniquely dependent on the hospital setting. In small, rural community hospitals, the hospitalist service not only provides the inpatient medicine coverage but also will often provide critical care services in the absence of a dedicated intensivist. This broad skill set is another attractive element for PAs seeking to use the breadth of their experience and training. The scope of practice for hospitalist PAs is no different than that of other PAs functioning in an inpatient environment. PA duties and responsibilities are clearly defined by state law and institution bylaws and would be identical to those of PAs on an internal medicine service with addition of the critical care skills mentioned earlier. Some HM services have sought out experienced surgical PAs for the added comfort with procedures (e.g., intubation, thoracentesis, paracentesis, central and arterial line placement). As in many other disciplines, PAs provide greater contact opportunities for nurses and patients, thus increasing satisfaction and improving outcomes.

The 2005-2006 SHM Survey provides the following statistics:

- Thirty percent of hospitalist groups employ PAs and/or nurse practitioners (NPs).
- Groups more likely to employ PAs/NPs include academic programs, groups in the eastern United States, and groups older than 5 years.
- Midlevel providers perform the duties outlined in Table 28-1.

Unlike the adage, "Don't sweat the small stuff," hospital medicine is *all* small stuff; SWEAT IT! It is attention to the details and coordinating the multifaceted inpatient management pathway that have set hospitalists apart from their outpatient colleagues. It would be unreasonable to expect an outpatient physician who sees more than 30 patients per day in the office to be readily available to deal with electrolyte abnormalities as soon as the inpatient laboratory work is processed. Immediate availability to evaluate

TABLE 28-1 Physician Assistant (PA)/Nurse Practitioner (NP) Function Table

PA/NP Function	HMGs (%)
Round daily on hospitalized patient	83
Write prescriptions for patients	82
Perform H&P on admission	77
Act as initial responder (consult, admit)	66
Participate in discharge planning	66
Order specialty consultations	53
Assist in teaching students	33
Night or weekend call	30
Postdischarge follow-up calls	20
Emergency responses; Code Blue	14
Perform invasive procedures	11

From Society of Hospital Medicine 2005-2006 Survey. Use of PAs and NPs in hospital medicine groups. Hospitalist 2006;10:10.

H&P, history and physical examination; HMGs, hospital medicine groups.

a patient with worsening cardiopulmonary function is also nearly impossible for a physician grinding through a full office schedule. In that setting, specialist availability may also be delayed because specialists have their own office hours and procedures to manage. Larger hospitals may have house staff to manage these scenarios, but an expanding number of smaller hospitals are now turning to hospitalist programs to deal with the increasing acuity level of admitted patients.

In addition to the fast-paced challenges of admissions, discharges, and daily rounds, documentation has become a major factor of the hospitalist's impact on the fiscal health of the organization. Hospitalists have been called on to keep abreast of the latest coding and reimbursement requirements. Accurate and complete documentation for every patient has significantly improved the hospital's ability to maintain or increase reimbursement percentages in a rapidly changing health care environment. In addition to the financial impact, a key feature of this exacting documentation also affects patient safety. Medication reconciliation (MedRecon) is a time-consuming but essential element of hospital care. Although it is common for patients to see more than one outpatient health care provider, it is NOT common for all of these encounters to be documented in the same record. PCPs increasingly use electronic health records (EHRs) to maintain an accurate overview of the patient's active and chronic problems, as well as medications. Review and reconciliation is a crucial aspect of management in the acute setting, and hospitalists are at the forefront of gathering, reviewing, and adjusting the often extensive medication regimen of patients with multiple comorbidities. It is then vital that any changes, deletions, or additions to the regimen be explained to the patient and family, as well as clearly described to the PCP at the time of discharge.

When considering the expansive per-patient workload of an average HM service, it becomes clear how PAs provide considerable leverage to accomplish the daily management requirements. With an older and more acute inpatient population, focused attention to laboratory and radiology results, gastrointestinal and urinary function, skin integrity, deep vein thrombosis prophylaxis, incentive spirometry, occupational and physical therapy evaluations, and social service/discharge planning are elements that must be evaluated and managed to achieve consistently good outcomes. Of equal importance is the component of keeping family members and PCPs advised of the patient's progress and anticipated outpatient transition.

The PA role on the hospitalist team will be demanding, stressful, and rewarding. It provides an opportunity for both new grads and experienced clinicians to develop and expand their roster of skills. The hospitalist patient care model has had an enormous impact on the way inpatient care is provided in many regions. As in most other areas of patient care, hospitalist leaders have embraced the advantages that midlevel providers bring to a team. They often rely on them to provide the subtle but often crucial pieces of patient information that facilitate the patient's smooth journey into and out of the hospital setting.

CASE STUDY 28-1

Mr. S is a 58-year-old male with an 8- to 10-year history of hypertension and diabetes. He is a nonsmoker who presented to the emergency department (ED) with complaint of anterior chest pressure that is distinctly different from his gastroesophageal reflux disease (GERD) symptoms and began approximately 6 hours ago while he was at his sedentary office job. His initial workup in the ED reveals marked hypertension, with a blood pressure (BP) of 186/100 mm Hg; mild tachycardia, heart rate (HR) 110; hyperglycemia, with a blood glucose of 412 mg/dL; a normal electrocardiogram (ECG); and normal cardiac biomarkers (troponin I, creatine phosphokinase [CPK], and isoenzyme of creatine kinase with muscle and brain subunits [CKMB]). He is currently pain free after receiving aspirin, sublingual nitroglycerin, and supplemental oxygen. The hospitalist service is contacted for admission to evaluate possible acute coronary syndrome (ACS).

A complete history and physical examination (H&P) shows that the patient has not felt well recently and has had 24 to 48 hours of malaise with nausea and intermittent diarrhea. He has not taken any of his antihypertensive or oral hypoglycemic medications. His laboratory work is consistent with prerenal azotemia. The patient is admitted to the cardiac step-down unit, and serial cardiac enzymes are ordered. He is placed on frequent blood glucose monitoring and is given short-acting insulin coverage until his blood sugar approaches normal range. Given his hypertension and tachycardia, he is given an intravenous (IV) beta-blocker, for the antihypertensive benefits and for ACS. He is continued on topical nitrates, therapeutic low-molecular-weight heparin, a proton pump inhibitor, and IV fluids.

The following day, the patient's troponin I remains negative and his blood glucose has descended to below 200 mg/dL, although a glycosylated hemoglobin shows poor long-term control with results of 9.6%. The patient's renal status corrected, and his blood pressure descended to 150/80 mm Hg. He has remained pain free, and given his risk factors he is scheduled for a stress echocardiogram. This evaluation reveals no evidence of inducible ischemia to 12.5 metabolic equivalents (METS) (>80% maximum predicted heart rate [MPHR]). After discussing the results of the tests with both the patient and his wife, the patient is released with instructions for an early follow-up with his PCP to discuss his hypertension and glycemic control. The patient was continued on his angiotensin-converting enzyme inhibitor for both hypertension and diabetes benefits. Daily low-dose enteric-coated aspirin is added to his regimen. Repeat laboratory work to evaluate renal function and potassium level was ordered for the day of outpatient follow-up. A call is placed to the PCP's office, and a dictated discharge summary is provided within 24 hours.

Note: This scenario is a typical example of patient management on a hospitalist service. Because the diagnostic and therapeutic goals were well defined, there was no specific need to further consult Cardiology (other than for the echocardiogram and interpretation) or Endocrinology. The patient's length of stay (LOS) was less than 48 hours and, in many cases, may have qualified for observation status. Patient education and PCP notification were completed before discharge.

CASE STUDY 28-2

Ms. L is a 61-year-old female with a poorly defined history of occasional lightheadedness and a syncopal episode a few weeks ago for which she did not seek medical attention. Earlier in the day, she experienced yet another episode of near-syncope and finally called her PCP, who directed her to go to the ED for further evaluation. On arrival, she was noted to have a weak pulse, mild diaphoresis, and nausea. Heart monitor showed a high-rate atrial fibrillation with ventricular response of 160-170. Ms. L's blood pressure (BP) was 106/62, and her respirations were 22 with 95% saturation on room air. An IV line was initiated, and she was given a bolus dose of IV calcium-channel blocker followed by a drip. Initial laboratory work was unremarkable, including cardiac biomarkers, renal function, and thyroid-stimulating hormone (TSH). The HM service was consulted for admission. The patient was admitted to the Cardiac Step-Down Unit, and serial cardiac enzymes were ordered. She had a modest drop in systolic BP to 92/50, which resolved with a 500-mL bolus of normal saline. Her heart rate had improved with the calcium-channel blocking drip, and this was titrated downward to address her mild hypotension. Approximately 6 hours after admission, the patient spontaneously converted to sinus rhythm. Her hemodynamics stabilized, and her drip was subsequently transitioned to oral medication. She was noted to have a minimal elevation in her cardiac troponin I, which normalized by the following morning. Her TSH, renal function, and fasting lipid panel were all within normal limits. Her $CHADS_2$ score[4] was 1, and the patient was continued on the antiplatelet therapy initiated on admission because she did not want to begin full systemic anticoagulation with warfarin sodium. She was educated about stroke risk and new anticoagulation therapies currently available and will discuss this with her PCP. She was discharged on her existing medication regimen with the addition of aspirin and calcium-channel blocker. Standard documentation and communication with the PCP office were completed at the time of discharge.

CASE STUDY 28-3

Mr. P is a 72-year-old white male who was feeling well until earlier on the day of admission. He presented to the ED after noticing bright red blood with his last bowel movement. He is hemodynamically stable and has initial hemoglobin of 9.4 g/dL (his normal is 12 g/dL). His blood urea nitrogen-creatinine ratio was within normal limits. He only takes aspirin, an angiotensin receptor blocker (ARB) for hypertension, and a multivitamin. He had two more bowel movements in the

ED, and the hospitalist service was consulted for admission. The patient was admitted to a medical floor given his lack of significant comorbidities, and a gastroenterology consult was requested. His antihypertensive was held, and he was given IV fluids at 100 mL/hour. The patient underwent serial hemoglobin tests and was scheduled for lower endoscopy the next morning. His hemoglobin dipped to 8.6 g/dL with IV hydration but did not require a transfusion. Endoscopy revealed marked diverticulosis with stigmata of recent bleeding but no active hemorrhage. The patient was monitored for an additional 24 hours to watch for rebleed, but none occurred. His hemoglobin remained stable above 9.0 g/dL. His aspirin was discontinued, and a call was placed to the PCP with follow-up in 3 to 5 days and a repeat complete blood count (CBC).

Note: This case highlights a typical HM scenario in which hospitalist service admits patients whose chief complaint will clearly require specialist intervention. Much like the outpatient physicians, many specialists find the hospitalist model an efficient way to maximize their time between the procedural laboratory and office schedule. By having the hospitalist group oversee the "standard elements" of the admission, specialists can concentrate on the specific issue requiring their expertise while knowing the adjunct medical issues are being overseen by the admitting service. This technique has helped expedite patient care and increase the productivity of the specialist team.

CASE STUDY 28-4

Ms. F is a 78-year-old female with history of worsening pain and disability in her right knee from progressive degenerative joint disease (DJD). She has chronic and well-controlled medical problems including hypertension, coronary artery disease, hypothyroidism, hyperlipidemia, GERD, DJD, and osteoporosis. The patient underwent an elective total knee replacement (TKR) earlier in the day under spinal anesthesia and is currently recovering in the Joint Replacement Center (JRC) specialty unit. The Orthopedic Service has consulted HM for management of her medical comorbidities. The preoperative evaluation, operative anesthesia, and recovery room records are all reviewed, the patient is examined, and her medications are restarted appropriately. The patient begins the JRC rehabilitation activities on postoperative day 1, and the HM service is paged midmorning with a report of mild lightheadedness and positive orthostatic vitals. The patient is ordered a 500-mL bolus of normal saline and is seen later in the afternoon. She has no complaints, and her hemoglobin dropped 1.5 g from preadmission. No transfusion is required, and the remainder of her hospital stay is uneventful. The patient is discharged to home with family on postoperative day 4.

Note: This case highlights a common utilization of HM services. With many practice models providing 24-hour in-house coverage, surgical patients can have medical problems expediently handled, including urgent evaluation and transfer to a monitored or critical care unit if indicated.

CLINICAL APPLICATIONS

1. Project BOOST is a national initiative managed by the SHM.
   a. How does your facility manage ongoing quality issues?
   b. What aspects of daily clinical practice would benefit from a focused quality improvement (QI) project?
   c. In what ways can PAs become an integral part of the QI team?
2. HM is a delicate balance between meticulous attention to "the small stuff" and efficiently moving the patient from admission to discharge.
   a. What are the available tools, both technology and process, that improve accuracy and efficiency in the clinical setting?
3. Handoffs are a critical aspect of HM.
   a. What are the elements of safe and effective handoffs between HM team members during admission?
   b. Between HM team and primary care team at discharge?

KEY POINTS

- Primary focus is on the acute admission problem(s)
- Know and apply latest "best practice" methodology
- Become proficient and comfortable using multiple EHRs
- Surgical comanagement is an increasing component of HM practice
- Close attention to medication reconciliation at admission and discharge
- Close attention to focused discharge summary and PCP communication
- SWEAT the small stuff!

References

1. Kuo YF, Sharma G, Freeman JL, Goodwin JS. Growth in the care of older patients by hospitalists in the United States. N Engl J Med 2009;360:1102.
2. Wachter RM. The emerging role of "hospitalists" in the American health care system. N Engl J Med 1996;335:514.
3. Society of Hospital Medicine website. *http://www.hospitalmedicine.org/AM/Template.cfm?Section=Home&TEMPLATE=/CM/HTMLDisplay.cfm&CONTENTID=27659*; Accessed January 3, 2012.
4. Wikipedia website. *http://www.wikidoc.org/index.php/CHADS_Score*; Accessed January 3, 2012.

The resources for this chapter can be found at www.expertconsult.com.

CHAPTER 29

ORTHOPEDICS

Patrick C. Auth

CHAPTER CONTENTS

Orthopedics is the surgical specialty dealing with musculoskeletal disorders, including trauma, sports medicine, and degenerative joint disease. The word *orthopaedic* was introduced from a French physician, Nicolas Andry, in 1741 from the title of his book: *Orthopaedia: or, The Art of Correcting and Preventing Deformities in Children: By such means, that may easily be put into practice by parents themselves, and all such as are employed in educating children.*[1] The word *orthopedics* is derived from the Greek *orthos pais* and means "straight child." Additionally, Andry designed the symbol that is now recognized as the logo for orthopedic surgery. The "tree of Andry" is taken from an engraving in *Orthopaedia* and shows a crooked tree tied to a stake in order to straighten it (Figure 29-1).

Physician assistants (PAs) who work in orthopedic surgery appreciate the mixture of office-based practice, the opportunity to participate in surgical procedures, and caring for patients who range in age from the neonate to the elderly. PAs with backgrounds as athletic trainers or physical therapist assistants and physical therapists find orthopedic practice a particularly appealing employment niche. In this chapter the utilization of PAs in orthopedics is explored, an overview of the approach to the orthopedic patient is presented, selected common problems are reviewed, and the challenges and rewards of orthopedics for PAs are discussed.

PHYSICIAN ASSISTANTS IN ORTHOPEDICS

According to the 2008 Census of the American Academy of Physician Assistants, 10% of PAs nationwide work in orthopedic surgery, compared with 25.9% in family/general medicine.[2] Orthopedics is the largest of the surgical subspecialties, employing almost three times as many PAs as the next most frequent

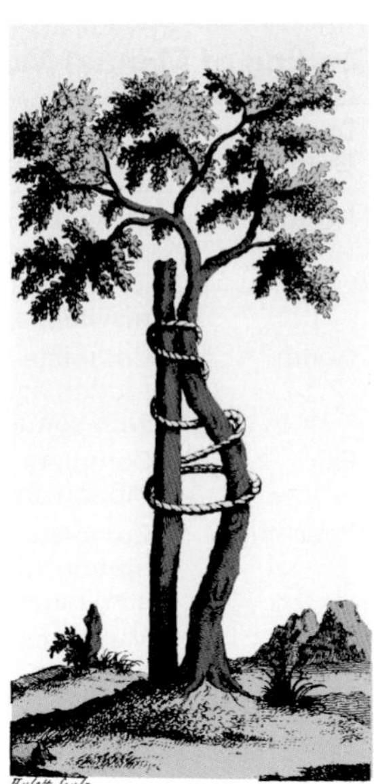

FIGURE 29-1 ■ The Tree of Andry. (By kind permission of the Wellcome Institute Library, London.)

choice—cardiovascular surgery—which employs 3.1% of PAs nationwide.[2]

The utilization of PAs in orthopedic surgery is increasing, by both the percentage of PAs in the job market and in absolute numbers. Compared with 2001, when 1416 PAs (8.2%) worked in orthopedics, 2528 PAs (10%) were employed in orthopedics in 2009.[2,3] By comparison, during the same period, PAs in cardiovascular surgery decreased from 760 in 2001 (4.4%) to 681 (3.2%) in 2006. In addition, PAs in orthopedic surgical practices conduct more than 18.6 million patient visits, an average of 70 per week per PA.[4]

Orthopedic PA roles vary from strictly office-based to primarily hospital-based, although the most typical role includes both outpatient and inpatient responsibilities. In the office, PAs evaluate patients and initiate treatment, including splints, casts, and other orthopedic devices. Typical outpatient problems include activity-related injuries, degenerative or chronic use conditions, and follow-up after surgical procedures. Orthopedic PAs may first-assist at surgery and may follow orthopedic patients through the course of their hospitalizations.

The foundation of evaluating any patient with an orthopedic problem is the history and physical examination because these result in the diagnosis of as much as 80% to 90% of orthopedic conditions. The core competencies of orthopedic history, musculoskeletal physical examination, and special orthopedic tests are discussed in the following sections.

ORTHOPEDIC HISTORY

A thorough and accurate orthopedic history provides the necessary information for the clinician to make an accurate preliminary diagnosis. PAs use the orthopedic history for important information about the disorder, its prognosis, and treatment.

The orthopedic history includes the following[5,6]:

- The patient's age and lifestyle
- Occupational history
- Sports and training habits
- Hobbies
- Dominant hand
- Past joint disorders
- Medical history, including previous injuries, surgeries, and treatments
- Current medications and allergies

The chief complaint must be thoroughly explored according to the PQRST format. The following questions also provide invaluable information in the diagnosis of orthopedic conditions.[5,6]

- What is the patient's age? Many orthopedic conditions are age related. For example, congenital hip dysplasia, Osgood-Schlatter, and Legg-Calvé-Perthes are diseases known to occur in a younger patient population. Arthritic conditions, such as degenerative joint disease and osteoarthritis, are noted more often in an older patient population.
- What is the occupation of the patient? Occupations that involve repetitive activities, such as lifting, typing, reaching, grasping, and pulling, predispose the joints and spine to injuries. As a result of poor body mechanics and repetitive use, muscles and joints become over-stressed, which can result in overuse injuries such as carpal tunnel syndrome, low back sprain/strains, rotator cuff tendonitis, and deQuervain tenosynovitis.
- What was the patient doing at the time pain first started? Information surrounding the onset of the pain helps the PA understand the mechanism of injury and if there was a specific episode in which a body part was injured.
- Has the patient experienced the pain before? An answer to this question helps the PA determine if this is a new or recurrent injury. If the pain is recurrent, the PA will explore the site of the original pain and radiation, duration and frequency of the symptoms, previous diagnostic studies, recovery time, and treatment that alleviated the symptoms. This information will help the PA determine if the condition is acute or chronic and allows assessment of the patient's tolerance to pain.

- Is the pain associated with activities, rest, time of day, and posture? Insidious onset of morning pain, fatigue, and polyarthritis is associated with rheumatoid arthritis. Peripheral nerve entrapments and thoracic outlet syndrome are typically worse at night. Chronic pain is often associated with posture, fatigue, and activity. Pain in only one joint suggests bursitis, tendonitis, or injury.
- Is the pain associated with symptoms elsewhere in the body? A butterfly rash on the cheek is associated with systemic lupus erythematosus. A scaly rash and pitted nails of psoriasis are associated with psoriatic arthritis, and red, burning, and itchy eyes are associated with reactive arthritis.
- How does the patient describe the pain? Muscle pain is typically dull and aching, aggravated by a particular joint or spine range of motion; nerve pain is sharp and burning and radiates in a specific nerve distribution. Bone pain is described as deep and boring. Vascular pain is diffuse and aching and is referred to other parts of the body.
- Does the patient experience a "locking," "clicking," or "giving way" or a "pop" or "shift" in the joint? A history of "locking" or "clicking" sensation is associated with a meniscal tear or loose body. A history of "giving way" is associated with a patellar dislocation, and "pop" or "shift" is associated with a cruciate or collateral ligament knee rupture.
- Is the patient experiencing any life, work/school-related, or economic stressors? Job security, academic issues, and marital and financial problems can all contribute to increasing pain because of psychological stress.

MUSCULOSKELETAL PHYSICAL EXAMINATION

The musculoskeletal physical examination is similar to the evaluation of other organ systems. The examination is systematic and includes inspection, palpation of bony landmarks, assessment of range of motion, muscle testing, sensory evaluation, and special maneuvers.

During inspection, the PA looks for symmetry of joints, joint deformities, or malalignment of bones. During inspection and palpation, the joint, surrounding tissues, and bony landmarks are assessed for swelling, ecchymosis, muscular atrophy, skin changes, subcutaneous nodules, and crepitus, which is an audible and/or palpable crunching during movement of tendons or ligaments over bone.[7]

TABLE 29-1 **Grading of Manual Muscle Testing**

Numeric Grade	Descriptive Grade	Description
5	Normal	Complete range of motion against gravity with full or normal resistance
4	Good	Complete range of motion against gravity with some resistance
3	Fair	Complete range of motion against gravity
2	Poor	Complete range of motion with gravity eliminated
1	Trace	Muscle contraction but no or limited joint motion
0	Zero	No evidence of muscle function

From American Academy of Orthopaedic Surgeons. Essentials of Musculoskeletal Care, Section 1, General Orthopaedics, Table 1.

The next step in the physical examination is to assess the range of motion of the joint to demonstrate limitations in range of motion or increased mobility and joint instability from ligamentous laxity. Measuring joint motion provides an index for limitations, as well as important information concerning the results of treatment.[7]

Muscle testing provides a semiquantitative measurement of muscle strength (Table 29-1). A sensory evaluation must be done if the patient presents with a motor and/or sensory deficit. Evaluation of peripheral nerves is outlined in Table 29-2.

SPECIAL ORTHOPEDIC TESTS

Once the PA has completed the history and physical examination, special orthopedic tests can be performed to assess a disease or condition in a particular joint. The results of orthopedic tests are used in combination with a thorough history, physical examination, and diagnostic studies to arrive at a diagnosis. Table 29-3 lists some of the more common orthopedic tests.[7,8]

COMMON ORTHOPEDIC PROBLEMS

This section of the chapter addresses selected common orthopedic problems, with discussion of typical patient presentation, preferred diagnostic studies, treatment goals, and approach to treatment.

TABLE 29-2 **Evaluation of Peripheral Nerves**

Nerve	Muscle	Sensory
Upper Extremity		
Axillary	Deltoid shoulder abduction	Lateral aspect of arm
Musculocutaneous	Biceps-elbow flexion	Lateral proximal forearm
Median	Flexor pollicis longus–thumb flexion	Tip of thumb, volar aspect
Ulnar	First dorsal interosseous abduction	Tip of little finger, volar aspect
Radial	Extensor pollicis longus–thumb extension	Dorsum of thumb web space
Lower Extremity		
Obturator	Adductors-hip adduction	Medial aspect, midthigh
Femoral	Quadriceps-knee extension	Proximal to medial malleolus
Peroneal Deep branch	Extensor hallucis longus–great toe extension	Dorsum of first web space
Superficial branch	Peroneus brevis–foot eversion	Dorsum of lateral foot
Tibial	Flexor hallucis longus–great toe flexion	Plantar aspect of foot

From American Academy of Orthopaedic Surgeons. Essentials of Musculoskeletal Care, Section 1, General Orthopaedics, Table 42.

Shoulder

Impingement Syndrome

An impingement syndrome results from compression of the rotator cuff tendons and the subacromial bursa between the greater tubercle of the humeral head and the undersurface of the acromial process.[8] The patient's symptoms include shoulder pain aggravated by overhead motions and/or inability to move the shoulder because of pain. The hallmark physical examination finding is pain reproduced by the painful arc maneuver.[9] There is also subacromial tenderness and a positive impingement test but no signs of tendon inflammation on physical examination. Magnetic resonance imaging (MRI) is indicated for chronic cases to rule out a rotator cuff tear. Treatment goals include increasing the subacromial space to reduce the degree of impingement and prevent the development of tendonitis and tendon rupture. Pendulum stretching exercise combined with prescription of a nonsteroidal anti-inflammatory drug (NSAID), restrictions on overhead reaching and positioning, and physical therapy for toning exercise are the treatments of choice.[9,10]

Biceps Tendonitis

Biceps tendonitis refers to inflammation of the long head of the tendon as it passes through the bicipital groove of the anterior humerus. The patient reports shoulder pain aggravated by lifting or overhead reaching. Physical examination reveals local tenderness in the bicep groove, pain aggravated by flexion of the elbow isometrically, a positive Yergason test, and a painful arc maneuver.[9] MRI is indicated if concurrent rotator cuff tendon tear is suggested by examination. The treatment goal is to reduce inflammation and swelling in the bicep tendon through restriction of lifting and reaching, application of ice, phonophoresis, weighted pendulum stretching, and toning exercise for the short head biceps and brachioradialis tendon.

Glenohumeral Osteoarthritis

Glenohumeral osteoarthritis is wear and tear of the articular cartilage of the glenoid labrum and humeral head. It is often preceded by trauma. Injuries associated with the development of osteoarthritis include rotator cuff tear, shoulder dislocation, humeral fracture, and rheumatoid arthritis. The patient has gradual onset of shoulder pain and stiffness. Physical examination reveals local tenderness under the coracoid process, restricted abduction and external rotation range of motion, crepitation on range of motion, swelling of the infraclavicular fossa, and/or general fullness to the shoulder. Radiographs reveal osteophyte formation at the inferior humeral head, flattening and sclerosis of the humeral head, narrowing of the articular cartilage, irregularities at the inferior glenoid fossa, and spurring of the humeral head. Treatment combines exercise to improve range of motion and muscular support with ice applications and the use of an NSAID to reduce the inflammation.

Elbow

Olecranon Bursitis

Olecranon bursitis is inflammation of the bursal sac located between the olecranon process of the ulna and the overlying skin. Most cases are caused by repetitive trauma in the form of pressure.[9] The patient has pain and swelling behind the elbow. Physical examination reveals swelling, heat, and

TABLE 29-3 **Common Orthopedic Tests**

Structure Tested	Orthopedic Test	Procedure	Rationale
Cervical spine	Foraminal compression (Spurling test)	Patient bends head to one side; examiner carefully presses straight down on the head.	Pain that radiates into the arm toward which the head is flexed during compression indicates pressure on a nerve root.
	Valsalva maneuver	Patient seated, instruct patient to bear down as if moving his or her bowels.	Localized pain of the spine indicates a space-occupying lesion (herniated disk protrusion, tumor).
	Jackson compression test	The patient rotates the head to one side; examiner exerts downward pressure on the head. Performed bilaterally.	The test is positive if on testing, pain radiates into the arm, which is indicative of pressure on the nerve root.
Shoulder	Adson maneuver	Patient seated, establish radial pulse, instruct patient to rotate head and elevate chin to the side being tested. Examiner laterally rotates and extends patient's shoulder. Patient instructed to take a deep breath and hold it.	Decrease or absence of the radial pulse—a positive test for thoracic outlet syndrome.
	Supraspinatus tendinitis test	Patient is seated, instruct patient to abduct arm. Examiner resists abduction.	Pain over the insertion of the supraspinatus tendon is indicative of supraspinatus tendinitis test.
	Yergason test	Patient's elbow flexed to 90 degrees and stabilized, against the thorax, forearm pronated. Examiner resists supination, while the patient also laterally rotates the arm against resistance.	Tenderness of the bicipital groove, or tendon may pop out of the groove—indicative of bicipital tendinitis.
	Impingement test	Patient's arm is forcibly elevated through forward flexion by the examiner.	The patient's face shows pain, reflecting a positive test result. This is indicative of overuse of the supraspinatus.
Elbow	Cozen test	Patient seated, examiner stabilizes the patient's forearm. Patient is instructed to make a fist and extend it. Examiner forces extended arm into flexion against resistance.	Pain in the area of the lateral epicondyle—indicative of lateral epicondylitis.
	Golfer elbow	Examiner palpates the patient's medial epicondyle, the patient's forearm is supinated, and the elbow and wrist are extended by the examiner.	Pain in the area of the medial epicondyle—indicative of medial epicondylitis.
	Tinel sign	Patient seated, examiner taps the groove between the olecranon process and the medial epicondyle with a reflex hammer.	Tingling sensation in the ulnar nerve distribution is a positive sign—indicates neuritis or neuroma of the ulnar nerve.
Wrist	Tinel sign	Examiner taps over the palmar surface of the wrist.	Paresthesia in the median nerve distribution—indicative of carpal tunnel syndrome.
	Phalen test	Examiner flexes the patient's wrists and holds this position for 1 minute.	Paresthesia in the median nerve distribution—indicative of carpal tunnel syndrome.
	Finkelstein test	Patient instructed to make a fist with the thumb across the palmar surface of the hand and then to stress the wrist ulnarward.	Pain distal to the styloid process of the radius—indicative of de Quervain disease.

TABLE 29-3 **Common Orthopedic Tests—cont'd**

Structure Tested	Orthopedic Test	Procedure	Rationale
Hip	Ortolani click test	Pediatric patient is supine, examiner grasps both thighs, thumbs on the lesser trochanters, and flexes and abducts the thighs bilaterally.	A palpable and/or audible click—positive signs for a displacement of the femoral head into or out of the acetabular cavity.
	Patrick test (FABER)	Patient is supine, the examiner places the patient's test foot and leg on top of the knee of the opposite leg; the examiner lowers the test in abduction.	A positive test is indicated by the test leg's remaining above the opposite leg—indicative of hip disease.
	Trendelenburg test	Patient is standing, the examiner grasps the patient's waist and places his thumbs on the posterior superior iliac spine on each ilium. The examiner instructs the patient to flex one leg at a time.	This test assesses the stability of the hip and the ability of the hip abductors to stabilize the pelvis on the femur. If the posterior superior iliac spine of either side fails to rise when the leg is flexed, it indicates a weak gluteus medius on the opposite side of flexion.
	Anvil test	Patient is supine, the examiner taps the inferior calcaneus with his or her fist.	Pain localized in the thigh is indicative of a femoral fracture or joint pathology.
Lumbar spine	Straight leg raising test	Patient is supine, examiner raises the patient's leg to point of pain or 90 degrees, drops the leg slightly until there is no pain; examiner then dorsiflexes the patient's foot.	Radiating pain with ankle dorsiflexion—stretching of the dura mater of the spinal cord (disk lesion, sciatic).
	Bragard test	Patient is supine, examiner raises the patient's leg to the point of pain, drops the leg 5 degrees; examiner then dorsiflexes the patient's foot.	Posterior thigh and/or leg pain is indicative of sciatic radiculopathy.
	Bowstring test	Patient supine, examiner places the patient's leg atop of his shoulder. Firm pressure from the examiner's thumb is applied to the popliteal area.	Pain in the lumbar region or radiculopathy—indicative of tension or pressure on the sciatic nerve.
	Sacroiliac yeoman test	Patient prone, the examiner stabilizes the pelvis and flexes the patient's leg and extends the thigh.	Deep sacroiliac pain indicates a sprain of the anterior sacroiliac ligaments; lumbar pain indicates lumbar involvement.
Knee	McMurray test	Patient supine, knee flexed at 90 degrees, examiner externally rotates the leg as examiner extends the leg; repeat for internal rotation.	A palpable or audible click—indicative of a meniscal tear.
	Apley compression test	Patient prone, knee flexed at 90 degrees, examiner stabilizes the patient's thigh with his knee. The examiner places downward pressure on the patient's heel while internally and externally rotating the foot.	Pain on either side of the knee at the level of the joint line is indicative of a torn meniscus on the respective side.
	Anterior/posterior drawer sign	Patient supine, hip flexed to 45 degrees, knee flexed to 90 degrees, patient's foot on table held in place with examiner sitting on the foot; examiner grasps behind flexed knee and exerts pulling and pushing pressure on the leg.	Gapping when the leg is pulled is indicative of anterior cruciate ligament laxity; gapping when the leg is pushed is indicative of posterior cruciate ligament laxity.
	Abduction (valgus stress) and adduction (varus stress) tests	Patient is in supine position, examiner applies valgus stress at the knee, ankle is stabilized in slight lateral rotation; repeat with examiner applying varus stress.	Laxity with valgus stress is indicative of medial collateral ligament instability; laxity with varus stress is indicative of lateral collateral ligament instability.

Continued

TABLE 29-3 **Common Orthopedic Tests—cont'd**

Structure Tested	Orthopedic Test	Procedure	Rationale
Ankle	Anterior drawer sign	Patient supine, examiner grasps the foot and exerts a pulling and pressure on talus; tibia and fibula are stabilized with examiner's hand.	Laxity when the tibia is pushed is indicative of anterior talofibular ligament instability. Laxity when the tibia is pulled is indicative of posterior talofibular ligament tear.
	Tinel sign	Examiner taps over the posterior tibial nerve.	Paresthesias radiating to the foot—indicative of tarsal tunnel syndrome.
	Lateral and medial stability tests	Patient in supine position, examiner grasps the patient's foot and passively inverts; repeat with eversion.	Laxity with inversion indicative of anterior talofibular and/or calcaneofibular ligament instability; laxity with eversion indicative of deltoid ligament instability.

redness over the olecranon process, but range of motion is not affected. Diagnosis is confirmed by aspiration of bursal fluid and analysis to differentiate acute traumatic bursitis from gout and infection. The goals of treatment are to reduce swelling and inflammation and to prevent chronic bursitis. Treatment includes aspiration, drainage, and laboratory analysis of bursa fluid, neoprene elbow sleeve, corticosteroid injection, and antibiotics for infection.

Wrist

de Quervain Tenosynovitis

de Quervain tenosynovitis is an inflammation of the extensor and flexor tendons of the thumb. The tenosynovitis develops as a result of repetitive or unaccustomed use of the thumb (gripping and grasping), which leads to friction of the tendons as they pass over the distal radial styloid. The patient has wrist pain and difficulty with grasping. Physical examination reveals tenderness and swelling at the radial styloid process; inflammation and swelling of the extensor pollicis longus, extensor pollicis brevis, and abductor pollicis longus tendons; and decreased range of motion of the thumb. Tenderness is noted over the distal portion of the radial styloid; pain is aggravated by resisting thumb extension and abduction and by a positive Finkelstein maneuver. Treatment goals include reducing inflammation in the tenosynovial sac, thereby preventing adhesions from forming and tendonitis from recurring. Treatment includes a thumb spica splint; physical therapy (ice, phonophoresis with hydrocortisone gel, stretching exercises); and NSAIDs. Corticosteroid injections may be indicated for patients experiencing symptoms for longer than 6 weeks.[9,11]

Carpal Tunnel Syndrome

Carpal tunnel syndrome is a neuropathy of the median nerve that results from compression under the transverse carpal ligament at the wrist. The patient has a loss of sensation in the median nerve distribution (thumb, index, and medial half of the long fingers). Physical examination reveals decreased sensation (light touch, sharp/dull) of the median nerve distribution, a positive Tinel sign, and a positive Phalen sign. Thenar muscle atrophy is a late finding. The nerve conduction velocity test is the test of choice to confirm median nerve compression. The goal of treatment is to reduce compression of the median nerve and prevent recurrence of carpal tunnel syndrome through improved ergonomics. The treatment includes wrist splint, reduction of repetitive wrist motion, NSAIDs, ergonomics, physical therapy (stretching exercises for the flexor tendons), and corticosteroid injection. Surgical release is considered if motor symptoms have developed or symptoms fail to improve.[9]

Dorsal Ganglion

Dorsal ganglion is an overproduction of synovial or tenosynovial fluid and its accumulation into the subcutaneous tissue from abnormalities in the wrist or

CASE STUDY 29-1

HISTORY

A 44-year-old female secretary presents to the primary care office with an 8-week history of increasing right hand pain. The pain is associated with numbness of the right thumb and index and long fingers, and it is worse after an 8-hour day at work. The patient reports that she frequently drops objects and is having difficulty opening doors with her right hand. Recently, the patient has awakened at night with the numbness and needs to shake her hand to get relief from the numbness.

PHYSICAL EXAMINATION

The patient is right hand dominant.

Inspection: Hand reveals no thenar atrophy, skin is warm and moist.

Sensation: Decreased sensation to light touch of the median nerve distribution of the hand. Two-point discrimination and vibratory sensation of the hands are intact bilaterally.

Motor: Thumb opposition against resistance reveals no weakness of the thenar muscles.

Peripheral pulses: Radial, ulnar, and brachial pulses are strong and equal bilaterally.

Special tests: Positive Phalen and Tinel tests.

DIAGNOSTIC TESTS

Radiographs of the wrist are normal. Electromyogram (EMG) and nerve conduction velocity (NCV) studies confirm carpal tunnel syndrome.

DIAGNOSIS

Carpal tunnel syndrome.

TREATMENT

Carpal tunnel syndrome is the most common compression neuropathy in the upper extremity; it affects adults of all ages, women more than men. It is common during the last trimester of pregnancy and often resolves after childbirth. When associated with distal radius fractures, it must be recognized and treated emergently with carpal tunnel release. In this case, the patient should be treated conservatively with splinting of the wrist in neutral position, a course of NSAIDs, and avoidance of repetitive activities of the right hand and wrist. The patient should wear the splint all day and while sleeping. Work-related carpal tunnel may be improved with ergonomic modifications, such as using keyboard supports and antivibration padded gloves, repositioning the wrist at the keyboard or assembly line, and avoiding holding the wrist in a flexed position. Corticosteroid injection into the carpal ligament is used as an adjunct treatment. Decompressive surgery is considered with persistent hand pain that does not resolve with nocturnal splinting, when conservative therapy fails, or with rapidly developing motor or sensory deficits.

the extensor tendon sheath. The patient has a painless lump at the wrist. Physical examination reveals a highly mobile, fluctuant cyst overlying the wrist, with minimal tenderness and full range of motion of the wrist. The goals of treatment are to reassure the patient that it is not cancer and then to aspirate the cyst to prevent recurrence. Treatment includes aspiration, reassurance and education of the patient, a wrist brace to limit repetitive motions, and surgical excision of the cyst and sinus if treatment is refractory.[9]

Hand

Trigger Finger

Trigger finger is an inflammation of the flexor tendons of the finger as they cross the metacarpophalangeal (MCP) head in the palm. As a result of repetitive gripping, pressure over the palm causes swelling and inflammation of the flexor tendons. As the swelling and inflammation increase, the flexor tendons lose their smooth motion under the A1 pulley, the specialized ligament that anchors the tendon to the bone. The patient has a painful finger and a loss of smooth motion of the finger when gripping.[12] Physical examination reveals tenderness at the base of the finger, increased pain with tendon extension, and clicking or locking with active flexion of the proximal interphalangeal (PIP) joint (fingers) and the interphalangeal (IP) joint (thumb). Treatment goals involve reduction of swelling and inflammation in the flexor tendon sheath, which allows smoother movement of the tendon under the A1 pulley, and the prevention of recurrence. Treatment includes ice, restricted gripping, buddy-taping or metal finger splint, and corticosteroid injection for persistent cases. Surgical release is considered if symptoms are not relieved with injection.[9,12]

Chest

Costochondritis

Costochondritis is inflammation of the cartilage at the junction of the rib and the costal cartilage. Patients complain of anterior chest pain. Physical examination reveals local tenderness, either 1 inch from the midline of the sternum or at the costochondral junctions, and reproducible pain by chest wall compression. Radiographs of the chest are normal. The goals of treatment are to reassure the patient that this is not a cardiac condition and to reduce inflammation. Treatment includes reassurance, restriction of strenuous activity, NSAIDs, and local anesthetic injection.[8]

Hip

Trochanteric Bursitis

Trochanteric bursitis is an inflammation of the lubricating sac located between the midportion of the trochanteric process of the femur and the gluteus medius tendon/iliotibial tract, caused by repetitive flexing of the hip. A disturbance in gait is the most common cause of a trochanteric bursitis. The patient has hip pain over the outer thigh or difficulty on walking. Physical examination reveals local tenderness of the greater trochanter, increased hip pain at the extremes of internal and external rotation and with resisted hip abduction, and normal range of motion of the hip. Findings of underlying lumbosacral or sacroiliac diseases, gait disturbance, or leg length discrepancy may also be noted.

Radiographs of the hip are recommended to evaluate for underlying disease. The goals of treatment are to reduce inflammation of the bursa, correct disturbances of gait, and prevent recurrence with hip and back stretching exercises. Treatment includes application of heat; passive stretching of the gluteus medius tendon, lumbosacral spine, and sacroiliac joint; and the use of NSAIDs, therapeutic ultrasound, and the transcutaneous electrical nerve stimulation (TENS) unit for chronic bursitis, as well as corticosteroid injection.[9,12,13]

Knee

Chondromalacia Patellae

Chondromalacia patellae is the pathologic entity of cartilage softening on the underside of the kneecap. Typically, this condition is an overuse syndrome. Poor muscle tone, overdeveloped vastus lateralis, flexibility deficits, pes planus, and blunt trauma to the knee predispose to the condition. The patient complains of anterior knee pain and a "noisy" or "clicking" or "catching" sensation of the knee, infrequently associated with swelling. The patient may complain of the knee "locking." Physical examination reveals painful retropatellar crepitation, the patella may be visibly subluxed, and a palpable patellar click and positive apprehension sign may be noted. Radiographs of the knee should include a sunrise view to evaluate for lateral subluxation, narrowing of the patellofemoral articular cartilage, and osteoarthritic changes. Treatment goals are to improve patellofemoral tracking and alignment, reduce pain, and slow down the development of arthritis. Treatment includes NSAIDs to improve quadriceps strength and endurance, knee sleeve for pelvic muscle strength, and, for persistent cases, local corticosteroid injection.[9]

Prepatellar Bursitis

Prepatellar bursitis is an inflammation of the bursal sac located between the patella and the overlying skin. The most common cause is blunt trauma resulting from a fall. The patient complains of swelling of the knee and pain in front of the knee. Physical examination reveals swelling and inflammation over the inferior portion of the patella, bursal sac tenderness, and normal range of motion. Chronic prepatellar bursitis has a cobblestone-like roughness or a palpable thickening. Treatment goals are to identify the cause of the bursitis and reduce the inflammation. Treatment approaches include padding and protection of the bursa, as well as aspiration and drainage for diagnostic studies.[9,13]

Baker's Cyst

Baker's cyst is an abnormal collection of synovial fluid in the fatty layers of the popliteal fossa. The fluid escapes from the synovial lining, resulting in a fibrotic reaction in the subcutaneous tissue and cyst formation. The patient complains of tightness behind the knee. Physical examination reveals a palpable cystic mass in the medial aspect of the popliteal fossa. No signs of peripheral vascular insufficiency are noted. A large cyst may impair knee flexion. Diagnostic ultrasound can assess the size of the cyst, but definitive diagnosis requires aspiration. The goal of treatment is to correct the abnormal accumulation of fluid. Treatment includes advising that the cyst may resolve on its own; restricting squatting, kneeling, and repetitive bending; applying a knee sleeve; and providing local aspiration and corticosteroid injection. Surgical removal may be advised if the cyst interferes with full function of the knee.[9]

Meniscal Tear of the Knee

A torn meniscus is a disruption of the fibrocartilage pads between the femoral condyles and the tibial plateaus. The main function of the menisci is shock absorbency of the knee joint. The mechanism of injury involves rotatory stress on a weight-bearing knee. The patient complains of the knee "locking," "clicking," or "giving way." Physical examination reveals joint line tenderness, a positive

McMurray's test, joint effusion, decreased passive range of motion, and inability to squat or kneel. Radiographs of the knee may show degenerative changes. MRI confirms the presence of a meniscal tear. Goals of treatment are to define the type and extent of the tear, strengthen the muscular support of the knee, and determine the need for surgery. Treatment includes ice, elevation, and physical therapy to strengthen the knee. Isolated meniscal tear in a repairable zone in a young patient should be repaired; symptomatic meniscal tear in a nonrepairable zone or a complex meniscal tear should be arthroscopically débrided.[9,12,13]

CASE STUDY 29-2

HISTORY

A 25-year-old female soccer player presents to the primary care physician with a sudden onset of left knee pain while playing soccer. The patient states that she twisted her left knee while playing soccer and heard a "pop"; the knee suddenly gave way. The patient states the knee immediately swelled and she was not able to continue in the game. She has no medical history of knee injury.

PHYSICAL EXAMINATION

Inspection: Swelling of the left knee.
Palpation: No tenderness of the meniscus or patellofemoral and collateral ligaments.
Sensory: Intact sensation to light touch and sharp/dull.
Peripheral pulses: Femoral, popliteal, dorsalis pedis, and posterior pulses are strong and equal bilaterally.
Range of motion: Passive and active motion of the left knee decreased with flexion and extension.
Special tests: Positive bulge sign, positive patellar ballottement test; positive Lachman test and anterior drawer sign, negative posterior drawer sign; negative McMurray sign and varus and valgus stressing.

DIAGNOSTIC TESTS

Anteroposterior and lateral radiographs of the knee are negative.
MRI positive for anterior cruciate ligament tear.

DIAGNOSIS

Anterior cruciate ligament tear.

TREATMENT

The anterior cruciate ligament (ACL) is a primary stabilizer of the knee, and a tear of the ACL results from a twisting or hyperextension force applied to the knee joint. Initial treatment includes rest, ice, knee immobilization, NSAIDs, and crutches. An arthrocentesis in this case will most likely reveal hemarthrosis of the knee. In the absence of a distended knee joint, there is no need for aspiration of an acutely injured knee. Definitive treatment of an ACL tear for a young, active patient is reconstruction and referral to the physical therapy department for rehabilitation. Female athletes, particularly those playing soccer, gymnastics, and basketball, are at the highest risk for ACL injury. Older or less active patients can be treated more conservatively with physical therapy, with the goal to control instability.

Ankle

Plantar Fasciitis

Plantar fasciitis is inflammation of the origin of the longitudinal ligament that forms the arch of the foot. Predisposing conditions include obesity, flatfeet (pes planus), working on concrete, poorly fitted shoes, and prolonged standing. The patient has heel pain aggravated by weight bearing. Physical examination reveals tenderness of the plantar fascia, pain with calcaneal compression, and limited flexibility of the Achilles tendon. Radiographs and bone scan are indicated to rule out stress fractures. Radiographs are indicated to rule out pressure-aggravated heel spur. Treatment goals are to reduce inflammation and increase the flexibility of the heel and ankle. Treatment includes reduction of weight bearing, padded arch supports, NSAIDs, stretching exercises, corticosteroid injection, and surgery for recurrent fasciitis.[9,10]

Foot

Bunion

Bunion is a bony prominence and valgus deformity of the great toe. Asymmetric pressure over the articular cartilage caused by narrow shoes occurs over years. The patient complains of abnormal-looking toes, pain of the great toe, and shoes that do not fit. Physical examination reveals metatarsophalangeal (MTP) joint tenderness and enlargement, hallux valgus deformity of the great toe, crepitation of the joint, and limited range of motion. Radiographs assess the valgus angle and degree of arthritic changes. Treatment goals are to reduce joint inflammation and prevent arthritic deterioration and further valgus deformity. Treatment includes advising the patient to wear loose-fitting shoes and prescribing NSAIDs. Bunionectomy may be considered to improve alignment, reduce medial joint line pressure, and improve function.[9,10]

Hammer Toe

Hammer toe describes the toe deformity caused by contracted extensor tendons of the foot. The hammer toe deformity is a result of years of tight, inflexible extensor tendons. The patient complains of pain over the ball of the foot, calluses, or abnormal-looking toes. Physical examination reveals tight extensor tendons, tenderness directly over the MTP joint, corns, and calluses. Treatment goals are to stretch the dorsal extensor tendons and reestablish normal toe alignment. Treatment includes loose-fitting shoes, padding for corns and calluses, stretching exercises, and flexor tenotomy or arthroplasty if symptoms and deformity are persistent.[9]

Fractures

A significant portion of the PA's scope of care in an orthopedics practice involves the evaluation, diagnosis, and management of fractures. A fracture refers to a broken bone and is a result of direct or indirect violence to the bone. Table 29-4 lists definitions of fractures. The history should include a detailed account of the mechanism of injury; the position of the joint at the time of injury; the motion of the joint that exacerbates or relieves pain; neurologic symptoms; previous musculoskeletal injuries; past illness (e.g., asthma, heart disease, peripheral vascular disease, diabetes mellitus, bleeding disorders); last meal; medications taken (e.g., steroids, anticoagulants); and history of smoking.[12]

Physical examination must be a meticulous head-to-toe examination that includes the following:

- The joint above and below the injured joint
- Neurologic examination (range of motion, sensory, motor)
- Peripheral vascular

The emergent treatment of the patient with potential injury to more than one organ system is handled by a team of specialists, including an orthopedic practitioner. Treatment is organized in three stages: primary survey, secondary survey, and definitive management. The primary survey is concerned with the ABCs (airway, breathing, and circulation). The secondary survey includes a careful account of the accident, a description of the mechanism of injury, a thorough physical examination, and radiologic studies. Radiographs of the joint above and below the injury site and comparison views should be considered. Special views may be ordered after consultation with the radiologist.[12]

TABLE 29-4 **Definitions of Fractures**

Closed	Fracture site does not communicate with the exterior of the body
Open	Fracture site communicates with the exterior of the body
Articular	Fracture that involves the joint surfaces
Undisplaced	Hairline fracture without loss of normal anatomic configuration
Displaced	Separation of fracture fragments has occurred with loss of anatomic configuration
Angulated	Fracture with a bending or angular deformity (Figure 29-2)
Comminuted	Fracture involves bone fragment in more than two pieces
Avulsed	Bone fragment pulled off by attached ligaments (Figure 29-3B)
Oblique	The fracture line site runs obliquely to the axis of the bone
Compression	The fracture is common in cancellous flat bones because of the spongy consistency (Figure 29-3C)
Impacted	Fracture that is produced by severe violence that drives the bone fragment firmly together (see Figure 29-3A)
Spiral	Fracture produced by a twisting or rotatory force
Segmental	Fracture with a single, large, free-floating segment of bone between two well-defined fracture lines
Stress	The bone may undergo a "fatigue" fracture from repetitive forces
Pathologic	Fractures that occur from relatively minor trauma to diseased bones (Figure 29-3D)
SALTER-HARRIS CLASSIFICATION (FIGURE 29-4)	
Fractures involving the epiphyseal plate at the end of the long bone of a growing child	
Salter Type	
I	The growth plate is fractured
II	The growth plate and the metaphysis are fractured
III	The growth plate and the epiphysis are fractured
IV	The metaphysis, growth plate, and epiphysis are fractured
V	Nothing "broken off," compression injury of the epiphyseal plate

The definitive management of fractures—after serious injuries to the head, abdomen, and chest have been stabilized—includes the following:

- Elevation of the extremity
- Cold compress to reduce swelling
- Immobilization (splinting, cast)
- Analgesics
- Manual or surgical reduction

Table 29-5 lists some of the most common orthopedic fractures seen in a primary care office.

Pediatric Orthopedics

This section provides an overview of selected problems in pediatric orthopedics, including etiology, patient presentation, diagnostic studies, treatment goals, and approach to treatment.

Osteochondritis Dissecans

Osteochondritis dissecans of the knee results from repetitive stress that causes osteonecrosis of the underlying bone and ultimately a subchondral stress fracture. The most common location is the medial femoral condyle. Symptoms usually present during childhood, including pain and stiffness after running and sport activities. Physical examination may be unremarkable or may reveal mild effusion or quadriceps atrophy. Management involves modifying activity to prevent symptoms. The patient may not be involved in sports for 3 to 12 months. Indications for operative treatment include an unstable knee, a loose body, or persistent symptoms after nonoperative management has been implemented.[14]

Developmental Dysplasia of the Hip (DDH)

Developmental dysplasia of the hip encompasses all dysplastic hip disorders. DDH is associated with ligamentous laxity and is detectable at birth. DDH is

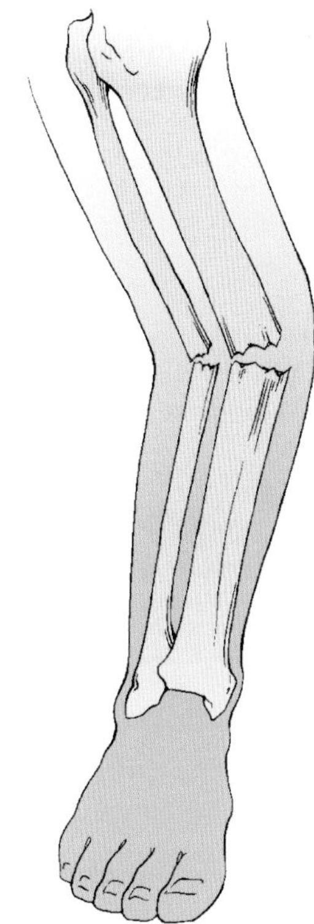

FIGURE 29-2 ■ Fracture type, angulated fracture. (From Eiff MP, Calmbach WL, Hatch R. Fracture Management for Primary Care, 2nd ed. Philadelphia: WB Saunders, 2003.)

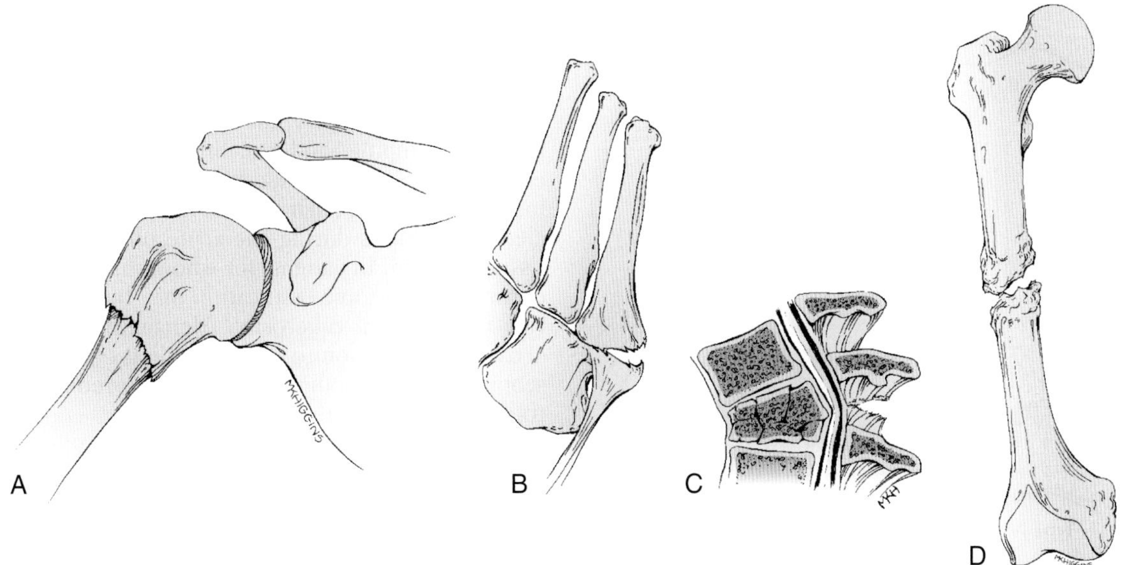

FIGURE 29-3 ■ Fracture types. **A,** Impacted. **B,** Avulsion. **C,** Compression. **D,** Pathologic. (From Eiff MP, Calmbach WL, Hatch R. Fracture Management for Primary Care, 2nd ed. Philadelphia: WB Saunders, 2003.)

more common among females and is more likely to be noted in the left hip in breech presentation. There is an increased incidence in North American Indians and whites of northern European ancestry. Most afflicted neonates are detectable at birth and are asymptomatic. Parents may notice a limp, a waddling gait pattern, or a limb-length discrepancy when the infant begins to walk. Physical examination reveals a positive Ortolani click test. In older children, secondary adaptive changes may be evident, including waddling gait and symmetry of the gluteal thigh and labial folds. The goal of treatment is to contain the femoral head within the acetabulum while the acetabulum develops and the hip stabilizes. An abduction brace is usually sufficient for newborns and infants. The brace should be continued until acetabular development and joint stability have occurred.[14]

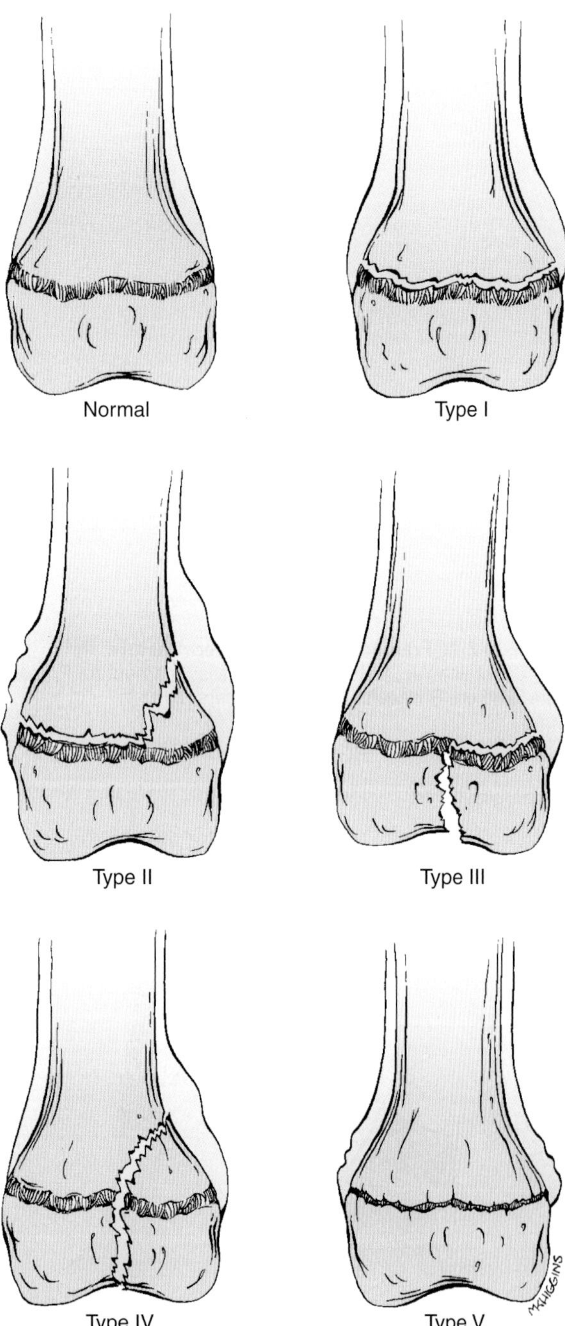

FIGURE 29-4 ■ The Salter-Harris classification. (From Eiff MP, Calmbach WL, Hatch R. Fracture Management for Primary Care, 2nd ed. Philadelphia: WB Saunders, 2002.)

Pes Planus (Flatfoot)

Flatfoot is an abnormally low or absent longitudinal arch. It may be congenital or may result from trauma or tendon degeneration. Flexible flatfoot is more common and involves a normal foot shape in infants. Flexible flatfoot is usually painless. Physical examination reveals the heel in valgus alignment, an abducted forefoot, and a loss of longitudinal arch on weight bearing. The range of motion is normal, but secondary contracture of the Achilles tendon may develop in older children. Management is usually not required. Modifications to shoe and orthotic devices have not been proven to alter the natural development of a longitudinal arch. If fatigue symptoms or activity-related discomfort persists, shoe modification may provide support and, thus, relief.[12,14]

Osgood-Schlatter Disease

Osgood-Schlatter disease results from repetitive injury or small avulsion injuries at the bone-tendon junction where the patellar tendon inserts into the secondary ossification center of the tibial tuberosity. The typical history includes pain exacerbated by running, jumping, and kneeling activities. Physical examination reveals tenderness and swelling at the insertion of the patellar tendon into the tibial tubercle. Radiographs during the acute phase reveal soft tissue swelling. In patients for whom this condition is chronic, heterotopic ossification may be noted anterior to the tibial tuberosity. Management involves activity modification to permit healing of the microscopic avulsion fractures. Athletes may return to full training in 6 to 7 months.[14]

Arthritic Disorders

Rheumatoid Arthritis

Rheumatoid arthritis (RA) is a systemic autoimmune disease and results from a cellular-mediated immune response (T cell) that incites inflammatory response initially against the soft tissue and later against cartilage and bone, which leads to joint destruction. The female-to-male ratio is 2.5:1. It appears that female hormone influences the development of rheumatoid arthritis because there is an increased risk in nulliparous women, decreased incidence with the use of oral contraceptives, and remission of symptoms during pregnancy. The typical history involves an insidious onset of morning stiffness, fatigue, and

TABLE 29-5 **Types of Fractures**

Bone/Joint	Fracture Description	Mechanism of Injury	Complication(s)
Clavicle	Most common location is middle third of the clavicle, common in children and young adults	Indirect through a fall on the lateral shoulder or an outstretched hand or a direct blow to the clavicle	Uncommon, rarely subclavian vessels trapped
Humerus	Proximal humerus fracture, common in elderly patients	Young adults high-energy trauma, fall onto arm or elbow	Loss of motion, nonunion, nerve and vascular damage
Elbow	Supracondylar fractures most common in children and elderly patients	Fall on extended or flexed elbow	Loss of motion, ulnar nerve palsy, varus or valgus deformity
Wrist	Colles fracture, fracture of the distal radius, common in elderly patients, related to osteoporosis in this age group	Fall on the outstretched hand with wrist in extension	Stiffness of the finger joints and shoulders, carpal tunnel syndrome, rupture of tendons (Figure 29-5)
	Scaphoid fracture	Fall on the outstretched hand or direct blow to hand	Delayed union, nonunion, avascular necrosis
Fingers	Boxer fracture of the 5th metacarpal neck (Figure 29-6A and B)	Direct impact on metacarpal head with hand in clenched position	Prominent metacarpal head in palm, rotational malunion
	Mallet finger, avulsion fracture of the distal phalanx	Forced flexion of fingertip actively extended	Mallet finger deformity
Rib	Nondisplaced rib fractures most common	Blunt trauma or severe paroxysms of coughing	Pneumothorax, trauma to internal organs and vessels
Pelvis	Pelvic fracture	Automobile passenger, pedestrian accidents, or minor fall in older patients	Hemorrhage, rectal injuries, ruptured diaphragm, nerve root injury
Hip	Femoral neck fracture	Minor trauma secondary to a fall, common among older adults owing to osteoporosis, women more than men	Avascular necrosis
Knee	Tibial plateau	Direct blow or twisting injury	Loss of range of motion, early degenerative joint changes, infection, nerve and vascular injuries
Ankle	Ankle fractures are intra-articular injuries	Plantar flexion and inversion injury—"twisted ankle"	Associated 5th metatarsal fracture
Foot	Calcaneal fracture	Fall from a height and lands on the heels	Associated compression fractures of lumbar spine, compartment syndrome
Toes	Phalangeal fractures	Blunt trauma	Maceration secondary to taping
		Type I: Fracture of growth plate Type II: Fracture of growth plate with fracture of metaphysis Type III: Fracture of growth plate and portion of epiphysis Type IV: Single fracture through growth plate, metaphysis, and epiphysis Type V: Nothing fractured, crushing injury to growth plate	Potential for growth disturbances

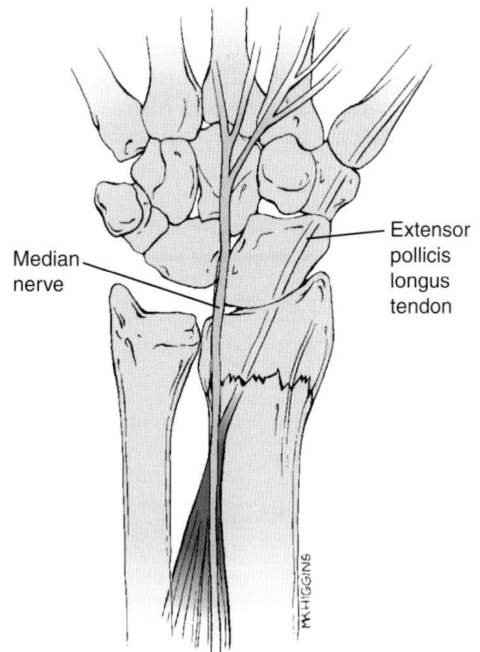

FIGURE 29-5 ■ The median nerve may be associated with a distal radius fracture. (From Eiff MP, Calmbach WL, Hatch R. Fracture Management for Primary Care, 2nd ed. Philadelphia: WB Saunders, 2003.)

polyarthritis. The joints most commonly involved are the hands, feet, knees, elbows, shoulders, ankles, and neck. Physical examination may reveal chronic swelling; thickening of the metacarpophalangeal (MCP) and proximal interphalangeal (PIP) joints; pannus ingrowth, which gradually denudes articular cartilage; limited range of motion; ulnar deviation of the MCP joint; rheumatoid nodules of the bony prominences; and hand deformities such as swan-neck and boutonnière deformities. Additionally, there may be systemic involvement of other organs such as lung, heart, skin, and eye or involvement of the gastrointestinal or genitourinary systems. Diagnostic studies reveal elevated erythrocyte sedimentation rate, C-reactive protein, positive rheumatoid titer, and a hypochromic, normocytic anemia. Radiographs reveal periarticular erosions and osteopenia of the MCP and PIP joints, carpal bones, and cervical spine. The goal in management is to control the synovitis and pain, maintain joint function, and prevent deformities. **Drug therapy will begin with NSAIDs; additional drugs include antimalarials, methotrexate, sulfasalazine, gold salts, penicillamine, and steroids.** Physical therapy may be used to improve the patient's function, and splints and braces can be used on affected joints to prevent joint destruction.[15-17]

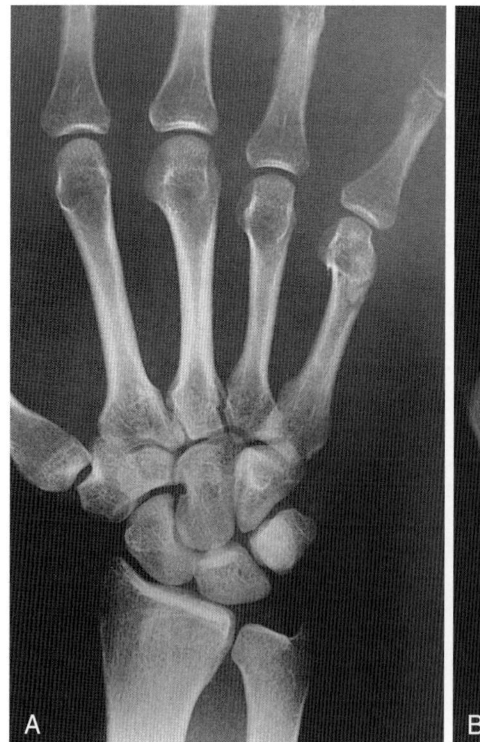

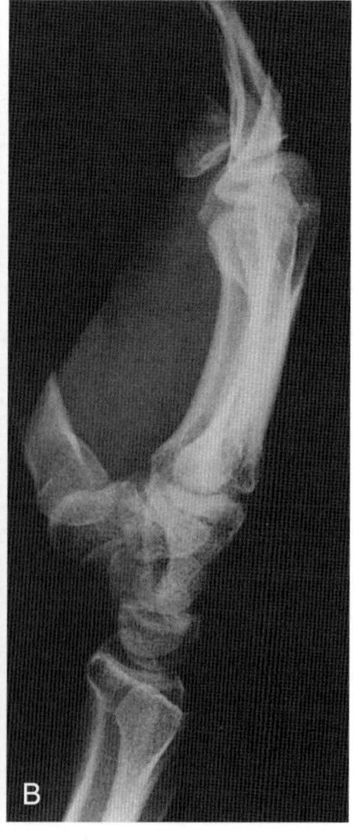

FIGURE 29-6 ■ **A,** Anteroposterior view. **B,** Lateral view of a boxer's fracture. (From Eiff MP, Calmbach WL, Hatch R. Fracture Management for Primary Care, 2nd ed. Philadelphia: WB Saunders, 2003.)

Osteoarthritis (Degenerative Joint Disease)

Osteoarthritis is the most common form of arthritis, and 85% of adults 65 years of age and older radiographically demonstrated changes of osteoarthritis. Osteoarthritis results from the failed attempt of chondrocytes to repair damaged cartilage, characterized by increased water content, alterations of proteoglycans, collagen abnormalities, and binding of proteoglycans to hyaluronic acid. The joints undergo degenerative changes including subchondral bony sclerosis. The physical examination reveals insidious onset of joint pain, usually pain after exercise or use of the joint. The common joints involved are the hand (DIP, PIP); wrist; hip; knee; and cervical/lumbar spine. Hand deformities include Heberden nodes, hard and painless nodules of the dorsolateral aspects of the DIP joint secondary to overgrowth, and Bouchard node, hard painless nodules of the PIP. Radiographic studies reveal osteophytes and "joint space" narrowing, subchondral cysts from microfractures, and bone repair. The management treatment begins with supportive measures (i.e., activity modification, cane); NSAIDs; and application of heat. Surgical procedures ranging from arthroscopic débridement to total joint arthroplasties may be useful and advance patients to resistant nonoperative treatment.[15-17]

Reactive Arthritis

Reactive arthritis is characterized by sterile inflammation of joints from infections originating at nonarticular sites. *Chlamydia trachomatis* is usually the causative organism of the postvenereal variety, as well as *Shigella*, *Salmonella*, *Yersinia*, and *Campylobacter* following enteric bacterial infection. The triad of features for reactive arthritis include oligoarticular arthritis, conjunctivitis, and urethritis or cervicitis. The physical examination may reveal a seriously ill–appearing patient (i.e., fever, rigors, tachycardia, exquisitely tender joints). The arthritis is most commonly asymmetric and frequently involves large, weight-bearing joints (usually knee and ankle). Mucocutaneous symptoms are balanitis, stomatitis, keratoderma, and blennorrhagica. The diagnostic studies reveal positive human leukocyte antigen (HLA)-B27, elevated white blood cell count and sedimentation rate, moderate normochromic anemia, and hypergammaglobulinemia. Synovial fluid reveals a negative bacterial culture, positive cultures or serology for *C. trachomatis*, or stool cultures positive for *Shigella*, *Yersinia*, or *Campylobacter*. Radiographs reveal periosteal proliferation, thickening, spurs, erosions at articular margins, residual joint destruction, syndesmophytes (spine), and sacroiliitis. The mainstay of therapy is NSAIDs. No treatment is necessary for the conjunctivitis and mucocutaneous lesions. Iritis may require treatment. Physical therapy during the recovery phase and prompt treatment of the precipitating process reduce one's chances of developing reactive arthritis.[14-16]

CHALLENGES AND REWARDS FOR PHYSICIAN ASSISTANTS IN ORTHOPEDICS

PAs working in orthopedic surgery encounter a number of challenges. Although some patients demonstrate improvement and/or cure of their problems, other orthopedic patients have chronic disabling conditions that do not improve. PAs may find it difficult to help patients make the behavioral changes needed to improve their musculoskeletal status. For example, obesity exacerbates most orthopedic problems, but losing weight constitutes one of the more difficult challenges for patients and clinicians.

As with any subspecialty practice, PAs in orthopedic surgery may find limited opportunities to use the full range of their primary care skills. However, PAs in orthopedic surgery will find themselves working collaboratively with physicians and PAs in other specialties who also treat patients who have orthopedic injuries. Some of the specialties include rheumatology, plastic surgery, trauma, neurology, and gerontology.

Rewards for orthopedic PAs include the satisfaction of helping patients regain function and improve their quality of life. Many PAs find it particularly satisfying to see athletes resume their training and succeed in their sports (often the PAs who choose this field enjoy participating in athletic activities themselves). Additionally, there is a wide range of conditions and ages of patients that offer orthopedic PAs a diversity in scope of care that is not offered in other specialties.

CONCLUSION

PAs in orthopedics must develop a thorough knowledge of anatomy and must sharpen their history and physical examination skills because most diagnoses are based on this foundation. In addition to helping patients and exercising their clinical skills, orthopedic PAs enjoy participating in outpatient, inpatient, and surgical care. As the U.S. population ages, this surgical subspecialty is likely to continue to offer a wide range of opportunities for PAs.

CLINICAL APPLICATIONS

1. Practice the orthopedic special tests listed in Table 29-3.
2. If you accepted a position in an orthopedic surgery practice, what knowledge and skills would you need to update?
3. Interview a patient who has recovered from an orthopedic injury. What rehabilitation approaches were successful for this patient? Why?

KEY POINTS

- The utilization of PAs in orthopedic surgery continues to increase each year.
- PAs in orthopedic surgical practices conduct more than 18.6 million patient visits, an average of 70 per week per PA.
- It is estimated that 80% to 90% of orthopedic conditions can be diagnosed based on thorough and accurate orthopedic history and physical examination.
- An example of common orthopedic conditions a PA will diagnosis and treat in a primary care setting include impingement syndrome, bicep tendonitis, glenohumeral osteoarthritis, olecranon bursitis, de Quervain tenosynovitis, carpal tunnel syndrome, dorsal ganglion, trigger finger, costochondritis, trochanteric bursitis, chondromalacia patellae, prepatellar burisitis, Baker cyst, and plantar fasciitis.
- As the U.S. population ages, the orthopedic surgical subspecialty will continue to grow and offer a wide range of opportunities for PAs.

References

1. Dandy DJ, Edwards JD. Essential Orthopaedics and Trauma. 5th ed. Philadelphia: Elsevier Churchill Livingstone, 2009.
2. American Academy of Physician Assistants. 2008 PA Census. *www.aapa.org*; Accessed July 9, 2011.
3. American Academy of Physician Assistants. 2001 PA Census. *www.aapa.org*; Accessed April 19, 2007.
4. American Academy of Physician Assistants. Number of patient visits made to physician assistants and number of medications prescribed or recommended by physician assistants in 2008. *www.aapa.org/images/stories/iu08visitsandrx.pdf*; Accessed July 9, 2010.
5. Magee DJ. Orthopedic Physical Assessment. 5th ed. Philadelphia: Elsevier Saunders, 2008.
6. Griffin WB. Essentials of Musculoskeletal Care. 3rd ed. Rosemont, Ill: American Academy of Orthopaedic Surgeons, 2006.
7. Bickley LS. Bates Guide to Physical Examination and History Taking. 10th ed. Philadelphia: Lippincott Williams & Wilkins, 2009.
8. Cipriano JJ. Photographic Manual of Orthopaedic Tests. 4th ed. Baltimore: Lippincott Williams & Wilkins, 2006.
9. Anderson BC. Office Orthopedics for Primary Care Diagnosis and Treatment. 3rd ed. Philadelphia: Elsevier Saunders, 2006.
10. Matsul M. The painful shoulder: is it impingement syndrome? J Am Acad Physician Assistants 2000;13(18):23–30.
11. O'Neil DM. Understanding inflammatory disorders of the upper extremity. J Am Acad Physician Assistants 2001;14(16):23.
12. Swiontkowki MF (ed). Manual of Orthopaedics. 6th ed. Philadelphia: Lippincott Williams & Wilkins, 2006.
13. Puffer JC. 20 Common Problems in Sports Medicine. New York: McGraw-Hill, 2002.
14. Bergaman AB. 20 Common Problems in Pediatrics. New York: McGraw-Hill, 2001.
15. Skinner HB. Current Diagnosis and Treatment Orthopedics. 4th ed. New York: McGraw-Hill, 2006.
16. Malagna GA, Nadler SF. Musculoskeletal Physical Examination: An Evidence-Based Approach. Philadelphia: Elsevier Mosby, 2006.
17. Brinker MR. Review of Orthopedic Trauma. Philadelphia: Saunders, 2001.

The resources for this chapter can be found at www.expertconsult.com.

CHAPTER 30

DERMATOLOGY

Kristine J. Kucera

CHAPTER CONTENTS

In this chapter, an overview of dermatology is presented for physician assistants (PAs) in training and new or experienced graduates who may be contemplating dermatology as a clinical specialty. Dermatology is a visually oriented specialty that offers a unique perspective on health care and includes patients from every age and demographic group. Dermatology can be an unexpectedly complex specialty, and the breadth and depth of dermatologic diagnoses can be daunting. The number of dermatologic conditions experienced tends to increase by middle age to the point that many people intermittently seek care for differing types of skin, hair, and nail disorders. Dermatology is a rewarding specialty that enables the clinician to become adept in a number of surgical procedures while establishing longstanding clinician-patient relationships because of the chronicity of many dermatologic disorders that may require decades of follow-up care.

HISTORY OF DERMATOLOGY

Since the beginning of recorded history, physical and written reference is made to the adornment and ailments of the skin, hair, and nails. Mummified bodies from Egypt and ancient papyrus documents reflect the presence of assorted lesions, tattoos, and piercings. The Hebrew Bible of 2700 years ago describes dermatologic diseases and therapies, suggesting that disorders were of divine infliction. Centuries later, the ancient Greek and Roman civilizations attempted to distinguish dermatologic diseases by external and internal causes. More than 200 years ago, modern dermatology evolved among groups of Austrian, English, French, and German dermatologists, who developed the origins of the modern-day nosography of dermatologic disorders.[1] As the specialty evolved, dermatology was combined with syphilology owing to the variable cutaneous manifestations of syphilis. Before the formation of the American Board of Dermatology in 1932, dermatologists were recognized by the Section on Dermatology and Syphilology of the American Medical Association.[2]

Dermatology in the United States began in the 1830s with Henry Daggett Bulkley and Noah Worcester. Bulkley established the first dermatology clinic, Broome Street Infirmary for Diseases of the Skin, in New York in 1836. He also developed and presented the first series of lectures on dermatology in North America. Worchester joined the faculty of the Medical School of Ohio and wrote America's first dermatology textbook, *Diseases of the Skin*.[3]

WHAT IS DERMATOLOGY?

Dermatology includes the diagnosis and treatment of pediatric and adult patients with benign and malignant disorders of the skin, mouth, external genitalia, hair, and nails, as well as a number of sexually transmitted diseases. To be certified as a dermatologist, a physician must have had at least 4 years of postgraduate residency training accredited by the Accreditation Council for Graduate Medical Education. The first broad-based general clinical (internship) year is followed by 3 years of intensive training in dermatology, including dermatopathology and dermatologic surgery.

A certified specialist in dermatology may subspecialize and become certified for Special Qualification as follows:

- **Dermatopathology** (Special Qualification in Dermatopathology)—Although all dermatologists have training and experience in dermatopathology, Special Qualification in Dermatopathology, signifying advanced competence, can be obtained by either a board-certified dermatologist or a pathologist. Special Qualification involves additional extensive training and experience in the evaluation of tissue specimens submitted from dermatologic patients.
- **Immunodermatology** (Special Qualification in Dermatological Immunology/Diagnostic and Laboratory Immunology)—An immunodermatologist is a dermatologist who, through additional specialty training, has developed expertise in the study of the cause, diagnosis, treatment, and outcome of skin diseases involving the immune system. These physicians have a basic understanding of such diseases from the perspective of anatomic and clinical pathology, as well as from the interpretation of immunologic analyses of tissue cells and body fluids.[4]

DERMATOLOGY ORGANIZATIONS

Society for Dermatology Physician Assistants

The Society for Dermatology Physician Assistants (SDPA), founded in 1994, represents full-time dermatology PAs practicing under board-certified dermatologists. The mission of the SDPA is to provide continuing medical education that enhances members in the practice of dermatology, form a leadership structure that provides services and advocacy for its members, advance the utilization of PAs in the practice of dermatology, and develop resources for supervising physicians on the hiring of PAs in dermatology. The SDPA website (*http://www.dermpa.org*) provides a wealth of current and useful information for the PA who may be interested in dermatology. The site includes many helpful links to hundreds of other relevant sites; major topics of these include academies and organizations, continuing medical education opportunities, journals and publications, commercial sites, disease-specific information, searchable sites/search engines, skin cancer–related sites, dermatology practice/dermatology PA websites, and information on universities, colleges, schools, and scholarships.

Dermatology Demographics

According to the National Center for Health Statistics, in 2008, approximately 34.4 million office visits were made to dermatologists, and approximately 12.7 million visits to office-based physicians occurred because of skin rash.[5] The 2009 Census Report from the American Academy of Physician Assistants[6] reports that 3.8% of PAs practice in dermatology. The U.S. dermatology workforce, which is affected by a physician shortage, has reportedly seen a rapid and substantial influx of PAs.[7] Currently, the demand for dermatology PAs exceeds the supply, particularly for PAs with dermatology experience.

The range of services provided by dermatology PAs is extensive and includes general dermatology with a concentration on common skin, hair, and nail disorders; skin cancer surgery, including shave, punch, and excisional biopsies; cryosurgery; electrodesiccation and curettage; lesion excision; and Mohs micrographic surgery. LASER (light amplification by stimulated emission of radiation) use by dermatology PAs is commonplace; carbon dioxide, ruby, alexandrite, neodymium:yttrium-aluminium-garnet (Nd:YAG), argon, tunable dye, pulsed tunable dye, potassium titanyl phosphate (KTP), NLite, and erbium LASERs are used for treatment of a variety of cutaneous conditions. Dermatology PAs may also provide a variety of cosmetic services, including sclerotherapy, injections with Botox or dermal fillers, microdermabrasion, and chemical peels.

CLINICAL DERMATOLOGY

Dermatologic Interview

In addition to the standard medical history elements of chief complaint, current problem or illness, medical history, family history, personal and social history, and review of systems, the dermatologic interview often requires the clinician to concentrate on other details. The history of skin lesions is essential and includes seven key questions: time of onset, site of onset, symptoms, evolution of individual lesions, pattern of spread, aggravating or alleviating factors, and previous treatment.[8] Medical history should include previous skin conditions or skin cancers and indicators of atopy. Atopy indicators may include a history of hay fever, allergic rhinitis, asthma, sinusitis, keratosis pilaris, ichthyosis vulgaris, dry skin, wool insensitivity, removal of collar labels from clothing due to irritation, Dennie-Morgan folds, and palmar hyperlinearity. Family medical history should include information on any skin conditions such as psoriasis or eczema and any previous skin cancers.

Dermatologic Examination

A proper dermatologic examination consists of several elements. Following a thorough history and review of systems, sectional draping and exposure with appropriate chaperone presence as needed allows the clinician to visualize the entire body without compromising patient modesty. One of the most important elements of the examination is the distribution of lesions. A fully clothed patient who rolls up one sleeve or one pant leg to reveal a "rash that is all over my body" is getting an inadequate examination. Patients typically do not examine their scalp, back, buttocks, or posterior legs, and the presence and distribution of lesions in these areas may provide substantial clues to the correct diagnosis. Dispensing medication requires complete visualization of the lesion distribution so that sufficient medicinal quantities can be estimated and prescribed.

Skin Examination Tools

A centimetre ruler is necessary to measure lesions for documentation and to track changes in size, shape, and configuration. A Wood's lamp is useful in examining patients suspected of having conditions that may fluoresce in different colors, including *Microsporum*-related tinea capitis (green) and erythrasma (coral red). A handlight or penlight is necessary to inspect orifices, particularly the oral mucosa, for associated findings such as Wickham striae in lichen planus. A magnifying lens enhances subtle lesion features, and skilled dermatologic clinicians are adept at using epiluminescence microscopy for differentiating pigmented lesions.

Skin Lesion Distribution

Lesion distribution is one of the most important elements in correctly diagnosing a patient's condition. Many diseases have similar clinical appearances, but their distribution influences the differential diagnoses.

- **Generalized**—covering much of the body surface in a regular arrangement pattern.
- **Localized**—restricted to one particular body area.
- **Symmetric**—lesions appear to be distributed in a similar arrangement on both sides of the body.
- **Asymmetric**—lesions are not distributed in a symmetric pattern.
- **Discrete**—lesions are distinctly separate from each other with identifiable borders.
- **Grouped**—lesions appear in clusters or groups.
- **Confluent**—lesions are coalesced together from smaller into larger areas where the borders may become ill-defined.
- **Sun-exposed**—lesions appear on areas of the body that are more sun-exposed than others.
- **Intertriginous**—appearing within the skin folds.

Skin Lesion Configuration

- **Annular**—round or circular with areas of central clearing.
- **Arciform**—a partial circle.
- **Circinate**—round, circular.
- **Iris or targetoid**—targetlike (bull's eye) lesions of annular configuration with central color contrast.
- **Linear**—straight.
- **Margination**—defining lesion borders by degree of sharpness and definition.
- **Serpiginous**—wandering, uneven borders.
- **Zosteriform**—in a dermatomal distribution.

Primary Lesions

A primary skin lesion is a cutaneous change that is directly caused by the presenting disease process. The key to accurate description and interpretation of cutaneous disease is identification of the primary lesion. Table 30-1 lists primary skin lesions.

Secondary Lesions

Secondary skin changes result from external factors, such as infection, trauma, scratching or friction, and changes caused by healing (Table 30-2).

Text continued on p.481

TABLE 30-1 **Primary Skin Lesions**

Description	Examples
A flat, circumscribed area that is a change in the color of the skin; <1 cm in diameter	MACULE Freckles, flat moles (nevi), petechiae, measles, scarlet fever 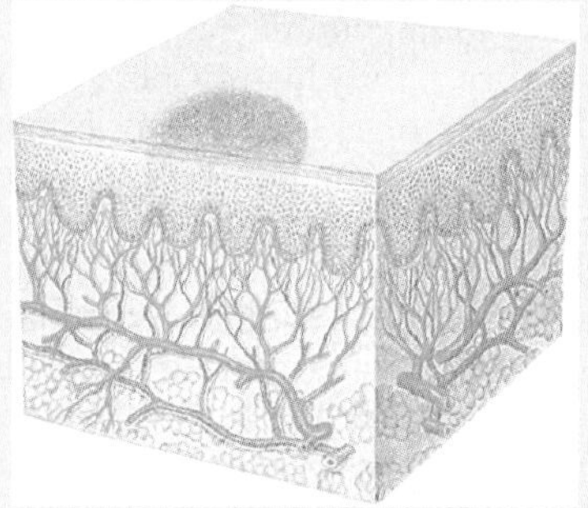
An elevated, firm, circumscribed area <1 cm in diameter	PAPULE Wart (verruca), elevated moles, lichen planus 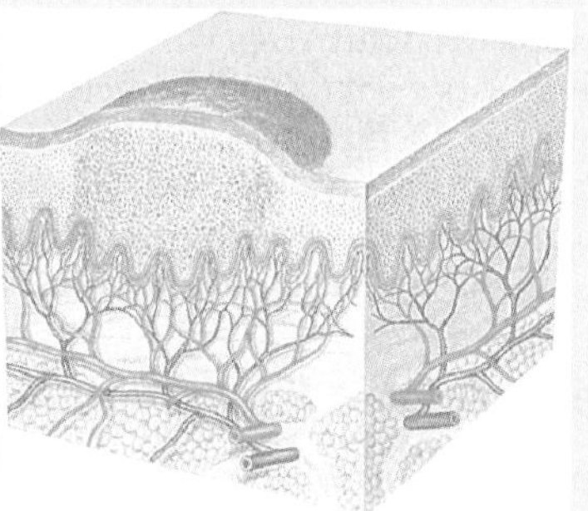
A flat, nonpalpable, irregularly shaped macule >1 cm in diameter	PATCH Vitiligo, port-wine stains, Mongolian spots, café au lait spots 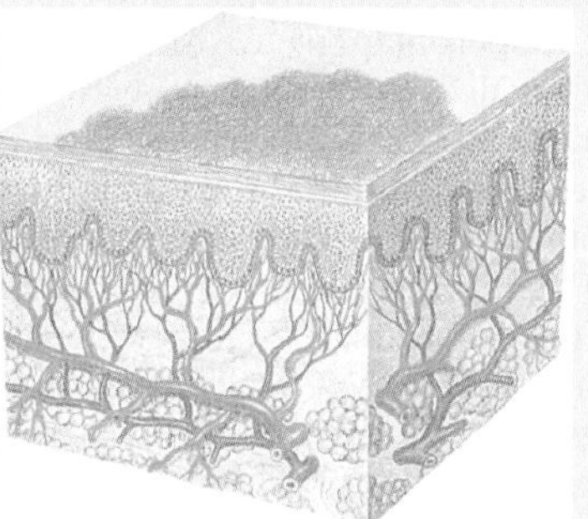
Elevated, firm, and rough lesion with flat-top surface >1 cm in diameter	PLAQUE Psoriasis, seborrheic and actinic keratosis 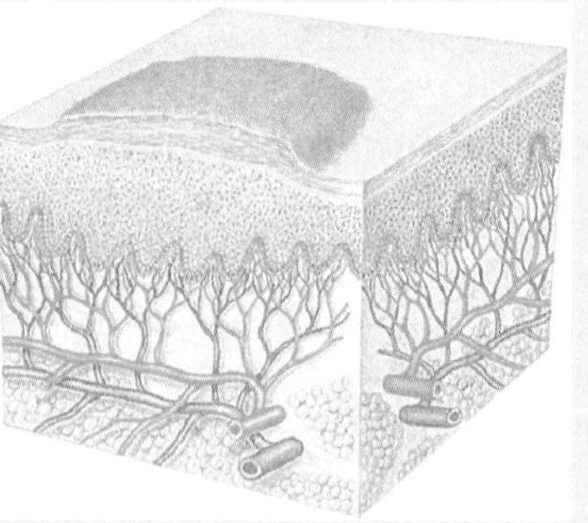

TABLE 30-2 **Secondary Skin Lesions—cont'd**

Description	Examples
CRUST	
Dried serum, blood, or purulent exudate; slightly elevated; size varies; brown, red, black, tan, or straw.	Scab on abrasion, eczema
ATROPHY	
Thinning of skin surface and loss of skin markings; skin translucent and paperlike	Striae; aged skin

Modified from Thompson JM, Wilson SF. Health Assessment for Nursing Practice. St. Louis: Mosby, 1996.

COMMON PROCEDURES IN DERMATOLOGY

Skin Biopsy

Skin biopsy requires the PA to choose the best surgical technique that will gain the most useful information using the least amount of tissue, resulting in the best cosmetic outcome. The three common categories of skin biopsy are shave, punch, and excisional. For an excellent discussion on skin biopsy procedures for PAs, see DiBaise in the Resources section at the end of this chapter.

Shave

The shave biopsy technique can serve the dual purpose of either a biopsy or an excision, depending on the size and depth of the lesion. The shave technique is primarily indicated for epidermal and superficial lesions when a portion of the tissue is sufficient for dermatopathologic examination. If dermal depth is required, or if the lesion extends to subdermal tissue, a punch, excision, or incisional biopsy is recommended.

Punch

For full-thickness specimens or larger surface area lesions requiring only a small amount of tissue for diagnostic purposes, the punch biopsy technique is preferred. Additionally, if special studies such as light or electron microscopy, immunofluorescence, or cell cultures are required, the punch technique is usually used.[9]

Excisional

Excisional biopsies are indicated when complete removal of the lesion is desired, for a suspicious lesion of relatively small size, or for pigmented lesions with atypical features.[9]

Electrosurgery

The most common form of electrosurgery used in dermatology is electrodesiccation, which is typically accompanied by curettage of electrodesiccated lesions. Diagnostic certainty must be a factor because there is no residual tissue for dermatopathologic evaluation following electrosurgery. With the lowest possible power setting that results in tissue destruction, electrodesiccation is frequently used for elimination of spider and vascular (cherry) hemangiomas, verrucae, superficial nonmelanoma skin cancer, and actinic keratoses.[1]

Cryosurgery

Cryosurgery has several indications and advantages over other surgical modalities in selected dermatologic patients with appropriate lesions. The portability and ease of cryosurgical application render it advantageous for most body areas. Cutaneous lesions with more sharply demarcated borders are typically more responsive to cryosurgery, and the rapid healing is an additional advantage. Although cryosurgery is contraindicated in patients with cryoglobulinemia, cold intolerance, or cold urticaria, it is especially useful in elderly, high-risk surgical patients and patients with coagulopathies and pacemakers because of its ease of application and the relatively minimal associated risks (Table 30-3).[10]

Potassium Hydroxide Test

All patients who present with a scaly rash require a potassium hydroxide (K^+OH^-) test to rule out the presence of dermatophyte (fungal and yeast) infections. The K^+OH^- test is performed by gently scraping across the advancing edge of a scaly rash with a glass slide or a No. 15 surgical blade and collecting the cellular debris and scale on a glass slide. One to three drops of 20% K^+OH^- solution is applied to the scale to dissolve the cell walls, and a glass coverslip is applied. Using K^+OH^- with dimethyl sulfoxide (DMSO), gently heating the slide, or waiting 10 to 15 minutes will hasten the dissolution of the keratin and make it easier to see the fungal elements. Begin by examining the slide under low microscope power with the condenser lowered. In a dermatophyte (tinea) infection, look for branching hyphae. In candidiasis, look for budding yeast.

TABLE 30-3 **Cryogens and the Centigrade Temperature**

Cryogen	Temperature (°C)
Ice	0
Salt ice	−20
CO_2 slush	−20
CO_2 snow	−70
CO_2 solid	−78.5
Liquid nitrous oxide	−89.5
Liquid nitrogen	−20 (swab)
Liquid nitrogen	−195.8 (spray/probe)

From Jones PE. Cryosurgery. In: Asprey DP, Dehn RW (eds). Clinical Procedures for Physician Assistants. Philadelphia: Saunders, 2001, p 385.

Scabies Prep Test

All patients presenting with intractable nocturnal pruritus and a typical burrowlike rash or papules in the interdigital web spaces between the fingers or in the waist, axillae, buttocks, or external genitalia warrant a skin scraping examination to rule out scabies. Burrows or unexcoriated papules are vigorously scraped with a No. 15 blade coated with mineral oil, and the cellular debris is transferred to a glass microscope slide. A glass coverslip is applied, and the findings are examined under low power to detect the diagnostic presence of mites, eggs, or fecal pellets (scybala).[1]

Tzanck Smear

The Tzanck smear is helpful in the diagnosis of herpetic lesions such as herpes simplex, varicella zoster virus, and herpes zoster. The procedure involves gently unroofing an intact vesicle with a No. 15 blade and scraping the underside of the vesicle in a perpendicular fashion with the edge of the blade. The material is smeared onto a glass microscope slide and is allowed to air-dry, or is rapidly fixed with alcohol (ETOH). After it has dried, the slide is stained with either a Wright or Giemsa stain and is gently rinsed. When it has been air-dried again, the slide is examined under low power for multinucleated giant cells.[1]

Acetowhitening

To facilitate the diagnosis of condylomata acuminata lesions, moisten a gauze pad with 3% to 5% acetic acid (vinegar is 5%), and apply the pad to suspected genital warts for 5 to 10 minutes. Condyloma lesions will whiten and appear as circumscribed macular/papular lesions with a granular surface and a punctate vascular pattern.[11]

Dermoscopy

Dermoscopy is a noninvasive diagnostic technique that magnifies the skin and allows inspection of the deeper layers of skin. A dermatoscope is used, which is a hand lens with built-in lighting and magnification. With proper use, the dermatoscope can increase the clinical diagnosis of melanocytic, nonmelanocytic, benign, and malignant skin lesions.[12]

Mohs Micrographic Surgery

Developed by Frederic E. Mohs, MD, in the 1930s, the Mohs micrographic surgical procedure has been refined and perfected for more than half a century. Dr. Mohs developed a unique technique of color-coding excised specimens and created a mapping process to accurately identify the location of remaining cancerous cells. Clinical studies have shown that Mohs micrographic surgery has a 5-year cure rate of up to 99% in the treatment of basal cell and squamous cell carcinomas. Mohs micrographic surgery is primarily used to treat basal and squamous cell carcinomas, but it can be used to treat less common tumors, including melanoma.[13]

CASE STUDY 30-1

A 40-year-old man presents with a scalp lesion that has been present for approximately 20 years, according to the patient. A maternal aunt died from malignant melanoma 5 years earlier. He reports having a "mole in his scalp" that his barber thought had been changing over the past 8 months. The patient is a nurse who had heard that "moles with hair growing from them" were always benign. Examination of the scalp reveals a 2-cm asymmetric, multicolored nevus with an irregular border and papular elevation on one side. An excisional biopsy reveals a malignant melanoma.

Patients with a positive family history of melanoma, one or more blistering sunburns, excess cumulative lifetime sun exposure, and lighter hair, eye, and skin coloration are more susceptible to developing malignant melanoma. Complete skin examinations (to include hair-bearing areas) are necessary for the evaluation of changing or suspicious lesions. Any lesion that changes in size, shape, or color or becomes symptomatic should be evaluated as soon as possible, even if the lesion has been present for many years. Melanomas arising from previously benign-appearing nevi are not uncommon. In Case Study 30-1, the patient suffered from inoperable metastatic disease and died 11 months after diagnosis.

CASE STUDY 30-2

A 44-year-old woman with a long-standing history of psoriasis reports for follow-up care. She had developed "new lesions" on her thighs and self-treated twice daily with Ultravate (halobetasol) ointment, a group I topical steroid previously prescribed for plaque psoriasis of the elbows and knees. She asks about the presence of "stretch marks" and bleeding near the new lesions.

Although the patient thought she was doing the right thing by applying Ultravate to the lesions that she assumed were psoriatic, she had not been told to avoid using superpotent steroidal preparations in areas of thinner skin, such as the groin, intertriginous spaces, and face. A complete evaluation of the new lesions, including a punch biopsy, revealed a new diagnosis of erythema annulare centrifugum, a condition unrelated to the previously established diagnosis of psoriasis. Striae with scattered shallow ulcerations developed because of the thinness of the intertriginous skin on the proximal thighs and the occlusive effect of the thighs rubbing together. The shallow ulcerations healed with topical antibiotic therapy, but the striae remain a permanent reminder of the potential adverse effects of misused topical steroids.

CONCLUSION

Dermatology is a medical subspecialty that attracts the visually oriented clinician who is interested in a variety of patient conditions and age ranges. The growing interest in laser therapy, cosmetic dermatology, and extended surgical opportunities makes the specialty particularly attractive to clinicians who have or desire advanced psychomotor skills. The patient evaluation element requires advanced skills in gathering a detailed and often elusive history to determine allergic or occupational origins of skin lesions. Dermatology is a rewarding specialty that challenges the mind while simultaneously honing cutaneous surgical skills.

References

1. Freedberg IM, Eisen AZ, Wolff K, et al. Fitzpatrick's Dermatology in General Medicine. 5th ed. New York: McGraw-Hill, 1999.
2. The History of Dermatology Society website. *http://www.dermato.med.br/hds/*. Accessed April 26, 2011.
3. Crissey JT, Parish LC, Holubar K. Historical Atlas of Dermatology and Dermatologists. New York: Parthenon, 2002.
4. American Board of Dermatology website. *http://www.abderm.org/*. Accessed June 3, 2011.
5. National Center for Health Statistics website. *http://www.cdc.gov/nchs/data/ahcd/namcs_summary/namcssum2008.pdf*; Accessed April 26, 2011.
6. 2008 AAPA Physician Assistant Census Report. Alexandria, VA: American Academy of Physician Assistants. *http://www.aapa.com*. Accessed May 17, 2011.

7. Resneck JS, Kimball AB. Who else is providing care in dermatology practices? Trends in the use of nonphysician clinicians. J Am Acad Dermatol 2008;58:211.
8. Wolff K, Johnson RA, Suurmond D. Color Atlas and Synopsis of Clinical Dermatology. 5th ed. New York: McGraw-Hill, 2005.
9. O'Sullivan RB, Padilla RS. Excision. In: Ratz JL (ed). Textbook of Dermatologic Surgery. Philadelphia: Lippincott-Raven Publishers, 1998.
10. Jones PE. Cryosurgery. In: Asprey DP, Dehn RW (eds). Clinical Procedures for Physician Assistants. Philadelphia: Saunders, 2001.
11. Habif TP. Clinical Dermatology: A Color Guide to Diagnosis and Therapy. 3rd ed. St. Louis: Mosby, 1996.
12. Johr R, Soyer HP, Argenziano R, et al. Dermoscopy: The Essentials. New York: Mosby, 2004.
13. American Society of Mohs Surgery website. *http://www.mohs.net/about.html*. Accessed June 3, 2011.

The resources for this chapter can be found at www.expertconsult.com

CHAPTER 31

ONCOLOGY

Debra S. Munsell

CHAPTER CONTENTS

Cancer: A term for diseases in which abnormal cells divide without control. Cancer cells can invade nearby tissues and can spread throughout the bloodstream and lymphatic system to other parts of the body.[1] The collection of diseases commonly called cancer has been in existence for centuries. Hippocrates (460-370 BC), the Greek physician considered by many to be the "Father of Medicine," is credited with the first use of the term *karkinos.* Legend has it that he applied the term *karkinos* to lesions because "the disease has the veins stretched on all sides as the animal the crab has its feet."[2] Egyptian papyri from 300 to 1500 BC refer to breast tumors. The oldest specimen of a human cancer was found in the remains of a female skull dating to 1900-1600 BC (the Bronze Age).[3] Findings in mummified skeletal remains of Peruvian Incas, more than 2400 years old, show abnormalities that are suggestive of malignant melanoma.

The earliest documented cancer treatment is noted in the Edwin Smith Papyrus, which describes conditions consistent with breast cancer, treated with the "fire drill" (cauterization). Also suggested in the papyrus is the removal of surface tumors (surgery). These writings also reveal the use of compounds of barley, pigs' ears, and other local material for the treatment of stomach and uterine cancer. Scottish surgeon John Hunter (1728-1793) advocated the surgical removal of tumors that were mobile on examination. Advances in pathology after the discovery and use of the microscope and radiographs have led to the modern treatments we currently use in the treatment of cancer patients.[3] Cancer therapy today includes many therapies besides surgery, chemotherapy, and radiation. Not only does cancer affect the physical aspect of the patient, but it also affects social, emotional, and spiritual aspects. Physician assistants (PAs) can develop a challenging and rewarding career in cancer therapy, a career that stimulates intellectual curiosity and rewards the soul. The oncology PA can choose to subspecialize in the surgical, radiation, or medical treatment of any cancer type. Opportunities also exist for PAs in clinical cancer research. The field of oncology care is a growing field that combines the use of specialized medical knowledge and skills with intuitive and compassionate interpersonal skills. It allows the PA to provide primary care in a specialized setting.

DEMOGRAPHICS

The American Cancer Society projects the diagnosis of 1,638,910 new cases of cancer and 577,190 deaths from cancer in the United States in 2012.[3a] These figures do not include basal cell carcinomas and squamous cell carcinomas of the skin. The American Cancer Society reports that more than 2.2 million people will have been treated for nonmelanoma skin cancer in 2011.[4] Cancer as a cause of death in the United States is currently second only to heart disease. Cancer is the cause of death in one out of four people in the United States. The risk for developing cancer increases with age, with most cases affecting adults who are middle-aged and older. The National Institute on Aging predicts that the population aged 65 and older in the United States will double in size over the next 25 years.[5] Oncology is a field that cares disproportionately for the aging population. The 5-year survival rate for all cancers diagnosed between 1995 and 2001 is 65%, an increased survival from 50% in 1974 to 1976. This translates to an increase in both the numbers of people diagnosed with malignancies and the number of people who are cancer survivors. In a recent comprehensive analysis of the supply and demand for oncology services through 2020, the American Society of Clinical Oncologists (ASCO) predicts a shortage of oncologists and recommends the increasing use of PAs to meet the increasing demand for oncology services.[6]

Cancers of the breast, lung and bronchus, and colon and rectum are predicted to be the most common cancers affecting women in 2011. The three leading cancer sites predicted to affect men are prostate, lung and bronchus, and colon and rectum. Cancers of the lung and bronchus are estimated to be the leading cause of cancer death in men and women in 2011, with an estimated 156,940 individuals affected.[4]

The economic impact of cancer is staggering. The National Institutes of Health[4] projected overall cancer-related costs at $263.8 billion in 2011. This includes $102.8 billion for direct health costs, $20.9 billion for indirect costs (lost productivity secondary to illness), and $140.1 billion for indirect mortality costs (loss of productivity secondary to early death).

Approximately 11.7 million Americans with a history of cancer were estimated in January 2007, according to The National Cancer Institute.[4] Cancer patients are surviving longer due to positive trends in early diagnosis, as well as innovative cancer therapies. These patients are often returned to their primary caregivers after definitive therapy. This means that millions of people are living today with the sequelae of their particular cancer therapy and are seeking care from their primary care practitioners. These sequelae range from skin changes to life-changing physical disabilities. Knowledge of oncology therapy and its sequelae will aid the PA in the day-to-day treatment of cancer survivors. With a fundamental knowledge of current cancer therapy, the PA will be able to provide quality health care to all patients whose lives have been touched by cancer.

PATIENT CARE

The first visit a patient makes to his or her health care provider is critical in the establishment of a trusting, caring provider-patient relationship. These patients are experiencing a myriad of emotions ranging from acceptance to shock, disbelief, and denial. The initial visit for cancer treatment is often frightening for the patient. Patients seeking care have often had a preliminary diagnosis given to them by the referring health care provider and are confused. Others may have done independent research before the initial visit with the oncologic specialist. It is important to acknowledge the patient's knowledge level and anxiety; this will help establish a good foundation for the remainder of the visit.

The initial setting of the visit should be a room that is comfortable for the patient and any accompanying guests. Ideally, the initial comprehensive history should be taken from patients before they have been asked to change into an examination gown. This will allow the patient to remain clothed and comfortable while sharing the detailed information. The patient's wishes regarding the presence of guests should be elicited and upheld. Often patients need the support of others during these sessions, and many find that someone else remembers important treatment information best. Allowing the patient to record the conversations may also be helpful.

A comprehensive history pertinent to the chief complaint must be recorded. For instance, if a patient presents with the preliminary diagnosis of colon cancer, a comprehensive review of the gastrointestinal system should be performed. In addition to organ or disease-specific site questions, questions regarding anorexia, pain, insomnia, nausea, vomiting, unexplained weight loss, bruising, fatigue, hair loss, constipation, diarrhea, and masses or lesions that are slow to heal should be asked. Often these somewhat vague symptoms are the initial signs of malignancy. Included in the initial examination should be a comprehensive review of all systems to ensure a comprehensive review of the patient's status. Many times the review of systems will reveal other areas of concern. The patient's general health status and any specific medical conditions must be taken into account before the development of a definitive treatment plan. Family history, social history, and medical history should be recorded, specifically detailing any personal or immediate family history of cancer. Some cancers are known to occur in familial patterns, and others besides the patient may be at risk. Patients with a personal history of cancer are more likely to develop another. A thorough social history should be elicited. This should include a tobacco and substance abuse history, as well as a history of alcohol use. The patient's occupation and prior exposure to environmental agents should be recorded. Specific questions regarding prior radiation exposure must be asked because many individuals were treated with external beam radiation for acne before the 1970s. The social history should include questions regarding the social support available to the patient during cancer therapy. Decisions regarding a definitive treatment

TABLE 31-1 **Oncologic Emergencies**
Spinal cord compression
Increased intracranial pressure with herniation
Superior vena cava obstruction
Seizures
Hypercalcemia
Hypernatremia
Tumor lysis syndrome
Disseminated intravascular coagulation
Venous thromboembolism
Neutropenic fever

plan should include all aspects of the patient's life. Financial and social support may need to be arranged for the patient.

All medications the patient is currently taking must be recorded. Significant reactions between medications and cancer therapies will be avoided if this is done. Include all complementary and alternative therapies that the patient is using because many common over-the-counter remedies may affect medications.[7] Saw palmetto, often used for prostate health, increases the anticoagulant effects of warfarin. Ginkgo biloba, taken to improve memory, interacts with anticoagulants including aspirin, warfarin, ticlopidine, clopidogrel, and dipyridamole. St. John's wort, a popular therapy for depression, has photosensitizing properties and significant interactions with prescription antidepressants. Kava, used as an herbal sedative, has additive effects with central nervous system depressants and antipsychotics.

Careful attention to detail at the initial patient visit will alert the clinician to any impending medical or cancer-related emergencies (Table 31-1). Familiarity with the signs and symptoms of oncologic emergencies is essential for the PA practicing in any field of oncology.

CASE STUDY 31-1

Mr. G is a 46-year-old man who reports tenesmus and rectal bleeding over 3 months. He had no anorexia, weight loss, fatigue, constipation, or change in stool caliber. Family history was negative for cancer in parents, siblings, grandparents, or other members.

On physical examination, a firm mass was palpated in the rectum with moderate discomfort and slight bleeding. The lungs were clear, and no organomegaly, abdominal tenderness, or hyperactive bowel sounds were noted.

Colonoscopy was performed, which revealed a 1.8 cm × 5.6 cm mass in the anterior wall of the distal rectum near the anal verge. A biopsy of the mass was positive for moderately differentiated adenocarcinoma. Transrectal ultrasound revealed the mass to be nearly circumferential, with involvement of the muscularis propria near the level of the prostate. This mass was noted on magnetic resonance imaging of the abdomen and pelvis, with no involvement of the seminal vesicles or the prostate gland. There was no evidence of metastatic disease in the lungs, liver, or abdomen. Chest radiograph was negative, and blood counts, chemistries, and carcinoembryonic antigen were all within normal limits.

This cancer was staged as T2N0M0. Multimodality therapy using preoperative chemoradiation and surgical resection was discussed with the patient and his wife, and they were provided information for both standard therapy and research protocol options. The probability of cure with surgery alone is approximately 50%; the addition of chemoradiation increases this to 65% for patients with resectable disease.

The patient opted for standard therapy and received daily continuous-infusion fluorouracil by portable pump with radiation therapy for 5 to 6 weeks. Four weeks after completion of chemoradiation, he underwent an abdominal perineal resection with surgical closure of the anus and formation of a colostomy. He then received 4 months of adjuvant chemotherapy with daily continuous-infusion fluorouracil alone. This therapy was generally well tolerated with mild-to-moderate fatigue, anorexia, diarrhea, neutropenia, and skin irritation in the radiation field. The only major long-term complication was severe erectile dysfunction.

Submitted by Michael E. Poole, PA-C, MPH

FOR THE STUDENT

Before beginning a clinical rotation in an oncology setting, the ideal student will have had prior internal medicine and surgical experience. This experience will allow the student to feel more comfortable in dealing with the often-complex oncologic patient. You should contact your preceptor before the first day of the rotation for instructions. Ask about the type of practice and your role in patient care. Professional dress, including your white coat, is required unless explicitly expressed. You will need your basic physical examination tools: reflex hammer, penlight, stethoscope, and eye chart. Your preceptor may suggest specific reading material or texts appropriate to your setting. A good general text for the student is *Cancer Facts: A Concise Oncology Text* by James F. Bishop, MD.

Depending on your rotation setting, you may be assigned to a PA preceptor or a physician preceptor. Other members of the team may include nurses, fellow students, and administrative staff. It will be important for you to arrive on time (or a little early), introduce yourself, and make a point of getting to know the routine of the setting. Remember that you are a guest in the practice. This is the time to find out the general layout of the facility, the hours of operation, and your personal role on the team.

The oncology field, like other specialties, has a unique medical language and set of approved abbreviations. Ask your preceptor for a list of approved abbreviations before you begin documentation; this will assist you in learning the new terminology. You will be exposed to new medical treatments and equipment on the rotation. You may observe fine-needle aspirations, bone marrow biopsies, and ultrasound-guided biopsies. Surgical oncologists may be using state-of-the-art stereotactic equipment in the treatment of brain tumors. A rotation in Radiation Oncology will allow you to observe external beam radiotherapy administered by linear accelerators or proton beam therapy delivered in specialized treatment centers (Figure 31-1). You may witness a team of surgical oncologists and radiation oncologists deliver brachytherapy treatment or implant radioactive "seeds."

The field of oncology is both challenging and rewarding. You will be caring for vulnerable patients and their family members. You will be challenged by the immense amount of knowledge that you must assimilate in a short period of time. You may experience the sorrow of caring for a patient who has not responded to therapy. You may experience the thrill of sharing the news that the patient has reached the 5-year mark without a recurrence of disease. A rotation in the field of oncology is a rollercoaster ride of adventure and reward. You will find that you gain much more than education about cancer care; you may develop a love for the care of the patient with cancer.

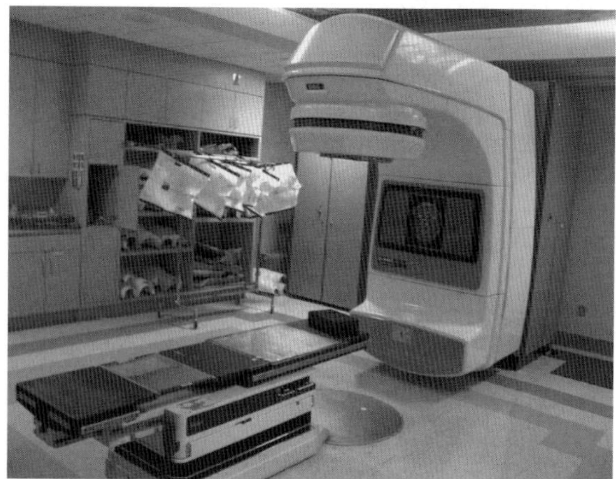

FIGURE 31-1 ■ Linear accelerator. (From Abeloff M. Clinical Oncology, 3rd ed. Philadelphia: Elsevier Churchill Livingstone, 2004.)

TIP BOX

- Cancer patients are often sensitive to odors. Wear scents, hairspray, soaps, lotions, and perfumes SPARINGLY.
- Have an outlet for your frustrations—a hobby or interest that refreshes you when times are tough.
- You are a vital part of the health care team, and you will need respite care—take periodic "mental health days" to restore your focus.
- Cancer patients are like all other patients—they respond to genuine signs of caring—a smile, a handshake, a hand gently placed on a shoulder.

The field of oncology is growing rapidly. Cancer research is rapidly discovering novel treatment options for many types of cancers. The population in the United States is aging, and with that aging comes an increase in the number of patients diagnosed with cancer. Patients are surviving initial therapy for cancers and are living longer, with an increased risk for developing additional malignancies. There will continue to be a need for caring, well-trained PAs in oncology.

PAs have been accepted as vital participants in the cancer care team. Patients and physicians both appreciate the role that PAs play in the care of the patient with cancer. There will be steady, rewarding growth of the PA who chooses to work in oncology.

CASE STUDY 31-2

Mr. P is a 49-year-old married father of three who works as an electrician. He was referred to the multidisciplinary lung cancer clinic by his primary care provider. Mr. P had been in good health all of his life. Approximately 4 months before presentation, Mr. P developed right shoulder pain. Treatment with nonsteroidal antiinflammatory drugs (NSAIDs) brought a brief period of relief, but the pain returned and continued to worsen. He then developed pain in his right forearm and fourth and fifth fingers, with associated numbness.

Mr. P had noted increased fatigue and decreased stamina but had continued to try to work. His appetite was good, although he had a 5-lb weight loss in the past month. He denied shortness of breath, dyspnea on exertion, cough, sputum production, or hemoptysis.

Medical history was remarkable for hypertension diagnosed 3 years previously. He did not have any drug allergies. He had smoked one pack of cigarettes a day for 25 years and stopped 3 years ago. Review of systems was negative for headaches, fever, chills, and night sweats. He had no chest pain, abdominal pain, constipation, diarrhea, nausea, or vomiting. He had no numbness or tingling in his extremities, other than the numbness and pain in his right fourth and fifth fingers. He presented to his primary care physician (PCP), who noted a right Horner syndrome.

On physical examination he appeared well, and vital signs were stable. Karnofsky performance status was 80%. His skin was without rashes, and there was no cervical, supraclavicular, axillary, or inguinal adenopathy. He had a right-sided Horner syndrome. There were no oral lesions. No abnormalities in the lungs, heart, and abdomen were found. Extremities showed no clubbing, edema, or cyanosis. Neurologic examination revealed the cranial nerves to be grossly intact, the reflexes symmetric and 2+, and the strength 5+/5. He had decreased sensation in an ulnar distribution of the right forearm and hand. Chest radiography revealed a mass in the right superior sulcus. Chest computed tomography (CT) confirmed a 6 × 6-cm superior sulcus tumor. There was no evidence of mediastinal node enlargement.

Mr. P was scheduled for a brain CT and bone scan to complete his staging workup. Both of these were negative for distant disease. A whole-body positron emission tomography (PET) scan showed a large area of hypermetabolic activity in the right upper lobe, but no other focal abnormalities were seen and there was no evidence of mediastinal, hilar, or axillary abnormalities.

Mr. P was referred to thoracic surgery and underwent bronchoscopy and cervical mediastinoscopy. The bronchoscopy revealed no endobronchial lesions. The mediastinoscopy was negative for evidence of malignancy at 2R, 4R, 4L, and level 7 lymph nodes. Mr. P underwent pulmonary function tests, which were adequate for surgery. He returned to the multidisciplinary thoracic oncology clinic a week following his mediastinoscopy. He was seen in conjunction with the radiation oncology department and in follow-up by surgical oncology team members.

Mr. P was thought to be a good candidate for neoadjuvant treatment before resection of the superior sulcus tumor. He was also a good candidate for treatment in a clinical trial and met with the research nurse to discuss the current neoadjuvant trial of concurrent chemotherapy and radiation. Mr. P agreed to treatment on this protocol, and informed consent was obtained. He received 6 weeks of concurrent radiation and chemotherapy. During this treatment, he experienced mild nausea, which was treated with antiemetics; moderate esophagitis treated with narcotics and viscous lidocaine; mild radiation dermatitis; and moderate fatigue, but only a 5-lb weight loss. Erythropoietin injections were given to maintain his hemoglobin above 12 g/dL.

At the completion of his adjuvant chemotherapy and radiation, he underwent repeat staging with chest CT, which showed that the right upper lobe mass had decreased in size, measuring approximately 4.5 cm in largest dimension. A repeat brain CT was negative for metastatic disease.

Mr. P was taken to the operating room approximately 4 weeks after completing his neoadjuvant therapy. He underwent right thoracotomy, right upper lobectomy with chest wall resection, and removal of ribs 1 to 3. Final pathology showed a residual poorly differentiated adenocarcinoma as dispersed mild clusters of cells within a 2.5 × 2 × 2-cm mass containing fibrosis and necrosis, typical of treated tumor. There was no lymphatic or vascular invasion. There was extension to the parietal pleura, but the chest wall margin was free of tumor. The posterior rib margins were free of tumor, and the anterior rib margins were negative for tumor following decalcification. Additional lymph node dissection, including level 11 and level 7, was negative for malignancy.

Mr. P had an uneventful postsurgical hospital course and was discharged without incident. He returned to the multidisciplinary clinic 2 weeks after surgery, at which time he was doing well, although he was experiencing postthoracotomy pain and continued shoulder and right arm pain. He noted some slight weakness in his right hand and was referred for physical therapy and occupational therapy. He continued to require narcotics for pain control. The management plan for Mr. P included follow-up in the multidisciplinary thoracic oncology clinic monthly for 4 months, where he would be evaluated by the surgical and medical oncology teams. After that, he would be seen in the medical oncology department every 3 months for the first year, every 6 months for 5 years, and yearly thereafter.

By Susan Blackwell and Lee A. Daly

SALARY RANGES

The American Academy of Physician Assistants[8] annually releases a census report for PAs practicing in a specialty setting. The 2009 PA census report for PAs was completed by 19,608 PAs, 27% of those eligible to practice. Four hundred ten participants identified themselves as practicing in radiation oncology, surgical oncology, pediatric oncology, or medical oncology. In 2006, the mean salary reported for PAs practicing in radiation oncology was $78,514, with a standard deviation (SD) of $15,234. Surgical oncology PAs salaries were reported to have a mean of $82,571 with an SD of $15,046. Pediatric oncology PA salaries had a mean of $77,047 and SD of $12,901. Those practicing in medical oncology had salaries with a mean of $78,972 and SD of $14,801.

CASE STUDY 31-3

Ms. J is a 43-year-old premenopausal woman who presented with a right breast mass that was self-detected 2 weeks previously. Previous mammograms 9 months earlier were unremarkable. Repeat mammogram revealed new architectural change in the right upper outer quadrant. Ultrasound demonstrated a solid mass. Initially, fine-needle biopsy was nondiagnostic. She underwent excisional biopsy for a 2.5-cm invasive ductal carcinoma with negative surgical margins. Estrogen and progesterone receptors were positive. She opted for breast-conserving surgery and had an axillary node dissection with 3 of 17 lymph nodes involved with cancer. Radiologic evaluation, including bone scan and chest/abdomen CT, was within normal limits, ruling out distant disease.

Ms. J was otherwise healthy, except for an active 20-pack-year smoking history. Family history was remarkable for a living, 87-year-old maternal grandmother with a history of mastectomy for breast cancer at age 57 and two maternal great aunts who had breast cancer late in life. Her mother and two sisters are alive and well. She was nulliparous. She lived alone, with supportive family nearby.

Her tumor size, three involved lymph nodes, and premenopausal status placed her in an intermediate–to–high-risk category for recurrence. An estimated 40% risk for systemic recurrence within 10 years was discussed. Chemotherapy and the use of tamoxifen are shown to increase disease-free and overall survival in women with similar histories. The chemotherapy and tamoxifen benefit was estimated at a relative 50% reduction of her risk, or an absolute 20% reduction. The short-term and long-term risks of chemotherapy were reviewed with Ms. J, and chemotherapy options were presented.

She decided to enroll in a multicenter treatment trial and was randomly assigned to the standard treatment arm of four cycles of doxorubicin and cyclophosphamide over 12 weeks. She tolerated her chemotherapy with only minimal nausea. She received radiation to her breast and lower axilla over 6 weeks. Ms. J completed 5 years of oral tamoxifen this year and is without evidence of disease.

By Susan Blackwell and Lee A. Daly

CANCER CARE

Recent advances in technology and medicine have vastly improved the quality and practice of cancer care. Many institutions have adopted a multidisciplinary approach to cancer therapy. This method organizes care in disease-specific sites, offering the patient the expertise of all clinicians who may be involved in their care. For instance, a new patient with head and neck cancer may initially be evaluated by the head and neck surgeon for staging. The patient may then be scheduled for consultations with the medical oncologist, radiation oncologist, audiologist, nutritionist, physical therapist, speech pathologist, and dental oncologist. All of these disciplines would be housed together in close proximity for patient convenience and optimal communication among the treating teams. The teams ideally meet regularly to jointly discuss the new patients and optimize available therapies. The value of a team approach to cancer care lies in the individual treatment plans initiated for each patient. The PA working in such a multidisciplinary setting has the advantage of participating in comprehensive care.

For many years, surgical treatment of solid tumors was considered standard of care. The objective of cancer therapy is to offer the patient the treatment modality that will offer the best likelihood of cure, and this initial treatment was often surgical in nature. Innovations in cancer detection and imaging now allow clinicians to diagnose cancer at earlier stages, opening the door to advances in medical and radiation oncology. Early-stage cancers may now be treated primarily with chemotherapy, radiation therapy, or a combination of the three modalities. PAs have a long history of practicing in the surgical theater, and many surgical oncology subspecialties employ PAs in both the clinical and operating room settings. If the treatment plan initially calls for radiation or chemotherapy, the surgical team may still be involved in obtaining appropriate biologic specimens for diagnosis.

Medical oncologists are specialty-trained physicians who use systemic therapies to treat cancer. These oncologists traditionally relied on chemotherapeutic agents to treat malignancies, but innovations in cancer care now make use of other systemic agents in addition to chemotherapy. Biologic therapy—the use of the body's own immune system to fight cancer—is a relatively new concept in cancer care. Biologic response modifiers (BRMs) are substances produced in the human body in small amounts and can now be produced in a laboratory setting. These laboratory-produced BRMs are now being used to stimulate the body's response to disease or infection, with promising results. Vaccines (therapeutic and prophylactic) have also been developed for use in cancer therapy. Examples of prophylactic vaccines are the hepatitis B vaccine and Gardasil, the new vaccine being used to prevent infection with two of the strains of human papilloma virus (HPV) associated with cervical cancer. Melanoma patients are among the patients currently being investigated for treatment with tumor-specific vaccines.[9] Recently, the U.S. Food and Drug Administration (FDA) approved a new medication, vemurafenib, as treatment for those with metastatic melanoma who also have the gene mutation BRAF (V600E). This advancement in care is just one example of the progress being made in the care of cancer patients.[10]Practitioners in medical oncology often offer adjuvant or concomitant therapy along with radiation oncology and surgical resection. Palliative therapy for patients whose malignancies are not responding to conventional therapy is often provided by the medical oncology service.

Radiation therapy, the use of ionizing radiation to treat cancer or other benign disease, is a relatively new field when compared with surgical and medical oncology. Patients undergoing radiation therapy are treated by a team of experts who are trained in the biology of cancer and the effects of ionizing radiation. The team consists of the radiation oncologist, the medical physicist, the dosimetrist, radiation technologists, and nursing personnel. Recently, many radiation oncologists have discovered the utility of including a PA in their practice. The PA serves a unique role, assisting the team in caring for the patient while undergoing specialized radiation therapy. Radiation therapy, like chemotherapy and surgery, has sequelae of treatment that are often troubling and life threatening for the patient. The PA is often the clinician who evaluates and treats the side effects of therapy and educates patients about their progress. Like chemotherapy, radiation therapy is often used palliatively in cancer care.

Rapid increases in technology have given clinicians many new diagnostic and treatment options for malignancies. The field of oncology is a rapidly growing field, with innovative therapies being introduced daily. PAs who choose to practice in oncology can have a rewarding and intellectually stimulating career, a career that will allow them to influence positively the lives of their patients.

GOALS OF TREATMENT

The goal of cancer therapy is to offer the patient the best option for cure. This option must include consideration of the patient's performance status. The patient must be aware of the risks and benefits of the treatment plan and must be an integral part of the discussion. The PA is often the clinician who will manage the treatment effects and advise the patients of their treatment options. The PA should fully inform all patients about their diagnosis, treatment options, and survival expectations. Informed consent must include any adverse effects of the treatment modality (Table 31-2). Giving

TABLE 31-2 **Common Complications of Cancer Therapy**

Chemotherapy	Surgery	Radiation Therapy	Bioimmunotherapy
Nausea, emesis	Disfigurement	Fatigue	Fatigue
Fatigue	Loss of function	Osteoradionecrosis	Severe flulike symptoms
Photosensitivity	Pain—immediate and long-term	Mucositis of involved mucosal surfaces	Slowed mentation
Extravasation of chemotherapeutic agent	Postoperative complications	Development of radiation-induced second malignancies	Reactions at injection sites
Anemia	Changes in sexual function, desire	Alopecia in radiated area	Short-term hematologic changes
Mucositis of involved mucosal surfaces	Changes in fertility	Skin changes (atrophy, telangiectasia, ulceration)	Appetite changes
Thrombocytopenia	Psychological changes, depression	Changes in sexual function, desire	Altered taste
Neutropenia		Changes in fertility	
Alopecia		Psychological changes, depression	
Skin changes		Anemia	
Changes in sexual function, desire		Neutropenia	
Changes in fertility			

TABLE 31-3 Major Reasons for Therapeutic Inadequacies in the Management of Cancer Pain

Patient Barriers
- Limited expectations regarding the ability to provide pain relief
- Excessive concern about addiction, tolerance, and toxicities of opioids
- Legitimate concern that more pain signifies progressive tumor

Health Care Provider Barriers
- Inaccurate perceptions of patient pain intensity
- Failure to determine the etiology of pain and apply specific therapy
- Lack of knowledge regarding opioid equivalencies and pharmacology
- Excessive concern about addiction, tolerance, and toxicities of opioids
- Excessive concern regarding the regulatory oversight of opioids

From Abeloff M. Clinical Oncology, 3rd ed. Philadelphia: Elsevier Churchill Livingstone, 2004.

TOP 20 CLINICAL PROBLEMS

- Management of cancer pain
- Breast cancer
- Lung cancer
- Colorectal cancer
- Leukemia
- Lymphoma
- Bioimmunotherapy for malignancies
- Treating the long-term cancer survivor
- Cancer screening and early detection
- Development of cancer vaccines
- Melanoma
- Cutaneous malignancies
- Prostate cancer
- End-of-life care of cancer patients
- Complementary and alternative care in the treatment of cancer
- Childhood cancers
- Brain tumors
- Myelodysplastic syndromes
- Ovarian cancer
- Pancreatic cancer

patients this information will allow them to participate fully in their care, empowering them to be involved in their treatment. If the intent of treatment is palliative, inform patients of all options and allow them to choose those options that they feel are appropriate to their beliefs and lifestyle. The patient must be reassured that the clinicians will not abandon them if they seek palliative care, and that their symptoms and needs will be fully addressed at all times. Address issues of pain management at every patient visit. PAs can play a vital role in the appropriate management of cancer-related pain (Table 31-3). Discuss quality-of-life issues with all patients undergoing cancer care, curative or palliative.

Perform regular evaluations of the patient with cancer to monitor treatment effects and response to treatment. Early recognition of impending complications or lack of response to treatment will allow the clinician to halt or revise the treatment plan to improve the outcomes. The patient, the family, and significant others should all be included in the treatment plan from the beginning. It is important to address all questions regarding the diagnosis and treatment options. All parties involved must clearly understand survival issues, to give the patient and the family time to prepare social, spiritual, and financial concerns.

CLINICAL APPLICATIONS

1. Review your patient population with regard to risk factors for cancer. What cancer types are most prevalent in your community? Develop a list of the most prevalent cancer types noted and then develop a plan to address the risk factors associated with these cancers with all of your patients.
2. Review your patient population and identify those individuals who are cancer survivors. Develop a plan to address their needs regarding follow-up, sequelae of treatment, possible recurrence and second primaries.
3. Identify an issue such as cancer prevention or cancer awareness that is lacking in your community. Develop a plan to address this issue that includes a cross section of the community, especially including persons or populations at high risk. Make this issue a permanent part of your health education discussions with patients.

KEY POINTS

- There is a continuous and increased demand for practitioners in the field of oncology.
- Physician assistants are well suited to the practice of oncology.
- There is a wide variety of clinical and research opportunities for PAs interested in caring for patients with malignancies.
- Current investigation is being conducted in the use of complementary and alternative therapies as adjunct treatment for malignancies.
- Rapid advances in cancer research are allowing more people to sustain a good quality of life while undergoing therapy and as cancer survivors.

References

1. MD Anderson Cancer Center Patient Information. *http://www.mdanderson.org*. Accessed August 19, 2011
2. Moss RM. Galen on Cancer: How Ancient Physicians Viewed Malignant Disease. *http://www.cancerdecisions.com*. Accessed August 19, 2011.
3. Rare Cancer Alliance Cancer History. *http://www.rare-cancer.org/history-of-cancer.php*. Accessed August 19, 2011.

3a. American Cancer Society. Cancer facts & figures 2012. Atlanta: American Cancer Society. *http://www.cancer.org/acs/groups/content/@epidemiologysurveilance/documents/document/acspc-031941.pdf*. Accessed November 6, 2012.

4. American Cancer Society. Cancer Facts and Figures 2011. Atlanta: American Cancer Society, 2011.
5. U.S. Census Bureau News. *http://www.nia.nih.gov/sites/default/files/nia-who_report_booklet_oct-2011_a4__1-12-12_5.pdf*. Accessed August 19, 2011
6. Erickson C, Salsberg E, Forte G, et al. Future supply and demand for oncologists. J Oncol Pract 2007;3:79.
7. American Cancer Society's Guide to Complementary and Alternative Cancer Methods. Atlanta: American Cancer Society, 2000.
8. American Academy of Physician Assistants. 2011 AAPA Physician Assistant Census Report. *http://www.aapa.org*. Accessed August 19, 2011
9. National Cancer Institute Cancer Topics. *http://www.cancer.gov/cancertopics*. Accessed August 19, 2011
10. FDA Approves Zelboraf for Melanoma. *http://www.cancer.org/Cancer/News/fda-approves-zelboraf-for-melanoma*. Accessed August 19, 2011.

The resources for this chapter can be found at www.expertconsult.com.

CHAPTER 32

Infectious Disease

Durward A. Watson • L. Jill Jones-Hester

CHAPTER CONTENTS

The physician assistant (PA) concept emerged during the 1960s in response to demands for more accessible and affordable health care.[1] Likewise, the selection of the infectious disease (ID) practice by PAs reflects the response of these individuals to the demands resulting from the advent of the acquired immunodeficiency syndrome (AIDS) epidemic in the 1980s. The 1990s demonstrated small yet steady increases in the absolute numbers of PAs involved in the medical care of an exploding population of patients who have human immunodeficiency virus (HIV), hepatitis B, and hepatitis C. In this decade, the role of the PA in ID has further expanded to assist in management of general ID-patient issues, including, although not exclusive of, fevers of unknown origin (FUOs), neutropenic fever, sepsis syndrome in the intensive care unit (ICU) setting, bacteremia, ventilatory-assisted/nosocomial pneumonia, posttransplant infection, infective endocarditis, skin and soft tissue infections, osteomyelitis, septic arthritis, and postoperative infections. In addition, the PA plays an increasingly vital role in outpatient clinical management of HIV and chronic hepatitis, particularly as viral resistance to therapies, access to medications, and ongoing clinical research issues place increasing demands on the medical community as a whole. Because no studies have been done to date on the utilization of PAs in ID, in this chapter anecdotal information concerning the scope of practice of PAs who select ID as their practice is provided. Additional goals of this chapter are to discuss the following:

- The historical development of ID as a specialty
- Common roles of the PA within the specialty
- Mentoring of the PA student through an ID clinical rotation
- Problem-based clinical assessments in the ID setting
- In-depth discussion of three common clinical issues, including chronic comorbid viral infection, sepsis syndrome, and infective endocarditis
- Representative case studies

HISTORY OF INFECTIOUS DISEASE

Infectious disease emerged as a specialty in the past century after significant advances had been made in the field of antibiotic therapies to treat life-threatening contagious, postoperative, and trauma-related infections. Especially during the years after World War II, the industrialized world benefited from the development of chemotherapeutic agents, the expansion of public health practices, and profound discoveries in the field of microbiology and immunology, all of which led to significant decreases in the incidence of mortality and morbidity due to infectious processes. It was in this exciting and changing environment that the ID specialty, as it is recognized today, had its beginnings. Kass,[2] in providing a historical perspective, suggested three distinct phases in the rise of ID as a specialty area of medicine. In the earliest phase, all clinicians were by default ID specialists in that a large proportion of problems addressed in an ordinary practice setting involved infectious processes. There was little to provide in terms of effective preventive measures or treatment for infections during this phase, and the medical research was focused primarily on the description of clinical syndromes and the natural history of processes rather than on treatments. Advances in public health measures and the prosperity characterizing the early 19th century heralded the second phase in the history of ID. Microbes were recognized as a cause of disease, and target vaccines were developed.

These advances began the trend toward decreasing mortality and morbidity secondary to infectious disease. A shift in the disease management focus of the general practitioner slowly took place as the scientific community was able to provide objective tools for disease recognition, vaccine, and other strategies for disease prevention, as well as applicable treatments for an expanding number of disease-causing pathogens and conditions. These advances allowed clinicians who were specifically drawn to ID to focus their attention on new approaches to disease management and to emerge as clinicians whom the general practitioner could rely on to manage previously common infections, as well as emerging infections resulting from the expansion of a global economy and collapsed travel time in nearly all parts of the world. Thus, this third phase saw the differentiation of the ID specialist from other types of clinicians. As a result, the ID specialist today serves as a consultant to other clinicians in the treatment of patients affected by a myriad of infectious diseases.

The World Health Organization (WHO) collects information on global deaths by International Classification of Diseases (ICD) codes.

The table below lists the top infectious disease causes of morbidity of greater than 100,000 deaths in 2002 (estimated). For comparison, 1993 data are included.

The top three single-agent/disease killers are HIV/AIDS, tuberculosis, and malaria. Although the number of deaths due to nearly every disease have decreased, deaths due to HIV/AIDS have increased fourfold. Childhood diseases include pertussis, poliomyelitis, diphtheria, measles, and tetanus. Children also make up a large percentage of lower respiratory and diarrheal deaths.

COMMON ROLES OF THE PA IN AN INFECTIOUS DISEASE PRACTICE

Census data from the American Academy of Physician Assistants (AAPA) suggest that less than 1% of responding PAs indicated involvement in the ID subspecialty in 1991, the first year that data were collected. Over the past decade, more have chosen this area as their primary practice focus, but the percentage of PAs in ID practices has remained steady at less than 1%.[3] However, these numbers do not reflect the vast number of primary care PAs who treat patients affected by the problems generally seen in an ID practice.[4] Although ID practices, both public and private, vary somewhat in the manner in which the PA is used, the PA will be considered a member of the medical team and, as such, will be expected to fulfill a number of clinical management and organizational assignments. The PA normally holds a daily roster of clinic outpatient appointments and may additionally, as a result of particular interest or expertise, be

Worldwide Mortality Due to Infectious Diseases

Rank	Cause of Death	Deaths 2002 (In Millions)	Percentage of All Deaths	Deaths 1993 (In Millions)	1993 Rank
N/A	All infectious diseases	14.7	25.9%	16.4	32.2%
1	Lower respiratory infections	3.9	6.9%	4.1	1
2	HIV/AIDS	2.8	4.9%	0.7	7
3	Diarrheal diseases	1.8	3.2%	3.0	2
4	Tuberculosis (TB)	1.6	2.7%	2.7	3
5	Malaria	1.3	2.2%	2.0	4
6	Measles	0.6	1.1%	1.1	5
7	Pertussis	0.29	0.5%	0.36	7
8	Tetanus	0.21	0.4%	0.15	12
9	Meningitis	0.17	0.3%	0.25	8
10	Syphilis	0.16	0.3%	0.19	11
11	Hepatitis B	0.10	0.2%	0.93	6
12-17	Tropical diseases	0.13	0.2%	0.53	9, 10, 16-18

Note: Other causes of death include maternal and perinatal conditions (5.2%), nutritional deficiencies (0.9%), noncommunicable conditions (58.8%), and injuries (9.1%).

primarily responsible for clinical management of a subset of patient issues within the outpatient setting. Examples include offering routine gynecologic examinations for Pap smears and sexually transmitted disease (STD) surveillance for female HIV patients; performing anal Pap surveillance examinations for human papilloma virus (HPV) and risk assessment for squamous cell carcinoma (SCC) in male HIV patients who have a history of male-to-male rectal intercourse; and conducting close clinical follow-up, including safety laboratory surveillance of hepatitis C patients who are on interferon-based regimens. The efficient PA will learn how to effectively delegate tasks to nursing support staff in ordering special imaging studies, arranging consults to other medical and surgical specialists, and referring patients to social and pharmaceutical-assistance programs when necessary. The PA will be expected to work closely with ambulatory infusion nursing personnel to ensure clinical oversight of patients coming out of the hospital on parenteral therapies. In a practice that conducts clinical research, the PA will be relied on as a subinvestigator to maintain a working knowledge of the various research protocols and to work closely with clinical research personnel in overseeing safety and clinical management issues with respect to research subjects. Increasingly, the PA is asked to maintain Allied Health Care hospital privileges so that he or she may assist in the initial evaluation and ongoing clinical management of hospitalized patients for whom the practice has been consulted. As the physician assistant gains knowledge base and presentation skills, he or she may elect to present topics in local journal clubs, grand rounds, and inpatient or community education forums. Additionally, the PA will, as in other medical or surgical settings, likely be asked by local training programs to supervise PA student clinical rotations throughout the academic year.

STUDENT MENTORING

Briefly, the challenges and responsibilities involved in student mentoring will be similar to those required in other clinical settings. Students should be exposed to routine daily clinical responsibilities of the mentoring PAs. Students can be expected to initially observe and then conduct history-taking and physical examination of patients in a variety of clinic and hospital settings. Patient presentations made to mentoring PAs and supervising physicians should be problem focused around ID issues. The clinician should assist in sharpening the student's assessment skills and help the student formulate practical short- and long-term treatment planning. In addition, once or twice during the rotation, it is instructive to assign the student a topic to read overnight and be prepared to discuss in depth the next day during clinic or hospital rounds.

PROBLEM-BASED CLINICAL ASSESSMENT IN THE INFECTIOUS DISEASE SETTING

PAs working in an ID setting need to have a basic understanding of the pathophysiology, clinical presentation, and treatment of viral, bacterial, fungal, and parasitic infections. Although dramatic progress has been made over the past several decades in the treatment and prevention of these infections, infectious diseases continue to be responsible for significant morbidity and mortality in both the developed and the developing regions of the world. In the United States, infections frequently encountered in clinic and hospital settings include viral infections caused by agents including HIV, herpes simplex virus (HSV), hepatitis B (HBV), hepatitis C (HCV), influenza virus, cytomegalovirus (CMV), Epstein-Barr virus (EBV); bacterial and mycobacterial infections responsible for pneumonias, endocarditis, meningitis, colitis, pyelonephritis, cystitis, and various STDs; skin and soft tissue infections; osteomyelitis; septic arthritis; fungal infections such as *Cryptococcus* and histoplasmosis affecting the pulmonary tree, the skin, and/or the cerebrospinal fluid; *Candida* species, which can adhere to indwelling catheters and shunts; and parasitic infections of the skin and gastrointestinal system.

Whether the initial patient presentation occurs in the hospital setting or outpatient clinic, evaluation of the patient is based on the established principles of obtaining a medical history, performing a thorough examination, and ordering pertinent laboratory, radiographic, and skin antigen/antibody testing to support a working clinical assessment. Concern for the immune status of a patient is raised on the basis of the frequency or severity of infections; the finding of an unusual, opportunistic infectious agent; and, of course, in the transplant setting. One screening approach to a patient with suspected infectious disease is provided in Table 32-1.[5]

History

Initial evaluation of the patient includes an extensive history to draw out the patient's general health status, past medical conditions (including antimicrobial treatments for serious infections), surgeries

TABLE 32-1 **Patient Screening History and Physical Examination (H&P)**

History	Medications, medical allergies
	Frequency, severity, distribution, type of infections
	Causative infectious agents, outcome of treatments
	Medical history, surgeries
	Vaccination history, foreign travel, sexually transmitted disease, pet exposure
	History of transplantation, shunt placement, grafting, metal plate/screw devices
Physical	Weight, height, vital signs
	Hair: sheen, pigmentation
	Oropharynx: thrush, oral hairy leukoplakia, ulcers, gingivitis, dentition
	Sinus: percussion over sinus cavities
	Lymphatic survey: cervical, supraclavicular, axillary, inguinal
	Chest: adventitious breath sounds, diaphragmatic excursion, anteroposterior diameter
	Cardiovascular: rhythm, rate, murmurs, gallops, carotid/peripheral pulses
	Abdominal: bowel sounds, tenderness, organomegaly, mass, ascites
	Musculoskeletal: strength, range of motion, fractures
	Neurologic: central nervous system assessment, focal neuropathy, sensory discrimination
	Skin: wounds, dehiscence, abscess, rash, eczema, nodules, cellulitis, edema, telangiectasias
Laboratory	Complete blood count with WBC differential
	Complete metabolic panel
	Hepatic panel
	Coagulopathy panel
	Lipid panel
	Thyroid panel
	Inflammatory panel including erythrocyte sedimentation rate, C-reactive protein, and SPEP
	Serologies for HIV, chronic hepatitis, syphilis
	Genotypic resistance panel in newly diagnosed HIV
	Immunoglobulin panel
	Cerebral spinal fluid (CSF) cell counts
	Specialized serologies including toxoplasmosis, histoplasmosis, *Cryptococcus*, cytomegalovirus, Epstein-Barr virus, West Nile virus
	Cultures including aerobic/anaerobic blood culture (cx), urine cx, CSF cx, wound cx, and cultures obtained from paracentesis, thoracentesis, and percutaneous nephrostomy tubes
	Stool assays for routine C/S, *Cryptosporidia*, ova and parasites, *Clostridia difficile* toxin, WBC, RBC
Imaging	Pertinent to the case
Pathology	Pertinent to the case

Modified from Mandell G, Bennet J, Dolin R. Principles and Practice of Infectious Disease, 5th ed. Philadelphia: Churchill Livingstone, 2000.

C/S, Cerebrospinal fluid; RBC, red blood cell count; SPEP, serum protein electrophoresis; WBC, white blood cell count.

(including whether or not the patient has had stabilizing metal implants, autografting, and/or native or prosthetic valve placements); illicit drug, alcohol, and smoking history; history of tattooing/body piercing; STD history; current/past sexual behaviors; vaccinations; and history of medical/food allergies. A list of current medications, both prescribed and over-the-counter, should be obtained. Inquire regarding foreign travel, household pets/animal exposure, current employment/residence, and household members.

Physical Examination and Laboratory/Imaging Database

A comprehensive physical examination should be completed, with documentation of weight, height, vital signs, and fundoscopic, oral, skin, lymphatic, cardiopulmonary, abdominal, genitourinary, rectal, and neurologic findings. The results of laboratory, pathology, and imaging databases are reviewed, and additional pertinent studies are ordered on the basis of clinical assessment and working diagnoses.

CASE STUDY 32-1

A 51-year-old black single mother employed as a detective in a large metropolitan police department transferred her care for management of her comorbid HIV and HCV infections in May 1999, after her previous physician retired. Her husband died of complications of AIDS in 1995. In May 1999, her HIV viral load measurement by PCR was 122 copies/mL and her CD4 count was greater than 900 cells/mm^3; her hepatitis C viral load was more than 5 million copies, she had genotype 1a virus on genotypic testing, and her biopsy revealed grade 2 inflammation and moderate bridging fibrosis. Her serum glutamate pyruvate transaminase (SGPT) was 49, and she had no hepatic stigmata; her liver span was not appreciated on percussion. She was naïve to treatment for her comorbid chronic viral infections. The patient has a medical history of hypertension. She has had one tubal pregnancy and a subsequent tubal ligation. Her 7-year-old daughter is HIV infected, clinically stable, and under physician management at a regional children's health care center that has a large, well-funded treatment clinic for pediatric HIV. The daughter is not coinfected with hepatitis C.

DISCUSSION: CHRONIC COMORBID VIRAL INFECTION

This patient represents a growing number of patients encountered in an HIV-oriented outpatient practice who are comorbidly infected with hepatitis C. Approximately 25% of the 800,000 people living with HIV in the United States are infected with hepatitis C.[6] With respect to her HIV infection, the patient has been fortunate; she has maintained stable low viral loads and high CD4 cell counts over the subsequent 3 years since her initial evaluation in the clinic. Although the Department of Health and Human Services (DHHS) guidelines from January 2011 may support delaying treatment regimens in clinically stable HIV-infected individuals in whom CD4 cell count measurements remain greater than 500 cells/mm^3, because of the patient's comorbid hepatitis C status, HIV therapy initiation would be favored by many ID clinicians because HAART is thought to attenuate liver disease progression in coinfected patients with hepatitis B/hepatitis C "by preserving or restoring immune function and reducing HIV-related immune activation and inflammation."[7]

Likewise, a "wait-and-see" approach cannot be taken with regard to the patient's comorbid hepatitis C infection. HCV is a "flavivirus" that was identified in the mid-1980s.[8] HCV is usually transmitted by percutaneous exposure, but rates of sexual and perinatal transmission of HCV are significantly higher among HIV-positive patients. Approximately 25% of HCV-infected patients spontaneously clear the virus, usually within a few months of infection. Those who do not are considered to be chronically infected, with a 2% to 20% incidence of progression to cirrhosis within 20 years.[9] Factors leading to increased rate of progression include age, level of alcohol intake, and HIV coinfection.

Once properly staged for therapeutic intervention of HCV, the patient may qualify for treatment, which may include newly approved protease inhibitor therapy targeting specific hepatitis C virus enzymes. These oral agents, when added to traditional pegylated interferon and oral ribavirin, have shown promise in trial data of significantly increasing the likelihood of overall response and shortening time frames for therapy.[10] This patient would, therefore, benefit from being referred to clinical trial participation found at many university hospital medical centers throughout the United States.

CASE STUDY 32-2

A 58-year-old black woman who has a history of insulin-dependent diabetes mellitus (IDDM), end-stage renal disease (ESRD), and ulcerative colitis status post partial colectomy 6 months ago, is now 10 days post colon reanastomosis and removal of colostomy bag. In the past 48 hours, new fever (101.2°F), painful abdominal distention, and leukocytosis with a whole blood cell count (WBC) = 17,500/mm^3 and 10% bands have developed. Her husband reports to the nurses that his wife is acting confused.

After an abrupt fall in her systolic blood pressure, she has been transferred to the ICU, where she has been intubated and stabilized on intravenous fluids, bicarbonate, and norepinephrine (Levophed). Her abdominal computed tomography (CT) scan demonstrates small fluid collection with air at the site of her anastomosis.

Following the collection of two sets of aerobic/anaerobic blood cultures, a new triple lumen catheter is placed and she receives parenteral vancomycin and piperacillin-tazobactam ordered by the ID consultant. Both antibiotics are dosed on the basis of renal clearance after discussion with the nephrologist. The patient undergoes anastomosis repair, and at surgery, *Escherichia coli* sensitive to piperacillin-tazobactam and quinolones is found; the same organism is found in 2/4 blood culture bottles. Vancomycin is discontinued, and her gram-negative coverage is switched to parenteral fluoroquinolone (Levaquin), dosed for renal clearance; parenteral metronidazole is added to cover anaerobic growth. She is transitioned successfully from parenteral nutrition to oral soft diet. At 3 weeks, a repeat abdominal CT scan demonstrates resolution of abscess. The percutaneous Jackson-Pratt drain, placed at the time of her anastomotic repair surgery, is removed, and her antibiotics are discontinued.

DISCUSSION: SEPSIS SYNDROME

In the ICU setting, sepsis syndrome will be the most common reason for ID consultation. However, because sepsis syndrome may be caused by microbial circumstances other than infection, other services including pulmonary, cardiology, and nephrology may also be involved in patient care management. Sepsis syndrome is best characterized as systemic inflammatory response syndrome (SIRS), which results in multiple-organ failure. Sepsis is the widespread inflammatory response to a variety of clinical insults. Early sepsis may be associated with acute respiratory alkalosis due to stimulation of ventilation.[11] As respiratory function declines, lactic acidosis develops, signaling septic shock. Septic shock is sepsis with hypotension despite adequate fluid resuscitation and requires vasopressor support. Shock liver is implied by sudden and dramatic transaminase elevations. Approximately 40% of sepsis syndrome can be attributed to systemic microbial infection, and the majority of these infections will be from gram-negative organisms.[12] This condition can be described as bacteremia. However, an identified organism is not found in the majority of sepsis events. Sepsis is the systemic or host response to infection. Sepsis syndrome is triggered by host defense inflammatory and coagulation mechanisms in response to organ tissue damage at the cellular level. The bacterial products that trigger inflammatory and coagulant defense mechanisms that, in turn, lead to sepsis syndrome include cell-wall *endotoxins* (lipopolysaccharides) of gram-negative rods and similar polypeptide chains on the surface of gram-positive cocci; these products lead to the recruitment of macrophages and monocytes. Gram-positive cocci can also produce *exotoxins,* which "bypass" macrophages and directly stimulate T cell production. Figure 32-1 and Table 32-2 illustrate the inflammatory and coagulant response to microbial triggers resulting in sepsis syndrome.

CLINICAL PRESENTATION

Fever, marked tachycardia, hypotension, hypercapnia, and abrupt altered mental status, the latter especially in the elderly, are all signs consistent with the onset of sepsis syndrome in a patient who may be postoperative, bed bound, or under treatment for preceding serious infection or other life-threatening condition such as myocardial infarction, stroke, or tumor. The patient may, in fact, be hypothermic, which is thought to be a poor prognostic sign in a septic patient and suggests poor host response. Examination is likely to demonstrate cool, clammy skin; poor respiratory effort; flaccid muscle; and skin surface hemorrhage. Lactic acidosis associated with respiratory alkalosis will occur early in sepsis syndrome; progression of shock will lead to metabolic acidosis and death if acid-base abnormalities are not quickly addressed. The patient will be oliguric, and pulmonary edema will most often appear on chest radiographs. Leukocytosis with bandemia will be present; however, leukopenia may occur as a result of poor inflammatory response in an immune-compromised patient.

TREATMENT CONSIDERATIONS

This case study illustrates a number of questions that will help frame a treatment plan for the septic patient.

- Fever?
- Leukocytosis?
- Anemia?
- Acid-base fluid balance?
- Respiratory function?
- When were the patient's lines/Foley catheters last changed?
- Microscopy (including Gram stains/fungal smears from pending culture)?
- Imaging database?
- Operative report?
- Prior antibiotics?
- Duration of stay in hospital or health care facility?

Through careful history and physical examination, clues to the source of sepsis may be found. Gram stain of suspicious fluids will often yield early guidance for treatment. As examples, urine should be routinely Gram stained and cultured, sputum should be examined in a patient with productive cough, and intraabdominal collection in a postoperative patient should be percutaneously sampled under radiologic guidance. Blood cultures should be taken from two distinct sites for aerobic and anaerobic analysis. Intravenous antibiotic therapy should be initiated immediately after obtaining appropriate cultures. The choice of antibiotics can be complex; and the patient's history, comorbidities, clinical syndrome, and Gram stain data should be considered. A couple of guiding principles are worth keeping in mind when choosing empirical antimicrobial therapy for the septic patient. First, systemic infections caused by gram-negative bacilli, particularly *Pseudomonas aeruginosa, Candida* species, and polymicrobials, are responsible for high rates of mortality.[13] Secondly, *Staphylococcus aureus* is associated with significant morbidity if not treated early in the course of infection.[14] There is growing evidence that methicillin-resistant *S. aureus* (MRSA) is a cause of sepsis in hospitalized patients and should be covered until proven otherwise. Therefore, broad-spectrum coverage directed at gram-positive and gram-negative bacteria is most often used as initial therapy while awaiting results of blood, urine, sputum, soft tissue, and/or surgical cultures. Furthermore, consideration should be given to the known susceptibility patterns of organisms under suspicion as seen in the community, hospital, and, if available, ICU setting. Finally, the susceptibility pattern of any previously isolated organism in the patient ought to inform the clinician's choice of new therapy.

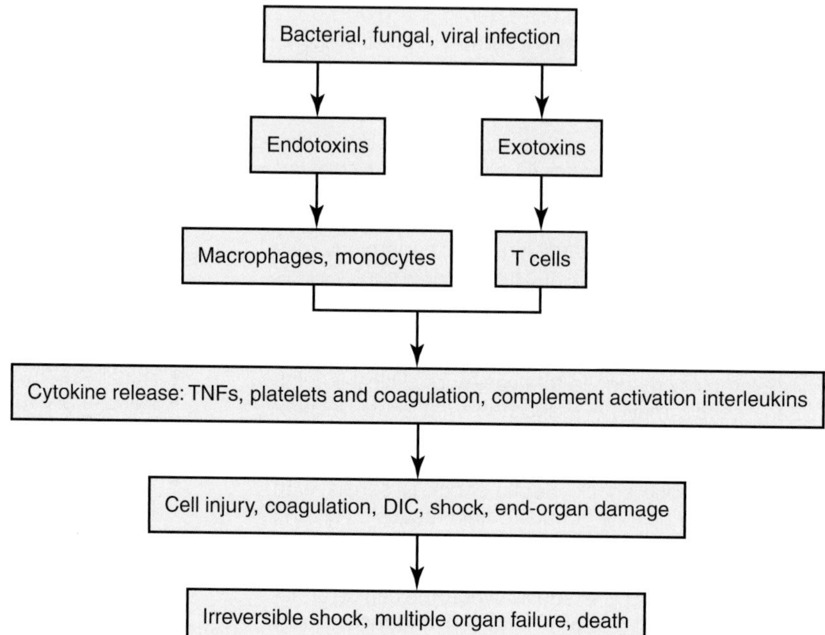

FIGURE 32-1 Inflammatory and coagulant response in sepsis syndrome. DIC, disseminated intravascular coagulation; TNFs, tumor necrosis factors.

TABLE 32-2 **Evaluation of Common Sources of Sepsis**

Suspect Site	Symptoms/Signs	Microbiologic Database
Upper respiratory tract	Pharyngeal swelling plus exudates, lymphadenopathy	Throat swab
Lower respiratory tract	Productive cough, pleurisy, adventitious breath sounds	Sputum, bronchoalveolar lavage
Urinary tract	Fever, urgency, dysuria, groin pain	Urinalysis with > 50 WBC/hpf + midstream urine > 100,000 CFU/mL Catheter urine > 100,000 CFU/mL Suprapubic aspirate > 1000 CFU/mL
Wound or burn	Inflammation, edema, blister, erythema, purulent drainage	Superficial wound cx not considered reliable (need débrided wound tissue)
Skin	Erythema, edema, lymphangiitis	As above, although débridement avoided
Central nervous system	Signs of meningeal irritation	CSF microscopy, protein, glucose, bacterial/viral serologies
Gastrointestinal	Abdominal pain, distention, diarrhea, vomiting	Stool for cx and sensitivity (C&S), ova and parasites, *Clostridia difficile* toxin, AFB/fungal
Intraabdominal	Abdominal pain, distention	Cx percutaneously of surgically drained fluid
PPD	Cloudy PD fluid, abdominal pain, fever	Cell count, cx of PD fluid
Genital tract	Low abdominal pain, vaginal discharge	Endocervical and high vaginal swabs into selected media

Modified from Cohen J. Microbiologic requirements for studies of sepsis. In: Sibbald WJ, Vincent JL, eds. Clinical Trials for the Treatment of Sepsis. New York: Springer-Verlag, 1995, p 73.

AFB, acid-fast bacillus; CFU, colony-forming unit; cx, culture; hpf, high-power field; PD, peritoneal dialysis.

CASE STUDY 32-3

A 78-year-old hypertensive retired male is admitted originally for shortness of breath and bilateral ankle swelling. He had undergone dental work 3 months earlier. He recalls that about 2 weeks after his dental surgery, he began experiencing dyspnea on exertion. Later, he developed fatigue, night sweats, and intermittent low-grade fever. A grade II/VI diastolic murmur was noted along the left sternal border. He was treated as an outpatient with diuretics for left-sided congestive heart failure. On the day before admission, he began experiencing increasingly severe shortness of breath. He also began coughing frothy pink phlegm and arrived in the emergency department gasping for air.

Physical examination (PE): lethargic in appearance, in moderate respiratory distress. Vital signs (VS): Temperature, 101.5°F; blood pressure, 106/66 mm Hg; heart rate, 85 per minute; respirations, 36 per minute. Eye, ear, nose, and throat (EENT): no dentition abnormalities. No retinal hemorrhages or exudates. Neck: supple. Sitting up at 30 degrees, jugular vein distention (JVD) noted to the level of his jaw bilaterally. Chest: diffuse wheezes, rales lower two thirds of lung fields. Cardiovascular (CV): loud S3 gallop, II/VI holosystolic murmur left sternal border radiating to the apex. Abdomen: no hepatosplenomegaly. Ext: 2+ pitting edema of the ankles extending midway up the thighs. Nail beds without splinter hemorrhages. 2+ bilateral distal phalangeal (DP) pulses.

Laboratory database: WBC 11,700/mm^3 (69% polymorphonuclear neutrophils [PMNs], 4% band forms, 22% lymphs, 3% monos), hemoglobin (Hgb) 12.1, normochromic, normocytic. Urinalysis (U/A) with 1+ protein 10-20 RBC, 5-10 WBC. Erythrocyte sedimentation rate 67. Electrocardiogram (ECG) normal sinus rhythm, PR prolongation, left bundle branch block (LBBB). Chest radiograph diffuse pulmonary edema. 4/4 blood cultures positive for *Staphylococcus viridans*.

DISCUSSION: INFECTIVE ENDOCARDITIS

Infective endocarditis (IE) is caused by bacterial or fungal infection of the endocardial surface of the heart (Table 32-3). Certain predisposing conditions allow formation of platelets and fibrin, commonly called "vegetation," to deposit at the "low pressure" side of the mitral, aortic, and, less commonly, the tricuspid and pulmonary valves. These conditions include injection drug use, prosthetic heart valves, and structural heart disease. Other risk factors include invasive procedures or vascular device placement, a history of infective endocarditis, and HIV infection. Finally, routine dental procedures, gastrointestinal endoscopy procedures, and urologic cystoscopies all pose a small risk for infective endocarditis.

Transient bacteremia will sometimes develop following dental, upper respiratory, urologic, and lower gastrointestinal procedures. *S. aureus* now accounts for 31% of all infective endocarditis attributable to nosocomially acquired infections and intravenous drug use, as well as to community-acquired infections. Common oral and skin flora *S. viridans* accounts for 18% of infective endocarditis.[15] Other bacterial causes include *Enterococcus,* commonly seen in patients who have had urologic or gastrointestinal procedures.[16] *Streptococcus bovis* IE is associated with colonic neoplasia or other gastrointestinal lesions. Gram-negative bacteria of the HACEK group *(Haemophilus, Acinetobacter, Corynebacterium, Eikenella, Kingella)* are involved less often.

CLINICAL PRESENTATION

Patients with IE may present with a constellation of symptoms, summarized in Table 32-4. However, others may present with only intermittent fever of several days to weeks. Patients who have IE secondary to *S. aureus* will generally have acute-onset and rapidly progressive symptoms.[17] Be aware that patients with IE are at risk for septic emboli and that signs of abrupt-onset dyspnea, chest pain, confusion, and limb pain should be promptly investigated.[18] Elderly patients may present with mental status changes, poor appetite, and malaise. Fever may be the only clinical complaint in an intravenous drug user. Patients may present with new murmur. Vascular lesions such as conjunctival hemorrhages and Janeway lesions (painless macular red spots on palmar/plantar surfaces) may be present. Additionally, Osler nodes (painful, red nodules on fingertips and lower extremity surfaces) and Roth spots (exudative retinal lesions) may also appear.

Diagnosis of IE is often problematic given the variety of presentations. However, persistent bacteremia without an identified source is often the common thread leading to accurate diagnosis. The standard diagnostic tool for IE remains the Duke Criteria (Table 32-5), which has an estimated 80% sensitivity in the diagnosis of native-valve endocarditis (NVE); a much lower diagnostic sensitivity is expected from Duke Criteria in patients with prosthetic valve endocarditis (PVE) or pacemaker lead IE. Using the Duke Criteria, diagnosis of IE is *definite* when two major criteria, one major and three minor criteria, or five minor criteria are met. Diagnosis is *possible* in patients with one major and more minor criteria or three minor criteria.

TREATMENT CONSIDERATIONS

Before the availability of antimicrobial therapy, IE was usually fatal. Approximately 80% of patients with IE now survive their infection; however, an estimated one in six patients will not survive their initial hospitalization for IE and up to a third of patients with highly virulent organism (*S. aureus*) will expire.[19] Infective endocarditis requires a team approach, including the patient's primary care physician, cardiologist, ID consultant, and, possibly, a CV surgeon.

Following diagnosis of IE, bactericidal antimicrobial therapy should be administered on the basis of culture identity and sensitivity testing, including in vitro determination of the minimum inhibitory concentration (MIC). Initial microbiologic response to therapy should be obtained by repeat blood cultures 48 to 72 hours after antibiotics have begun. Monitoring the patient for heart failure, emboli, or other complications is especially important in the first days of antimicrobial intervention and throughout the course of therapy. Finally, duration of therapy must be adequate to clear vegetative valve infection. A summary of recommendations for treatment of adult IE and duration is found in Table 32-6.

Up to 30% of patients with active IE require valve repair or immediate replacement surgery.[20] Surgical intervention is recommended if the patient has severe valvular dysfunction leading to heart failure; infective endocarditis is due to fungal or highly resistant organisms; complications such as heart block, annular abscess, or destructive lesion has occurred; or when emboli are recurrent despite adequate antimicrobial therapy, particularly with large vegetations.

TABLE 32-3 Etiologies of Infective Endocarditis

Native Valve Endocarditis

a. *Staphylococcus viridans* (most common), *Streptococcus faecalis* (enterococcus), *Streptococcus bovis* (associated with colon cancer)
b. *Staphylococcus aureus* (second most common)
c. HACEK group (uncommon)—hold blood culture for >7 days

Intravenous Drug-Associated Endocarditis

a. *S. aureus* (most common)
b. GNB often *Pseudomonas aeruginosa*
c. Fungi
d. Polymicrobial

Prosthetic Valve Endocarditis

a. Early: nosocomial pathogens: *S. aureus*, *Staphylococcus epidermidis* (and other coagulation-negative staphylococci), GNB, fungi
b. Late (12 mo postoperative): mouth and skin flora: *S. viridans*, *S. aureus*, *S. epidermidis*, GNB, fungi

GNB, gram-negative bacilli; HACEK, *Haemophilus, Acinetobacter, Corynebacterium, Eikenella, Kingella*.

TABLE 32-4 Signs and Symptoms of Infective Endocarditis

Fever	Nausea/Vomiting
Fatigue	Anorexia
Malaise	Headache
Chills/Sweats	Chest pain
Arthralgia	New heart murmurs (regurgitation)
Splenomegaly	Heart failure
Petechiae	Sepsis
Conjunctival hemorrhages	Septic emboli
Janeway spots	Dyspnea
Osler nodes	Confusion
Roth spots	

TABLE 32-5 Duke Criteria for Infective Endocarditis

Major Criteria

IE-positive blood culture (*Staphylococcus viridans, Streptococcus bovis,* HACEK, *Staphylococcus aureus,* ECOC) or persistently positive blood cultures or single positive blood culture for *Coxiella burnetii* (i.e., "Q fever IE")

Echocardiographic (transthoracic echocardiography, transesophageal echocardiography) findings of vegetations, abscesses, or new dehiscence of a prosthetic valve

New murmur (valve regurgitation)

Minor Criteria

Predisposing condition (structural heart disease, intravenous drug use)

Temperature >100.4°F

Vascular phenomena (arterial emboli, intracranial hemorrhage, Janeway lesions, mycotic aneurysm, septic pulmonary infarct)

Immunologic phenomena (glomerulonephritis, Osler nodes, Roth sport, rheumatoid factor)

Microbiologic evidence (positive blood cultures not meeting major criteria)

ECOC, enterococcus; HACEK, *Haemophilus, Acinetobacter, Corynebacterium, Eikenella, Kingella*; IE, infectious endocarditis.

From references 16, 17, 21, and 22.

TABLE 32-6 **American Heart Association Initial Intravenous Therapy/Duration for Infectious Endocarditis**

Microorganism	Antibiotic	Duration
Streptococcus NVE	Penicillin G or ceftriaxone plus gentamicin*	4-6 wk 2 wk*
Streptococcus PVE	Penicillin G or ceftriaxone w/wo gentamicin	6 wk 2 wk
	Penicillin G or ceftriaxone plus gentamicin†	6 wk
MSSA NVE	Nafcillin or oxacillin w/wo gentamicin	≥ 6 wk 3-5 d
MRSA NVE	Vancomycin	≥ 6 wk
MSSA PVE	Nafcillin or oxacillin plus rifampin	≥ 6 wk ≥ 6 wk
MRSA PVE	Vancomycin plus rifampin plus gentamicin	
ECOC NVE or PVE	Ampicillin-sulbactam or penicillin G plus gentamicin	4-6 wk
HACEK NVE or PVE	Ceftriaxone or ampicillin-sulbactam or ciprofloxacin	4 wk

From Baddour LM, Wilson WR, Bayer AS, et al. Infective endocarditis: diagnosis, antimicrobial therapy, and management of complications: a statement for healthcare professionals from the Committee on Rheumatic Fever, Endocarditis, and Kawasaki Disease, Council on Cardiovascular Disease in the Young, and the Councils on Clinical Cardiology, Stroke, and Cardiovascular Surgery and Anesthesia, American Heart Association. Circulation 2005;111:e394.

ECOC, enterococcus; HACEK, *Haemophilus, Acinetobacter, Corynebacterium, Eikenella, Kingella;* MRSA, methicillin-resistant *Staphylococcus aureus;* MSSA, methicillin-sensitive *S. aureus;* NVE, native valve endocarditis; PVE, prosthetic valve endocarditis.

*Patients with NVE who do not have evidence of intracardiac/extracardiac complications, or preexisting renal or otic disease may be treated with shorter courses of combination therapy.

†When streptococcus is relatively or fully resistant to penicillin.

References

1. Carter RD. Sociocultural origins of the PA profession. J Am Acad Phys Assist 1992;5:655.
2. Kass EH. History of the specialty of infectious diseases in the United States. Ann Intern Med 1987;106:745.
3. Census report. Alexandria, VA: American Academy of Physician Assistants, 2006.
4. Zmigrodski JA. The lonely road. Primary care providers coping with AIDS. Physician Assist 1995;19:21.
5. Mandell G, Bennet J, Dolin R. Principles and Practice of Infectious Disease. 5th ed. Philadelphia: Churchill Livingstone, 2000.
6. Chung A, Kim A, Polsky B. HIV/hepatitis B and C co-infection: pathogenic interactions, natural history and therapy. Antivir Chem Chemother 2001;12(Suppl. 1):73.
7. DHHS Guidelines. *http://www.dhhs.gov*. Accessed January 2011.
8. Craven D, Nunes D. Managing hepatitis C infection in HIV-positive patients. AIDS Clin Care 2000;12:71.
9. DHHS Guidelines. *http://www.dhhs.gov*. Accessed October 2006.
10. Pockros PJ. Ther Adv Gastroenterol 2010;3:191.
11. Simmons DH, Nicoloff J, Guze LB. Hyper-ventilation and respiratory alkalosis as signs of gram-negative bacteremia. JAMA 1960;74:2196.
12. Young LS. Sepsis syndrome. In: Mandell GL, Bennett JE, Dolin R, (eds). Principles and Practice of Infectious Diseases. 5th ed. Philadelphia: Churchill Livingstone, 2000.
13. Young LS (as above).
14. McDonald JR, Friedman ND, Stout JE. Risk factors for ineffective therapy in patients with bloodstream infection. Arch Intern Med 2005;165:308.
15. Fowler Jr VG, Miro JM, Hoen B, et al, for the ICE Investigators. *Staphylococcus aureus* endocarditis: a consequence of medical progress. JAMA 2005;293:3012.
16. Hill EE, Herjgers P, Herregods MC, Peetermans WE. Evolving trends in infective endocarditis. Clin Microbiol Infect 2006;12:5.
17. Habib G. Management of infective endocarditis. Heart 2006;92:124.
18. Baddour LM, Wilson WR, Bayer AS, et al. Infective endocarditis: diagnosis, antimicrobial therapy, and management of complications: a statement for healthcare professionals from the Committee on Rheumatic Fever, Endocarditis, and Kawasaki Disease, Council on Cardiovascular Disease in the Young, and the Councils on Clinical Cardiology, Stroke, and Cardiovascular Surgery and Anesthesia, American Heart Association. Circulation 2005;111:e394.
19. Unpublished data from the International Collaboration on Endocarditis Prospective Cohort Study, 2006.
20. Hill EE, Herligers P, Herregods MC, Peetermans WE. Evolving trends in infective endocarditis. Clin Microbiol Infect 2006;12:5.
21. Fournier PE, Casalta JP, Habib G, et al. Modification of the diagnostic criteria proposed by the Duke endocarditis service to permit improved diagnosis of Q fever endocaritis. Am J Med 1996;100:629.
22. Durack DT, Lukes AS, Bright DK. New criteria for diagnosis of infective endocarditis: utilization of specific echocardiographic findings. Duke Endocarditis Service. Am J Med 1994;96:200.

CHAPTER 33

Occupational and Environmental Medicine

Maryann Ramos

CHAPTER CONTENTS

Occupational and environmental medicine (OEM) is a clinical specialty that addresses worksite and environmental concerns that affect health. The specialty encompasses workplace illnesses and injuries and their prevention, as well as several community health disciplines and policy issues.

The World Health Organization (WHO) adds, "Occupational Health should aim at the promotion and maintenance of the highest degree of physical, mental and social well-being of workers in all occupations; the prevention among workers of departures from health caused by their working conditions; the protection of workers in their employment from risks resulting from factors adverse to health; placing and maintenance of a worker in an occupational environment adapted to his physiological and psychological equipment and, to summarize, the adaptation of work to people and of each person." An updated version of the WHO statement is to promote the improvement of working conditions. In 2007, the World Health Assembly endorsed the WHO Global Plan of Action on Workers' Health (GPA) (2008-2017), which is a follow-up of the WHO Global Strategy on Occupational Health for All endorsed by the World Health Assembly in 1996.

The main objectives of the GPA are to do the following:

- Strengthen the governance and leadership function of national health systems to respond to the specific health needs of working populations.
- Establish basic levels of health protection at all workplaces to decrease inequalities in workers' health between and within countries and strengthen the promotion of health at work.
- Ensure access of all workers to preventive health services and link occupational health to primary health care.
- Improve the knowledge base for action on protecting and promoting the health of workers and establish linkages between health and work.
- Stimulate incorporation of actions on workers' health into other policies, such as sustainable development, poverty reduction, trade liberalization, environmental protection, and employment.[1]

Environmental medicine takes a broader look at contaminants in the workplace, in the ambient environment, and at home. In a perfect world, various hobby exposures that include toxins, exposures to air and water pollution, as well as negative impact of the impaired food chain are evaluated. Occupational medicine clinicians would serve their patients' best interest by taking both their ambient environment and total exposure into consideration.

Physician assistants (PAs) fit into the OEM specialty well. Because the discipline requires a solid basis of general medicine, and all PAs are trained in basic general medicine, they have only to ask the question occupational medicine practitioners pose in addition to the history of the present illness.[2] That question is, "What is your work?" Acknowledging the workplace and its dangers, those who work in OEM seek the work-relatedness of injury or illness. Knowing how to ask about work and considering the implications and suspicions of exposure, illness, and injury are the bases of occupational medicine.[3]

One PA who conducts research has accomplished much in the world of ergonomics, the science of person and work interface. In the recent back injury research published in the *Journal of Occupational and Environmental Medicine*, the article entitled "Survey of Acute Low Back Pain Management by Specialty Group and Practice Experience" is enlightening because it focuses on cost containment of this ubiquitous work injury.[4] Another prolific PA considers the roles and utility of PAs in occupational medicine and occupational physicians.[5]

KEY POINTS TO CONSIDER

1. The team approach: Health care providers such as physicians, PAs, occupational health nurses, industrial hygienists, and safety managers work together to address the prevention and treatment mission.
2. PAs in the workplace: PAs care for various work-related injuries such as back injuries from incorrect lifting, tendonitis of the wrists leading to carpal tunnel syndrome, muscle injuries, fractures, lacerations, and hearing loss. The preventive aspect of injuries is an integral part of occupational health care delivery. In many cases, assessing the injury and its future prevention is part of patient education at the end of the visit that may involve the safety manager.
3. Occupational medicine PAs see work-related illnesses caused by poor indoor air quality. Inadequate fresh air intake or poor exhaust systems may allow toxins, pollutants, and infection-causing bacteria or viruses to circulate in closed spaces that can lead to disease or death. Carbon monoxide from improperly vented internal combustion engines can cause asphyxiation. Other indoor pollutants such as mold, bacteria, or volatile inorganic chemicals can cause serious breathing difficulties such as asthma, bronchitis, tuberculosis, or latent problems such as cancer.
4. Treatment of immediate injuries and illnesses is accomplished for many workers by providers in an OEM clinic. It might be advisable to refer facial lacerations to a plastic surgeon. Life-threatening injuries or illnesses should be quickly referred to a tertiary medical center.
5. Prevention is practiced by using surveillance and screening. Surveillance is accomplished by following a group of people identified as exposed to hazards. An example of surveillance is hearing conservation's annual audiogram. Screening is done by examining work groups that may have been exposed to a toxic substance, such as providing blood tests to painters or demolition crews to detect lead intoxication.

WHAT SHOULD YOU KNOW BEFORE YOU START THE ROTATION?

Students contemplating a rotation in an OEM clinic would benefit from general preparation in primary care or general medicine. Basic knowledge of toxicology would help differentiate exposures and routes of such exposures. Examples of routes of exposures are via the lung, stomach, or skin: the inhalation, ingestion, and dermatologic routes, respectively. Armed with that preliminary knowledge would make the practical experience more meaningful. In addition to patient evaluation of lung dysfunction listening for rales, rhonchi, and wheezes, foreknowledge of toxins and their target organs will help the provider focus on the occupational history. This understanding should enable the clinician to differentiate routine upper respiratory infections from occupational exposure. Useful procedures or skills for students would include patient evaluation, ability to list differential diagnoses, provide computer searches, follow sterile technique in the ambulatory setting, and suture minor wounds.

The following history of the profession provides students a perspective about the field.

HISTORY OF OCCUPATIONAL MEDICINE

Medical care in the workplace dates back to ancient history. The Egyptian, Imhotep, made the connection between work and illness in 2980 BC. In about 350 BC, Hippocrates, the father of medicine, admonished followers to observe the environment of their patients. Luke, an apostle of Christ, later noted the same connection. Agricola and Paracelsus studied the effects of gold and mercury on certain workers in the 1500s.

Bernardino Ramazzini is considered the father of occupational medicine. His book, *Diseases of Tradesmen*, was published in 1713. This work gave us profound insight into occupation-related illnesses. Dr. Ramazzini was a physician who stressed the importance of a person's ability to work without the hindrance of a disease that makes labor a curse rather than a pleasure. He described the diseases of metal diggers, painters, midwives, glassmakers, potters, sewer workers, those who inhaled noxious gas, and those who held their bodies in improper postures while they worked. He amended Hippocrates' list of medical history questions by adding the one about the patient's occupation.

The following is taken from *Diseases of Tradesmen:*

> The arts that men practice are various and diverse and from them may arise various diseases. Accordingly, I have tried to unearth in the shops of craftsmen, for these shops are schools whence one can depart with more precise knowledge, whatever may appeal to the taste of investigators, and, which is the main thing, to suggest medical precautions for the prevention and treatment of such diseases as usually affect the workers a doctor should question carefully, "What occupation does he follow?"[6]

It became clear to London physician Percival Pott that illness was related to habits or work exposure, especially occupational or environmental cancer. In 1775, Dr. Pott perceptively reported the first occupational cancer—an increased prevalence of scrotal cancer among chimney sweeps heavily exposed to soot or coal tar in their work. Dr. Pott also described tuberculosis of the bone, a condition that bears his name.[7]

Other types of skin cancer were noted in the 1800s to be linked to occupational exposure to inorganic arsenic and to tar and paraffin oils containing polycyclic aromatic hydrocarbons. In the same era, an association between bladder cancer and occupational exposure to certain dyes was made. Not until 1935 was the first case report of bronchogenic carcinoma in a patient with asbestos exposure published. Some types of cancer occurring earlier in the 1930s had not yet reached the public eye. It was noted later that radium watch dial painters who licked their radium-tipped brushes to obtain a fine point contracted work-related cancer.[8]

LABOR ORGANIZATIONS' CONTRIBUTION

In the United States, during the Industrial Revolution, labor organizations' concerns brought safety problems to the forefront. Massachusetts created the first factory inspection department in the country in 1867 and enacted the first job safety law, requiring metal guards on textile spinning machinery. In the 1870s and 1880s, the Knights of Labor, the leading labor organization, demanded "the adoption of measures providing for the health and safety of those engaged in mining and manufacturing, building industries, and for indemnification . . . for injuries." The U.S. Bureau of Labor was created in 1888. In 1910, the Labor Commissioner led an investigation of the match industry in the first major public act to control occupational disease.

In Great Britain, during the same period, a centralized system of factory inspection was established in 1878. Sir Thomas Morison Legge became the first Medical Inspector of Factories in 1898. Legge wrote *Lead Poisoning and Lead Absorption* with K.W. Goadby in 1912 and described the entities of anthrax, glassblowers' cataract, work-related skin cancer, toxic jaundice, and poisoning by phosphorus, arsenic, and mercury. He lectured extensively in many hospitals where he stressed the need to educate medical students about occupational diseases. Legge was knighted for his work in 1925.[9]

Alice Hamilton was the first American physician to devote a lifetime to occupational medicine. She was also the first woman professor at Harvard Medical School, where she made great contributions to the cause of preventing workplace injury and illness. She wrote her first article concerning workplace safety in 1907, urging Americans to join "every civilized country" in making workers immune from the "sacrifice of life and health." Hamilton went on to write *Industrial Poisons in the United States* in 1925, *Industrial Toxicology* in 1934 (5th edition 1998, edited by R.D. Harbison), and *Exploring the Dangerous Trades* in 1943. She studied the problems of lead poisoning and, working with the American Association for Labor Legislation, helped reduce that disease among bathtub enamellers in 1906. Her recommendations concerning matchmakers' phossy jaw, which led to jawbone breakdown, led to substitution of dangerous white phosphorus with safer phosphorous sesquisulfide in "strike-anywhere" matches. The U.S. Bureau of Labor published a document based on her work, prompting passage of the White Phosphorus Match Act, which prohibited the export and import of matches made of white phosphorus. This was one of the most effective reforms and is an excellent example of substitution of a safe component for one that caused unnecessary disease and death. Hamilton later studied the effects of carbon monoxide in steelworkers, carbon disulfide–causing neurologic disease in the viscose rayon industry, and mercury in hat makers.[10] Hat makers in Danbury, Connecticut, gained the appellation of "mad hatters" because of the neurologic and mental changes of mercury disease.

LEGISLATION

The real burst of activity and concern for occupational health and safety, as well as accompanying legislation, began after 1900, once the modern industrial economy gained full steam and labor became more of a political force.

By 1900, most states had enacted minimal legislation dealing with employment hazards. More than 200 publications concerning occupational disease appeared before that year. Implementation of the workers' compensation system was an important step in the health care of workers. Workers' compensation is a government-driven no-fault system that enables employees to receive benefits for medical care and lost wages incurred through work-related injury and illness. Before enactment of workers' compensation, common law governed. An employee who was injured had to prove negligence on the part of his or her employee to recover damages. In addition, three common law defenses known as contributory negligence, assumption of risk, and the fellow servant rule had to be overcome as well. The result was a time-consuming, uncertain process that was expensive to worker and employer. The no-fault system eliminated the need to prove negligence and permitted the employee to receive benefits more easily, but it set limits on the benefits granted.

Workers' compensation was first enacted in Germany in the late 1800s. Around 1900, Great Britain adopted its own workers' compensation laws. In 1911, Wisconsin enacted the first U.S. workers' compensation law based on the British concept of a no-fault system of benefits provided to most workers who had incurred work-related injury. Then other American states began to enact workers' compensation laws. New York's law was at first declared unconstitutional and then was passed. By 1948, all states had workers' compensation legislation.

In 1913, the National Safety Council was organized and began its "safety first" educational program. In 1914, the U.S. Public Health Service established the Office of Industrial Hygiene and Sanitation for research in occupational health. This agency was the forerunner of the National Institute for Occupational Safety and Health (NIOSH).[11] NIOSH, a part of the Centers for Disease Control and Prevention, is the federal agency responsible for conducting research and making recommendations for the prevention of work-related injury and illness.

In 1936, the Walsh-Healey Public Contracts Act was passed requiring compliance with health and safety standards by employers receiving federal contracts over $10,000. Shortly thereafter, the federal government provided funds to states for industrial health and safety programs, and the Bureau of Mines was authorized to inspect and investigate mine hazards. The Atomic Energy Act was passed in 1954, establishing radiation safety standards. The Nuclear Regulatory Commission currently provides oversight of these standards.

Enforcement of these laws was sketchy, and those with occupational disease rarely received compensation for work-related disabilities because of the difficulty in proving causal effect and the lack of exposure data. In addition, the role of toxins ingested, inhaled, or absorbed through a person's skin, as well as those that may accumulate outside a workplace, may confuse the picture of workplace exposures. This is sometimes called a confounding variable. These confounders also make the diagnosis of occupational cancer for a cigarette-smoking worker exposed to a workplace lung toxin quite difficult. In addition, increased pollution of the working environment and a concurrent 29% increase in industrial accident rates raised more doubts about the reliability of workplace exposure data.

The death of 78 miners in a 1968 coal mine explosion in Farmington, West Virginia, paved the way for the 1969 Coal Mine Health and Safety Act. In 1970, the federal Occupational Safety and Health Act (OSH Act) was passed. In 1972, the Black Lung Benefits Act was passed. The Toxic Substances Control Act (TOSCA) became law in 1976. TOSCA provided for extensive restriction of the hazards of the chemical industry.

The OSH Act has at its core the general duty clause, which holds that businesses, with the exception of railroads, mining, and weapons manufacturing industries, must promote a safe and healthy workplace. All but the smallest workplaces such as domestic sites are covered under this overarching piece of legislation. The intent of the legislation is to control risk by setting specific safety and hygiene standards, enforceable by inspectors who respond to complaints from workers (whistleblowers) or after a major disaster such as workplace death (Figure 33-1).

An addition to OSH Act, the Occupational Exposure to Bloodborne Pathogens Act, was passed in 1992. This initiative was aimed at preventing transmission of hepatitis B virus and human immunodeficiency virus in the workplace, as well as at preventing more than 200 deaths per year from hepatitis alone. Those with potential exposure to blood or body fluids must receive training, and employers must make

Text continued on p.515

ASBESTOS MEDICAL QUESTIONNAIRE

1. Name ______
2. Social Security Number ______
3. Present Occupation ______ Company ______
4. Address ______
   ______
5. Telephone Number ______
6. Interviewer ______
7. Date ______
8. Date of Birth ______
9. Place of Birth ______
10. Sex: Male ______ Female ______
11. Marital Status: Single ______ Married ______ Widowed ______ Separated/Divorced ______
12. Race: White ______ Black ______ Asian ______ Hispanic ______ Am.Indian ______ Other ______
13. What is the highest grade completed in school? ______
    (For example, 12 years is completion of High School)

OCCUPATIONAL HISTORY

14. a. Have you ever worked full-time (30 hours per week or more)? Yes ______ No ______

    b. Have you ever worked for a year or more in any dusty job? Yes ______ No ______ Does not apply ______

    Specify job/industry ______ Total years worked ______

    Was dust exposure: Mild ______ Moderate ______ Severe ______

    c. Have you ever been exposed to gas or chemical fumes in your work? Yes ______ No ______

    Specify job/industry ______ Total years worked ______

    Was exposure: Mild ______ Moderate ______ Severe ______

    d. What has been your usual occupation or job (the one you worked longest at)?

    1. Job occupation ______
    2. Number of years employed in this occupation ______
    3. Position/job title ______

FIGURE 33-1 Sample of an asbestos exposure questionnaire. (Courtesy Medicus, P.C., 1245 Route 9, Wappingers Falls, NY 12590. Material Safety Data Sheets: *http://www.atsdr.cdc.gov/csem/exphistory/docs/sample_msds.pdf.*)

e. Do you bring up phlegm like this on most days for 3 consecutive months or more during the year? Yes___ No___

f. For how many years have you had trouble with phlegm? # of years___

33. a. Have you had periods or episodes each day of (increased) cough and phlegm lasting for 3 weeks or more? (For those who usually have cough and/or phlegm.) Yes___ No___

IF YES TO PART a:

b. For how long have you had at least one such episode per year? # of years___

34. Does your chest ever sound wheezy or whistling:

a. When you have a cold? Yes___ No___

b. Occasionally apart from colds? Yes___ No___

c. Most days or nights? Yes___ No___

IF YES TO 34a, b, or c:

For how many years has this been present? # of years___

35. a. Have you ever had an attack of wheezing that has made you feel short of breath? Yes___ No___

IF YES TO PART a:

b. How old were you with your first attack? Age in years___

c. Have you had two or more such episodes? Yes___ No___

d. Have you ever required medicine or treatment for the(se) attack(s)? Yes___ No___

36. If disabled from walking by any condition other than heart or lung disease, please describe and proceed to question 38a.

Nature of condition(s) ____

37. a. Are you troubled by shortness of breath when hurrying on the level or walking up a slight hill? Yes___ No___

IF YES TO PART a:

b. Do you walk slower than people of your age on the level due to breathlessness? Yes___ No___

c. Do you ever have to stop for breath when walking at your own pace on the level? Yes___ No___

d. Do you ever have to stop for breath after walking about 100 yards or after a few minutes on the level? Yes___ No___

FIGURE 33-1, cont'd ■ For legend see opposite page.

e. Are you too breathless to leave the house or breathless on dressing or climbing one flight of stairs? Yes___ No___

38. a. Have you ever smoked cigarettes? (*No* means less than 20 packs of cigarettes or 12 oz. of tobacco in a lifetime or less than 1 cigarette a day for 1 year.) Yes___ No___

IF YES TO PART a:

b. Do you still smoke cigarettes? (As of 1 month ago.) Yes___ No___

c. How old were you when you first started regular cigarette smoking? Age ______

d. If you have stopped smoking cigarettes completely, how old were you when you stopped? Age ______

e. How many cigarettes do you smoke per day? packs/day___

f. On the average of the entire time you smoked, how many cigarettes did you smoke per day? packs/day___

g. Do or did you inhale the cigarette smoke? Yes___ No___

h. If yes, how much? ___Slightly ___Moderately ___Deeply

39. a. Have you ever smoked a pipe regularly? (*Yes* means more than 12 oz. of tobacco in a lifetime.) Yes___ No___

IF YES TO PART a:

b. How old were you when you started to smoke a pipe regularly? Age ______

c. If you have stopped smoking a pipe completely, how old were you when you stopped? Age ______

Still smoking ______

d. On the average over the entire time you smoked a pipe, how much tobacco did you smoke per week? (Average pouch contains 1 1/2 oz.) Oz. per wk. ___

Does not apply ______

e. How much pipe tobacco are you smoking now? Oz. per wk. ___

None ______

f. Do you or did you inhale the pipe smoke? Yes___ No___

g. If yes, how much? ___Slightly ___Moderately ___Deeply

FIGURE 33-1, cont'd Sample of an asbestos exposure questionnaire. (Courtesy Medicus, P.C., 1245 Route 9, Wappingers Falls, NY 12590. Material Safety Data Sheets: *http://www.atsdr.cdc.gov/csem/exphistory/docs/sample_msds.pdf*.)

40. a. Have you ever smoked cigars regularly? (*Yes* means more than 1 cigar a week for 1 year.) Yes___ No___

IF YES TO PART a:

b. How old were you when you started smoking cigars? Age ________

c. If you have stopped smoking cigars completely, how old were you when you stopped? Age ________

Still smoking ________

d. How many cigars did you smoke per week over the entire time you smoked? (Average) # per wk. _____

e. How many cigars are you smoking now? # per wk. _____

None ________

f. Do you or did you inhale the cigar smoke? Yes___ No___

g. If yes, how much? _____Slightly _____ Moderately _____Deeply

SIGNATURE ______________________________ DATE ______________

FIGURE 33-1, cont'd For legend see opposite page.

provisions for environmental controls such as hand washing facilities, hepatitis B vaccine, and protective equipment for the health care worker.[12]

WHAT TO EXPECT

Preceptor's Plan

Preceptors for a rotation in OEM would show students their clinical worksites, as well as the patients' screening areas. Furthermore, students who see the occupational team in action during screening, work-related evaluations, or walking through a worksite, would be enlightened. Students who perform hands-on encounters at an OEM site would learn to evaluate and treat the occupational patient in a very real way. The approach to the patient may differ slightly depending on the type of practice, whether it is a hospital-based consulting practice, a free standing clinic, or an industrial clinic, but the basic workup would be similar.

Patient Examinations

Clinical work-related evaluations are varied in occupational medicine. Some examples include preplacement, screening, surveillance, and executive health examinations.

Preplacement examinations are done before exposures and are focused on such work-related hazards as environmental noise, infectious diseases, or toxins. One component might be a blood test for hepatitis or a tuberculosis skin test in food service workers as part of the examination.

Screening examinations evaluate those workers who may have come into contact with a toxic substance. An example of a mass screening is that for anthrax done in 2001 on postal workers and those in congressional offices in Washington, D.C.

Surveillance examinations are focused examinations based on a person's job title and ongoing exposures. Targeting intervention activities might follow the examinations. Examples include police and firefighter personnel requiring annual examinations that include hearing conservation (a hearing screening in the office, compared with their first, baseline examination, as well as the previous year's examination) and cardiovascular fitness that includes blood pressure and lipid evaluations. Some facilities may require exercise stress testing for certain workers at certain intervals. Pulmonary function testing may be required of firefighters or others with exposures to inhaled toxins. Tuberculosis skin testing is done in most surveillance cases, especially for health, food service, and child care workers.[13]

TIP BOX

Use the "Little Suzy Rule" for doing Department of Transportation physical examinations: When in doubt about your decision to clear a driver to get behind the wheel of an 18 wheeler, ask yourself if you'd be uncomfortable having this driver share the road your children and grandchildren might be on.

JONATHAN GREEN, PA-C

If you get abnormal lab values in a heavy metal screening evaluation, first repeat the lab work before you attack the problem at full speed. In 90% of the cases the lab work comes back normal and a lot of unnecessary work is avoided.

JACK LASOSKI, PA-C

Executive examinations might include laboratory testing for diabetes, elevated lipids, anemia, blood pressure/vital sign evaluation, and an electrocardiogram. These tests would be reviewed by the physician or PA who would follow with a hands-on physical examination including digital rectal prostate screen for prostate cancer in males. Laboratory testing might also include an exercise treadmill test for cardiovascular fitness, an audiogram, and an age-dependent colon screen.

Immunizations

As part of the examination process, immunizations for hepatitis B might be given to health care workers, prison guards, and child care workers. Service workers might be scheduled to get influenza vaccinations as part of the occupational health encounter.

Referrals

As in other specialties, PAs in OEM should think of the patient who might best referred to consultants. Examples include the case of a metal foreign body in the conjunctiva in which the ophthalmologist might remove the object and some of the surrounding tissue; the patient with facial lacerations, and the patient in pulmonary or cardiac distress who should be transported to a hospital emergency department. Some practices prefer that the PA confer with the charge OEM physician before referrals, whereas others prefer that the PA simply follow the clinic guidelines and refer immediately.

Team Players

The **occupational medicine physician** has been trained in a School of Public Health in the medical specialty area of OEM. He or she is the head of the OEM team. It is likely the OEM physician has gone through residency, including a Master's in Public Health (MPH), and is likely board certified in the field. The specialty has been recognized since 1916.[14]

Many **occupational PAs** have also been trained in schools of public health and have earned the MPH designation as well. However, many PAs have learned the specialty on the job.

Occupational health nurses are often certified occupational health nurses (COHNs). This certification reflects special education and testing.

Case managers are usually nurses with special training in tracking and intervening with occupational injuries that come under federal workers' compensation laws.

Safety managers assess the company's positions, evaluate the possibility of on-the-job injury and illness, establish training programs focused on exposures, and put preventive measures in place. Safety managers may also be company engineers. Engineering controls (change in the air handling equipment or other parts of the structure) are put into place by the safety manager, who must coordinate this work with the company's maintenance department. If toxins are unable to be contained using engineering controls, personal protection equipment is necessary. It falls under Safety or Industrial Hygiene to train and ensure compliance for hearing protection, hard hats, gloves, steel-toed boots, and face masks. Fit testing is required periodically for certain masks and respirators.

Industrial hygienists plan, perform, and document field investigations using sensitive instruments that usually measure parts per million of a substance in the air. Exposure documentation and teamwork is an important part of this position. Industrial hygienists' duties sometimes overlap those of the safety managers[15] (Tables 33-1 to 33-3).

Settings

OEM clinic settings vary. A large company usually supports its own clinic and ensures that all those exposed get timely appointments. Free-standing clinics may have other business, such as general or family practice. Hospital clinics generally have their beginnings in employee health. Hospital practices generally combine outpatient facilities and cater to hold contracts to care for workers in nearby companies. Hospital-based groups have the benefits of 24-hour emergency service and support from departments such as radiology and physical therapy. They are more likely to have full-time case managers.

TABLE 33-1 Job Description: Occupational Medical Program Specialist, Human Resources Department

Objective

Plans, directs, and coordinates medical services, including medical service contracts, cost accounts, and preventive medicine services; offers expert opinions concerning exposures to hazards; and provides and evaluates medical services for the company.

Dimensions

Supervises the company's contracts for employee physical examinations and consulting medical director services. Interfaces with the consulting medical director in matters concerning occupational medicine. Provides the company with technical and administrative expertise for compliance with legal standards (i.e., applicable Nuclear Regulatory Commission, State Department of Labor, and federal safety and health regulations and standards).

Principal Accountabilities

Develops contract specifications and policies and procedures to execute medical programs on a company-wide basis.

Supervises the execution of the company's physical examination program to maintain compliance with the Nuclear Regulatory Commission and the State Department of Labor regulations and commitments.

Advises and educates workers and managers about hazards in the workplace and their health effects by searching the literature and compiling data relating to workplace exposures.

Initiates literature searches of toxic hazards by supervising literature searches, then synthesizes a position paper with input from the consulting medical director.

Personally provides clinical support to employees in monitoring chronic health problems

Offers medical counseling and referral to medical or surgical services

Coordinates clinical screening services, such as those for cholesterol and blood pressure.

Promotes healthy habits and activities by introducing wellness education, describing risks for workplace, while traveling, and at home.

Works in conjunction with the Consulting Medical Director to expedite workers' compensation claims and lost-time injury issues.

TABLE 33-2 Job Description: Physician Assistant in Employee Health

Summary

This position is accountable for ensuring quality medical care for employees.

Nature and Scope

Reports to the Medical Director of Employee Health Service. The PA is responsible for giving complete, comprehensive preemployment examinations to establish a health survey and database for every employee candidate, including all employees and full-time students.

Functions as a health care provider for employees with minor emergencies. Maintains medical records using a problem-oriented approach and ensures confidentiality for all patients seen.

Provides instruction in safety and good health practices and is responsible for immunizations as approved and recommended by the Centers for Disease Control and the hospital's Infection Control Committee. The incumbent will be actively involved in the wellness program endorsed by the hospital and any other projects under the supervision of the Medical Director.

Works directly or indirectly with the emergency department physician, as indicated by privileges. He or she is expected to recognize and interpret signs and symptoms and initiate appropriate diagnostic and therapeutic measures.

This position requires a minimum of a bachelor's degree and a certificate from an accredited PA program, as well as certification by the National Commission on Certification of Physician Assistants, plus appropriate state licensure as required.

Principal Accountabilities

The PA will work cooperatively with the employee health physician in the identification, treatment, and management of epidemiologic problems. Initiates requests for consultations for problems out of the scope of the employee health service.

Provides urgent care for conditions that would not reasonably require the PA to seek immediate management by the physician, including but not limited to suturing superficial lacerations, immobilizing trauma victims before radiographs are taken, and removing a foreign body superficially embedded in the cornea. Initiation of emergency treatment for cardiopulmonary arrest is started by the PA as the physician is being called.

Other duties may be delegated by the physician, depending on experience and training and as hospital or clinic privileges allow.

Culture of the Setting

The culture of the occupational health setting resembles an emergency department at times, when walk-in patients arrive unannounced. These visits are generally a small proportion of the occupational health business, unless the philosophy of the company is to treat all illness that prevents a person from working; if such is the case, the clinic may care for some primary care patients. Examples might be treating coughs expeditiously to prevent upper respiratory illness from spreading though a company or before airplane travel.[16]

TABLE 33-3 Employee Health Coordinator: Occupational Health

Position Summary

This position is accountable for ensuring quality medical care for employees.

Nature and Scope

Reports to the Director of Employee Health. This incumbent oversees all phases of the occupational health clinical program. Implements program goals and policies that have been established by the medical and administrative directors. Works in coordination with the business manager in matters concerning budget, marketing, and personnel management.

Facilitates the coordination of occupational health clinic services with the other services offered in the entire occupational health program.

Maintains liaison with client companies to provide a continuum of interest and credibility through personal communication efforts.

Is responsible for the quality assurance program of the employee health service, such as monthly statistics on exposure and screening for tuberculosis (TB), hepatitis, rubella, and AIDS of employees seen in the employee health clinic. He or she is an active participant in the hospital safety and infection control committees and must interface with the personnel responsible for those committees.

Is responsible for developing and implementing a wellness program for the employees of the hospital and other organizations as appropriate and for coordinating the activities of such programs.

Coordinates the daily activities of the employee health clinic to allow for routine physical examinations; treatment of acutely ill employees; epidemiologic follow-ups; routine screenings for tuberculosis, hepatitis, rubella, and AIDS; employee education; and wellness-related activities.

Is responsible for giving complete and comprehensive preemployment physical examinations and for documenting findings in a systematic manner on a problem-oriented medical record. The incumbent shall maintain the privacy of the patient and the confidentiality of the medical record. He or she is responsible for immunizations as recommended by the Centers for Disease Control (CDC) and the Infection Control Committee. The incumbent must also be able to accurately assess those employees who present for treatment and must initiate appropriate diagnostic and therapeutic measures according to protocol. In addition to the previously listed responsibilities, the incumbent is responsible for any other duties as deemed appropriate.

Directs and assigns work to clinicians and secretaries and provides managerial support, such as personnel counseling, recruitment and/or dismissal, and general performance reviews for these workers, including day-to-day disciplinary needs.

Endeavors to provide state-of-the-art expertise and counsel to client companies in matters of occupational health and safety, workers' compensation, and any other relevant areas of occupational medicine.

Facilitates the whole health care rendering process for the client's employees, from entry to return to duty.

With the assistance of the program's Business Manager or Marketer, obtains new clients and develops new services for clients.

The Code of Ethical Conduct for Physicians Providing Occupational Medical Services, published by the American College of Occupational and Environmental Medicine, will be followed in carrying out all previously listed duties and responsibilities.*

Principal Accountabilities

The incumbent is a permanent member of the Safety Committee and the Infection Control Committee. He or she will work cooperatively with the Physician Director and Infection Control Nurse/Epidemiologist.

Generates monthly statistical reports on TB, rubella, hepatitis, and AIDS, as well as other epidemiologic investigative reports to be presented to the Director of Emergency Services and the Infection Control Committee.

Is responsible for treatment and/or referrals for problems of employees presenting to the employee health clinic.

Coordinates a wellness program for employees and other organizations as appropriate.

Initiates a weekly meeting with the emergency department Medical Director to discuss medical care rendered and other timely issues.

Reviews and revises policies and procedures on at least an annual basis.

The Employee Health Coordinator must possess a bachelor's degree in health care (master's preferred) and must have a background in public health, industrial, or ambulatory care settings. He or she must possess management skills as demonstrated by education and/or experience. He or she must possess appropriate licensure as required.

*Code of Ethical Conduct, Board of Directors of the American College of Occupational and Environmental Medicine. Adopted October 25, 1993.

AIDS, acquired immunodeficiency syndrome.

TIP BOX

PAs working in occupational medicine should not forget their primary care roots. Many times workers can't easily access their own primary care providers. A PA in the workplace setting can often afford those patients an opportunity not only to have a positive impact on occupational issues but also to integrate preventive care, chronic care management, and health promotion activities.

KENNETH K. WISCOMB, PA-C

Most occupational health interactions are scheduled annual surveillance and preemployment, screening visits. Site visits are generally accomplished with the occupational health care team and the company management, industrial hygienists, union leaders, and engineers. Stress levels for the staff are generally minimal, unless there are busy companies that may have poor safety practices, unexpected injuries leading to many walk-in patients, and a small staff. On-call situations are rare in occupational health practice. Most OEM companies have agreements with emergency departments. The best scenario has an educated emergency department taught to care for the worker's immediate injury after the occupational health business hours. The patient will be referred back to the OEM clinic for follow-up and case management.

Terminology

Many acronyms are used in OEM:

OSHA—Occupational Safety and Health Administration. The federal group provides watchdog and legal interdictions if a plant is operating to the determinant of its workers. The OSH Act (29 USC 654) general duty clause of the OSHA legislation states that each employer shall furnish to each of his or her employees employment and a place of employment that are free from recognized hazards that are causing or are likely to cause death or serious physical harm to his employees and shall comply with occupational safety and health standards promulgated under the OSH Act.[17]

Whistleblower—a person who calls OSHA to report a dangerous work situation. This person is sheltered by a provision in the OSH Act from any negative impact after calling OSHA.

Case Management (CM)—involves the review of medical records, communication with employer and employee, injured employee, medical provider, and a return-to-work plan.

MRO—a medical review officer, charged with evaluating drug and alcohol abuse in employees.

RTW—return-to-work plan scheduled for a limited duration that may involve light duty or a less arduous position that allows for worker recovery.

OTJ—"on the job" may refer to injuries or training.

Medical Risk Assessment—a report that evaluates a situation with negative health implications, investigates its causes, and suggests corrective action.

Equipment to Which Workers and Students on Rotation Are Exposed

Those in OEM clinics would use general tools of patient evaluation, such as the stethoscope, sphygmomanometer, pulmonary function test, audiometer hearing test booth, color blindness plates, and vision test equipment. Sophisticated clinics may operate physical therapy equipment, whereas others may evaluate ergonomic factors such as back and hand strength using specialized ergonomic test equipment.

Challenges and Rewards

The challenge for an OEM provider is to put prevention to work and have the fewest injuries and illnesses due to planning, worker education, immunization programs, screening and surveillance, and a safe workplace. Rewards include limitation of lost worker time and a strong economic bottom line for a company because of better productivity from a healthy workforce.

Emerging Issues

Health care costs in the workplace make companies less competitive. Costs for the manufactured product will escalate on the basis of the lack of health cost containment. General Motors Corporation and other automakers have been searching for ways to stem rising health care expenditures for years. GM says health care costs add between $1500 and $2000 to the sticker price of every automobile it makes. Health benefits for unionized auto workers became a central issue derailing the 2008 congressional push to provide a financial bailout to GM and its ailing Detroit rival, Chrysler.[18]

Salary Range

Results of the 2011 American Academy of Physician Assistants Census Survey indicate that the mean total income from primary employers for PAs who are not self-employed and who work at least 32 hours per week for their primary employer is $90,000. This is an increase over PAs who graduated in 2009 of 2.8%. The statistics available from the U.S. Bureau of Labor Statistics for PAs' mean annual wage posted in May 2010 is $87,140, with a range of $57,450 to $117,720. The Bureau predicted much more rapid growth than average for all occupations in this field, with a forecast of 39% job growth between 2008 and 2009.[15]

Typical Day

- The typical day may begin with a patient evaluation for preplacement examination. This would be followed by notifying the hiring manager of fitness for duty, perhaps through the occupational health office administrator.
- A carpenter may walk in with a wood splinter in his hand. He would have been triaged by the occupational health nurse, the wound would have been cleansed, and he would be presented for the PA to manage. After soaking the hand in a warm povidone iodine and water solution, the splinter would be removed. Tetanus inoculation evaluation would be done, and the patient would be inoculated if his or her last inoculation was more than 5 years ago.
- There may be a meeting with the manager of the police unit to check on the increased number of musculoskeletal injuries among officers. An evaluation of suggested fitness exercises is done, and arrangements made to encourage officers to attend physical training exercise classes on the worksite.
- A worksite visit to a leased property might be done to decide where to hang an automated defibrillator in a remote site that employs 9000 of our personnel. Managers would be given the overall responsibility to ensure the unit is checked daily for battery recharge life and that local staff is trained in basic life support and defibrillator use.
- A person from an area where a flood occurred during renovation comes in with complaints of wheezing. After a history is taken that reveals some pollen and dust allergies and a propensity for sinusitis infections, an examination of her chest is done. An office-based pulmonary function test shows decreased function. She may be given a bronchodilator and referred immediately to the nurse case manager. After the nurse takes the pertinent information and files the preliminary report, the patient is sent home and then to her private physician for long-term follow-up. She is asked to report back to our clinic in 3 working days for back-to-work evaluation. Plans to visit her worksite with an industrial hygienist and a building manager/maintenance foreman follow. If there is mold on the walls, a recommendation may be made to the patient's manager to relocate her until cleanup is complete.

CASE STUDY 33-1

CHIEF COMPLAINT

A 25-year-old black male laborer comes in for his first visit. "I get tired, I feel nervous, food doesn't taste right, and I can't sleep. I have stomach pain, and I've taken Tums but they don't help. I've felt so jittery that I've been snapping at everyone. I can't even stand being around myself! This has been going on for about 4 months."

MEDICAL AND FAMILY HISTORY

A review of his medical history form reveals that he has received vaccinations for diphtheria, tetanus, and polio and has not been exposed to tuberculosis. He has been in good general health all his life. There is no history of surgery or accidents. There is no family history of neurologic or cardiac disease. His father died in an auto accident 10 years ago.

SOCIAL HISTORY

He denies cigarette smoking or other tobacco use. He admits drinking two beers a day. He denies psychological pressures. He denies illegal drug use. He is a heterosexual, practices safe sex, and reports no sexual problems. He lives with his mother and brothers.

WORK HISTORY

The patient has worked for 4 years for a construction firm as a laborer. Until 6 months ago, his jobs had been limited to working on new building construction. For most of that time, he was a hod carrier, using a wheelbarrow to transport wet cement from the large cement truck to areas of a building site inaccessible to a truck with an automatic cement chute. He says he was reassigned to general labor division, helping with gutting and reconstruction of old buildings, 6 months ago. He goes down to the building basement and retrieves parts of the wooden framing removed by carpenters who bang it down and saw up partitions to make way for the new framing. He says that conditions are dusty, his clothes get covered with white powder, and that he sometimes coughs at work. He says his cough is much better on weekends. He denies a chronic cough or shortness of breath.

Physical Examination

Vital signs: blood pressure, 120/80 mm Hg; pulse, 80 per minute; respirations, 16 per minute. An unplanned weight loss of 10 lb is noted.

Notable physical findings include anxious and fidgety demeanor, fingernail pallor, increased deep tendon reflexes, and tremor of outstretched hands.

Diagnosis

Suspicious of lead dust in the old building, disturbed by the demolition, a blood lead and zinc protoporphyrin (ZPP) level was drawn and found to be elevated. He was diagnosed with lead toxicity.

Treatment

The worker was removed from the current job site and reassigned. He was treated with chelation and followed with blood levels at monthly intervals.

Other workers were screened for lead exposures and treated as needed. The state toxicity laboratory was notified.

CASE STUDY 33-2

Chief Complaint

A 45-year-old white woman has pain in her wrists and hands, sometimes radiating into the forearm. It sometimes wakens her at night.

History of Present Illness

This woman has been working at an automobile parts plant for 3 years. During the past 4 months, there were layoffs at the plant and her quota of parts was increased. She denies any hobbies or home activities that involve twisting pressure on her wrists.

Social and Family History

The patient works on an assembly line and has a daily quota. Her work involves pressing an "O" ring onto a rod with pliers to make a part for an auto window mechanism. She has been a two-pack-a-day cigarette smoker for 20 years and is a social drinker (takes two drinks at an occasional party). She states that she had the usual childhood diseases and complete vaccinations. She is married with no children.

Medical History

The patient has been in good health all her life with the exception of lumbosacral strain that required a 1-week convalescence 2 years ago. She complains of occasional back pain when she overworks or does not lift using the appropriate muscles. She reports diabetes mellitus, rheumatoid arthritis, and thyroid problems.

Physical Examination

Positive findings include decreased sensation in the median nerve distribution tested by sharp-dull discrimination. Pain is noted on direct pressure of the carpal tunnel bilaterally. (The carpal compression test, performed by applying direct pressure on the carpal tunnel, is probably the most sensitive test.) Pain is exacerbated by dorsiflexion of the wrist. Tinel sign is positive (tingling or shock-like pain is elicited on volar wrist percussion). Phalen sign is positive (pain or paresthesia in the distribution of the median nerve when the patient flexes both wrists to 90 degrees, with the dorsal aspect of the hands held in apposition for 60 seconds).

Diagnosis

Tendonitis of wrists; carpal tunnel syndrome to be ruled out.

Treatment

Removal of the worker from the assembly line. Splinting of the hand and forearm at night. Referral to an orthopedic surgeon to seek alleviation of symptoms, which may require the injection of corticosteroids into the carpal tunnel for some patients.

TOP 21 CLINICAL PROBLEMS ENCOUNTERED AND BEST RESOURCES FOR THE PROBLEMS

- **Asbestos-causing diseases** Occupational Safety and Health Administration *http://www.osha.gov/SLTC/asbestos/index.html*
- **Avian flu—protecting poultry workers** Occupational Safety and Health Administration *http://www.osha.gov/dts/shib/shib121304.html*
- **Back pain** Centers for Disease Control and Prevention *http://www.cdc.gov/nchs/pressroom/06facts/hus06.htm*
- **Biosafety including communicable diseases** HIV and Hepatitis, New York Committee on Safety and Health *http://www.iaff.org/hs/resi/infdis/Learn_More.htm*
- **Protecting health care personnel from HIV** Centers for Disease Control and Prevention. Guidelines, 2007 *http://www.cdc.gov/HAI/organisms/hiv/hiv.html*

- **Diseases and organisms in health care settings** *http://www2a.cdc.gov/niosh-Chartbook/ch2/ch2-2.asp*
- **Carpal tunnel syndrome** National Institutes of Health. *http://www.ninds.nih.gov/disorders/carpal_tunnel/carpal_tunnel.htm*
- **Ears, altitude, and airplane travel** American Academy of Otolaryngology—Head and Neck Surgery. *http://www.entnet.org/HealthInformation/ears-Altitude.cfm*
- **Ergonomics** Occupational Safety and Health Administration *http://www.osha.gov/SLTC/ergonomics/index.html*
- **Health promotion** Centers for Disease Control and Prevention *http://www.cdc.gov/HealthyLiving/*
- **Indoor air quality** Environmental Protection Agency *http://www.epa.gov/iaq/*
- **Latex allergy** Occupational Safety and Health Administration *http://www.osha.gov/SLTC/latexallergy/*
- **Motor vehicle safety standards** Occupational Safety and Health Administration. *http://www.osha.gov/SLTC/motorvehiclesafety/standards.html*
- **Noise-induced hearing loss** National Library of Medicine, National Institutes of Health *http://www.nlm.nih.gov/medlineplus/noise.html or http://www.nycosh.org/workplace_hazards/PhysicalHazards/noise_hearing_protection.html*
- **Privacy rights in the workplace** Health Insurance Portability and Accountability Act *http://www.hhs.gov/ocr/hipaa/*
- **Privacy rights** Disclosure of Employee Fitness for Duty examinations for Department of Transportation drivers to the employer *http://www.fra.dot.gov/downloads/safety/hazmatch7.pdf*
- **Reproductive health of females** Effects of Workplace Hazards, Centers for Disease Control and Prevention *http://www.cdc.gov/niosh/docs/99-104/*
- **Silicosis and other dust diseases of miners, quarry workers, grinders** Centers for Disease Control and Prevention *http://www.nlm.nih.gov/medlineplus/ency/article/000138.htm*
- **Travelers' health** Centers for Disease Control and Prevention *http://www.cdc.gov/travel/*
- **Tuberculosis in health care workers** Centers for Disease Control and Prevention. *http://www.cdc.gov/niosh/topics/tb/*
- **Workers' compensation** U.S. Department of Labor *http://www.dol.gov/dol/topic/workcomp/index.htm*

All URLs were accessed March 5, 2012.

CLINICAL APPLICATIONS

1. History taking—always ask, "To what are you exposed at work?" That way you will not miss an exposure that may be an underlying cause of the presenting complaint. If you follow that question with one such as, "Is anyone else sick at work?" you are on your way to solving group problems like an epidemiologist! *http://www.osha.gov/SLTC/occupationalepidemiology/index.html*
2. Another important clinical aspect of the job is that you may see your hospital-based colleagues who have finger sticks with contaminated needles or scalpels. pAs in occupational medicine, employee health, or the emergency department should acquaint themselves with the protocol for early antiviral medication and learn how to get information from the index patient, as well as follow the health care provider. *http://www.cdc.gov/niosh/topics/bbp/*
3. Prevention is a key concept in this field. Just two musculoskeletal applications of prevention in the workplace are providing correct ergonomic information for computer use to avert carpal tunnel syndrome and giving tips on lifting patients and materials that currently challenge ubiquitous back injuries in patient care technicians, nurses, emergency medical technicians, manual laborers, and PAs. *http://www.cdc.gov/niosh/topics/ergonomics/*

KEY POINTS

- The effective team approach: Health care providers such as physicians, PAs, occupational health nurses, industrial hygienists, and safety managers work well together to address prevention and treatment.
- PAs in the workplace care for varied work-related injuries such as back injuries from incorrect lifting, inflammatory pain of the wrists (carpal tunnel syndrome), muscle injuries, fractures, lacerations, and hearing loss. The preventive aspect of injuries is an integral part of occupational health care delivery. In many cases, assessing the injury and its future prevention is part of patient education at the end of the visit.
- PAs in the workplace see work-related illnesses caused by poor indoor air quality. Poor indoor air introduces pollutants and infection-causing bacteria or viruses in closed spaces that can cause immediate problems such as asphyxiation, asthma, bronchitis, or latent problems such as tuberculosis and cancer.
- Treatment of immediate injuries and illnesses is accomplished for many workers by providers in an OEM clinic.
- Prevention is practiced by using surveillance, screening, and health promotion. Surveillance is accomplished by following a group of people identified as exposed to hazards. Screening is done by examining work groups that may have been exposed to a toxic substance, such as laboratory tests focused on lead in the blood of painters or demolition crews.
- Students of medical sciences who learn about OEM are likely to sustain their own good health while serving others.

References

1. World Health Organization (WHO) website. *http://www.who.int/ http occupational_health/publications/emhealthcarework/en/index.html*; Accessed August 13, 2012.
2. Ramos M. Occupational medicine. An overview for physician assistants. Physician Asst 1989;13(79):85.
3. Lax MB, Grant WD, Manetti FA, Klein R. Recognizing occupational disease—taking an effective occupational history. J Am Acad Fam Pract. September 15, 1998. *http://www.aafp.org/afp/1998/0915/p935.html*; Accessed March 2, 2012.
4. Webster BS, Courtney TK, Juang Y-H, et al. Survey of acute low back pain management by specialty group and practice experience. J Occup Environ Med 2006;48(7):723. *http://journals.lww.com/joem/Abstract/2006/07000/Survey_of_Acute_Low_Back_Pain_Management_by.16.aspx*; Accessed March 2, 2012.
5. Hooker RS. Physician assistants in occupational medicine: how do they compare to occupational physicians? Occup Med (Lond) 2004;54:145. *http://www.ncbi.nlm.nih.gov/pubmed/15133137*; Accessed March 2, 2012.
6. Gochfeld MJ. Chronological history of occupational medicine. J Occup Environ Med 2005;47:96.
7. Waldron HA. On the history of scrotal cancer. Ann Royal Coll Surg Engl 1983;vol. 65. *http://www.ncbi.nlm.nih.gov/pmc/articles/PMC2494418/pdf/annrcse01522-0070.pdf*; Accessed March 2, 2012.
8. Tomaselli KP. Collecting clues: cancer registries might have an answer. Am Med Assoc News April 17, 2006. *http://www.ama-assn.org/amednews/2006/04/17/hlsa0417.htm*; Accessed August 13, 2012.
9. Waldron T. Thomas Morison Legge (1863-1932): the first medical factory inspector. J Med Biogr 2004;12:202. *http://www.ncbi.nlm.nih.gov/pubmed?term=thomas%20morison%20legge%20%281863-1932%29%3A%20the%20first%20medical%20factory%20inspector*; Accessed March 2, 2012.
10. History of Alice Hamilton, M. D. CDC/NIOSH website. *http://www.cdc.gov/niosh/awards/hamilton/hamhist.html*. Accessed March 2, 2012.
11. U.S. Department of Labor, Occupational Safety & Health Administration. OSHA 35-year Milestones. July 20, 2006. *http://www.osha.gov/as/opa/osha35yearmilestones.html*; Accessed March 2, 2012.
12. OSHA Standards for Bloodborne Pathogens. *http://www.osha.gov/pls/oshaweb/owadisp.show_document?p_table=STANDARDS&p_id=10051*; Accessed March 2, 2012.
13. Occupational Health Surveillance Program. State of Massachusetts. *http://www.mass.gov/eohhs/gov/departments/dph/programs/occupational-health-surveillance.html*; Accessed March 2, 2012.
14. American College of Occupational and Environmental Medicine website. *http://www.acoem.org/*; Accessed March 2, 2012.
15. PA Professional, October 2011. *https://www.aapa.org/uploadedFiles/content/Research/Todays_PA(2v).pdf*; Accessed March 5, 2011; U.S. Bureau of Labor Statistics, physician assistant wages. *http://bls.gov/oes/current/oes291071.htm*; Accessed March 2, 2012.
16. American Industrial Hygiene Association. Definition and Background of the Profession. *http://www.aiha.org/Content/AccessInfo/consumer/AIHACareerWorks.htm*; Accessed March 5, 2012.
17. American Academy of Otolaryngology. Head and Neck Surgery. Ears, Altitude and Airplane Travel. *http://www.entnet.org/HealthInformation/earsAltitude.cfm*; Accessed March 5, 2012.
18. OSHA Fact Sheet on Job Safety and Health 2002. *http://www.osha.gov/OshDoc/data_General_Facts/jobsafetyandhealth-factsheet.pdf*; Accessed March 5, 2012.

The resources for this chapter can be found at www.expertconsult.com.

SECTION V

PROFESSIONALISM

CHAPTER 34

PROFESSIONALISM

William C. Kohlhepp • Anthony Brenneman

CHAPTER CONTENTS

Trust between the patient and clinician is central to the therapeutic relationship. Without this requisite level of trust, patients will not reveal information about themselves nor will they follow treatment recommendations.[1-3] Trust builds from the belief that the clinician possesses expert knowledge (that will be applied to the benefit of individuals and society) and will avoid self-interest while acting on behalf of those served. Growing from that public trust, a level of autonomy to self-regulate is afforded to medicine. However, the autonomy extended to the profession must be in balance with medicine's priority of advancing the public welfare. This combination of commitment to service, the possession of a specialized body of knowledge, and the ability to self-regulate are the key components of professionalism.[4]

Some have questioned whether the shared body of medical knowledge and participation in a supervised practice qualifies physician assistants (PAs) for consideration as professionals.[5] Others have clearly demonstrated that PAs should be considered as professionals. Soon after PAs began to practice, Tworek[6] applied the standards of professionalism to PAs and concluded that those in the occupation had become professionalized. Picking up that distinction later, Gianola[7] concluded that the evolution to the modern role of PAs has resulted in our becoming a full profession.

Thus, when the four leading PA organizations adopted the *Competencies for the Physician Assistant Profession*,[8] they followed the lead of our physician colleagues and included professionalism as one of the six "general competencies."

Recognition as a profession brings with it opportunities and responsibilities. In recent years, a variety of pressures resulting from changes in the health care delivery system have made it more difficult for medicine to live up to those responsibilities. As a result, the professional tenets of medicine have been called into question.[2,4] A return to professionalism depends on clearly defining the term and identifying ways to foster and assess this competency. Lessons for PAs can be learned from the physician experience.

UNDERSTANDING ITS IMPORTANCE

Early in the history of medicine, the promises of the Hippocratic Oath grounded medicine and instilled in physicians a strong commitment to service. As attention later shifted to the science of medicine, the specialized knowledge associated with medicine became the central focus. Consequently, the understanding of and commitment to the service responsibilities diminished with significant consequences to the overall impression of physicians as professionals.[1]

Compounding the consequences of that shift in focus, the business aspects of medicine also began to impact medicine's image. Some have suggested that medicine used its significant knowledge base to find ways to manipulate the market to increase the demand for services, dramatically increasing costs for health care. In this scenario, physicians were thought to have put their own economic interests above the needs of patients and society—an action that goes against the precepts of professionalism.[4,9]

As health care costs escalated, government and insurer involvement in health care increased with resulting tighter controls over medicine. Precertification and utilization review efforts by the government and insurers reduced the ability of health professionals to make autonomous medical decisions. Credentialing efforts by insurers that evaluated the performance of health professionals adversely impacted self-regulation efforts. As constraints over decision-making and self-regulation have increased, the influence of medicine has decreased and the image of physicians as professionals has been affected.[4,9]

As changes in the health care system challenge the professionalism associated with medicine, today's clinicians must understand what it means to be a professional and must be willing to abide by the expectations that result. However, questions have been raised concerning the uniform existence of that understanding of and commitment to professionalism. After 2 years of observations during medical school interviews, as well as class discussions and exercises, Hafferty[10] voiced concerns about the existence of the core values central to professionalism. He noted that medical students might feel less of an obligation to be bound by the expectations set forth in a code of ethics. He also suggested that they might not feel a need to ascribe to the values outlined in professional oaths that are generally part of most medical school graduations. He also observed that even White Coat Ceremonies, despite all their symbolism, seem to fail to remind medical students of the values and obligations of professionals.

Reinforcing the tenets of professionalism during medical education is critical because there is a strong link between what is learned about professionalism in medical school and what one exhibits later in practice. In a landmark study, Papadakis and colleagues[11] at the University of California–San Francisco School of Medicine conducted a case-control study that compared medical school graduates who were disciplined by the Medical Board of California with controls matched by medical school graduation year and specialty. Of those graduate physicians disciplined by the Medical Board, 95% experienced a violation associated with a professionalism lapse. When compared with controls, the physicians who experienced professionalism lapses during medical school were twice as likely to later experience an adverse medical board action while in practice.[11]

ELEMENTS OF THE PA COMPETENCY OF PROFESSIONALISM

Recent efforts to define professionalism have shifted from the sociologic definition to a focus on values associated with professionals. The most commonly appearing elements identified in a recent literature search included a number of ill-defined concepts, such as "altruism, accountability, respect, integrity, ethic[ism], lifelong learn[ing], honesty, compassion, excellence, self-regulating, service," that provide little guidance to the clinician who aspires to professionalism.[12]

Van de Camp and colleagues[13] provide an understandable overarching structure that brings together key values with service delivery concepts. The latest model includes four areas of professional behavior: toward the patient, toward other professionals, toward the public, and toward oneself. The authors note that their behavior-based focus intentionally avoided the use of vaguely understood elements that have been associated with professionalism. Another improvement in the recent model is that it included elements that grew from the models of competency developed by the Accreditation Council on Graduate Medical Education in conjunction with the American Board of Medical Specialties.[14,15]

The Competencies for the PA Profession incorporate nearly all of the top 10 constituent elements of professionalism mentioned most frequently in the literature and fit well into the structure outlined by Van de Camp and colleagues[13] (Table 34-1). In addition, a number of other, less frequently mentioned elements are included.

BEHAVIOR TOWARD THE PATIENT

Values—Respect, Compassion, Integrity

Respect, compassion, and integrity are the hallmarks of being an admirable PA. Professionalism first and foremost involves respect for one's patients, meeting them as equals no matter the situation. It requires a commitment to truly caring for and about another human being. Respect for others (e.g., the patient's families, co-workers, physicians, nurses, residents), as stated in the American Board of Internal Medicine's Medical Professionalism Project,[16] is the essence of humanism, and humanism is central to professionalism and fundamental to the collegiality of medical providers. Compassion, like respect, embodies the ideals of a caring practitioner. Like the Norman Rockwell pictures of the kindly physician caring for the young child and also demonstrating concern for the parents, we are charged with providing that same compassion in all of our interactions with our patients and others. We must treat each person as an individual, not allowing lifestyles, beliefs, idiosyncrasies, or family systems to influence or shape our respect or compassion. This unconditional compassion for patients serves as the foundation for another key element needed in patient care, empathy. Compassion and empathy are essential elements of a positive relationship with patients. Faced with a compassionate and empathetic clinician, patients are more likely to follow treatment plans and to be satisfied with the care received.[17]

Integrity is the base from which respect and compassion grows. The definition of integrity is to be forthcoming with information and to not withhold or use that information for power.[18] Integrity requires that we admit to our errors, use resources appropriately, and exercise discretion, especially in areas of confidentiality. In addition to these three, there are other humanistic values that foster positive relationships with patients. These include accountability, taking responsibility, punctuality, being organized, politeness, courtesy, patience, positive demeanor, and maintaining professional boundaries.[19] These qualities demonstrate our respect and compassion for ourselves, our patients, their families, and our fellow health care providers.

TABLE 34-1 **Physician Assistant (PA) Competencies**

Professional Behavior Toward the Patient

- PAs must prioritize the interests of those being served above their own
- PAs must demonstrate a high level of ethical practice
- PAs must demonstrate a high level of sensitivity and responsiveness to a diverse patient population, including culture, age, gender, and disabilities
- PAs are expected to demonstrate respect, compassion, and integrity

Professional Behavior Toward Other Professionals

- PAs are expected to demonstrate professional relationships with physician supervisors and other health care providers

Professional Behavior Toward the Public

- PAs are expected to demonstrate responsiveness to the needs of patients and society
- PAs are expected to demonstrate commitment to ethical principles pertaining to provision or withholding of clinical care, confidentiality of patient information, informed consent, and business practices
- PAs are expected to demonstrate accountability to patients, society, and the profession
- PAs must demonstrate adherence to legal and regulatory requirements, including the appropriate role of the PA

Professional Behavior Toward Oneself

- PAs are expected to demonstrate commitment to excellence and ongoing professional development
- PAs must know their professional and personal limitations
- PAs must practice without impairment from substance abuse, cognitive deficiency, or mental illness
- PAs are expected to demonstrate self-reflection, critical curiosity, and initiative

Content from Physician Assistant Competencies (2005).[12] Structure adapted from Van de Camp K, Vernooij-Dassen M, Grol R, Bottema B. How to conceptualize professionalism: a qualitative study. Med Teach 2004;26:696.

Primacy of Patient Welfare

Altruism is central to professionalism, but the concept is both controversial and difficult to understand. Definitions of altruism include a focus on actions that benefit others and are voluntary without promise of external rewards.[20]

Arguing that the actions of health professionals are not altruistic, critics note that health professionals experience both external and internal rewards from their efforts. They note that the knowledge and skill applied by health professionals often bring wealth, status, and power to those individuals. The critics also point to the internal rewards gained (the gratitude from patients served, satisfaction from being involved in the lives of those patients, feeling good about growing knowledge and skills, and the satisfaction of curiosity, the acquisition of wisdom, and attainment of the respect of colleagues for those achievements). Those who believe the actions of health professionals are indeed altruistic counter that, although those rewards do accrue, they follow the service, are secondary to them, and are not conditions that are set before services are delivered. Those proponents also remind us that health professionals attempt to deliver the highest quality service even when no reward is anticipated.[21]

It seems logical then that gaining rewards through service does not invalidate altruism for health professionals. However, what is equally clear is that clinicians must avoid conflicts of interest that result from financial or organizational arrangements.[1] For example, referral decisions cannot be influenced by managed care agreements that return bonuses when visits to specialists fall below projections.

In addition to meeting the needs of patients, altruism also means advocating for patients. Some have even suggested that the PA acronym should stand for "patient advocate." In this environment of preauthorization before the use of diagnostic studies or treatment modalities, it often takes a lot of effort to assist patients in understanding the system and overcoming the obstacles it presents. Another dimension of altruism relates to making yourself available to patients, even if it means your personal plans might be affected.[22] Wilkinson believed that the responsibilities of meeting such an expectation were lost in the broader term of altruism, which led this dimension to be characterized as "balance availability to others with care for oneself."[18]

Ethical Principles and Practice

Ethical components are evident in approximately 25% of all clinical decisions that occur in the inpatient setting. In outpatient settings, estimates of the involvement of ethical components have ranged from 5% to 30%.[23,24] The ethical components result from value judgments regarding the consequences of decisions made by the decision-maker and fulfillment of the rights of others. Usually, the ethical aspect is not explicitly considered because it is a garden-variety ethical conflict for which universal agreement on the resolution exists. To develop skills in applying ethical principles, PAs should make a habit of recognizing the presence of ethical dilemmas that surface even when they are a minor component of the decision-making. (See Chapter 35 for further exploration of ethics.)

Sensitivity and Responsiveness to a Diverse Population

The U.S. Census Bureau highlights dramatic changes in our country's ethnic makeup over the next 45 years. For example, the portion of the population identified on the census as "White alone, not Hispanic" is expected to drop from the current level of 69% to 50% by 2050.[25] As a result of these changes, health care professionals will be practicing in an increasingly diverse cultural environment and will be called on to provide services to individuals from cultures other than their own. In addition, increasing attention is focused on existing racial/ethnic disparities in health care delivery that are affecting outcomes.[26]

The success of the health care encounter depends primarily on accurate and effective communication between patient and clinician. Failures of communication can result from differences in language, culture, and perspectives regarding health. Communication between patient and clinician affects "patient satisfaction, adherence to medical instructions, and health outcomes."[27] It is clear that the education of health professionals must address cultural competence. (See Chapter 39 for further exploration of Health Disparities.)

BEHAVIOR TOWARD OTHER PROFESSIONALS

Professional Relationships with Physicians and Other Health Care Providers

The physician-PA team relationship is fundamental to the PA profession and enhances the delivery of high-quality health care. In its 1998 report, the Pew Health Professions Commission highlighted the relationship between PAs and physicians, noting, "The frequent consultation, referral, and review of PA practice by the supervising physician is one of the strengths of the PA profession. The characteristics of this relationship are also considered to be the elements of professional relationships in any well-designed health system."[28]

Team practice is an essential component of the effort to improve the quality of health care. The Institute of Medicine (IOM) has called for a campaign of "Cooperation among Clinicians." Effective teams require that team members work together with clear goals and expectations. Leadership, communication, and conflict management are key to that clarity. Matching the roles and training of team members to the tasks at hand will promote cohesiveness in interdependent teams.[29] (See Chapter 53 for further exploration of the physician-PA relationship.)

BEHAVIOR TOWARD THE PUBLIC

Responsiveness to Patient Needs and Needs of Society

At first glimpse, this principle seems straightforward, without need of explanation—"I will be responsive to the needs of my patients." Similar language is used in the Hippocratic Oath, as well as in the *Guidelines for Ethical Conduct for the PA Profession*,[30] but are we responsive and do we act on those needs? For instance, is being responsive to your patients simply filling that antibiotic prescription or casting a broken arm? Or is it the aforementioned plus actively listening and being "in the moment" with your patient instead of thinking about the next item on the review of systems. Do your actions speak louder than your words when meeting with your patients? Will they say you are responsive to my needs, even if they do not get what they think they need (an antibiotic for a 2-day history of a sore throat) or will they say you are distracted, not listening, and ultimately not caring or responsive about them as individuals?

In the same way, we need to be responsive to society's needs. On the surface this again seems clear, that we devote a part of our time to serving society (working in a free clinic or homeless shelter).[31] However, it also includes monitoring our actions and the impact they have on society. It is being responsive and working with local, state, and national leaders to address health care needs, whether through access to health, coverage for care, or developing healthy lifestyle programs. It is advocating for individuals who have no health insurance by working at the state and national level to change or effect policy. We bring to light the individuals of society who have little voice in how they receive health care. We are given a white coat to wear when we graduate from a PA program that tells those around us that we have specialized knowledge. Even when we are not "officially" wearing the white coat, we are still health care providers and, as such, must always be ready to respond to society at large or to those immediately beside us.

Accountability to Patients, Society, and the Profession

Accountability includes commitment, dedication, duty, legal/policy compliance, self-regulation, service, timeliness, and work ethic.[19] The inclusion of accountability demonstrates that once the white coat is placed on the new professional, it remains on at all times. One cannot choose to be timely in care of patients sometimes and not at other times, just as we cannot be committed to the profession part of the time. By being accountable to the profession, society, and our patients, the profession itself will be better able to provide care, advance its status, and drive changes needed for the future of health care.[4]

Examples of accountability include coming to class on time, participating in class, completing assignments, arriving to work on time, and meeting deadlines. It also means being accountable to the profession by paying your dues on time, keeping your licensure up to date, complying with state filing laws, and accepting and performing under state practice laws as currently stated. Additionally, accountability to society includes reporting errors. The importance of this responsibility is well documented in the Institute of Medicine's *To Err is Human*, which quantifies the cost to society, patients, and the profession if errors go unreported.[32] It also involves reporting poor behavior in peers, practicing medicine in an ethical and responsible manner, being aware of your own limits, and identifying developmental needs and ways to improve.

There is much overlap between responsiveness to society, patients, and the profession and accountability, but each has distinct attributes as well. We must constantly strive to be responsible (in many ways an inward approach) and accountable (an outward approach) to how we practice medicine, participate in our community, and interact within our profession.

Adherence to Legal and Regulatory Requirements

State laws and regulations dictate who may practice as a PA, the medical services a PA may perform, and the requirements for supervision. It is the responsibility of each PA to make sure that you have a valid and current state license and have met any additional state requirements before you begin to practice. It is your responsibility to ensure that everything you do is within the limits of your state law and regulations.[33] (See Chapter 7 for further exploration of the adherence to legal and regulatory requirements.)

BEHAVIOR TOWARD ONESELF

Commitment to Excellence and Professional Development

Excellence has been defined as "a conscientious effort to exceed ordinary expectations and to make a commitment to lifelong learning."[16] Professionals must also be committed to lifelong learning, maintaining our medical knowledge, and the provision of quality clinical care. As a profession, we must strive to keep all our members competent and to ensure appropriate mechanisms are in place to accomplish this goal.[34]

Not only is professional development the ongoing maintenance of a current certificate, the maintenance of continuing medical education, or the learning of new procedures, but it also goes beyond self and out to the profession as a whole. We are committed to maintaining and advancing our knowledge, and by this standard we are also committed to "work collaboratively to maximize patient care, be respectful of one another, and participate in the process of self-regulation, including remediation and discipline of members who have failed to meet professional standards."[12] We also have an obligation to participate in these processes by volunteering for review boards, working on educational and standard-setting processes, and accepting external review of everything that we do.

Examples of excellence and professional development include, but are not limited to, mastering techniques (whether new or already learned), developing and setting goals, teaching self and others, and helping to develop or maintain a climate that fosters professionalism. Wilkinson defines this as having a commitment to autonomous maintenance and continuous improvement of competence.[18] Professional development also extends to working on local, state, or federal levels to promote the profession and access to health care; giving back to society, which helped educate us through being our patients/care receivers/teachers; and teaching the next generation of care providers by mentoring new students and demonstrating professionalism first hand.

Demonstrate Self-Reflection, Critical Curiosity, and Initiative

A key part of lifelong learning is the ability to reflect on performance in practice. Self-reflection starts with the identification of an incident that challenged one's values, beliefs, or understanding. Learning from the incident involves accessing resources to increase understanding followed by considering how the situation might have been handled differently. In many situations, things are made more challenging by the complexity and uncertainty that is an ever-present part of caring for patients. Often, it leads to making plans for future learning.[35]

Another aspect of lifelong learning is self-assessment, which involves assessing one's strengths; identifying areas for additional learning; and then showing initiative to pursue appropriate learning experiences.[36] Self-regulation is a hallmark feature of professionalism, and self-assessment is essential to that process.[37]

Know Professional and Personal Limitations

One specific aspect of self-assessment is to know one's limitations. During the process of patient care, PAs may be challenged by situations in which they may need to judge whether or not they possess the knowledge and skill necessary to address the patient's needs. The quality of care delivered and patient safety depend on the PA engaging in effective self-assessment. Simply put, it is essential that you know what you do not know and know where to get help. With the physician-PA team, immediate access to assistance is built in the patient care delivery model.

Practice without Impairment

When identifying strengths and weaknesses in the self-assessment, one needs to be aware of any limitations from impairment. Such assessments also extend to being aware of impairment in other members of the team. Impairment has been defined as "any physical, mental, or behavioral disorder that interferes with the ability to engage safely in professional activities."[38] Other conditions that may ultimately result in impairment include fatigue, stress, and burnout. It is a professional obligation to ensure the public that its practitioners are capable of practicing safely. It is the responsibility of the PA to self-identify or for colleagues to intervene. A key goal is to remove the PA from practice either temporarily or permanently, which may ultimately mean placing the profession ahead of personal and professional relationships.

FOSTERING PROFESSIONALISM

Professionalism has been identified as the most difficult of the six competencies to foster and assess.[2] Many methodologies are currently in use to teach professionalism, including courses, workshops, problem-based learning, role playing, simulated patients, and trigger films.[39,40] Professionalism can best be taught when students see positive examples of this competency modeled by their instructors and clinical preceptors. Conversely, what is learned in the classroom can be undermined by the "hidden curriculum," when unprofessional practices by preceptors are observed by students in clinical settings.[2,41]

Powerful symbolic tools can be used to reinforce the importance of professionalism in clinical practice. The White Coat Ceremony, with its imagery of putting on the white coat, can be used to remind students of the need to incorporate professionalism into their patient interactions.[2] Similarly, the graduation oaths taken by students signify entry into the profession of medicine with an associated commitment of the graduate to adopt the tenets of professionalism.

A number of effective ways to assess professionalism exist, including one-on-one counseling, role playing, case simulation review, peer assessment, objective structured clinical examinations (OSCEs), critical incident reports, and learner-maintained portfolios. To date, the most effective assessment tool is having preceptors directly observe student behavior in real-life clinical situations. However, the 360-degree evaluation shows promise as a tool for effectively evaluating professionalism, and multiple methods should always be used when assessing professionalism.[39-43] Another way of thinking about assessing professionalism is along a continuum similar to "Bloom's Taxonomy." One progresses from basic knowledge or Knowing (does the student know/understand the principles of professionalism) through to advancing levels of Doing (can the practitioner use all he or she has learned and advocate for the patient in complex systems?). With this continuum in mind, Hawkins and colleagues show how assessment activities can be appropriately targeted. For example, Knowing can be assessed through testing methods or discussions and Doing through chart review.[44] Areas that remain difficult to assess and do not have clear methodology for assessment include self-assessment (can the student/clinician self-assess and correct over time?), lifelong learning (does it occur and how often), advocacy (for patients, families and the profession), balancing availability and care for oneself, and advancing knowledge at many levels, not just medicine.[18] It remains incumbent on all PAs, whether in the learning phase or during practice, that every effort to assess, advance, and reflect on professionalism and all that it means is done regularly, because by doing so, we advance ourselves, our practice, and our profession.

CONCLUSION

With the defining of competencies for the PA profession, the competency of professionalism is receiving increased attention. In fact, the National Commission on Certification of Physician Assistants (NCCPA) is giving serious consideration to revising the certification maintenance process to include the completion of self-assessment modules. PAs are reminded of the importance of developing a "professional self," one that maintains a commitment to practicing in accordance with the values of medicine, particularly caring for the patient, and not just focusing on knowledge and skills. Caring for the patient means focusing on the needs and welfare of that patient rather than the PA's self-interest.[45,46]

CLINICAL APPLICATIONS

1. Think of a time when a "professional" treated you with unprofessional behavior. How did that make you feel and how could the situation have been handled more appropriately?
2. Discuss with a classmate how you might handle a clinical encounter when a patient requests something that you feel morally opposed to? Which of the Physician Assistant Competencies concerning professionalism might apply to this situation?
3. Think about areas in your own professional development that might need to be worked on and how you might approach these areas in a positive manner.

CASE STUDY 34-1

Your daughter is scheduled to graduate from high school this afternoon. As you are completing morning rounds and are preparing to sign out to a colleague, one of your long-time patients enters the emergency department (ED) with substernal chest pain. The ED physician believes that a workup for acute myocardial infarction (MI) is warranted. You enter the ED and find another PA from your practice preparing to evaluate the situation. You know the PA to be competent and conscientious, so you plan to get home to assist in preparations for the event. When you see the patient to reassure him that he is in good hands, he pleads with you to stay and oversee his care. Apprehensively, he says, "I will feel so much better if you are here."

- Which of the four areas of professional behavior does this situation illustrate?
- What are your thoughts on an appropriate course of action?

This case is used with permission from the American Board of Internal Medicine's Project Professionalism.[16]

CASE STUDY 34-2

An unscheduled follow-up office visit awaits you. You learn that the patient whom you are seeing for the first time is returning because her urinary symptoms have not resolved. During your interaction with the patient, you discover that the electronic medical record contains an inaccurate reference to a pelvic examination that was documented as having been done during the earlier examination by a PA colleague. On further questioning of the patient, you determine that a pelvic examination was not done and the patient was apparently treated on the basis of a cursory history by that PA.

- Which of the four areas of professional behavior does this situation illustrate?
- What are your thoughts on an appropriate course of action? Would your course of action change if the person involved was your supervising physician?

This case is used with permission from the NCCPA Foundation's *Concepts in PA Excellence: Exploring Ethics.*[47]

KEY POINTS

- Professionalism is incorporated throughout the training and professional careers of all health care providers.
- It is incumbent on each member of the PA profession to uphold and foster the tenets of professionalism as described in the *Competencies for the Physician Assistant Profession.*
- Professionalism embodies behavior toward the patient, behavior toward other professionals, behavior toward the public, and behavior toward oneself.
- Being part of the profession means always being aware that you will be recognized as a PA no matter what the situation is, whether in the role of a care provider or in everyday activities.
- Society grants different groups the privilege and status of a profession, but if the tenets are not upheld, society has the right to remove that status.

ACKNOWLEDGMENT

The authors recognize the contributions of the late Paul Robinson to the initial version of this chapter.

References

1. Swick HM. Toward a normative definition of medical professionalism. Acad Med 2000;75:612.
2. Cohen JJ. Professionalism in medical education, an American perspective: from evidence to accountability. Med Educ 2006;40:607.
3. Swick HM, Bryan CS, Longo LD. Beyond the physician charter: reflections on medical professionalism, perspectives in biology and medicine. Perspect Biol Med 2006;49:263.
4. Cruess RL, Cruess SR, Johnston SE. Renewing professionalism: an opportunity for medicine. Acad Med 1999;74:878.
5. Hooker R, Cawley J. Current Status: A Profile of the Profession in Physician Assistants in American Medicine. St. Louis: Churchill-Livingstone, 2003, p. 67.
6. Tworek RK. Professionalization of an allied health occupation: the physician's assistant. J Allied Health 1981;10:107.
7. Gianola FJ. Mortality, professionalism, and clinical ethics. Perspect Phys Assist Educ 2004;15:135.
8. Accreditation Review Commission for Education of the Physician Assistant (ARC-PA), American Academy of Physician Assistants (AAPA), National Commission on Certification of Physician Assistants (NCCPA), Physician Assistant Education Association (PAEA, formerly Association of Physician Assistant Programs). Competencies for the Physician Assistant Profession (website). *http://www.nccpa.net/pdfs/Definition%20of%20PA%20Competencies%203.5%20for%20Publication.pdf*; Accessed November 30, 2011.
9. Sullivan WM. What is left of professionalism after managed care? Hastings Cent Rep 1999;29:7.
10. Hafferty FW. What medical students know about professionalism. Mt Sinai J Med 2002;69:385.
11. Papadakis MA, Hodgson CS, Teherani A, Kohatsu ND. Unprofessional behavior in medical school is associated with subsequent disciplinary action by a state medical board. Acad Med 2004;79:244.
12. Van de Camp K, Vernooij-Dassen M, Grol R, Bottema B. How to conceptualize professionalism: a qualitative study. Med Teach 2004;26:696.
13. Van de Camp K, Vernooij-Dassen M, Grol R, Bottema B. Professionalism in general practice: development of an instrument to assess professional behavior in general practitioner trainees. Med Educ 2006;40:43.
14. Accreditation Council on Graduate Medical Education. Common Program Requirements- IV.A.5: ACGME Competencies (website). *http://www.acgme.org/acWebsite/dutyHours/dh_dutyhoursCommonPR07012007.pdf*; Accessed November 30, 2011.
15. Hawkins RE, Weiss KB. American Board of Medical Specialties. Maintenance of Certification Program (website). *http://www.abms.org/About_Board_Certification/MOC.aspx*; Accessed November 30, 2011.
16. American Board of Internal Medicine. Project Professionalism (website). *http://www.abim.org/pdf/publications/professionalism/pdf*; Accessed July 20, 2011.

17. McGaghie WC, Mytko JJ, Brown WN, Cameron JR. Altruism and compassion in the health professions: a search for clarity and precision. Med Teach 2002;24:374.
18. National Board of Medical Examiners. Embedding Professionalism in Medical Education: Assessment as a Tool for Implementation (website). *http://www.nbme.org/PDF/Publications/Professionalism-Conference-Report-AAMC-NBME.pdf*; Accessed November 30, 2011.
19. Wilkinson TJ, Wade WB, Knock LD. A blueprint to assess professionalism: results of a systematic review. Acad Med 2009;84:551.
20. Piliavin JA, Charng H. Altruism: a review of recent theory and research. Annu Rev Sociol 1990;16:27.
21. Racy J. Professionalism: sane and insane. J Clin Psychiatry 1990;51:138.
22. Cruess R, McIlroy J, Cruess S, et al. The professionalism mini-evaluation exercise: a preliminary investigation. Acad Med 2006;81:S74.
23. Connelly JE, DalleMura S. Ethical problems in the medical office. JAMA 1988;260:812.
24. Kollemorten I, Strandberg C, Thomsen BM, et al. Ethical aspects of clinical decision making. J Med Ethics 1981;7:67.
25. U.S. Census Bureau. U.S. Interim Projections by Age, Sex, Race, and Hispanic Origin (website). *http://www.census.gov/population/www/projections/usinterimproj/*; Accessed November 30, 2011.
26. Betancourt J. Cross-cultural medical education: conceptual approaches and frameworks for evaluation. Acad Med 2003;78:560.
27. Betancourt J, Green A, Carrillo JE, Park E. Cultural competence and health care disparities: key perspectives and trends. Health Affairs 2005;24:499.
28. The PEW Health Care Commission. Charting a Course for the Twenty-First Century: Physician Assistants and Managed Care. San Francisco: University of California San Francisco Center for the Health Professions, 1998.
29. Leavitt M. Institute of Medicine Committee on Quality of Health Care in America. Crossing the Quality Chasm: A New Health System for the 21st Century. Landover, MD: National Academies Press, 2001.
30. American Academy of Physician Assistants. Guidelines for Ethical Conduct (website). *http://www.aapa.org/your_pa_career/becoming_a_pa/resources/item.aspx?id=1518&terms=ethics*; Accessed November 30, 2011.
31. Hilton S, Slotnick H. Proto-professionalism: how professionalisation occurs across the continuum of medical education. Med Ed 2005;39:58.
32. Kohn LT, Corrigan JM, Donaldson MS, (eds). To Err Is Human: Building a Safer Health System. Washington DC: National Academy Press, 1999, Committee on Quality of Health Care in America. Institute of Medicine.
33. American Academy of Physician Assistants. From Program to Practice. A Guide to the PA Profession. Alexandria, VA: American Academy of Physician Assistants, 2007.
34. ABIM Foundation, ACP-ASIM Foundation, European Federation of Internal Medicine. Medical Professionalism in the New Millennium: A Physician Charter. Ann Intern Med 2002;136:243.
35. Stark P, Roberts C, Newble D, Bax N. Discovering professionalism through guided reflection. Med Teach 2006;28:25.
36. Westberg J, Jason H. Fostering learners' reflection and self-assessment. Fam Med 1994;26:278.
37. Eva KW, Regehr G. Self-assessment in the health professions: a reformulation and research agenda. Acad Med 2005;80:S46.
38. American Medical Association. PolicyFinder Database: H-95.955, Substance Abuse among Physicians (website). *http://www.ama-assn.org/go/policyfinder*; Accessed November 30, 2011.
39. Ber R, Alroy G. Teaching professionalism with the aid of trigger films. Med Teach 2002;24:528.
40. Stephenson A, Higgs R, Sugarman J. Teaching professional development in medical schools. Lancet 2001;357:867.
41. Duff P. Teaching and assessing professionalism in medicine. Obstet Gynecol 2004;104:1362.
42. Stern DT. Measuring Medical Professionalism. Oxford, England: Oxford University Press, 2006.
43. Stern DT, Papadakis M. The developing physician—becoming a professional. N Engl J Med 2006;355:1794.
44. Hawkins RE, Katsufrakis PJ, Holtman MC, Clauser BE. Assessment of medical professionalism: Who, What, When, Where, How, and ... Why? Med Teach 2009;31:385.
45. Hafferty FW. Professionalism—the next wave. N Engl J Med 2006;355:2151.
46. Orr R, Pang N, Pellegrino E, Siegler M. Use of the Hippocratic Oath: a review of twentieth century practice and a content analysis of oaths administered in medical schools in the U.S. and Canada in 1993. J Clin Ethics 1997;8:377.
47. Lombardo P, Cohn R, Goldgar C, (eds). Concepts in PA Excellence: Exploring Ethics. Duluth, GA: National Commission on the Certification of Physician Assistants Foundation, 2006.

The resources for this chapter can be found at www.expertconsult.com.

CHAPTER 35

CLINICAL ETHICS

F. J. (Gino) Gianola • Keren H. Wick

CHAPTER CONTENTS

Physician assistants (PAs) need comprehensive, thoughtful introductions to not only the issues [ethics and professionalism] but also their reaction to them if they are to provide individuals and their relatives with the assistance they require.[1]

What exactly are ethics and moral agency? Can they be taught, and can they be learned? A common question students ask is: "Isn't medical ethics just an add-on course? We need to know real medicine to practice. We need more hard science and pharmacology." This chapter addresses these concerns and gives the student and practicing PA a framework to contemplate and engage in clinical ethical analysis.

A 2004 column explained that "bioethics is simply truth-telling and advocating for your patients, even when you don't agree with their choices. Ethical decisions rarely involve options that are clearly right or wrong—instead they are the complicated choices that appear to pit one right against another."[2] Truth-telling is essential in developing a trusting relationship with patients. Moreover, we need to tell the truth to ourselves as well. Reflecting on and evaluating personal values are foundational in the development of a professional and clinical ethic. The concept of one "right" versus another seems too rigid and assumes a legal construct. The conundrum arises when moral values or principles collide.

Issues of human fetal tissue transplantation, cloning, stem cells, face transplants, genomic medicine, and microrobotics fuel intriguing class discussion, and they will be concerns in future practice. Scientific discoveries are coming fast, and in many cases they surpass ethical analysis or clinical application for everyday practice. Many of the advances have created major societal distress, and legal precedents have affected medical care. Examples include the legalization of abortion with the *Roe v Wade* Supreme Court decision. The Karen Ann Quinlan case brought to light three ethical concerns: the right to die; the creation of formal ethics committees in hospitals, nursing homes, and hospices; and advance health directives. Also of concern is the concept of informed consent, which was absent in the Tuskegee Syphilis Study conducted between 1932 and 1972 in Tuskegee, Alabama. Black sharecroppers were denied treatment for syphilis, enrolled in the study, and unable to give informed consent because they were not informed of their diagnosis. Clinical knowledge and skills cannot address these questions adequately without the application of bioethical principles.

Ethical matters have been a concern since the inception of the profession. Should a person without full medical school training be allowed to practice medicine? Some physicians thought it was unethical to allow someone other than a physician to perform the duties of a physician. This person would be an interloper in the doctor-patient relationship. Those concerns were assuaged by assuring physicians that PAs were augmenting the physician's practice and that the PA would receive education and training in the medical model. The tasks performed were to be delegated and supervised by the physician.

The essentials for this humanistic medical model of education for PAs are well described by Heikkinen and Moson.[1] As noted in the introductory quotation, PAs need to be prepared with an awareness of the ethical and professional nuances that may arise in clinical practice and also how they might react consciously or unconsciously, which will impact their overall ability to deliver appropriate and thoughtful care to their patients.[1] This article was written more than 35 years ago, and the authors' insight still holds true today.

Clinical ethics cannot be addressed adequately in a single book chapter. The conundrums and dilemmas that PAs encounter on a daily basis while carrying out their professional obligations and responsibilities can sometimes seem overwhelming. Consequently, this chapter does not attempt to answer all potential ethical questions. It will address basic clinical ethical concepts and a limited number of individual ethical issues. It will provide a brief description of several historical and contemporary events that have contributed to the modern environment of clinical ethics. Resources for health care ethics are also included. The chapter's ultimate goal is to help the PA to become a self-aware ethical practitioner, colleague, and professional.

PHYSICIAN ASSISTANTS AS PROFESSIONAL MORAL AGENTS

Before moving on to the common types of ethical challenges in clinical medicine, one might ask why PAs have the authority and responsibility to initiate and engage in these ethical discussions and decisions. The features that typically characterize a profession include extensive training; a significant intellectual component; provision of an important service to society; certification; organization of members; and individual exercise of autonomy and judgment. PAs as a group and as individuals fulfill these criteria and thus are viewed as professionals.

PAs must be mindful of the two fundamental processes of professional growth:

- The continued improvement of technical skills and medical knowledge through education and experience
- A self-directed reflective process that advances appropriate character traits, attitudes, and virtues.

To be a good moral agent is to act consistently and dutifully for the patient's welfare and best interests.

As professionals, PAs are expected to work within the bounds of acceptable standards of practice and to exercise responsibility with a significant degree of dependent autonomy and personal judgment when interacting with and for patients. Patients come to clinics and hospitals because they have certain physiologic or psychological needs that require PAs to act as or to be an agent. The intimate interpersonal nature of the PA-patient relationship gives the PA's agency its moral element.

SKILLS, COMPETENCE, AND CONFIDENCE

There may be a proclivity to view knowledge and skills as simply clinical requirements and to be casual about the moral dimension. The engaged interview and dialogue used while obtaining a history and the application of physical examination techniques are moral, as well as clinical, interventions because they contribute to the health, well-being, and dignity of all patients. The proper exercise of a PA's professional moral agency depends on technical proficiency, competence, general knowledge, and the skills required to perform clinical duties to benefit the patients.

National certification and recertification and the agreement on a set of core competencies[3] demonstrate that PAs keep up with the rapid changes in medicine and consequently are worthy of trust. Continuing medical education is fundamental to the proper exercise of our moral agency. The *Guidelines for Ethical Conduct for the Physician Assistant Profession* include the directive that "PAs . . . strive to maintain and increase the quality of their health care knowledge, cultural sensitivity, and cultural competence through individual study and continuing education."[4] Time and resources must be designated for attendance at professional conferences, workshops, and for reading and study of clinical, ethical, and legal literature.

CHARACTER AND VIRTUE

The health care provider's moral agency for the good of patients is based on not only clinical competency and command of technical skills but also integrating and suffusing a technical competency with individual character, qualities, and attitudes, including empathy, respect, honesty, kindness, and fairness. As medical professionals, PAs should strive to be virtuous, that is, continually thoughtful and reputable in their private, professional, and social lives.

Patients expect unambiguous and empathetic interaction, including an appreciation of their worries and fears and respect for their values and goals. In most cases, patients want to bring the story of their hopes and goals to the PA-patient relationship to create trust. With that trust, they assume that the PA will provide courtesy and kindness.

In this professional relationship, patients will raise questions about their losses and grief, their pain and suffering, the significance of the illness to their lives, and, sometimes, the significance of life itself. The PA may not have expertise in "spiritual" or philosophic issues but is obliged to provide an opportunity for patients to discuss spiritual concerns or to refer patients to others (such as chaplains) for spiritual support. Although these core personal issues are stressful for the patient and the PA, one should not avoid discussing these complex issues with patients. The challenge lies in how to frame these conversations carefully and respectfully. This engaged conversation can provide the context needed for each individual life.

ETHICS AND MORALS AND THEORIES

Ethos (Greek) and *moralis* (Latin) both mean "custom" and are often used interchangeably. Common Western medical moral traditions include the following: Do not murder, do your duty, do not cheat, keep your promises, do not deceive, do not cause pain, do not disable, obey the law, do not deprive of freedom, and do not deprive of pleasure. Jonsen describes the difference between morality and ethics. "[M]orality describes the practices and conduct that arise from customs; ethics describes the choices arising from reasonable examination of morality."[5] It can be frustrating to separate the two. However, this chapter examines some of the choices that arise from the modern moral issues science has created for those who care for patients. A number of ethical theories can be applied to any ethical puzzle. Although this chapter does not explore all the theories, Table 35-1 identifies and briefly describes the normative Western ethical approaches.

TABLE 35-1 **Ethical Theories**

- **Utilitarianism** Consequence-based: consequentialism as good ends rather than right means; achieving the greatest good for the greatest number of people (Bentham, Mills).
- **Deontology** *deon* (Greek) Obligation- or duty-based: life is governed by unbreakable rules such as the Ten Commandments (Kant).
- **Virtue** Character-based: courage, justice, wisdom, charity (Aristotle, Plato, Thomas Aquinas).
- **Rights** Theory of liberal individualism: rights provide protection of life, liberty, expression, and property. Moral, legal, and institutional rules are created to distinguish valid from invalid rights (Locke).
- **Communitarianism** Community-based: social contract tradition; a person's moral and/or political obligations are dependent on a contract or agreement between them to and from society (Socrates, Rousseau, Hobbes).
- **Feminist** Ethics of Care relationship-based: willingness to act on behalf of one with whom there is a significant relationship. The value of intimate personal relationships, sympathy, compassion, fidelity, discernment, and love (Gilligan, Baier).
- **Casuistry** Case-based reasoning: practical decision-making and reflection to specific cases by use of analogic analysis; social consensus paradigm (Jonsen, Toulmin).
- **Principlism** Common morality–based: pluralistic ordinary shared moral beliefs and *prima facie* duties, "at first glance" duty that is binding (obligatory) other things being equal, that is, unless it is overridden or trumped by another duty or duties. Fidelity, reparation, gratitude, noninjury, harm-prevention, beneficence, self-improvement, justice (Sedgwick, Ross, Beauchamp, Childress).

SHORT HISTORY OF CLINICAL BIOETHICS

The 1960s were a turbulent time of social change and tremendous technologic transformation within science and medicine. The medical community saw the beginning of genetic engineering, organ transplantation with a successful heart transplant, common use of intensive care units, contraceptive pills, and medically safe abortions. These developments all occurred during the 1960s and early 1970s. These advances put considerable pressure on traditional medical ethics. The divisions between scientific facts and moral values were becoming increasingly evident.

Two statements in *The Encyclopedia of Bioethics* bring into focus the issues for clinical ethics. First is a definition of bioethics. In the introduction to the 1995 revised edition of the *Encyclopedia*, the Editor-in-Chief defined bioethics as "the systematic study of the moral dimensions—including moral vision, decisions, conduct, and policies—of the life sciences and health care, employing a variety of ethical methodologies in an interdisciplinary setting."[6] The second creates the inner tension for PAs. The first task of bioethics was to erase the supposedly clear line that could be drawn between facts and values, and then to challenge the belief that those well trained in science and medicine were as capable of making the moral decisions as the medical decisions.[7]

The encyclopedia further defines four fields of bioethics: theoretical bioethics, clinical bioethics, regulatory and policy bioethics, and cultural bioethics. The focus of this chapter is clinical bioethics. In-depth information on the other fields will not be presented, although they often overlap and will be mentioned as appropriate.

An example of the tension in clinical bioethics was the development of hemodialysis. In 1960, technology had improved enough to make long-term dialysis possible. This new artificial kidney was one of the first life-prolonging, high-technology treatments, and it captured the public's attention. In the early 1960s, Dr. Belding Schribner developed an indwelling arteriovenous shunt, which allowed patients with end-stage renal disease to be connected to dialysis machines as outpatients. The first outpatient dialysis clinic was opened at the Seattle Artificial Kidney Center at Swedish Hospital. The demand for this treatment was immense, but resources were scarce.

Swedish Hospital and the King County Medical Society established an anonymous seven-member Admissions and Policy Committee. The committee members were chosen to represent "society at large." The members included a minister, a lawyer, a housewife, a labor leader, a state government official, a banker, and a surgeon. One reason for the formation of the committee was to supplant some of the responsibility otherwise exercised by the doctors. The task of the committee was to select candidates to receive dialysis. The committee developed shared criteria with which to identify appropriate patients (Table 35-2). The group became the first medical ethics committee.

The members were *not* chosen by physicians. They were "seven humble laymen . . . all high-minded, good-hearted citizens."[8] Members remained

TABLE 35-2 How the "God" Committee Worked: Criteria Used in Selection

Two nephrologists would describe the situation. All prospective patients would be prescreened by a board of physicians who identified medical or psychiatric conditions that might make patients unsuitable candidates. Given that all patients would die without the treatment, all patients were to be considered of equal urgency regardless of their life expectancy. The criteria the physicians recommended:

- Automatic rejection of older patients because they were too likely to develop other serious complications
- Rejection of children (a) because the procedure might generate uncontrollable suffering and (b) due to the significant medical uncertainties of dialyzing children

Despite these recommendations, physicians offered advice; however, they acknowledged "frankly, there were no guidelines."

Factors that members weighed in making their selections:

- Age and sex of patient
- Marital status and number of dependents
- Income
- Net worth and emotional stability with particular regard to the patient's capacity to accept treatment
- Educational background
- Nature of occupational past performance and future potential
- Names of people who could serve as references

From Blagg CR. Development of ethical concepts in dialysis: Seattle in the 1960s. Nephrology 1998;4:235.

on the committee voluntarily, anonymously, and without pay. The Admissions and Policy Committee acted autonomously and never met any of the candidates personally. One year after the committee was formed, Shana Alexander wrote a story for *Life* magazine titled "They decide who lives, who dies."[8] The article had national reverberations. The treatment's high monetary cost and the shortage of dialysis machines were brought to the public's awareness. This committee was later referred to as "Seattle's God Committee." In an effort to be somewhat open about their decision-making methods, the committee prepared public transcripts of actual deliberations. However, they did not reveal precisely how many meetings were held or the number of patients reviewed.

By 1972, the federal government had taken notice, and Senator Warren Magnusson (D-WA) introduced legislation to amend the Social Security Act to include medical coverage for all patients with end-stage renal disease. This ended the rationing of dialysis and the accompanying controversy. This remains the only chronic disease with full governmental coverage for care and treatment.

In 1971 André Hellegers founded the Kennedy Institute of Ethics at Georgetown University. In doing so he brought together two scholars, James Childress and Thomas Beauchamp. Childress, a Protestant theologian, and Beauchamp, an analytic philosopher, coauthored *Principles of Biomedical Ethics*, one of the first major texts on clinical bioethics. The latest edition was published in 2008.[9] In reviewing each edition, one can watch the evolution of clinical bioethics from the end of the 20th century to the beginning of the 21st. The text is based on four principles: autonomy, beneficence, nonmaleficence, and justice. In presenting this text, Beauchamp and Childress provided a tool that has become common language in the field of clinical ethics. There are many ways to evaluate ethical dilemmas, but in the clinical arena, these four principles are discussed most often.

DATA TO COLLECT FOR A CLINICAL ETHICAL ANALYSIS

When examining a patient, clinicians use specific tools. A PA will take a history of the present illness to look at specific data: onset, duration, location, what makes it better, and what makes it worse. When examining an ethical issue, PAs also need to collect specific data. Common principles have been developed, and information-gathering relies on using these principles. Most clinicians, regardless of their theoretic, philosophic, or religious positions, have agreed with the Beauchamp and Childress principles. These generalized principles are important professional values and are repeatedly woven into codes of ethics, ethics policies, and guidelines.

Autonomy

The principle of autonomy consists of the concepts of privacy, freedom of choice, and self-determination. These are major values in countries such as the United States, where the democratic process established the concepts of "life, liberty, and the pursuit of happiness" and constitutional protection. The practical application for PAs is that each patient should be viewed and treated as an autonomous, or self-governing person who is allowed to act in accordance with freely chosen *informed* goals, as long as those actions do not obstruct or violate the autonomous actions of others. A common example is an adult's choice to use tobacco only in the privacy of his or her own home or automobile to demonstrate respect for other persons and their autonomy. If the value of respect for patients and their autonomy is to be upheld, patients must be free to make their own decisions about smoking.

Nonmaleficence

In the Hippocratic Oath, nonmaleficence and beneficence are articulated as part of a continuum. "I will use treatment to help the sick according to my ability and judgment, but will never use it to injure or wrong them."[10] Beauchamp and Childress describe this relationship: "in nonmaleficence one ought not inflict evil or harm, while in beneficence, one ought to prevent evil or harm, one ought to remove evil or harm and finally one ought to do or promote good."[9]

For the PA providing health care, the injunction to "not inflict evil or harm" can be more easily understood in association with and relative to the principle of beneficence. The practice of medicine can frequently cause pain or at least discomfort and expose patients to the risk of harm. Obtaining blood for a blood chemistry can be uncomfortable, and there is a possibility of iatrogenic infection. Similarly, radiographic procedures expose the patient to radiation. Prescribing medications may have side effects and the possibility of an allergic reaction. The harm or risk for harm can be justified by the benefits of the procedures and treatments. In the practice of medicine, the PA is always balancing—maximizing possible benefits while minimizing possible harms.

In the tobacco scenario, the PA should educate the patient about the harms of smoking tobacco.

Beneficence

The principle of beneficence described earlier means the PA must actively make safe the well-being of patients and actively keep them from harm's way. This principle establishes the responsibility of the PA and other health care professionals to benefit their patients and always act in the best interest of the patient. The patient's benefit is contextual and is inclusive of physical and mental health. It also consists of other components of health such as active employment, meaningful relationships, and participation in pleasurable activities. Frequently this principle is the altruistic force that propels many individuals into the PA and other health professions. In the tobacco scenario, the PA should tell the patient not to smoke.

Justice

Justice is the moral obligation to treat people fairly, providing equal access to resources according to their needs, merit, and contribution. Of the four principles, justice is the most complex in description, understanding, and application. Needs, merit, and contribution are frequently in conflict as patients interact with the health care system. The principle of justice requires that for the burdens and benefits associated with health care to be distributed or allocated fairly, equals must be treated equally. When access and resources are scarce or inadequate to meet the needs of everyone, the difficulty of distributive justice is most apparent. Who determines the distribution of the resources and how? Who gets what in each situation? Similar to autonomy and the value of the person, justice is a culturally appreciated principle in societies such as Canada, western Europe, and the United States. Nevertheless, the application of the principle of justice is complex and challenging. Additionally, in the tobacco scenario, the PA should tell the patient that the money (about $96 billion annually)[11] paid by the federal government and private insurance for the treatment of disease and illness caused by smoking could go toward preventive and other health services needed by fellow citizens.

The four-principle method, or the Georgetown Mantra, to address ethical dilemmas is not the only analytic approach to clinical ethics, but as Jonsen has pointed out frequently, the model has been widely adopted as the usual basis for analyzing bioethical concerns.[5] Application of the principles will not solve ethical dilemmas easily but will provide a common language to engage in a dialogue with health care colleagues and patients. Clouser and Gert[12] note that "the principles are located just below theories and just above rules."

HOW TO COLLECT DATA FOR A CLINICAL ETHICAL ANALYSIS

Now the challenge is how to move from contemplating the broad spectrum of principals to clinical application. The classic casuistic method was used for centuries in Catholicism and, to some extent, Judaism and Islam to search context, text, and traditional rhetoric for cases similar to the specific case that presented itself.[13,14] The "new" casuistry must be more than talking about a case. It must be an articulated art (i.e., it must be able to discuss the singular in unique terms that can be generally understood and appreciated). It must have the quality of moral discourse, that is, its judgments about particulars must reflect the features of universality and prescriptivity now commonly appreciated as essential to moral thought.[13]

Jonsen, Siegler, and Winslade[15] provide a down-to-earth, planned, clinical, accessible approach to recognize, assess, and make reasoned moral judgments on the ethical issues seen in clinical medicine. More often than not, these decisions need to be made in a timely manner. Their four-topic paradigm consists of concerns that are fundamental and essential in every clinical encounter in which an ethical concern may be identified. The topics are as follows (see also Table 35-3).

- Medical indications:
  - What is the clinical presentation, including prognosis, diagnosis, and treatment?
- Patient preferences:
  - What are the patient's goals? What would the patient like to be done in this situation?
- Quality of life:
  - What symptoms will affect the patient's quality of life? The objective of all clinical encounters is to improve, or at least address, quality of life for the patient.
- Contextual features:
  - What is the context for this clinical encounter? Medical personnel must consider the patient's family, insurance coverage, hospital policy, legal constraints, and additional matters outside their control and the patient's control.

PAs can approach ethical data-gathering by using this paradigm in a way that is similar to how they collect data for a history of present illness and physical examination. By collecting the data in the same way each time while considering the context that the patient presents, a clinician will not exclude data that may seem unimportant at the time of collection. In so doing, the paradigm becomes a valuable and powerful clinical tool.

Collecting these data allows the case analysis to begin. The first task is to identify the ethical question. What is the dilemma or disagreement? Although this seems straightforward, identification of the dilemma—moving it from an uncomfortable feeling to a definable issue—can often clarify the problem. Then one can ask whether the case is analogous to other cases that have been encountered. What are the resemblances and distinctions? Are there similar cases where there have been societal and professional agreement? This may help, but the final outcome will, of course, depend on the facts of the specific case.

The decision-making process when addressing ethical dilemmas requires consistent and thoughtful behavior. Ethical issues in clinical medicine are not simple. But if a health care team first collects all the information needed to make a decision and then applies a standard approach to the decision-making process, that process can become both less problematic and more reliable.

RECOGNITION OF ETHICAL ISSUES IN PRACTICE

What is the nature of the ethical issues that health care providers perceive in daily practice? What ethical issues might not be recognized by the clinical team? Jeremy Sugarman, MD, director of the Center for the Study of Medical Ethics and Humanities at

TABLE 35-3 **Four-Topic Paradigm**

Medical Indications	**Patient Preferences**
Principles of Beneficence and Nonmaleficence 1. What is the patient's medical problem? Is the problem acute? chronic? critical? reversible? emergent? terminal? 2. What are the goals of treatment? 3. In what circumstances are medical treatments not indicated? 4. What are the probabilities of success of various treatment options? 5. In sum, how can this patient be benefited by medical and nursing care, and how can harm be avoided?	Principles of Respect for Autonomy 1. Has the patient been informed of benefits and risks, understood this information, and given consent? 2. Is the patient mentally capable and legally competent, and is there evidence of incapacity? 3. If mentally capable, what preferences about treatment is the patient stating? 4. If incapacitated, has the patient expressed prior preferences? 5. Who is the appropriate surrogate to make decisions for the incapacitated patient? 6. Is the patient unwilling or unable to cooperate with medical treatment? If so, why?
Quality of Life	**Contextual Features**
Principles of Beneficence and Nonmaleficence and Respect for Autonomy 1. What are the prospects, with or without treatment, for a return to normal life, and what physical, mental, and social deficits might the patient experience even if treatment succeeds? 2. On what grounds can anyone judge that some quality of life would be undesirable for a patient who cannot make or express such a judgment? 3. Are there biases that might prejudice the provider's evaluation of the patient's quality of life? 4. What ethical issues arise concerning improving or enhancing a patient's quality of life? 5. Do quality-of-life assessments raise any questions regarding changes in treatment plans, such as forgoing life-sustaining treatment? 6. What are plans and rationale to forgo life-sustaining treatment? 7. What is the legal and ethical status of suicide?	Principles of Justice and Fairness 1. Are there professional, interprofessional, or business interests that might create conflicts of interest in the clinical treatment of patients? 2. Are there parties other than clinicians and patients, such as family members, who have an interest in clinical decisions? 3. What are the limits imposed on patient confidentiality by the legitimate interests of third parties? 4. Are there financial factors that create conflicts of interest in clinical decisions? 5. Are there problems of allocation of scarce health resources that might affect clinical decisions? 6. Are there religious issues that might influence clinical decisions? 7. What are the legal issues that might affect clinical decisions? 8. Are there considerations of clinical research and education that might affect clinical decisions? 9. Are there issues of public health and safety that affect clinical decisions? 10. Are there conflicts of interest within institutions and organizations (e.g., hospitals) that may affect clinical decisions and patient welfare?

Reproduced with permission from: Jonsen AR, Siegler M, Winslade WJ. Clinical Ethics: A Practical Approach to Ethical Decisions in Clinical Medicine, 7th ed. New York: McGraw-Hill, 2010.

Duke University, wrote an invaluable book in 2000 titled *20 Common Problems: Ethics in Primary Care.*[16] As described in a recent article, Sugarman divided his book into four sections, a structure that offers a practical design to consider ethical problems.

> *Problems in practice that may be inconspicuous*
>
> The ethical issues present may not be immediately obvious problems. They include inappropriate requests for treatment and tests, medical exemptions or privileges, genetic testing, preventive medicine, complementary and alternative therapies, and adherence.
>
> *Problems related to systems of care*
>
> Ethical concerns surround managed care, hospice and home care, consultation and referral, conflict of interest, and PAs' obligation to their patients.
>
> *Problems related to the process of care*
>
> Ethical challenges related to a provider's course of action might involve issues of refusal of care, truth-telling, confidentiality, treating minors, pain control, suspected abuse and neglect, and finally, treatment at the end of life.
>
> *Preventive ethics*
>
> This area includes advance directives and other aspects of care planning, informed consent, and decision-making capacity.[17]

The five case studies that follow address the major areas described by Dr. Sugarman. Each case is presented in the four-topic paradigm approach. The cases are outlined, but the answers are open for you to contemplate, ponder, apply the four-topic method, and, with the resources provided at the end of each case, discover a solution within the context of the case and your analytic abilities. We encourage you to discuss the cases with fellow students or colleagues. Alas, there are few black and white answers, only plenty of gray. Ethical conundrums are rarely right versus wrong but instead occur when two moral rights collide. Remember: Each ethical case encountered should be viewed in the context of the patient's situation. This analytic method provides a tool for not only clinicians but also patients and families to identify the ethical features present in potentially confusing clinical encounters.[15]

CASE STUDY 35-1

The following case is an example of the application of the analytic method. Use this as a sample to guide how you address the four subsequent case problems. This sample case was first published in the inaugural column of the feature PA Quandaries in the *Journal of the American Academy of Physician Assistants.*[2]

MR. T

Mr. T is a 50-year-old Vietnam veteran who receives his health care outside of Veterans Administration (VA) facilities. Seven years ago, he received a diagnosis of hepatitis C virus (HCV) infection, which was assumed to be secondary to past intravenous (IV) drug use. He has also been treated for bipolar disorder and posttraumatic stress disorder (PTSD). He has had three major depressive episodes in the past 25 years, with suicidal ideation (but no suicide gestures or attempts) in two of the three episodes. His last major episode was 3 years ago and was without suicidal ideation.

Mr. T's liver enzymes are elevated up to two times the upper limits of normal. His renal function and glucose levels are normal. The HCV viral load is 480,000 eq/mL of genotype 3 HCV. A liver biopsy showed mild chronic hepatitis without bridging fibrosis or cirrhosis. HIV test results are negative. Mr. T was divorced 5 years ago. His medical history includes the abuse of multiple drugs and alcohol and a 20 pack-year smoking history. He stopped smoking 20 years ago, has not used "hard"drugs for the past 12 years, and has not drunk alcohol for 5 years.

After discussion of treatment options and side effects, Mr. T agrees to see a gastroenterologist to discuss combination ribavirin and pegylated interferon treatment for hepatitis C. However, the gastroenterologist refuses to treat Mr. T, citing his history of depression, suicidal ideation, and alcohol abuse.

Ethical Question

The primary care provider asks, "How can I carry out my ethical duty to provide the best care for the patient (beneficence) by initiating interferon therapy when the gastroenterologist favors no treatment because it may cause severe depression and because he is concerned about the patient's ability to adhere to therapy (nonmaleficence)?"

Medical Indications (Beneficence and Nonmaleficence)

The first section of the paradigm includes the diagnosis, prognosis, and treatment of the patient's medical problem, as well as the goals of treatment. In Mr. T's case, the treatment is combination therapy with ribavirin and pegylated interferon and the goal is to eliminate all measurable levels of HCV, decreasing the need for liver transplant. The treatment also decreases the risk for hepatocellular carcinoma. The side effects include influenza-like symptoms, hematologic abnormalities, and neuropsychiatric symptoms. Depression is common in patients with hepatitis C, and severe depression is a common side effect of interferon therapy.

Mr. T's viral genotype, low viral load, favorable liver biopsy, and HIV-negative status are factors that make him a good candidate for combination therapy. However, he has a history of significant previous drug and alcohol abuse, bipolar disorder, and PTSD. This may worsen his prognosis, increase his risk for severe side effects, and influence his ability to adhere to treatment.

The consulting gastroenterologist cites the National Institutes of Health (NIH) 1997 consensus statement on the management of hepatitis C, which says that the "treatment of patients who are drinking significant amounts of alcohol or . . . actively using illicit drugs should be delayed until these habits are discontinued for at least 6 months."[18] The consensus statement also says that "such patients are at risk for the potential toxic effects" of treatment and also may not be compliant. Depression is one contraindication to treatment with interferon that must be considered.

In response, the primary care team presents updated recommendations from the 2002 National Institutes of Health (NIH) consensus statement on the management of hepatitis C, which states that "many patients" with chronic HCV infection "have been ineligible for trials because of injection drug use, significant alcohol use, age, and . . . comorbid medical and neuropsychiatric conditions. Efforts should be made to increase the availability of the best current treatments to these patients."[19]

According to the 2002 consensus statement, therapy for hepatitis C can be successful for patients who continue to use alcohol, drugs, or methadone. "However, few data are available on HCV treatment in active [injection drug users] who are not in drug treatment programs. Thus, it is recommended that treatment of active injection drug use be considered on a case-by-case basis and that active injection drug use in and of itself not be used to exclude such patients from antiviral therapy."[19]

The gastroenterologist and primary care provider discussed both sets of NIH recommendations. The gastroenterologist maintained that he could not in good conscience recommend treatment for Mr. T.

Patient Preference (Autonomy)

The second section of the paradigm includes information that supports the patient's right to choose within ethics and law. What is the patient's preference for treatment? Has the patient been informed of benefits and risks? Does the patient comprehend the information, and has the patient given consent? Mr. T has repeatedly expressed his wish for combination therapy for his hepatitis C. He is well aware of the risk of interferon-induced severe depression and is willing to take an antidepressant if necessary for this side effect.

Quality of Life (Beneficence, Nonmaleficence, and Autonomy)

The third section of the paradigm includes information that describes the restoration, maintenance, or improvement of the quality of life for Mr. T. Information includes the likelihood that he will return to a normal life with or without treatment. Are there any deficits (physical, mental, or social) that the patient may experience if treatment succeeds? Are there any preconceived notions that may prejudice the provider's assessment of the patient's quality of life? With successful treatment, Mr. T could return to a normal life with continued evaluation and close monitoring. Without treatment, his liver disease will likely continue to progress.

Contextual Features (Justice)

The fourth section of the paradigm includes information about social, legal, economic, or institutional circumstances specific to this case. Are there family issues that might influence decisions on treatment? Religious or cultural factors? Problems with allocation of resources? Are there provider issues that could influence treatment decisions? Is there any conflict of interest on the part of the providers or institution? A significant contextual issue in assessing Mr. T's ability to participate in the HCV treatment is his history of bipolar disease, PTSD, and past alcohol and drug abuse.

Recommendations and Analysis

The primary care provider's opinion is that treatment is necessary for this patient (beneficence). The gastroenterologist has significant apprehension and does not want to cause harm (nonmaleficence). How does the clinician use the consultant's data to make decisions when there is a conflict regarding recommended treatment?

Generally, the primary care provider is responsible for directing and coordinating care of the patient. The ethical principle of beneficence obligates the clinician to act in the patient's best interest, weighing the risks and benefits of therapies within the patient's biopsychosocial circumstances. In the clinician's judgment, the treatment benefits in this case outweigh the risks that interferon will cause severe depression and that the patient will fail to adhere to treatment. The clinician trusts the patient not to abuse drugs and alcohol because Mr. T has been abstinent for years. The relationship between them has developed to the point where the clinician believes that Mr. T is willing to take an antidepressant if needed to treat any depression that may ensue with treatment.

The gastroenterologist does not want to expose Mr. T to the potential side effect of severe depression (nonmaleficence) given his bipolar disease. A considerable number of his patients have experienced severe depression while receiving interferon treatment. The consultant is also concerned that, when stressed by the intense treatment, Mr. T may relapse and abuse alcohol.

The primary care provider's responsibility is to provide to the patient accessible, comprehensive, coordinated, continuous, accountable care. Part of this is managing consultative care. In this case, the gastroenterologist has failed to use the most recent guidelines for care, a decision that is inconsistent with ethical practices. At this point, the primary care provider should refer Mr. T to a VA facility for consultation and care or send him to another consultant.

CASE STUDY 35-2

Problems in Practice that Might Be Inconspicuous

Ms. A is a 32-year-old woman who has been a patient in a primary care practice for 10 years. She has been seen by the PA in the practice for the past 5 years. She has been in good health, with the occasional seasonal viral infection. She is a single parent with two children—a 10-year-old daughter and an 8-year-old son. She is a faculty member at a small liberal arts college in town. At the age of 18, she noted a palpable lump in her breast. After a clinical examination and mammogram, she was told she had fibrous breasts. The breast lump was thought to have been secondary to increased caffeine intake while studying for tests. She has not had any return of lumps, masses, or tenderness. Family history indicates her mother had breast cancer 20 years ago that was treated without sequelae.

Ms. A's mother has just undergone genetic testing for *BRCA I/II* and was found to be a carrier of the *BRCA I* gene. Ms. A is in clinic considering a test looking for the *BRCA I/II* gene. She would like her 10-year-old daughter to be tested, too. **The ethical question the PA asked:** Should I order this test and give her the results? Should she have it now or wait and see if she gets breast cancer and then test? Should I never test because there is no "treatment"? Should her daughter be tested?

The four-box paradigm is used in a structured analytic case-based approach to the ethical questions. We will look at specific questions that must be answered. We need all the data for a complete critical analysis. We will ask the questions and provide direction for the reader to arrive at an analytic answer.

Medical Indications (Beneficence, Nonmaleficence)

In this case what is the probability for developing breast cancer if Ms. A has the *BRCA I* gene? What is the possibility of having the *BRCA II* gene? What are the data regarding false-positive or false-negative tests? How reliable are the tests? What are the cancer preventions Ms. A can access to decrease her chances of developing breast cancer? What do the facts show if she has a positive test? And if she has a negative test? How successful are the preventive measures? How will Ms. A benefit from this test? What are the harms from the test results?

Patient Preference (Autonomy)

Is Ms. A legally competent? Does she have the mental capacity to make decisions about herself? Has she been informed of the benefits and risks of testing? Does she understand the information? Has she given consent for testing? Can she give consent for her daughter?

Quality of Life (Beneficence, Nonmaleficence, Autonomy)

How has the knowledge of her mother's positive test affected her life? How will a positive or negative test result impact her life? How would not having a test affect her life? What specific events can she foresee as a result of either test outcome? What are her worst fears? What is the best outcome? How will testing her daughter affect her relationship with her daughter?

Contextual Features (Justice, Loyalty, Fairness)

What are the family issues that influence her decision for testing? Are there cultural or religious concerns that may be at issue? What are the limits of confidentiality about her test results? Will her health insurance company have access to the results? Will her employer have access to the results? Will the insurance company pay for the test? Does she have the financial ability to cover the costs of the test? As the PA who is caring for Ms. A, do you have the expertise to be her genetic counselor? Is your supervising physician competent in genetic counseling? If not, is there a referral system for her? Are there any state or federal laws that influence her testing?

Recommendations and Analysis

The case analysis incorporates the significant and supportive data sustaining an ethical position from each section of the paradigm. Address the data within the provisions of autonomy, beneficence, nonmaleficence, and justice. One or more of these principles are incorporated within each section of the Jonsen paradigm.

We should also consider whether the data obtained from this patient appear similar to any previous cases that have been observed either in current clinical setting or in the general medical community. Are there any precedents for the case?

CASE STUDY 35-3

Problems Related to Systems of Care

Mr. B is a 71-year-old gentleman with a history of hypertension, hyperlipidemia, hypertriglyceridemia, type 2 diabetes, and retinopathy. His medications include lisinopril, hydrochlorothiazide, lovastatin, gemfibrozil, metformin, and NPH insulin; he takes his medications meticulously as prescribed and rarely misses a dose. His out-of-pocket expenses for medications and supplies are about $600 per month. He is a retired schoolteacher and lives with his wife of 55 years. Mr. B was able to retire from his job at age 56 after 30 years as a science teacher. He has five children, seven grandchildren, and two great-grandchildren. Mr. B and his wife recently moved to a small apartment. Mr. B is able to accomplish his tasks of daily living, cooking, bathing, and golf at public courses. He no longer drives his car because of his deteriorating vision and gas prices. In the past 5 years, living expenses and medical costs have increased dramatically for Mr. B and his wife while his retirement income has not increased. Mr. B intends to purchase his medications in Canada and would like to know what you think about this plan. **The ethical question the PA asked:** What do I do as a PA when a patient asks me for a prescription that I know he intends to fill outside the United States?

Medical Indications (Beneficence, Nonmaleficence)

Mr. B's hypertension, hyperlipidemia, hypertriglyceridemia, type 2 diabetes, and retinopathy are well controlled by his medications. What would happen if his regimen changed? His goal is to maintain his health and physical activity as long as possible.

Patient Preference (Autonomy)

Mr. B continues to score a 30/30 on his mini-mental status examinations over the past 10 years. He is legally competent and has the capacity to make his medical decisions. He currently wants to continue his medication regimen. He understands the benefits and risks of all his medications. He has no side effects from any of his medications. He has demonstrated good judgment in adjusting his insulin dosages on the basis of his blood glucose levels.

Quality of Life (Beneficence, Nonmaleficence, Autonomy)

Mr. B's current quality of life is very good. However, if he had to stop his medication, his future quality of life would be poor, considering the complications from his health conditions. If he continues his treatments, he should face fewer physical or mental deficits.

Contextual Features (Justice, Loyalty, Fairness)

A core component of this case involves the context of the situation. Mr. B has chosen to have his prescriptions filled outside the country to save money. The savings on his medication costs will provide enough funds for food or rent. If he cannot get less expensive medication, he may need to stop one or two of his medications. Questions that should be answered in this section include issues of law, other financial support, and medical liability.

Recommendations and Analysis

Again, the case analysis incorporates the data sustaining an ethical position from each section of the paradigm. Review the data in terms of the principles of biomedical ethics as described by Beauchamp and Childress. What issues of beneficence and nonmaleficence present themselves? What are the issues of distributive justice? If you refuse to write the prescriptions, what are the consequences? If you go ahead and write the prescriptions, what may transpire? What is the ethical principle you apply for your decision?

CASE STUDY 35-4

Problems Related to the Process of Care

Mrs. C is 38-year-old woman being treated for chronic headaches, anxiety, and depression. Her medical history includes four surgeries: an appendectomy, cholecystectomy, hysterectomy, and resection of a bowel obstruction. She has also had endometriosis, panic attacks, migraine headaches, and a recent suicide attempt. Medication history includes meprobamate, alprazolam, atenolol, gabapentin, amitriptyline, and sertraline. Mrs. C has a history of abusing cocaine and marijuana. She had abstained from use for a number of years. Two months ago she attempted suicide, and the toxicology screen was positive for alcohol, benzodiazepines, cocaine, and amitriptyline. After her recovery it was determined her attempted suicide was due to her uncontrollable headache pain.

In an attempt to control her headaches, she was started on a fentanyl patch, meperidine, and hydroxyzine for breakthrough pain. Her current medication list includes venlafaxine, gabapentin, and atenolol. Mrs. C is in clinic today with breakthrough headache pain uncontrolled by her fentanyl patch. The PA who is her primary care provider will not be in the clinic for another 3 hours. The providers present in the clinic refuse to see her because of unpleasant experiences with her in the past.

Mrs. C is employed at a software company as a programmer. She enjoys her job, is on track to be a project manager, and when at work performs her job exceptionally well. She is respected by her office contemporaries when she is not in uncontrolled pain. At this time she lives alone with her pets in her condominium overlooking the city. She enjoys playing chess, doing crossword puzzles, and sudoku. Her family lives a significant distance from her. She attends church occasionally and had been a member of the social justice committee at her parish.

When the PA arrives, she finds Mrs. C in her examining room with dimmed lights. She is scruffy, crying, and curled up on the examination table with a blanket over her head. She tells the PA of her excruciating headache. After a thorough neurologic examination, which is normal, **the PA's ethical question is:** How do I determine if Mrs. C requires more pain medication? Is she exhibiting behaviors of addiction? Is there a time not to treat or meet the pain control needs of a patient?

Medical Indications (Beneficence, Nonmaleficence)

Mrs. C's medical problem is a severe head pain described as occipital neuralgia and muscle tension. Depression and anxiety accompany her chronic pain, as well as her suffering, expressed by her suicide attempt. What is her prognosis for chronic nonmalignant pain control? What are the goals of treating nonmalignant pain? Are narcotics used for control of chronic pain? Is there a distinction between addiction, abuse, and dependence? How do you treat chronic pain in a patient who has an addiction, abuse, or dependence history? Can or should you prescribe a narcotic for long-term chronic pain control for a patient who has such a history?

Patient Preference (Autonomy)

Mrs. C wants to be pain free. Is she fully competent while taking opioid medication? Will chronic narcotic pain therapy affect her capacity to make informed decisions? Is Mrs. C's right to choose her therapy being valued?

Quality of Life (Beneficence, Nonmaleficence, Autonomy)

What is Mrs. C's current quality of life? If not engaged in pain therapy, what would her quality of life be like? Do the providers have biases that may affect their assessment of Mrs. C's quality of life? What could those biases be? What adverse events could transpire if Mrs. C's pain therapy is not successful?

Contextual Features (Justice, Loyalty, Fairness)

What specific issues may possibly influence the PA's treatment decisions? How will the rules and regulations of the practice of medicine in your state affect the pain therapy for Mrs. C? How will the Drug Enforcement Agency and other federal agencies' rules and law enforcement affect the treatment of Mrs. C's chronic pain?

Recommendations and Analysis

As with the previous cases, the case analysis incorporates the data from each section of the paradigm. What issues present themselves in terms of beneficence and nonmaleficence? What are the issues of autonomy in this case? Is drug addiction, abuse, or dependence the moral failure of a patient or a medical ailment? Are there any cardinal cases similar to Mrs. C's?

CASE STUDY 35-5

Preventive Ethics

Mr. D is an 80-year-old with a history of paranoid schizophrenia, dementia, dyskinesia, dysphasia, hypertension, and chronic obstructive pulmonary disease (COPD). He is in the clinic today to discuss with the PA his general health and an advance directive specifically regarding cardiopulmonary resuscitation. He has several medical conditions and currently lives in a long-term care facility. He has lived at this home for the past 12 years since his wife died. Five years ago he was deemed incompetent to make long-term health decisions by the county mental health psychiatrist. An advocate's corporation was appointed by the court to be his guardian for health care decisions.

Mr. D had been an active member of his community and was employed as a train engineer for 35 years. Before his illness and his wife's death, he and his wife traveled by train around the United States, Canada, and parts of Europe. On visits to the PA, he continues to wear his bib overalls, always pressed and clean, and his engineer's cap with his Railroad Union pins.

During the visit, Mr. D was asked if he wanted cardiopulmonary resuscitation (CPR) if he had a cardiac arrest. His answer was "yes." Because of his medical condition, he most often responded in monosyllables such as yes, no, and why. The guardian who accompanied Mr. D agreed with his affirmative answer. **The ethical question:** When can we ignore the patient and the court-appointed guardian and not perform CPR?

Medical Indications (Beneficence, Nonmaleficence)

Do Mr. D's advanced age, COPD, hypertension, and dementia increase the probability of cardiac arrest or cerebral vascular accident? What is the morbidity from CPR in chronically ill elders? What is the benefit (beneficence) to harm (nonmaleficence) balance?

Patient Preference (Autonomy)

Is Mr. D competent to make this decision? Had Mr. D discussed the end of life choices prior to his dementia? Is the guardian making medical decisions that are in the best interest of the patient?

Quality of Life (Beneficence, Nonmaleficence, Autonomy)

How does Mr. D perceive his quality of life in the present time? If Mr. D experiences cardiac arrest and undergoes CPR, what are the best and worst physical, psychological, and social deficits he will face after resuscitation? When will Mr. D's dementia and other medical conditions now and in the future be considered disadvantageous when considering CPR? Additionally, what could the provider biases be that may affect the evaluation of Mr. D's quality of life?

Contextual Features (Justice, Loyalty, Fairness)

Mr. D has no family that will participate in his health care decisions. It is not clear what Mr. D's religious background has been. Mr. D is financially sound and will be for the remainder of his life due to prudent investments and a sound pension. The concern of some of Mr. D's health care team is the court-appointed advocate's corporation. It appears to some members of the team that the advocate's corporation has a history of keeping its clients on full code status irrespective of the age or medical condition. The corporation receives a payment from the state for each client as long as the client is alive.

Recommendations and Analysis

Again, the case analysis incorporates the data sustaining an ethical position from each section of the paradigm. What issues of beneficence and nonmaleficence present themselves? What are the issues of distributive justice? When can medical futility be used as the basis for not performing CPR? Is the patient's autonomy the deciding factor in this ethical analysis? Are there precedents or cases that are similar to Mr. D's situation? After looking at the information from this case and the resources provided, how would you answer the question asked of the PA: When can we ignore the patient and the court-appointed guardian and not perform CPR?

CONCLUSION

As moral agents, PAs have the opportunity to practice medicine every day in an ethical manner. Clinicians may often overlook an ethical issue because they are unaware that an issue exists. When a conundrum is recognized, the difficulty of addressing the challenge can be tremendous. However, there is a practical, user-friendly, and accessible approach to make a reasoned professional moral judgment. This chapter offers the tools to identify and assess situations and then make the professional moral judgments that will be presented to PAs as science moves swiftly into the future.

CLINICAL APPLICATIONS

1. Describe the four principles that underlie our approach to bioethical decision-making.
2. Discuss the four parts of Jonsen's paradigm for analyzing medical ethical dilemmas.
3. Identify one clinical scenario that you have seen or heard about for each of Sugarman's four broad categories of ethical problems.
4. Analyze these scenarios using Jonsen's paradigm.
5. Does your local hospital or other clinical facility have a bioethics committee? If so, how have they structured their operating principles?

KEY POINTS

- Physician assistants are moral agents. They have the right and responsibility to engage in the processes of identifying, discussing, and making recommendations in response to questions of clinical ethics.
- Professional ethics are inseparable from clinical ethics because a clinician's approach to one will both inform and be influenced by the other.
- Several general moral theories have been applied to questions of medical ethics over time. The field has evolved to focus on methods that incorporate principles of respect for patient participation in the decision-making process.
- The principlism of Beauchamp and Childress has become a central theme in bioethics and lies at the core of methodologies for applied medical ethics as well as many institutional codes of ethics. It includes the principles of beneficence, nonmaleficence, justice, and autonomy.
- The applied clinical ethics of Jonsen, Siegler, and Winslade provide a framework for clinicians to address the immense variety of ethical dilemmas that arise in clinical practice. This approach takes into account not only medical technicalities but also the case context, patient preferences, and quality of life.
- Ethical issues in clinical practice must be identified, analyzed in an objective fashion, and addressed with full respect for the patient.

References

1. Heikkinen CA, Moson PF. Whither the PA? PA J 1975;5:234.
2. Gianola FJ. A practical, case-based approach to healthcare ethics and the case of Mr. T. J Am Acad Phys Assist 2004;17:13.
3. National Commission on Certification of Physician Assistants. Competencies for the Physician Assistant Profession (website). *http://www.nccpa.net/PAC/Competencies_home.aspx*; Accessed November 10, 2011.
4. Guidelines for Ethical Conduct for the Physician Assistant Profession: American Academy of Physician Assistants (website). *http://www.aapa.org/your_pa_career/becoming_a_pa/resources/item.aspx?id=1518*; Accessed November 10, 2011.
5. Jonsen AR. Bioethics Beyond the Headlines. Who Lives? Who Dies? Who Decides? Lanham, MD: Rowman & Littlefield, 2005.
6. Post S. Introduction. In: Post S (ed). 3rd ed. Encyclopedia of Bioethics. vol. 1. New York: Macmillan Reference, 2004. p. xi.
7. Callahan D. Bioethics. In: Post S (ed). 3rd ed. Encyclopedia of Bioethics. vol. 1. New York: Macmillan Reference, 2004. p. 278.
8. Alexander S. They decide who lives, who dies. Life 1962;53:102.
9. Beauchamp TL, Childress JF (eds). 6th ed. Principles of Biomedical Ethics. New York: Oxford University Press, 2008.
10. Jonsen A. Do no harm: axiom of medical ethics. In: Spicker SF, Englehardt HT (eds). Philosophical Medical Ethics: Its Nature and Significance. Dordrecht, Netherlands: D. Reidel Publ, 1977. p. 27.
11. Centers for Disease Control and Prevention. Smoking-attributable mortality, years of potential life lost, and productivity losses—United States, 2000–2004. MMWR Morb Mortal Wkly Rep 2008;57:1226.
12. Clouser K, Gert B. A critique of principalism. In: Jecker NS, Jonsen AR, Perlman RA (eds). 2nd ed. Bioethics: An Introduction to the History, Methods, and Practices. Sudbury, MA: Jones and Bartlett, 2007. p. 153.
13. Jonsen AR, Toulmin S. The Abuse of Casuistry: A History of Moral Reasoning. Berkeley, CA: University of California Press, 1988.
14. Jonsen AR. Casuistry and clinical ethics. In: Jecker NS, Jonsen AR, Perlman RA (eds). 2nd ed. Bioethics: An Introduction to the History, Methods, and Practices. Sudbury, MA: Jones and Bartlett, 2007. p. 171.
15. Jonsen AR, Siegler M, Winslade WJ. 7th ed. Clinical Ethics: A Practical Approach to Ethical Decisions in Clinical Medicine. New York: McGraw-Hill, 2010.
16. Sugarman J. 20 Common Problems: Ethics in Primary Care. New York: McGraw-Hill, 2000.
17. Gianola FJ. Public safety versus patient interest: which to choose? J Am Acad Phys Assist 2007;20:49, 51.
18. Consensus Statements: NIH Consensus Development Program, Management of Hepatitis C, 1997 (website). *http://consensus.nih.gov/1997/1997HepatitisC105html.htm*; Accessed September 19, 2011.
19. Consensus Statements: NIH Consensus Development Program, Management of Hepatitis C, 2002 (website). *http://consensus.nih.gov/2002/2002HepatitisC2002116main.htm*; Accessed September 19, 2011.

The resources for this chapter can be found at www.expertconsult.com.

CHAPTER 36

MEDICAL MALPRACTICE AND RISK MANAGEMENT

R. Monty Cary • James L. Cary

CHAPTER CONTENTS

Many unrecognized pitfalls that could trigger a medical malpractice lawsuit exist in the daily practice of medicine. You will learn that one cannot predict which case will come back to "bite you." As a physician assistant (PA) you will find that lawsuits infrequently result from the cases in which something was obviously missed or those concerning patient misunderstandings. More than likely, a lawsuit will result from an incident that did not raise any suspicion or red flags. Therefore, it is important for the PA student to learn the pitfalls of medical malpractice.

The shock of being named in a medical malpractice lawsuit and the stress of going through the entire process from discovery to deposition to preparation for the trial and conclusion can change your views on medicine and the way you practice medicine in the future. You may choose to continue to practice medicine; however, with two or more allegations or successful medical malpractice lawsuits against you, the decision may not be yours. The insurance company, the physician, or the clinic or hospital may make the decision for you.

PHYSICIAN ASSISTANT'S REACTION TO NOTIFICATION OF A LAWSUIT

When one is named in a medical malpractice lawsuit, the first reaction is usually that of denial and surprise. It is much the same as when a patient is told that he may have cancer or diabetes. Your reaction to the devastating news of an allegation of medical malpractice would be similar to that of a patient receiving the news of a life-changing medical condition. You would say, "It can't be happening to me." You would not be able to believe it and would think, "I'm too young." "My career is over." "I have been careful, and I know that I did not do anything wrong."

Maybe you have been careful, and maybe you did not do anything wrong; however, you would still have to defend the allegations of medical malpractice or negligence. Furthermore, as a PA you are never too young or too old to be sued because these allegations can come at any time during your practice career.

Soon, you would recognize that this is not a dream and that you really are being sued. You then have to start the process of learning an entirely new area of practice in which you have little or no experience. It would quickly become apparent that the courtroom is not the same as the operating room, the office, or the clinic. In the operating room, office, or clinic, you have at least some level of control. But in the courtroom, you would be like a duck out of water.

An alleged medical malpractice lawsuit can have a significant impact on your life. You would not be able to practice as you have in the past. You would suddenly find yourself asking, "How do my co-workers feel about me?" You would be distraught and angry with the patient, yourself, and with nearly anyone you come in contact with. You might question the very idea of someone questioning your ability! What would you do the next time you see the patient in the waiting room—make sure that he or she is not on your schedule or avoid him or her by taking a long lunch?

This process is an emotional roller coaster that can last up to 55 months. From notification to verdict can take a long time. Some cases have lasted more than 10 years. Can you imagine that emotional roller coaster ride for 10 years?

In addition, throughout the proceedings you would have a "higher degree of self-doubt." You will be asking yourself, "Why do I feel so guilty?" "Did I cause the problem, and am I going to win or lose this case?"

REASONS THAT PHYSICIAN ASSISTANTS ARE SUED

1. **Lack of Adequate Supervision**[1]**:** As a PA you must ensure that the legal requirements of the state in which you are practicing are met. Inadequate supervision may occur if a PA has too limited physician supervision or if documentation of such physician supervision is incomplete or not documented at all. When a PA and supervising physician discuss a case, the chart notations must reflect such a discussion. It is always better to document the discussion; your case will be much easier to defend if such a note is in the chart. An easy way to accomplish this is to place a simple statement in the chart such as the following: "*In consultation with, name of doctor*, the following was discussed." Then discuss the conversation including the history, physical examination, assessment, and treatment plan.
2. **Untimely Referral**[1]**:** All providers must recognize the need for timely consultations. The PA is not the only one who will be expected to refer in a timely manner. You must remember that discussing your patient with your supervising or alternate supervising physician is a referral. In addition, document the fact that you discussed the patient's case with your supervising or alternate supervising physician or with another consulting physician. Referring a patient to the emergency department (ED) or Urgent Care center when appropriate is just as important as discussing the case with your supervising physician. In some cases ordering a STAT radiograph, laboratory studies, or other testing is considered a referral.
3. **Failure to Diagnose**[1]**:** Here are some examples of situations in which there have been failures to diagnose properly:
   - Misinterpreted information
   - Uncertainty about a diagnosis
   - Lack of skills in managing a case
   - Uncertainty about the assessment of a patient (most misdiagnoses come from cases that present atypically)
   - Patient's condition does not follow the anticipated course

   All of these lead to misdiagnosis. If this occurs, consultation with the supervising or alternate supervising physician should occur immediately and should be documented in the medical record.
4. **Inadequate Examination**[1]**:** The PA must always confirm and expand on the history of the chief complaint. The focus of the physical examination should be determined by the patient's history but also focus on any abnormal findings discovered during the examination. The physical examination should always include inspection, auscultation, palpation, and percussion where necessary. Never rely on other medical staff members' interpretations of

what the patient said. It is your responsibility to personally evaluate your patient appropriately on the basis of the concerns identified within the encounter.

5. **Lack of Documentation**[2]**:** If someone reads the medical record on a patient you saw recently, would that person get an accurate picture of the care and treatment you provided for the patient or would missing information from the record speak louder than what is noted? Malpractice suits can be indefensible if there are significant problems with the medical record. Remember: A practitioner can never document enough. Include both the negative and positive findings in the history and physical examination, as well as laboratory, radiology, and other studies that have been ordered for the patient.
6. **Lack of Communication**[2]**:** Although one will not find "poor communications" listed anywhere as an official cause of malpractice claims, it underlies almost every malpractice action. Insurance claims administrators and medical malpractice defense attorneys estimate that communications failures are a contributing factor in 80% of all professional claims and lawsuits.[1] The use of appropriate communication skills with your patient can mean the difference between a subpoena and a thank you note.

COMMONSENSE RISK MANAGEMENT STRATEGIES

Fortunately, many of these risks can be prevented or minimized by a few commonsense risk management strategies, which can be easily incorporated into the office, clinic, or hospital practice. The key is to consciously make these tactics part of your everyday standard operating procedure so that they become second nature. Incorporating risk management strategies into your practice pays dividends. These risk management strategies will reduce medical liability exposure.[1] They will ultimately provide better care to the patient and improve the overall efficiency of the practice. In addition, important details have less chance of "falling through the cracks."

Documentation

Five years from now, if someone reads your records or notes on a patient who was treated today, will he or she get an accurate picture of the care given? The medical record has been called the "the witness whose memory never fades."

The medical record serves a number of purposes:

1. It serves as a record of what **you** have done **to** and **for** the patient.
2. It serves as a record to **other** health care professionals as to what has been done **to** and **for** the patient.
3. It is a legal document.

Medical malpractice lawsuits can be indefensible if there are significant problems with documentation in the medical record. Lawrence Weed's problem-oriented medical record developed in the 1950s is still regarded as a valuable tool.[3,4] S.O.A.P. (Subjective, Objective, Assessment, and Plan) has been used for many years in documentation of medical encounters. Today there is an even better method than using S.O.A.P. It is S.O.A.P.E.R., where the "E" indicates that the patient has been *educated* on what to do (e.g., *rest, apply ice, elevate the foot and ankle, take the medication as instructed*). The "R" represents the RESPONSE that the patient gives when he or she understands the instructions given by the health care provider (e.g., *"The patient has been given a treatment plan and understands the instructions."*)

Suggestions for Strengthening Your Medical Record

Establish a consistent method of charting and organizing the medical record. Here are a few suggestions:

1. Note all conversations with patients, including telephone calls. Failure to record and document the substance of a telephone conversation with or about a patient is universally recognized by risk management experts as an especially vulnerable area of medical liability.[5] Courts can and do choose to ignore verbal testimony that is not supported by the written medical record. Make it a habit to take notes of a conversation during the telephone call, and then dictate the conversation immediately afterward. You will better remember important details if you dictate immediately after the telephone conversation. If you do not dictate your medical record, make sure that it is documented somehow.
2. Initial and date the document you review. All diagnostic studies and records from other physicians and facilities should be initialled and dated before they are filed in the chart. Instruct and insist that your staff put all laboratory and radiology reports, as well as other reports and consultations, on the chart and put them on your desk for your review before they are refilled. Check if your office, clinic, or hospital requires your supervising physician to initial the reports as well.

3. The history and physical examination should address all systems that are appropriate for the complaint, and documentation should reflect that review. The medical record should include all relevant examinations performed on the patient. It is also important to include pertinent negative and positive findings in the record.
4. When charting, write a full note, and not simply a short comment, such as "medication refill." The provider should document which medications were refilled, the quantity, and the directions for taking the medications. Avoid only placing a single notation in the chart for prescription refills, such as "Xanax refilled." Prescription refill notations should be complete (e.g., "Xanax 1 mg #60, take one tablet P.O. Q 12 H or twice daily with one refill.") For the record, also dictate when and who filled the last prescription.
5. Limit the use of abbreviations. Some institutions will require that you use their approved list of abbreviations. Do not make up abbreviations that no one else will understand.
6. Establish a consistent method of charting and organizing the records. Review your office medical record for ways to improve efficiency and decrease the potential for errors.

Confidentiality and Professionalism

Confidentiality and professionalism go hand in hand. Whether you are in a clinical or nonclinical area, the nature of your work is such that from time to time you may have access to private, sensitive, and personal information that your patients, customers, and employees expect you to keep confidential. Professionalism is one of the pillars on which your success is based, and one of the key elements of professionalism is discretion.

Discretion is having and using sound judgment in one's speech and behavior while being respectful of the wishes and requests of your patients.

CASE STUDY 36-1

A woman wanted to keep the fact that she was pregnant private. She instructed the doctor not to tell her husband or any other family member. Her mother-in-law lived in the same town and knew that her daughter-in-law was not feeling well and visited with the family doctor. A pregnancy test was done at the local hospital. The mother-in-law asked one of the doctor's office staff about the results of the visit and pregnancy test but was not given the information. She knew a laboratory worker at the hospital. She inquired and was given the results to the pregnancy test. It was positive. The pregnant woman found out about the inquiry, sued the hospital, and won the case. She sued both the hospital and the laboratory worker for breach of confidentiality.

CASE STUDY 36-2

Professionalism in the health care workplace is paramount to the cohesive nature of a health care team. Each member of the team is an integral part of a successful team and should be treated with respect. The following example is an unfortunate exchange between team members. These comments were written in a patient's chart during her hospitalization. A physician wrote: "If the nurses around this hospital would read the medication orders, we wouldn't have medical emergencies like this one." In response, a nurse wrote: "If the physicians around this hospital would learn to write so we could read it, there wouldn't be medication errors like this one."

As noted throughout this chapter, developing and using effective communication skills are an important aspect of medical practice. When issues arise within a team situation, address these concerns directly with the team. It is inappropriate and ultimately embarrassing to use a legal document to air disputes between members of the health care team.

Dictation

Dictating is perhaps one of the best modes to document care:

1. It is the easiest and best way to document medical information.
2. It eliminates the inaccuracy of writing messages on slips of paper.
3. It encourages a more complete entry.
4. It simplifies documentation of telephone conversations.
5. It reduces the risk that an important communication will be overlooked.
6. Dictating will produce 175 words/minute on average, whereas written documentation will produce only 87 words per minute for the same encounter.

Legibility

If handwritten, the entry must be legible and easy to read. If an entry is not legible, some courts will consider the documentation as incomplete. If noted as incomplete, the court may choose to ignore the entry.

Alteration of the Medical Record

Do not for any reason ever alter the medical record! Here is a good rule to remember with making a mistake in writing in the chart. Use the word "SLIDE."

SL—Single line through the mistake.
I—Initial the entry as an error.
D—Date the entry.
E—Note "error" in the area.

Although it is natural to wish the records had been more complete or detailed than they are, resist the urge to change or delete any entry in the record after the fact. Doing so will virtually guarantee that your care will be rendered questionable. An item in the record, which to the defendant physician or medical practitioner seems certain to doom a case, may in reality be explainable at deposition or trial. If you think your alterations in the record will not be detected, think again. Finding alterations in the medical record is just like finding a DNA match. Today with the large sums of money for rewards, the plaintiff's attorney will hire a "document sleuth" to review the record. These medical record professionals will use infrared and ultraviolet microscopic techniques to look for composition of the age of the ink, slant of the script, and depressions made in the paper by the writing instrument, to identify entries that were made at different times.

INTERPERSONAL COMMUNICATIONS

Experts in the field of interpersonal communications have established that much of the emotional content of a message comes through body language. It is therefore necessary to listen with your entire body, not just with your ears. When patients speak, let them know that you are interested in what they have to say. You can do this by making periodic eye contact and maintaining an active body position.

If the patient knows that you are interested, he will work harder to communicate. You should also learn to listen objectively, not subjectively. Here are some suggestions:

1. Close the examination room door completely.
2. Stop ALL phone calls except true emergencies.
3. Show sincere concern for every patient.
4. Do not complain to the patient about your workload; after all, the patient you are talking to is your workload.
5. Treat the family with respect and kindness.
6. Do not make promises you cannot keep. Do not promise that studies such as a magnetic resonance image or computed tomography scan will be done the same day.
7. Do not talk to the patients condescendingly.
8. Remember: If you are kind to your patients, you are more likely to receive a thank you card versus a subpoena.

Communication Successes

1. Providers who spend less than 15 minutes are more likely to be sued than providers who spend an average of 18 minutes with each patient.[1]
2. Providers who use more humor and laugh with their patients are more successful in patient communication. In most cases you can tell within just a few seconds how you will be able to interact with a patient when you enter the room.
3. Successful providers are more careful to explain what they are doing before they do it. This includes abdominal examinations and pelvic examinations. This also applies to children and examining their ears. You can extrapolate this to many other areas as well.
4. The successful provider encourages patients to talk. Patients who are more communicative are more likely to be compliant with your suggestions and recommendations.[1]

Poor Communications

Here are some examples of communications for which patients have expressed their dissatisfaction.

1. Poor service or not enough service.
2. Automated voice systems—not hearing a human voice.
3. An office appointment waiting time that is longer than 45 minutes. If an emergency occurs, let the patient know the reason for the delay.
4. Staff not acting compassionately.
5. Being treated rudely by the staff or provider.

The next time you see a patient, think how you can improve communications with the patient and family and "document, document, document." The saying in real estate is "location, location, location." In medicine it is "communication, communication, communication" and "document, document, document!"

DISCOVERY RULE

The discovery rule states that the statute of limitations does not begin until the occurrence of the event puts the plaintiff on notice. This means when the plaintiff knows or should have known that an error occurred. The court's reason for this is that the plaintiff should not be faulted for "blameless ignorance." This is especially true if the problem is "inherently unknowable." The average claim takes 22 months to be reported after the medical incident and then an additional 34 months for the claim to be resolved. That is a total of 55 months, which is a long time to be on the emotional roller coaster that we have previously described.

CASE STUDY 36-3

The plaintiff brought suit against a physician 4 years after he had been discharged from the hospital. Four years earlier while in the hospital, his radiographs were interpreted as normal. Four years later, a malignant tumor was revealed. The plaintiff's attorney simply retrieved the radiograph that was taken 4 years earlier and indeed, a small tumor was seen. The statute of limitations began when the plaintiff noted the original radiograph was read incorrectly and not on the day the radiograph was taken 4 years earlier.

CASE STUDY 36-4

In another case, a surgeon left a rolled-up towel inside his patient's chest. When she died 7 years later, an autopsy was performed and the towel was found. The family filed a lawsuit against both the hospital and surgeon. It was noted by the family and supported by the medical records that the patient had complained of chest pain from time to time, but no one ever ordered a chest radiograph to evaluate.

MEDICAL MALPRACTICE DEFINED

Medical malpractice can be defined as negligence on the part of a physician, allied health care professional, or hospital that causes physical or emotional damage to the patient.

There are four elements to a medical malpractice lawsuit.

1. Duty
2. Breach
3. Causation
4. Injury—damages

The *duty* to care arises from the provider-patient relationship, which is an implied contract. Once a health care provider or hospital agrees to treat the patient, the provider has assumed the duty to treat the patient with that degree of skill, care, and diligence possessed or exercised by a competent and careful provider or hospital.

Breach of duty is the second element of negligence that a plaintiff must prove in a medical malpractice suit. A health care provider's treatment of a patient is measured against an acceptable standard of care. A breach of duty occurs when a provider's behavior falls below the accepted standard of care.

Two types of standards exist:

1. External: This is set by a national standard such as a national accrediting body or professional organization (e.g., the American College of Obstetrics and Gynecology's standards for interpreting Pap smears).
2. Internal: Standards are developed and implemented at a local level. These types of standards are more likely to be used in a medical malpractice lawsuit (e.g., the protocols set up by the office or hospital, including what we now call the job description).

Causation is the third and perhaps most difficult element to prove. Even if the plaintiff can prove that a health care provider did not meet the standard of care, the damages cannot be collected unless the plaintiff can show that the provider's negligence caused an injury or that a reasonable close connection existed between a provider's conduct and the patient's injury. Establishing legal causation requires a plaintiff to prove that the conduct of a provider was the "cause in fact" of the patient's injury or that some or all of the patient's injury would not have occurred "but for the provider's negligence."

Injuries/damages: How or what injuries or damages did the patient suffer from because of the deviation from the standard of care? Here are some examples:

1. Death—disability—deformity—severe pain
2. Special: medical expenses—lost wages—out-of-pocket expenses
3. General: intangible losses of pain—suffering—emotional distress
4. Punitive damages: oppressive—fraudulent or malicious damages

NATIONAL PRACTITIONER DATA BANK

The quality of health care became of interest to many people in the 1980s. As a result, the 1986 Congress passed public law 99-660—the Health Care Quality Improvement Act. The National Practitioner Data Bank, which is not accessible to the public, was established in the midst of the malpractice crisis of the 1980s. The National Practitioner Data Bank became operational in September 1990. Its primary objective was to reduce the incidence of medical malpractice by restricting the ability of incompetent practitioners to move freely from hospital to hospital, as well as from state to state. Public Law 99-660 covers physicians, dentists, and allied health care professionals, including PAs who are licensed, certified, or registered by a state. Medical malpractice payments are required to be reported to the National Practitioner Data Bank regardless of the settlement or award amount.

CASE STUDY 36-5

For 3 days a cattle rancher had been moving cattle from one pasture to another. On the second day of moving cattle he began having chest pain while working. When he was resting, taking a break, and driving to and from the pastures, there was no chest pain or other associated symptoms.

On the third day the severity of the chest pain increased and he began having some nausea without vomiting, shortness of breath, and diaphoresis. Around noon on the third day he decided to go to the Urgent Care center, which was about 5 miles away from where he was working.

Because it was around noon, there were no other patients in the Urgent Care center. He was lucky in that he was taken in right away and seen by the PA on duty at the time. The physician was at lunch but had remained in the Urgent Care center.

The patient was a 54-year-old white male who had the classic substernal chest pain with exercise/work. On the third day he started having associated symptoms of nausea without vomiting, diaphoresis, and radiation of pain to the left jaw and left arm. Vital signs were blood pressure of 160/98, pulse 110, respirations of 24, temperature of 101.2° F. The electrocardiogram showed an ST elevation in limb lead 2. He was indeed diaphoretic and looked anxious.

The PA recognized that the patient was indeed having a myocardial infarction. He notified the physician working in the Urgent Care center immediately. In addition, he gave the patient an aspirin, started an intravenous line, and placed a nitroglycerin patch on the patient. The nurse called 911, and he was prepared to transport as soon as the ambulance arrived. A call was also placed to the local hospital notifying them the patient was coming. The patient was transported to the hospital in stable condition.

Unfortunately, that night the patient had another myocardial infarction and died.

The man's wife and three teenage sons sued with the following complaints against the PA, physician, and Urgent Care center: (1) the PA did not follow the standards of care for treatment of a myocardial infarction, (2) failed to transfer the patient in a timely manner, and (3) the physician in the Urgent Care center did not see the patient.

During the deposition of the PA, it was determined that the standard of care in the treatment of a myocardial infarction was followed. Also during the deposition, it was found that the PA saw the patient in a timely manner and the patient was diagnosed quickly by obtaining an accurate history, conducting a complete physical examination as it relates to a myocardial infarction, and doing an electrocardiogram that showed an acute myocardial infarction. It was determined that the patient was transferred from the Urgent Care center to the hospital in a timely manner. The PA was exonerated.

The patient's wife stated during her deposition that once she arrived at the Urgent Care center, she talked to the physician in the examination room while he was in with her husband, thereby disproving the claim that the physician did not see the patient. She also stated that her husband was transferred to the hospital in a timely manner. At the end of the physician's deposition, he was also exonerated.

RISK MANAGEMENT ISSUES: The PA did a good history and physical examination, made the correct diagnosis, consulted with the supervising physician on duty, and documented well. There was also good communication among the PA, the physician, and the patient and his wife, which was all documented. The Urgent Care center had called 911, and the patient was transported to the hospital in a timely manner. It was well documented that the patient was stable when transported.

The issues in a medical malpractice case were all satisfied. The appropriate documentation included the history and physical examination, the correct diagnosis, and the timely referral. In addition, there was good communication among the PA, the physician, and the patient and his wife. As a result of these factors, both the PA and physician were exonerated.

CASE STUDY 36-6

The patient was a 64-year-old white male who was walking on his treadmill at home. He was accustomed to doing so for the past several months and had no previous problems. After walking for approximately 15 minutes, he developed a sudden onset of back pain. The pain was in the right lower lumber area with radiation to the right buttocks, hip, and right posterior thigh. The pain was sharp and severe enough to cause him to stop walking. He did not suffer any associated symptoms of numbness, tingling, or weakness of the lower extremities and did not identify any problems with his bowel or bladder.

He took two Tylenol without relief of pain.

The next day, his son made an appointment with the family doctor but instead was seen by the PA at 11:00 a.m.

The PA obtained the following: The **Chief Complaint** was back pain with some radiation to the right buttocks and right leg.

History: Sudden onset of back pain with exercise with radiation to the right leg, hip, and buttocks. No relieving factors. The pain was worse with leaning and bending forward. Tylenol was not helpful in relieving the pain. No prior history of back pain.

Physical Examination: The PA recorded that there was a right-sided lumbar muscle spasm. Reflexes were equal bilaterally in the lower extremities. There was some pain in the right buttocks and posterior right thigh with palpation. It was recorded that there was some difficulty with ambulation and difficulty with getting on and off the examination table.

Assessment: Right lower lumbar strain and muscle spasm with right leg sciatica.

Plan: Toradol 10 mg injection. Lortab 10/500 mg one tablet every 4 to 6 hours as needed for pain. Moist heat to the right lumbar area 4 times a day for 20 minutes. Rest for 24 hours and no treadmill. To follow up as needed.

The next day, the patient was no better. He had no relief of his pain with the treatment previously mentioned. He was again seen in the same office as the day before. He was seen by the PA covering the walk-in clinic. He was seen at approximately noon. His family physician was out of the office on both days.

The following was noted by the second PA: he first reviewed the medical record from the day before.

History: The back pain had not improved. There was no numbness, tingling, or weakness of the lower extremities. There was no abdominal pain, and there were no bowel or bladder habit changes. The pain medication did not help.

Physical Examination: Basically no difference from the day before. The patient continued to have lumbar muscle spasm and sciatic notch tenderness. The reflexes were equal bilaterally. There was difficulty with ambulation and getting on and off the table.

Assessment: Right lower lumbar muscle spasm with right leg sciatica. This is basically the same diagnosis as the day before.

Plan: An injection of Toradol 10 mg IM, add Flexeril 10 mg one tablet 3 times a day. Return as needed.

The next day the patient passed out at home. His family called 911, and he was taken to the local hospital.

In the ambulance he was suspected of having a ruptured abdominal aortic aneurysm (AAA) by the EMT. Despite resuscitation attempts of massive fluids and CPR, the patient was pronounced dead 20 minutes after arrival at the ED.

The patient's daughter, who was an attorney, filed a medical malpractice law suit within days after the funeral.

This case is bad and gets ugly for all of the reasons a PA or any health care provider might be sued for. The **risk management issues** include the following:

Untimely Referral: Neither PA consulted with the supervising physician. To complicate matters further, they did not consult with the other physicians in the group who were in the office at the time the patient was seen. They did not refer the patient to the ED or Radiology for radiographs of the lumbar spine. The office was attached to the hospital by a third-floor walkway.

It would be wonderful to diagnose a "triple A" by discussing it with your supervising physician or sending the patient to the ED and having the ED doctor call and say how wonderful you are by diagnosing an AAA or having the radiologist call and tell you that the patient has an AAA. In this case the untimely referrals were not talking to the physician in the office at the time of the patient's visit and not referring the patient to the ED or Radiology.

Inadequate History: Neither PA obtained an adequate history as it relates to back pain. The patient's brother had an aneurysm years earlier. The patient was a long-time smoker of two packs a day. The history of back pain was not specific. The first PA did not ask about abdominal pain. The second PA did ask about abdominal pain but failed to do an abdominal examination because there were no complaints of abdominal pain. As a general rule, any patient who is older than the age of 50 should have an abdominal examination performed if their complaint is back pain. Even if the answer is "no" to "are you having abdominal pain?" you should perform an abdominal examination.

Inadequate Examination: The examination of the back was incomplete. A complete back examination always includes an examination of the abdomen whether there is complaint of abdominal pain or not. This is especially true if the patient is older than 50 years of age. One of the PAs may have noticed diminished or absent pulses of the lower extremities if an examination of the lower extremities had been performed. One of the PAs stated in the deposition that the patient was obese and an abdominal examination would not have been of value. The patient was not obese. In fact, he was 5′11″ tall and weighed only 143 lb.

Failure to Diagnose: The failure to diagnose was due to the following: (1) inadequate history, (2) inadequate physical examination, (3) failure to refer, and (4) failure to order the proper radiographs.

Inadequate Supervision: Neither PA consulted with the supervising physician or with the physician seeing patients in the office the days the patient was seen. The supervising physician stated in his deposition that the first time he knew of the patient's death was when he was served notice of the pending lawsuit. The patient was associated with the supervising physician's practice for the past 15 years.

A malpractice case could have been avoided if the PA had performed a more complete history and physical examination, consulted with an office physician, or referred the patient to the ED or Radiology for further evaluation. Perhaps if an abdominal examination would have been done, there would have been the discovery of an AAA and the patient would have been referred to the ED of the hospital that was attached to the medical office building.

Unfortunately, both PAs were sued and the plaintiff won the case. For one PA, this was the second successful medical malpractice case against him. He was unable to obtain medical malpractice insurance coverage and was forced to find another profession.

The supervising physician was also successfully sued for inadequate supervision of a PA.

The combined monetary value of this case was over $1 million. Both the physician and the two PAs were entered into the National Practitioner Data Bank.

CASE STUDY 36-7

PW has been a PA for 13 years and feels really good about his fund of knowledge regarding the PA profession and the treatment of primary care issues. He is confident in his medical care and consults with his physician as needed, and he does not hesitate to give his own recommendations. His primary care physician, Dr. J, is also confident in him, trusts his judgment, and does not "look over his back." PW orders testing when necessary, but he withholds testing when he believes that it is not indicated. His theme was "do no harm" and "don't put people through unnecessary testing." He has said in the past that "unnecessary testing is what is wrong with medicine today."

Mrs. G came to PW for a checkup. She was a regular patient of the practice and saw PW for what she considered an urgent complaint. Dr. J was gone that day from the office. Mrs. G had a history of anemia and has her blood analyzed in the office on a regular basis. She was called by the office staff and notified that her most recent hemoglobin blood test was 11.6. PW thought that this was adequate for her. PW said, "We will just watch it." After all, PW thought that she had no other symptoms and she felt good. No follow-up was made at this time, and although Mrs. G wanted more testing, she trusted PW. Despite the fact that Mrs. G is 62 years old and had a family history of cancer, PW did not advise her to get a colonoscopy or sigmoidoscopy. He had never performed a digital rectal examination on her, assuming that the OB-GYN doctor would do it during her annual examination.

Approximately 9 months later, Mrs. G again complained of fatigue and weakness with some mild abdominal pain. PW thought that with her mild symptomatology and fairly sudden onset of symptoms, she had an acute viral illness. PW wanted her to "wait it out" and return if no better. She did return again to see him and she felt a little better. PW again thought that the viral illness was running its course. Two weeks later Mrs. G went to the ED with chest pain and shortness of breath. The emergency physician performed a full workup. A chest radiograph showed a large right lung mass, and a computed tomography (CT) scan showed multiple liver masses. A liver biopsy was ultimately performed and revealed metastatic cancer. Her attending hospital physician thought that the cancer had originated in her colon and spread to her lungs and liver. A colonoscopy in the hospital confirmed this. A general surgeon who was consulted explored her abdomen and found that most of it was filled with tumor. The surgeon informed Mrs. G that nothing could be done at this point and she should be placed in hospice to try to make her comfortable. She died 3 weeks later.

Two weeks after Mrs. G's diagnosis, PW and Dr. J were served with a lawsuit. Dr. J and PW were sued for medical malpractice. They both met with their defense attorney, and he warned them that a malpractice trial would be a long and unpleasant experience. Both of them were deposed before the plaintiff's attorney. PW was asked if he had ever discussed ordering a screening colonoscopy with Mrs. G. He had not. He was asked whether he was aware of a history of cancer in Mrs. G's family. PW said that he was aware of her family history. He was also asked if he had performed any screening on Mrs. G for cancer (e.g., digital rectal examination, breast examination) or whether he had ever recommended that she get such screenings. PW replied no. Dr. J, as the supervising physician, was also questioned vigorously by the plaintiff's attorney and admitted that he had not seen the patient and was not aware of Mrs. G's condition. There were several days of depositions and finally the defense attorney pulled PW and Dr. J aside and said it was time to discuss a settlement offer. The case was settled for the limit of the policy, which was $1 million.

RISK MANAGEMENT ISSUES

Depositions are part of the discovery process, and it is important for all practitioners to be familiar with this process. The deposition gives a "preview" of a court proceeding and provides attorneys on both sides an idea of how the defendant will hold up under questioning should the suit lead to a trial. The deposition allows insight into the testimony and an opportunity to identify any differences in statements made during discovery.

Screening tests can be a controversial issue, especially in our cost-conscious society. Some practitioners order every screening test to "cover" themselves. Although this is a somewhat "safe" way to go, it is also expensive for the patient and society. Performing screening tests based on national guidelines and related to age, family history, and other identified risk factors is an effective method of limiting unnecessary testing in patient populations. In this case PW ***never*** suggested a screening colonoscopy despite her gastrointestinal symptoms, age, and his knowledge of her family history. PW is also liable because he never discussed the case or had his supervising physician see and evaluate the patient. However, if the screening colonoscopy had been ordered and the patient did not comply, the risk to the practitioners would have been low.

In general, age-specific and symptom-specific screening should be done regardless of patient symptoms. Examples would be prostate-specific antigen testing, mammography, and colonoscopy as a minimum. Other screenings should be done on the basis of the patient's age, risk factors, and symptoms. If screening tests are ordered, they should be documented in the medical record. If the patient does not comply with your recommendations, you should also document this in the medical record.

CLINICAL APPLICATIONS

1. Evaluate a recent S.O.A.P note that you have completed for possible omissions or incomplete data that could lead to misinterpretation of the encounter.
2. Describe the proper way to adjust the medical record when an error is made when writing in the chart. How might this be handled in an electronic medical record?

KEY POINTS

- Developing a respectful and open patient-provider relationship is important to minimize the potential of lawsuits.
- It is your responsibility to completely understand your practice environment, at the state, local, and hospital levels.
- When in doubt, ask for help or assistance from your supervisor or refer the patient in a timely manner.
- Document, document, document!
- Work hard to be a good team member and support the other members of your team.

References

1. Davidson J. Issues in quality care: a look at leading malpractice risk issues. J Am Acad Phys Assist 1996;9:23.
2. Cary RM. Six key principles to avoiding malpractice lawsuits. Arthritis Pract 2007;3:28.
3. Weed LL. Medical records, patient care and medical education. Ir J Med Sci 1964;17:271.
4. Weed LL. Medical education and patient care. N Engl J Med 1968;2788:593.
5. Gorney M, Dixon LA, Shepard S. Telephone communication for doctors (website). *http://www.thedoctors.com/KnowledgeCenter/PatientSafety/articles/CON_ID_003859*; Accessed December 21, 2011.

CHAPTER 37

Postgraduate Residency Programs

David P. Asprey • Maura Polansky

CHAPTER CONTENTS

In the early 1970s, formal educational programs were developed to provide physician assistants (PAs) with a postgraduate specialty education experience using the physician internship or residency training model of education. These residency programs provided the graduate PA with an opportunity to gain additional didactic and clinical experience in a specialty area of medicine that would build on the primary care PA or surgical assistant (SA) training acquired from the entry-level PA program. Furthermore, the training typically provided an accelerated learning curve in part due to the formalized and structured didactic education component and in part due to the required number of work hours during the residency being greater than most typical PA jobs. Most residency programs are located within larger teaching hospitals or clinics throughout the United States. Many of these PA residency programs were developed in response to the call to reduce the number of physician residents in training. As the number of physician residents available to hospitals decreased, PAs were viewed as a desirable substitute for the traditional house staff. Consequently, PA residencies developed to respond to the need for additional house staff in the hospitals.

PA residency programs vary in length, area of specialty training, amount of didactic education, credential awarded on completion, and number of residents admitted each year. In response to the wide degree of variety in the residency programs, some individuals expressed the need for accreditation and standardization.[1,2] After carefully studying the issue, the Accreditation Review Commission on Education for the Physician Assistant (ARC-PA) voted in favor of establishing an accreditation process in 2006 and implemented accreditation services for postgraduate programs in 2007. As of November 2011, six residency programs have obtained accreditation.[3]

Although the residency programs could generally be viewed as successful during their first 40 years, their growth and development have recently been modest due to an increased interest from PA graduates and residency medical doctor (MD) programs. Initially many PA educators speculated that their growth was affected in part by the delay in developing an accreditation process and the tenuous nature of PA residency program funding. Now that an accreditation process has been established, we will observe with interest the impact on the growth of postgraduate residency programs.

HISTORY OF POSTGRADUATE RESIDENCY EDUCATION

The first postgraduate PA program began in 1971 by Montefiore Medical Center in affiliation with the Albert Einstein School of Medicine in New York. Montefiore Medical Center began employing and educating PAs to replace surgical house officers. These PA residents were employed and trained alongside physician surgery house officers and were substituted in place of surgical physician residents. In 1975, Norwalk Hospital and the Department of Surgery at the Yale School of Medicine established a 1-year surgical residency program exclusively structured for PAs, which combined didactic and clinical instruction. By 1980, six postgraduate residency programs were known to exist. The exact number of programs has not been known due to the lack of a consistent means of tracking programs. The most accessible information regarding the number of programs has been based on membership into the Association of Postgraduate Physician Assistant Programs (APPAP) established in 1987 by seven programs, three in surgery.[4] Since then, additional programs have been established in various surgical and medical specialities. The most recent membership roster of the APPAP lists 53 programs in 17 specialties.[5]

The number of PAs having undergone training in postgraduate residency programs has also been difficult to determine. The 1996 census was the last time that the American Academy of Physician Assistants (AAPA) reported data on residency programs attended by its responders. At that time, the data indicated that of 13,256 respondents, 708 (5.3%) PAs reported having attended a PA postgraduate residency program.[6] In 2009, one author suggested that only approximately 2% of PA graduates participate in postgraduate education, although the source of this estimate was not reported.[7] Recent data presented at the Physician Assistant Education Association conference indicated that 109 PAs participated in 43 nonmilitary programs during 2011.[8] Although comprehensive data regarding the number of current PA residents and graduates is limited, it seems apparent that even with the expansion of PA postgraduate residency programs, the percentage of PAs trained in such programs remains small.

Over the years, some of the most important issues addressed by those involved in PA postgraduate education and others in the PA profession included questions related to the potential value of such programs for PAs, the impact on the profession that may occur from expansion of postgraduate training, and whether or not program accreditation would be beneficial or potentially detrimental. Despite these questions, relatively little research has been conducted regarding PA residency programs.

In 1998 Asprey and Helms conducted a survey of currently enrolled PA residents.[9] All 17 member programs of the APPAP were contacted to participate requesting distribution of the survey to the PA residents. Forty-five PAs from 14 programs were surveyed. They found that the most common reason PAs decided to pursue residency training was to be able to compete for jobs in the specialty reported by 89% of respondents. Other important reasons reported included the interest in additional clinical knowledge and skills before going into practice (84%) and improved future earning potential (80%). Other common reasons included the potential to improve future earnings, their current level of competency in the specialty, flexibility to change specialty area, and obtaining an advanced degree. PAs learned about PA residency programs primarily from their PA school (41%) or from a fellow student or colleague (26%). (Of interest, a study of PA students published in 2002 reported that only one third of PA students were provided information regarding residency programs by their PA school.) The majority (84.7%) applied to a single program, although it is important to note that only a limited number of programs were available at that time.

Program directors from 16 of the APPAP 17 programs also participated in a program directors survey in 1998.[10] They reported that the primary reasons for developing programs included an identified need for additional training for PAs in the specialty (50%), a need to replace physician residents or house officers (25%), and the need to recruit additional PAs to the institution (19%). Given the subsequent restriction to work hours for physician interns and residents, it is likely that more programs will need PAs to replace physicians in training now. All programs required PA residents to have graduated from an accredited PA program, and most required that they be certified by or eligible for National Commission on Certification of Physician Assistants (NCCPA) (63% and 81%, respectively). Only half required state licensure. The most frequently reported factors influencing selection of candidates were interest in the specialty (100%), interviews (94%), letters of recommendation (94%), academic performance (88%), desire to continue education (81%), and possession of a degree (56%).

A study published in 2007 compared surgical postgraduate PAs with those who sought a surgical position without having completed a residency.[11] Surgical residency graduates reported working more hours per week and a higher salary; however, when the salary was adjusted for hours worked, the salary per hour was similar between the two groups.

In addition to these studies of programs and PA residents, a few individual programs have also reported their experiences, most dating back 20 or more years.[13,14] Two recent articles have been published, both describing programs in specialties that have not traditionally used PAs. Reynolds and Bricker[15] reported their neonatal invasive care program at the University of Kentucky in Lexington. In this article from 2007, they discuss the history of extensive utilization of nurse practitioners in the neonatal intensive care unit and their efforts to incorporate PAs into their practice setting. PAs were identified as a potential resource for increasing their non-physician clinician staff at the University of Kentucky. They state their goal to "essentially . . . attempt to cover the entire clinical component of a neonatology fellowship in 1 year instead of 3 years, which is the current standard for physicians." They also reported their results of surveying pediatric (physician) residents regarding their acceptance of PA residents, finding that most had a favorable impression of the PA residents and believed they had served as a valuable teaching resource for the PAs. The majority (70%) also reported that the PA resident had served as a valuable teaching resource for them. In 2010, Will and colleagues[16] from the Department of Medicine, Mayo Clinic, Phoenix, described their experience with developing and running a hospitalist program for PAs. They indicated the increasing demand for hospitalists as a primary reason for program development along with the impact of workforce restrictions on physician residents by the Accreditation Council for Graduate Medical Education (ACGME). Their program began in 2007 and accepts one fellow per year. The goals are to include nurse practitioners in the hospitalist program and to validate educational efforts with measurable outcome data. These single institution reports begin to explore some of the additional, largely unanswered questions regarding PA resident education, related to the impact of other health care providers in the educational setting.

ASSOCIATION OF POSTGRADUATE PROGRAMS

At the AAPA Annual Meeting in Los Angeles in May 1988, a group of representatives of postgraduate PA residency programs met to formalize a national postgraduate PA program organization. Bylaws were written and approved by the eight founding programs, and subsequently the APPAP was formed to further the specialty education of PAs.[17]

APPAP's bylaws state the association's purpose:

> *The Association is organized and shall be operated for charitable, educational and scientific purposes. In accordance with these purposes the Association shall:*
>
> 1. *Serve as an information center to physician assistants, programs training physician assistants at the entry level, other medical and health care disciplines and to the public with respect to post-graduate educational curricula and programs for physician assistants.*
> 2. *Assist in the development and organization of postgraduate educational curricula and programs for physician assistants.*
> 3. *Assist in the development of evaluation methodologies for postgraduate educational curricula and programs.*
>
> *APPAP's business meetings are open to all PA students, educators, administrators and health professionals interested in postgraduate PA education.*[10]

APPAP maintains liaisons with the AAPA, ARC-PA, and the Physician Assistant Education Association (PAEA) and works with these organizations on mutual goals to further the PA profession and postgraduate PA education. Additional information regarding current member residency programs, bylaws, and general information can be viewed at the website *http://www.appap.org*.

APPAP took the initial step in developing standards for postgraduate programs by adopting its own set of program essentials, which were intended to identify the desirable elements of a PA residency program. These essentials were developed and approved in 1991 by the member programs. Compliance with the essentials was voluntary and was neither reviewed nor enforced by any external entity in its initial format. However, APPAP member programs were asked to agree to adhere to the essentials as a condition of membership. Currently the APPAP responsibilities of membership include the expectation that programs will "adhere to sound educational principles and support other member programs in the pursuit of such principles."

Given the current availability of accreditation for postgraduate PA programs, the profession will observe with great interest the impact that this component of PA education will have on the profession.

APPAP MEMBERSHIP

APPAP currently has five classes of membership:

- **Active Program Members**—Active Program Members shall be postgraduate programs with a curriculum, including didactic and clinical components, which trains NCCPA eligible/certified PAs for a defined period of time, usually a minimum of 12 months in a medical/surgical specialty. Programs must award a certificate or graduate academic credit or degree.

- **Provisional Program Members**—Provisional Program Members shall be newly developing postgraduate PA programs that have not yet graduated their first class. When such programs have graduated their first class, they will be eligible for and may be advanced to membership as Active Program Members. Provisional Program Members may have the privileges of the floor and may serve on committees, but they may not vote or hold office.
- **Inactive Program Members**—Inactive Program Members shall be those formerly Active Program Members or Provisional Program Members that have temporarily suspended educational activities. Upon reinstitution of their former educational program that was previously approved for membership, membership at the former designation will be reinstituted on recommendation of the Board and vote of the Assembly. Inactive Program Members may have the privileges of the floor and may serve on committees, but they may not vote or hold office.
- **Affiliate Members**—Affiliate Members shall be those institutions, organizations, agencies, or programs that have demonstrated interest in postgraduate PA education. Affiliate Members may have the privileges of the floor and may serve on committees, but they may not vote or hold office.
- **Individual Members**—Individual Members shall be persons who have demonstrated an interest in postgraduate PA education. Individual members may have the privileges of the floor and may serve on committees, but they may not vote or hold office.[17]

Currently, 17 areas of specialization are available at 53 APPAP member programs. The most commonly represented specialty areas are emergency medicine, surgery, critical care, orthopedics, and cardiovascular surgery. The current APPAP member programs and their areas of specialty training may be reviewed at the APPAP website.

PA postgraduate residency programs may be categorized as two basic types.[8] The first type is the traditional physician residency model or apprenticeship model. These programs possess a modest amount of practically oriented didactic curriculum combined with an intense clinical-rotation experience that leads to a certificate of completion. The second type is an academic model program. These programs combine a highly structured and formalized didactic education (through courses taken for academic credit) with an intense clinical-rotation experience that typically leads to a master's degree (or credit toward a master's degree) on completion. APPAP member programs follow several models of training with varying titles, including fellowships, master's degree programs, and residencies. All APPAP member programs must award a certificate or a degree or provide graduate academic credit.

RESIDENCY PROGRAM ACCREDITATION

Dating back to 1980, the PA accreditation agencies (Joint Review Committee, which predated the ARC-PA) and PA educational organizations considered the possibility of establishing an accreditation process for PA residency programs as a means of ensuring educational standards were used by programs.[4] A formal task force with representatives from the ARC-PA and APPPA was established in 1999 to consider this issue in more detail. In 2001, representatives of the AAPA and APAP (currently names PAEA) joined the task force with meetings continuing until 2005. The potential implications on PA education and the profession were explored over time. Although some members of the task force identified accreditation as a means of ensuring core educational standards were met, others expressed concern about the potential for unintended consequences that could result from an accreditation process—specifically the concern that the existence of accredited programs might limit opportunities for PAs not trained in accredited programs to work in specialty practices (i.e., lack of mobility across specialties). Because of these concerns, in 2005 the AAPA House of Delegates adopted a policy statement opposing accreditation.

After years of consideration, in March 2006 the ARC-PA voted in favor of offering optional accreditation to PA residency programs. The first version of the accreditation standards was published in 2007.[3] The standards address a wide range of educational administration issues including ensuring programs have adequate faculty and staff, funding, and patient care experiences. Programs must be full-time programs of a minimum of 6 months in duration offering in-residency clinical training and didactic instruction. Programs must have matriculated PAs before applying for accreditation. Programs must adhere to work-hour restrictions as used by the ACGME. As part of the accreditation review process, the program curriculum must be reviewed by a medical review committee of experts in the discipline to determine if program objectives can be met by the established curriculum. After curriculum review has occurred, programs must complete a full application documenting how each accreditation standard is met. The ARC-PA then conducts a site visit to verify application information. If programs are found to adhere to the accreditation Standards, programs may receive accreditation for a maximum of 3 years. An annual report is required each year, and programs must reapply for accreditation after 3 years to maintain their accreditation status.

The ARC-PA has emphasized that accreditation is optional, and to date few programs have applied for accreditation. The first of two programs were granted accreditation in March 2008. As of fall 2011, six programs have been accredited (including reaccreditation of the first two programs). A list of accredited programs is available on the *www.arc-pa.org* website. Given the brief period of time that accreditation has been offered, the impact on programs, PA residents, or the profession cannot be determined.

CURRENT AVAILABLE PROGRAMS

As previously mentioned, the exact number of programs is unknown with earlier studies relying on membership data from the APPAP. The term "postgraduate" education has often applied to include both residency programs and academic programs that may or may not provide onsite clinical training. The use of membership data by the APPAP has its limitations because membership does note ensure consistency in the type of education offered, may be inclusive of programs not actively enrolling PAs, and may not be inclusive of all available programs because membership in APPAP is optional. However, the use of APPAP membership data has provided general information regarding the scope of postgraduate education. The current membership of the APPAP was discussed earlier. Further information can be found on the organization's website and by accessing individual program material via published links *(www.appap.org)*.

In 2008, Wiemiller and Somer[18] sought to identify all "postgraduate PA programs" to address the bias of omitting programs that were not members of the APPAP. They identified 55 programs in 19 specialties, but only 44 programs (76%) were members of the APPAP. The most common specialties represented in this study were surgery (n = 14), emergency medicine (n = 7), and orthopedics (n = 6). Most programs (67%) reported enrolling one to five PAs annually. Thirty-eight percent of programs were described as adopting an "academic model," with 11.4% reporting charging tuition. Because this study sought to include all postgraduate programs, it is likely that it included programs that might not be clinical training programs consistent with the physician residency model. A study conducted in 2011 sought to identify only those programs that provided in-house clinical training for PAs at the postgraduate level.[8] Investigators identified 43 nonmilitary and 7 military programs meeting this criterion with active PA enrollment in early 2011. Twenty-six programs had enrolled their first PA in 2008 or later, suggesting a recent growth in PA clinical postgraduate program development.

Our understanding of the scope and characteristics of postgraduate programs is limited to data from these recent studies along with the current APPPA membership data with online information provided by programs. Therefore, while reading the following available program information, readers should consider the limitations of this data in understanding PA postgraduate residency programs.

GENERAL CHARACTERISTICS OF EXISTING PROGRAMS

Class sizes vary from as few as 1 student to as many as 18 with most programs accepting 2 to 3 PAs annually. No data on applicant-to-enrollee ratios are available. A 1998 study of enrolled residents revealed a balanced sex distribution and the average age of 34.4 years (range 24 to 57). The average amount of prior health care experience before PA school was 57 months (range 6 to 240). Most residents (61%) had worked as PAs at the time of enrollment in the program, with the remaining having a mean of 51 months of PA practice experience.[9,10] More recent data on demographics and health care prior experience have not been published. Given the trends in PA education with younger and less experienced students in PA school, it is likely that there have been substantial changes in these characteristics since these prior studies.

Admission Requirements

Residency programs may vary in their specific requirements for eligibility for the programs. All require graduation from an accredited PA program. In addition, a majority of programs require NCCPA certification or eligibility for the NCCPA examination for admission. Some programs also require state licensure or eligibility; in other cases, a specific degree may be required. Admission requirements are typically published online by each program.

Application Process

PA residency program selection is generally considered to be competitive, and admission requires the completion of a program application package. No centralized application service is available (e.g., CASPA, which is used by most entry-level PA programs). The application material required typically includes submission of a program application form, a copy of the certificate of completion from the PA program (or diploma), a copy of the NCCPA certification (if applicable), transcripts, educational and work history or résumé, letters of recommendation, and a narrative describing the candidate's interest in the residency and the specialty area. In addition, nearly all residency programs require a personal interview. Residency directors have reported using many different criteria in making admissions decisions for their programs. Commonly used measures include interest in the specialty, the interview, letters of recommendation, level of motivation, academic performance, interpersonal skills, desire to continue education, and possession of a degree.

Curriculum

PA residency programs vary in length from 6 to 24 months, although the majority (80%) of programs are 12 months in length.[8,18]

All residencies should offer didactic instruction, either at the beginning of the residency or incorporated throughout the program.[18] In a study published in 2000, residents estimated their total number of hours of didactic education associated with the residency program they attended to be 350.4 hours for residents in internship model programs and 413.4 hours for residents enrolled in an academic model program.[9] All programs reported by Wiemiller provided lectures to PA residents, and most also included attendance at conferences and grand rounds.[18] Some programs also offer skills labs and journal clubs. The most recent data on hours of didactic curriculum are available from a study conducted in 1999 when surveyed residency directors reported the average number of hours of didactic curriculum in their program to be 249 hours for internship model programs and 531 for academic model programs.[10]

Clinical Hours Worked

The number of clinical hours required by programs varies dramatically from specialty to specialty and from program to program, but residents tend to work more than a traditional 40-hour workweek. Data from a study of surgical PAs from 2007 reported residents in academic model programs reported working 44.1 clinical hours per week, whereas those enrolled in internship model programs reported working an average of 72.3 clinical hours per week.[11] Wiemiller and Somer[18] found that 31% of surveyed programs reported requiring in-house call as part of their program. For accredited programs, work-hour restriction includes limiting work hours (including clinical and academic activities) to a maximum of 80 hours averaged over a 4-week period.[3] Other restrictions addressed by the ACGME include requiring a minimum of 1 day in 7 free from all educational and clinical responsibilities and 10 hours off from all daily duty periods, including being on call.

Stipend/Fringe Benefits

Compensation depends on the nature of the residency (internship vs. academic model) and the total benefits package. In 2008 Wiemiller[18] reported a stipend range of \$12,000 to \$63,000 including programs that also charged tuition (3.6%). Data from 2011 indicate that most programs provide an annual stipend between \$40,000 and \$60,000.[8] Benefits packages vary but generally include such items as health insurance, malpractice insurance, and paid vacation time.

Credential Awarded

The most commonly awarded credential is the certificate of completion or training. In some instances, the residency program is also linked to an academic institution that grants academic credit or leads to a master's degree. The Wiemiller study[18] reported that 78% of programs offered a certificate of completion, 9% offered a master's option, and two programs reported offering no credential or certificate. Data from the 2011 study including only clinical programs indicated that none offer academic credit or degrees.[8]

In recent years, military programs have begun offering a clinical doctorate degree. In 2006, the U.S. Army Emergency Medicine PA residency program was expanded from a 12-month program to an 18-month program.[19] The program worked with Baylor University in Waco, Texas, to provide academic credit for their training program that leads to a doctor of science in PA studies (DSc). Since this time, additional military programs have begun offering a DSc with six programs identified in a 2011 study.[8] No civilian residency programs offer doctorate degrees.[8]

RESIDENT PERCEPTIONS OF TRAINING

Residents' perceptions of their training in general are positive. Table 37-1 presents findings about residents' levels of satisfaction with various aspects of their training.[9] It also categorizes the data on satisfaction into high and low categories for broader comparisons. All residents reported satisfaction in the summary evaluations of their residency training experiences and substantial satisfaction in the areas of degree of responsibility and didactic and clinical education. Residents were least satisfied with the salary and benefits packages. When asked if they would recommend their residency program to other PAs interested in their specialty, 71.7% (*N* = 33) answered "definitely" and 28.3% (*N* = 13) said "probably." None replied that they would not recommend their training program.

Included in this chapter is an interview with two PAs who attended a residency. The interview explores the PAs' perceptions of their residency experience and their reasons for electing to attend a residency program.

In 1987, Keith and Doerr[12] completed a study and published data regarding their experience in surgical PA postgraduate residencies. They conducted a survey of the graduates of the Montefiore Medical Center Surgical Residency Program. The results of this survey from the 110 respondents showed that 86% remained employed as PAs. Of the 110 respondents, 86 (78.2%) were employed by institutions and 24 (21.8%) were employed by physicians in private practice. This survey also included a salary analysis, which indicated that graduates of postgraduate residency programs earned significantly higher pay than PAs practicing in the same specialty who had not completed a postgraduate residency program. The average salary of the respondents was 21% greater than the national average salary of PAs. The graduate residents were asked to comment on their perceptions about the degree to which their training prepared them for their jobs. About 72% indicated satisfaction with the preparation they had received, 20% believed they were overprepared, and 8% felt inadequately prepared for the positions they held.

RESIDENCY GRADUATE EMPLOYMENT OPPORTUNITIES

Employment opportunities and roles for PAs are rapidly expanding to include a high proportion of specialty areas. Because of this diversity and specialization, formal postgraduate training is assuming a greater importance as an adjunct to PA primary care education. Postgraduate curricula are designed to build on the knowledge and experience acquired in PA school, enabling the PA to competently assume a role as PA on a specialty health care team. Many postgraduate programs have pioneered the role of the PA in these specialty areas and offer experienced role models, as well as formalized instruction. Little objective information has been published comparing the number of employment opportunities and

TABLE 37-1 **Summary of Residents' Satisfaction Levels**

Educational Experience	Very High	High	Low	Very Low
Clinical supervision received	15 = 32.6%	24 = 52.2%	6 = 13%	1 = 2.2%
▪ High vs. low satisfaction	High = 84.8%		Low = 15.2%	
Degree of responsibility	19 = 43.2%	24 = 54.5%	1 = 2.3%	0 = 0%
▪ High vs. low satisfaction	High = 97.7%		Low = 2.3%	
Degree of autonomy	14 = 31.8%	22 = 50.0%	8 = 18.2%	0 = 0%
▪ High vs. low satisfaction	High = 81.8%		Low = 18.2%	
Salary or stipend	3 = 7.3%	20 = 48.8%	14 = 34.1%	4 = 9.8%
▪ High vs. low satisfaction	High = 56.1%		Low = 43.9%	
Benefits package	10 = 24.4%	17 = 44.7%	7 = 18.4%	4 = 10.5%
▪ High vs. low satisfaction	High = 69.1%		Low = 28.9%	
Didactic education	15 = 32.6%	25 = 54.4%	3 = 6.5%	3 = 6.5%
▪ High vs. low satisfaction	High = 87.0%		Low = 13.0%	
Clinical education	16 = 35.6%	23 = 51.1%	3 = 6.7%	3 = 6.7%
▪ High vs. low satisfaction	High = 86.7%		Low = 13.4%	
Overall residency training	16 = 34.8%	30 = 65.2%	0 = 0%	0 = 0%
▪ High vs. low satisfaction	High = 100%		Low = 0.0%	

Modified from Asprey D, Helms L. A description of physician assistant post-graduate residency training: the resident's perspective. Perspect Physician Assist Educ 2000;11:79.

TABLE 37-2 Mechanism by Which Residents Learned about Physician Assistant Residency

Mechanism	*N*	Percentage
Information provided to me by the PA program I attended	19	41.3
From a fellow student or colleague	12	26.1
Journal advertisements	4	8.7
Other	4	8.7
By interactions with a residency graduate	3	6.5
By a mailing sent to me	2	4.3
Website	1	2.2
Journal article about the residency	1	2.2
Totals	46	100

Modified from Asprey D, Helms L. A description of physician assistant post-graduate residency training: the resident's perspective. Perspect Physician Assist Educ 2000;11:79.

the salaries commanded between residency-prepared and nonresidency-prepared PAs. However, there is anecdotal information and a general belief that the residency-prepared PA has a competitive edge over nonresidency-trained PAs when applying for PA positions and commands additional salary.

Selecting a Residency Program

Residents have often indicated that the way they learned about the residency program was either through information provided by the PA program they attended or from a fellow student or colleague. The complete list is presented in Table 37-2. Residents identify improved ability to compete for a job in their specialty, interest in acquiring additional knowledge and skills before entering practice, improved future earning potential, and the desire for increased competence in the specialty area as the items that had the greatest influence on their decision to attend residency. The majority of enrolled residents reported that they had applied to a single residency program.[9]

CASE STUDY 37-1

Age: 33
Gender: Female
PA program attended and year you graduated: Rosalind Franklin University, 2009
Residency program attended and year started: Illinois Bone and Joint Institute—Orthopedic Residency, 2009

Q: Why did you elect to attend a residency program after graduating from PA school?
A: To gain confidence functioning in a clinical atmosphere. I also wanted to build my résumé with some postgraduate experience in orthopedics to increase my chances to compete for a job in that specialty.
Q: Why did you elect to attend a residency program after graduation as opposed to getting your specialty training on the job?
A: The residency program exposed me to the multiple subspecialties of orthopedics.
Q: What exposure to the specialty you completed your residency in did you receive in your entry-level PA program education?
A: The PA program taught me sterile operating room (OR) technique, suturing, and hand tying. We had a casting and splinting lab. We also had lectures in various orthopedic topics.
Q: Briefly describe the curriculum in your residency program.
A: The curriculum consisted of morning rounds, grand rounds, surgical cases, emergency department trauma call in-house, and weekly morning lectures.
Q: What types of procedural activities did you gain experience with?
A: Suturing in the OR and closing of traumatic wounds, digital and field blocks, joint aspiration, casting/splinting, traction, etc.
Q: Was there a research element in your residency program?
A: No
Q: How was your performance in the residency program evaluated?
A: Not formally
Q: What unique knowledge and skills do you feel you acquired that were beyond what you received in your PA program education?
A: How to manage specific orthopedic injuries, OR techniques for repair of fractures, how to triage injuries, how to read various types of images
Q: Who served as your teachers in the residency?
A: Physicians, senior PAs, and medical residents from other specialties
Q: What compensation did you receive during the residency? Did you receive benefits, too?
A: The stipend was $50,000 with full benefits.
Q: What is/was the length of your residency?
A: 12 months
Q: How many hours did/do you work during an average week with the residency?
A: 80 to 100
Q: How many residents were enrolled in your program?
A: Four to seven; it depended on the time of the year. The admission was a rolling process.
Q: What job opportunities did you find were available when you had completed the

residency? Or what is your perception of job opportunities awaiting you?

A: There were plenty of job opportunities in the Chicago area. Physicians loved to hear about the residency program.

Q: What are/were the most positive aspects of being a PA resident?

A: I had a ton of exposure to trauma. The IBJI residency was at Lutheran General Hospital, a level 1 trauma center.

Q: What are/were the negative aspects of being a PA resident?

A: The time commitment; there was very little time that year for other aspects of my life outside of work.

Q: What advice would you have to PAs considering attending a residency?

A: If you choose a residency, make sure you want a job in that field when you finish. The program can be very time consuming. You need to be able to commit yourself to this field entirely for 1 year.

CASE STUDY 37-2

Age: 41

Gender: Female

PA program attended and year you graduated: Baylor College of Medicine, 2007

Residency Program attended and year started: MD Anderson Cancer Center, 03/08–03/09

Q: Why did you elect to attend a residency program after graduating from PA school?

A: I knew when I applied to PA school (a second career for me) that I wanted to work in oncology. Even though I knew I could get a job in oncology without the residency experience, I felt that it would be a great opportunity to get some incredible experience in a short amount of time and would really benefit me in the long run.

Q: Why did you elect to attend a residency program after graduation as opposed to getting your specialty training on the job?

A: I could not get the same type of specialty training through on-the-job experience. I was able to do rotations in all aspects of oncology, attend lectures, and do a research project, none of which I can do in my current position.

Q: What exposure to the specialty you completed your residency in did you receive in your entry-level PA program education?

A: I did an elective rotation in oncology while in PA school. Otherwise, oncology was only covered as a part of each didactic lesson (e.g., gynecologic cancers covered in our lectures on women's health).

Q: Briefly describe the curriculum in your residency program.

A: Curriculum was 2- to 4-week rotations in different oncology areas (medical, surgical, radiation oncology for all major types of cancer), regularly scheduled lectures/grand rounds throughout the year with additional specific lectures for each rotation, reading list for each rotation, regular meetings with program director, end-of-rotation evaluations with preceptors, journal clubs (presented 4 throughout the year), and research project.

Q: What types of procedural activities did you gain experience with?

A: I first- and second-assisted in various surgical oncology areas (breast, urology, gastrointestinal, neurology, head and neck) plus I was trained and performed 10 bone marrow aspiration/biopsy procedures.

Q: Was there a research element in your residency program?

A: Yes, I wrote a paper on the prognostic markers in chronic lymphocytic leukemia.

Q: How was your performance in the residency program evaluated?

A: I had a postrotation evaluation by each rotation preceptor, plus regular meetings with evaluation and feedback from the program director.

Q: What unique knowledge and skills do you feel you acquired that were beyond what you received in your PA program education?

A: Obviously, in-depth knowledge in oncology that went way beyond what is taught in PA school. Plus, hands-on work experience in a large cancer hospital, where I was able to work as a privileged PA (i.e., able to see patients on my own, write orders, etc.). Plus, being at a prestigious academic cancer research institution and working side by side with some of the world's most renowned physician faculty is an awesome experience. I gained a foundational understanding of the common principles of oncology—pathophysiology, chemotherapy, molecular pathways and targeted therapy, side effects of treatment, survivorship issues, infectious disease, pain control, and palliative care.

Q: Who served as your teachers in the residency?

A: Preceptors were PAs for the most part along with some nurse practitioners. Others who served as teachers included physicians, pharmacists, nurses, social workers, and of course the patients themselves.

Q: What compensation did you receive during the residency? Did you receive benefits, too?

A: I received a salary that was about one half to two thirds what I could have earned as a PA right out of school. I also received benefits. This was the hardest thing—I came out of PA school with loans that had to be deferred until I finished the residency. Once I started work, I really got no financial benefit as a result of doing the residency (i.e., higher starting salary). I think my starting salary was perhaps $1000 more than for someone right out of school, but I had to fight for that.

Q: What is/was the length of your residency?

A: 1 year

Q: How many hours did/do you work during an average week with the residency?

A: Average 40 hours per week, plus time required each evening for reading/studying

Q: How many residents were enrolled in your program?

A: 2 per year

Q: What job opportunities did you find were available when you had completed the residency? Or what is your perception of job opportunities awaiting you?

A: I remained at MD Anderson following my residency, so job opportunities were plentiful. I had my pick of which department I wanted to go work. Most rotations ended with an offer to come work in that department when I finished the residency (pending availability of positions, of course). However, I did not do any searching outside of MD Anderson, so I cannot say how the residency influenced job opportunities I might have had beyond MD Anderson.

Q: What are/were the most positive aspects of being a PA resident?

A: Positive: meeting so many new people, learning so many different things; being able to take advantage of all the lectures, grand rounds, conferences, etc. that I never am able to do now that I am working; being able to find out which area of oncology I wanted to work in.

Q: What are/were the negative aspects of being a PA resident?

A: Physicians and others often had no idea what my position and privileges were—there are so many people in training at MD Anderson but so few PA residents, that I was often mistaken for a student. Also, just when I got comfortable in a particular area—knew the people, processes, disease info, etc.—I would move to the next rotation. Lastly, the low salary compared with what I could have earned my first year out of school.

Q: What advice would you have to PAs considering attending a residency?

A: Make sure you are committed to this specialty. If you see yourself working in this specialty for the foreseeable future, then it is worthwhile for the experience you will gain that you simply cannot get through on-the-job training. Do not do a residency simply because you think it will help you get a job or to find out whether you really like that specialty.

CONCLUSION

PA residency education continues to evolve and mature as they reach the 40-year milestone of existence. The postgraduate programs can generally be considered successful in preparing graduate PAs to practice effectively in a variety of specialty areas within medicine. Considerable interest has been demonstrated by applicants to the residency programs and by institutions interested in developing new PA residency programs. The PA profession is unique in that it has both academic model-type residencies and more commonly, the internship model residency. It seems reasonable to conclude that as more entry-level PA programs offer a master's degree on completion, level of interest in the residency programs granting a master's degree (academic model programs) may decline. PA residents in general are satisfied with their educational experiences and would recommend the residency program to others.

PA residency programs have fairly recently implemented an accreditation system. This important step in the maturation of the postgraduate programs may serve to address issues related to the stability of the programs. The specific role that postgraduate residency program education will have on the profession continues to be a topic of considerable interest. Some individuals have expressed the concern that postgraduate training in the form of residency programs may evolve to a point where some institutions will expect or require PAs to complete a residency to be considered for employment; however, to date this does not seem to have occurred. This evolving form of education in the PA profession will be closely monitored for its potential effects on the profession.

CLINICAL APPLICATIONS

1. If you were interested in PA residency education, how would you find out about the distinctive features of each program?
2. What are some of the pros and cons associated with attending residency programs?
3. Would you choose a residency program with a certificate or a master's degree? Why?
4. What impact do you think the accreditation process for postgraduate programs has had on the programs? The PA profession?
5. Interview two PAs working in the same specialty—one who attended a residency program and one who did not. Ask them to describe their PA careers and how they acquired the knowledge and skills related to their specialties. What similarities and differences did you identify?

References

1. Katterjohn KR. Legislation: the increasing interest by hospitals in substituting PAs for housestaff. Physician Assist Health Pract 1979;3:8.
2. Timmer S. Call for uniform guidelines for postgraduate surgical residency programs. J Am Acad Physician Assist 1991;4:453.
3. Accreditation Review Commission for Physician Assistants website. *http://www.arc-pa.net/postgrad_programs/*; Accessed November 1, 2011.
4. Polansky M. A historical perspective on postgraduate physician assistant education and the Association of Postgraduate Physician Assistant Programs. J Physician Assist Educ 2007;18:100.
5. Association of Postgraduate Physician Assistant Programs website. *http://www.appap.org/Membership/tabid/67/Default.aspx*; Accessed November 1, 2011.
6. American Academic of Physician Assistants census report (website). *http://www.aapa.org/research/data_and_statistics.aspx*; Accessed November 1, 2011.
7. Hooker RS. Assessing the value of physician assistant postgraduate education. J Am Acad Physician Assist 2009;22:13.
8. Polansky M, Garver G, Wilson L, et al. The Current State of Affairs: Defining Postgraduate Clinical PA Education. Abstract presentation November 4, 2011, PAEA Education Forum.
9. Asprey D, Helms L. A description of physician assistant postgraduate residency training: the resident's perspective. Perspect Physician Assist Educ 2000;11:79.
10. Asprey D, Helms L. A description of physician assistant postgraduate residency training: the director's perspective. Perspectives Physician Assist Educ 1999;10:124.
11. Brenneman T, Hemminger C, Dehn R. Surgical graduates' perceptions on postgraduate physician assistant training programs. J Physician Assist Educ 2007;18:1.
12. Keith DE, Doerr RJ. Survey of a physician assistant internship concerning practice characteristics and adequacy of training. J Med Educ 1987;62:517.
13. McGill F, Kleiner GJ, Vanderbilt C, et al. Postgraduate internship in gynecology and obstetrics for physician assistants: a 4-year experience. Obstet Gynecol 1990;76:1135.
14. Brandt LB, Beinfeld MS, Laffaye HA, et al. The training and utilization of surgical assistants: a retrospective study. Arch Surg 1989;124:348.
15. Reynolds EW, Bricker JT. Nonphysican clinicians in the neonatal intensive care unit: meeting the needs of our smallest patients. Pediatrics 2007;119:361.
16. Will KK, Budavari AL, Mishark K, Hartsell ZC. A hospitalist postgraduate training program for physician assistants. J Hospital Med 2010;5:94.
17. Association of Postgraduate Physician Assistant Programs website; *http://www.appap.org/Resources/ByLaws/tabid/63/Default.aspx*. Accessed November 1, 2011.
18. Wiemiller MJ, Somers KK, Adams MB. Postgraduate physician assistant training programs in the United States: emerging trends and opportunities. J Physician Assist Educ 2008;19:58.
19. Salyer SW. A clinical doctorate in emergency medicine for physician assistants: postgraduate education. J Physician Assist Educ 2008;19:53.

The resources for this chapter can be found at www.expertconsult.com.

CHAPTER 38

DEALING WITH STRESS AND BURNOUT

Ruth Ballweg

CHAPTER CONTENTS

As part of physician assistant (PA) training, students receive extensive information about stress. PAs learn that almost all change creates stress, and most clinicians optimistically believe that stress can be "managed." Typical classroom presentations include the concepts of "good" and "bad" stress, the Holmes-Reye Stress Scale as a teaching and evaluation tool for patients, and recommended treatment plans (exercise, decreased caffeine intake, improved nutrition, and even short-term psychotherapy) for patients with stress. This chapter does not attempt to duplicate that information. Rather, the focus of the chapter is to identify and discuss the specifics of stress and burnout as they apply to PAs, recommend strategies for prevention, and suggest a range of treatment interventions.

DECISION TO BECOME A PHYSICIAN ASSISTANT

Ironically, whether we choose to look at it this way or not, PAs all become personal experts on stress as part of our medical education. The consideration of any medical career creates stress. The prospect of long hours; personal sacrifice; a commitment to care of patients, sometimes at the expense of family; and the recognition of the intensity of a medical career demand serious consideration. Many PAs at some point considered becoming physicians. This consideration was at least understandable to our teachers, mentors, family, and friends. Becoming a nurse also made some sense ("You'll always have a job"). The relatively new career of PA commonly may still not be either understood or supported. Fortunately, the admissions process for most PA programs has favored the selection of risk-taking and pioneering individuals who see the PA profession as a unique opportunity. Candidates are often referred to practicing PAs who are willing to provide firsthand exposure to the PA profession.

Nevertheless, the first stress for successful candidates to PA programs has been the job of answering the question, "You're going to become a what!?" Even the most understanding friend may still ask, "When will you be a doctor?" The most supportive friend, employer, or parent may still not understand why being a PA is a separate and different career with its own satisfactions and rewards.

EXPERIENCE OF STRESS IN TRAINING

Next come the adventure and stress of PA training. Asked about the difference between PA and physician training programs, many of the founders of PA education are quick to point out that both PA and nurse practitioner (NP) programs, although designed to train new types of primary care providers, were also intended to be a proving ground for new concepts in medical education. Problem-based learning, the use of simulated patients, and videotaping to teach patient interviewing skills, and new types of clinical training experiences were used early on in PA and NP programs, before their more recent appearance in medical schools. Objectives and competency-based learning also were used to make PA training extremely efficient. As a result, the curriculum of most PA programs is intended to present a large amount of information in a short time. PA program directors often say, "It's not that the material is so hard, but that it comes in truckloads." Students often say the intensity of PA classroom training is "like drinking from a fire hydrant." As programs have moved to the graduate levels, PA curricula have also added significant research and management content, which places further demands on each PA student.

In addition to simple acquisition of information, the relatively short duration of PA training, compared with that of physicians, demands that the PA student develop a professional identity in an extremely responsible role quickly. This rapid role transition actually accounts for much of the stress PA students experience. Students entering the PA profession as a first career choice generally have a successful college career as a foundation for their PA training but may have had little exposure to patient care. Thus, the stress for these students is often that of developing a way of relating to patients and seeing themselves as decision-makers on the health care team. People who enter PA programs as second-career students, former registered nurses (RNs), licensed practical nurses (LPNs), military corpsmen, paramedics, surgical/respiratory/radiology/laboratory technicians, and other allied health personnel may have had identities as members of the health care team but generally find that they have to relinquish their former identities to assume their new role of PA.

Recognizing these concerns, PA program admissions committees often seek and choose applicants who are flexible, trainable, proactive, and proficient in multiple tasks. Students less adaptable to the extremely rapid didactic and clinical experiences required of them in PA training may become alienated from classmates who are enthusiastically moving ahead on an exciting career path.

Another unique aspect of PA training that often creates some short-term stress, but may actually decrease long-term stress, is the emphasis on sensitive issues and interpersonal skills as part of training. Included in this training has been extensive small-group work, with faculty feedback, to teach interviewing and physical examination skills. Course work is also required to include primary care topics dealing with sexuality, parenting, death and dying, cross-cultural issues, and family dynamics. In studying these topics, students are forced to confront their personal opinions and biases as they apply to interactions not only with their colleagues but also with their future patients.

Current trends in health professions education include an emphasis on professionalism and opportunities for interdisciplinary education. Learning to give and receive feedback are critical skills in new educational environments.

Although stressful at first, these new skills are designed to increase clarity regarding expectations and performance. As a result, stress can be decreased by minimizing misunderstanding and confusion.

One solution for stress in the didactic year is to focus on planning for the future in the clinical year. This diversionary tactic is probably most appealing for students with prior clinical experience, who may feel that they are "just putting in time" in the classroom until they can "really perform" in the clinical setting. In contrast, students with more extensive academic experience and less clinical identity may approach the clinical year with increasing anxiety. Regardless of each group's anticipatory viewpoint, the clinical year brings certain predictable stresses:

- No matter how well the program has prepared the site and used it in the past, some members of the physician, nursing, and administrative staff, in at least some sites, still will not know what a PA is or does.
- Medical students assigned the same clinical placements still may not understand the PA role and may at first perceive the PA student as a threat.
- The process of relocating from site to site is disorienting. The health care system may, for the first time, appear extremely fragmented to the PA student, who may not have realized that medicine is practiced so many different ways in so many different settings.
- The demand for documentation (charting) as to both detail and timeliness is much greater than the student had expected. New electronic health record (EHR) systems are still under development, and the transition to these new processes creates stress for all clinicians—but especially

health care professionals, but because of confidentiality and a lack of specific shared experiences, it is difficult and sometimes even inappropriate for them to "debrief" their health care professional, family member, or friend about specific patient care stresses. Some employment settings provide support groups for their health care providers. In addition to formal support networks, social events with co-workers also effectively reduce stress. Although many PAs use other PAs for support in patient care issues, it is valuable to see all members of the health care team as part of a support network because different viewpoints may bring different insights to a situation or incident.

One of the best published resources on stress in the helping professions is Christina Maslach's *Burnout: The Cost of Caring.*[2] In reviewing patient care stresses, Maslach believes that a large part of the problem is that health care professionals, as students and as practitioners, are often so busy acquiring facts and proficiency in procedures that they do not learn the relatively simple interpersonal skills that will carry them through difficult situations and reduce stress on the job.

Surprisingly, interpersonal skills are often not recognized as a major necessity for providers. They are considered secondary to other professional skills: extras rather than essentials, the "icing on the cake" rather than the cake itself. This viewpoint is sadly in error because it trivializes an essential aspect of the relationship between provider and recipient. It fails to recognize that both of them are human beings whose personal attitudes and feelings can affect not only the delivery of care but also how and even whether it is accepted.[2]

Recognizing that health care professionals may have been taught to deal with specific crisis situations, Maslach is concerned that it is in fact the daily encounters, producing incremental stress, for which daily "garden variety" interpersonal skills should be gained. Maslach lists three of these skills as examples:

1. **How to Start, Stop, and Keep Things Going:** Just like true love, the course of helping relationships does not always run smoothly. Getting things started on the right foot often depends on how you greet the other person, whether there is any initial social talk to reduce tension and "break the ice." Similarly, bringing things to a successful halt depends on whether you interrupt the person (and how you do so), how you announce that time is up, whether you evaluate the progress that has been made, how you say good-bye, and so on.
2. **How to Deal with Different People:** The infinite variety of human beings is what makes working with people so interesting, exciting, and challenging. It is also what makes it so difficult at times. The approach that a practitioner uses with one client may not work with someone else because of differences in sex, age, cultural backgrounds, personality, values, attitudes, and so forth. Although practitioners often long for a single strategy that will work well with everybody, the truth is they need to have several different strategies in their hip pocket, ready to be used when appropriate.
3. **How to Talk about Unpopular Topics:** All too often in helping relationships, what needs to be said is what one person does not want to say and the other does not want to hear. Practitioners dread these difficult moments, and it is here, more than anywhere else, that they express a need for additional interpersonal skills. The topics that are most difficult to handle are how to ask tough questions, how to discuss sensitive issues, and how to deliver bad news. Special skills training for these problems would go a long way toward alleviating the emotional exhaustion of burnout.[2]

Formal Professional Issues

Formal professional issues are potential stressors for PAs. Although significant progress has been made in many areas of the country, medical practice acts in some states are still restrictive of PA practice. Reimbursement policies also vary dramatically from state to state and region to region. Institutions that have not previously employed PAs may need help in adapting their credentialing processes for the effective utilization of PAs. Relatively new graduates may have a poor appreciation of the rapid progress that has been made by the PA profession in removing barriers to practice. As a result, new PAs may feel helpless and hopeless. One of the best solutions is political involvement. State PA academies are always seeking the energies of PAs willing to serve on a wide range of committees, all ultimately dealing with the expansion of PA practice. Although some PAs have initially believed that they did not have either the time or the skills for such involvement, almost all PAs who have become engaged in these activities have found that the sense of "making a difference" is a strong deterrent to stress and burnout.

One stress that may be somewhat more pressing for PAs than for other providers is keeping up with new developments to maintain one's professional competence. Initially trained in a primary care model with broad skills, PAs are first certified by an examination that tests primary care knowledge. Changes in the recertification process, along with the development of new "Certificates of Added Qualification" (CAQs) for PAs in some specialties, add to the stress for new graduates considering options for their developing careers.

Although it is difficult for most health care professionals to keep up with continuing developments in the medical field, PAs are among the few health care professionals who must undergo periodic recertification by examination at 6-year intervals. In addition, the profession is the only one in which recertification is tied directly to state registration and the right to work.[1]

Role Ambiguity Issues

Aside from the specifics of regulation, certification, and credentialing, the ambiguity of the PA profession is both the good news and the bad news. Many PAs have chosen the profession because of its limitless aspects. Other PAs are distressed by the fact that the PA career lacks precise definition with clearly delineated standards of practice, consistent legislation, and reimbursement standards throughout the country.

Trying to meet society's expectations for high-quality medical care in a time of rapid change in the health care system is both exciting and terrifying. Because it is a relatively new career, new opportunities for PAs are constantly being developed, often by creative and innovative members of the profession. Here, expectations are the critical factors. It is to be hoped that:

- PA program applicants have researched the profession as part of their entry process into training.
- PA programs have given the students exposure to practicing PAs serving as role models and providing realistic insights into both the frustrations and satisfactions of their jobs.
- PA students in their clinical rotations have sought to achieve an understanding of the emotional context of their jobs as part of their training.
- Practicing PAs regard questions from consumers about PAs as opportunities to educate them not only about PAs but also about the variety of health care professions that exist today.

BURNOUT

We are all concerned when stress turns to burnout. Originally thought of as a syndrome characterized by emotional depletion and exhaustion, burnout is now better understood as a state and process that begin as a response to work-related stressors.[3] Holmes and Fasser[1] describe the process as moving through tedium ("the experience of physical, emotional, and mental exhaustion precipitated by stress and characterized by feelings of strain, emotional and physical depletion, and negative attitudes toward self, environment, and life") into burnout. "The cumulative effects of sustained tedium in the work environment produce tension, irritability, and fatigue, which end in a defensive reaction of detachment, apathy, cynicism, or rigidity, referred to as burnout."[1]

Personal Characteristics

Some individuals seem more prone to burnout than others. According to Maslach,[2] "burnout is more likely if the person is younger, less mature, and less self-confident; is impulsive and impatient; has no family commitments but needs other people who can provide approval and affection; and has goals and expectations that are not in tune with reality." Armstrong and colleagues[4] list four types of individuals most susceptible to burnout: "those who assume too much responsibility and feel driven to achieve goals; those who view their jobs as the major reason for living and fail to develop outside activities; those who place a heavy emphasis on completing the task regardless of the cost; and those who are truly overworked."

Identifying Burnout

One of the biggest problems with burnout is that we are least able to identify it in ourselves until it is a critical problem. Thus, we must rely on our friends, family members, and colleagues to be our "early warning systems." Similarly, we must provide this same assistance to other friends in health care. Colon[3] suggests that clinicians should always "maintain a high index of suspicion . . . for symptoms of burnout." Complications can include depression, substance abuse, and even suicide. Appropriate and supportive referrals for assessment and treatment are particularly important.

Maslach[2] also believes that employers should be on the alert for burnout. The organization should institute standard reviews, or preburnout "checkups" at periodic intervals (1 month after starting the job, then every 3 months or so). When such reviews are a ritualized and regular procedure for all staff, then no one person has to accept the burden of alerting you to the fact that he or she is beginning to get singed around the edges.

Assessment and Treatment

In assessing individual situations of burnout, three questions are important[2]:

- What is the individual's role?
- What roles do other people play?
- What role does the institution play?

Answers to these three questions will give some direction to a treatment plan.

On an individual level, Maslach describes the physical and psychological dysfunction accompanying burnout. "Exhaustion, illness, depression, irritability, increased use of alcohol and drugs, these are some of the personal costs."[2] Personal strategies might include a redefinition of work style and the search for a better balance between professional and private life.

In terms of patients and co-workers, interpersonal symptoms are changes in relationships with clients, such as callous and insensitive behavior. Colon[3] describes the "clues" of burnout in PAs:

> A classic example is when the clinician jokes about patients' illnesses, calls patients by symptoms, and becomes less trusting and less sympathetic toward them. Another sign is overall loss of concern and feeling for patients. Occasionally, however, the opposite is true: A burned-out clinician becomes too involved with patients or overidentifies with them and commits a considerably greater number of hours than required for their care.

Strategies for interpersonal aspects of burnout most often include the assistance of others in the same or similar situation to offer perspectives and solutions. In some situations, the best treatment plan might also call for the assistance of a therapist experienced in the concerns of health care providers.

Burnout at the institutional level may be the result of unrealistic workloads, barriers to practice, inefficient staffing patterns, and poor management. Maslach[2] describes the effects of burnout at the institutional level as being "reflected in high rates of absenteeism, turnover, and complaints about staff performance." Strategies for a dysfunctional employment setting include "redesigning jobs, changing organizational policies, devising explicit structures and contracts, establishing flexible leaves and support services, and improving the training programs for staff."[2]

"One of the most important aspects of burnout treatment (and prevention) is increasing an individual's sense of personal power, because it is "powerlessness" that makes one feel most trapped. Maslach discusses "ways in which the individual exerts some active control in a situation rather than just passively acquiescing to it. The person changes the work routine, redefines goals, uses downshifts, takes breaks, seeks out positive feedback, engages in decompression activities, and so forth. All of these activities involve choice and initiative—the hallmarks of freedom and autonomy."[2] Believing that individual health care providers (PAs in this case) generally have more power than they realize, Maslach further notes that "by wiggling around in the job and finding out what can change and what cannot, the practitioner can counteract the helplessness and 'the hell with it all' attitude associated with burnout."[2]

The other well-known strategy for treating burnout is working toward the goal of reestablishing some balance in one's life. At the simplest level, this includes eating balanced meals and establishing realistic sleep and exercise patterns. Further activities include developing interests outside work and cultivating friendships and relationships away from the health care environment. Placing greater emphasis on family and leisure time has been effective for some individuals. Others have chosen to seek additional education or training as a way of expanding their horizons. Many health care providers see therapists as needed for help in balancing their lives.

CASE STUDY 38-1

Dennis is a 34-year-old paramedic enrolled in the first year of a PA program. It is now halfway through the didactic year of training. His classmates are concerned that he has become increasingly "negative" toward the program in which he is enrolled. This seems particularly unusual to them because he had been working toward getting into this specific program for longer than 5 years before admission, expanding his clinical experience, enrolling in basic science coursework to fulfill the prerequisite requirements for program admission, completing his bachelor's degree, and volunteering in community programs serving the homeless.

When his faculty advisor meets with him, Dennis says he feels that much of the coursework is either "too soft and a waste of time" or "not appropriate to what PAs need to know." He feels that he is "not getting what he has paid for" from the program. The faculty advisor, who was also a former paramedic, suggests that he meet with some practicing PAs from similar backgrounds to find out their opinions on these issues. He provides him with three contacts, and they plan to meet again in a week.

The student meets with two of the graduates who are available that week. One works in a general internal medicine outpatient clinic, and the other is employed in a rural private practice. They both describe similar concerns during didactic training and independently share with him that, in retrospect, they feel that their frustration during didactic training was actually more related to their own role transition. One PA says that during his didactic training, he did not really understand the broad roles that PAs are expected to play within the health care system. Therefore, he kept trying to "manage" his learning by focusing it down to specific areas (what he thought PAs "needed" to know). This strategy had worked during his paramedic career but turned out to be ineffective for a PA student. This PA suggests that the student look at the "bigger" picture and try to be less resistant and more flexible in his approach to the curriculum.

The second PA specifically wants to talk about the "softer stuff" in the curriculum. She says that she initially thought the behavioral science content of the program was totally unnecessary, until she got into her clinical year. In the first week of her first rotation (general internal medicine), she was "blown away" to find out how many of her patients had some behavioral science component to their illness. Not only that, but they also expected her to be comfortable talking about these issues. Even more surprising was the fact that she had gained competency in these skills during the didactic year, despite her resistance to these issues. Now she says it would almost be fun to take the behavioral science course again, if only she had the opportunity.

The student returns to meet with his advisor. He reports on his contact with the graduates, and they discuss the findings. Although Dennis says he still has concerns about what he is learning, he seems much less hostile and anxious. He says that he plans to try to be more flexible about his approach to the curriculum and his own learning. He also has made plans to keep in contact with both the graduates he has met. One of them has offered her clinic to him as a potential training site. He says that he really feels good about this. The student and his advisor schedule a follow-up appointment at the end of the quarter, or sooner if needed.

CASE STUDY 38-2

Jo is a senior student who has only three more clinical clerkships before her graduation. She has been a strong student throughout both the didactic and clinical years but suddenly seems to be behind in submitting her written assignments, including chart notes, patient care logs, and a research paper on "the perfect PA job." Her faculty advisor contacts her and arranges to visit Jo in her clinic, a Veterans Health Administration outpatient site.

In meeting with Jo at the start of the day, the faculty advisor asks her how things are going and gets the following response: "I can't seem to get caught up. I can't sleep. I just can't do this!" She also says that she has a hard time fitting in regular meals, has totally abandoned her daily exercise routine, and has been too busy to even e-mail her fellow classmates. Further conversation reveals that Jo is also engaged in negotiations with four potential employers, all in sites where she has previously been assigned for clinical rotations. She is receiving almost daily calls from all of these sites and believes that she has to make a decision immediately. At the same time, she notices that she is having trouble making decisions about even the simplest patient care issues.

The faculty advisor suggests that she needs to prioritize her concerns. If she spends too much time on future employment negotiations, she may not successfully complete the program. If she is ill, from not eating, not sleeping, and abandoning her social contacts, she will probably not be able to fulfill her job responsibilities in a new employment setting. In addition, she may be at risk for board examination failure if she continues to be distracted from her learning during the remaining 3 months of training. The student says, "Of course, why do you think I'm not sleeping!?"

They discuss a variety of strategies, including even a timeout from the program. Finally, they agree on the following actions:

- Complete any outstanding assignments as the highest priority, beginning with the copies of chart notes and patient care logs.
- Eat breakfast and lunch on a more regular schedule, attempt to reinstitute an exercise routine, and decrease caffeine consumption.
- Delay job negotiations at least until the completion of this rotation.
- Reestablish contact with at least two fellow students.
- Plan for weekly follow-up with faculty advisor.
- Consider referral for supportive therapy if not improved.
- Consider a brief leave of absence, with no penalty, if not improved.

CONCLUSION

Given the complexity and intensity of the health care system within which we work, it is normal to expect that we will all be regularly subjected to significant amounts of stress. It is also important to acknowledge that we generally have anticipated this stress as part of our career choice. We may not, however, have always gauged accurately the emotional costs of pioneering what still is a relatively new career. We also may not always have recognized the importance that good interpersonal skills, strong support systems, and well-chosen jobs play in job satisfaction.

Unfortunately, it is not unreasonable to predict that everyone in health care will experience some form of burnout during his or her professional life. As Colon[3] points out, "Stress is a particularly urgent problem for PAs. Their unique position in health care delivery can intensify other stressors of medical practice. Consequently, PAs must be especially on guard against burnout: in themselves, in other PAs, in supervising physicians, and in support staff."

Although PAs are generally satisfied with their career and actively promote it to individuals choosing health care careers, we must be realistic in recognizing the sources of stress and satisfaction. It is only by recognizing those stresses and satisfactions that we are best able to evaluate our current professional and personal lives and make the ongoing choices that will sustain our health as individuals.

CLINICAL APPLICATIONS

1. Begin a personal "stress" log to document your progress in the program. On a daily or weekly basis, list all of those issues and concerns that you believe are contributing to your stress. Divide your list into two categories: (1) things you can do something about and (2) things you cannot do anything about. Develop a strategy for attacking and resolving the items on the first list.
2. Interview at least one preceptor to whom you are assigned in your clinical year. Ask about his or her perception of common stresses in professional practice and abilities to resolve these stresses. Discuss what involvement he or she has with colleagues for mutual support.

KEY POINTS

- Regardless of any prior clinical experience, all students experience significant stress during both the didactic and clinical phases of PA training. One reason for this is the need for the rapid assumption of an extremely responsible clinical role.
- An effective and supportive relationship with a supervising physician is one of the great "stress relievers" for practicing PAs.
- Burnout is more likely to be recognized by friends and colleagues than it is by the person experiencing it.
- Greater public acceptance of the PA role has reduced the stress levels of practicing PAs.

References

1. Holmes SE, Fasser CE. Occasional stress among physician assistants. J Am Acad Physician Assist 1993;6:172.
2. Maslach C. Burnout: The Cost of Caring. Englewood Cliffs, NJ: Prentice-Hall, 1982.
3. Colon EA. Burnout. Physician Assist 1986;10:18.
4. Armstrong M, King M, Meller B. Avoiding orientation burnout: a practical guide designed to help inservice instructors. Nurs Manage 1982;13:27.

The resources for this chapter can be found at www.expertconsult.com.

SECTION VI

PRACTICE-BASED LEARNING AND IMPROVEMENT

CHAPTER 39

HEALTH DISPARITIES

Diane D. Abercrombie

CHAPTER CONTENTS

After decades of improvements in preventive health care and significant declines in disease mortality for many Americans, disparities in health and health care continue to persist in the United States.[1-3] As such, reducing and ultimately eliminating health disparities remains a focus of national attention. Racial and ethnic minorities, those with disabilities, women, economically and educationally disadvantaged, and the medically underserved, among others, continue to suffer a disproportionate burden of disease. The reasons for health disparities appear to be multifactorial, still poorly understood, and complex. Compelling evidence indicates that among minorities, race and ethnicity correlate strongly with health disparities. Minority populations, typically classified as African Americans, Hispanic Americans, Asian Americans/Pacific Islanders, American Indians (AIs), and Alaska Natives (ANs), are much more likely to experience poorer health outcomes, decreased life expectancy, higher mortality, and premature deaths. These groups are also less likely to be recipients of health care services geared toward health promotion, disease prevention and early detection of disease, and high-quality medical treatments.[1-3]

There are a host of key factors, or determinants, of health disparities. These include but are not limited to insurance status, socioeconomic status, residential and geographic segregation, English as a second language (ESL), cultural and racial bias, and stereotyping (Table 39-1).[1,2,4] Racial and ethnic minority groups comprise more than 50% of those uninsured, representing for some (e.g., African Americans, Hispanics, AIs) two to five times that of white Americans. In January 2010, the U.S. Senate passed the Patient Protection and Affordable Care Act (Affordable Care Act). This legislation seeks to address health care disparities through programs that would benefit most Americans, including racial and ethnic minority groups. Its greatest impact is thought to come from the general provisions aimed at reducing financial barriers to care, thereby increasing access to care and providing access to health insurance for an additional 32 million Americans who are not eligible for a group insurance plan.[5,6]

There is also strong evidence indicating a correlation between low health literacy and health disparities among minorities. The Institute of Medicine (IOM) defines health literacy as the degree to which individuals can obtain, process, and understand basic health information. Also included in this definition is the capacity to which an individual can ascertain services prerequisite to make appropriate health decisions. America's low health literacy rate among our more vulnerable groups threatens the well-being of the American health care system and adds billions of dollars to health care costs.[7,8]

The Office of Minority Health (OMH) was created by the Department of Health and Human Services (DHHS) in 1986 as a direct response to the landmark 1985 Report of the Secretary's Task Force on Black and Minority Health. This report documented health disparities among minorities and placed their disadvantaged health status on the forefront of U.S. health policy agenda. In conjunction with DHHS, OMH works to improve the health and health care of racial and ethnic minorities.[9] In 2003, the Agency for Healthcare Research and Quality (AHRQ) introduced its first published report with regard to health care equality and health care disparities. The most recent report, the *2011 National Healthcare Disparities Report*, was released in March 2012 and combines both qualities of health care and health care disparities as a single report. It provides a comprehensive national overview of health care quality and disparities in health care, identifies recent changes, and monitors the success of interventions that target a reduction in health disparities while enhancing health care quality in the United States.[10]

This chapter serves as an introduction to health disparities and low health literacy. Physician assistant (PA) education is an important component of an overall strategy to eliminate health disparities, while raising awareness regarding the causes and definition of low health literacy. It is imperative that current and future generations of PAs become knowledgeable about the disproportionate burden of disease and poorer health outcomes that exist in the United States among minority populations. Any efforts to improve quality of health care, reduce the cost of health care, and reduce and/or eliminate disparities in health should be coupled simultaneously with improvements in health literacy. PAs are challenged to develop new skill sets that will allow for effective, culturally inclusive patient care. Students must comprehend the underlying causes of low health literacy and health care disparities in order to provide efficient health care for America's diverse patient population. Rick Rhors, president of the American Academy of Physician Assistants in 2005, stated it best: "... each PA has the opportunity—no, the obligation—to take action. Few other issues of such magnitude can be so effectively addressed by one PA—and one patient—at a time."[11] This belief is supported by the ground-breaking 2002 Institute of Medicine Report (IOM), *Unequal Treatment: Confronting Racial and Ethnic Disparity in Health Care*, which calls for the cross-cultural education of health care providers as a fundamental element in eliminating racial and ethnic disparities in health care (Table 39-2).[8]

TABLE 39-1 **Causes of Health Care Disparities**

- Health care access
- Health care resources
- Unequal treatment
- Poorer health outcomes
- Health status for racial and ethnic minority patients
- Patient-physician relationship
- Health care delivery system
- Language and cultural barriers
- Lack of provider cultural competence
- Patient beliefs
- Provider biases and prejudice
- Stereotyping
- Low health literacy
- Poverty, racism, discrimination
- Lack of health insurance or limited health insurance plans
- Personal, geographic, residential, socioeconomic, and environmental factors

TABLE 39-2 **Ethnic and Racial Disparities Summary***

Infant mortality	Infant mortality rate per 1000 live births (2007) for non-Hispanic black (13.35) represents 2.4 times that of non-Hispanic white (5.58). The overall U.S. infant mortality rate was 6.68. African Americans are four times more likely to die at infancy because of complications related to preterm and low birthweight as compared with non-Hispanic white infants.
Cancer screening	Cancer is the second leading cause of death for most racial/ethnic minorities. For Asian and Pacific Islanders, cancer represents the number one killer. African American men are 2 times more likely to die from prostate cancer, and African American women are 36% more likely to die from breast cancer, despite the fact that breast cancer is diagnosed 10% less frequently in African American women.
Cardiovascular disease (CVD)	Heart disease is the leading killer across most racial/ethnic populations, accounting for 26% of all deaths in 2006. African American men are 30% more likely to die from heart disease and 32% have hypertension compared with 23% of whites.
Diabetes	Among adults, African American are twice more likely, Indian/Alaska Natives 2.1 times more likely, Native Hawaiians 5.7 times more likely, and Mexican Americans 1.9 times more likely than non-Hispanic white adults to be diagnosed with diabetes.
HIV/AIDS	Racial/ethnic minorities account for nearly 71% of newly diagnosed HIV/AIDS cases in 2008. In 2008, 73% of babies born with HIV/AIDS were born within minority groups. The disease is an epidemic among minority populations with African Americans accounting for 52% of all HIV/AIDS cases diagnosed in 2008.
Immunizations	African Americans and Hispanics are less likely to receive the influenza vaccine (51%, 56%) as compared with whites (70%). These minority groups are also less likely to receive the pneumococcal vaccine than whites. In 2008, Asian/Pacific Islanders had more than 23 times the rate of newly diagnosed tuberculosis than whites.

From Graham G, Gracia JN. Department of Health and Human Services. Office of Minority Health. Eliminating Racial and Ethnic Health Disparities. *http://minorityhealth.hhs.gov/templates*. Accessed August 1, 2011.

*The DHHS has selected six focus areas in which racial and ethnic minorities experience a disproportionate burden of disease.

WHAT ARE HEALTH DISPARITIES?

According to *Unequal Treatment*, health disparities are differences in the incidence, prevalence, mortality, and burden of diseases and other adverse health conditions that exist among specific population groups in the United States.[6] Disparities in health care exist even when controlling for gender, condition, age, and socioeconomic status. The *Healthy People 2020* initiative is a set of health promotion and disease prevention objectives for the nation. It endeavors to improve the health of all groups. *Healthy People 2020* states if a health outcome is seen in a greater or lesser extent between populations, a disparity exists. *Healthy People 2020* emphasizes that the term "disparities" refers to more than mere racial or ethnic disparities. Gender, sexual identity, age, disability, socioeconomic status, and geographic location all play a pivotal role in the achievement of good health. Thus, recognizing the impact of social determinants is crucial to understanding the definition of health disparities.[12]

One of the important missions of the National Institutes of Health (NIH) is the utilization of research that identifies factors that play an important role in the discovery and detection of innovative knowledge regarding the prevention, detection, diagnosis, and treatment of disease and disability. That mission is central to the expanding efforts to eliminate health disparities. In 2003, the NIH clarified its 2000 definition of health disparities to include a method research component to its previous definition. The NIH now defines health disparities as health disparities research (HD): basic, clinical and social sciences aimed at identifying, understanding, preventing, diagnosing, and treating health conditions, diseases, disorders in socioeconomically disadvantaged subpopulations (e.g., low literacy, living in medically underserved, rural, and urban communities).[13] In 2006, Braveman proposed a definition of health disparity/inequality as a "particular type of difference in health or in the most important influences on health that could potentially be shaped by policies. It is a difference in which disadvantaged social groups systematically experience worse health or greater risks than more advantaged groups."[14]

On January 14, 2011, the Centers for Disease Control and Prevention (CDC) released its *Health Disparities and Inequalities Report, United States, 2011*. This report is the first in an anticipated series of serial, consolidated assessments highlighting health disparities by gender, race and ethnicity, income, education, disability, and additional social determinants of health in the United States. This report defines health disparities as those differences in health outcomes between groups reflective of social inequalities and calls for innovative intervention strategies that incorporate social and health programs.[15]

Numerous other definitions of health disparities exist. In the United States, health disparities are well documented among minority populations. In essence, health disparities are population-specific differences in the presence of disease, health outcomes, mortality, and access to health care. Literature continues to acknowledge that the leading disparities for preventable conditions often exist among racial and ethnic minority populations.[2,10,15] At present, research has shifted to include transdisciplinary multilevel research on the social determinants of health disparities, community-based participatory research, and public health approaches to eliminating health disparities. The literature states that innovative and creative, broad-based approaches are necessary to address the multiple complex factors that result in the disproportionate burden of certain diseases and poorer health outcomes for minority populations. New research investigates the combination of population, clinical, and basic science to elucidate the complex determinants of health disparities (Table 39-3).[2-4,16-17]

HEALTH LITERACY AND ITS IMPACT ON HEALTH DISPARITIES

Parker and Kindig[18] stated that any efforts seeking to reduce and/or eliminate health disparities must take into simultaneous account the issue of health literacy. The Affordable Care Act (2010), Title V, defines health literacy as the degree to which an individual has the capacity to obtain, communicate, process, and understand basic health information and services to make appropriate health decisions. This definition mirrors the *Healthy People 2010* definition of health literacy with the exception of the word "communicate."[6,19]

Data depict clear-cut links between poor health outcomes and low literacy skills.[20] Individuals with low literacy skills possess decreased health knowledge and awareness, inferior self-management skills, increased hospitalization rates, inadequate physical and mental health, and increased health care costs and mortality.[7] Reports from the 1992 National Adult Literacy Survey (NALS), the 2003 National Assessment of Adult Literacy (NAAL), and the 2004 Prudential Medicare Study all show that limited health literacy skills affect individuals of all ages and races. In particular, those who are socioeconomically disadvantaged, immigrants, elderly, residing in rural areas, and racial/ethnic minorities represent those at greatest risk for limited health literacy.[21-23] In 2000, *Healthy People 2010* identified low health literacy as

TABLE 39-3 **Definitions of Health Disparities**

Agency	Definition
2002, IOM, *Unequal Treatment*	"Health disparities are differences in the incidence, prevalence, mortality, and burden of diseases and other adverse health conditions that exist among specific population groups in the United States."
Healthy People, 2020	"... A particular type of health difference closely linked with social, economic, and/or environmental disadvantage. Health disparities adversely affect groups of people who have systemically experienced greater obstacles of health based their racial or ethnic group; religion; socioeconomic status; gender; age; mental health; cognitive, sensory, or physical disability; sexual orientation or gender identity; geographic location; or other characteristics historically linked to discrimination or exclusion."
National Institutes of Health (2003)	"... Health disparities research (HD) includes basic, clinical, and social sciences studies identifying, understanding, preventing, diagnosing, and treating health conditions, diseases, disorders, and other conditions that are unique to, more serious, or more prevalent in subpopulations in socioeconomically disadvantaged (i.e., low education level, live in poverty) and medically underserved, rural, and urban communities."

a public health, widespread problem. According to the 2010 National Action Plan to Improve Health Literacy, most health information is not presented in a user-friendly format. Only 12% of English-speaking American adults have adept health literacy skills, and at least 9 out of 10 adults cannot comprehend how to use common health information. This results in a multitude of negative health outcomes: lack of necessary primary disease prevention and health promotion services, inappropriate use of the health care system, medication errors, poor comprehension of nutrition labels, poor patient compliance, increased health care costs, decreased self-esteem, and difficulties managing chronic conditions such as diabetes mellitus and hypertension, to name a few.[19,24,25] *Healthy People 2020* states that health literacy is an important part of its goal to use strategies in health communications and health information technology (IT) to improve population health outcomes, as well as enhance health care quality and health equity.[12]

In 2004, a pioneer report by the IOM, *Health Literacy*, issued several recommendations to combat low health literacy to include increased research on health literacy, creating other ways by which health literacy can be measured and incorporating health literacy content in our professional programs.[26] Current literature states that health literacy is one of the critical factors contributing to the epidemic of health disparities. Empowering individuals and changing our health care system to meet the needs of our low health literate population are considered paramount in the quest to reduce health disparities. It is difficult for at-risk populations to alter their health behaviors without clear communication that accommodates for the patients' skill level.[25]

HEALTH DISPARITIES: SCOPE OF THE PROBLEM

It has become increasingly evident that underrepresented minorities experience racial disparities in health in the United States. Many initiatives have taken place, but progress has been slow.[27] According to Census 2010 results, the U.S. population has increased from 281.4 million people (Census 2000) to 308.7 million people, a 9.7% increase.[28,29] According to the U.S. Census Bureau, data collected on race and Hispanic origin (Cuban, Mexican, Puerto Rican, South or Central American, or other Spanish culture or origin regardless of race) were based on published guidelines from the U.S. Office of Management and Budget's (OMB) 1997 Revisions to the Standards for the Classification of Federal Data on Race and Ethnicity. Race and Hispanic ethnicity (origin) are considered separate and distinct concepts. Therefore, two separate questions must be asked during data collection regarding self-identification. It should also be noted that individuals have been allowed to self-identify with more than one race since Census 2000. There are 57 possible multiple race combinations.[29]

According to Census 2010, there are 27.3 million more people residing in the United States as of April 1, 2010. Most of this growth was due to an increase in those identifying as Hispanic or Latino. Hispanic Americans constitute the nation's largest minority group (16.3%), black or African American (12.6%), American Indian and Alaska Native (0.9%), Asian (4.8%), Native Hawaiian and Other Pacific Islander (0.2%), Some Other Race (6.2%), and Two or More Races (2.9%). Although issues have been raised regarding the factors that influence the reporting of race (overestimation of Two

TABLE 39-4 **Census 2010**

Race	Number	% of Total Population	% Change 2000 to 2010
Total population	308,745,538	100.0	9.7
White	223,553,265	72.4	5.7
Hispanic or Latino	50,477,594	16.3	43.0
Black or African American	38,929,319	12.6	12.3
American Indian and Alaska Native	2,932,248	0.9	18.4
Asian	14,674,252	4.8	43.3
Native Hawaiian and Other Pacific Islander	540,013	0.2	35.4
Some Other Race	19,107,368	6.2	24.4
Two or More Races	9,009,073	2.9	32.0

or More Races, which involved Some Other Race category in Census 2000), it is noteworthy that the great majority of the U.S. population reported only one race during Census 2010, and those data are more comparable (Table 39-4).

These disproportionate groups are expected to continue to grow as a proportion of the total U.S. population; therefore, the future health of America as a whole will be substantially influenced by our success in improving the gaps in health of these groups. The reduction, and ultimately, elimination of health disparities is a major goal in the United States, with race and ethnicity being of major focus.[8,12,15]

The 2005 report titled *The Commission to End Health Care Disparities* states, "Racial and ethnic disparities pose moral and ethical dilemmas that are among the most significant challenges of today's rapidly changing health care system." When compared with whites, minority groups have higher incidences of chronic diseases, higher mortality, and poorer health outcomes.[30] In its 5-year summary report (2010), the commission states they have noted some growth and established awareness of the need to eliminate racial and ethnic disparities in health care. They continue to remain optimistic of a health care system that provides effective, high-quality medical care for all Americans. Toward that effort the commission set forth provider awareness and education, data collection, quality improvement, policy and advocacy, and workforce diversity as priorities for its strategic objectives for 2009-2011.[31]

In its *Racial and Ethnic Disparities in Health Care Updated 2010* report, the American College of Physicians (ACP) reverberate the literature regarding the poorer health status of minorities in the United States as compared with white Americans. They also reiterate much of the new literature that calls for structural changes within America's health care system to meet the needs of America's multicultural population and recognize the critical role of social determinants of health status and their contributions to health disparities. Residential segregation, lack of equal access to quality education, and obstacles to economic opportunity are equally important in determining one's health status. The ACP report suggests the most significant variable influencing health disparities is insurance status. Insured Americans are more likely to have access to health care. It is well established that minorities are less likely to have insurance, even when adjusting for work status. Lack of insurance affects an individual's ability to participate in preventive health care measures, as well as manage chronic disease states. It is estimated that almost 32% of Native Americans/Alaskan Natives are uninsured, with 31% of Hispanics uninsured, compared with roughly 11% of whites uninsured. Minorities receiving dual coverage from both Medicare and Medicaid may be vexed by variations in federal and state spending and policy choices. Of those minorities enrolled in federal and state programs such as Medicaid and Children's Health Insurance Program (CHIP), more are eligible for coverage but are not enrolled (e.g., lack of awareness, language barriers, complex enrollment process). Within those uninsured, racial and ethnic minorities are still less likely to have equal access to health care.[32]

Those with ESL often receive poorer quality of care and have worse access to care than those fluent in English. This barrier to effective health care was highlighted in the 2002 IOM report and has worsened in some ethnic groups. Unfortunately, legislation requiring the use of interpreters for patients with limited English proficiency is loosely enforced, resulting in significant barriers of communication between the patient and physician.[8,32]

Among some minority groups (Hispanic, African American, and Asian), there exists an element of mistrust of the health care provider. Evidence also shows that these minority groups express feeling less respect from their physicians than white patients. Although ongoing, cultural competency training in professional programs is promising as an effective strategy to enhance the minority patient-provider relationship.[32]

The fragmented, disorganized health care system in America contributes significantly to health disparities among minorities. Quality of care is often suboptimal. For those residing in communities of color, typically there are fewer health care workers per person. Studies document that minority patients are often more comfortable with health care providers of similar race/ethnicity. But these providers are overworked and underpaid as compared with white physicians. Furthermore, African Americans are far more likely to use an emergency department, community health clinic, or hospital as their routine source of health care.[32]

According to AHRQ's *2008 National Healthcare Disparities* report, African Americans are more likely to experience inadequate provider-patient communication than white patients and are less likely to receive patient education on exercise and preventive measures against acute myocardial infarction. Compared with white Americans, Native Americans and Alaskan Natives are not screened for colorectal cancer as often, whereas Asian Americans are not appropriately hospitalized as often for pneumonia as white Americans. Finally, African Americans fared significantly worse on 19 of 38 core quality-of-care measures in the 2008 report.[33] The 2010 AHRQ combines data from both the *National Healthcare Quality Report* and the *National Healthcare Disparities Report.* The report highlights four themes as it relates to health care disparities, expands its report to include data from urban versus rural areas, and summarizes information on eight national priorities identified by the IOM Committee:

- Minorities and low-income groups continue to experience suboptimal health care quality and access to health care.
- Although quality of care seems to be improving for minority groups, access and health disparities are not improving.
- Urgent improvements are necessary in such areas as cancer screening, diabetes management, inner-city and rural health care, preventive services, access to care, and disparities based on geography (central United States).
- Finally, progress has been found to be lagging in several areas such as population health, safety, and access. Other priority areas such as health system infrastructure, overuse, and care coordination require more research. However, AHRQ's 2010 report concludes that all eight priority areas reveal disparities related to race, ethnicity, and socioeconomic status.[10]

Orsi, Margellos-Anast, and Whitman conducted a study to evaluate whether the black-white disparity among each of 15 health status indicators had widened, narrowed, or remained the same within a 15-year period both nationally and locally (Chicago). Investigators also evaluated if there was a general shift toward widening, narrowing, or remaining the same, if all 15 indicators were looked at together for both the United States and Chicago. This investigation represented a 7-year update to previous reports in the literature,[34-36] which assessed health status indicators among blacks and whites in Chicago and the United States. Their analyses found that even after 15 years of interventions devoted to reducing and eliminating disparities both nationally and locally, health disparities persist and in some areas seem to be getting worse. Compared with non-Hispanic whites, the non-Hispanic black all-cause mortality has widened to 42% by 2005 versus 36% in 1990. There is nearly a 99% higher mortality from breast cancer in non-Hispanic black women from 1990 to 2005. Disparity in mortality from heart disease, the number one killer of Americans, has also increased. In 2005, non-Hispanic blacks were 24.3% more likely to die from heart disease compared with 8.4% in 1990. Although progress is being made, it is slow. The authors conclude the reduction/elimination of health disparities both nationally and locally is more of a myth than fact. Despite its best efforts, America is either stagnant in its efforts or moving in a negative direction. The decline in the national economy may further exacerbate racial disparities in health.[27]

New Research: Reducing and/or Eliminating Racial/Ethnic Disparities in Health

It is unlikely that a single, predominant cause of health and health care disparities exists. Thus, it is unlikely that a single intervention strategy will suffice. It is crucial that future health disparities research moves from prior disease-focused efforts. New literature examines the impact of the social determinants of health and our health service delivery system and their impact on health disparities. The health disparities agenda is expansive and includes continued research and interventions regarding quality of care provided to racial and ethnic minorities; patient/provider interaction or relationship; linguistic and/or cultural competency of providers and organizations serving minority communities; applicability, planning, and implementation of developing e-health technologies in minority communities; and workforce diversity.

Despite research efforts, gaps between racial and ethnic groups persist and appear to be widening. Health disparities began to receive national attention in 1998, with the Racial and Ethnic Health

Disparities Initiative. Since then, there has been extensive literature in this area. *Healthy People 2010* called for focus on federal research and policy interventions. In 2007, Chin and colleagues[37] stated that new research needed to investigate health disparities from a "multifactorial, culturally tailored" viewpoint. Interventions should target the various causes of disparities.[37] What have emerged are new research paradigms integrating theories from both social and behavioral sciences. The latest research combines social, behavioral, clinical, and basic sciences in its understanding of the determinants of health.[2]

The use of community-engaged research (CEnR) is known as an effective research strategy successful in improving health outcomes among minorities. The CEnR approach uses a diversity of approaches that focus on creating a working and learning environment between academic researchers and community stakeholders to include community-partnered participatory research, tribal participatory research, and community-based participatory research (CBPR). These approaches hold promise in the elimination of health disparities because each approach engages community members and community needs assessment in its understanding of health problems within the community. Through focus group sessions, community involvement allows investigators to ask the right questions and choose appropriate outcome measures. The result is methodologically sound research allowing for the design and implementation of multilevel interventions that are realistic for the target population (e.g., California Breast Cancer Research Program, 2010).[4]

A midcourse review of *Healthy People 2010* found little success had been made toward reducing health disparities in the United States. The prevalence of hypertension, a major risk factor for coronary heart disease, stroke, kidney disease, and heart failure, approaches 40% greater risk in African Americans than whites. Asian/Pacific Islander men and women experience liver cancer at three times the rate of non-Hispanic whites. In recognition of these despairing results, the Federal Collaboration on Health Disparities Research (FCHDR) formed in 2006 believed that an integrated, coordinated approach to the elimination of health disparities was lacking. The FCHDR noted much of the previous research on health disparities was conducted by various agencies under the umbrella of the Department of Health and Human Services (DHHS). However, by use of a wide range of federal departments and agencies, the FCHDR has created a transdisciplinary, systems-thinking approach to investigate the multifaceted and complicated factors that contribute to health disparities. The overarching goal is the reduction and ultimately elimination of health disparities. Perhaps with a closing of the gap between health and health care, health equity can be achieved. The strength and uniqueness of FCHDR is multifarious: (1) be able to connect both federal and nonfederal partners, (2) manipulate limited funding and resources, (3) integrate research with practice, (4) promote effectiveness and efficiency, and (5) create new multiagency approaches that bridge different perspectives, extensive experience, and subject matter expertise on health disparities. This unique approach will allow FCHDR to disseminate and implement new findings on health disparities on a much larger scale for minorities and others. Like the CeNR approach, members from the community that represent the affected population are included as a viable component of FCHDR research initiatives and interventions.[3]

Addressing health disparities as a public health goal emerges as a strong stimulus for a new approach to closing the health care gap experienced by minority populations. The public health approach chooses to look at population-level determinants of health outcomes rather than individual health outcomes, in part, because population characteristics affect health outcomes independent of individual characteristics. The Centers for Population Health and Health Disparities (CPHHDs) was established in 2002. Eight such agencies were launched in 2003, to explore the determinants of health disparities and develop and conduct multilevel, transdisciplinary research combining population, social, behavioral, clinical, and biologic theory and methods. Several investigations are under way. Researchers at Ohio State University are conducting a case-control study to examine the impact of social, behavioral, and biologic factors and the increased risk of developing cervical abnormalities among Appalachian women. Investigators at the University of Texas Medical Branch in Galveston are linking social, geographic, behavioral, and biologic data to understand the impact that stress has on the health of Hispanics. Early results suggest socioeconomic status and ethnic disparities in stress and health are consistent across psychosocial and biologic analyses.[17]

The medical profession must serve as a catalyst to improve health care not just for minority populations but all Americans. PAs can play a pivotal role in this agenda and in expanding access to quality medical care for all individuals. The American Academy of Physician Assistants (AAPA) is an active partner in national campaigns to improve patient care and help in the cause to eliminate health disparities. One such effort in this national campaign was the selection of health disparities as the Host City Prevention Campaign (HCPC) at the AAPA Annual Conference in San Francisco in 2006. More recently, in his candidacy speech as president-elect in March 2010, Robert Wooten, PA-C, referred to The Heads Up Project, created by the AAPA Committee on Diversity as an excellent educational tool that PAs can use to help raise awareness about health disparities. PAs can also use Heads Up to enhance their abilities to identify and eliminate these disparities. You will also find valuable literature resources on the elimination of health disparities in the *Journal of the American Academy of Physician Assistants*.

Finally, recent health care reforms may provide timely opportunities to create a more equitable health care system and have a powerful, positive impact on health disparities. Although not scheduled for enactment until 2014, Fiscella presents research investigating health care reform provisions within six domains:

1. *Access related to insurance coverage and costs*: Via expanded coverage for up to 32 million uninsured Americans, reducing the cost barriers and stigma associated with mental health, and eliminating co-payments for evidence-based preventive care.
2. *Strengthening primary care*: Via improving payment reform for physicians, eliminating Medicare-Medicaid payment differences, and providing financial incentives for providers to work in shortage areas, to include state-operated health insurance exchanges.
3. *Improvements in health information technology*: Improvement in health information technology for both providers and patients.
4. *Changes in physician payment*: Consider payment based on value versus volume and bundling payments but monitoring this impact on those residing in underserved areas.
5. *Adoption of a national health care quality strategy*: Integrate multiple elements of health reform with improved accountability for programs serving underserved populations.
6. *Improved monitoring of health care disparities and accountability*: Improved detection of disparities, which translates to best practices, and holding federally sponsored programs that research health disparities accountable for progress in implementing interventions, which propel forward efforts to reduce and/or eliminate health disparities (Table 39-5).[38]

TABLE 39-5 Eliminating Health and Health Care Disparities

- Define and describe issues related to health care disparities.
- Define the role of low health literacy and health disparities.
- Identify areas of strengths, gaps, opportunities, and priorities to address low health literacy and health care disparities in research and intervention development.
- Facilitate the adoption and implementation of new transdisciplinary, community, and public health disparity research, and evaluate their impact on the reduction of health care disparities.
- Evaluate the impact of health care reform on health disparities and the creation of an equitable health care system.
- Ensure unbiased access to continuous quality health care by culturally competent health care providers.

CLINICAL APPLICATIONS

- Choose a health disparity and describe how a transdisciplinary, collaborative, or public health research project could address the health disparity. What would a potential intervention look like?
- Describe how low health literacy directly affects health disparities.
- Contact your local Public Health Department and determine what the health disparities are for your region. What type of innovative approaches might you use to help in reducing or eliminating the disparities in your area?

KEY POINTS

- Despite decades of improvements in preventive health care services and declines in disease mortality, health disparities persist in the United States. Efforts toward reducing and/or eliminating health disparities have been slow and resulted in minimum progress.
- Numerous definitions of health disparities exist. The Institute of Medicine in 2002 defined health disparities as differences in the incidence, prevalence, mortality, and burden of disease and other adverse health conditions that exist among specific population groups in the United States.

- *Healthy People 2020* emphasizes that "disparities" refers to more than race/ethnicity. Current research echoes the importance of the social determinants of health (e.g., gender, sexual identity, age, disability, socioeconomic status, geographic location, language, education, disability) and their impact on health disparities.
- Strong evidence indicates a correlation between low health literacy and health disparities among minority groups. Individuals with low health literacy experience decreased health knowledge, poor self-management skills, increased hospitalization rates, inferior physical and mental health, and increased health care costs and mortality.
- New research approaches to investigating and designing interventions that target health disparities are focusing on transdisciplinary, community-engaged, public health, and collaborative designs.

References

1. Ramos E, Rotimi C. The A's, G's, C's, and T's of health disparities. BMC Med Genomics 2009;2:29, *http://www.biomedcentral.com*; Accessed July 18, 2011.
2. Dankwa-Mullan I, Rhee KB, Williams K, et al. The science of eliminating health disparities: summary and analysis of the NIH Summit recommendations. Am J Public Health 2010;100 (Suppl. 1):S12.
3. Rashid JR, et al. Eliminating health disparities through transdisciplinary research, cross-agency collaboration, and public participation. Am J Public Health 2009;99:1955.
4. Gehlert S, Coleman R. Using community-based participatory research to ameliorate cancer disparities. Health Soc Work 2010;35:302.
5. Errickson SP, Alvarez M, Forquera R, et al. What will health-care reform mean for minority health disparities? Public Health Rep 2011;126:170.
6. Patient Protection and Affordable Care Act. Public Law No.111–148 (2010).
7. Parker RM, Wolf MS, Kirsch I. Preparing for an epidemic of limited health literacy: weathering the perfect storm. J Gen Intern Med 2008;23:1273.
8. Institute of Medicine. Unequal Treatment: Confronting Racial and Ethnic Disparities in Healthcare. Washington, D.C. The National Academies Press 2002, p. 552.
9. Centers for Disease Control (CDC). Report on the Secretary's Task Force on Black and Minority Health. MMWR Morb Mortal Wkly Rep 1986;35:109.
10. Agency for Healthcare Research and Quality.2011 National Healthcare Disparities Report. *http://www.ahrq.gov/qual/nhqr11.pdf*; Accessed on August 1, 2012.
11. Rohrs RC. Eliminating health disparities—an opportunity, and an obligation. J Am Acad Phys Assist 2006;19:14.
12. U.S. Department of Health and Human Services. Healthy People 2020. *http://www.healthypeople.gov/2020/about/disparitiesAbout.aspx*; Accessed July 26, 2011.
13. U.S. Department of Health and Human Services. National Institutes of Health. NIH-Health Disparities Definition. *http://www.nida.nih.gov*; Accessed July 20, 2011.
14. Braveman PA. Health disparities and health equity: concepts and measurement. Ann Rev Public Health 2006;27:18. 1.
15. Frieden TR. Centers for Disease Control and Prevention. CDC Health Disparities and Inequalities Report—United States, 2011. MMWR Morb Mortal Wkly Rep 2011;60(Suppl):1.
16. Satcher D, Higginbotham EJ. The public health approach to eliminating disparities in health. Am J Public Health 2008;98:400.
17. Warnecke RB, Oh A, Breen N, et al. Approaching health disparities from a population perspective: the National Institutes of Health Centers for Population Health and Health Disparities. Am J Public Health 2008;98:1608.
18. Parker RM, Kindig DA. Beyond the Institute of Medicine Literacy Report: are recommendations being taken seriously? J Gen Intern Med 2006;21:891.
19. Suellentrop K, Morrow B, Williams L, D'Angelo D. Centers for Disease Control and Prevention (CDC). U.S. Department of Health and Human Services. (2000). *Healthy People 2010*, 2nd ed. [with Understanding and Improving Health (vol. 1) and Objectives for Improving Health (vol. 2)]. Washington, D.C: U.S. Government Printing Office.
20. Yin HS, Johnson M, Mendelsohn AL, et al. The health literacy of parents in the United States: a nationally representative study. Pediatrics 2009;124:289.
21. Kirsch I, Jungeblut A, Jenkins L. Adult literacy in America: a first look at the results of the National Adult Literacy Survey. Washington, D.C: United States Department of Education; 1993.
22. Kutner M, Greenberg E, Baer J. A first look at the literacy of America's adults in the 21st century (NCES 2006-470). U.S. Department of Education. Washington, D.C. National Center for Education Statistics, 2005.
23. Wolf MS, Gazmararian JA, Baker DW. Health literacy and functional health status among older adults. Arch Intern Med 2005;165:1946.
24. U.S. Department of Health and Human Services. Office of Disease Prevention and Health Promotion. National Action Plan to Improve Health Literacy. Washington, D.C. Author, 2010.
25. von Wagner C, Steptoe A, Wolf MS, Wardle J. Health literacy and health actions: a review and a framework from health psychology. Health Educ Behav 2009;36:860.
26. Institute of Medicine. Health Literacy: A Prescription to End Confusion. In: Nielsen-Bohlman I, Panzer A, Kindig DA (eds). Washington, D.C. National Academies Press, 2004.
27. Orsi JM, Margellos-Anast H, Whitman S. Black-white health disparities in the United States and Chicago: a 15-year progress analysis. Am J Public Health 2010;100:349.
28. U.S. Census 2000 (website). *http://www.census.gov*; Accessed July 27, 2011.
29. U.S. Census 2010 (website). *http://www.census.gov*; Accessed July 27, 2011.
30. Commission to End Health Care Disparities (website). *www.ama~assn.org/go/enddisparities;* Accessed July 22, 2011.
31. Commission to End Health Care Disparities: five-year summary (website). *www.ama-assn.org/ama1/pub/upload/mm/433/cehcd-five-year-summary.pdf*; Accessed August 1, 2011.

32. American College of Physicians. Racial and Ethnic Disparities in Health Care, Updated 2010. American College of Physicians; 2010: Policy Paper. *http://www.ama-assn.org/resources/doc/public-health/acp-disparities-health-care.pdf*; Accessed August 1, 2011.
33. Agency for Healthcare Research and Quality. 2007 National Healthcare Disparities Report-At-a-Glance. Rockville, MD; February 2008. *http://www.ahrq.gov/qual/nhdr07/glance.htm*; Accessed July 28, 2011.
34. Department of Health and Human Services. Office of Minority Health. Eliminating racial and ethnic health disparities. *http://minorityhealth.hhs.gov/templates*; Accessed August 1, 2011.
35. Keppel KG, Pearcy JN, Wagener DK. Trends in racial and ethnic-specific rates for the health status indicators: United States, 1990-98. Stat Notes 2002;Jan:1.
36. Margellos H, Silva A, Whiteman S. Comparison of health status indicators in Chicago: are Black-White disparities worsening? 2004;94:116.
37. Chin M, Walters AE, Cook SC. Interventions to reduce racial and ethnic disparities in healthcare. Med Care Res Rev 2007;54(Suppl. 5):7S.
38. Fiscella K. Health care reform and equity: promise, pitfalls, and prescriptions. Ann Fam Med 2011;9:78.

CHAPTER 40

PATIENT SAFETY AND QUALITY OF CARE

Torry Grantham Cobb

CHAPTER CONTENTS

Late January 2001, 18-month-old Josie King turned on the hot water and climbed into a scalding-hot bathtub. She suffered second-degree burns on 60% of her body and was admitted to Johns Hopkins Medical Center. On February 22, 2001, two days before her planned discharge home, Josie's parents held their brain-dead daughter for the last time as she was disconnected from the ventilator. Her death was the result of severe dehydration and a narcotic overdose—a series of medical errors that occurred in one of the best medical centers in the country.[1]

QUALITY CARE MOVEMENT IN AMERICA

In 2000, the Institute of Medicine (IOM) Committee on the Quality of Health Care in America published a landmark report entitled, *To Err Is Human, Building a Safer Health System*.[2] The report cited a study that estimated 98,000 people died every year in U.S. hospitals as a result of medical errors.[3] This is analogous to crashing a jumbo jet every day for a year and killing all the passengers on board. Until this report, the magnitude of the medical error problem in the U.S. health care system was largely unrecognized.

On the basis of these numbers, every 6 months more American lives are lost as a result of medical errors than were lost during the entire Vietnam War. If the Centers for Disease Control and Prevention (CDC) ranked medical errors as a cause of death in the United States, it would rank sixth, higher than the number of deaths due to diabetes, pneumonia, Alzheimer disease, renal disease, and influenza. Furthermore, more people die from medical errors annually than die from motor vehicle crashes, breast cancer, or human immunodeficiency virus/acquired immunodeficiency syndrome.[2] However, public awareness and public efforts for these latter problems are significantly more than for the medical errors that occur in the health care system. Raising awareness of the problems and setting national, state, and local agendas to address the issues has been the focus of the quality care movement.

In addition to the cost in human lives, preventable medical errors have been estimated to result in total costs (additional care, lost income, lost productivity, and disability) of between $17 billion and $29 billion annually.[4] The less quantifiable toll of physical and psychological pain, reduced patient and provider satisfaction and trust, and poorer health status of communities and society are a significant outcome of medical errors as well.

The jumbo jet analogy provides a stirring, concrete image for the magnitude of the death toll. If a jumbo jet were crashing daily in the United States, Americans would not believe it safe to fly, and public outcry would demand that the problems be fixed. The call to action would most likely be tremendous. Unfortunately, the patient safety crisis has not been elevated to the same level of public awareness, much less outrage. Over the past decade however, tremendous strides have been made to investigate the problems and search for solutions.

Determining the Magnitude of the Problem

In 2002, the Agency for Healthcare Research and Quality (AHRQ), in collaboration with the University of California–Stanford Evidence-Based Practice Center, developed a collection of patient safety indicators (PSIs) to screen data for patient safety concerns.[5] These PSIs can be readily identified in hospital discharge data and are deemed potentially preventable patient safety incidents. In 2003, this set of 20 evidence-based PSIs was released to the public to aid in assessing and improving patient safety in hospitals throughout the United States.

A study published in 2004 reviewed patient safety–related incidents from approximately 37 million Medicare patients from 2000 to 2002.[6] Excluding obstetric deaths and extrapolating this to the general public, the researchers estimated that the patient safety incidents resulted in an additional $19 billion in inpatient costs and more than 575,000 preventable deaths in the United States from 2000 to 2002. Table 40-1 summarizes additional findings. Although determining the exact magnitude of the problem is difficult, it is clear that serious problems must be addressed.

Why Errors Occur

Historically, medical errors have been hidden from the public. The IOM reports that "The biggest challenge to moving toward a safer health system is changing the culture from one of blaming individuals for errors to one in which errors are treated not as personal failures, but as opportunities to improve."[7] The modern patient safety movement has replaced the secrecy and "blame and shame" of medical errors with a systems approach used in other high-risk

TABLE 40-1 **Patient Safety in American Hospitals Study Released by HealthGrades**

1. Approximately 1.14 million total patient safety incidents occurred among the 37 million hospitalizations in the Medicare population from 2000-2002.
2. The PSIs with the highest incident rates per 1000 hospitalizations at risk were failure to rescue, decubitus ulcer, and postoperative sepsis. These patient safety incidents accounted for almost 60% of all patient safety incidents among Medicare patients hospitalized from 2000-2002.
3. Of the total 323,993 deaths among patients who experienced one or more PSIs from 2000-2002, 263,864, or 81%, of these deaths were potentially attributable to the patient safety incident(s).
4. Failure to rescue (i.e., failure to diagnose and treat in time) and death in low mortality DRGs (i.e., unexpected death in a low-risk hospitalization) accounted for almost 75% of all mortality attributable to patient safety incidents.
5. Of the remaining 65,972 deaths attributable to the other 14 patient safety indicators (excluding failure to rescue and death in low mortality DRGs), almost 75% were in patients with decubitus ulcer (34,320), postoperative pulmonary embolism, or deep vein thrombosis (8445) or postoperative respiratory failure (6320).
6. There were small variations in PSI incident rates across hospitals and regions.
7. Overall, the Central and Western regions of the United States performed better than the Northeast and Sunbelt.
8. Teaching hospitals and larger hospitals (>200 beds) had slightly higher patient safety incident rates per 1000 as compared with nonteaching hospitals across most PSIs.
9. Patient safety incidents were more prevalent among medical admissions compared with surgical admissions.
10. Overall, the best performing hospitals (hospitals that had the lowest overall PSI incident rates of all hospitals studied, defined as the top 7.5% of all hospitals studied) had 5 fewer deaths per 1000 hospitalizations compared with the bottom 10th percentile of hospitals. This significant mortality difference is attributable to fewer patient safety incidents at the best performing hospitals. Fewer patient safety incidents in the best performing hospitals resulted in a lower cost of $740,337 per 1000 hospitalizations as compared with the bottom 10th percentile of hospitals.
11. The 16 PSIs studied accounted for $8.54 billion in excess inpatient cost to the Medicare system over 3 years, or roughly $2.85 billion annually. Decubitus ulcers ($2.57 billion), postoperative pulmonary embolism or deep vein thrombosis ($1.40 billion), and selected infections due to medical care ($1.71 billion) were the most costly and accounted for 66% of all excess attributable costs from 2000-2002.

From Healthgrades website. *http://www.healthgrades.com/media/english/pdf/HG_Patient_Safety_Study_Final.pdf.* Accessed July 2004.

DRGs, diagnostic-related groups; PSIs, patient safety indicators.

industries such as airlines and nuclear power plants. This paradigm acknowledges humans as fallible and seeks to create strategies to anticipate, prevent, or catch unsafe events before they cause harm. The systems approach for safety in other industries has well-known and proven strategies, but those approaches have not been applied to medicine until recently.

The Swiss cheese model of organizational accidents developed by British psychologist James Reason is a good way to illustrate how medical errors occur (Figure 40-1).[8] Rather than errors being the result of a single incident, they are viewed as multiple layers of fail-safes in which the holes align to produce a medical error. For example, there are several layers of protection for a patient whose provider orders the wrong dosage of a home medication in the hospital. First, the order must be received by the pharmacist and not recognized as an error. Next, the nurse administering the medication must also fail to recognize the dosage error. Finally, the patient would need to accept the error as well. The model seeks ways to shrink the holes in each layer of protection, thus making the alignment less likely and resulting error less likely to occur. It also emphasizes the need to identify the root causes that make the medical errors possible.

Human Mistakes

The overwhelming majority of medical mistakes are not made due to lack of knowledge, training, or information. They are made by honest, hard-working individuals who have demanding and often stressful jobs. They often occur during automatic tasks as unintentional performance lapses in an environment where faulty processes, systems, or conditions fail to catch or prevent the error.[9] The medical profession is often compared with other high-risk occupations whose members must perform under a high degree of stress with a high degree of accuracy. The difference is that medical professionals must combine complex decision-making with customer interactions and automatic behaviors.[9] The training for medical providers has emphasized decision-making with significantly less of a focus on customer interaction and essentially no training in how to manage risky automatic behaviors.

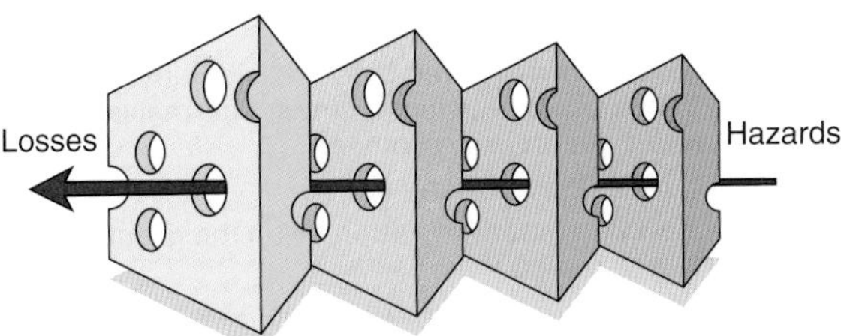

FIGURE 40-1 Swiss cheese model of medical errors. (From BMJ 2000;320:768. *http://www.bmj.com/content/320/7237/768.full.* Accessed on May 24, 2012.)

Safety versus Quality

The IOM defines quality of care as "the degree to which health services for individuals and populations increase the likelihood of desired health outcomes and are consistent with current professional knowledge."[7] In the 2002 report *Crossing the Quality Chasm*, the IOM advanced six aims for providing quality health care: patient safety, patient-centered care, effectiveness, timeliness, efficiency, and equitability.[7] Safety is thereby considered a component of quality. Rather than the focus of quality being entirely on practicing evidence-based medicine, the IOM recognizes a broader definition and acknowledges aspects of quality health care provision that are important to patients and society.

TYPES OF MEDICAL ERRORS

In 2001, the former chief executive officer of the National Quality Forum (NQF) coined the term "never event" to identify especially egregious medical errors (such as wrong-site surgery) that should never occur.[10] Since that time, the list of never events has been expanded and grouped into six categories: surgical, product or device, patient protection, care management, environmental, and criminal (Table 40-2).

The Joint Commission has also compiled a list of events that signal the need for immediate investigation. These so-called sentinel events are defined by the Joint Commission as "unexpected occurrence[s] involving death or serious physical or psychological injury, or the risk thereof."[11] Serious injury is further defined as including the "loss of limb or function," and the phrase "or the risk thereof" includes any actions or events that would increase the risk of a serious adverse outcome if it occurred again.[11]

Sentinel events also include the following:

- Infant abduction or discharge to the wrong family
- Unexpected death of a full-term infant
- Severe neonatal jaundice (bilirubin >30 mg/dL)
- Surgery on the wrong individual or wrong body part
- Surgical instrument or object left in a patient after surgery or another procedure
- Rape in a continuous care setting
- Suicide in a continuous care setting, or within 72 hours of discharge

- Hemolytic transfusion reaction due to blood group incompatibilities
- Radiation therapy to the wrong body region or 25% above the planned dose[11]

The Joint Commission's top 10 most frequently reported sentinel events from 1995 to 2010 were as follows:

- Unintended retention of foreign body
- Delay in treatment
- Wrong patient, wrong site, wrong procedure
- Operative/postoperative complication
- Suicide
- Patient fall
- Medical error
- Other unanticipated events
- Perinatal death or injury
- Criminal events[12]

The Joint Commission makes a point that the terms "sentinel event" and "medical error" are not synonymous. Not all medical errors result in sentinel events, and not all sentinel events are the result of medical errors.

Medication Errors (Figure 40-2)

Medication errors account for more than 770,000 injuries and deaths each year.[13-15] This results in an estimated $5 billion in additional costs for the

TABLE 40-2 **National Quality Forum's Health Care "Never Events," 2006**

Surgical Events

Surgery performed on the wrong body part

Surgery performed on the wrong patient

Wrong surgical procedure performed on a patient

Unintended retention of a foreign object in a patient after surgery or other procedure

Intraoperative or immediately postoperative death in an American Society of Anesthesiologists Class I patient

Artificial insemination with the wrong sperm or donor egg

Product or Device Events

Patient death or serious disability associated with the use of contaminated drugs, devices, or biologics provided by the health care facility

Patient death or serious disability associated with the use or function of a device in patient care, in which the device is used for functions other than as intended

Patient death or serious disability associated with intravascular air embolism that occurs while being cared for in a health care facility

Patient Protection Events

Infant discharged to the wrong person

Patient death or serious disability associated with patient elopement (disappearance)

Patient suicide, or attempted suicide resulting in serious disability, while being cared for in a health care facility

Care Management Events

Patient death or serious disability associated with a medication error (e.g., errors involving the wrong drug, wrong dose, wrong patient, wrong time, wrong rate, wrong preparation, wrong route of administration)

Patient death or serious disability associated with a hemolytic reaction due to the administration of ABO/HLA-incompatible blood or blood products

Maternal death or serious disability associated with labor or delivery in a low-risk pregnancy while being cared for in a health care facility

Patient death or serious disability associated with hypoglycemia, the onset of which occurs while the patient is being cared for in a health care facility

Death or serious disability (kernicterus) associated with failure to identify and treat hyperbilirubinemia in neonates

Stage 3 or 4 pressure ulcers acquired after admission to a health care facility

Patient death or serious disability due to spinal manipulative therapy

Environmental Events

Patient death or serious disability associated with an electric shock or electrical cardioversion while being cared for in a health care facility

Any incident in which a line designated for oxygen or other gas to be delivered to a patient contains the wrong gas or is contaminated by toxic substances

Patient death or serious disability associated with a burn incurred from any source while being cared for in a health care facility

Patient death or serious disability associated with a fall while being cared for in a health care facility

Patient death or serious disability associated with the use of restraints or bedrails while being cared for in a health care facility

Criminal Events

Any instance of care ordered by or provided by someone impersonating a physician, nurse, pharmacist, or other licensed health care provider

Abduction of a patient of any age

Sexual assault on a patient within or on the grounds of the health care facility

Death or significant injury of a patient or staff member resulting from a physical assault (i.e., battery) that occurs within or on the grounds of the health care facility

ABO/HLA, blood group consisting of groups A, AB, B, and O/human leukocyte antigen.

health care system.[16,17] Common errors related to medication include illegible prescriptions and orders (see Figure 40-1). Fortunately, the advent of electronic medical record systems has made a significant impact.

Other medications problems stem from the lack of standardization and presence of ambiguity in labeling of medications used in hospitals. For example, the epinephrine that is used in medical emergencies for cardiac arrest and anaphylaxis is packaged in the same vial with a similar label but in different concentrations. For anaphylaxis, a lower concentration of the medication should be given intramuscularly, whereas for cardiac arrest, a higher concentration should be given intravenously. Inadvertently, giving the wrong concentration of the medication has led to fatal outcomes.[18] In an effort to decrease the risk of this medical error, some hospitals are stocking prefilled intramuscular dose syringes for anaphylaxis on their crash carts. Efforts used at the development and manufacturing level, such as removing or limiting the number of drugs that look alike or sound alike (e.g., Celebrex and Cerebyx), are approaches that should reduce medical errors.

FIGURE 40-2 Illegible prescription. Can you discern the name of the first medication on this prescription? If you said Plendil, then you agreed with the pharmacist who filled the prescription. Unfortunately, the physician intended for the patient to get Isordil. This error resulted in a fatal overdose for the 42-year-old patient. A jury in Texas attributed the patient's death to the illegible prescription. The physician and the pharmacist each paid $225,000 in compensation to the patient's family. This was the first reported case of medical malpractice due to illegible handwriting. (From Charatan F. Compensation awarded for death after illegible prescription. West J Med 2000;172:80. *http://www.ncbi.nlm.nih.gov/pmc/articles/PMC1070756/*. Accessed May 24, 2012.)

Another strategy designed to reduce medication errors is the ban on the use of certain words and abbreviations when ordering medications. The "do not use" list was developed by the Joint Commission in 2004 during a 1-day summit of representatives from more than 70 professional medical organizations and special interests groups.[19] The goal of the summit was to identify abbreviations, acronyms, and symbols that have the potential to cause errors and propose a method to eliminate or reduce the threat. The result was the official "do not use" list (Table 40-3).

Surgical Errors (Figure 40-3)

The National Quality Forum, a nonprofit organization that sets national priorities and goals for health care quality and safety, lists surgical events as one of the six major categories of "never events."[10] Three of the top 10 sentinel events reported by the Joint Commission from 1995 to 2010 were surgical events (wrong-site surgery, unintended retention of foreign body, and operative/postoperative complications).[11]

To address surgical errors, the Joint Commission developed a universal protocol for preventing wrong-site, wrong-procedure, and wrong-person surgery.[20] Endorsed by more than 40 professional

TABLE 40-3 **Official "Do Not Use" List**

Do Not Use	Potential Problem	Use Instead
U, u (unit)	Mistaken for "0" (zero), the number "4" (four) or "cc"	Write "unit"
IU (International Unit)	Mistaken for IV (intravenous) or the number 10 (ten)	Write "International Unit"
Q.D., QD, q.d., qd (daily)	Mistaken for each other	Write "daily"
Q.O.D., QOD, q.o.d, qod (every other day)	Period after the Q mistaken for "I" and the "O" mistaken for "I"	Write "every other day"
Trailing zero (X.0 mg)	Decimal point is missed	Write X mg
Lack of leading zero (.X mg)		Write 0.X mg
MS	Can mean morphine sulfate or magnesium sulfate	Write "morphine sulfate"
MSO4 and MgSO4	Confused for one another	Write "magnesium sulfate"

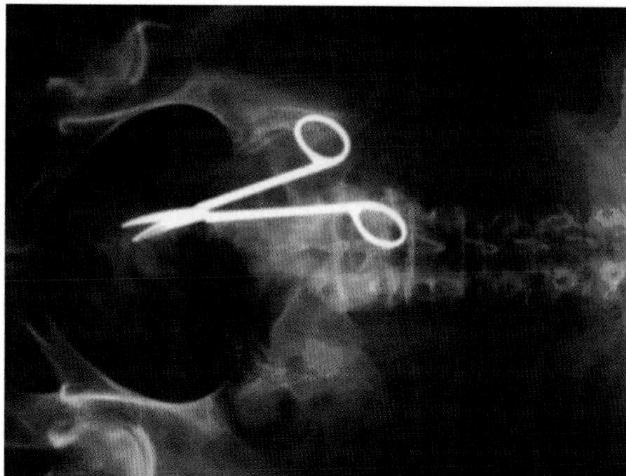

FIGURE 40-3 ■ Retained surgical object. (From *http://www.msnbc.msn.com/id/4788266/ns/health-health_care/t/scissors-left-woman-after-surgery/#.T71khl4yeS0.* Accessed May 23, 2012.)

medical organizations, the protocol mandates active involvement and effective communication among all members of the surgical team. It involves a verification process, marking of the surgical site, and a time-out procedure (Table 40-4).

The unintended retention of foreign objects ranked fourth among the most common sentinel events reported in 2008.[21] Although the exact number cannot be determined, it has been estimated that more than 1500 cases of retained surgical objects (RSO) occur annually.[22] Studies have estimated that needles, sponges, or other surgical objects are inadvertently left in a patient's body once in every 7000 surgical procedures with the estimate for abdominal procedures being as high as 1 in every 1000 to 1500 operations.[23,24] Strategies to prevent unintended retention of foreign objects include manual counting and intraoperative/postoperative radiographs, bar coding sponges and instruments, electronic article surveillance tags, and radiofrequency identification tags.[25]

Transition and Communication Errors

Lack of continuity of care is a well-recognized problem in health care systems. No one can provide around-the-clock coverage, so inevitably patients are cared for by many providers. This discontinuity provides an opportunity for the inaccurate transfer of data and thus increases the risk of medical errors. The Joint Commission reports that up to 80% of serious medical errors occur as a result of miscommunication between providers during transitions of care.[26] In an effort to reduce hand-off errors, the Joint Commission's 2006 National Patient Safety Goals require all health care providers to implement a standardized approach to handing off patients.[27] The mandate contains guidelines for this process, many of which are drawn from other high-risk industries. The following criteria must be met:

- Interactive communications
- Up-to-date and accurate information
- Limited interruptions
- A process for verification
- An opportunity to review any relevant historical data[26]

To further aid in a safe and effective sign-out process, the AHRQ has developed a structured sign-out protocol called **ANTIC**ipate.[27]

TABLE 40-4 **Universal Protocol for Preventing Wrong-Site, Wrong-Procedure, Wrong-Person Surgery**

Preoperative Verification Process

- Purpose: To ensure that all of the relevant documents and studies are available before the start of the procedure and that they have been reviewed and are consistent with each other and with the patient's expectations, as well as with the team's understanding of the intended patient, procedure, site, and, as applicable, any implants. Missing information or discrepancies must be addressed before starting the procedure.
- Process: An ongoing process of information gathering and verification, beginning with the determination to do the procedure, continuing through all settings and interventions involved in the preoperative preparation of the patient, up to and including the "time-out" just before the start of the procedure.

Marking the Operative Site

- Purpose: To identify unambiguously the intended site of incision or insertion.
- Process: For procedures involving right/left distinction, multiple structures (such as fingers and toes), or multiple levels (as in spinal procedures), the intended site must be marked such that the mark will be visible after the patient has been prepped and draped.

"Time-Out" Immediately before Starting the Procedure

- Purpose: To conduct a final verification of the correct patient, procedure, site, and, as applicable, implants.
- Process: Active communication among all members of the surgical/procedure team, consistently initiated by a designated member of the team, conducted in a "fail-safe" mode (i.e., the procedure is not started until any questions or concerns are resolved).

Modified from The Joint Commission. Universal Protocol for Preventing Wrong Site, Wrong Procedure, Wrong Person Surgery. Oakbrook Terrace, IL: The Joint Commission, 2003.

- **A**dministrative data (e.g., patient's name, medical record number, and location) must be accurate.
- **N**ew clinical information must be updated.
- **T**asks to be performed by the covering provider must be clearly explained.
- **I**llness severity must be communicated.
- **C**ontingency plans for changes in clinical status must be outlined, to assist cross-coverage in managing the patient overnight.

A 2005 study of a computerized and structured sign-out process at an academic medical center demonstrated increased efficiency and continuity of care.[28] An investigation of sign-out protocols adapted from Formula 1 auto racing and aviation has also been shown to reduce communication errors.[29]

Traditionally, medical teams have had steep authority gradients. Fear and intimidation prevented others from expressing concerns about patient safety. The patient safety movement however, has focused on teamwork and the leveling of responsibility to make all team members equally responsible for patient safety. A strategy originally developed by the U.S. Navy to improve communication on nuclear submarines, SBAR (situation, background, assessment, recommendation), was introduced into health care settings in 1990.[30] Since then, it has become a widely used tool to effectively communicate between caregivers. The following is an example of a telephone communication using SBAR.

Introduction

- PA Smith, this is Donna Reynolds, RN. I am calling from XYZ Hospital about your patient Janet Hall.

Situation

- Here's the situation: Mrs. Hall is complaining of chest pain and having increasing shortness of breath.

Background

- The supporting background information is that she had a lumbar fusion 2 days ago. About an hour ago she began complaining of chest pain. Her pulse is 122, and her blood pressure is 140/64. Here oxygen saturation was 80% on room air. She appears ashen and has increased work of breathing.

Assessment

- My assessment of the situation is that she may be having a cardiac event or a pulmonary embolism.

Recommendation

- I have started her on oxygen and would like to get a STAT ECG. I recommend that you see her immediately. Do you agree?

TABLE 40-5 Ten Categories of Preventable Hospital-Acquired Conditions

1. Foreign object retained after surgery
2. Air embolism
3. Blood incompatibility
4. Stages III and IV pressure ulcers
5. Falls and trauma
   - Fractures
   - Dislocations
   - Intracranial injuries
   - Crushing injuries
   - Burns
   - Electric shock
6. Manifestations of poor glycemic control
   - Diabetic ketoacidosis
   - Nonketotic hyperosmolar coma
   - Hypoglycemic coma
   - Secondary diabetes with ketoacidosis
   - Secondary diabetes with hyperosmolarity
7. Catheter-associated urinary tract infection (UTI)
8. Vascular catheter-associated infection
9. Surgical site infection following:
   - Coronary artery bypass graft (CABG)—mediastinitis
   - Bariatric surgery
     - Laparoscopic gastric bypass
     - Gastroenterostomy
     - Laparoscopic gastric restrictive surgery
   - Orthopedic procedures
     - Spine
     - Neck
     - Shoulder
     - Elbow
10. Deep vein thrombosis (DVT)/pulmonary embolism (PE)
    - Total knee replacement
    - Hip replacement

Modified from Centers for Medicare and Medicaid CMS Hospital-Acquired Conditions (HAC) and Present on Admission (POA) Indicators (website). *http://www.premierinc.com/quality-safety/tools-services/safety/topics/guidelines/cms-guidelines-4-infection.jsp.* Accessed July 11, 201.

Hospital-Acquired Conditions

The CDC estimates that 1.7 million health care–associated infections occur annually and result in 99,000 deaths.[31] For U.S. hospitals, the added financial burden may exceed $45 billion.[32] To address this problem and other health care–acquired conditions, the Centers for Medicare and Medicaid Services (CMS) initiated a new payment policy for certain hospital-acquired conditions (HACs) in October 2008.[33] The CMS has identified 10 categories of HAC they consider "reasonably preventable" (Table 40-5). As such,

CMS now refuses to pay hospitals for the increased cost of care that results from preventable HACs.[33] Commercial insurance companies are expected to follow suit, thus placing further restrictions on the reimbursement of services that result from preventable HACs.

PATIENT SAFETY STRATEGIES

The Department of Health and Human Services National Strategy for Quality Improvement in Health Care for March 2011 outlines strategies to improve the quality of care, make people healthier, and make health care more affordable. A major component of the quality improvement plan is increased patient safety.[34] The goal is to eliminate preventable health care–acquired conditions, such as infections and medication errors (Table 40-6).

TABLE 40-6 **Examples of Federal Initiatives Making Care Safer**

Michigan Keystone Intensive Care Unit Project: Nearly 1 in every 20 hospitalized patients in the United States each year acquires a health care–associated infection while receiving medical care. Central intravenous line–associated bloodstream infections are among the most deadly types, with a mortality rate of 12% to 25%. In this AHRQ-funded project, a research team at Johns Hopkins University partnered with the Michigan Health and Hospital Association to implement CDC recommendations to reduce central line bloodstream infections in 100 intensive care units throughout the state. The initiative, known as the "Keystone Project," reduced the rate of these central line bloodstream infections by two thirds within 3 mo. Over 18 mo, the program saved more than 1500 lives and nearly $200 million. These dramatic improvements have been sustained for 5 years, and the approach used is now being spread to all 50 states and the District of Columbia. For more information, go to *www.ahrq.gov/about/annualmtg07/0928slides/goeschel/Goeschel.ppt.*

Safe Use Initiative: Today, tens of millions of people in the United States depend on prescription and over-the-counter medications to sustain their health—with as many as 3 billion prescriptions written annually. Too many people, however, suffer unnecessary injuries, and even death, as a result of preventable medication errors. The U.S. Food and Drug Administration (FDA) has launched the Safe Use Initiative to create and facilitate public and private collaborations within the health care community with the goal of reducing this preventable harm. The Safe Use Initiative will identify specific, preventable medication risks and then develop, implement, and evaluate cross-sector interventions to reduce these risks. For more information, go to *http://www.fda.gov/Drugs/DrugSafety/ucm187806.htm.*

Reprinted from Report to Congress: National Strategy for Quality Improvement in Health Care March 2011, *http://www.healthcare.gov/center/reports/quality03212011a.html#s2-1ex.*

AHRQ, Agency for Healthcare Research and Quality; CDC, Centers for Disease Control.

Health Information Technology

Other initiatives designed to make health care safer are electronic medical records and medical informatics. Instant access to patient information and the ease of sharing that information with other providers has improved medical care. The advent of electronic order entry and computerized prescriptions has significantly reduced the number of medication errors.[35]

Role of the Patient

In 2002, the Joint Commission and CMS launched a national campaign advocating that patients assume a larger role in preventing medical errors by becoming active, involved, and informed participants in the health care system.[36] The program, called Speak Up, encourages patients to speak up if they have questions or concerns. The program advocates asking questions when patients and their families do not understand (Table 40-7).

The World Health Organization (WHO) is also leading the way in patient safety efforts. The

TABLE 40-7 **The Joint Commission and CMS Speak Up Initiative**

- **S**peak up if you have questions or concerns. If you still don't understand, ask again. It's your body and you have a right to know.
- **P**ay attention to the care you get. Always make sure you are getting the right treatments and medicines by the right health care professionals. Do not assume anything.
- **E**ducate yourself about your illness. Learn about the medical tests you get and your treatment plan.
- **A**sk a trusted family member or friend to be your advocate (advisor or supporter).
- **K**now what medicines you take and why you take them. Medicine errors are the most common health care mistakes.
- **U**se a hospital, clinic, surgery center, or other type of health care organization that has been carefully checked out. For example, The Joint Commission visits hospitals to see if they are meeting The Joint Commission's quality standards.
- **P**articipate in all decisions about your treatment. You are the center of the health care team.

From *http://www.jointcommission.org/assets/1/18/Facts_about_Speak_Up1.pdf.* Accessed August 25, 2012.

program WHO Patient Safety seeks to coordinate and promote improvements in patient safety worldwide. The WHO Patients for Patient Safety program encourages consumers of health care to become partners with their health care team to make medical care safer.[37]

The American College of Physicians (ACP) also advocates for patients playing a role in their own safety as patients.[38] The ACP summarizes the rights and responsibilities of patients as follows:

At the Appointment

Rights:

- To be an active participant in discussions
- To have understandable, legible instructions and prescriptions
- To have an explanation of why a particular course of treatment is recommended

Responsibilities:

- To be open and honest about symptoms, drugs he or she might be taking, medical history
- To voice concerns
- To speak up if he or she does not understand
- To check back on test results

At the Pharmacy

Rights:

- To receive the correct prescription
- To receive verbal and written information about how to use the drug
- To have information on drug interactions, side effects, and what to do about them

Responsibilities:

- To check the prescription to make sure it is what the doctor ordered
- To remind pharmacists about other drugs or allergies
- To ask questions if necessary

At Home

Right:

- To research his or her condition using the library, Internet tools, etc.

Responsibilities:

- To know the validity of the source of health information
- To verify health information with the physician

Medical Error Disclosure

Since July 2001, the Joint Commission has required disclosure of adverse outcomes.[39]

The Sorry Works! Coalition, founded in 2005, is dedicated to promoting apologies and full disclosure for medical errors.[40] The Sorry Works! Coalition advocates that providers and health care institutions apologize for medical errors (Table 40-8). They believe that apologies combined with up-front compensation serve to reduce the anger felt by patients and their families when errors occur. They also believe that this results in fewer medical malpractice lawsuits and reduced legal costs. The approach is believed to result in expedient justice for victims (Table 40-9). The Sorry Works! Coalition believes that medial errors can be reduced through honesty and full disclosure.

During a 7-year period in which the Lexington Veterans Administration Hospital (VA) practiced the principles set forth by the Sorry Works! Coalition, the average payout for malpractice claims was $16,000 relative to the national average of $98,000. The Lexington VA reported the full disclosure reduced the number of pending lawsuits by half and reduced litigation costs from $65,000 to $35,000 per case, an annual savings of $2 million.[39]

TABLE 40-8 Three-Step Disclosure Process

Sorry Works! is a program that needs to be administered by a team of medical, risk, insurance, and legal professionals within a medical, hospital, or insurance setting.

The Sorry Works! program is predicated on a three-step disclosure process:

- Initial disclosure
- Investigation
- Resolution

Step 1—Initial disclosure is all about empathy and reestablishing trust and communication with patients and families in the immediate aftermath of an adverse event. Providers say "sorry," but no fault is admitted or assigned. Providers take care of the immediate needs of the patient/family (food, lodging, counseling, etc.) and promise a swift and thorough investigation. The goal is to make sure the patient/family never feels abandoned. In the spirit of good customer service, pull the patient or family closer to the providers and institution.

Step 2—Investigation is about learning the truth. Was the standard of care breached or not? We recommend involving outside experts and moving swiftly so that the patient/family does not suspect a cover-up. Stay in close contact with the patient/family throughout the process.

Step 3—Resolution is about sharing the results of the investigation with the patient/family, as well as their legal counsel. If there was a mistake, apologize, admit fault, explain what happened and how it will be prevented in the future, and discuss fair, upfront compensation for the injury or death. If there was no mistake, continue to empathize ("we are sorry this happened"), share the results of investigation (hand over charts and records to patient/family and their legal counsel), and prove your innocence. However, no settlement will be offered and any lawsuit will be contested. Sorry Works! is compassion with a backbone.

From *http://sorryworks.net/threestep.phtml*. Accessed July 8, 2011.

TABLE 40-9 **Sorry Works! Coalition: Five Things Every Provider Should Know about Disclosure**

1. **Disclosure is good for doctors, as well as nurses, hospitals, and insurers.** An enormous and growing body of data is showing that disclosure coupled with apology (when appropriate) actually reduces lawsuits, litigation expenses, and settlements/judgments. The key is anger—disclosure and apology keep a lid on anger, whereas traditional deny-and-defend risk management strategies increase anger felt by patients and families and increase the likelihood of costly litigation.
2. **Five-star customer service, informed consent, and good communication lay the groundwork for successful disclosure.** For disclosure to work, you have to be credible. You also have to begin building positive evidence early in the process. Patients and families want to be treated with respect at all times, and they also want to see doctors and nurses treating each other with respect. Absent these feelings, disclosure after an adverse event might appear to a patient/family as a form of manipulation. "Why is Dr. McGod being nice to me now?" will be the skeptical question rolling around the heads of your patients/families. Also, procedure-specific informed consent will aid in credible disclosure discussions, especially where there was no error. Unfortunately, sending your nurse in 5 minutes before the procedure with a bunch of forms to sign does not count! You have to invest the time and energy upfront.
3. **Empathetic "I'm sorry" immediately after the adverse event.** Doctors should provide an empathetic apology immediately after an adverse event coupled with a promise of an investigation and customer service assistance such as food, lodging, phone calls, transportation, etc. *"I'm so sorry this happened Mrs. Jones, . . . I feel bad for you and your family."* Notice: Doctors should NOT prematurely admit fault or assign blame. Also, do NOT get defensive. Simply say you are sorry the event happened (as you should be!) and that you feel bad for the patient/family, acknowledge their feelings, promise an investigation, and take care or assist with any immediate needs of the patient/family. Show you care! And document the chart accordingly without emotion or speculation. Write down what you said, what you promised, and any questions or comments by the patient/family.
4. **Call somebody!** Call your risk manager, insurance company, defense counsel, etc., immediately after the empathetic apology with the patient/family. Inform this person of the situation and ask for assistance with an investigation that will lead to a resolution of the situation, which may include a real apology (I'm sorry I made a mistake) coupled with fair, upfront compensation (paid for by your insurer) or more empathy if no error occurred.
5. **Train nurses and staff on disclosure!** Nurses and staff must understand their role in disclosure. No, it does not mean that nurses will be apologizing for doctors, but it does mean that nurse and front-line staff should know that it's OK for them to empathize; say "sorry" and stay connected with patients and families after the adverse event. In fact, we want the nurses and staff to take service to a new, higher level with patients/families after an adverse event. We want nurses to be part of our effort to save and restore relationships. This is so important because for far too long nurses have literally been told to "shut up" after an adverse event and are forced to run from their patients and families, making the doctors and hospital look guilty, even if no mistake happened!

CLINICAL APPLICATIONS

1. What is the name of the landmark report published in 2000 that launched the patient safety movement in America?
2. Explain the Swiss cheese model of organizational accidents.
3. What is a sentinel event?
4. What are the top 10 sentinel events as defined by the Joint Commission?
5. What are some of the strategies that have been implemented in the health care system to improve patient safety?

KEY POINTS

- Medical errors occur in every health care setting. The IOM report, rather than laying blame, focused on establishing systems to make processes safer.
- The magnitude of the medical error crisis is difficult to measure but results in significant cost in human lives, lost productivity, and mistrust in the health care system.
- Medical errors are the result of failures in a system that should catch or prevent human errors from occurring.
- A variety of health care agencies are actively involved in projects and programs aimed at improving patient safety.
- Patient sign-outs and handoffs are a significant source of medical errors, accounting for up to 80% of serious medical errors.
- Health information technology is paving the way for improved patient safety.
- Organizations, such as the Sorry Works! Coalition, that advocate for full disclosure for medical errors are reducing litigation costs and promoting honesty in patient safety matters.

References

1. Pronovost P, Vohr E. Safe Patients, Smart Hospitals: How One Doctor's Checklist Can Help Us Change Health Care from the Inside Out. New York: Hudson Street Press, 2010.
2. Kohn L, Corrigan J, Donaldson M, (eds). To Err Is Human: Building a Safer Health System. Washington, DC: Committee on Quality of Health Care in America, Institute of Medicine: National Academy Press, 2000.
3. Brennan TA, Leape LL, Laird NM, et al. Incidence of adverse events and negligence in hospitalized patients. Results of the Harvard Medical Practice Study I. N Engl J Med 1991;324:370.
4. Johnson WG, Brennan TA, BrennanNewhouse JP, et al. The economic consequences of medical injuries. JAMA 1992;267:2487.
5. Department of Health and Human Services Agency for Healthcare Research and Quality. March 2003, Revision 2 (October 22, 2004). AHRQ Pub. No. 03–R203 (website). *http://www.qualityindicators.ahrq.gov*; Accessed June 10, 2011.
6. HealthGrades 2004. Patient Safety in American Hospitals (website). *http://www.healthgrades.com/media/english/pdf/HG_Patient_Safety_Study_Final.pdf*; Accessed June 10, 2011.
7. Institute of Medicine. Crossing the Quality Chasm: a New Health System for the 21st Century. Washington, D.C.: National Academy Press; 2001.
8. Reason JT. Human Error. New York: Cambridge University Press; 1990.
9. Wachter RM. Understanding Patient Safety. New York: McGraw-Hill; 2008.
10. National Quality Forum. Serious reportable events in healthcare 2006 update (website). *http://www.qualityforum.org/Publications/2007/03/Serious_Reportable_Events_in_Healthcare%E2%80%932006_Update.aspx*; Accessed June 12, 2011.
11. Joint Commission. Sentinel Event 2011 (website). *http://www.jointcommission.org/sentinel_event.aspx*; Accessed June 14, 2011.
12. Joint Commission. 2011 Sentinel Event Trends Reported by year. *http://www.jointcommission.org/Sentinel_Event_Trends_Reported_by_Year/*; Accessed June 14, 2011.
13. Classen DC, Pestotnik SL, Evans RS, et al. Adverse drug events in hospitalized patients. JAMA 1997;277:301.
14. Cullen DJ, Sweitzer BJ, Bates DW, et al. Preventable adverse drug events in hospitalized patients: a comparative study of intensive care and general care units. Crit Care Med 1997;25:1289.
15. Cullen DJ, Bates DW, Small SD, et al. The incident reporting system does not detect adverse drug events: a problem for quality improvement. J Qual Improve 1995;21:541.
16. Bates DW, Spell N, Cullen DJ, et al. The costs of adverse drug events in hospitalized patients. JAMA 1997;277:307.
17. Bates DW, Cullen DJ, Laird N, et al. Incidence of adverse drug events and potential adverse drug events. JAMA 1995;274:29.
18. Kanwar M, Irvin CB, Frank JJ, et al. Confusion about epinephrine dosing leading to iatrogenic overdose: a life-threatening problem with a potential solution. Ann Emerg Med 2010;55:341.
19. Joint Commission. 2010 Facts about the Official "Do Not Use" List (website). *http://www.jointcommission.org/assets/1/18/Official_Do%20Not%20Use_List_%206_10.pdf*
20. Joint Commission. 2011 Facts about the Universal Protocol (website). *http://www.jointcommission.org/assets/1/18/Universal%20Protocol%201%204%2011.PDF*
21. Joint Commission on the Accreditation of Healthcare Organizations. 2008 top 10 sentinel events by type (website). *http://www.jointcommission.org/NR/rdonlyres/67297896-4E16-4BB7-BF0F-5DA4A87B02F2/0/se_stats_trends_year.pdf*; Accessed June 20, 2011.
22. Gawande A, Studdert DM, Orav EJ, et al. Risk factors for retained instruments and sponges after surgery. N Engl J Med 2003;348:229.
23. Egorova N, Moskowitz A, Gelijns A, et al. Managing the prevention of retained surgical instruments: what is the value of counting? Ann Surg 2008;247:13.
24. Allen G. Evidence for practice. AORN J 2008;87:833.
25. Cobb TG. Iatrogenic retention of surgical objects: risk factors and prevention strategies. J Am Acad Phys Assist 2010;23:33.
26. Joint Commission Center for Transforming Healthcare. 2011 Facts about hand-off communications. *http://www.centerfortransforminghealthcare.org/projects/about_handoff_communication.aspx*; Accessed June 2, 2011.
27. Department of Health & Human Services Agency for Healthcare Research and Quality Patient Safety Network. Handoffs and signouts. *http://psnet.ahrq.gov/primer.aspx?primerID=9*; Accessed June 20, 2011.
28. Van Eaton EG, Horvath KD, Lober WB, et al. A randomized, controlled trial evaluating the impact of a computerized rounding and sign-out system on continuity of care and resident work hours. J Am Coll Surg 2005;200:538.
29. Catchpole KR, de Leval MR, McEwan A, et al. Patient handover from surgery to intensive care: using Formula 1 pit-stop and aviation models to improve safety and quality. Paediatr Anaesth 2007;17:470.
30. Hohenhaus S, Powell S, Hohenhaus JT. Enhancing patient safety during hand-offs: standardized communication and teamwork using the 'SBAR' method. Am J Nurs 2006;106:72A.
31. Centers of Disease Control and Prevention. Preventing healthcare-associated infections. Retrieved from *http://www.cdc.gov/washington/cdcatWork/pdf/infections.pdf*; Accessed June 25, 2011.
32. Scott, RD. The Direct Costs of Healthcare-Associated Infections in U.S. Hospitals and the Benefits of Prevention. 2009 Centers for Disease Control and Prevention Report (website). *http://www.cdc.gov/ncidod/dhqp/pdf/Scott_CostPaper.pdf*; Accessed June 25, 2011.
33. Centers for Medicare and Medicaid Services. Eliminating serious, preventable, and costly medical errors—never events (website). *http://www.cms.hhs.gov/apps/media/press/release.asp?Counter=1863*; Accessed June25, 2011.
34. Report to Congress: National Strategy for Quality Improvement in Health Care March 2011 (website). *http://www.healthcare.gov/center/reports/quality03212011a.html#s2-1ex*; Accessed June 25, 2011.
35. Anderson JG, Jay SJ, Anderson M, Hunt TJ. Evaluating the impact of information technology on medication errors: a simulation. J Am Med Inform Assoc 2003;10:292.
36. Joint Commission. 2011 Facts about Speak Up™ Initiatives. *http://www.jointcommission.org/facts_about_speak_up_initiatives/*; Accessed June 25, 2011.
37. World Health Organization. 2011 Patient Safety. *http://www.who.int/patientsafety/patients_for_patient/en/*; Accessed June 25, 2011.
38. American College of Physicians. The Role of the Patient in PatientSafety.*http://www.acponline.org/running_practice/patient_care/safety/patient.htm*. Accessed June 25, 2011.
39. Wojcieszak D, Banja J, Houk C. The Sorry Works! Coalition: Making the case for full disclosure. Joint Commission Forum 2006;32(6).
40. Sorry Works! Coalition. About Sorry Works! Coalition. *http://www.sorryworks.net/about.phtml*; Accessed July 2, 2011.

The resources for this chapter can be found at www.expertconsult.com.

CHAPTER 41

Population-Based Health

Theresa V. Horvath • Harry Pomeranz

CHAPTER CONTENTS

Population-based medicine is the approach to patient care that involves the family and community in the treatment of individual patients. By considering the environmental, occupational, and social context of disease and by integrating health promotion and preventive measures into routine health care, health disparities are reduced and costs diminished.[1] A population-based approach also improves adherence to national treatment guidelines, promotes the application of evidence-based approaches, and improves the utilization of resources. It further improves the health outcomes of those with the greatest need for care because of chronic disease and confounding features such as poverty or disability.

Although there is no consensus on precisely what constitutes "population health," Nash and colleagues[2] define it as "the distribution of health outcomes within a population, the health determinants that influence distribution and the policies and interventions that impact the determinants." Members of a population share risk factors, designated by characteristics such as age, gender, disease state, social status, ethnicity, or geographic location. By identifying the characteristics of those at greatest risk for morbidity and mortality and implementing strategies to curtail those risks, the need for tertiary-level care is reduced. Chronic diseases are an important focus of population-based preventative measures due to the social and economic burden they engender. Because more than 133 million people currently have chronic disease, and that number is expected to increase over the next decade by 15%, health policies that affect the amount and distribution chronic disease can best cut health care costs nationwide.[2,3]

Lastly, population-based practice is driven by the ideal of health justice. Health justice is the recognition that the burden of disease, disability, and death is unequally distributed across groups of people, and that those with the most severe disease often have less access to care. The quest to rationally distribute financial and human resources to those most at need is at the heart of population-based health care.

HISTORY

The need to practice population-based medicine was identified more than a century ago by Abraham Flexner in his ground-breaking study of medical education in the United States. As early as 1910, Flexner saw that the needs of national health care delivery had outgrown the traditional model of medical practice that focused solely on the individual.[4] In his study, Flexner wrote that the traditional model was "remedial" and that treating patients in isolation of the community in which they live was inadequate. Instead, he advocated for an approach that would incorporate social and preventive elements of care.

In 1961, Kerr White's "The Ecology of Medical Care" provided a second important argument for a population-based approach. White's model developed a visual paradigm of a population whereby the proportion of patients at each level of care was represented as a nested box. This schematic presented both the relative numbers of patients at each level and the interrelation of each level to the entire population. Kerr and his colleagues[5] were the first to define other key concepts in population-based medicine such as "primary medical care" and "health statistics and epidemiology."

The most important change in the thinking about the population-based provision of health care in the United States began in 1979 with then Surgeon General Julius B. Richmond's *Healthy People: the Surgeon General's Report on Health Promotion and Disease Prevention*. This report proposed that the U.S. Department of Health and Human Services (HHS) set an agenda for improving the health of the nation. This challenge was met, and in 1990 the first *Healthy People*, a comprehensive set of health care objectives, was published. Revised *Healthy People* agendas have been developed for every decade since, each incrementally more detailed than its predecessor. For instance, *Healthy People 2000* contained 15 topics and 226 objectives, whereas *Healthy People 2020* listed 42 topics and almost 600 objectives.[6] This increase is due to the growing awareness of the impact of social and environmental factors, as well as the role that social inequality plays in population health. The specific objectives of *Healthy People 2020* are further discussed in a later subsection.

WHAT IS POPULATION-BASED MEDICINE?

Population-based medicine is both an approach to medical care and a field of study.[2] As a medical approach, it addresses the needs of groups of people that share common demographic features, risk factors or diseases.[1,7] It is practiced in both clinical and community settings and aims to reduce disparities in the distribution of acute disease, as well as prevent or slow the progression of chronic disease. The shift from the traditional model of health care to the focus on populations does not replace the one-to-one clinician-patient relationship, but rather considers the role of health care systems, health policy, patient education and interdisciplinary care for those with preventable illness or complications.

As a field of study, the three major components of health determinants, patient outcomes and health policy, are impacted through the overall goals of population-based medicine, which are fourfold[1,8]:

1. **Reduce need** through implementing preventive measures
2. **Reduce demand** through health education and decision-making assistance
3. **Reduce overuse and underuse of resources** through efficient office management systems and better communication with patients
4. **Increase delivery** of health promotion and disease prevention strategies through evidence-based guidelines, good quality improvement activities, and collaboration with public health systems.

These goals are operationalized through four "pillars" of population-based practice: chronic care management, quality and safety, health policy, and public health (Figure 41-1).[2] Although participation in the health policy and public health realms require specialized training, clinically practicing physician assistants play an important role as members of the interdisciplinary teams that deliver chronic care management and often in the teams that ensure quality and safety. Interdisciplinary medical teams are at the root of population-based care because a coordinated approach can best deliver care that includes medical, psychosocial, and community factors that contribute to illness. The interdisciplinary team also makes better use of subspecialty medicine because the most effective health care management avoids repetition of care, inappropriate care, or ineffectual care. The use of evidence-based guidelines provides the best strategy for prioritizing resources and ensuring that the largest numbers of at-risk individuals receive preventive care.

PAs also join teams that create patient-centered medical homes (PCMHs). The patient-centered medical home is a practice modality that emerged in response to the need for primary care that included the coordination of psychosocial and disease management services. PCMHs use evidence-based guidelines to promote prevention strategies including patient self-care and behavior change.[9] They work on the principle that the most effective care is delivered when patients develop an ongoing relationship with a personal clinician, who is able to address all aspects of care throughout the life cycle. Care within a PCMH is accessible, affordable, and integrated within the patient's community.[2] Within the four pillars scheme, prevention is a driver of health for chronic care management, quality and safety, and public health. Preventive medicine occurs at three levels: primary, secondary, and tertiary prevention.

Primary prevention targets an at-risk healthy population to prevent the acquisition of a specific condition. Examples include wide-scale immunization campaigns to prevent or eradicate infectious disease, laws concerning helmet or seat belt use, and national advertising campaigns to prevent fetal alcohol syndrome or illness due to second-hand smoke.

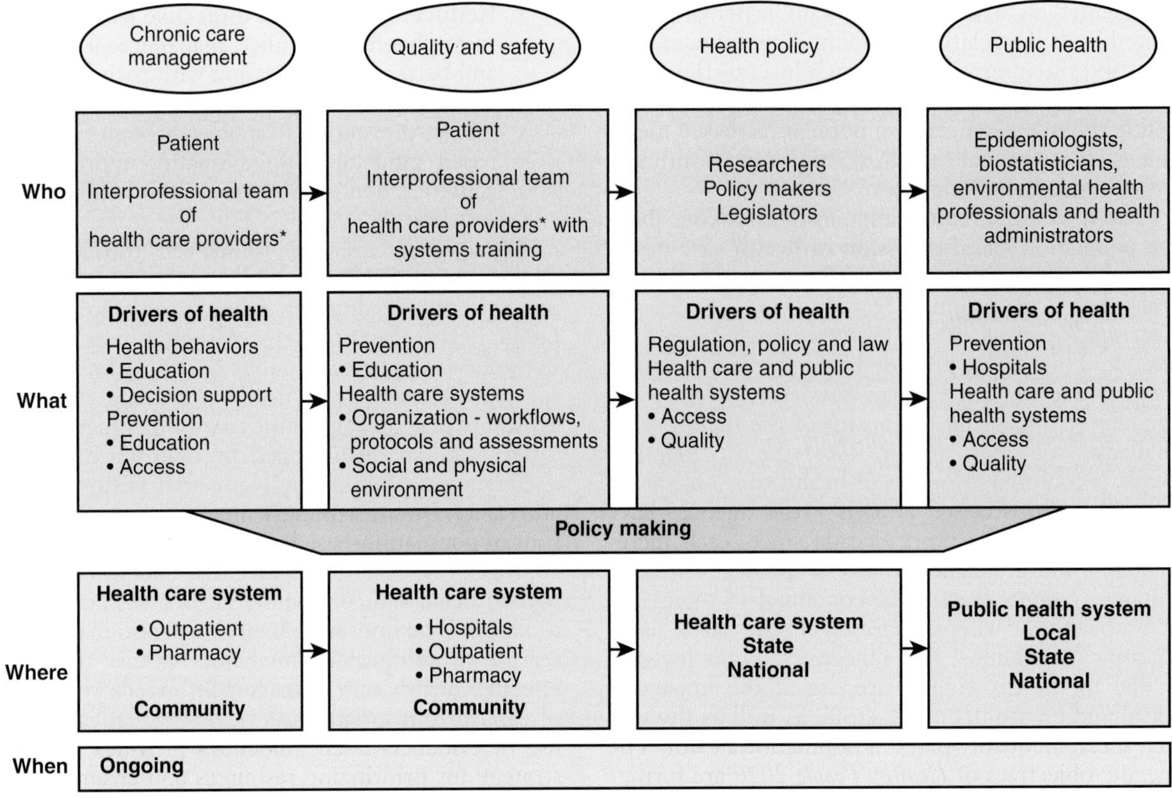

FIGURE 41-1 The four pillars of population health. (From Nash DB, Reifsnyder J, Fabius RJ, Pracilio VP. Population Health. Creating a Culture of Wellness. Ontario: Jones and Bartlett Learning, 2011.)

Secondary prevention identifies and treats individuals who have a risk factor for a disease or who have a disease and are asymptomatic or unaware. Routine screenings for hypertension, diabetes, and breast cancer are examples of secondary prevention.

Tertiary prevention prevents further complications for those diagnosed with a disease. Routine ophthalmologic and podiatric examinations for diabetics and cholesterol and weight reduction programs for hypertensive patients are examples of tertiary prevention.

Because one goal of population-based medicine is to reduce cost, the true cost-effectiveness of chronic management programs and preventive measures including the PCMH has resulted in a debate that remains unresolved.[2] Although preventive measures may require an initial outlay of capital, the PCMH is associated with improved quality of care, reduced medical errors, and increased patient satisfaction.[10] Proponents of the PCMH assert that judicious management of all levels of prevention, from preillness to advanced chronic disease, is an ultimate cost savings because the use of human and material resources is reduced as use of tertiary care is diminished.

PREVENTION OF MEDICAL ERRORS

After the 1999 groundbreaking report of the Institute of Medicine (IOM), *To Err Is Human*, revealed that medical errors alone may account for 44,000 to 98,000 deaths annually, or about 2% to 4% percent of all deaths,[11] the prevention of medical errors became a target of national concern. Fragmented care and the lack of protocols and assessment mechanisms were cited as two important factors for this high rate. Medical error is also cited as a source of unnecessary health care costs. One easy-to-implement response to this problem is the use of the checklist, which has been well received in many medical disciplines, from preventive medicine to critical care. Atul Gawande popularized this method after learning of the success of checklist in the aviation industry to prevent airline crashes. The checklist is made up of a line item for

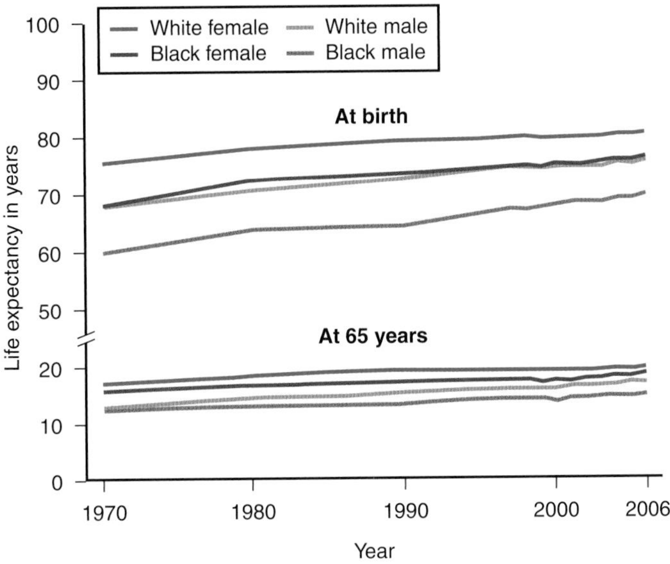

FIGURE 41-2 Life expectancy by gender and race. (From the National Vital Statistics System. CDC/NCHS, Health, United States, 2009.)

every step in a procedure or protocol. By using the team approach and by identifying a team leader who takes ultimate responsibility for delivering patient care, medical error caused by forgetfulness, or laziness, would be dramatically reduced, as it has been in pilot studies.[12] Nash and colleagues[2] further recommend that an interdisciplinary team approach in patient safety would lead to relational coordination, where the principles of teamwork were made explicit. The culture or belief system of those in health care delivery would be ultimately changed, as although one individual is identified as the leader, the whole team is responsible for the prevention of errors.

The four-pillar model underscores the objectives of population-based medicine, from preventing disease in healthy individuals to decreasing the rate of complications in chronic illness; it delineates the actors in the implementation and administration of a population-based approach and the objectives of each sphere or "pillar." Lastly, it presents a scheme that illustrates the interrelationships between the patient, the provider, the health care delivery system, and health policy regulation. It shows that only a coordinated effort among all stakeholders can produce the aim of better patient outcomes at lower cost.

DETERMINANTS OF HEALTH

Determinants of health are measured by indicators such as morbidity and mortality. Life expectancy, a measure of the overall health of a population, represents the average number of years that can be expected if current death rates were constant. Life expectancy also accentuates differences between populations. For example, from 1900 through 2006, life expectancy at birth in the United States increased from 46 years to 75 years for men and from 48 years to 80 years for women. But although life expectancy has improved for all groups over time, the difference between rates for African Americans and whites has remained disparate, with African American rates consistently lower than whites (Figure 41-2).[13] Life expectancy is an important indicator of global health as well, where the influence of poverty places a decisive role in life expectancy. For example, the life expectancy in a nonindustrialized country like Sierra Leone is 45 years, whereas it is 85 years in an industrialized country such as Japan.[14] Epidemiologic rates can be used as a basis of comparison between U.S. communities as well, as data are collected by country, state, county, and on occasion by census track. These can be used as benchmarks by which the study population can be measured.

The social determinants of health are the conditions under which one is born, lives, and dies (Table 41-1). Unlike other determinants, social determinants are directly reflective of the distribution of money and other resources within the population. Poverty, for instance, lowers access to resources such as education, employment, and adequate housing. These factors all increase the likelihood of mortality due to population-attributable factors. In a recent meta-analysis, Galea and colleagues[15] found that approximately 245,000 deaths in the United States in 2000 were attributable to low education, 176,000 to racial segregation, 162,000 to low social support, 133,000 to individual-level

TABLE 41-1 Examples of Social and Physical Determinants

Examples of Social Determinants
- Availability of resources to meet daily needs, such as educational and job opportunities, living wages, or healthful foods
- Social norms and attitudes, such as discrimination
- Exposure to crime, violence, and social disorder, such as the presence of trash
- Social support and social interactions
- Exposure to mass media and emerging technologies, such as the Internet or cell phones
- Socioeconomic conditions, such as concentrated poverty
- Quality schools
- Transportation options
- Public safety
- Residential segregation

Examples of Physical Determinants
- Natural environment, such as plants, weather, or climate change
- Built environment, such as buildings or transportation
- Worksites, schools, and recreational settings
- Housing, homes, and neighborhoods
- Exposure to toxic substances and other physical hazards
- Physical barriers, especially for people with disabilities
- Aesthetic elements, such as good lighting, trees, or benches

From *Healthy People 2020* website. *http://www.healthypeople.gov/2020/about/new2020.aspx*. Accessed July 17, 2012.

poverty, 119,000 to income inequality, and 39,000 to area-level poverty. These findings show the importance of social factors in both individual and population-based health and demonstrate the need for multileveled interventions.

PREMATURE MORTALITY

Estimates of early death in the United States point to five types of predictors: Behavioral patterns account for 40%; gestational and genetic factors 30%; social circumstances 15%; access to and quality of medical care 10%; and environmental conditions 5% (Figure 41-3).[16] More than any individual domain, the intersection of domains accentuates the effect of each contributing component. Furthermore, the relative impact of these factors affects individuals differently, depending on their stage of life and preceding or subsequent factors.[17] Each domain contains modifiable and nonmodifiable variables. Population-based medicine addresses only the modifiable factors, which are identified by

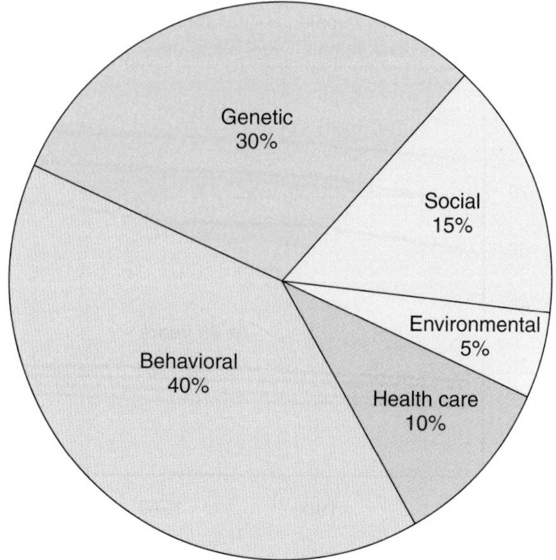

FIGURE 41-3 The determinants of health. (From McGinnis MJ, Williams-Russo P, Knickman JR. The case for more active policy attention to health promotion. Health Affairs 2002;21:78.)

the presence of risk factors and the ability to use preventive measures.

1. **Behavioral choices.** Lifestyle and behavior patterns represent the single most important influence over health in the United States.[10] Behavior choices regarding diet, alcohol and drugs, smoking, sex, and recklessness such as speeding and weapon use cause premature death in and of themselves or can contribute to the incidence and complications of potentially fatal diseases such as heart disease, cancer, human immunodeficiency virus (HIV), and stroke. Meta-analysis of the estimate burden of premature death attributable to behavioral choices approaches 1.2 million annually, which is nearly half of all yearly death in the United States.[18] Of all the behavioral causes of death, tobacco use is the greatest threat to health. When smoking is combined with poor diet and inactivity, it contributes to more than a third of the total death rate each year, whereas the combined effect of all other causes such as alcohol, infectious disease, toxic agents, motor vehicle accidents, firearms, and illicit drug use accounts for only a little more than one seventh (Figure 41-4).[18] The importance of national smoking cessation and healthy eating campaigns is underscored by these data.

   Health behavior is, in essence, the result of individual health knowledge and the desire to put that knowledge into practice. Yet the

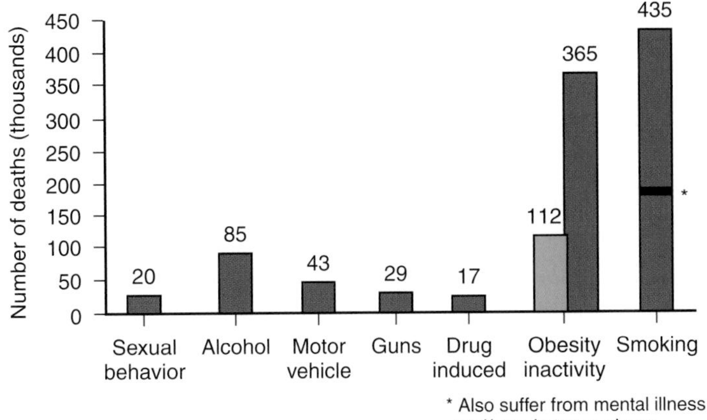

FIGURE 41-4 Estimated deaths attributable to social factors in the United States in 2000. (Data from Mokdad AH, Marks JS, Stroup DF, Gerberding JL. Actual causes of death in the United States, 2000. JAMA 2004; 291:1238.)

ability to make healthy choices can sometimes extend beyond the conditions of individual control. For instance, the lack of options for fresh, affordable food or safe places to exercise makes adherence to lifestyle treatment plans especially difficult. Furthermore, not all populations have the same access to information or the ability to comprehend that information, especially if it is written. The lack of health literacy can be associated with risky behavior choices, especially when confounded by other health disparities such as poverty.[19] The efficacy of written health education material and oral health counseling cannot be measured when the population literacy level is not accounted for.

2. **Genetics.** Familial disease, the best example of a nonmodifiable variable, plays a small role in premature death, accounting for less than 2% of death in the United States.[20] Yet when combined with behavioral factors, the effect of some inherited disorders is either potentiated or diminished. The detection and treatment of gestational diabetes is an example. The national campaign to prevent hyperglycemia during pregnancy begun in the mid-1970s resulted in a marked decrease in gestational diabetes. This advance also reduced the number of children with type 1 diabetes with familial aggregation on the maternal side.[21] Furthermore, the prevention of gestational diabetes reduces fetal exposure to hyperglycemia and resulting insulin resistance, thereby decreasing the likelihood of developing non–insulin-dependent diabetes in later life. Therefore, the screening, detection, and treatment of hyperglycemia during pregnancy have had a direct effect on not only pregnancy outcomes but also the incidence of both type 1 and type 2 diabetes among some offspring. Although pregnancy offers particular challenges and opportunities for prevention, the screening, detection, and treatment of other familial conditions such as high blood pressure and high cholesterol also mitigate the untoward effects of inherited disease.
3. **Social factors.** Social factors refer to the effect of social cohesion or active social relationships and connectedness found within family or community life. Support for discontinuing drug, alcohol, or tobacco use or in changing diet can be critical to success; lack of support can likewise make the challenges overwhelming. Communities formed of individuals with similar health concerns may be especially beneficial because the common bond can optimize information sharing, emotional support, and material support.

One example from Africa exemplifies the compounded benefits of social cohesion. High mortality from HIV disease in Tete Province, Mozambique, was found to be associated with the inability of infected individuals to reach the clinic for antiretroviral therapy in that rural part of the country. A team from Doctors without Borders devised a plan whereby one member of a self-forming group of patients would make the trip into town each month and deliver the full prescription to the rest of the members. This strategy cut the cost and inconvenience of a trip to the clinic from 12 trips per year to 2 for each patient, decreased the need for physician consultation fourfold, and reduced the death rate from 20% to 2%.[22] This project also demonstrates the power of social capital, or the social and political advantages that stem from social connections. Social capital as a factor in illness and in health is considered more frequently among practitioners of population-based medicine.[23] The integration and participation of the ideas of non–health community leaders for health education campaigns can be critical in fostering trust and ensuring success, especially if the clinicians are not members of the target population.

The absence of social cohesion, called *social isolation*, is a risk to health. Socially isolated persons have a death rate two to five times higher than that of those who maintain close ties to friends, family, and community.[24] Social isolation is often the result rather than the cause of other problems such as old age, disability, and mental illness. When these factors are compounded with medical illness, this subgroup becomes of special interest for population-based practitioners.

4. **Medical care.** Improvements in the quality or use of medical care in the United States have had a relatively limited impact in reducing mortality.[10] This is a stark distinction from other countries, especially those that have severe shortages of technology, equipment, and human resources to treat their populations. The two areas most amenable to population-based initiatives are in reducing health disparity and, to a lesser degree, in the prevention of medical errors.

TABLE 41-2 **Disparity in Mortality Rates**

Infant Mortality
- Infant mortality rates are higher for infants of black, Puerto Rican, and American Indian mothers (13.6, 8.2, and 8.3 deaths per 1000 live births) than for infants of other race groups
- Infant mortality decreases as the mother's level of education increases

Homicide
- Homicide is the leading cause of death for black males 15-25 years old and the second leading cause of death for young Hispanic males
- Rate for young black males is 17 times the rate for non-Hispanic white males

HIV Disease
- HIV disease is the leading cause of death for black males 25-44 years old and third leading cause of death for Hispanic males aged 25-44

Motor Vehicle-Related Injuries
- Vehicle injuries for young American Indian males 15-24 years old is about 80% higher than for young white males

Stroke
- Stroke rates for Asian American males aged 45-54 and 55-64 are 31%-40% higher than for white males in these age groups

Suicide
- Rate for American Indian males is double the rate for young white males

From Centers for Disease Control and Prevention (CDC): Forward: CDC Health Disparities and Inequalities Report–United States, 2011. MMWR 2011. *http://www.cdc.gov/mmwr/pdf/other/su6001.pdf*. Accessed August 28, 2012.

DISPARITY IN HEALTH

Health disparity refers to differences in the incidence, prevalence, mortality, and other adverse health conditions that exist among specific population groups. Therefore, although gains have been made in the overall health of the population in the United States, the gap among subpopulations, especially between racial and ethnic groups, persists (Table 41-2). A population-based approach can determine if disparity exists within a population, and if so, the degree and causes of the disparity. Three areas of population-based care can increase the likelihood of disparity: individual demographics, health behavior, and the accessibility of the health care delivery system, including the cultural sensitivity of providers.

a. **Individual Demographics:** Old age, presence of a disability, and low socioeconomic status, defined as the combined effect of education, occupation, and income, are examples of characteristics shared by subpopulations with a disproportionate burden of disease. Living in high-density urban areas or remote rural areas is predictive of having higher disease rates as well.[25] State and national programs to incentivize providers to work in high-risk communities, such as the National Health Service Corps, is an example of a response to curtail the magnitude of disparity due to individual demographics.
b. **Provider sensitivity to the cultural beliefs of the patient** affects patient ability to agree with or comply with treatment. Cultural competence is developed over time and typically includes a defined set of values, principles, and behaviors that facilitate a provider's ability to work effectively cross-culturally. Lack of provider sensitivity could be due to not having knowledge or understanding of patient or population belief systems. This is more likely if the provider and patient are ethnically discordant. Second, unconscious bias or blatant racism can contribute to ineffective health care delivery.[26] Integrating cultural competence curricula into the training programs of health care providers, including physician assistants, is an approach to combat interpersonal bias.

c. **Health Care Delivery System** affects disparity through denial of care as a result of lack of insurance. Working families denied insurance by either their employers or by national programs such as Medicaid make up a large segment of those who cannot receive care due to inability to pay. A sad irony is that low-income families contribute a disproportionately high proportion of their income to health expense regardless of insurance status. Health-related payment, including out-of-pocket expenses, direct payment for health insurance, and contribution to taxes, constitute 20% of family income for those in the lowest quintile; the proportion of family income directed toward private and public health care is no more than 16% in any other quintile.[27]

The Affordable Care Act is aimed at bridging the gap between the access to health care received by insured versus uninsured patients by subsidizing expansion of Medicaid, filling the "donut hole" of coverage for Medicare, reducing or eliminating the proscription of coverage for preexisting illness, and removing annual and lifetime limits of coverage. The implementation of this Act is likely to address some, but not all, of the disparity due to insurance coverage. Without population-based measures to identify and treat the health needs of the uninsured or underinsured, health disparity based on insurance status will persist.

Environmental Conditions. Toxic substances, microbial agents, and structural hazards found in the home or workplace can contribute to preventable mortality and morbidity. Estimates of the mortality due to toxic-agent exposures alone are 60,000 deaths per year.[8] Contaminants found in food and water have been associated with skin disease, cancer, and allergy. Airborne pollutants such as particulates, sulfur dioxide, and carbon monoxide have been associated with transient increases in mortality and morbidity rates, as well as an increase in pulmonary and cardiovascular conditions.

Environmental and occupational causes of morbidity and mortality lend themselves to evidence-based analysis and programmatic solutions, in part because they are determined by place, a discrete variable. This provides unique opportunities for population-based campaigns, assessment of the outcomes, and refinement of the interventions.

Integrating Population-Based Strategies—*Healthy People 2020*

For clinically practicing physician assistants, integrating evidence-based guidelines for population health into patient care first requires the identification of the main risks to health within the target population. The *Healthy People* agendas can aid in developing a strategy to improve care because they present a national set of target goals for a large array of preventable illness, providing benchmark goals that communities throughout the country strive to achieve.

The *Healthy People* project was developed after HHS requested the Institute of Medicine (IOM) develop a mechanism that would shift the delivery of health care so that improved health outcomes would be achieved. Every decade, agendas are created that reflect the most current priorities for preventable illness and injury. For the current agenda, the Committee on Leading Health Indicators for *Healthy People 2020* has defined four categories in an effort to organize and prioritize each entry:

Topic—General category, such as "chronic disease."

Indicator—Measurement of the rates of disease, including incidence and prevalence.

Objective—The quantification of an indicator, for example, the reduction of the prevalence of a certain disease by a given percent.

Leading health indicator—Measurement of a major health concern, such as infant mortality rate or life expectancy at birth.

Furthermore, the HHS charged *Healthy People 2020* with three additional tasks: first, revisit and refine the mission; second, identify overarching goals; and third, sharpen the focus of the agenda by identifying 12 key indicators, 12 topics, and 24 crucial objectives.[28]

The **mission** of *Healthy People 2020* is to do the following:

1. Identify nationwide health improvement priorities
2. Increase public awareness and understanding of determinants of health, disease, disability, and opportunities for progress
3. Provide measureable objectives and goals applicable at national, state, and local levels
4. Engage multiple sectors to take actions to strengthen policies
5. Improve practices that are driven by the best available evidence and knowledge
6. Identify critical research evaluation and data collection needs

The **overarching goals** of *Healthy People 2020* are to do the following:

- Attain high-quality, longer lives free of preventable disease
- Achieve health equity; eliminate disparities
- Create social and physical environments that promote good health
- Promote quality of life, healthy development, and healthy behaviors across life stages

TABLE 41-3 ***Healthy People 2020*** **Topics, Indicators, and Objectives**

Topics	Indicators	Objectives
Access to Care	Proportion of the population with access to health care services	1. Increase the proportion of persons with health insurance 2. Increase proportion of persons with a usual primary care provider 3. (Developmental) Increase the proportion of persons who receive appropriate evidence-based clinical preventive services
Healthy Behaviors	Proportion of the population engaged in healthy behaviors	4. Increase the proportion of adults who meet current federal physical activity guidelines for aerobic physical activity and for muscle-strengthening activity 5. Reduce the proportion of children and adolescents who are considered obese 6. Reduce consumption of calories from solid fats and added sugars in the population aged 2 years and older 7. Increase the proportion of adults who get sufficient sleep
Chronic Disease	Prevalence and mortality of chronic disease	8. Reduce coronary heart disease deaths 9. Reduce the proportion of persons in the population with hypertension 10. Reduce the overall cancer death rate
Environmental Determinants	Proportion of the population experiencing a healthy physical environment	11. Reduce the number of days the Air Quality Index (AQI) exceeds 100
Social Determinants	Proportion of the population experiencing a healthy social environment	12. (Developmental) Improve the health literacy of the population 13. (Developmental) Increase the proportion of children who are ready for school in all five domains of healthy development: physical development, social-emotional development, approaches to learning, language, and cognitive development 14. Increase educational achievement of adolescents and young adults
Injury	Proportion of the population that experiences injury	15. Reduce fatal and nonfatal injuries
Mental Health	Proportion of the population experiencing positive mental health	16. Reduce the proportion of persons who experience major depressive episodes (MDE)
Maternal and Infant Health	Proportion of healthy births	17. Reduce low birth weight (LBW) and very low birth weight (VLBW)
Responsible Sexual Behavior	Proportion of the population engaged in responsible sexual behavior	18. Reduce pregnancy rates among adolescent females 19. Increase the proportion of sexually active persons who use condoms
Substance Abuse	Proportion of the population engaged in substance abuse	20. Reduce past-month use of illicit substances 21. Reduce the proportion of persons engaging in binge drinking of alcoholic beverages
Tobacco	Proportion of the population using tobacco	22. Reduce tobacco use by adults 23. Reduce the initiation of tobacco use among children, adolescents, and young adults
Quality of Care	Proportion of the population receiving quality health care services	24. Reduce central line–associated bloodstream infections

From Institute of Medicine website, March 3, 2011. *http://www.iom.edu/Reports/2011/Leading-Health-Indicators-for-Healthy-People-2020/Table.aspx*. Accessed July 17, 2012.

The lead indicators can be found in Table 41-3.

The *Healthy People* paradigm is helpful in setting goals and objectives for a small population such as a clinical practice. The agenda aids in setting realistic targets and providing national benchmarks by which the progress of an intervention can be assessed. By presenting a national perspective, *Healthy People* can also call attention to health issues that are unidentified or under-reported in a population (Figure 41-1).

Integrating Population-Based Medicine into Clinical Practice

Because population-based medicine is an approach that augments rather than substitutes for one-to-one care, developing ways to assess the evidence, develop the tools, and identify responsible personnel may require the formation of new tracking systems and the acquisition of resources when integrated into clinical practice. Once that transition is made, using population-based techniques is relatively easy. Guidelines for accomplishing this include the following:

1. **Define the population.** The definition of a population is any group of individuals who share specific characteristics. The population of interest in a clinical practice may include patients with a common demographic such as age, disease state, or insurance status, or it could be broad enough to include the whole patient panel. For interventions at the community level, data to develop inclusion criteria can be obtained from local health departments, hospitals, or health insurance plans.
2. **Create an information system.** The identification and tracking of those individuals with the characteristics of interest must be established. In the clinical setting, the electronic medical record greatly facilitates the gathering of this information.
3. **Identify and prioritize into patient groups.** Depending on available resources, those for whom a population-based intervention would be most medically appropriate and cost-effective are identified. Criteria most often include those patients with preventable diseases or complications from chronic diseases. Those individuals who are most at risk for serious health consequences or the most costly health consequences can also be considered, even if they are relatively few in number.
4. **Identify the intervention.** An intervention is developed using evidence-based guidelines for prevention strategies, disease identification, or management protocols. Smoking cessation, cholesterol reduction, and diabetes detection are examples of population-based interventions.
5. **Adapt an office system.** Develop policies and procedures that include goals and performance indications. Determine how monitoring will occur and by whom.
6. **Monitor and assess.** Periodic assessment determines if the desired outcomes are within reach. Feedback from all participants is solicited, and problem areas identified and addressed.

These six steps are clear-cut and can aid a clinical team to better patient outcomes, especially among the chronically ill. Learning the techniques of population-based care can also be learned as part of regular medical training. Community Oriented Primary Care (COPC) is especially popular among family medicine training programs of both physicians and physician assistants. COPC uses the analogy that the identification and implementation of a community-based health strategy uses the same steps as the diagnosis and treatment of an individual patient:

Step 1: The community or target population is defined.

Step 2: An assessment of the community is made, which includes the collection of both quantitative and qualitative data. For instance, vital statistics are analyzed at the local and national levels, as well as those specific to the population of interest. Qualitative assessment includes observational and descriptive data collected from multiple visits to the community, interviews with key informants, and an inventory of community resources such as parks, libraries, houses of worship, transportation, and housing availability. Other information, such as the availability of fresh fruits and vegetables and prices of groceries, may be included in this assessment. This step is similar to the history and physical examination of a patient.

Step 3: A community "diagnosis" is made, leading to the formulation of a plan of action.

Step 4: A detailed assessment of the selected health problem is conducted.

Step 5: Implementation of the intervention is the "treatment."

Step 6: Program evaluation is the "follow-up care."

Although COPC is a practical way to teach population-based medicine, the model was developed to be a continuous process of integrating primary care delivery and public health. COPC is practiced with that aim, both in the United States and abroad.[29]

CLINICAL APPLICATIONS

The following three examples show the range of ways that population-based practices can be implemented. The first is an office-based primary prevention; the second a hospital-based secondary prevention; and the third a system-based practice modality for tertiary care. Although different, they demonstrate the far-reaching influence a population-based approach can bring.

1. **Standing orders for immunizations:** In an effort to increase immunization rates among high-risk adults, the Task Force on Community Preventive Services of the Centers for Disease Control recommends the implementation of a standing order for immunizations. By eliminating the need for individual orders, all adults meeting high-risk criteria for age or underlying medical condition would be vaccinated. Used in conjunction with a provider

reminder system, community demand for and access to vaccines would be increased. This cost-effective, easily implemented intervention would only reach those already enrolled in the health care system, which is its one drawback. See *http://www2a.cdc.gov/vaccines/ed/whatworks/strategies_list.asp.*

2. **Increased referral for cardiac rehabilitation:** Cardiac rehabilitation (CR), a comprehensive approach to address the modifiable complications after cardiac surgery, reduces morbidity and mortality to a similar degree as statins, aspirin, and beta-blockers. Yet CR is under-referred and underutilized. In a recent population-based study, a mortality reduction of 21% to 34% was demonstrated among elderly cardiac patients who had been the subjects of automatic referral mechanisms for CR.[30] The benefits of automatic referral cut across sociodemographic lines. Wider adoption of automatic referral for CR is predicted to reduce postsurgery complications including mortality by up to 45%.[30]
3. **Integrated Health Care Delivery Systems.** The integrated health care systems use interdisciplinary teams that involve the patient in shared decisions. Its hallmarks are high medical quality, low costs, and high patient satisfaction due to the focus on well-being, as well as physical and mental function.[31] The most well-known example of integrated health care is the Mayo Clinic. The ability of the Mayo Clinic to keep costs low yet provide individualized health care to its patients speaks to its enduring popularity and its potential as a model for integrated care.

SUMMARY

Population-based practice uses evidence-based treatment and prevention guidelines to curtail costs and effectively use resources to groups of individuals sharing the same risk factors or disease states. While not discounting the obvious benefits of the one-to-one relationship between the clinician and the patient, population-based care can be more effective in reducing the incidence of primary disease and the effects of chronic disease. Health disparity can be reduced with the identification and implementation of programs for those with special or greater risk. By using interdisciplinary teams and evaluation of the social and environmental factors that may be at play, a more efficient and responsive model of health care delivery can be implemented.

KEY POINTS

- Population health is defined by the health outcomes within a population regarding:
  - Distribution
  - Policies
  - Interventions
- The major components of population-based medicine are:
  - Reduce need
  - Reduce demand
  - Reduce mismanagement of health resources
  - Increase delivery of health promotion and disease prevention strategies
    - Prevention of medical errors is best accomplished through an interdisciplinary team approach to patient safety
    - Determinants of health become manifest through differences in:
      - Life expectancy
      - Premature mortality
- Determinants of health
  - Behavioral choices (40%)
  - Genetics (30%)
  - Social factors (15%)
  - Health care (10%)
  - Environmental (5%)

References

1. Peters KE, Elster AB. Roadmaps for Clinical Practice: A Primer on Population-Based Medicine. Chicago: American Medical Association Press, 2002.
2. Nash DB, Reifsnyder J, Fabius RJ, Pracilio VP. Population Health. Creating a Culture of Wellness. Ontario: Jones and Bartlett Learning, 2011.
3. Bodenheimer T, Chen E, Bennett HD. Confronting the growing burden of chronic disease: can the U.S. health care workforce do the job? Health Affairs 2009;28(1):64.
4. Flexner A. Medical Education in the United States and Canada. New York, NY: Carnegie Foundation for the Advancement of Teaching, 1910. Bulletin No. 4.
5. University of Virginia, Historical Collections of the Claude Moore Health Sciences Library. Biography: Kerr Lachlan White, MD, CM, FACP. *http://historical.hsl.virginia.edu/kerr/bio.cfm;* Accessed September 1, 2011.
6. Institute of Medicine. Leading Health Indicators for Health People 2020. Letter Report. Washington D.C. The National Academy of Sciences, March 2011.
7. Lipkin M, Lydrand WA (eds). Population-Based Medicine. New York: Praeger Publishers, 1882.
8. Fries JF. Reducing the need and demand for medical services. Psychol Med 1998;60:140–142.
9. Carney PA, Eiff MP, Saultz JW, et al. Aspects of the patient-centered medical home currently in place: initial finding from preparing the personal physician for practice. Fam Med 2009;41:632.
10. Rosenthal TC. The medical home: growing evidence to support a new approach to primary care. Am Board Fam Med 2008;21:427.
11. Institute of Medicine. To err is human. Building a safer health system. November 1999. *http://www.iom.edu/Reports/1999/To-Err-is-Human-Building-A-Safer-Health-System.aspx*; Accessed September 15, 2011.
12. Gawande A. Check List Manifesto. How to Get Things Right. New York: Metropolitan Books, 2009.
13. Kochanek KD, Xu JQ, Murphy SL, et al. Deaths: preliminary data for 2009. National Vital Statistics Reports; 59(40). Hyattsville, MD: National Center for Health Statistics, 2011.
14. United Nations Statistics Division. Social Indicators, Estimates for 2010-2015. *http://unstats.un.org/unsd/demographic/products/socind/health.htm*; Accessed October 1, 2011.
15. Galea S, Tracy M, Hoggatt KJ, et al. Estimated Deaths Attributable to Social Factors in the United States; Am J Public Health 2011;101:1456.
16. McGinnis MJ, Williams-Russo P, Knickman JR. The case for more active policy attention to health promotion. Health Affairs 2002;21:78.
17. Institute of Medicine. Health and Behavior: The Interplay of Biological, Behavioral, and Societal Influences. Washington: National Academy Press, 2001.
18. Mokdad AH, Marks JS, Stroup DF, Gerberding JL. Actual causes of death in the United States. JAMA 2000;2004(294):1238.
19. Weiss BD, Hart G, Pust RE. The relationship between literacy and health. J Health Care Poor Underserved 1991;1(4):351.
20. Muller H. Hereditary colorectal cancer: from bedside to bench and back. Ann Oncol 2000;11(Suppl).
21. Dorner G, Plagemann A, Reinagel H. Familial diabetes aggregation in type I diabetics: gestational diabetes an apparent risk factor for increased diabetes susceptibility in the offspring. Exp Clin Endocrinol 1987;89:84.
22. Decroo T, Telfer B, Biot M, et al. Distribution of antiretroviral treatment through self-forming groups of patients in Tete Province Mozambique. J Acquir Immune Defic Syndr 2011;56:e39.
23. Lomas J. Social capital and health: implications for public health and epidemiology. Social Sci Med 1998;47:1181.
24. Berkman LF, Glass T. Social integration, social networks, social support, and health. In: Berkman LF, Kawachi I (eds). Social Epidemiology. New York: Oxford University Press, 2000. p. 137.
25. Eberhardt MD, Panuk ER. The importance of place and residence: examining health in rural and non-rural areas. Am J Public Health 2004;94:1682.
26. Burgess D, van Ryn M, Dovidio J, Saha S. Reducing racial bias among health care providers: lessons from social-cognitive psychology. J Gen Intern Med 2007;22:882.
27. Ketsche P, Adams ER, Wallace S, et al. Lower-income families pay a higher share of income toward national healthcare spending than higher-income families do. Health Affairs 2011;30:1637.
28. Committee on Leading Health Indicators for *Healthy People 2020*. Board on Population Health and Public Health Practice. Institute of Medicine of the National Academies. National Academies Press. Washington, D.C. *www.nap.edu. Accessed* June 16, 2011.
29. Mullen F, Epstein L. Community-oriented primary care: new relevance in a changing world. Am J Public Health 2002;92:1748.
30. Grace SL, Russell KL, Reid RD, et al. Effect of cardiac rehabilitation referral strategies on utilization rates. A prospective, controlled study. Arch Intern Med 2011;171:235.
31. Boon H, Verhoef M, O'Hara D, Findlay B. From parallel practice to integrative health care: a conceptual framework. BMC Health Serv Res 2004;4:15.

The resources for this chapter can be found at www.expertconsult.com.

SECTION VII

SYSTEMS-BASED PRACTICE

CHAPTER 42

HEALTH CARE DELIVERY SYSTEMS

Ruth Ballweg

CHAPTER CONTENTS

Most Americans laugh if asked to consider the U.S. health care "system." They will say that it is "nonexistent," "flawed," "broken," or "needs healing." Overall, they will agree that it " just doesn't work!" Recognizing that the word "system" should meet the *Merriam-Webster Dictionary* definition of "a regularly interacting or independent group of items functioning as a unified whole,"[1] Americans say that "there's nothing systematic about it." Instead, the United States has multiple entities including delivery systems, insurance companies, governmental agencies, medical training facilities, clinician groups, and cottage-industry-type businesses all providing care with little coordination and much confusion. As a result, the cost of health care in America continues to rise at an alarmingly high rate and poses the threat of destabilizing American business and the entire economy.

In contrast, other developed countries keep costs down and quality up through the use of systems that organize care, and they provide access to everyone. Although we may criticize other countries' health care systems for perceived delays in care or decreased availability of services, the people in these countries report less stress than Americans due to the assurance that health care will always be available without risking a family's economic stability. Although the health reform legislation passed in 2010 has the major goal of increasing access to health insurance—and thus access to health care—for many in America who were previously "uncovered," the legislation will also create many initiatives that are designed to create and enhance *systems* of care.

The "systems" idea is not a new one. In 1929 a Committee on the Costs of Medical Care sought to respond to the concern that health care expenditures were at 4%, "a sum that was believed to threaten the country's financial recovery."[2]

The committee recommended that "medical services should be more largely furnished by groups of physicians and related practitioners so organized as to maintain high standards of care and to retain the personal relations between patients and physicians."[2]

The systems approach—as compared with "independent" private physician practice—is now necessary given the complex health care environment, which will include requirements for detailed and "compliant" billing processes, assessment of quality indicators, and "report cards" for physician practices. In addition, the upcoming requirements for electronic medical records that record data, interface with complex institutions and services, aid in decision-making, and have the potential to communicate with patients will be difficult to maintain without inclusion in larger systems.

Larger health care delivery systems create complex issues including questions about the mix of types of providers, tensions between primary and specialty care, and power struggles between physicians and administrators. All of these play out to create opportunities—and barriers—for physician assistants (PAs). As a result, it is important for PAs to understand rapidly evolving health care systems and how they work.

HEALTH CARE SYSTEMS

Governmental policies played a large part in the creation of larger health care "systems" in the United States. Certificate of need laws were designed to restrict uncontrolled growth in hospital beds and new technologies. By 1982 diagnostic related groups (DRGs) were introduced to decrease hospital costs by identifying standard lengths of stay for designated conditions and putting hospitals at financial risk for longer hospitalizations.

> To maintain profitability, hospitals sought to capitalize on economies of scale, to increase their patient base and to leverage purchasing opportunities.[4]

As health care became more complex and expensive, rural and community-based hospitals either closed, merged, or were bought up by larger systems. Similarly, physician practices were purchased by these systems in order to keep them in business.

Ultimately these growing systems came to be about establishing structured referral—or "feeder"—systems to guarantee the patient volumes that were necessary to maintain stability and to fund the acquisition of new technologies. In addition, large systems offered more cost-effective centralized services such as billing, purchasing, marketing, human resources, compliance services, and access to specialty care and procedures.

Increasing numbers of patients without health insurance, problems with geographic access, and maldistribution of the health workforce led to the development of parallel systems of federally funded community health centers.[5] Designed to provide broad primary care services—including oral health care, patient education, and outreach—the community health centers grew and expanded during the past 20 years and will receive further funding for expansion under health reform legislation.

As a specific type of large health care system, health maintenance organizations (HMOs) such as Kaiser Permanente[6] and Group Health Cooperative recruit physicians, PAs, and nurse practitioners (NPs) who work under a salaried model and provide care with structured, evidence-based guidelines. Staff model HMOs—such as Kaiser[6]—are essentially a "closed system" that maintains both clinics and hospitals. Mixed-model HMOs such as Group Health[7] operate their own delivery systems but also purchase services from external hospitals and specialty groups and contract with providers outside their facilities to provide care in smaller communities.

Finally, the federal government operates its own large delivery systems for veterans,[8] military personnel,[9] and incarcerated individuals in federal prisons.[10] Each of these closed systems relies on salaried clinicians (including significant numbers of PAs and NPs), as well as structured processes and guidelines to provide care to large numbers of patients.

INTEGRATED SYSTEMS

The term "integrated health system" refers to "a network of organizations that provides or arranges to provide a coordinated continuum of services to a defined population and is willing to be held clinically and fiscally accountable for the outcomes and health status of the population served."[11] With the development of large systems, the next step has been to consider how those systems can improve patient care while at the same time reducing costs. A more descriptive definition of integrated systems refers to structures that were formed with the goals of providing high-quality, low-cost care to populations of patients in broad geographic areas, eliminating duplication of services and providing care across the continuum (referred to as "seamless" health care).

Horizontally Integrated Systems

Probably the easiest to set up, horizontally integrated systems were created—usually across a single specialty such as family medicine—to allow private practices to remain in business while creating volume (more patients, more physicians) for a centralized billing process, acquisition of technology such as electronic health records, marketing, and the creation of more efficient call systems. In some settings these horizontally integrated systems were configured and managed by regional hospitals as a strategy to retain community physicians in their practices—but also as a feeder system for the hospital's services.

Other horizontally integrated systems were organized and led by physicians.

These systems—called independent practice associations (IPAs)—moved on to partner with insurance companies to create HMO products for their patients.

These HMOs were based on managed care concepts but were different from the traditional staff model HMOs such as Kaiser and Group Health, which were both insurance companies AND delivery systems.

Physicians and organized medicine were fond of IPAs and other developing structures that kept physicians in charge. A major advantage of the early IPAs was that individual physicians did not have to negotiate contracts with insurance companies.[12] Things got confusing, however, when individual practices (which were still owned by individual physicians or physician groups) joined more than one IPA and attempted to sort out the requirements of multiple insurance contracts. Practices with PAs and NPs faced additional complexities on the basis of the insurers' policies on reimbursement for these two groups.

Obviously there are advantages to large medical groups. Describing the situation in California, where IPAs and IMGs are well developed, Robinson and Casalino[13] say that "small independent practices cannot stand alone in California; the advantages of belonging to a large integrated medical group or IPA are overwhelming. The immediate reason why primary care physicians link their fate to that of larger organizations is that contracts with health plans are available only through these organizations. Beyond this, however, we suggest four reasons why integrated medical groups and IPAs have advantages over small independent practices: economies of scale; ability to spread the financial risk of capitation payment; reduction in the transaction costs of negotiating, monitoring, and enforcing agreements; and creation of an organizational context for continuous process innovation."

Some horizontal systems took on a more structured form by becoming integrated medical groups. Individual physicians sold their practices and became employees of the group. Like the IPAs, these groups also managed contracts from multiple payers and ultimately became the building blocks for the vertically integrated or virtually integrated systems, which now define large segments of the U.S. health care system.

Both IPAs and integrated medical groups rely on gatekeepers, physicians, PAs, or NPs, to manage primary care and to make appropriate referrals to specialists. In addition, the systems benefit from insurance contracts that designate their systems and their physicians as "preferred providers," which opens their doors to larger numbers of patients. In exchange, the system gives discounted rates for the care of the insurance company's subscribers. By this arrangement, only noninsured patients (called "self-payers") pay full price for health care services.

Vertically Integrated Systems

Vertical integration refers to consolidating under one organizational roof and common ownership all levels of care, from primary care to tertiary care and the facilities and staff necessary to provide this full spectrum of care.[14]

Although systems such as Kaiser were originally closed, vertically integrated systems were later created by academic medical centers, large urban hospital systems, and regional medical centers. Despite advantages for patients, a major incentive for the development of vertically integrated systems is the creation of "market share" made up of loyal consumers who are used to receiving their care continuously over time by a familiar system.

Again, describing the situation in California, Robinson and Casalino[13] point out, "Cooperation between physicians and hospitals can encourage efficient use of services for hospitalized patients and a smooth transition to postacute care. Integration can discourage the duplication of clinical services such as radiology and administrative services, such as utilization management-agreement and discharge planning. Ideally, an integrated organization can function as a seamless system within which patients can move freely from outpatient to inpatient to subacute to home health services. Vertical integration also facilitates cooperation in contexts in which financial incentives are misaligned."

Virtually Integrated Systems

Although the primary differences between vertically and virtually integrated systems relate to their structure (shared ownership as compared to relationships based on contractual arrangements), the ideal unifying feature for both groups is a shared electronic health record.

These integrated systems are still a work in progress. The 2010 Health Reform legislation will influence the structure of the U.S. health care system as it supports integrated delivery systems in a variety of forms. Robinson and Casalino[13] remarked: "Market forces are creating both vertically integrated firms and virtually integrated networks. In turn, the new forms of organizations and contracts are transforming markets and the nature of competition in health care. The advantages of virtual integration through contractual relations, compared with vertical integration through unified ownership, lie in the potential for autonomous adaptation to changing environmental circumstances."

PATIENT-CENTERED MEDICAL HOMES

Although there have been many similar primary care models in the past, the "medical home" movement originated with the American Academy of Pediatrics (AAP), which promoted a central location for archiving a child's medical record. In its 2002 policy statement, the AAP expanded the medical home concept to include these operational characteristics: accessible, continuous, comprehensive, family centered, coordinated, compassionate, and culturally effective care. Eventually pediatricians (AAP), family physicians (American Academy of Family Practice), internists (American College of Physicians), and the osteopaths (American Osteopathic Association) signed on to the concept and developed the following Joint Principles of the Patient-Centered Medical Home[17,18]:

PRINCIPLES

Personal physician—each patient has an ongoing relationship with a personal physician trained to provide first-contact, continuous, and comprehensive care.

Physician-directed medical practice—the personal physician leads a team of individuals at the practice level who collectively take responsibility for the ongoing care of patients.

Whole person orientation—the personal physician is responsible for providing for all the patient's health care needs or taking responsibility for appropriately arranging care with other qualified professionals. This includes care for all stages of life; acute care; chronic care; preventive services; and end-of-life care.

Care is coordinated and/or integrated across all elements of the complex health care system (e.g., subspecialty care, hospitals, home health agencies, nursing homes) and the patient's community (e.g., family, public and private community-based services). Care is facilitated by registries, information technology, health information exchange, and other means to ensure that patients get the indicated care when and where they need and want it in a culturally and linguistically appropriate manner.

Quality and safety are hallmarks of the medical home:

- Practices advocate for their patients to support the attainment of optimal, patient-centered outcomes that are defined by a care planning process driven by a compassionate, robust partnership among physicians, patients, and the patient's family.
- Evidence-based medicine and clinical decision-support tools guide decision-making.
- Physicians in the practice accept accountability for continuous quality improvement through voluntary engagement in performance measurement and improvement.
- Patients actively participate in decision-making, and feedback is sought to ensure patients' expectations are being met.
- Information technology is used appropriately to support optimal patient care, performance measurement, patient education, and enhanced communication.
- Practices go through a voluntary recognition process by an appropriate nongovernmental entity to demonstrate that they have the capabilities to provide patient-centered services consistent with the medical home model.
- Patients and families participate in quality improvement activities at the practice level.

Enhanced access to care is available through systems such as open scheduling, expanded hours, and new options for communication among patients, their personal physician, and practice staff.

In addition to principles for care, the patient-centered medical home is also a reimbursement strategy having the intent of stabilizing primary care by incentivizing physicians and systems for providing quality care as described below.

Payment appropriately recognizes the added value provided to patients who have a patient-centered medical home. The payment structure should be based on the following framework:

- It should reflect the value of physician and non-physician staff patient-centered care management work that falls outside of the face-to-face visit.
- It should pay for services associated with coordination of care both within a given practice and among consultants, ancillary providers, and community resources.
- It should support adoption and use of health information technology for quality improvement.
- It should support provision of enhanced communication access such as secure e-mail and telephone consultation.
- It should recognize the value of physician work associated with remote monitoring of clinical data using technology.
- It should allow for separate fee-for-service payments for face-to-face visits. (Payments for care

management services that fall outside of the face-to-face visit, as described earlier, should not result in a reduction in the payments for face-to-face visits.)

- It should recognize case mix differences in the patient population being treated within the practice.
- It should allow physicians to share in savings from reduced hospitalizations associated with physician-guided care management in the office setting.
- It should allow for additional payments for achieving measurable and continuous quality improvements.[18]

Although the Joint Principles of the Patient-Centered Medical Home has many attributes, it is silent on the utilization and reimbursement of PAs and NPs. On current practice situations, both groups believe that there are settings where others besides the physician can be the leader of a medical practice. This would include situations where the physician would choose not to assume a leadership position and would prefer to delegate this to the PA or NP. This was one of the concerns addressed at a Macy Foundation Conference in January 2010 with the following recommendation as an outcome of the conference:

> Coupled with efforts to increase the number of physicians, nurse practitioners and physician assistants in primary care, state and national legal, regulatory, and reimbursement policies should be changed to remove barriers that make it difficult for nurse practitioners and physician assistants to serve as primary care providers and leaders of patient-centered medical homes or other models of primary care delivery.[19]

Primary care leaders also see the medical home as a strategy for revitalizing primary care and also for "leveling the playing field" for reimbursement. Bruce Landon and his colleagues see the model of the patient-centered medical home as a policy shorthand to address the reinvention of primary care in the United States. They have identified a number of barriers to this innovation including developing new payment models, as well as the need for upfront funding to assemble the personnel and infrastructure required by an enhanced non–visit-based primary care practice and methods to facilitate Group Health Cooperative—as an early adopter of the medical home model—has begun to chronicle physicians'[20] experience with the transition. Group Health physician Dr. Harris Myers reported that "for doctors, it's often a hard journey." He also said: "Now that they've moved to the medical home, most Group Health doctors like the new digs and don't want to go back."[21]

ACCOUNTABLE CARE ORGANIZATIONS

In contrast to the medical home model, which addresses primary care, proposed accountable care organizations (ACOs) are designed to create structures with a hospital as the foundation. Dr. Elliott Fisher—well known for his leadership with the Dartmouth Health Atlas—describes his planned systems in "Creating Accountable Care Organizations: The Extended Hospital Medical Staff." His goal is to move away from traditional fee for service toward reimbursement based on performance and accountability. That cannot happen unless physicians are evaluated as groups rather than as individuals. "The provision of high-quality care for any serious illness requires coordinated, longitudinal care and the engagement of multiple professionals across different institutional settings. Also, many of the most serious gaps in quality can be attributed to poor coordination and faulty transitions."[22]

Fisher proposes "virtual" systems made up of physicians already affiliated with local acute care hospitals. The affiliations may be direct, through their inpatient work or through the care patterns of the patients they serve.[23] Terming this group an *extended hospital medical staff*, Fisher argues that improving quality and lowering cost should be realized by fostering greater accountability on the part of this "extended medical staff."[23]

From the PA/NP point of view, it is unclear how both groups would be included into ACOs and, more importantly, how this would affect their reimbursement. This is another area where "the devil is in the details" and PA and NP professional organizations will need to pay attention to ensure that their members are included.

IMPLICATIONS FOR PHYSICIAN ASSISTANTS

Although the original PA model of practice was designed around a one-on-one employment/supervisory relationship, usually with a single physician, large health systems create complexities that were never considered. In some cases these complexities are to the profession's advantage, and in other cases they require constant vigilance to prevent barriers to practice.

RECRUITMENT/HIRING/EMPLOYMENT ISSUES

In the initial development of PAs, a physician initially hired a PA singularly on the basis of his or her own judgment. Now it is more common to find that at least initial recruitment and screening is done by a human relations staff member. Unfortunately in today's large systems, the PA and physician may not actually meet until the late stages of employment negotiation or even after the employment contract is signed. This is a significant disadvantage to both the physician and the PA who really need to determine, both objectively and subjectively, whether the working relationship will be a good fit for each person. It is wise for the PA seeking employment to request time spent with the physician—and in the clinical setting—to fully assess the employment situation. This type of time also allows the PA to meet other members of the team and to get a better sense of the site's "attitude" toward PAs and the PA role.

As big systems get even bigger, it is important to pay attention to the "governance" of PAs within these large organizations. Because PAs work with physicians, the optimum place for their administration is under the medical staff or the medical director. Unfortunately, some institutions have believed that it is appropriate to place PAs under the nursing staff office. This is generally unworkable.

Large systems are also often unionized. Although PAs have traditionally not been seen as a unionized profession, specific circumstances in large systems may make this impossible to avoid. There are tremendous variables depending on the unions involved, their experience with PAs, and their relationships to nurses and physicians in the same employment setting. It is reasonable to expect that the creation of larger systems will result in greater unionization of the health care workforce.

STATE AND FEDERAL REGULATIONS

The regulatory framework for PAs varies widely from state to state and may not always fully support the optimum utilization of PAs in new settings. In 2010, for example, PAs were still not able to authorize hospice services. The Centers for Medicare and Medicaid Services also put in place new restrictions on the ability of PAs to order the services of respiratory therapists in inpatient settings. Although both of these appear to be close to resolution, they are examples of new types of issues that arise as PA practice is expanded. The American Academy of Physician Assistants (AAPA) has worked to maximize PA practice opportunities; however, there is no substitute for the interactions with state medical boards by other professional organizations, employing institutions and patient advocacy groups. As new roles emerge and expand, PAs cannot assume that this will be without struggle.

REPORTING PATTERNS

Legally a PA must have a relationship with a specific physician in order to practice. Most states, however, interpret this quite liberally and allow for actual supervision to be provided by other physicians within the clinic or practice group. Although this generally works well, there is the potential for the erosion of the physician-PA relationship if team members do not pay attention to each other's strengths, weaknesses, and areas of expertise. This is obviously much more difficult as systems get larger and more complex. Unfortunately, because physicians typically have received little, if any, training in building and maintaining relationships with PAs, it becomes the responsibility or obligation of the PA to provide the leadership in this area. Consultations, although less and less necessary over the length of the relationship, are still critical to the relationship as much as to direct patient care.

NEW DELIVERY SYSTEMS—MEDICAL HOMES

As new medical home models develop within delivery systems, it is important that PAs involve themselves in the planning process to ensure that they are fully used and appropriately compensated to be consistent with physician practice. This may include specific administrative time or reimbursement for e-mail communications with patients or accurate accounting of the contributions that they make in patient encounters outside of the face-to-face visit.

Interactions with Nurse Practitioners

Most settings now hire both PAs and nurse practitioners. In some settings the two roles are similar; in others, very different. Ideally the roles should be complementary and not competitive. Occasionally, and unfortunately, the culture of a particular clinical setting may have created dysfunctional relationships between the two groups. Often this culture is based on either which group was hired first in the institution or on a specific incident that divided the two groups.

Ideally, it is useful for members of both groups to find ways to work together to maximize patient care.

LEADERSHIP ROLES FOR PHYSICIAN ASSISTANTS IN HEALTH CARE SYSTEMS

Although most PAs chose their career because they wanted to take care of patients, it is important that some PAs assume positions of leadership in emerging and expanding health care delivery systems. One of the reasons that NPs have sometimes prevailed in big systems is that nursing administrators and nurse managers became their advocates. Although PAs have relied on their supervising physicians to carry out this advocacy role, new administrative structures in large systems require specific PA representation. Preparation for these roles can include additional academic preparation, such as degrees in health administration, public administration, or business, as well as focused certificates in specific topic areas such as quality, informatics, evidence-based medicine and reimbursement. Some PA leaders have received in-house, on-the-job training over time, preparing them for leadership roles.

PLANNING FOR THE FUTURE

Looking ahead, the most important strategy will be the inclusion of PAs on planning and implementation bodies within health systems and government. PAs should prepare themselves for these roles, recommend/nominate each other and themselves for these positions, and assume active and articulate roles in these groups. As a profession, PAs are still building the culture for this type of activity in terms of valuing and respecting time spent on such activities.

CONCLUSIONS/PROJECTIONS

As U.S. health care systems expand, evolve, and "remake themselves" in response to the 2010 health reform legislation, it is reasonable to expect that PA roles will further expand and develop. This will create a need for PA programs to continue to recruit candidates who have a flexible and open-minded view of the profession and an interest in pioneering new roles. In pursuit of "full utilization" of PAs in large delivery systems, increasing numbers of PAs will need to see themselves as leaders, to participate actively and visibly in planning, operations, and governance activities, and to work together with other health professionals to optimize patient care, make cost-effective decisions, increase access, and decrease disparities.

CASE STUDY 42-1: LARGE HEALTH MAINTENANCE ORGANIZATION

Group Health was one of the first employers of PAs in the Pacific Northwest. Since that time, PAs have been used in many service lines in the organization including primary care, urgent care/emergency medicine, orthopedics, and general surgery. Group Health is now developing and implementing its own primary care model. The first step has been to beta-test the model in one of Group Health's clinics in a suburb of Seattle. With that successful implementation, Group Health is now planning to expand this innovation system wide to its multiple primary clinics throughout Washington State. You have been identified as a PA leader within Group Health and have been asked to be the PA representative on a Group Health state-wide committee charged with further developing the model, developing policies for the clinicians, and creating training materials for use across the organization.

1. What are the issues you should be concerned with for the patients? For the clinical staff? For the nonclinical staff? For PAs and NPs specifically?
2. Because Group Health is both an insurance company and also a delivery system, what are the opportunities that exist for the system to develop models that might not be possible in a traditional fee-for-service system?
3. Are there specific tasks in the medical home model that are more appropriate, cost effective, or efficient when performed by nonphysician clinicians (e.g., PAs, NPs, PharmDs) in a medical home model? Should there be incentives for performing these tasks?
4. What is your own opinion on the issue of "leadership" within a medical home clinic? Given the fact that Group Health has many senior PAs and NPs, what roles and responsibilities should they have in the developing medical home models? How would you implement your suggestions?

CASE STUDY 42-2: REGIONAL RURAL HEALTH SYSTEM

You are working at Heartland Health—a new rural health network system serving several Midwestern states. You have actually been working in the same location for more than 15 years; however, what was formerly a single-physician private family practice has now become part of a large (and new) system when your physician sold the practice to the new group and became an employee of Heartland Health. Six other similar practices that employ PAs and NPs also became a part of the network at the same time.

All of the private practice physicians had been struggling with decisions about the purchase of electronic medical records and increasingly complicated billing systems, which were difficult to maintain at the solo-practice level. All of the physicians were also nearing retirement age and seeking respite from the heavy responsibilities of 24/7 on-call schedules.

While you were involved in this decision-making process (and even received a "retention bonus" as an incentive for you to stay), you are now surprised to hear of the system's policies regarding PAs and NPs. Heartland Health plans to hire more PAs and NPs—although they are seeking to find what they call "generic" practitioners who will not work consistently with the same physician or within the same clinic. Management's idea is that these "generic" PAs and NPs will substitute for physicians—particularly in the evenings and on weekends—and will be flexible generalists who will be able to work in any of the system's clinics as assigned. You and your other PA and NP colleagues became aware of this plan when you discovered that the hiring process for the new hires would not include interviews with the community physicians or the current PAs and NPs. Instead they would be screened by the human resources office and then interviewed by the associate medical director for Heartland Health, who would interview them and make hiring decisions. (The practice act in your state does allow PAs to work for a single system in multiple sites as long as there is a designated preceptor and an approved practice plan). Although it has not been announced yet, you and our colleagues are concerned that you, too, will be moved around to meet the needs of Heartland Health and that the continuity relationship you have with your patients, your preceptor, and your community will be disrupted.

1. What are the pros and cons of this situation for your patients, for the system, for your community-based practice, and for you?
2. Should you and/or your colleagues intervene? Why, or why not?
3. If you decide to get involved, how would you approach this? What would be your strategy? Whom would you involve?
4. On the basis of your analysis of this situation, what would be your recommendations to Heartland Health?

CASE STUDY 42-3: VETERANS ADMINISTRATION

You are the senior PA for the VA in a large U.S. city. Your region includes three large VA multispecialty hospitals/clinics, two domiciliaries, and a growing number of community-based outreach clinics in the smaller communities surrounding your city.

As a PA leader, you have been tasked with increasing the visibility of VA employment to civilian PAs and PA students. This assignment is based on the growing population of veterans from Iraq and Afghanistan. VA workforce projections demonstrate the expanded need for PAs and NPs to care for the general needs of veterans, as well as the specific needs of veterans with posttraumatic stress disorder, amputations, closed-head trauma, and other battle-specific conditions. As you have approached practicing PAs about their potential interest in PA jobs, you discover that many of them are poorly informed about the VA system. Sometimes, because of their own political views, they state that they would never consider a job in the VA. Some of them say that they are afraid of working with veterans. To make matters worse, the two PA programs in your community also do not see the value of rotations in the VA—despite a shortage of clinical rotations in general.

1. Consider solutions to this issue at the community level and at the national level. Identify incidents or situations in the popular culture (e.g., movies, TV shows) that might create or perpetuate these biases.
2. Recommend possible strategies for working with the AAPA or your state PA academy to provide better information about the VA system and VA employment.
3. Create a plan to work with the PA programs' clinical coordinators to better familiarize them with the benefits of rotations in the VA, including possible stipends and unique learning opportunities. If given the opportunity to present to PA students on the opportunities of VA training and VA practice, what are the areas you would highlight?
4. If you are unable to interest the local PA programs in VA rotations, consider how you might reach beyond your regions to other PA programs seeking relevant clinical rotations for their students.

CASE STUDY 42-4: COMMUNITY HEALTH CENTERS

The Tumbleweed Community Clinic Systems serves three rural Texas counties with one large all-purpose clinic (providing services in primary care, mental health, oral health, and prevention) and six other smaller satellite clinics, each of which employs three physicians and two PAs or NPs. This clinic system has rapidly expanded, and there are many new clinicians and administrators. Few of the new employees have experience with community health centers (CHCs), and none have worked in clinic systems that routinely use PAs and NPs. You and seven other PAs and NPs are new hires, although all of you are experienced providers who have worked in CHCs and other primary care settings.

As you begin your job you find that the staffing plan for the clinic is for PAs and NPs to have no scheduled patients but instead see only "walk-in" patients (a large number of patients typically seen in CHCs). In addition, the PA/NP providers will all be scheduled to cover evening and weekend clinics and will move between clinics in order to best meet the needs of the systems. All "walk-in" patients will be referred to physicians for follow-up. The supervision plan is that the medical director and two associate medical directors in the central clinic will serve as preceptors for the PAs and NPs. They will delegate on-site supervision to the local physicians but will periodically review charts, which are maintained on the clinic's electronic health record.

1. What are the advantages and disadvantages of this type of staffing?
2. How do you think the proposed staffing pattern will have the greatest effect on patients and patient satisfaction?
3. You meet with the other PAs and NPs to analyze the situation. What might you expect to hear from the group? Would you expect any difference in opinions between the PAs and the NPs?
4. How would you approach the clinic's management regarding your concerns? What recommendations would you make to the clinic management?

CASE STUDY 42-5: FAMILY MEDICINE RESIDENCY

The Hospital of the Eastern Shore houses a large family medicine residency, which has a mission to train primary care physicians for its local rural region. The program admits 10 residents a year into a 3-year program. Although the residency has regularly served as a training site for PA students, it has never before hired PAs as providers in the clinic. You and a fellow classmate from your program are beginning your jobs. Both of you have worked in other primary care clinics for the past 5 years and were recommended for your new jobs by your past supervising physicians—all of whom are graduates of this same residency program.

To begin with, you are both assigned to teams that are designed to eventually become "medical homes." You have been well accepted by the faculty, visiting attending physicians, and the residents. Now that you are settled in, the plan is for the residency to engage in discussions about the appropriate role of PAs and NPs in the clinic. For example, should PAs participate in the administration and leadership of the residency? Should PAs join the faculty in interviewing medical school candidates for admission to the residency? Should PAs have faculty status within the residency? Should PAs have their own panel of patients? What happens when patients would rather see the "permanent" PAs rather than the transient residents?

1. How is your role (and your potential role) in the residency different from your prior employment in a primary care clinic?
2. How can you affect the residents' perception of PAs and influence their choices about future employment/support of PAs in their practice setting?
3. What recommendations do you have about the residency's responsibilities for training PA and NP students?
4. What recommendations do you and your colleagues have to the residency about the best role for you right now? In 5 years? In 10 years?
   a. Large HMO (e.g., Kaiser or Group Health)
   b. Regional rural health systems
   c. Veterans Administration
   d. Community health center
   e. Academic medical center

KEY POINTS

- The cost of health care in America continues to rise at an alarmingly high rate and poses the threat of destabilizing American business and the entire economy.
- Other developed countries keep costs down and quality up through the use of systems that organize care and ensure access to everyone.
- The systems approach, compared with "independent" private physician practice, is now necessary given the complex health care environment that will include requirements for electronic health records, detailed and "compliant" billing processes, assessment of quality indicators, and "report cards" for physician practices.
- Policy makers describe integrated systems as being horizontally integrated, vertically integrated, and virtually integrated.

- The patient-centered medical home has been promulgated by primary care physician groups (e.g., pediatrics, family medicine, general internal medicine) as a strategy for providing care in a team-based model with physician leadership. PAs and NPs are considered to be key clinicians in the medical home model—partially due to the shortage of primary care physicians. In addition to being a care delivery model, the medical home model is also a reimbursement strategy with the ultimate plan of implementing a "pay-for-performance" system, which will reward clinics that keep their patients healthier.
- ACOs are large health care systems that—through their integration—aim to provide high-quality health care. A number of incentives—and disincentives—have been created to make ACOs work. PAs and NPs are also considered to be key components of an effective ACO.

References

1. Merriam-Webster Dictionary (website). *http://www.merriam-webster.com/dictionary/system.*
2. Crosson J. 21st century health care—the case for integrated delivery systems. N Engl J Med October 1, 2009;361:14.
3. Reference deleted in proofs.
4. Touchette MA, Zarowitz BJ. Integrated health care delivery systems. In: University of the Sciences in Philadelphia, Remington, (eds). The Science and Practice of Pharmacy. 21st ed. Philadelphia: Lippincott, Williams & Wilkins, 2005; 119.
5. Health care for all, serving West Marin. A history of community health centers, n.d. (website). *http://www.coastalhealth.net.* Accessed August 31, 2012.
6. Kaiser Permanente's history in health care reform, 2007; *http://xnet.kp.org/newscenter/pointofview/2007/062207*; Accessed March 1, 2012.
7. Crowley W. Group Health Timeline. Seattle: Group Health, 2007.
8. United States Department of Veterans Affairs. VA history, 2010. *http://www4.va.gov/about_va/vahistory.asp*; Accessed July 24, 2012.
9. U.S. Department of Defense Military Health System. History of the military health system, 2010. *http://xnet.kp.org/newscenter/point ofview/2007/062207kphchistory*; Accessed March 1, 2012.
10. Chavez, Scott R, Ballweg, et al. Correctional medicine. Physician Assistant: A Guide to Clinical Practice. 4th ed. Philadelphia: WB Saunders/Elsevier, 2008. p. 828.
11. Shortell S, Gillies R, Anderson D, et al. Remaking Health Care in America, Building Organized Delivery Systems. San Francisco: Jossey-Bass, 1996.
12. Bodenheimer T, Grumbach K. Understanding Health Policy: A Clinical Approach. 3rd ed. New York: Lange/McGraw-Hill, 1995. p. 67–77.
13. Robinson J, Casalino L. Vertical integration and organizational networks in health care. Health Affairs 1996;15(1):7–22.
14. Bodenheimer T, Grumbach K. Understanding Health Policy: A Clinical Approach. 3rd ed. New York: Lange/McGraw-Hill; 1995. p 72.
15. Reference deleted in proofs.
16. Reference deleted in proofs.
17. AAPA, Retrieved from *http://www.aapa.org/advocacy-and-practice-resources/trends/patient-centered-medical-home.*
18. American Academy of Family Physicians (AAFP), American Academy of Pediatrics (AAP), American College of Physicians (ACP), American Osteopathic Association (AOA), Joint Principles of the Patient-Centered Medical Home, March 2007, pp 1–3. *http://www.pcpcc.net/content/joint-principles-patient-centered-medical-home;* Accessed January 10, 2012.
19. Ballweg R, Macy Jr Josiah. Foundation. Who and How: Physician Assistant Educational Issues in Primary Care. New York: Josiah Macy Foundation. April 2010. 215–224.
20. Landon B, Gill J, Antonelli RC, Rich C. Prospects for rebuilding primary care using the patient-centered medical home. Health Affairs 29(5):827–835.
21. Meyer H. Report from the field. Group Health's move to the medical home: for doctors, it's often a hard journey. Health Affairs 2010;29(5):844–851.
22. Fisher ES, Staiger, Douglas O, Bynum, Julie PW, Gottlieb DJ. Creating accountable care organizations: the extended hospital medical staff. Health Affairs, December 5, 2006:44–57.
23. Cohen Jordan T. A guide to accountable care organizations, and their role in the senate's health reform bill. *http://www.healthreformwatch.com/2010/03/11/a-guide-to-accountable-care-organizations-and-their-role-in-the-senates-health-reform-bill/.*

The resources for this chapter can be found at www.expertconsult.com.

CHAPTER 43

REHABILITATIVE AND LONG-TERM CARE SYSTEMS

Kathy A. Kemle

CHAPTER CONTENTS

The physician assistant (PA) profession is rooted in primary care. Although increasing numbers of PAs are choosing specialty areas, 35% reported practicing in primary care (family and general medicine, internal medicine, pediatrics, and obstetrics/gynecology) in the 2009 American Academy of Physician Assistants national census. Thirty-eight percent of respondents reported that they function primarily in hospitals, and 9% indicated that they work in solo office practice with a physician supervisor.[1]

Most medical care is delivered in outpatient offices, ambulatory care centers, and acute care hospitals. However, there is a growing trend for care to take place in the patient's home, fueled by a need to decrease costs and by clients' desire to stay in their own homes. That home may be an individual domicile, congregate housing, an assisted living facility (ALF), an inpatient hospice, or a skilled nursing or other long-term care facility. The focus of this chapter is care delivery in this nonmedical setting, an area of immense opportunity for PAs who choose to embrace it (see Table 43-1 for information on various sites of care).

The "silvering" of the developed world is a well-established reality. This demographic shift will result in an aging "tsunami" of need for all kinds of care: medical, psychological, social, and functional. The disorders of aging do not conform to traditional medical approaches, which strive to find a single cause (diagnosis) to account for multiple symptoms. They are syndromes and thus multifactorial, requiring a holistic approach by an interdisciplinary team. PA programs have included geriatrics and geriatric syndromes in their curricula since the 1980s. With a generalist-training model, PAs are well prepared to assume a growing role in coordinating and directing care for older adults. In addition, PA education focuses on "hands-on" clinical skills, those most readily available and needed to provide services in a nonmedical environment. It incorporates a large amount of instruction in chronic disease management, a hallmark of aging. PA education emphasizes preservation of function and independence, both of which are core values of the geriatric population.

Most of the health care of the elderly and disabled younger individuals is financed by Medicare, administered by the Centers for Medicare and Medicaid Services. Since 1998, Medicare Part B has reimbursed PA employers in all settings at 85% of the physician allowable rate, if the services are medically necessary and would ordinarily be provided by a physician. The care must be provided by PAs working with physician supervision and must be within the scope of practice allowed by state law and regulations. Supervision may be via telecommunication and does not necessarily imply the physical presence of the physician, unless this is required by state law. PAs may bill any evaluation and management code except the initial comprehensive evaluation of the skilled nursing home (Part A) patient.

Table 43-2 lists the components of Medicare. Further information on reimbursement is provided in the section on each site of care.

TABLE 43-1 **Sites and Types of Long-Term Care**

Type/Site	Description	Payer
Inpatient rehabilitation hospital	Provide at least 3 hr of therapy/day; must make progress to continue	Medicare/Medicaid
Skilled nursing facility (SNF) postacute hospital; needs therapy	PT/OT, or speech must progress to continue	Medicare
Long-term hospital	Handle complex care such as ventilator patients	Medicare
Home health care	Nursing or therapy in the home; requires face-to-face encounter with physician, NP, or PA	Medicare/Medicaid
Hospice	May be in home, NH, ALF, or inpatient hospice; avoids hospitalization; usual prognosis <6 mo; concentrates on comfort	Medicare, other
Home care/ personal care	ADL/IADL care in the home	Varies but usually self-pay or Medicaid
Nursing home	Chronically ill patients who are not able tobenefit from rehabilitation and need nursing care	self-pay or private insurance, Medicaid
ALF	Institutional care; may serve small numbers or large; services vary widely and little regulation exists; patients usually less disabled than in nursing homes	Self-pay, few Medicaid
Day care	Provide limited services during day; some housed in ALF	Self-pay, Medicaid

ADL, activities of daily living; ALF, assisted living facility; IADL, instrumental activities of daily living; NH, nursing home; NP, nurse practitioner; OT, occupational therapy; PA, physician assistant; PT, physical therapy.

TABLE 43-2 **Medicare**

Component	Covers	Eligibility	Deductible
Part A	Hospital, hospice	Aged, disabled	Yes
	Home health medical equipment		
	Nursing home rehabilitation*		
Part B		Must elect and pay premium	Yes
	MD, PA visits		Yes
	Includes house calls, nursing home visits		Yes
Part C	Medicare Advantage plans, HMOs	Must elect	Varies
Part D	Prescription drug benefit	Must elect	Varies

*Nursing home after 3-day hospital stay; initial stay 20 days; 80 additional days with co-payment.

HMOs, health maintenance organizations; MD, medical doctor; PA, physician assistant.

HOME CARE—INFORMAL CAREGIVERS

The 65 million unpaid family caregivers are the largest source of long-term care in the United States. They may provide care on a full-time or part-time basis and may live with their care recipient or separately, some even at long distances. Most are women (usually wives or adult daughters), but there is an increase in the number of men serving in this role. Men are more likely to assume instrumental activities of daily living such as handling finances, whereas women tend to perform the "hands-on" activities of daily living (bathing, dressing, toileting, feeding, and mobility). Females are more likely to suffer emotional distress, anxiety, and depression related to their caregiving role. The majority of caregivers are middle-aged (35 to 64); however, many caregivers of older adults, especially spouses, are themselves elderly. Older caregivers tend to spend more hours providing care and are more likely to have their own health concerns.

About one fifth of the white and black populations in the United States are providing care, with slightly lower numbers of Asian and Hispanic Americans doing so. African Americans report less stress than white caregivers, and Hispanics and Asians experience more depression. Many caregivers find great fulfilment in their roles, enjoying closer relationships with their care recipients and satisfaction from providing what they believe is the best care for their loved ones. Most caregivers are employed outside the home, which, although it adds to stress in the workplace, may actually prove beneficial as a social outlet and a means of increasing income.[2] The 2009 economic downturn was especially difficult for homes in which caregiving took much of the family resources.[2]

Caregivers with higher incomes report less stress than those of more limited means.

Caregivers pay a high price emotionally and physically for their roles. Depression is the most common psychological disorder and is especially prevalent in those caring for a demented person. Elevated stress is associated with increased likelihood of harm to the recipient. Caregivers also suffer disproportionately from increased risk for cardiovascular disease, immune system dysfunction, and elevated blood pressure. Elderly spousal caregivers experiencing stress have a markedly higher mortality rate than their noncaregiving, age-matched peers.

The monetary value of informal caregiving is difficult to assess but has been estimated to far outweigh the combined cost of home health and nursing home care. Although some support services are available, many caregivers are unaware of their existence or how to access them. Use of support has been shown to reduce stress and depression and to delay institutionalization by as much as a year. A 2006 study of ethnically diverse caregivers of demented patients found that bimonthly in-home and telephone interviews of caregivers addressing depression, burden, self-care, and care-recipient problem behaviors improved quality of life, although no difference in institutionalization was observed.[3] As the economic contributions of informal caregivers have begun to be recognized, there has been a movement toward legislative and regulatory efforts to provide more support for individuals to remain at home. These include redirection of Medicaid dollars to informal caregivers rather than to institutions.

As primary care providers, PAs can impart an invaluable service to their caregiving patients by helping them to optimize their own health. The PA may be the only social and emotional outlet for the often-isolated caregiver. Recognizing and expressing appreciation of their efforts can be a positive incentive to continue in the role. Providing information on community support programs and assisting the family in locating respite may be an important therapeutic intervention for both care provider and recipient.

HOME CARE—HOME CARE ORGANIZATIONS

Home care organizations include home health agencies, home care aide organizations, and hospices.[4] Most agencies are Medicare certified and provide skilled nursing assistance. Although the enactment of Medicare in 1965 greatly accelerated growth in the industry, the changes that occurred in the 1997 Balanced Budget Act led to a decline in the home health agency sector. However, demand continues to increase and in 2000, each day, an estimated 1.5 million persons were enrolled in home care.[5] Medicare is the single largest payer, accounting for slightly less than one third of total payments. Other sources include private out-of-pocket, Medicaid, CHAMPUS, and the Veterans Administration. Medicaid home care expenditures vary on the basis of state eligibility rules and are oriented toward personal care activities such as bathing and dressing.

Of those patients who receive Medicare home health services, most have chronic diseases, which impact ability to perform activities of daily living. The most common primary diagnoses in 2009 were as follows:

Diabetes
Heart disease including congestive heart failure
Malignant neoplasm
Chronic obstructive pulmonary disease
Hypertension
Cerebrovascular disease

Recipients generally must have a skilled nursing need and meet Medicare's definition of homebound (i.e., unable to leave their homes without great difficulty, generally only for physician office visits or to go to church). Other therapists such as physical and occupational practitioners are available without a skilled nursing need but require a physician's order. Most clients are older than 85 years of age, female, and in poor health. The increasing use of Telehomecare, which uses telephone lines and Internet connections to link medical providers with homebound patients, has had positive effects on self-management of chronic illness.[6] Managed care is another source of financing for home health, usually via a negotiated prepaid rate. Most contracts are through employer-based insurance, but it is being used by states in an attempt to reduce unsustainable Medicaid expenditures.

HOSPICE

Most medical care is this country is delivered in the expectation or hope of attaining a cure. Palliative medicine is directed toward the relief of suffering in all of its manifestations, rather than an effort to cure disease. Although those at the end of life often desire a more palliative approach, care providers should always focus on symptom management, regardless of prognosis.

Hospice is a philosophy of care that concentrates on the comfort and dignity of the patient and their family. Most hospice care takes place in the home, but inpatient hospice care programs are available in some communities. Hospice may also care for patients who reside in nursing homes or assisted living facilities. In 2007, the average length of stay on hospice varied by age and gender with the oldest patients and females enjoying the longest length of service. Only 3% received care for at least 30 days, suggesting that the benefit is underutilized.[7] A 2002 survey of families revealed that longer stays were perceived as more beneficial, but even short hospice experiences were helpful.[2] To access the Medicare Part A Hospice Benefit, patients must choose a palliative approach, although contrary to common belief, they may continue to be resuscitated in the event of a cardiopulmonary arrest. A physician must certify that the patient's life expectancy is less than 6 months if his or her disease process follows its natural progression. This requirement has contributed to the myth that hospice is only for cancer patients because the trajectory of decline related to most neoplasm is relatively predictable, and survival in other diseases may be less well-defined. However, many other disorders qualify, and there is no penalty for longer survival, provided the individual is declining (see Table 43-3 for the most common hospice diagnoses). Hospice continues to provide bereavement support of the family up to 13 months after the death of the patient.

Hospice incorporates many of the same principles as home care: physical assessment, psychosocial support, disease and symptom management, use of an interdisciplinary care team, and patient and family education. Teams include hospice nurses, the hospice medical director, social workers, clergy, and volunteers. Promotion of the dignity of individuals and their ability to live their last days and months to the fullest extent possible are the goals.

Life closure is difficult to attain when physical symptoms interfere with concentration, and, therefore, relief of pain and discomfort is a core skill for team members. The patient's perception of symptoms is the basis for successful management but does not always coincide with the observations of team members. Suffering incorporates pain but is also a total experience influenced by family relationships, cultural background, religious belief system, and social supports of the patient. The clinician must be well versed in medical and nonmedical means of treating these symptoms. The American Academy of Hospice and Palliative Care Medicine produces a series of self-education materials, which promotes best-practice approaches in palliative care. Other self-directed learning materials are also cited in this chapter.

Caring for a dying loved one is extremely rewarding but can lead to exhaustion and burnout in family members. Symptom management may become impossible to achieve in the home setting. Hospices can provide continuous care by a registered nurse until symptoms are controlled or respite care in a hospital, nursing home, or an inpatient hospice setting may allow the caregivers a short vacation from their caregiving responsibilities. The hospice respite benefit is the only form of respite service covered under the Medicare program. A growing number of hospitals maintain specialized units for palliative care and/or palliative care consult teams, using PAs as core members of an interdisciplinary team.

Few PAs are involved in hospice care, but the increasing complexity of hospice patients is beginning to increase their use. PAs mirror the practice patterns of their supervising physicians, and as more physicians become comfortable with palliative medicine, greater numbers of PAs will choose this rewarding specialty. PAs may provide a vital link between the attending physician, the patient, and the hospice agency. Changes in the reimbursement structure of the hospice benefit may also allow more hospices to employ PAs in the future.

TABLE 43-3 Hospice Diagnoses in Order of Frequency in 2007

Malignant neoplasm (42.8%)
Nonmalignant diagnoses (57.2%)
Heart disease, including congestive heart failure
Dementia
Chronic obstructive pulmonary disease
Cerebrovascular disease

From Caffrey C, Sengupta M, Moss A, et al: Home Health Care and Discharged Hospice Care Patients: United States, 2000 and 2007. National Health Statistics Report, No. 38. April 27, 2011.

MEDICAL HOUSE CALLS

In the early 1900s, most physician services took place in the patient's home and diagnostic tools fit easily in the "black bag." Gradually, improvements in transportation and technologic advances led to centralized care in office-based practices, and house calls became a rare practice. Physician training became concentrated in inpatient units, so doctors had no role models in home care. Liability and safety concerns contributed to the decline. A further disincentive was poor reimbursement compared with office visits. Other reasons for the change were more personal. Clinicians may be uncomfortable with visiting certain neighborhoods or in the unfamiliar environment of another person's home. They may be unable to manage complex patients without their customary diagnostic and therapeutic tools or the immediate availability of the expertise of consultant colleagues. House calls remain an inefficient use of provider time because of the time lost in travel. House call clients often suffer from a complex array of chronic diseases. The time devoted to care tends to be greater. However, the inefficiency of providing care for these patients in the office is a hidden cost to the practice.

In recent years, house calls have enjoyed a resurgence of popularity. Tangible benefits of house calls are a more accurate assessment of functional status and environmental safety, a closer relationship with patients and their families (reducing liability concerns), and a better understanding of the challenges faced by both the patient and their caregivers. In 2010 nearly 200,000 home visits were billed to Medicare by PAs (G. Schwartz, oral communication from American Academy of Home Care Physicians, March 2012).

Technology has advanced to allow the provider to take the office to the patient. Portable laboratory devices, electrocardiograph machines, and pulse oximeters have augmented the house call provider's ability to assess the patient in the home. Mobile services are available for diagnostic studies in larger population centers. The use of an electronic medical record allows the provider to record the visit and access patient materials without the need for a bulky paper chart.

Medicare reimburses for physician services provided in the home by PAs. Patients do not have to meet the stringent housebound requirement needed for home care agency visits but must simply need medical care and have difficulty accessing the physician office. Many PAs and physicians maintain a small panel of their patients whom they see in the home. Some physicians and PAs have chosen to work exclusively as house call providers and may be in solo practice or employed by companies that specialize in medical house calls.

CASE STUDY 43-1

Mrs. A is a 96-year-old woman with severe congestive heart failure, osteoarthritis, hypertension, and coronary artery disease. She is cared for at home by her 78-year-old daughter. Mrs. A has been slowly declining and is only able to walk from her chair to her bed and bedside commode. She does not want to be hospitalized, understands that her prognosis is limited, and has chosen hospice. It is difficult for her daughter to bring her to the office because she cannot access the car.

Her daughter calls the physician's office to report that her mother seems more short of breath and more confused than usual. The hospice nurse has visited and believes the patient would benefit from diuresis. The physician asks his PA to go to the patient's home and evaluate her. The PA finds a woman in moderate respiratory distress with an oxygen saturation of 89% despite her home oxygen therapy, fever of 100.8° F, and right lower lobe rales; the diagnosis is pneumonia rather than an exacerbation of congestive heart failure. The hospice has provided a supply of palliative medications in the home, and the PA administers a small dose of oral morphine, which greatly relieves the patient's dyspnea. She teaches the daughter how to give the morphine and advises the use of a fan for further relief of the patient's distress. An appropriate antibiotic is called in to the local pharmacy. The PA requests hospice nurses to visit the following day and report on the patient's condition. The nurses monitor her symptoms and ensure continued comfort. Mrs. A recovers and is able to enjoy her 97th birthday 1 month later with her family, subsequently dying in her sleep. Her daughter expresses gratitude to the care team for helping her mother to live her last few months in her own home.

ASSISTED-LIVING FACILITIES

Another site of care for older and disabled adults is the ALF. Most are located in urban or suburban areas and provide assistance in activities of daily living. In 2006, between 600,000 and 1 million individuals resided in about 30,000 ALFs in the United States.[8] The facilities are usually funded via private payment from residents, but some are financed through state Medicaid programs and by charities. They may assist residents with medication management but are specifically prohibited from maintaining a medical director or skilled nursing services. Physicians or PAs may visit their patients in these facilities, if the visit is medically necessary and if it is difficult for the patients to access the physician office. Medicare has recognized the growing complexity of residents in ALFs and reimburses visits at the same rate as that provided for house calls. Because the growth in this industry has been exponential and the need for services is only expected to increase, it is likely that medical providers will be providing more care in ALFs.

NURSING HOMES

The mission of nursing homes has changed dramatically over the past two decades along with their patient populations. There are generally two types of patients: long stays (>6 months), who usually have multiple chronic disease and functional losses; and short stays, who are there for short-term rehabilitation after an acute hospitalization. Medicare provides a 20-day fully covered period after a 3-day hospital stay for skilled nursing services or for therapy. Patients must show progress over the duration of the stay to continue to use the benefit. An additional 80 days is available with a co-payment from the beneficiary. A physician, PA, or nurse practitioner must certify patients to receive this service.

A new and challenging reality is the rapid increase in the number of Americans who enter nursing homes as their final site of care. Patients require more intense medical management than ever, but physician involvement remains limited. Low reimbursement rates coupled with liability concerns have led many physicians to avoid long-term care facilities despite the rising medical intricacy of the patients housed there. According to the AAPA 2009 census, few PAs (5%) reported working primarily in a nursing home, although it is likely many see a limited number of nursing home patients as part of their practice.

PAs' employers are reimbursed for visits made by PAs in nursing homes at 85% of the physician rate, provided the care is medically necessary. PA participation in long-term care has been shown to reduce hospitalizations to a level even lower than that of community-dwelling Medicare recipients.[9] The presence of a PA reassures nursing staff, patients, and families that a well-trained clinician is available to evaluate and manage their symptoms. Patients must be seen every 30 days for the first 90 days of their stay and at 30- or 60-day intervals thereafter. PAs may alternate the required visits with their physician supervisors. Acute care visits may be made at any time by the PA, if warranted by the patient's medical condition. Medicare will usually pay for 18 visits per year without question; however, reimbursement for additional visits may be made if documentation supports their necessity.

One exception to care by PAs is the initial comprehensive visit required for those patients whose stay is covered by Medicare Part A (skilled nursing facility patients). The physician must complete this service, but should the patient need care before the physician's assessment, the PA may see the patient and manage the acute situation. Patients admitted as self-pays or as long-term clients (ICF patients) may be initially assessed by the PA. Nursing home patients must have a yearly comprehensive history and physical examination, which may be performed by either provider.

KEY POINTS

- The growth in the aged and disabled population will continue to fuel a demand for home care services.
- Informal caregivers provide most of the care of disabled persons and often experience stress as a result.
- Palliative medicine focuses on the relief of suffering in all of its forms.
- House calls are a viable option for physicians and PAs who wish to care for the vulnerable elderly and disabled population.
- Medicare reimburses for PA visits at alternative sites.
- PAs can be integral components of the care of patients in their homes, wherever that home may be.

References

1. 2009 AAPA Physician Assistant Census Report. Alexandria, VA: American Academy of Physician Assistants, 2009.
2. National Association for Home Care and Hospice. Basic Statistics for Home Care and Hospice. Washington, DC: National Association for Home Care and Hospice, 2009.
3. Belle SH, Burgio L, Burns R, et al. Enhancing the quality of life of dementia caregivers from different ethnic or racial groups: a randomized, controlled trial. Ann Intern Med 2006;145(10):727–738.
4. Landers S, Peterson L. Trends in home diagnostic testing for Medicare beneficiaries. J Am Geriatr Soc 2007;55(1):138–139.

5. Federal Interagency Forum on Aging Related Statistics. Older Americans 2000: Key Indicators of Well-Being. Washington, DC: US Government Printing Office, 2000.
6. Bowles KH, Baugh AC. Applying research to optimize tele-homecare. Cardiovasc Nurs 2007;22(1):5–15.
7. Caffrey C, Sengupta M, Moss A, et al. Home Health Care and Discharged Hospice Care Patients: United States, 2000 and 2007. National Health Statistics Report, 2011. No. 38. April 27.
8. Kerr T. American Association of Homes and Services for the Aging (website). *www2.aahsa.org*; Updated March 6, 2007: Accessed December 4, 2011.
9. Ackermann RJ, Kemle KA. The effect of a physician assistant on the hospitalization of nursing home residents. J Am Geriatr Soc 1998;46(5):610–614.

The resources for this chapter can be found at www.expertconsult.com.

CHAPTER 44

HEALTH CARE FOR HOMELESS POPULATIONS

Lois C. Thetford • Linda J. Vorvick • Keren H. Wick

CHAPTER CONTENTS

Poverty and homelessness are most visible during difficult economic times. During the Great Depression (1929–1939), 25% of the labor force was out of work, banks collapsed, factory output fell by one third, and many homes were lost to foreclosure. Hunger was epidemic; farmers were unable to grow food. Americans migrated from the hardest-hit areas, lived in packing crates in shantytowns, rode the rails in search of work, and split up families. Out of that experience came the establishment of unemployment insurance, the Social Security system, the Federal Deposit Insurance Corporation, and many other programs to help people survive hard times.[1] Subsequent economic depressions have been shorter and less severe, but additional social determinants have caused surges in homelessness over the past 30 years.

Institutionalized care for psychiatric patients was reduced in the early 1980s, and without adequate housing, work training, or social adjustment assistance, many simply became homeless. This deficit of services for the mentally ill has continued; they comprise 26% of the chronic homeless population living in shelters.[2] Substance abuse treatment is also scarce, especially for those with both mental illness and substance abuse. Wealthy people with substance abuse can access treatment, but the poor cannot. Many addicts die waiting for a treatment bed to open up.

A homeless individual is any person lacking fixed, stable, permanent housing, whether he or she lives on the street, in a van, in a shelter, or a single- room occupancy facility. The Homeless Emergency Assistance and Rapid Transition to Housing (HEARTH) Act[3] reaffirms the McKinney Act definition of a homeless person. This definition is as follows:

1. An individual who lacks a fixed, regular, and adequate nighttime residence; and
2. An individual who has a primary nighttime residence that is:
   A. A supervised publicly or privately operated shelter designed to provide temporary living accommodations (including welfare hotels, congregate shelters, and transitional housing for the mentally ill);
   B. An institution that provides a temporary residence for individuals intended to be institutionalized; or
   C. A public or private place not designed for, or ordinarily used as, a regular sleeping accommodation for human beings.[4]

The HEARTH Act expands the definition of homelessness by adding families who have unstable housing and individuals who will face homelessness in the next 14 days.[3]

The first episode of homelessness usually lasts from a few weeks to months, usually in persons younger than 30 years of age. Up to 80% of people make the transition to more stable circumstances within a year. Ten percent are episodically homeless, having 4.9 shelter episodes in 3 years with an average stay of 54 days. Chronically homeless individuals are primarily middle-aged males with mental illness or substance abuse problems.[5] People who are homeless as children have a higher rate of homelessness as adults; of homeless mothers, 44% lived outside a primary home as a child, according to the National Center on Family Homelessness.[6]

Families make up 37% of the homeless. They become homeless due to job loss, bankruptcy due to medical bills, intimate partner violence, flooding, accidents, or disability. Of all homeless individuals, 22% are younger than 18 and 1.4% are unattached youth.[2] Youth homelessness most often results from familial disruption: divorce, abuse, neglect, or rejection.[7] People who live on the street experience a high rate of both physical and sexual assault. The rates for men are 27% per year, 32% annually for women, and 38% annually for transgendered persons.[8]

ADULTS

Of all homeless adults, 11% are single women and 44% are single men. Women heading a homeless family with their children comprise 27% of all homeless adults, whereas only 18% of men report being in a homeless family.[2] Homeless people have high rates of hypertension, diabetes, peripheral vascular disease, respiratory problems, and chronic liver and renal disease. Tuberculosis and human immunodeficiency virus (HIV) are endemic; cellulitis, diphtheria, endocarditis, *Haemophilus influenzae* bacteremia, and septic arthritis are all much more common than in the general public.[9,10] Their lifespan is approximately 30 years less than the average American's lifespan.[11]

CASE STUDY 44-1

A new patient, 38, comes into the clinic for headache and hypertension. Mr. Miller's clothes are a little ragged, and he has difficulty making eye contact. He reports that he ran out of medication for his blood pressure. He is unemployed and has no insurance. He does not know his family medical history but reports that both his parents died young. He admits to drinking and smoking when he can afford it, and most of his food comes from community feeding programs or a food bank. Regarding exercise, he says, "I walk a lot, sometimes all day, sometimes all night." He believes his headache is from his high blood pressure. He last worked during the previous month for Labor Ready. His blood pressure is 165/121, and his pulse is 74. His examination shows arteriovenous nicking in the left eye, dental caries and missing teeth, taut sternocleidomastoid muscle, and an interdigital rash on both feet.

How does a clinician know when he or she is seeing a homeless patient? Homeless patients often do not self-identify, but they will access medical care in many settings. The patient in Case 44-1 has several indicators: body habitus, economic situation, lack of family support or connection, untreated medical problems, significant social history—especially walking all day or all night—and alcohol. Mr. Miller is one of 1.5 million people who used a homeless shelter at least once in 2010.[2] Although they are most visible to the medical system due to high emergency department use (72 visits per year per 100 individuals),[12] homeless individuals are seen in family practice and specialty settings, pediatric clinics, veterans' hospitals, and women's health care settings. Most medical problems of homeless patients are best handled by good primary care. Although they have many acute problems, particularly physical trauma, that send them to the emergency department, a connection to primary care is the most effective treatment plan for both the patient and medical system.[13] Housing decreases the rate of emergency department use, as does case management.[14,15]

The evaluation of Mr. Miller identifies many risks for heart disease: a 20-pack-year history of smoking, hypertension that is uncontrolled, retinal vasculitis, alcoholism, dental decay, possible depression, and sleep deprivation. This is a high priority for the clinician, but the headache needs to be addressed first because that is what brought Mr. Miller into the facility. The care provider can reassure him that muscle tension is the likely cause, but treating his hypertension is essential. He currently has no control over his diet; cannot afford medication for his hypertension or headache; and has no access to dental care, psychiatric care, physical therapy, or substance abuse treatment. At this point, the health care provider can build trust by congratulating him for coming in for treatment, reassuring him that the clinical staff can help him, and ensuring that he will be able to obtain medication at no cost. He also needs basic blood chemistries to evaluate liver or kidney damage and anemia.

If the clinical facility has a social worker, the next step is to implement a "warm handoff," which allows a personal introduction if possible, an opportunity to verify his addition to the social worker's case load, and arrangements for follow-up appointments. If there is no social worker, the clinical staff needs to pursue appropriate resources within the local community. There is often a nurse or medical assistant in the clinic who knows what is available. That individual can make the connections to help set up a plan of care for this patient. Finally, the clinician needs to emphasize to Mr. Miller how important it is that he return, even if he misses the follow-up appointment for some reason. This patient needs to return for follow-up care.

PEDIATRICS

There are 1.5 million homeless children annually. Forty-two percent of homeless children are younger than the age of 6 compared with 34% nationally; 12% are in foster care compared with 1% in the general population. Homeless children have more acute and chronic illnesses, more emergency department visits and hospitalizations, more developmental delays, more school failure, and more emotional and behavioral problems than housed poor children. The lack of private space in congregate living settings, the lack of safety and stability, and exposure to violence all affect the parent-child bond, as well as the child's developing mind and self-esteem.[6]

CASE STUDY 44-2

The next patient is a 3-year-old girl brought into urgent care for a possible ear infection. Her 27-year-old mother has an 18-month-old toddler with her as well. The 3-year-old is alternately crying and sleeping on her mother's lap as the mother tries to control the wandering toddler. The mother says that she has Medicaid coverage but does not have her card with her. She reports that the child began to pull at her right ear yesterday, but today she has a fever and will not eat. The child's temperature is 102.8° F, with a pulse of 88 and respiration of 17. The examination shows a red, bulging tympanic membrane on the right and pink left tympanic membrane with a fluid line, as well as bilateral preauricular and postauricular and submaxillary lymphadenopathy. Lung and heart examinations are noncontributory.

The heart, lungs, and lymph nodes are examined while the child is still sleeping. She wakes during the ear examination. The throat is observed while she is crying. The record shows that she is behind on immunizations. The mother reports that they have been moving a lot and lost touch with her former health care provider. This provides an opening; instead of moving on to the medical issues, the care provider needs to find out why. Do they have safe, stable housing? The mother should be encouraged to explain as much as she can, and the provider can offer to hold or distract the other child while she talks.

Homeless children have ear infections at twice the rate and respiratory infections at four times the rate of the general population. They are four times as likely to have asthma. They experience more gastrointestinal problems (five times the usual rate) and emotional and behavioral problems (three times the usual rate). They are twice as likely to go hungry. The stressors of hunger or poor nourishment, lack of safety and stability, and parental distress are exacerbated by their exposure to violence (25% have seen family violence). By the age of 12, 83% have witnessed serious violence.[6]

In one case, during a medical intake with a homeless mother and four children at a domestic violence shelter, the mother was greatly impeded by her 2-year-old crying, pulling at her, and pushing the pen away to stop her from completing the necessary forms. An older sister was holding the 1-year-old, who then got down to walk around. The 2-year-old watched her younger sibling for a minute and then went up to her, put her hands around her neck, and started to squeeze. The mother promptly intervened, soothed both children, and reported that the child was just imitating the behavior of the father. During their shelter stay, all of them stabilized well, but in the acute posttraumatic period, this child displayed disturbing and dangerous behavior.

Emotional, behavioral, and cognitive development are arrested by traumatic experiences in infancy or early childhood.[16] Homeless children exhibit many behavioral symptoms as a result of trauma and loss that are often misdiagnosed, such as attention deficit hyperactivity disorder. Common responses to trauma in children include fearfulness, sleep problems or nightmares, sadness, increased separation anxiety, poor social and school functioning, reexperiencing events, lack of emotion, distractibility, depression, guilt, and avoidance.[16] Many homeless children suffer discrimination and targeting at school related to "not fitting in," being behind their age group scholastically, old clothing, and requiring special help. This tends to increase withdrawal, anxiety, and depression, creating further barriers to attending and catching up at school.[6]

In treating this child (Case Study 44-2) for her right acute otitis media and left serous otitis media, it is important to make sure that the family has access to refrigeration for the amoxicillin. Most shelters include a common kitchen that is open only for limited hours. The clinician must be sure that the family has shelter and that they are able to fill the prescription.[13] Vaccines should be offered, as should independent visits for the toddler and mother. At some shelters, there is a public health nurse or other service provider who can perform immunizations. Clinic staff should be sure to obtain accurate contact information, including the name of a staff person at the shelter. The mother should be given the clinician's card so that follow-up can be arranged. Finally, a referral to behavioral health should be offered to the mother if she is not already accessing counseling services through the shelter.

The mother in Case Study 44-2 established a good connection with the care provider, and she agreed to come back for her own checkup because she was overdue for routine care and had a number of other concerns. The majority of homeless families have experienced divorce or domestic violence, extreme poverty due to falling wages, loss of benefits, and the lack of affordable housing. One third of homeless mothers have chronic health conditions, and half suffer a major depression after becoming homeless.[6] Only half of pregnant homeless mothers receive regular prenatal care. One third abuse drugs or alcohol.[17]

ADOLESCENTS

There are 1.6 million youth on the street every year; most leave home because of extensive abuse, family dissolution, or the instability of residential care (e.g., foster care, hospitalization). Homeless youth suffer from malnutrition, exposure, mental illness, violent assault and rape, and disrupted emotional development. They are quickly exposed to drug use and prostitution, resulting in the highest rates of all populations for sexually transmitted diseases. They are up to 12 times more likely to contract HIV and 7 times more likely to die from acquired immunodeficiency syndrome (AIDS) than the average teen. Approximately 34% engage in survival sex (which involves exchanging sex for food, money, or shelter); 75% of those do so only while homeless.[18,19]

CASE STUDY 44-3

During an evening shift in urgent care, an 18-year-old male comes in after an assault. He provides few details but thinks his wrist is broken. He was with a friend when they were jumped by three young men. He has visible cuts and contusions on the head, upper torso, and arms. He is holding his left wrist, trying to appear stoic, but clearly in great distress. When asked about the mode of injury to his wrist, he replies: "They threw me onto the ground and one of them stomped on my arm. I heard it snap."

The radiograph shows ulnar fractures in two locations. The arm will be immobilized and then casted once the swelling has decreased. Only some of the lacerations need stitches. As he moves from the table to a chair, some blood is noticeable where he was sitting. When asked about this, he turns away and his eyes tear up. The clinician then explains the need to examine the site of injury and take cultures and blood tests for baseline status on sexually transmitted diseases. The patient agrees reluctantly.

Although only 3% to 5% of the U.S. population self-identifies as lesbian, gay, bisexual, or transgender (LGBT), 20% to 40% of homeless youth do so. Half of LGBT youth report negative family reactions to coming out; 32% were physically assaulted, and 26% were kicked out. They experience greater degrees of depression and loneliness than other homeless youth and are three times more likely to engage in survival sex.[20] They frequently have to hide their identities, even in shelters, due to discrimination by other youth and some youth service agencies. This is especially true for transgender youth.

Homeless youth will not seek care in standard medical settings except in an emergency. They will access youth-only medical services, especially if they are allied with food, shelter, or drop-in youth agencies. Homeless youth older than 18 can stay at adult shelters, but it is frequently unsafe for them to do so. They need youth or young adult services that are appropriate to their needs. Many such clinics exist in cities around the country, but rural and suburban areas have few. Many youth need full medical, dental, and psychiatric care.

MILITARY VETERANS

Over a year's time, 136,000 veterans are homeless according to the most recent comprehensive report in 2009.[21] Of all homeless men 33% are veterans, and 26% of the overall homeless population are veterans. The demographics of homeless veterans are varied: 15% served before the Vietnam era, 47% served during Vietnam, and 17% served after. Thirty-three percent served in a war zone, 67% served at least 3 years, and 89% received an honorable discharge.[22] Most veterans are less likely to be homeless due to a higher education level than the general homeless population.

Homeless veterans were found to have a higher rate of early psychological and physical trauma, greater social isolation, and higher substance use than nonhomeless veterans. The combined rate of divorce or separation among homeless veterans is 57%, whereas among the homeless in general, the rate is only 32%. Seventy percent suffer from substance abuse, and 45% suffer from mental illness. Although posttraumatic stress disorder is a factor, it is the combination of these issues, plus a lack of jobs, affordable housing, or access to health care that has caused surges in the homeless veteran population, especially post-Vietnam.[23]

Only 25% have used homeless services through the Veterans Administration (VA). Homeless veterans have identified three factors that discourage accessing health care services through the VA: insensitive clinicians, negative policies, and inefficiency.[23] Three-hundred U.S. community-based veterans organizations have been successful serving homeless veterans with a peer approach. These "veterans helping veterans" groups feature transitional housing with structured, substance-free environments, case management support, employment training, and job placement services. They also sponsor 1- to 3-day relief events called Stand Downs. More than 200 of these take place each year around the country, and more than 200,000 veterans and family members have accessed services through these events. The nonprofits are most successful working in collaboration with federal, state, and local government agencies, as well as veteran service organizations. A sampling of these collaborations is included in the McMurray-Avila article,[23] and a full list of Stand Down events is provided by the VA.[24]

Veterans as a group are older than other homeless people, with an average age of 45, whereas only 20% of the total homeless population is 45 or older. Thus, heart disease, liver disease, kidney failure, lung disease, and physical disability require more varied and complex medical care. Fifty-two percent have one or more chronic health problems, compared with 44% of other homeless patients. A combat history is important to the medical history because the patient may have been exposed to agent orange or ionizing radiation or may suffer from Gulf War syndrome. Female veterans have the same incidence of mental illness and substance abuse as other female homeless patients.[23]

To care for this population, specialty care is necessary in addition to primary care and case management services. The task of handling medications for multiple conditions while living on the street in a wheelchair poses a significant challenge without the help of social services. The National Health Care for the Homeless Clinicians' Network has published a series of guidelines on adapting a clinical practice to facilitate caring for these complicated medical problems.[25]

CONCLUSION

Caring for homeless populations requires extra patience and compassion, but it is rewarding. Whether physician assistants are in primary care or a specialty practice, they will see patients whose traumatic life experiences have caused them to lose housing, jobs, social support, and health care. The care provided can literally give them new life: the respect they need to begin to recover and the health they need to be able to work and rebuild. Resources that are available nationwide facilitate the provision of appropriate care and follow-up for this challenging population. To win the trust of those who have lost all is to understand that these are survivors whose strengths and inner resources have been dismissed and unappreciated but who, with a physician assistant's help, can rise again.

CASE STUDY 44-4

Mrs. Taylor (introduced in Case 44-2), age 27, comes in with her toddler after finding day care for her 3-year-old. She needs a full physical examination with Pap smear and reports seasonal allergies, insomnia, and anxiety. The medical assistant distracts the child while assisting with the examination. This follow-up visit reveals a history of physical abuse that began with her pregnancies. Before that, there was conflict over her husband's drinking and rudeness. Her father was an alcoholic, with her parents divorcing when she was 11. She reports waking often during the night; having flashbacks, anxiety, and nightmares; and crying a lot. These are identified as symptoms of posttraumatic stress disorder. The patient minimizes the impact of her symptoms and has mixed feelings about the diagnosis: "The abuse wasn't that bad, not like some other people's." She is at an early stage of recognizing issues arising from both her family of origin and her history of experiencing domestic violence. It is usually not possible to press this concern without causing her to withdraw from the therapeutic relationship. Follow-up visits for her and the children will offer new possibilities to build that relationship. In the meantime, offering safe sleep medication and referrals to behavioral health resources could help.

PMH: fully immunized, menstrual headaches, urinary tract infections during pregnancy, one miscarriage and two normal vaginal births; Medications: none; Allergies: pollens, grasses; Contraception: none, previously used oral contraceptive pills and Depo-Provera

FH: hypertension, alcoholism—father, paternal grandfather
Depression—mother, maternal aunt
Breast cancer—maternal grandmother
SH: Parents divorced when she was 11 years old
No smoking, drugs, or alcohol
Separated, married 8 years, abuse began with pregnancies, living at domestic violence shelter for 2 months
Husband drinks, currently unemployed, some support from sister and mother
ROS: premenstrual headache 2 days, no visual changes, +rhinitis, palpitations, and shortness of breath when anxious; GI/GU: monthly menses last 4 days, insomnia—wakes often during the night, nightmares, flashbacks, +anxiety, +cries often
Vitals: Ht. 5'2", Wt. 131, BP 124/76, HR 78, R 17
Mrs. Taylor's physical examination showed no abnormalities except HEENT: maxillary sinuses mildly tender, cloudy tympanic membranes, red mucosa in nares bilaterally, turbinates swollen and boggy

QUESTIONS:

1. Assess six problems for this visit.
2. How do you prioritize these problems?
3. She states that she has no need for contraception. Do you pursue this issue or not?
4. Would you prescribe any medications?

CASE STUDY 44-5

Carlos is 58, complaining of pain, burning, and numbness in his legs, exacerbated by recent falling. He has a pack of belongings with him and reports no address. He was brought into the health center by a Health Care for the Homeless outreach worker concerned that he has barely been able to leave his tent for the past week or two, and he is incoherent at times in spite of drinking less.
PMH: hypertension, hepatitis, combat-related injuries, chronic cough, immunizations from military service; Medications: none at present; Allergies: none; Family history: none
SH: daily drinking and smoking, no contact with ex-wife or children in United States or family in the Philippines
ROS: fatigue, poor appetite, recent weight gain, dyspnea, burning pain in feet and legs, instability, memory loss
Vitals: Ht. 5'7", Wt. 204, BP 172/118, HR 68, T 97.6
PE: +rales, +rhonchi; scars, striae, dilated veins on abdomen, liver 23 cm, +fluid wave, +shifting dullness; lower extremities: scarring, edema, decreased range of motion in knees, loss of sensation in feet bilaterally; neuro-asterixis, incoordination, short- and long-term memory deficits

QUESTIONS

1. What is the primary diagnosis for this patient?
2. How do you counsel the patient on the workup for this?
3. Can he give informed consent in this condition?
4. What kind of housing would be appropriate for his condition?

CLINICAL APPLICATIONS

1. Sara is an 18-year-old who presents to your clinic following a street assault. She has been seen here a few times in the past 18 months with acute illnesses and injuries. She has been homeless since 15 years old.
   A. What are the skills needed to engage with this teen?
   B. How is her homelessness affecting her health?
   C. What resources would you use from inside your clinic in treating her?
   D. What is the best plan to promote health in this patient?
2. Harry Badia is a 48-year-old male from a nearby shelter with hypertension and early renal failure. He has just been accepted into a Housing First Program and wants to stop drinking. He is uninsured and has no VA benefits.
   A. How do you team with this patient to identify his highest priority issues and treat those issues with him?
   B. Who else is available to be part of his health care team?
   C. How do you address the long-term issues of hypertensive disease and alcoholism with this patient?
3. The public health nurse refers Sonya to you from the domestic violence shelter. Sonya has two children with bad colds and coughs and is having shortness of breath herself. She has missed two periods since arriving at the shelter.
   A. What issues are highest priorities for Sonya's health?
   B. How do you manage all three or four patients in this visit?
   C. What skills do you need to apply to make successful linkages with Sonya and her family at this visit?
   D. What are the barriers to providing care for this family?

KEY POINTS

- Homelessness is a product of large-scale economic and social processes.
- Homeless populations, regardless of demographics, all have higher health care needs than housed populations.
- Younger individuals and families move in and out of homelessness.
- Older populations have more chronic homelessness and more chronic illnesses.
- Engagement with homeless individuals requires specific skills beyond those needed for others in the health care system.
- Health care plans need to be tailored to the living situation of the patient.

References

1. Roosevelt facts and figures: the Great Depression. Franklin D. Roosevelt Presidential Library and Museum website. *http://www.fdrlibrary.marist.edu/facts.html*; Accessed August 19, 2011.
2. Office of Community Planning and Development. The 2010 annual homeless assessment report (AHAR). US Department of Housing and Urban Development website. *http://www.hudhre.info/documents/2010HomelessAssessmentReport.pdf*; Accessed August 19, 2011.
3. Homelessness assistance reauthorization: a summary of the HEARTH Act. National policy update. National Alliance to End Homelessness website. *http://www.endhomelelessness.org*; Updated 2009. Accessed August 26, 2011.
4. Federal definition of homeless. US Department of Housing and Urban Development website. *http://portal.hud.gov/hudportal/HUD?src=/topics/homelessness/definition*; Accessed September 13, 2011.
5. Paquette K. Current statistics on the prevalence and characteristics of people experiencing homelessness in the United States. Homelessness Resource Center, Substance Abuse and Mental Health Service Administration website. *http://homeless.samhsa.gov/*; Updated July 2011. Accessed September 6, 2011.
6. The characteristics and needs of families experiencing homelessness. The National Center on Family Homelessness website. Needham, MA: 2011. *www.familyhomelessness.org;* Accessed September 4, 2011.
7. Fact sheet: youth homelessness. National Alliance to End Homelessness website. *http://www.endhomelessness.org/content/article/detail/1659 youth homelessness*; Updated 2010. Accessed September 6, 2011.
8. Kushel MB, Evans JL, Perry S, et al. No door to lock: victimization among the homeless and marginally housed persons. Arch Intern Med 2003;163:2492–2499.
9. HCH Clinicians' Network. Homeless people at higher risk for CA-MRSA, HIV and TB. Healing Hands 2006;10(5):1–6 *www.nhchc.org*; Accessed August 29, 2011.
10. Diseases and conditions. National Health Care for the Homeless Council website. *http://www.nhchc.org/clinicalresources/diseasesandconditions.html*; Accessed September 6, 2011.
11. O'Connell JJ. Premature mortality in homeless populations: a review of the literature. National Health Care for the Homeless Council website. *http://www.nhchc.org*; Updated 2005. Accessed August 29, 2011.
12. Ku BS, Scott KC, Kertesz SG, Pitts SR. Factors associated with use of urban emergency departments by the U.S. homeless population. Public Health Reports 2010;125(3):398–405.
13. Montauk SL. The homeless in America: adapting your practice. J Am Assoc Fam Physician 2006;74:1132–1138.
14. Parker D. Housing as an intervention on hospital use: access among chronically homeless persons with disabilities. J Urban Health 2010;87(6):912–919.
15. Rinke ML, Dietrich E, Kodeck T, Westcoat K. Operation care: a pilot case management intervention for frequent emergency medical system users. Am J Emer Med 2012;30:352–357.
16. Perry B. Helping traumatized children: a brief overview for caregivers. ChildTrauma Academy, Caregiver Education Series (website). *www.ChildTrauma.org*; Updated 2002. Accessed September 4, 2011.
17. Little M, Shah R, Vermeulen MJ, et al. Adverse perinatal outcomes associated with homelessness and substance use in pregnancy. CMAJ 2005;173(6):615–618.
18. Unaccompanied youth: fast facts. The National Network for Youth website. *http://www.nn4youth.org*; Accessed September 6, 2011.
19. Unaccompanied youth: overview. The National Network for Youth website. *http://www.nn4youth.org*; Accessed September 4, 2011.
20. Ray N. Lesbian, gay, bisexual and transgender youth: an epidemic of homelessness. The National Lesbian and Gay Task Force Policy Institute, National Coalition for the Homeless website. *http://www.theTaskForce.org*; Updated 2006. Accessed September 4, 2011.
21. Khadduri J, Culhane D. Veteran homelessness: a supplemental report to the 2009 Annual Homeless Assessment Report to Congress. US Department of Housing and Urban Development Office of Community Planning and Development and US Department of Veterans Affairs National Center on Homelessness Among Veterans website. *http://www.hudhre.info/documents/2009AHARVeteransReport.pdf*; Updated 2009. Accessed September 4, 2011.
22. Homeless veterans fact sheet. National Coalition for Homeless Veterans website. *http://www.nchv.org*:Accessed September 8, 2011.
23. McMurray-Avila M. Homeless veterans and health care: a resource guide for providers. National Health Care for the Homeless Council website. *http://www.nhchc.org/veteranshealthcare.html*; Updated 2001. Accessed September 6, 2011.
24. Stand Down. US Department of Veterans Affairs website. *http://www.va.gov/HOMELESS/StandDown.asp*; Accessed September 14, 2011.
25. Practice adaptations. National Health Care for the Homeless Council website. *http://www.nhchc.org/clinicalresources/practiceadaptations.html*; Accessed September 5, 2011.

CHAPTER 45

Correctional Medicine

R. Scott Chavez

CHAPTER CONTENTS

Inmates have a higher prevalence of health problems than the general population, both acute and chronic. For instance, the overall rate of confirmed AIDS cases among the nation's prison population is five times the rate of the general population. This stems in part from the communities inmates come from. More than 60% of incarcerated individuals are African American or Latino. Typically they are from an underserved urban community. By screening and treating inmates for various diseases, we take the important first step of preventing their spread into the larger community. But I believe it is also possible to make progress on eliminating disparities through corrections-based interventions.

Vice Admiral Richard H. Carmona, MD, MPH, FACS, CCHP, U.S. Surgeon General, U.S. Department of Health and Human Services National Conference on Correctional Health Care, Austin, Texas, October 6, 2003

WORKING IN A CORRECTIONAL ENVIRONMENT

Why would a physician assistant (PA) want to work in a jail or prison? That is certainly an important question, but the wrong one. The question is, "Why would a PA NOT want to work in a jail or prison?" As former Surgeon General Richard Carmona observed, correctional medicine should not be quickly dismissed because it addresses public health issues that prevent the spread of disease into our communities. It is also an enormous opportunity to make progress on eliminating health disparities.

As the rates of incarceration have increased over the past 25 years, so have the importance and complexity of correctional medicine. For every 145 Americans, there is one person incarcerated. The total number of people involved in the criminal justice system is estimated at 2.3 million in custody,[1] with 10 million released annually from jails.[2]

Correctional institutions are a microcosm of society and, as such, require correctional medicine practitioners to be specialists in public health, primary care, infectious disease, and chronic disease. As a microcosm, correctional institutions reflect the way in which political leaders have addressed issues of race, poverty, addiction, mental illness, and the economically disenfranchised segments of our society.[3] The correctional populations are marginalized due to racial disparities, low socioeconomic status, substance abuse, and mental health disorders. The marked health status disparities and outcomes of incarcerated populations are well documented.[4]

The opportunity to practice in correctional institutions enables PAs to rebuild lives and make a difference. Correctional health often attracts individual professionals who see this as an important role in the overall health of the community. Some of our society's sickest individuals are among incarcerated populations, and PAs working in correctional medicine need special skills and attitudes. In fact, correctional medicine is one of the cornerstones of public health in this country. Through effective standardization of care we can have a tremendous impact on the public's health.[5] PAs wanting to work in the eye of the public health storm in this country or those who want to address health disparities should consider correctional medicine as a career venue. The role and relationship between PAs and their patients are unique. The problems of race, poverty, addiction, mental illness, and economically depressed communities create enormous problems for the physician-PA health care team.

This chapter covers the issues commonly found in correctional medicine, such as access and quality of care, staffing, environmental, safety, and ethical issues. The chapter also assesses an array of clinical duties that correctional PAs perform, including conducting health screenings and evaluations; evaluating and managing chronic disease patients in clinics or infirmaries; conducting daily sick call; making cell checks in segregated housing; reviewing laboratory and other diagnostic test results; developing, monitoring, and modifying individual treatment plans; and discharge planning activities.

PROVIDING HEALTH CARE IN CORRECTIONAL INSTITUTIONS

Access to Care

To provide health care in this environment requires an understanding and knowledge of governmental, bureaucratic, and paramilitary hierarchies. Many correctional health professionals are employed directly by correctional authorities. However, during the past 25 years, correctional health care models have evolved into several types. Contractual health care systems such as for-profit companies, academic medical centers, and public health agencies have assumed the administrative structure for health services in prisons and jails. Under this structure, recruiting, training, and retaining of health care professionals are often easier than when health care professionals are employed directly by the correctional authority. Having professional autonomy and judgment within organized health systems has helped to attract qualified professionals into correctional medicine. There is some evidence that such arrangements provide quality health care because of their access to resources not otherwise available to county jails or state prisons.[6]

Ensuring that inmates have access to health care services is a fundamental responsibility for correctional medical professionals. It means that every inmate, regardless of where he or she is located in the jail or prison, must be able to inform health staff of their need to be seen; and when notified, health staff must act in a timely fashion, provide a professional clinical judgment, and ensure that ordered care is delivered. Any unreasonable barrier to inmate health services access must be removed.

What makes correctional medicine different from other venues of health care delivery is the long line of legal cases that have established the incarcerated individual's rights to health care,[7-9] addressing the responsibilities of custody officials in the health, mental health, and dental treatment of inmates. As a result of these and other court cases, correctional medicine has evolved.

Estelle v. Gamble established the concept of deliberate indifference as the test to determine whether government acted appropriately in the medical care of its inmates. As was clearly articulated, deliberate indifference is defined by prison doctors in their response to the prisoner's needs or by prison guards in intentionally denying or delaying access to medical care or intentionally interfering with the treatment once prescribed. Regardless of how evidenced, deliberate indifference to a prisoner's serious illness or injury states a cause of action.[7]

The government must ensure that adequate medical, dental, and mental health services are provided to those whom it imprisons. To accomplish this, a responsible health authority is established. The responsible health authority (RHA) ensures that primary, secondary, and tertiary care is provided for the well-being of the inmate population. The RHA works with custody staff to eliminate barriers that might hamper inmates from receiving these services in a timely manner. For example, one barrier might be where an officer, hostile to inmates, denies an inmate access to the sick call notification system. Training custody and health staff to recognize emerging medical or mental health needs is an important RHA role. Sometimes, there are unreasonable delays in escorting inmates to see health professionals or to get to outside appointments to obtain necessary diagnostic workups. The RHA works to ensure that access-to-care procedures are flexible to accommodate the special health needs of inmates, such as chronic illness, serious communicable infections, physical disabilities, pregnancy, fragility, terminal illness, mental illness, potential for suicide, or developmental disability. Such special needs affect housing, work, and program assignments; disciplinary measures; and admissions/transfers to and from institutions. Correctional PAs and custody staff need to adequately communicate about these special needs inmates to ensure that government provides appropriate care.

What distinguishes correctional PAs from their civilian community colleagues is that they must be concerned with federal due process. The 8th Amendment to the Constitution prohibits cruel and unusual punishment, and the 14th Amendment ensures the right to due process and full protection under the law. The rights of prisoners cannot be abridged, and those with mental health problems have increased legal protections.[10] Issues such as involuntary hospitalization, transfers from prison to mental hospitals, and involuntary medication and self-harm restrictions are closely scrutinized in mentally ill inmates. Few PAs are prepared to address these thorny legal and ethical access-to-care issues and as a result do not pursue this career track.

Many PA programs offer clinical clerkships in jails, prisons, and juvenile detention centers and can provide PA students an entrance into correctional medicine; however, in general PAs are not exposed to the complexities of correctional health care.

More PA programs need to become vested in correctional medicine and the disenfranchised populations that are served.

Clinical Autonomy

Safety of inmates, staff, and visitors takes priority in a correctional institution. Many decisions that would seem inconsequential in the free world take on great import in corrections. For example, the choice to issue a pair of crutches for a patient with a non–weight-bearing injury takes on a different perspective when considering the safety precautions required in a jail or prison. As a result, correctional health clinicians face a number of pressures when assessing the health needs of their patients.

Inherent in a correctional institution is the power that security staff wields, deciding on what can or cannot be permitted in the institution. Decisions about staff utilization, inmate housing, work assignments, and disciplinary sanctions for both staff and inmates are under the purview of administrative security staff. For example, hiring a PA to work in a jail takes not only the approval of the responsible physician but also that of the jail administrator. The PA must pass a detailed security screening, which, in some jurisdictions, may take several months to complete. The PA must abide by the employment rules directed by the medical authority, but he or she must also abide by the directives of security.

Sometimes there is conflict between security and medical staff over clinical decisions and actions. However, custody staff should not interfere with the implementation of clinical decisions. Qualified health professionals should direct clinical decisions and actions regarding all health care provided to their patients. Case in point: the PA orders a knee magnetic resonance image (MRI) of a high security risk inmate. Security staff is reluctant to transfer the inmate to the hospital for the MRI, particularly because he is a dangerous escape risk and policy requires three officers to transport him. The jail administrator refuses to transport the inmate because of the threat to public safety. Most civilian health staff members are not accustomed to such denials of care. In this case, the clinical decision should be tempered with cooperation and consultation with administrative security staff. How urgent is the MRI to making a clinical decision? How long has the patient been complaining of his symptoms? Is the denial of care deliberately indifferent to the inmate's medical need? The answers to these questions influence the course of action that the PA should take. More important, the successful correctional PA is one who knows how to negotiate with custody staff to achieve the goals necessary to provide the best possible care for his or her patient.

Clinical autonomy cannot be jeopardized; however, in a correctional institution, diagnostic and therapeutic orders are not issued in a vacuum—they require a coordinated effort among custodial, administrative, and health staff.

To facilitate the implementation of health care orders and decisions, most facilities hold meetings between security and health staff. Through joint monitoring, planning, and problem resolution, health, correctional, and administrative personnel can facilitate the health care delivery system. Included should be discussions on the barriers to effective treatment and care. For example, evidence-based medicine has shown that disease progression is controlled when the patient is involved in monitoring his or her disease. Patients with asthma should have peak flow meters, and diabetic patients should have glucometers. However, custody policies often prevent such items in the housing units for fear of security breaches. Treating asthma in a correctional environment is problematic because many have inadequate ventilation systems or restrictive keep-on-person medication programs. Restricting opportunities for inmates with diabetes to self-test, self-prepare, and self-administer insulin presents additional barriers to improving disease control. Administrative problem-solving, corrective actions, timetables for proposed changes, and updates on changes proposed during previous meetings are important strategies toward implementing effective patient care.

Quality of Care

Correctional PAs have to be knowledgeable in continuous quality improvement (CQI) monitoring. CQI identifies problems; proposes, implements, and monitors corrective action; and studies the effectiveness of corrective actions in addressing problems. This multidisciplinary (i.e., medical, nursing, mental health, substance abuse) structured process examines outcomes, high-risk/high-volume, or problem-prone aspects of care and ensures that established standards of care are met. CQI committees should assess processes that affect the effectiveness and efficiency of staffing, continuity of care, and quality of services.

Patient Satisfaction

Health care organizations are interested in the quality of care provided to their patients. They are interested in what their patients perceive to be quality. Correctional health systems are no different. Patient satisfaction surveys have been conducted by health care organizations for quite some time now; however, this is a new concept in corrections and is not widely accepted by correctional administrators. After all, correctional institutions are predicated on having individuals who do not want to be there and who are mistrusted by staff. This distrustful environment does not support surveying techniques. Yet a few correctional institutions are conducting inmate-patient satisfaction surveys. For example, the Oregon Department of Corrections has been conducting patient satisfaction surveys for more than a decade and has found a positive, constructive way to implement change for patient care.

STAFFING IN CORRECTIONAL MEDICINE

Staffing Issues

The recruiting, training, and retaining of health professionals to work in correctional health care is difficult because prisons and jails do not have medical care as the primary mission. Jails and prisons are foreign working environments for most health care professionals. Yet correctional institutions have a mandate to provide adequate and timely evaluation, treatment, and follow-up care consistent with contemporary standards.

The numbers and types of health care professionals required depend on the size of the facility and the scope of on-site medical, mental health, dental, and substance-abuse treatment. There is a difference in the functions and responsibilities of jails and prisons. Jails detain individuals who have been accused of a crime and who are waiting adjudication by either a jury or judge. On average, jails will hold detainees for about a year, although in some cases jails will hold individuals a few years past adjudication. The point is that once conviction and sentence have been rendered, the individual is transferred to a prison. Prisons are long-term holding facilities for individuals who have been convicted and sentenced for their crimes.

Compensation and benefit packages are generally not competitive and are a disincentive for many PAs. The security clearance process is sometimes lengthy and dissuades individuals from staying with the process, taking other jobs that may be offered. Opposition and pressure from family members is another barrier that a PA faces in taking a correctional health care position. The patient clientele are vastly different. Many are recalcitrant, ungrateful, argumentative, and even combative. In spite of these drawbacks, correctional PAs find that being at the crossroad of medicine, public health, law, ethics, and criminal justice is challenging and rewarding.

To help attract health professionals, some institutions serve as clinical rotation sites for students. One such example is the Cook County Department of Corrections, Cermak Health Services in Chicago. This site has been a clinical rotation site for area PA programs for more than 20 years. The level of morbidity and mortality in this patient population is high, and PA students often find themselves in challenging clinical situations. Clinical rotations in correctional institutions provide unique and challenging opportunities to exercise one's clinical skills.

PAs generally find correctional employment working for the legal authority (the sheriff or department of corrections). Some jails and prisons contract for-profit companies, academic medical institutions, or public health agencies to provide health services. Using these models, correctional institutions can attract health staff through better compensation, faculty appointments, and continuing education opportunities.

Finding and retaining qualified health professionals to work in jails, prisons, and juvenile detention and confinement facilities is an important concern. The goal is to find professionals who are willing to establish and maintain a therapeutic relationship with inmates. Medical professionals are trained to advocate quality patient care; however, providing such services in an antitherapeutic environment is difficult.

When these two dynamics collide, conflicts about authority over health services decision-making and management occur. For example, health care professionals hold to a tenet that patients should have control over the health care decisions that affect their lives. However, in correctional institutions such autonomy creates problems for custody.

An inmate who refuses to take clinically ordered behavior-modifying medications (increasing the likelihood of disruptive behavior) or refuses to submit to a human immunodeficiency virus (HIV) blood test when a staff member has come into contact with the inmate's blood presents problems for custody. How custody responds in such situations is often not the way medical professionals would solve the problem. These frequent conflicts arising between custody and health staff require well-developed effective communication and problem-solving skills. Those health professionals who do not have the skills are often co-opted and are seen as an extension of security rather than as medical professionals.

PAs working in a correctional environment need to know that it is a constant balance between public safety and public health. They need to know that their environment is a paramilitary, organizational-based hierarchy and that public safety drives decision-making relative to patient services. For example, administering medication to patients at a given time of day during pill call is made more complicated when the facility goes into a lockdown status (due to a breach in security, inmates are kept in their cells). The method and manner in which medication is administered completely change to accommodate the public safety situation.

Clinical Performance Enhancement

The clinical performance enhancement process evaluates the appropriateness of a health clinician's services. The PA's clinical work is reviewed by another professional of at least equal training in the same general discipline, such as the review by the facility's medical director or chief PA. The purpose of this review is to enhance clinical competency and address areas that need improvement. It is different from an annual performance review or a clinical case conference in that it is a professional practice review focused on the professional's clinical skills.

Clinical performance enhancement reviews in a correctional environment are no different from any other institutional setting (e.g., the military or hospital). For example, treating HIV must follow certain clinical guidelines regardless of setting. However, a correctional clinical performance enhancement review has an additional component in the review of one's clinical judgment by assessing how one's clinical competency affects public safety. The clinical PA may indeed be effective in managing the health care of uncooperative or even malingering inmates by gaining their trust and respect. However, if the clinical PA receives information from such inmates that public safety might be jeopardized, the clinical PA has a responsibility and duty to report it, even to the point of damaging patient trust and confidence.

Staff and Inmate Safety

In January 2004, a 15-day hostage standoff between Arizona corrections officials and two inmates captivated the nation's attention. The hostage standoff ended peacefully through a negotiated surrender of the inmates and the release of a female officer. This event perpetuates the public perception that jails and prisons are dangerous places. Although that is true, it is important to remember that events such as this are not an everyday occurrence. Correctional institutions work to ensure staff safety through strict policies and procedures and by ongoing training of its staff. Staff and public safety is compromised when lapses in training or procedures occur. For example, once in Sacramento, California, a deputy U.S. marshal placed his weapon under the front seat of his vehicle before entering the jail to pick up a prisoner. When he returned with the prisoner, he forgot to retrieve the weapon. It subsequently slid back where the prisoner was sitting. The prisoner, handcuffed with his hands in front, grabbed the weapon, ordered the deputy to pull over, and escaped.[11] As this case reminds us, it is in the best interest of public safety to ensure that the health and well-being of staff are protected. When staff members forget or fail to abide by policy and procedure, harm can occur.

Risk and harm reduction create a working environment in which staff feel safe to do their work. There is no central repository for the collection of hazardous duty incidents incurred by correctional health professionals. There are no studies on inmate assaults on health staff, although anecdotally, staff members report that assaults on health staff rarely occur.

In 2001, Human Rights Watch released *No Escape*, a descriptive report on male prisoner-on-prisoner sexual abuse in the United States that outlined first-hand accounts of prisoner rape and sexual assault stories from 200 prisoners among 37 states.[12] This report reviews the conditions that contribute to prisoner rape, namely the rapid expansion of the incarcerated population during the past 20 years; the increasing government decisions to privatize its prisons and jails; and the dismantling of prisoners' legal rights through the Prison Litigation Reform Act of 1996 (an act that made prisoner lawsuits regarding conditions of confinement and deliberate indifference more difficult). As a result of the shocking claims made in *No Escape*, Congress passed the Prison Rape Elimination Act of 2003 (PREA).[13] PREA requires "the gathering of national statistics about the problem; the development of guidelines for states about how to address prisoner rape; the creation of a review panel to hold annual hearings; and the provision of grants to states to combat the problem."[13] PREA is the first U.S. federal law passed that deals with assault on prisoners and aims to improve correctional institutions' safety.

COMMUNICABLE DISEASE IN CORRECTIONAL INSTITUTIONS

Infection Control

Correctional facilities generally have an exposure control plan that describes staff actions to be taken to eliminate or minimize exposures to pathogens. In closed environments like prisons and jails it is important that health professionals maintain standard hygiene practices and precautions. They need to be aware of infection control matters and should receive orientation and annual updates to infection control policies and procedures. Facilities also have needlestick prevention programs that include the use of self-capping needles and functional sharps disposal containers.

Many correctional institutions have infection control committees that establish and maintain the exposure control plan, monitor communicable disease among inmates and staff, ensure prompt treatment for inmates and staff with infectious disease, ensure staff receive appropriate training and maintain procedures, ensure that personal protective equipment is available and used, and meet reporting requirements, laws, and regulations issued by local, state, and federal authorities.

Community-Acquired Methicillin-Resistant *Staphylococcus aureus*

A major problem occurring in many jails and prisons today is the increasing rate of community-associated methicillin-resistant *Staphylococcus aureus* (CA-MRSA). Jails and prisons are commonly overcrowded and do not have sufficient hygienic practices with soap, water, or clean laundry. These conditions foster environments in which contagions such as *S. aureus* and CA-MRSA can be transmitted from one person to another.

CA-MRSA infections are generally mild, self-limiting, minor skin infections that appear as pustules or boils.[14] Inmates often complain of "spider bites," and correctional staff too often dismiss their claims. Education is necessary for both groups so that health staff can intervene and begin treatment.

Other confounding issues complicate the matter of containing CA-MRSA outbreaks in correctional institutions. This includes comorbidities of substance abuse and mental illness, distrust of authority figures, reluctance to cooperate with health care staff, and resistance to rules of hygienic practice. Many inmates have issues of substance abuse or mental illness, complicating the ability to adequately respond to self-cleanliness. Prior to their incarceration, many inmates were either homeless or came from home environments that did not have adequate sanitation or did not stress personal hygiene. The hygienic practices of frequent hand washing with soap and water, avoidance of picking lesions, daily showers, and limitation of the number of personal items shared with other inmates should be emphasized to all inmates.[15]

Other significant risk factors that have been found include prison occupation, gender, comorbidities, prior skin infection, and previous antibiotic use.[16] Resistance to antibiotic therapy has added to this problem. Commonly, inmates have not sought regular and consistent health care from one primary care provider. Too often when they do obtain health care, inmates have sought their care from emergency departments and public health community clinics. This episodic approach to their health care without consistent or organized management complicates the individual's resistance to antibiotic therapy.

Another problem that complicates matters is that inmates, by nature, distrust authority and rules. When the outbreak occurs in a jail or prison, inmates are quick to blame jail administrators and health staff for the problem and not take responsibility for themselves. This distrust of authority creates a barrier to improving jail and prison conditions and eliminating the transmission of CA-MRSA.

CA-MRSA is not isolated to a particular part of the country. Outbreaks have been recorded in San Diego, Los Angeles, Atlanta, Phoenix, New York, and Chicago jails,[17] as well as in state and federal prisons.[18]

Tuberculosis

Tuberculosis (TB) in correctional facilities is a continuous problem affecting the health status of communities at large. "Although the incident tuberculosis case rate for the general population has remained at fewer than 10 cases per 100,000 persons since 1993, substantially higher case rates, some as high as 10 times that of the general population, have been reported in correctional populations."[19]

The control of TB in correctional facilities is a multifaceted problem with no easy answers. Correctional institutions have policies on staff surveillance; however, it is difficult to maintain mandatory and periodic screening of correctional staff members. Between 2001 and 2004, the Florida Department of Corrections had one HIV-infected correctional staff member who was nonadherent with TB treatment and infected five correctional staff members over 2½ years. Four of the five cases were caused by an identical strain, indicating a probable common source.

Correctional institutions have poor ventilation and have a transient population, which further complicates the control of TB. As a result, contact tracing is extremely difficult. In 2002 Kansas had a case in which a TB-infected inmate was transferred to three jails and one prison. In that process he came into contact with more than 800 individuals and was positively linked via identical-band RFLP to two inmates (cellmates in two different locations). In contact tracing, 318 of the 800 inmates were found—six had a negative prior tuberculin skin test (TST), and 196 inmates had no prior skin test information. Forty-one (21%) had a positive skin test.

Failure to control TB in jails and prisons is a threat to the community. From 1999 to 2000, the South Carolina Department of Corrections had a TB outbreak in which 31 prisoners and one medical student in the community's hospital subsequently developed TB. In upstate New York there was a multidrug–resistant (MDR)-TB outbreak involving several correctional facilities and a hospital. The MDR-TB outbreak resulted in at least 50 health care professionals being infected and the death of one prison guard.

Latent tuberculosis infection (LTBI) is four times higher among prison inmates than in the general population. Among jail inmates, LTBI prevalence is 17 times higher than the prevalence in the general population. It is estimated that 500,000 inmates with LTBI are released nationwide every year.

Active TB is 15 times higher among jail inmates than in the general population. Two studies estimate that one third of active TB cases have been recently incarcerated.

Pulmonary tuberculosis has been reported to be as high as 3.75 times more common among foreign-born inmates and federal prisoners than among the general population.[20] Foreign-born inmates were 5.9 times more likely to have a positive TST than U.S.-born inmates and accounted for 60% of recently diagnosed TB cases in the federal prison system.[21] Because the U.S. Public Health Service provides care to the majority of foreign-born inmates in federal prisons and in Immigration and Customs Enforcement (ICE), there is a significant concern. Many local jails house foreign-born inmates as well.

Screening for TB infection is a top priority for most jails and prisons, planting tuberculin skin tests, performing a chest radiograph if positive, and then referring for treatment. A study comparing screening and treatment practices for latent tuberculosis in the Michigan Department of Corrections demonstrated that nationally recommended guidelines were followed.[22] Yet TB outbreaks do occur in jails and prisons because many inmates do not complete their LTBI treatment, thus creating an ideal situation to disperse the contagion.

Correctional institutions usually screen all inmates entering their facilities for tuberculosis. The Cook County Department of Corrections (Chicago), the Rikers Island Department of Corrections (New York), and the Washington, D.C., jails are a few settings in which all incoming detainees receive routine radiographic screening for TB. Most jails and prisons conduct tuberculin screening tests. In addition, many facilities have TB coordinators who monitor the screening and treatment of TB among inmates (e.g., Oregon prison system, Chicago and New York jails). The high prevalence of TB in jails and prisons suggests that correctional PAs are at the forefront of this public health battle through surveillance, detection, and treatment.

Human Immunodeficiency Virus

A major portion of the HIV epidemic is seen in jails. Hammett and colleagues[2] estimate that approximately 25% of all U.S. HIV-infected persons passed through the correctional system in 1997. In 2002 the Bureau of Justice Statistics reported that only 21.6% of jail inmates had received an HIV test after admission.[23] There are no jails that conduct mandatory HIV testing, and the testing they do is less systematic than in prisons.[24]

The Corrections Demonstration Project (CDP), a multicenter study by the Centers for Disease Control and Prevention (CDC) and the Health Resources and Services Administration (HRSA) involving health departments and correctional facilities, as well as community-based organizations in California, Florida, Georgia, Illinois, Massachusetts, New Jersey, and New York, tested 1020 inmates for HIV infection and found 17% seropositive cases.[25]

Incarcerated women are 15 times more likely to be HIV infected compared with women in the general population. Black women, who bear a significant burden of the HIV epidemic, predominate in the nation's jails and prisons.

Acquired immunodeficiency syndrome (AIDS) is estimated to be three times greater in prison than in the community.[26] The stigma of HIV and AIDS is certainly an issue in the community, but it is even more pronounced in jails and prisons. Once information about an inmate's HIV status is disclosed, it spreads throughout the institution, ostracizing the HIV-infected inmate even further in an already oppressive environment. Correctional PAs must take extra steps to protect the confidentiality of their patient's HIV status.

Screening for HIV in correctional institutions remains one of the more important public health strategies protecting community health. The potential of finding more seropositive individuals from among high at-risk individuals and the potential of increasing HIV/AIDS awareness makes correctional institution HIV screening a valuable resource. The CDC recommends routine testing for HIV and that a patient is to be notified that the testing will be performed unless he or she decides to "opt out" from the screening process.[27] Routine testing has the potential advantage to decrease any associated stigma when an inmate requests HIV testing.[28] Routine HIV testing on admission to prison may be ideal. In fact, six prison systems do mandatory HIV testing of entering inmates; however, in jails this may be more problematic for a number of reasons.[29] The average jail detainee is released within 72 hours of booking, making it difficult to find an optimal time to implement routine HIV testing. In addition, many jails have limited resources to conduct such testing and may not be able to handle the volume of inmates at the intake center or support the costs for providing such screening services.[29]

Another problem that jails face in implementing the routine HIV testing model is that when individuals are first arrested they are stressed during the initial stages of incarceration. Issues such as addiction, potential suicide, and withdrawal from intoxication may cloud the individual's judgment and they may "opt out" of the screening without fully understanding the benefits to such a test.[29] Also, with the open HIV testing model, the uncertainty of whether or not test results can be given to jail detainees in a reasonable timeframe is an issue of concern.

There are unique barriers to the provision of health care to HIV-infected inmates in prisons and jails. Maintaining continuity of care is a major problem. A study by Bernard and colleagues[30] found a gross difference between correctional institutions and community-based HIV clinics. They analyzed 30 CB-HIV clinics against 90 correctional health professionals (representing 33 states). Approximately 43% of correctional institutions did not have access to HIV specialists compared with 93% in community-based HIV clinics. Disruption in highly active antiviral therapy (HAART) is reported in 71% of correctional institutions, compared with 33% in community-based HIV clinics. Plasma HIV viral load testing is available in 65% of correctional institutions and in 87% of the community-based HIV clinics.

Health services for HIV-infected inmates need to improve through better medication distribution schedules, better testing of CD4, viral load and genotyping needs, improved availability of HIV specialist access, and improved HIV information through peer education.[30] Improving the discharge planning of soon-to-be-released HIV-infected inmates, maintaining confidentiality, and gaining the trust of patients are other ways that the provision of health care to HIV-infected inmates can be improved.

There is also a need to improve harm reduction and HIV prevention efforts in jails and prisons. The health of our communities is jeopardized without such efforts. A study conducted by the CDC on the transmission of HIV among male inmates in the Georgia Department of Corrections from 1992 to 2005 found that 88 inmates acquired HIV during their incarceration.[27] This study raises important discussions on the spread of HIV within correctional settings and the appropriate measures to prevent such transmission. Harm reduction is hotly debated among even correctional health care experts.[31] Inmate access to condoms and sterile syringes is opposed by many who see such activity as a threat to public safety. They claim that such items can be used to carry contraband and promote illegal activity inside a correctional institution. The CDC study makes the public health argument that illegal activity does occur inside a prison or jail and that the responsible thing to do is to implement harm reduction strategies and HIV prevention strategies. Multimedia HIV and hepatitis intervention programming is available for correctional PAs to teach inmates and correctional officers.[32]

Sexually Transmitted Diseases

The four most common sexually transmitted diseases (STDs) treated in a jail setting are syphilis, gonorrhea, *Chlamydia*, and genital herpes. In prisons, STDs are seen with less frequency because inmates spend long periods of time in jails and get treatment. However, many detention centers fail to adequately screen for and treat STDs.[33] Many have policies for STD screening based only on symptoms or by arrestee request. Often, jails do not have the resources to increase their STD testing, or inmates are released within less than 48 hours before STD testing and treatment can occur.

Expanded STD services are needed for disadvantaged populations. The Institute of Medicine[34] has recommended that jails increase their efforts in the provision of STD screening, diagnosis, treatment, counseling and education, and partner notification. National Commission on Correctional Health Care standards require that within 14 days of admission to jails and within 7 days of admission to prison, inmates are screened for STDs. However, due to the lack of health staff and resources, many correctional institutions do not adequately manage STDs, whereas they may use "test results to diagnose and treat infections but do not routinely assess the burden of disease in their population."[35]

Syphilis

The positive test rate for syphilis is high among persons entering correctional facilities. The most high-prevention-value female cases have been found in jail settings.[35] Results for approximately 293,000 syphilis tests indicated that the median percentage of persons with reactive syphilis was 8.2% (range, 0.3%–23.8%) for women and 2.5% (range, 1%–7.8%) for men.[36]

All persons with a positive syphilis test should be tested for HIV because these diseases are epidemiologically linked. Patients who have latent syphilis should be evaluated for neurosyphilis. Careful evaluation and follow-up care for neonates born to syphilis-infected mothers is also recommended because the mother can transmit syphilis to her newborn.

Gonorrhea and Chlamydia

Due to their risky sexual behavior and lack of access to routine screening, jail inmates are at high risk for STDs, such as gonorrhea and *Chlamydia*. Urine testing has simplified screening techniques for chlamydial and gonococcal infections; however, because often medical staff and space are limited and there are large numbers of detainees to process, screening is not effectively accomplished. Policies that direct screening when the inmates complain of symptoms are ineffective because high rates of infected individuals do not report symptoms.[37] For those who are tested, gonococcal and chlamydial infection rates are high.

The prevalence of *Chlamydia* among juveniles is high, mainly due to their high-risk sexual behavior. A study of 508 charts showed 20.8% of female adolescents and 8.9% of male adolescents tested positive during routine screening for *Chlamydia*. Additional findings included 76% were treated according to national guidelines, and 10% received follow-up care from the Department of Public Health after release.[38] In another study, the range of positive results for chlamydial infection was 8%–19.5% for adolescent girls and 2.8%–8.9% for adolescent boys. The range of positive results for gonorrhea was 3.4%–10% for adolescent girls and 0.7%–2.6% for adolescent boys.[36] Although these studies are focused on adolescents in large urban juvenile detention centers, these analyses point to early screening and treatment as an important community strategy in reaching individuals infected with *Chlamydia*. Public health departments can also provide an important service of follow-up care to adults and youth who are discharged from correctional institutions while still under treatment for *Chlamydia*.

Genital Herpes

Rapid and accurate diagnostic testing for genital herpes simplex virus (HSV) is unavailable in most correctional facilities.[35]

Treating STDs in jails remains elusive and compounds a public health problem that could be remedied. The CDP study group found that 22% of inmates who test positive for one of the STDs either declined treatment, were released before notification of results, or were released before starting treatment.[25]

Economic modeling has found that routine screening for STDs in prisons and jails is cost-effective.[39] An opportunity to improve the public's health is missed when jail health staff do not screen and treat for STDs. Along with aggressive screening, diagnostic, and treatment practices, jail staff should use routine rapid STD screening and treatment and work with their local public health department to ensure that contact and partner testing and counseling are accomplished.

Hepatitis

Corrections populations have high rates of hepatitis C. Estimates indicate that 12%–39% of all Americans with hepatitis C have spent some time incarcerated. This clear and present public health threat requires consistent policies and programming. A number of programs have been successful. For example, the Hepatitis C Continuity Program of the New York Department of Corrections coordinates care between the prison system and community providers, effectively ensuring continuity of hepatitis C virus (HCV) treatment to prisoners on release to the community.[40] The Hepatitis C Continuity Program demonstrates how coordination of efforts among community organizations, a correctional prison system, and a network of health professionals can be effective with inmates before their release from prison, although the program is still working out issues such as data sharing and referral prioritization.

Another program that the New Mexico prison system participates in is Project Extension for Community Healthcare Outcomes (Project ECHO), a telemedicine and distance-learning program aimed at improving health services access for hepatitis C–infected inmates.[41]

Another important strategy is vaccination. The CDC recommends that incarcerated populations receive hepatitis B vaccination. This strategy has been shown to be widely accepted among inmates when given the opportunity to be immunized.[42] Enhanced multisession one-to-one education on sexual risk behavior just before release from prison appears to be a successful strategy as well.[43] However, barriers to fully accomplishing these strategies include cost, lack of staffing, and in the case of adolescents the issue of consent.[44]

CHRONIC DISEASE IN CORRECTIONAL INSTITUTIONS

Thirteen days after his arrest, a 68-year-old male who had a medical history significant for heart disease and diabetes mellitus was found dead, naked, and lying on his back on a mat in his cell next to a half-eaten orange and a sandwich. He was on a self-medication program and was expected to administer his own insulin. The medical examiner's office reported that the inmate died of diabetes and that heart disease may have contributed to his death.[45]

This case illustrates some of the difficulties associated with managing chronic disease in correctional institutions—the lack of health staff to adequately monitor chronic disease, insufficient policies and practices to ensure adequate care, and overall poorly managed chronic disease care. This section discusses common issues and problems related to asthma, diabetes, and hypertension in prisons and jails.

Asthma

Data from the CDC show that a large disparity exists between minority populations and whites with asthma. Of the approximately 16 million U.S. adults with asthma in 2002, only 7.6% of whites, 15.6% of non-Hispanic multiple races, 11.6% of non-Hispanic American Indian and Alaska Natives, and 9.3% of non-Hispanic blacks had the respiratory condition. Because correctional institutions have high percentage of minorities, they will have a disproportionate burden of asthma. The CDC recommends targeted public health interventions to address these disparities.

Although asthma affects about 5% of the U.S. population, the National Commission on Correctional Health Care estimates 8.5% of inmates have asthma.[4] The Bureau of Justice Statistics, in its 2002 Survey of Inmates in Local Jails, reports that 9.9% of inmates have a current condition of asthma.

Many factors hinder asthma care in correctional institutions. Some correctional institutions (except juvenile detention and confinement facilities) still permit cigarette smoking by inmates. Approximately 60% of correctional facilities do not permit smoking on the premises by inmates, but some do allow staff to smoke in designated areas.[46] Moreover, less than 25% offer smoking cessation programming to inmates.[46]

Other factors include environmental problems such as inadequate ventilation systems, poor temperature control, poor maintenance of air filters, and old physical structures with mold. As a result, exacerbation of asthma is high among inmates in these environments.

Many jails and prisons do not permit inmates to keep their inhalers, making it difficult for them to get timely access to their inhalers or, in some cases, timely access to urgent care. Many correctional institutions do not have adequate medication management systems that ensure medication continuity for asthmatic patients. Due to the nature of jails, where inmates bond out or are released within hours of their arrest, asthmatic care is episodic instead of a proactive chronic care approach. Finally, asthmatic inmates may be exposed to chemical means of chemical restraint and control such as mace, pepper spray, or use of a Taser or stun gun. This also exacerbates their asthmatic condition.

Correctional PAs can improve the quality of life of their asthmatic patients through steps that ensure appropriate categorization of the patient's disease control and status as soon as they are admitted into the jail or prison. This care includes monitoring the patient's use of beta-agonist inhaler canisters during the month, offering and ensuring that their patients receive flu vaccinations, and obtaining and documenting peak flow meter readings in assessing acute respiratory attacks.

One area in which correctional PAs can make a difference is tobacco control. Tobacco use before incarceration is a huge problem in this population. It is estimated that 80% of inmates used tobacco before their incarceration. Too often, inmates resume their tobacco addictions soon after release,[47] which, unfortunately, can lead to other addictive behaviors. Correctional PAs have an excellent opportunity to break the cycle by providing health education and guidance to inmates to cease tobacco use and other addictions and by referring inmates to appropriate counseling and addiction services.

Diabetes

The National Commission on Correctional Health Care estimates a prevalence of 4.8% of inmates with diabetes.[4] The Bureau of Justice Statistics, in its 2002 Survey of Inmates in Local Jails, reported that 2.7% of inmates had a current condition of diabetes.

Inmates with insulin-treated diabetes should be identified within 2 hours of intake into jail; however, too often, they languish in police lockups (without any medical services) and are then transferred to the jail. As a result, many do not receive health services for several hours. Rapid identification and treatment of inmates with diabetes do not universally occur.

Because inmates do not have easy access to medical staff or services, diabetic care is particularly difficult, especially with insulin-dependent diabetic individuals. Institutional schedules such as mealtimes, pill lines, court appearances, school, or offender programming often interfere with consistent and routine diabetic care. Correctional PAs should work with their patients with diabetes and custody staff to develop flexible treatment strategies that allow the inmate to work within the institutional schedule while maintaining diabetes control. This is especially true for patients with uncontrolled type 1 diabetes, who need extensive health care resources and institutional flexibility to manage their diabetes. Glucose control should be the priority. Facilities that cannot accommodate these patients' needs may not be the right place to house them. Inmates with uncontrolled type 1 diabetes should be housed in facilities with 24-hour nursing care.

The role of diet and exercise in maintaining glycemic control is well documented. Yet not all diabetic inmates have access to daily exercise or low-fat, low-carbohydrate diets. In fact, medical nutrition is one of the most difficult factors to control in correctional institutions. Diabetic diets may be ordered, but the lack of communication or follow-through in the kitchen often results in failure to ensure that the right diet gets to the right patient. Supplemental food items in institutional commissaries are limited in heart-healthy snacks or alternatives to high-calorie, high-carbohydrate choices.

Correctional PAs can play an important role in the management of diabetes. Working with custody administration and staff, PAs can ensure that their diabetic patients have appropriate opportunities for exercise and adequate diets and alternatives. Correctional PAs can take an active role in staff training and encouragement of patient self-management, as well as stressing the need to control carbohydrate consumption and participate in daily exercise.

Correctional PAs can be advocates for patient self-management, encouraging strategies for patients with diabetes to learn to control their disease. Due to security concerns, there are few opportunities for patients with diabetes to have access to self-testing equipment (supervised or unsupervised), self-preparation of insulin, and self-administration of insulin.

Correctional PAs can advocate for opportunities for their inmate patients with diabetes to have a better understanding of how to control their disease through self-management and regulation. Correctional PAs can make a difference by providing annual and routine training sessions to all correctional staff on diabetes emergency care. In addition, by monitoring the status of soon-to-be-released patients with diabetes, correctional PAs can ensure that appropriate information and support is given so that follow-up in the community occurs.

Hypertension

The National Commission on Correctional Health Care estimates a prevalence of 18.3% of inmates with hypertension.[4] The Bureau of Justice Statistics (2002) reported that 11.2% of inmates had a current condition of hypertension. In comparison, the National Health and Nutrition Examination Survey (NHANES) data cite that 24% of the U.S. population has hypertension, and although hypertension among inmates is lower, it is significant given the fact that inmates are a relatively young population whose lifestyle and risky behavior has significantly reduced their morbidity.[4]

The treatment of hypertension in correctional institutions is made more difficult because of the numbers involved and the lack of organizational capacity to manage it. For example, permission for an inmate to keep his or her medication with personal possessions is determined on a case-by-case basis and is often too restrictive. As a result, inmates lack timely access to medications to ensure continuity, they fail to receive timely follow-up assessment and treatment modification, and they lack opportunities to learn about self-management of their disease.

Correctional PAs can improve chronic hypertension care by ensuring that the patient's level of control and conditional status is properly categorized, and that the patient is encouraged to gain self-management of his or her disease. Monitoring patient adherence through medication distribution systems and assessment of disease control are important strategies correctional PAs can use in managing their patients with hypertension.

This section has described the common correctional barriers to the treatment of chronic disease such as asthma, diabetes, and hypertension. Correctional PAs can play an important role in working with custody staff while advocating for patient needs and encouraging self-management.

MANAGING MENTAL HEALTH IN CORRECTIONAL INSTITUTIONS

When prisons were first developed in the United States, rehabilitation and social control dominated the debate as to what the main focus of imprisonment should be.[48] Little attention was given to mental health; however, since the 1980s correctional institutions have evolved into repositories of mentally ill offenders. Today, approximately 64% of the inmate population has symptoms of a mental disorder that are based on criteria specified in the Diagnostic and Statistical Manual of Mental Disorders, fourth edition,[49] with about 20% having a serious persistent mental illness (SPMI).[50] Persons with SPMI deviate from social norms and acceptable behaviour, and as a result they come to the attention of the criminal justice system. By default, correctional institutions warehouse individuals with SPMI. Ditton's[50] national study found that approximately 19% of all jail and prison inmates had severe mental illnesses. Although this study was performed before the introduction of mental health courts, the estimate of 20% of SPMI remains constant with other studies.[51]

Mental Health Screening

A little more than a quarter of federal inmates with mental health diagnoses have been incarcerated for three or more prior incarcerations. This is because, often, mental health services efforts are directed toward stabilization rather than treatment. The role of mental health is often seen as prompting individuals to adjust to the realities of incarceration. This short-term stabilization is a partial explanation why recidivism rates are so high, because mentally ill inmates return to the community with little or no help, only to return to jail or prison.

The mental health capacities in U.S. jails are inadequate. In a study of correctional facilities,[4] it was found that 41.6% did not use a screening instrument to assess mental illness on newly arriving inmates. Rather, screening was generally performed by visual observation and inmate verbal report. Individuals who tested "positive" are referred to mental health for an in-depth and thorough mental health assessment, although some institutions did report that they use the Mental Health Screening Form–III and the Beck Depression Inventory II (27.4% and 23%, respectively) to screen inmates for mental illness.

Suicide

Inmate suicides were the leading cause of death in 1983 (56% of all deaths), but due to improved standards and training, suicide rates have steadily declined. In 2002, the jail suicide rate was 47 per 100,000 in 2002, compared with 129 per 100,000 inmates in 1983.[52] Prisons have steadily maintained their suicide rate of 16 per 100,000 since 1990 (from a high of 34 per 100,000 in 1980).[52] In comparison, jails have a suicide rate four times that of the national average, which in 2004 was 11.05 suicides per 100,000.[53]

Rates of inmate suicide are closely related to jail size. More than 40% of the nation's jails house fewer than 50 inmates, and in 2002 they had a suicide rate of 47 per 100,000 inmates.[52] These small jails had a suicide rate five times higher than the largest jail systems (an average daily population of at least 1500 inmates). Reasons for this phenomenon include lack of adequate staffing, insufficient training, inadequate housing, and failure to properly screen individuals into the jail.

Suicide prevention efforts begin with well-trained staff who aggressively conduct intake screening and provide ongoing assessment of all inmates entering the correctional facility. Five points in time are especially important in monitoring individuals for suicidal ideation during their confinement: initial admission into the facility, after adjudication when the inmate is returned to the facility from court, following receipt of bad news or after suffering any type of humiliation or rejection, confinement in isolation or segregation, and following a prolonged stay in the facility.[54]

Correctional PAs should take an active role in the screening and assessment process to identify inmate suicide risk. Being alert to behavioral cues that an inmate might be contemplating suicide is ultimately the strongest preventive measure that correctional staff can demonstrate. Correctional PAs can help to prevent inmate suicides by establishing trust with inmates, gathering pertinent information, and taking action through effective communication.

Co-occurring Disorders

The relationship between drugs and crime is well established, with about half of state inmates and a third of federal prisoners reporting that they committed their current offense while under the influence of alcohol or drugs.[55] In 2002, 68% of jail inmates reported symptoms in the year before their admission to jail that met substance dependence or abuse criteria.[56] Studies consistently report between 72% and 78% of inmates with mental illness had a co-occurring drug or alcohol abuse problem.[57,58] Yet despite this well-established relationship of mental illness, drugs, and crime, few jails and prisons use a formal validated screening instrument for drug abuse among their entering inmates.[59]

In a 2006 study, 81.9% of the jails and prisons surveyed reported that receiving screening (which constitutes observation and inquiring for alcohol or drug use) is the most often used method to assess for drug abuse.[59] About a third of the respondents indicated that they use the Addiction Severity Index (ASI) and the Alcohol Use Subscale (ASI-Alcohol) to screen for substance abuse disorders. Sadly, 16.4% of the respondents indicated that they use no instruments to screen for substance abuse. Correctional PAs should promote the use of accurate and timely screening instruments for substance abuse.

Some jail and prison health authorities have established their own licensed methadone opioid agonist treatment programs to treat opioid addiction. In these settings correctional PAs have an important role in treatment of opioid addicts through methadone programming. However, little is known about how PAs are used in jail and prison opioid addiction programs, which is an area that needs to be examined. Some health authorities even provide buprenorphine as an alternative to methadone in the treatment of inmates with opioid dependence. Correctional PAs should find additional guidance in treating inmates with drug abuse by reviewing *Principles of Drug Abuse Treatment for Criminal Justice Populations.* They will find support for comprehensive reentry services designed to minimize relapse and recidivism.[60]

SPECIAL ISSUES IN CORRECTIONS

Pain Management

One issue that challenges all corrections health professionals is how to differentiate between legitimate pain sufferers and those manifesting drug-seeking behavior. Nearly 70% of the incarcerated populations are charged with serious drug offenses and have some sort of drug-seeking behavior.[56] Distinguishing between a true chronic pain sufferer from an individual who is manipulating and seeking drugs is something that a correctional PA learns to do quickly.

The history is an important way to distinguish pain sufferers from manipulators. A true chronic pain sufferer is someone who has narrowed his or her selection of medications to actually find some, but not total, relief. The drug-seeking individual, on the other hand, will have a polypharmacy approach, often mixing classes of drugs, "without finding any relief."

Associated pain with movement is another way to distinguish legitimate chronic pain sufferers from those exhibiting drug seeking behavior. A legitimate chronic pain sufferer generally reports being pain free at rest, whereas the individual who expresses multifocal pain at rest may indeed have some drug manipulation issues.

Nonmalignant pain management in correctional institutions is complex. Because incarcerated populations have documented histories of trauma, mental illness, and substance abuse disorders, clinicians find it difficult to assess what and how much to prescribe to this population. Correctional PAs can find supplemental information by reviewing The National Commission on Correctional Health Care's (NCCHC's) *Position Statement on Chronic Pain Management*, which can be found at *http://ncchc.org/resources/statements/chronic_pain.html.*

End of Life

Several factors contribute to the incarcerated population death rate. Data on prisoner deaths remain sketchy; however, limited studies have indicated that, when compared with the same age groups of civilians (such as 55–65 and 65 and older), prisoners have significantly higher mortality rates due to malignant neoplasms, chronic liver disease, pneumonia, septicemia, HIV, and AIDS.[61]

How are terminally ill inmates managed? In general, there are two options to managing terminally ill inmates in prison. The first is to compassionately release the dying inmate to a community setting. A compassionate or early medical release program permits terminally ill patients to return to the community and be housed in a home care setting, a hospice, or a long-term care skilled nursing facility. In this way a terminally ill prisoner can return home to be near his or her family in the last stages of death. However, there are many barriers to the liberal use of compassionate release programming. A prisoner's criminal record, public safety concerns, statutory limitations, and public activism against release have prohibited the compassionate release of some prisoners. The lack of community resources to accept transferees from prisons or the lack of outside family support may in fact disqualify a prisoner for an early release. In addition, the approval process may be inordinately long. Approvals for early release may require an independent medical board, a judge, prosecutor, and even public input before a decision is made to allow an individual to be released early and die outside the prison setting. It is not uncommon for prisons to release an inmate hours before he or she dies.

The second option is to create a correctional hospice program. Less than 3% of the U.S. prisons have a hospice or palliative care program.[62] There are a number of barriers to developing a hospice program, which include a lack of funding, an untrained staff in hospice care, and a prison culture that fosters suspicion and insensitivity. Approximately 85% of hospice patients receive Medicare coverage for services. Yet prisoners are not Medicare or Medicaid eligible, so any hospice-type service that is provided in correctional institutions is absorbed within the department budget or through pro bono activity by community hospice agencies. Most departments of corrections do not have formal hospice programs. Nearly 70% of terminally ill inmates are kept in infirmaries, about 10% are compassionately released, and 20% are cared for in a hospice program.[63] Thus hospice training and experience among correctional health workers is limited. Finally, the prison culture hampers the implementation of hospice care. Many consider correctional institutions as places for harsh punishment, assuming an attitude that demonizes inmates, providing few services as possible. This includes hospice care. Some staff members believe that palliative or hospice care would be "coddling prisoners"[63] and, as such, does not provide an appropriate tone for a prison. Another barrier to overcome is that inmates have a dim view of death and dying behind the "walls" and would rather be transferred to an outside hospital or have a compassionate release so that they can be with family and friends during their last stages of life. State rules governing such releases are often not supportive for compassionate releases, so with an increase in the elderly inmate population and terminal illness, there will be more need for hospice services.

The correctional PA is often involved in hospice and end-of-life care issues. Providing clinical support for a dying inmate is one aspect of that involvement, but the correctional PA can also be involved in providing support to staff and inmate volunteer workers who are involved in hospice care. Training of staff and providing psychological support are some of the ways that correctional PAs can be involved in hospice care.

One area of death that correctional PAs should not be involved in is executions. The mandate from professional organizations is clear on this point. The American Academy of Physician Assistants (AAPA) policy prohibits PAs from participating in executions. The NCCHC standard and position statement for health care professionals prohibits the involvement of health staff in any aspect of the execution process.[64] The ethical conundrum of establishing a therapeutic relationship with a patient, only to participate in his or her termination of life, is one that few PAs face; nonetheless, many correctional PAs have had to face this and many other ethical dilemmas on a daily basis.

MANAGING ETHICAL CONFLICTS IN CORRECTIONAL INSTITUTIONS

Autonomy

Correctional health care is the nexus among criminal justice, public health, law, and ethics. And although the challenging ethical issues of the correctional health care field are similar to the community, the nature of prisons and jails limits autonomy and choice. Correctional medicine ethics is much more complex because there are no clear-cut guidelines for an ethical conduct of correctional health professionals.

The competing priorities between correctional interests and health interests continuously provide flashpoints of conflict and tension. For example, one cornerstone of medical ethics is patient freedom of choice. In a prison or jail setting a patient's choice of provider is limited. Their ability to choose or change health providers is limited and in many cases not an option. Likewise, if a PA is having difficulty communicating with a troublesome patient, there is little opportunity to change to a different health care professional. As a result, both patient and PA are stuck with each other and must resolve their issues.

Issues such as informed consent and refusal of treatment are complex in correctional settings. Inmates have the right to be informed of the risks and benefits of proposed procedures and therapies and may refuse. However, can an inmate refuse treatment for a health condition that poses a risk to others? Correctional health staff are obligated to ensure the safety and public health of institutions. Medical isolation is usually the first step to contain an infectious inmate who refuses treatment. If the inmate remains recalcitrant, correctional health clinicians will obtain a court order to enact appropriate care. However, system disincentives, such as payment of a fee for health services or programming conflicts between sick call and court visits, might be causes for inmate refusals and should be analyzed. Other possible alternatives should be investigated.

The ethical conundrum is that when inmates are protesting their condition of confinement, refusal, such as hunger strikes or refusal to abide by custody rules, may be their only alternative. The dilemma that correctional health clinicians find themselves in is protecting the patient's health and life while honoring his or her efforts to effectuate system change. In these situations, correctional PAs need to educate and communicate with their patients and custody officials to alleviate conflict and improve clinical outcomes.

Justice

One ethical tenet is that patients are to be treated equally. Health care professionals are taught that they must remain neutral in their perspective about the patients they encounter and treat them accordingly. That ethical principle is put to the test every day in correctional medicine. How would you feel about treating a child molester with diabetes? Would a rapist with *Chlamydia* be treated any differently? This can be a major deterrent for many PAs who are new to correctional health care, and it can put their professional objectivity to the test every day. Regardless of their criminality, inmates should receive health care that is at community care standards.

Beneficence

The ethical principle of acting only for the benefit of the patient is *beneficence*. Correctional clinicians are challenged with regard to what constitutes beneficence for the patient or obligations to the state. For example, contraband in a correctional institution is a serious problem because it jeopardizes the security and safety of everyone. Body cavity searches are one method that correctional administrators use to ensure that contraband is not entering the facility. This presents a conflict for the correctional clinician who should conduct his or her actions with beneficence and resist efforts to have them conduct body cavity searches on their patients. Of course, if there is sufficient medical indication to conduct a body cavity search, then it should be performed.

Another issue that challenges the principle of beneficence is competency for execution. Establishing a therapeutic relationship is contingent on a goal to restore the individual to full function and thus improve his or her quality of life. It is antithesis to cases where the goal is restoring an individual's competency in order to carry out an execution sentence. NCCHC position statement advises correctional clinicians that restoring an inmate to competency for the purposes of execution should be made by an independent expert and not by any health care professional regularly in the employ of, or under contract to provide health care with, the correctional institution or system holding the inmate.[64] This requirement does not diminish the responsibility of correctional health care personnel to treat any mental illness of death row inmates.

Confidentiality

In an environment where there are "no secrets," it is difficult to protect the confidentiality of inmates' health problems. Maintaining confidentiality and privacy of patient information is difficult under circumstances where control is not maintained by health staff. The use of per diem workers, visiting clinicians, or other temporary health care providers also complicates how confidentiality is maintained.

The principle of confidentiality ensures the patient that disclosure of specific information given to the provider during a course of treatment will remain confidential. Because this can be complicated in a jail or prison, correctional PAs have to work harder to gain patient trust in a therapeutic relationship. When an inmate tells the clinician that he broke his jaw "while slipping in the shower" or "tripping and hitting my bunk bed" the clinician needs to understand that pressing for more information could jeopardize the patient-clinician relationship. On the other hand, if an inmate tells the clinician, in the course of a clinical encounter, that his new tattoo was obtained in the cell block, the clinician has the responsibility of informing custody that there is a potential that contraband material (ink, needles) is present in the prison. Discerning the difference between patient-specific confidential information and information that must be shared with custody staff is a fine line that many correctional PAs must negotiate.

FUTURE DIRECTIONS

The Patient Protection and Affordable Care Act (PPACA) will increase access to health insurance via Medicaid for many low-income individuals. What is not known is how returning inmates, with untreated mental health and substance abuse needs, will affect the changing public health landscape. As the PPACA regulation unfolds, its impact on correctional health care and the reentry population will need to be closely watched.

CONCLUSION

Unlike their noncorrectional colleagues, PAs who work in jails and prisons have unique challenges to their professional ethics and personal beliefs. Some are well suited for this work environment, whereas others do not fare well. This chapter has described the areas that are unique in correctional medicine, which are often not discussed in PA educational programs.

Why would a PA want to work in a jail or prison? After all, working conditions in U.S. prisons and jails are what you would expect in developing countries' health care systems, where patients often present to the clinic late in the course of their disease; they have self-medicated with legend drugs or traditional treatments; the health facilities are so "poor" that they may delay diagnosis; referrals (if needed) are not easily arranged; there are problems with shortages of trained staff; there is poor infection control and lack of follow-up care; and the "patient may be unable (e.g., because of financial hardship) to fully adhere to treatment."[45]

Beyond the similarity between U.S. correctional institutions and developing countries, why would you want to provide health care to patients who are seeking to "game the system" or who are litigious?[65]

The answer lies in the PAs' role. Practicing correctional medicine creates an opportunity for PAs to advocate for individual and community health, two cornerstones of the profession.

As patient advocates, correctional PAs have the opportunity to make a difference in the lives of disadvantaged and disenfranchised populations who need specialists in public health, primary care, infectious disease, and chronic disease. Correctional PAs can advocate for improved conditions of confinement and improved health services, making improvements in clinical care and patient outcomes.

An average day in the life of a correctional PA is complete with clinical and administrative responsibilities (see Case Study 45-1). Seeing patients in a variety of settings such as segregation cells, sick call clinics, inpatient settings, and dialysis units is a dynamic that creates opportunities for correctional PAs to advocate for patient needs.

As advocates for public health, PAs working in corrections address issues that directly prevent the spread of disease into our communities and have an impact on eliminating health care disparity to disenfranchised populations.

CASE STUDY 45-1

A DAY IN THE LIFE OF A FEDERAL CORRECTIONAL PHYSICIAN ASSISTANT

7:00 am Arrive at work. Exchange chit for keys and radio. Enter through sally ports. Go to segregation (SEG) unit and conduct rounds—offer inmates an opportunity to address health issues. (The SEG unit is a small, six-cell seclusion unit that houses inmates restricted from the general population.)

7:20 am Visit the dialysis unit; check on things and make sure that they are going well. (The facility has an in-house dialysis unit that accommodates up to 12 inmates at a time.)

7:30 am Visit the ambulatory care area (drop lunch off to the fridge). Check in with the nurses and assess the sick call volume for the day. Review visits made by the hospitalists from the previous night and any other pending questions. Confer with the nurses to see what staffing will be like for the day; scan the appointment list for the day. (The unit has several consultants who come in to provide services on site, plus the in-house staff schedules appointments.) Visit Medical Records to see what paperwork has been set aside that needs attention.

7:45 am Stop by the office to scan e-mails and pick up stethoscope.

8:00 am (Monday, Wednesday, and Friday only) Morning report meeting to review complex-wide patient health issues. (The facility has five institutions on campus, and many overnight emergencies are sent to the medical center, so discussion of follow-up is a priority.) Health services staff announcements are also made.

8:30 am Clinics begin. First scheduled appointments begin. Three to four are scheduled at 8:30 and 9:30.

10:45 am Inmates begin lunch. Progress notes completed on morning patients. Consults are entered into the computer; labs, radiographs ordered; and medication orders are faxed to the pharmacy. Check e-mails.

12:00 pm Lunch.

12:30 pm Afternoon scheduled sick call appointments begin. By 3:00 PM have progress notes, consult orders, labs, radiographs, and medication orders to the pharmacy.

3:00 pm During the afternoon inmates return from out-of-institution trips. They stop in the ambulatory care unit for screening. Triage them to a specific housing area until they can go back to the general population.

3:30 pm Pre-op orders for inmates having procedures (in our operating room, for positron emission tomography scans, radiology, or those going out.)

In between all of that an employee may present with an injury for assessment. I am second call for inmates coming in through receiving and discharge (R&D) for admittance into the institution, again assisting with disposition in the building, and ensuring continuity of care with medications and, in cases of any emergency calls, stopping and running to the emergency. As the afternoon winds down, there are numerous reports waiting to be completed: prerelease paperwork, transfer paperwork responses to the courts for medical study cases, responses to inmate inquiries ("cop outs"), follow-up labs, test and consult reports, and any meetings called such as team meetings, staff meetings, and occasional continuing medical education (CME) lunch session. I meet with my supervising physician (mine is the clinical director) to review charts and obtain countersignatures. The nonclinical duties squeeze in when they can. I chair the diabetes center of excellence committee (DICE) that meets weekly. I am past chair for the intracomplex inmate movement workgroup that coordinated the services for moving inmates around the complex to meet with consultants and use the OR at the medical center building (our campus is 750 acres). I chaired the dialysis care meetings and quarterly workgroups, and I serve on a few other workgroups. As the day winds down, I take another look at e-mails, check voice mail, and check my mailbox. Although the usual 8-hour day is often extended to 9½, I generally leave by 5.

Courtesy Robin Hunter-Buskey, PA-C.

CLINICAL APPLICATIONS

1. Is the clinical management of infectious diseases like HIV or hepatitis C any different in a prison or jail setting?
2. Serious persistent mental illnesses are a great concern in prisons and jails. How can PAs be clinically prepared to manage these conditions?
3. Will it be safe to work or do a clinical rotation in corrections?

KEY POINTS

- Inmates have a higher prevalence of health problems than the general population, both acute and chronic.
- Correctional medicine should not be quickly dismissed because it addresses public health issues that prevent the spread of disease in our communities and the enormous opportunity to make progress on eliminating health disparities.
- Correctional medicine is one of the cornerstones of public health in this country, and through effective standardization of care we can have a tremendous impact on the public's health.
- Ensuring that inmates have access to health care services is a fundamental responsibility for correctional medical professionals.
- Safety of inmates, staff, and visitors takes priority in a correctional institution, and many decisions that would seem inconsequential in the free world take on great importance in corrections.
- Clinical autonomy cannot be jeopardized; however, in a correctional institution diagnostic and therapeutic orders are not issued in a vacuum. Instead, they require a coordinated effort among custodial, administrative, and health staff.
- The recruiting, training, and retaining of health professionals to work in correctional health care is difficult because prisons and jails do not have medical care as the primary mission.
- PAs working in a correctional environment need to know that it is a constant balance between public safety and public health.
- Many correctional institutions have infection control committees that establish and maintain the exposure-control plan, monitor communicable disease among inmates and staff, ensure prompt

treatment for inmates and staff with infectious disease, ensure staff receive appropriate training, and maintain procedures (that personal protective equipment is available, is used, and meets reporting requirements, laws, and regulations issued by local, state, and federal authorities).
- One problem in correctional medicine is that the inmates, by nature, distrust authority and rules.
- Correctional health care is the nexus among criminal justice, public health, law, and ethics.
- As patient advocates, correctional PAs have the opportunity to make a difference in the lives of disadvantaged and disenfranchised populations who need specialists in public health, primary care, infectious disease, and chronic disease.

ACKNOWLEDGMENTS

The author thanks Peter C. Ober, JD, PA-C, American Academy of Physician Assistants liaison to the National Commission on Correctional Health Care, for his review of the manuscript and valuable comments.

The author also thanks Robin Hunter-Buskey PA-C, Senior Clinical Physician Assistant, Diabetes Specialist, Federal Correctional Complex (FCC) Butner, North Carolina for her daily timeline.

References

1. Harrison PM, Beck AJ. Prison and jail inmates at midyear 2005 (Bureau of Justice Statistics Special Report, NCJ 213133). Washington, DC: National Criminal Justice Reference Service, 2006.
2. Hammett TM, Harmon MP, Rhodes W. The burden of infectious disease among inmates of and releases from U.S. correctional facilities. Am J Public Health 2002;92:1789–1794.
3. Kelley E, Moy E, Stryer D, et al. Agency for Healthcare Research and Quality. 2006 National Healthcare Disparities Report. Rockville, MD: U.S. Department of Health and Human Services, Agency for Healthcare Research and Quality, May 10, 2007. AHRQ Pub. No. 07–0012 *http://www.ahrq.gov/qual/nhdr06/nhdr06.htm*. Accessed June 15, 2007.
4. National Commission on Correctional Health Care (2002). Health status of the soon to be released inmate (Vols. I and II). *http://www.ncchc.org/pubs/pubs_stbr.html*. Accessed October 12, 2006.
5. Chavez RS. Improving the public's health through correctional health care standards. Public Health Pract Illinois 2005;6(1):33–39.
6. Chavez RS. Assessing correctional health care: correlations of quality health care services in correctional institutions. University of Michigan (Ann Harbor) Dissertations; 2003.
7. Estelle v. Gamble, 429 U.S. 97 (1976).
8. Farmer v. Brennan, 511 U.S. 825 (1994).
9. Tillery v. Owens, (1989). 719 F. Supp 1256, 1286 (W.D.Pa 1989) aff'd, 907 F.2d 418 (3rd Circ. 1990).
10. Johnson D. Legal Issues Related to Managing the Challenging Mentally Ill. Presented at the National Commission on Correctional Health Care Conference, Atlanta, October 2006.
11. Thornton RL. New Approaches to Staff Safety. 2nd ed. Washington, DC: U.S. Department of Justice, National Institute of Corrections, 2002.
12. Human Rights Watch. No escape: male rape in U.S. prisons. New York: Human Rights Watch; 2001.
13. Prison Rape Elimination Act of 2003. *http://www.ojjdp.ncjrs.gov/about/PubLNo108-79.txt*. Accessed April 10, 2007.
14. Centers for Disease Control and Prevention (2007). Community-Associated Methicillin Resistant *Staphylococcus aureus* (CA-MRSA). *http://www.cdc.gov/ncidod/dhqp/ar_mrsa_ca.html*. Accessed July 30, 2007.
15. Turabelidze G, Lin M, Wolkoff B, et al. Personal hygiene and methicillin-resistant *Staphylococcus aureus* infection. Emerg Infect Dis 2006;12(3):422–427.
16. Aiello AE, Lowy FD, Wright LN, Larson EL. Methicillin-resistant Staphylococcus aureus among U.S. prisoners and military personnel: review and recommendations for future studies. Lancet 2006;6:335–341.
17. Hradecky G. MRSA: The San Diego Jail Experience *http://www.sdsheriff.net/library/MRSA_SD_JAIL_EXPERIENCE.pdf*. Accessed February 27, 2007.
18. Federal Bureau of Prisons. Management of methicillin-resistant *Staphylococcus aureus* (MRSA) infections. Washington, DC: Federal Bureau of Prisons; 2005 *http://www.bop.gov/news/PDFs/mrsa.pdf*. Accessed June 15, 2007.
19. MacNeil JR, Lobato MN, Moore M. An unanswered health disparity: tuberculosis among correctional inmates, 1993 through 2003. Am J Public Health 2005;95:1800–1805.
20. Rao NA. Prevalence of pulmonary tuberculosis in Karachi central prison. J Pakistan Med Assoc 2004;54(8):413–415.
21. Saunders DL, Olive DM, Wallace SB, et al. Tuberculosis screening in the federal prison system: an opportunity to treat and prevent tuberculosis in foreign-born populations. Public Health Reports 2001;116(3):210–218.
22. Bruggers R. A comparison of screening and treatment for latent tuberculosis to national recommended guidelines in three correctional facilities [unpublished master's thesis]. Downers Grove, IL: Midwestern University; 2004.
23. Maruschak L. Medical problems of jail inmates. Bureau of Justice Statistics Bulletin, NCJ 210696 *http://www.ojp.usdoj.gov/bjs/pub/pdf/mpji.pdf*. Accessed January 2, 2007.
24. Spaulding AC, Jacob-Arriola K, Ramos KL, et al. Primary care in jail settings: report on a consultants' meeting. J Correctional Health Care 2007;13(2):93–128.
25. Arriola KR, Braithwaite RL, Kennedy S, et al. A collaborative effort to enhance HIV/STI screening in five county jails. Public Health Reports 2001;116(6):520–529.
26. Maruschak L. HIV in prisons, 2001. Bureau of Justice Statistics. Washington, DC: U.S. Department of Justice. NCJ 202293; 2004.
27. Centers for Disease Control and Prevention. Revised recommendations for HIV testing of adults, adolescents, and pregnant women in health-care settings. Morb Mortal Wkly Rep 2006;55:2–17.
28. Beckwith CG, Poshkus M. HIV behind bars: meeting the need for HIV testing, education, and access to care. Infect Dis Corrections Rep 2007;9(17):1, 3–4.
29. Kavasery R, Altice FL. Routine HIV testing in jails: addressing the challenges. Infect Dis Corrections Rep 2007;9(17):3, 5.
30. Bernard K, Sueker JJ, Colton E, et al. Provider perspectives about the standard of HIV care in correctional settings and comparison to the community standard of care: how do we measure up? Infect Dis Corrections Rep 2006;9(3):1–6.

31. Wohl DA. Letter from the editor. Infect Dis Corrrections Rep 2006;9(5):2–3.
32. National Commission on Correctional Health Care. Hepatitis Education for Inmates and Correctional Officers. Chicago: National Commission on Correctional Health Care, 2002.
33. Parece MS, Herrera GA, Voigt RF, et al. STD testing policies and practices in U.S. city and county jails. Sex Transm Dis 1999;26(8):431–437.
34. U.S. Institute of Medicine. The Hidden Epidemic: Confronting Sexually Transmitted Diseases (a report prepared by the Committee on Prevention and Control of Sexually Transmitted Diseases). Washington, DC: National Academy Press, 1997.
35. Kahn RH, Joesoef R, Aynalem G, et al. Overview of sexually transmitted diseases. In: Puisis M, (ed). Clinical Practice in Correctional Medicine. 2nd ed. Philadelphia: Mosby Elsevier, 2006. p 175–181.
36. Mertz KJ, Voigt RA, Hutchins K, et al. Findings from STD screening of adolescents and adults entering corrections facilities: implications for STD control strategies. Sex Transm Dis 2002;29(12):834–839.
37. Mertz KJ, Schwebke JR, Gaydos C, et al. Screening women in jails for chlamydial and gonococcal infection using urine tests: feasibility, acceptability, prevalence, and treatment rates. Sex Transm Dis 2002;29(5):271–276.
38. Frye JC. Assessment of the standard of care for *Chlamydia trachomatis* in a juvenile detention center as compared to the national guidelines [upublished master's thesis]. Chicago: Midwestern University, 2006.
39. Kraut JR, Haddix AC, Carande-Kulis V, Greifinger RB. Cost-effectiveness of routine screening for sexually transmitted diseases among inmates in United States prisons and jails. National Commission on Correctional Health Care. Health Status of the Soon To Be Released Inmate. vol. 2. Chicago: National Commission on Correctional Health Care, 2002. p81–108.*http://www.ncchc.org/stbr/Volume2/Report5_Kraut.pdf.* Accessed August 2, 2006.
40. Klein SJ, Wright LN, Birkhead GS, et al. Promoting HCV treatment completion for prison inmates: New York State's hepatitis C continuity program. Public Health Rep 2007; 122(Suppl. 2):83–88.
41. Arora S, Thornton K, Jenkusky SM, et al. Project ECHO: linking university specialists with rural and prison-based clinicians to improve care for people with chronic hepatitis C in New Mexico. Public Health Rep 2007;122(Suppl. 2):74–77.
42. Devine A, Karvelas M, Sundararajan V. Evaluation of a prison-based hepatitis B immunisation pilot project. Austr N Z J Pub Health 2007;31(2):127–130.
43. Wolitski RJ. Relative efficacy of a multisession sexual risk-reduction intervention for young men released from prisons in 4 states. Am J Public Health 2006;96(10):1854–1861.
44. Tedeschi SK, Bonney LE, Manalo R, et al. Vaccination in juvenile correctional facilities: state practices, hepatitis B, and the impact on anticipated sexually transmitted infection vaccines. Public Health Rep 2007;122(1):44–48.
45. Chavez RS. The incarcerated male. In: Heidelbaugh J (ed). Clinical Men's Health: Evidence in Practice. Amsterdam: Elsevier, 2007. p. 532–547.
46. Chavez RS, Porter J, McIlwain L. Tobacco cessation policies in correctional institutions. Poster presentation to the Tobacco or Health Conference. Boston, December 2003.
47. Cropsey KL, Kristeller JL. The effects of a prison smoking ban on smoking behavior and withdrawal symptoms. Addict Behav 2005;30(3):589–594.
48. Rothman DJ. Perfecting the prison: United States, 1789–1865. In: Morris N, Rothman DJ (eds). The Oxford History of the Prison: The Practice of Punishment in Western Society. New York: Oxford University Press, 1998. p 102–116.
49. James DJ, Glaze LE. Mental health problems of prison and jail inmates. U.S. Department of Justice, Bureau of Justice Statistics, Special Report NCJ 213600. *http://www.ojp.usdoj.gov/bjs/abstract/mhppji.htm.* Accessed August 7, 2007.
50. Ditton PM. Mental health and treatment of inmates and probationers. Washington, DC: Department of Justice; 1999.
51. Teplin LA. Psychiatric and substance abuse disorders among male urban jail detainees. Am J Public Health 1994;84:290–293.
52. Mumola CJ. Suicide and homicide in state prisons and local jails. U.S. Department of Justice, Office of Justice Programs. NCJ 210036 Bureau of Justice Statistics August 10, 2007. *http://www.ojp.usdoj.gov/bjs/pub/pdf/shsplj.pdf.* Accessed September 26, 2007.
53. Centers for Disease Control and Prevention. Suicide: facts at a glance, 2007. *http://www.cdc.gov/ncipc/dvp/suicide/SuicideDataSheet.pdf.* Accessed; September 26, 2007.
54. Hayes L. Guide to developing and revising suicide prevention protocols. NCCHC Standards for Health Services in Jails. Chicago: National Commission on Correctional Health Care, 2003. p 159–164.
55. Mumola CJ. Substance abuse and treatment, state and federal prisoners, 1997. U.S. Department of Justice, Office of Justice Programs. NCJ 172871. *http://www.ojp.usdoj.gov/bjs/pub/pdf/satsfp97.pdf.* Accessed September 26, 2007.
56. Karberg JC, James DJ. Substance Dependence, Abuse, and Treatment of Jail Inmates, 2002. Bureau of Justice Statistics Special Report No. NCJ 209588. U.S. Department of Justice Office of Justice Programs. *http://www.ojp.usdoj.gov/bjs/pub/pdf/sdatji02.pdf.* Accessed September 26, 2007.
57. Abram KM, Teplin LA. Co-occurring disorders among mentally ill jail detainees. Am Psychol 1991;46(10):1036–1045.
58. McNiel DE, Binder RL, Robinson JC. Incarceration associated with homelessness, mental disorder, and co-occurring substance abuse. Psychiatr Serv 2005;56(7):840–846.
59. Chavez RS. An assessment of U.S. jail and prison screening and treatment practices for drug abuse and co-occurring disorders. Poster presentation at the American Association for the Treatment of Opioid Dependence, Atlanta, 2006.
60. National Institute on Drug Abuse. *Principles of Drug Abuse Treatment for Criminal Justice Populations* (revised; NIH Publication No. 06–5316). *http://www.nida.nih.gov/PODAT_CJ/*; Accessed September 2007.
61. Mumola CJ. Medical causes of death in state prisons, 2001-2004. Data Brief U.S. Department of Justice, Office of Justice Programs. NCJ 216340. Bureau of Justice Statistics. *http://www.ojp.usdoj.gov/bjs/pub/pdf/mcdsp04.pdf*; Accessed April 10, 2007.
62. National Hospice and Palliative Care Organization. Directory of Hospice and Palliative Care Programs in Correctional Facilities. Alexandria, VA: National Hospice and Palliative Care Organization, 2007.
63. Maull FW. Delivery of end-of-life care in prisons and jails. In: Puisis M, (ed). Clinical Practice in Correctional Medicine. 2nd ed Philadelphia: Mosby Elsevier, 2006. p. 529–537.
64. National Commission on Correctional Health Care. Position Statement on Competency for Executions, 1988, p.195. Standards for Health Services in Prisons. Chicago: National Commission on Correctional Health Care, 2003.
65. Allen B, Bosta D. Games criminals play: how you can profit by knowing them. Sacramento, CA: Rae John Publishers, 1993.

The resources for this chapter can be found www.expertconsult.com

CHAPTER 46

Military Medicine

John L. Chitwood

CHAPTER CONTENTS

Shortages in U.S. health care systems (civilian and military) during the 1960s resulted in needs not being fulfilled by physicians. Shortfalls in military physician recruiting were made more serious by the unpopular war in Vietnam. The decrease in availability of health care providers to U.S. Department of Defense (DOD) beneficiaries became a reality, and physician scholarship programs were initiated to bring more physicians into the military services. This shortage was not helped by the length of time in the "training pipeline" it took for a physician to be educated. Even after a medical student had been selected to receive a scholarship that obligated him or her to military service, it took 5 years for a general medical officer (GMO, who has no residency training) to be educated and up to 9 years for a board-eligible physician to be trained. Physician assistants (PAs) and other physician extenders, such as nurse practitioners, were seen as the short-term answer to a potentially long-term problem.

PA training programs were established in the U.S. Army, the U.S. Navy, and the U.S. Air Force in 1971. Enlisted military members with broad military and medical backgrounds were selected for advanced training as new health care professionals. Each curriculum consisted of 1 year of didactic training at various military educational facilities and a 1-year rotational clinical practicum in a military hospital. After completion of the 2-year program, all new graduates were credentialed by either the military hospital to which they were assigned or the military hospital that had medical supervision over their clinical practice. These graduates were credentialed to provide routine and emergency primary care under the direct or indirect supervision of a physician. Secondary to manpower ceilings, these military training programs have been activated, deactivated, and then reactivated since 1977. When PAs had been initially trained in the military, they were used in the enlisted and warrant officer ranks. The Air Force began commissioning PAs as officers in 1978, the Navy in 1989, and the Army in 1992.

Originally, the military training programs awarded only certificates of completion because PA programs were viewed as advanced coursework for highly trained military corpsmen. Military PA graduates now receive a certificate that enables them to sit for the National Commission for Certification of Physician Assistants (NCCPA) certifying examination, along with a Master of Science degree from a sponsoring university. A competitive bid process determines the sponsoring university. Military programs continue to grant a certificate so that, should there ever be a problem with the degree-granting institution's accreditation status, graduates of a military program would still be eligible to sit for the NCCPA examination.

Before 1996, the Navy PA program trained students in one class annually in San Diego, California. The Air Force PA program educated 75 students in three classes annually, and the Army had 50 students enrolled in two classes each year. The U.S. Coast Guard relied on recruiting civilian PAs or sending enlisted personnel to a variety of civilian PA educational programs. In 1990 the U.S. Air Force School of Health Care Sciences began training Coast Guard PA students who received commissions as officers upon graduation. Early on, the Navy also enrolled students in the Air Force program. In 1996 all military PA training programs were consolidated into a single program located within the U.S. Army Medical Department Center and School (AMEDDC&S) at Fort Sam Houston, San Antonio, Texas. In the Interservice Physician Assistant Program (IPAP), there is a mixed faculty for didactic and clinical instruction that comprises PAs, science officers, and physicians representing each uniformed service. Civilian personnel are also employed by the program. From 1996-2002 IPAP graduated PAs with a Bachelor of Science degree. Beginning in 2002 IPAP graduates earned a "generic" bachelor degree at the end of phase 1 and a Masters of Physician Assistant Studies (MPAS) degree at the end of phase 2.

Because of wartime need for PAs in the DOD and Department of Homeland Security (DHS), IPAP increased the throughput to up to 240 students per year (up to 80 entering in three classes). This leads to a total yearly enrollment of up to 480 (240 in phase 1 and 240 in phase 2), making IPAP the largest PA program in existence. These enrollment numbers are the projected number needed to maintain a strength of approximately 1700 PAs in the DOD.

Since the Services began training PAs, the length of the course had remained 24 months. Unarguably the amount and complexity of medical information, as well as didactic delivery methods, have increased exponentially. The IPAP curriculum confers 95 semester hours in the didactic phase at Fort Sam Houston and 50 hours during the clinical phase. Two thirds of the didactic phase hours are coded at the graduate level by the University of Nebraska (the affiliated university). All of the clinical phase hours have been coded as graduate level. This means that graduates of IPAP have a minimum of 91 semester hours of undergraduate work (60 are from prerequisite course work) and 113 graduate-level hours. After the didactic phase, the students return to their host services' medical treatment facilities for clinical preceptorships. Nonmilitary students from other federal agencies in the past have attended IPAP, but none since 2002.

Beginning in 2009, IPAP was organizationally moved from the "PA branch" to the newly created Graduate School located at the AMEDDC&S. The Graduate School is composed of graduate programs in physical therapy, nursing anesthesia, social work, pastoral care, and health care administration. This has led to a dynamic graduate-level environment. When the *U.S. News and World Report (USN&WR)* rankings were published in 2011 ("Best Graduate Schools in America"), all of the programs in the Graduate School (which are in ranked disciplines) were ranked among the best in the country. IPAP is currently ranked thirteenth.

The military services continue to rely heavily on IPAP to meet their respective PA inventory shortfalls. The recruitment of civilian PAs into active duty or into the National Guard or Reserve components is problematic for several reasons.

First, the United States is currently participating in two active wars and has been since 2001, the longest time in our history; this means that all PAs are guaranteed that they will be tapped for hazardous duty within 6 months of graduating or being commissioned into the military. This volunteering for harm's way is analogous to writing a check for "everything up to and including my life." In addition are the following reasons:

- Overall disparity in pay between the military services and the civilian sector:
  - The base pay of an O1 (second lieutenant) with less than 2 years of creditable service is $33,408 (DFAS, 2011).
  - The base pay of an O2 (first lieutenant) with less than 2 years of creditable service is $38,487 (DFAS, 2011).
  - A PA accession may be brought into the military as an O2 if he or she has a master's degree as a PA.
  - Since 2009, DOD PAs have been on more competitive footing; by signing a 4-year multiyear contract, after completion of an initial service contract, PAs may receive up to $25,000 per year of Incentive Special Pay and Multiyear Specialty Pay. Also, all DOD PAs who have a medically related master's degree and NCCPA certification receive an additional $6000 per year of board certification pay.
- Military PAs must have a bachelor's degree as a PA and must be NCCPA certified.
- The average (mean) starting salary of a civilian PA in 2008 was $71,004 (AAPA, 2009).
- The military is authorized by law, but not funded, to repay up to $50,000 of "qualified debt" for a PA accession; the services are funded to repay up to $32,000 of qualified debt (AFIT, 2011). The military began offering the Thrift Savings Plan in January 2002, and more than 30% of officers elected to participate during the first month. This 401(k)-type plan has not affected recruitment and retention. Some civilian-trained PAs may be overwhelmed by military productivity standards, coupled with the military's clinical support system and rules. The productivity expected (25+ patients per day) is not excessive; however, the support

infrastructure (physical, fiscal, and personnel) is not as flexible and efficient as in civilian health care models.

- Adaption to the role of a professional military officer first, and to the role of medical provider second, may appear to be too demanding and stressful. The application of these two standards can be disconcerting.
- The scope and demands of military practice may be broader than some PA roles in civilian practice. Military PAs often practice fairly autonomously in remote and austere situations. It is expected that they will function by providing quality care with minimal support and consultation. It is not uncommon for the PA to rarely see the preceptor and to have only telephonic/radio contact on an as-needed basis.

Because the attrition of PAs continues in each branch of the uniformed services, the Army and Air Force have begun recruiting fully qualified civilian PAs. The Army had great success in recruiting PAs during 2006 (Scott, 2007). The Air Force began civilian recruiting efforts in 2006 and is offering scholarship money to PA students who sign a contract to serve after graduation. This program funded $69.3 million for tuition/fees and $55.5 million for loan repayment for all Air Force Medical Service (AFMS) programs in 2011.

The credentials committees of the various medical treatment facilities (MTFs) recommend to the MTF commander the individual clinical privileges of student and graduate military PAs, who are assigned to or provide care within the medical support areas of the MTF. Hospital commanders define in writing the scope and limits of the clinical practice for each PA and designate the supervising physicians. Clinical privileges for PAs are determined on initial assignment, are reevaluated after any change of assignment, and are reviewed annually, unless more frequent evaluation is necessary.

Uniformed services PAs have continued to climb the ladder of rank and responsibility within DOD and the Public Health Service:

- In 2003 the first DOD PA assumed command in a fixed (nontent/mobile) hospital.
- In 2006 the Air Force selected the first PA to command a medical group.
- In 2005 the first PA to serve as the Deputy Major Command (MAJCOM) Surgeon was selected.
- In 2006 the first PA to hold "flag officer" rank in the Public Health Service attained the Rank of Rear Admiral.

In 2011, there were approximately 1700 PAs in all components of the uniformed services. A majority of these PAs are working in primary care, family practice, emergency departments, troop medical clinics, or dispensaries. PAs are considered to be the "gatekeepers" of the DOD health care system. Having repeatedly been proven cost-effective, PAs are providing quality medical care while increasing accessibility to medical care for all types of DOD beneficiaries.

SCOPE OF PRACTICE

Military PAs principally work in primary care and family practice. They can also be found in acute care ("fast track") and emergency services. Military PAs may specialize in aviation medicine, bone marrow transplant, cardiovascular perfusion, education, emergency medicine, occupational medicine, orthopedics, otolaryngology, oncology, public health, and general surgery. However, procedures performed by a PA must not exceed his or her authorized competency level. As military PAs progress in rank, they often assume nontraditional provider roles in leadership, administration, and research.

The military PA must keep abreast of innovations in primary patient care and combat medicine. Eighty-percent of Army PAs are assigned to combat or field maneuver units, the remainder being assigned to outpatient care at installation hospitals or to administrative positions. A majority of Air Force and Navy PAs are assigned to family practice or primary care clinics, but more combat operational roles are opening up to them at remote air bases and aboard ships because of their participation in Operations Desert Shield, Desert Storm, Iraqi Freedom, Enduring Freedom, and the Global War on Terrorism. Specialty-trained PAs must keep their skills current in the ever-changing technologies of their respective specialties and in family practice to maintain their NCCPA certification.

PAs in the U.S. Coast Guard must also be included in any discussion of military PAs. The Coast Guard is more than 200 years old and is a part of the U.S. Department of Homeland Defense during peacetime and the DOD during war. PAs in the Coast Guard have the same rank structure as PAs in the Navy. During wartime, they are federalized under the operational direction of the Department of the Navy. Coast Guard PAs are assigned to each Polar Class or Wind Class Icebreaker ship as the sole health care provider. They are also used as general medical officers in shore assignments. In addition, Coast Guard PAs perform medical administrative duties (such as serving as consultants to the U.S. Coast Guard Health and Safety Directorate) and are assigned as senior medical officers to post security units for worldwide deployment (e.g., in Korea, Turkey, and other operations areas). Coast Guard PAs, similar to other military PAs, may attend the Army flight surgeon training course and are designated as aviation medical officers. They attend the Tri-Service Combat Casualty Care Course, and are certified in advanced cardiac life support (ACLS) and advanced trauma life support (ATLS). They can also attend graduate specialty training and can earn graduate degrees. For this purpose, a Coast Guard PA instructor is permanently assigned to the IPAP school in San Antonio. Coast Guard PAs can be either members of the Coast Guard or members of the Public Health Service with duty assigned to the Coast Guard.

ROLE OF PHYSICIAN ASSISTANTS IN THE MILITARY

Military PAs roles are flexible and are not designed solely either for peacetime or wartime. Most military PAs deploy for 6 to 18 months (in a wartime role) and then return to home station to perform peacetime duties for up to 18 months.

Peacetime

Like their civilian counterparts, PAs in military service improve the productivity of a physician's practice, reduce patient waiting time, manage emergencies effectively, reduce pressure on the physician, improve patient access to professional care, and lower the costs of that care. It must be noted that when PAs see patients, they are personally productive but also allow the physicians in their practice setting to see more difficult patients. It has been hypothesized that PAs can see more than 80% of the patients in a given practice. This figure can be further defined by stating that PAs can effectively manage 80% of the disease/injury processes of their physician colleagues. Moreover, these 80% of disease processes may account for more than 90% of the patients seen.

Wartime

PAs have played extensive roles in all areas of responsibility (AORs) the United States is involved in. It is impossible to name all roles that PAs have filled, so here is a sample:

- Hospital commander
- Provincial reconstruction team (PRT) medical chief (includes tribal and government official liaison duties)
- Clinic commander
- Medical representation for all echelons of care
- Joint chiefs of staff duty
- Consultants to major commanders
- Consultants to the surgeons general
- Clinicians on humanitarian missions
- Liaison/advisor to health education professionals in the AORs (medical schools, technician schools, and midlevel provider initiatives)

Wartime military PAs provide routine and resuscitative unit-level medical care and evacuation to sick, wounded, and injured personnel from forward combat locations. In the past, PAs were primarily assigned to second echelon care positions. Currently PAs can be found at every echelon of care, from the battlefield to tertiary care facilities in the United States. Specialty-trained PAs, especially those trained in orthopedics and emergency medicine, may be used in nearly every echelon of care. In wartime, PAs often perform the following functions:

1. Conduct and/or supervise training of unit personnel in first aid, sanitation, personal hygiene, medical evacuation procedures, and the medical aspects of injury prevention.
2. Arrange for a unit preventive psychiatry program that includes unit leader training in methods of preventing psychiatric disorders and combat stress casualties.
3. Perform triage on and treat sick, wounded, or injured persons.
4. Refer patients who require additional treatment to a facility capable of that care.

With the current battlefield being more fluid, PAs have adapted to the vertigo of change. It is remarkable that during recent combat operations, injuries that resulted in a 25% mortality rate in the 1960s now result in less than 10% mortality. And more than 80% of all injuries are returned to duty by PAs).

Service Impact

Although PAs in uniformed services have been largely used in primary care and for troop care in maneuver units, they are also educated in the care of every type of DOD beneficiary. The additional use of specialty-trained PAs is cost-beneficial and represents an optimal utilization of a health care resource to extend the capabilities not only of the primary care physician but also of the highly trained specialist physician. Although the military has been in the forefront of creating formalized residency training programs for PAs, the DOD has been severely lagging in the utilization of PAs in specialty areas. The Army has taken the lead in enhancing its residency training by partnering with a civilian accredited university (currently Baylor University) to grant a doctorate degree to their residency graduates. New training opportunities are becoming available as a result of the creation of the San Antonio Military Medical Center (SAMMC), which is composed of the Air Force's flagship hospital, Wilford Hall Medical Center (WHMC), and the venerable Brooke Army Medical Center (BAMC), which includes the famous burn unit (WFBU) and the Center for the Intrepid (a world-class rehabilitation facility). SAMMC also led to the creation of the San Antonio Uniformed Services Healthcare Education Consortium (SAUSHEC), which combined San Antonio–based residency programs. Because of this the Air Force and Army in SAMMC began training together in 2010.

The daily working relationships of physician/PA partnerships foster unity of thought and medical logic that permit relative autonomy of practice by PAs when the military situation so dictates. PAs may be independently assigned to units that are deployed to remote areas of the world. In such instances, the medical decisions made by PAs follow accepted guidance and standards in that they are the senior medical officers on site.

Military PAs can be justifiably proud to be members of this relatively new health care profession that provides an innovative level of medical care previously unavailable. No other health care provider can be substituted for a PA, just as a PA cannot substitute for any other health care provider. PAs are the only midlevel providers who are educated according to the medical model to extend the capabilities of physician services in all treatment settings. Any discussion of the substitution of health care that PAs provide can be addressed only at the level of health care delivered—either increased, as with a physician, or decreased, as with a corpsman. Proper utilization of health care extenders such as PAs, along with nurses and corpsmen, creates a health care team capable of delivering routine and emergency primary care under the direct or indirect supervision of a physician. Each team works toward the common goal of improving the quality, accessibility, and cost-effectiveness of health care. The utilization of PAs with corpsmen in such health care teams enhances the availability of care and provides an excellent role model for enlisted personnel who might be considering health care careers.

COST-BENEFIT ANALYSIS

Patient care provided by PAs cannot be distinguished from physician care in the primary care setting. Although most studies suggest that PAs can perform 80% of the services performed by doctors, the percentages vary with the location of the PA's practice, the practice setting, and the specialty. Because of this equality of outcome, when cost-benefit comparisons are made for PA services, the benefit is the same, regardless of whether a physician or a PA cares for the patient.

In a valid cost-benefit analysis, a reliable method for determining the costs (salary and benefits) and benefits (costs of patient care elsewhere if purchased) must be used. Currently, the DOD does not determine actual manpower costs for individuals or identifiable groups of providers. The actual cost per provider should be readily available on the basis of the medical officer's Social Security Administration Number (SSAN). For a valid cost-benefit comparison between different providers (by groups or as individuals), a ratio must be computed. Because ratios are the purest form of analytical comparison, it would be useful if the DOD used them in making health care manpower decisions. If the actual cost of a PA were used (actual salary and benefits costs), the cost portion of the formula would be substantially lower than that of other providers who receive their salary on the basis of a higher pay grade and with more extensive monetary benefits, such as professional pay and bonuses. The number of patient visits, categorized by beneficiary type and diagnosis, would accurately determine the benefit figure used in the ratio and would determine the value of the services represented.

Because access to valid information as outlined earlier (by SSAN or provider group) is not available secondary to privacy act restrictions, a simpler method for determining value will be used: value of services rendered less the most common military salary/benefits figure. See the following analysis.

CASE STUDY 46-1

BENEFIT

- The average relative value unit (RVU)/military provider is 14.9/day (TRICARE Report, 2011).
- Military PAs earn 30 days (i.e., 4 weeks, including weekends) of leave (vacation) a year.
- Military PAs usually travel on temporary duty (TDY or TAD) orders for an average of 2 weeks a year.
- A workweek is defined as 5 days.
- Therefore, military PAs produce 3427 RVUs per year (52 weeks per year − 4 weeks' leave − 2 weeks TDY) = 46 (weeks worked in outpatient care per year) × 14.9 (RVUs per day) × 5 (days per week).
- The TRICARE Management Activity has determined that each beneficiary, on average, consumes 14.1 RVUs/year (TRICARE Report, 2011).
- The TRICARE Management Activity has determined that the average RVU cost/beneficiary is $1638/year (TRICARE Report, 2011).

- Accordingly, the cost of RVUs for TRICARE is $116.19.

Therefore, the economic impact of a military PA is:

3427 RVU × $116.19 (RVU cost) = *$398,183.13*

COST

This needs to be offset by the direct cost of employing the military PA. DOD PAs range in rank from O1 ($2784/mo = $33,408.00 direct taxable compensation per annum) to O6 ($10,391.10/mo = $124,693.2 direct taxable compensation per annum) (DFAS, 2011). More PAs hold the rank of O3 than any other ($5286/mo = $63,432 direct taxable compensation per annum) (DFAS, 2011).

This does not take into account nontaxable housing allowances and subsistence allowances. It also does not factor in board certification pay for which many PAs are eligible (requires a graduate degree relevant to PA practice and NCCPA board certification). It is conceded that the most accurate way to determine the costing of a PA is by having access to the actual cost accounting numbers based on all DOD PAs' SSANs.

Given this concession, the comparison salary used here for DOD PAs is for an O3 with 6 years of service = ***$62,265.60***.

NET value of a military PA to DOD
= *$398,183 − 62,265.60 = $335,917.40.*

This leads to an enviable cost-benefit ratio of 0.18.

The military PA works and practices in unique settings and with unique demands. Schafft and Cawley have stated that the medical provider is standing in the middle of the struggle among increases in demand for health services, quality of care, and cost containment. These demands are, and will continue to be, placed on all PAs, both civilian and military. Military PAs have committed to their challenges historically and will continue to meet the demands of patient care and operational readiness now and in the future. Their job satisfaction and superb morale come with their commitment to doing the best job possible under any conditions.

CLINICAL APPLICATIONS

1. Describe the changes in the training of military PAs since 1996.
2. Describe the "typical" day for a military PA. Compare that day with a typical day for a civilian PA in primary care.
3. Discuss the contribution of active duty and reserve PAs in past and present military operations.
4. Describe how to determine the cost-benefit ratio of a military PA.

KEY POINTS

- Military PAs provide high-quality, cost-effective medical care.
- PAs are a valued and accepted part of the military medical team.
- The number of PAs in the military fluctuates with the needs of the country.
- The working environment/mission/focus of military PAs varies by the needs of the service employing them.
- Coast Guard PAs' mission has changed with the fielding of the Department of Homeland Security.
- PAs in the military have risen to new heights of leadership opportunities.

DISCLAIMER

The author is solely responsible for the contents of this chapter. It is not a position paper representing the Department of Defense or any governmental entity.

ACKNOWLEDGMENTS

Many thanks to all civilian and military PAs, contributing daily to our patients' quality of life.

The resources for this chapter can be found www.expertconsult.com

CHAPTER 47

INNER-CITY HEALTH CARE

F. J. (Gino) Gianola • Howard Straker • Terry Scott • Keren H. Wick

"Of all forms of inequality, injustice in health is the most shocking and most inhumane."
DR. MARTIN LUTHER KING, JR.

CHAPTER CONTENTS

Providing health care in the neighborhoods that lie at the center of America's cities presents the physician assistant (PA) with a unique set of challenges and opportunities, demanding a special set of attitudes and skills. There is no more complex environment in which to practice, nor is there one in which there is a higher risk for heartbreak and frustration. There are few places, however, in which a dedicated practitioner can make as great a difference in the life of a community. If PAs and the academic institutions in which they are trained select and mentor applicants who reflect the patients cared for in the inner city, they can make a significant difference in these urban communities throughout the nation. They will have succeeded in affirming and understanding the cultures and lives of citizens who make the inner city their home. This chapter describes the challenges and opportunities of inner-city practice in the context of the unique forces that have shaped America's central cities over the past several decades.

CAN YOU ANSWER THESE QUESTIONS?

- In your city, who lives in the inner city? Are there new Americans? Do you know anyone personally who lives in the inner city? Have you become involved in any community activities? If not, how will you get involved?
- Do you know how welfare in your state works? Have you ever been in a welfare office? Do you know where the Social Security Office is in your city? Have you ever visited the office?
- Do you know the components of case management? What are they? Have you ever worked with a case manager? How would you find out what the case manager would need to know to help you provide the best care for your patients? How would you discover the culture of case managers?
- Do you know the amount of money an average person receives as assistance in your state? Could you create a budget for a family of four receiving assistance in your state?
- Do you know how your state has shifted from welfare toward workfare? How would you find out how this will affect your patients and community?

At the conclusion of this chapter, you should be able to formulate a course of action to answer these questions.

WHAT DO WE MEAN BY INNER CITY?

Inner city is a term that is used to describe the neighborhoods that lie closest to the historical center of a city, where a convergence of rivers, a deep harbor, or other natural features provided the city with a reason for being. By virtue of their location nearest the city's industrial and commercial activity, these neighborhoods had the advantage of proximity to employment but many disadvantages as well. Subject to the noise, traffic, and pollution that attend industry, these neighborhoods generally housed the working classes, while more affluent families resided in neighborhoods "uptown" or "on the other side of the tracks."

Throughout the 19th and early 20th centuries, these inner city neighborhoods played a critical role in the development of urban America. These districts provided the first homes for the numerous waves of immigrants who reshaped America's cities and, in turn, provided a ready source of labor for the factories, ports, and warehouses nearby. Although many of the residents were poor and lived in terribly overcrowded conditions, many were able to use the inner city as a place to gather strength, to learn the new language, find employment, and save enough money to have better choices.

When they could afford to, many made the choice to leave the inner city for nearby neighborhoods that were less crowded. There, a little farther from the center of the city, a family might have a row house instead of an apartment, and the children might have a place to play other than the streets. Through this process, the housing in the inner cities constantly opened up again for the next wave of newcomers, while those who had succeeded remained in better neighborhoods nearby as living symbols of the reality of the American dream.

In the midst of the 20th century, a number of significant changes took place in America's cities that severely altered the role and character of the inner cities. With the end of the Great Depression and World War II, a large domestic migration began. In this population shift, the immigrants came not from overseas but from rural areas of the southern United States that had been devastated by the Depression. Poor whites and blacks who had suffered greatly during the 1930s and early 1940s now streamed into the inner cities of the north in search of new opportunities in the factories nearby. For a time, it appeared as if these latest newcomers would succeed in repeating the now-familiar cycle. By working hard and saving their wages, they hoped to move up and out within a generation or two. The symbiotic relationship among the inner cities, nearby industry, and middle class urban neighborhoods, however, was nearing its end.

Ironically, this change was caused in large part by the very economic boom these new residents were helping to create. The new wealth enjoyed by ordinary Americans meant that many more could afford luxuries such as the automobile. Gradually, the private automobile replaced public transportation as the way in which the middle class got to work. This in turn undermined the financial health of the transit services upon which most inner city residents still had to rely. Meanwhile, new government programs were making it possible for returning servicemen to buy homes, provided the homes were built to certain standards that the older housing in the inner city could not meet. Both of these forces worked against the inner cities by encouraging the newly affluent to leave the city altogether for new suburban developments beyond the city's borders. This trend accelerated dramatically in the late 1950s as the federal government spent billions of dollars to construct a system of expressways designed to carry automobiles long distances at high speed. These new highways enabled the middle and upper classes to move even farther from their jobs in the city, and soon the lifeblood of the cities began to spill out across the countryside.

Inner city neighborhoods suffered severely from these changes. Not only were they drained of their middle class, but they also were seen as the path of least resistance for the construction of the expressways. In city after city, historic inner city neighborhoods that had nurtured generations of working-class Americans were sliced apart by highways, and hundreds of thousands of units of affordable housing were lost in the process.

As the middle-class workers abandoned the city, their jobs began to follow them. Commercial enterprises quickly followed their customers, and many industries concluded it was cheaper to build new factories in the countryside than to rebuild in the cities. Over time, this out-migration severely eroded the municipal tax base, leaving few resources to heal the wounds of the inner cities. Sadly, these demographic trends exacerbated class and racial tensions that have afflicted the nation throughout its history. For a host of reasons ranging from discrimination in the real estate industry to fears of school busing, those who left the cities during this period were predominantly white, while those who remained were disproportionately persons of color.

As the postwar dreams of millions of American families were coming true in the suburbs, the frustration of those who had been left behind in the inner cities was growing. Beginning in Detroit in the summer of 1967, an epidemic of rioting broke out in the nation's inner cities, resulting in many deaths and the destruction of millions of dollars in property. The true extent of the damage of those riots is incalculable because they provided those with resources with one more excuse to leave the central cities.

For its part, the federal government responded to the unrest with a mix of policies that encouraged tougher law enforcement and created a wide range of social and health programs such as Model Cities and Community Health Centers. Although some of these measures initially showed positive results, the government's War on Poverty was short-lived. Faced with the human and economic toll of the war in Vietnam in addition to the deaths of prominent political leaders and civil rights champions, the nation turned away from the problems of the inner cities.

A portrait of the inner cities during this period is deeply etched in America's consciousness. It is a portrait of boarded-up buildings and decrepit schools, of children left to play in alleys and men idle on the street corners, of a place where drugs and alcohol are prevalent and violence is always nearby. It is a place where there are too few choices, and no good ones.

Poverty and economic hardship continue to be all too common. Today, there is still truth in this portrait, but only half-truth. It shows only the weakness of these neighborhoods and none of the resilience. It shows nothing of the spirit that knows the odds and beats them anyway, of parents who work three jobs so that a child can go to college, of ministers and community leaders who keep hope alive among their followers, of women who struggle to raise children alone and do it well. In short, it is a portrait that shows all of the problems and none of the possibilities. The health care provider who chooses to practice in the inner city today will enter a world in which both of these realities are present on the same stage, and he or she will have the opportunity to change, if ever so slightly, the balance between those forces.

DIVERSITY IN THE INNER CITY

The population of the inner cities today is far more diverse than it was during the late 1960s when the images of the inner city became fixed in the American psyche. New waves of immigration from every corner of the globe have brought millions of new residents to the nation's ports of entry, where many have settled in the inner cities. The ethnic composition of these enclaves varies widely across America. Hispanics predominate in the southern tier of major cities, while the immigrant populations in northern cities are more diverse. They include large refugee populations from Southeast Asia, East Africa, and Central Europe, as well as Hispanic populations. In Seattle, for example, the public school children speak more than 100 different languages at home.[1] The immigrant population of the United States has more than tripled since 1970.[2] Twenty-three percent of the U.S. population in 2010 was foreign-born or first-generation American,[3] with the majority living in cities and their centers, up from 20% just 10 years ago.

This new explosion of diversity has created both challenges and opportunities for America's cities and for health care providers. In addition to the barriers to health care that grow from economic disadvantage, they must now confront barriers that grow from differences in language and culture as well. Before turning to those challenges, it may be useful to understand the character of the health care delivery system as it currently operates in most of America's inner cities. In general, that "system" differs markedly from systems of care in rural or suburban settings, and these differences have important effects on the way inner city residents use health services.

HEALTH DISPARITIES

In 2002 the Institute of Medicine published a groundbreaking report entitled *Unequal Treatment: Confronting Racial and Ethnic Disparities in Healthcare*.[4] This report documents racial and ethnic health care disparities described by more than 100 studies and also offers recommendations. Disparities have been verified in health status, health care screening, testing, and treatment for many diseases and conditions. People of color generally have less favorable outcomes than whites.[4] Some examples of health disparities follow:

- African Americans die from asthma at rates three times higher than white Americans.[5]
- Asian Americans have hepatitis B at twice the rate of white Americans.[6]
- Both African Americans and American Indians are roughly twice as likely as white Americans to suffer from diabetes.[7]
- Puerto Ricans suffer from asthma at twice the rate of white Americans.[8]
- African American, Hispanic/Latino, and Asian patients with the same condition are less likely to be referred for or receive kidney transplantation than whites.[4]
- African Americans and Hispanics/Latinos with the same conditions are less likely to receive advanced cardiac procedures such as angioplasty.[4]
- African American diabetic patients are less likely to have the appropriate glycosylated hemoglobin test, ophthalmologic visits, or influenza immunizations than whites.[4]

America's urban areas or cities are places that demonstrate the extremes of American society. Cities have people who are rich and poor, highly and poorly educated, and living in mansions or slums. Of course there are those who live in between. Cities also have extremes of health statistics. Washington, D.C., the nation's capital, is such an example. Washington, D.C., has the highest concentration of physicians per capita in the nation, yet it has some of the worst health statistics. The infant mortality rate for the city is 12.8 per 1000 live births, while the nation overall has a rate of 6.8. Further examination demonstrates the disparities across the city. The rate for white infant mortality is 4.19 compared with the rate for African Americans, 18.63,[9] a rate comparable to that of developing countries.

The population of an inner city is most likely to be concentrated with people of color with low economic means.[10] Social situations that affect health such as undereducation and unemployment are increased in the inner-city communities. At the time of this writing, there are more than 49 million Americans (18.5% of the population nationally) without health insurance. Uninsured rates are highest for Hispanics/Latinos (32%) and American Indians (30%), followed by rates for African Americans (22%).[11] Looking at racial and ethnic health disparities can offer insight into the health issues of the inner city. In Washington, D.C., the highest mortality rates are seen in the inner city, which is predominately African American, while lower rates affect the upper class areas of the city that are predominately white. Across the United States, life expectancy differs by not only race but also geographic location. In some cases, white males are more likely to reach the age of 65 than urban African American males are to reach 45.[12]

HEALTH CARE IN THE INNER CITY

Some of the differences in health care systems can be traced to the period of out-migration from the inner cities that occurred several decades ago. As the middle class left for the suburbs, most private practitioners went with them. Some hospitals moved out of town as well, although significant past investments in their facilities made this more difficult than for doctors who simply had to relocate their offices. Those hospitals that remained faced a difficult prospect. With their base of paying patients moving farther away, they could either ally with teaching hospitals and the training subsidies they received or attempt to become specialty centers capable of attracting patients from the suburbs.

Economics drove most private hospitals to become specialty centers, which dictated policies that had the effect of shutting out those who could not afford to pay the full cost of their care. Over time, inner city populations became more and more dependent on public teaching hospitals for their care. The advent of public health insurance programs such as Medicaid and Medicare mitigated this trend for a short time, but as the rates paid by these programs began to fall behind the costs of care, the trend accelerated.

As the population of the inner cities became more concentrated with poor people, private medical office practices faced increasing operational difficulties. More people were uninsured. The fees that Medicaid and Medicare paid the practices were too little to cover costs. Many practices were forced to shut down or relocate to other areas.

RECENT TRENDS IN THE INNER CITY

Although there has been an influx of immigrants from around the globe to urban areas, there is an overall loss of population in the inner cities. An increase in minorities, especially Hispanics, has caused a "minority majority" in the some of the nation's largest inner city populations. In the past two decades, inner city residents had been able to purchase homes in greater numbers than in previous decades. Unfortunately, the recent mortgage crisis and subsequent financial meltdown has had devastating effects on the inner city, gutting already economically fragile neighborhoods and displacing families.[13]

Many inner suburbs are becoming new inner city–like neighborhoods also. These areas offer public transportation systems that are less extensive or sophisticated than those established in the inner city. Stores, schools, and services are farther apart and more difficult to access. The displaced residents can become disconnected from their traditional health care services.

ROLE OF PUBLIC TEACHING HOSPITALS

The importance of America's urban public hospitals in providing care to inner city populations cannot be overstated. Simply put, if it had not been for these institutions, many millions of Americans would be without any access to care except that which private hospitals are required to provide in emergencies. In addition to the provision of care to those who could not otherwise afford it, these hospitals are major employers, often the cornerstone of the inner city's economy. Many of the patients of these hospitals have inadequate primary care. They present to the hospitals with later and more severe manifestations of disease than those with good primary care. Thus their care is complex and costly.

However great their contributions, urban public hospitals are also faced with severe constraints. By virtue of caring for large numbers of uninsured patients and even larger numbers whose public insurance does not cover the full cost of care, these hospitals suffer chronic budget shortages. These shortages frequently manifest themselves in overcrowding, outdated equipment, and rundown facilities.

There are also inherent contradictions in the multiple roles an urban public hospital must play. As a teaching institution, the hospital must organize services in a way that best provides instruction for the students and residents who rotate among the hospital's various departments. It must also give emphasis to specialty care procedures the students might otherwise never have an opportunity to learn. These teaching requirements are important, but they are often at odds with the hospital's role as a community institution responsible for providing its patients with continuity of care.

Although most public teaching hospitals are extraordinarily well suited for emergent care and acute illness, they are generally less well designed for the management of chronic illness and poorly suited to provide preventive care. When one author of this chapter worked in a community clinic, it was not unusual for patients to report that they had been seen numerous times for the same health problem at the nearby public hospital, never seeing the same provider, and had been subjected to the same battery of tests repeatedly. In some cases, they had been offered markedly different diagnoses and prescriptions. One elderly man presented a bag of 11 different medications he had been given for hypertension, uncertain which to take.

Some public teaching hospitals have made remarkable efforts to resolve these contradictions in their roles by establishing primary care departments and satellite clinics or by working with networks of community health centers. However, these efforts have often been cut short of their full potential by funding problems, leaving the populations of the inner cities overly dependent on the emergency department as their major source of care.[14]

ROLE OF PUBLIC HEALTH DEPARTMENTS

Urban public health departments have long played a vital role in the inner cities, especially in efforts to improve environmental health and sanitation and to control the spread of communicable disease. During the short-lived War on Poverty, some urban health departments used federal funds to expand their role to include providing new services to the inner cities. Unfortunately, most of these services were funded through "categorical grants" targeted to a specific health care problem such as sickle cell anemia or family planning, and the service delivery was also organized according to these categories. This meant that health departments might be able to provide a number of screening services and immunizations for a child but might not be able to care for the child's ear infection or other needs for which no categorical funding was available.

At times, this pattern of service delivery became absurd. In the late 1970s, for example, it was not uncommon for women to be required to visit three different health department programs and undergo three different examinations in order to piece together basic gynecologic services that could easily have been provided in one primary care visit. This fragmentation occurred because services for sexually transmitted disease screening, birth control, and cervical cancer screening were organized categorically to make it easy to comply with federal reporting requirements.

In the recent past, many urban health departments have decategorized their services to more closely reflect the needs of their patients. A few have ventured into primary care either by offering services directly or through alliances with other providers. With the onset of the acquired immunodeficiency syndrome (AIDS) epidemic and the increased incidence of other communicable diseases in the inner cities, health departments have also worked hard to expand their capacity to fulfill their traditional mission of protecting the public health through education, prevention, and the control of communicable diseases.

ROLE OF COMMUNITY HEALTH CENTERS

One of the few lasting legacies of the War on Poverty is the community health center movement, which plays a significant role in the health care of the majority of America's inner cities. Unlike public teaching hospitals and urban health departments, community health centers were expressly designed to meet the challenges of the inner cities as they existed in the late 1960s. They were intended to be governed by the communities they served, to offer relatively comprehensive preventive and primary care, and to provide services on a sliding-fee scale according to the patient's ability to pay. Community health centers were also intended to be an integral part of a larger effort to encourage community development on a much broader scale, but that larger initiative has yet to materialize.

Measured in terms of their initial goals, community health centers have had great success in many ways and have fallen short in others. They have reestablished the concept of primary care in many inner city neighborhoods in which the family doctor had all but disappeared. They have cared for millions of inner city residents in a way that is generally held to be more beneficial and cost-effective than other modes of care, and they have pioneered new innovations in caring for disadvantaged populations. These clinics use various types of clinicians including physicians, PAs, and nurse practitioners. They provide care in internal and family medicine, pediatrics, obstetrics and gynecology, mental health, and sometimes dental services.

Today many community health centers are faced with the growing ethnic diversity of their patients. The patients come with new languages and different cultural beliefs and practices. Many community health centers are challenged with a diffusion of their patients to outer neighborhoods, and many patients must travel long distances to return to their original community health center for care. Many of the community health centers have plans to expand to these outer neighborhoods. Like their colleagues in public teaching hospitals and urban health departments, those who practice in inner city health centers also face serious barriers to success, including chronic funding shortages and the challenges of dealing with an increasingly complex patient population (see Case Study 47-1).

CASE STUDY 47-1

The city had fallen on bad times. The major employer had just laid off thousands of employees, both blue and white collar, salaried and hourly workers. People were literally leaving their homes with unpaid mortgages. Small businesses were closing in all the neighborhoods. People who had been covered by adequate health insurance were now uninsured. The public hospitals were overwhelmed with many more visits. The working poor were now poorer, and city services were being overwhelmed. A famous billboard announced to people leaving the city by the only freeway, "Would the last person leaving please turn off the lights?" It was not a good time for the city.

The Vietnam War was still being waged. There were many returning veterans and others disillusioned by the years of death and destruction to both countries. In the city that was so devastated by layoffs and a poor economy, a group of disgruntled young people aged 20 to 26 wanted to make a lasting change. With hard work and the support of the community, they built a community clinic. It was a challenge to find health care providers, especially physicians, who had time to provide care. Eventually, a small cadre of physicians was found. However, as the community clinic developed and the patient load increased, the hours needed to be expanded. Full-time staff had to be found.

The clinic had a number of medical assistants and "patient advocates" who volunteered at the clinic in the evenings. The clinic decided to train some staff to become eligible for PA education. In 1976 two applicants from this clinic were accepted to the local PA program. The clinic provided the clinical training site, and the two graduated in 1977. They continued to practice at the same clinic for their entire careers, and one of the PAs became the medical director before retiring.

This experience has been repeated over and over again in community health centers in underserved areas throughout the country. Educating people from the community in PA programs and having them return to the community is one way to keep providers in the underserved areas of inner cities.

This community health center appears to have had good community support. How would you get the community involved in a community health center concept? What are some of the skills taught in your PA program that would help with community work?

This community clinic was able to identify community members to prepare for application to a PA program. How would you go about identifying potential candidates who would work and stay at a community health center? How would you assist as a graduate in identifying this type of candidate?

Are there any community health centers in an inner city near you? Is there a PA on staff? If yes, have you ever spoken with the PA? Have these PAs ever lectured for you in your PA program? Have they lectured at your state continuing medical education program?

What is it that keeps a person in the inner-city community clinic for an entire career?

INCREASING COMPLEXITY OF INNER-CITY PRACTICE

The face of the inner city has changed dramatically in the past three decades, reflecting a series of waves of immigration from all corners of the globe.

Hospitals and community health centers in Seattle, for example, which once cared for patients in one or two languages, now routinely provide care in more than 10 languages, and dozens more can be heard in the clinic. The challenges this presents begin with the need to bridge the language gap. To meet this need, inner city providers have responded in a variety of ways. Some have relied heavily on family members to translate between the doctor and the patient, whereas others have used staff members who have other roles within the organization but are called in to translate when the need arises. As the number of patients grows, most providers begin to contract with professional interpreters, and a few hire full-time interpreters as part of the organization's staff.

The quality of medical interpretation varies widely among these methods. Even among those interpreters who are employed by health care providers on a full-time basis, there are significant gaps in their understanding of health care technology and terminology. There are certainly enormous gaps in clinicians' understanding of how best to use medical interpreters. Some inner-city providers, such as Pacific Medical Clinics and Harborview Medical Center in Seattle, have begun experimenting with ways to improve cross-cultural care through training programs for both clinicians and interpreters. Funding for such efforts, or even for basic medical interpretation, however, remains difficult to find (see Case Study 47-2).

CASE STUDY 47-2

A 24-year-old recent Vietnamese immigrant comes to the clinic with her 6-month-old son with a complaint of "constant crying." The young woman does not speak English, and her 8-year-old daughter is translating for her. You obtain a history consistent with colic. The physical examination is consistent with your diagnosis. While performing your physical examination, you note unusual linear markings on the child's skin, with erythema and discoloration of the skin surrounding the markings. You note the child has not had any immunizations.

You also note during your discussion that the child interpreting asks the mother questions and the mother responds with lengthy answers, but what the child tells you she said is a much shorter response. You ask the child when she was last seen at the clinic, and she says she has never seen an American doctor. You also discover that she has had no immunizations.

Is it appropriate to have children interpret for their parents? How common is this practice? Are there any alternatives in your community?

In this case, you note some unusual skin markings on the child that are bruiselike scrapes. What do you think it is? Could there be cultural aspects to these findings? If yes, what? If you do not know, how would you find out?

There are many cultural norms in each ethnic community. How would you identify community resources to help you understand a specific culture?

Are there any other troubling issues in this case? What are they? How would you address them?

The challenge of caring for refugees and other recent immigrant communities goes well beyond the issue of interpretation. There are also enormous differences between the basic beliefs of these communities and the underlying values of American medical practice. For example, among certain Vietnamese, it is believed that if parents imagine that their child may become ill and it happens, they have caused it. Is it any wonder, then, that a Vietnamese mother may resist enrolling her child in a health insurance program that, in effect, requires her to imagine that her child may become ill?

UNIQUE HEALTH CONCERNS

The demographic change in America's inner cities is not the only change affecting the nature of health care delivery. There are also severe changes in the circumstances of the poorest members of inner-city communities that make it exceedingly difficult to provide care. One such trend is the increase in homelessness. Health centers designed to serve relatively stable low-income families now find themselves caring for large numbers of homeless families, with little chance of providing continuity of care as patients move from one shelter to another or from one city to another. In response, Health Care for the Homeless Projects have been created in many inner cities, providing on-site health care in shelters and sometimes on the streets.

A study of homeless mothers and children in New York found increased depression in the mothers compared with nonhomeless mothers. Behavioral problems were also higher for the children, particularly for boys (up to three times higher) compared with their nonhomeless classmates.[15] Providers in the inner cities are also seeing increases in communicable diseases such as tuberculosis that seemed all but nonexistent in urban America just a few years ago. Together with the continuing crisis of human immunodeficiency virus (HIV) and AIDS, these infectious diseases, partly as a byproduct of immigration and homelessness, pose special challenges for the inner city.

Health care providers working in the inner city and their professional associations are addressing some of these unique health issues. The American College of Physicians (ACP) commissioned Andrulis[16] to investigate inner city health care. Andrulis's paper and the resulting policy paper[17] bring to light Greenberg's concept of the urban health penalty. This is defined as "a condition that exists when healthier, more affluent persons leave the city and the remaining and new residents experience health problems that interact with the city's physical and economic deterioration."[18] He describes poverty zones where minorities are overrepresented, jobs are in short supply, and significant health problems result in premature death.[18] House and colleagues[19] studied this effect further, finding a mortality hazard ratio of 2.25 for urban males compared with those in rural or small town settings.

Inner city health care providers, whether they are large teaching hospitals, health departments, community health centers, or private physicians, have had to struggle against long odds to continue providing care to people in the inner cities. They have demonstrated remarkable staying power and creativity in the face of the problems we have described. Now they are faced with new challenges arising not only from changes in demographics, social conditions, and new epidemics, but also from reforms in health care financing and the welfare system. Some of these reforms, implemented with the intention of cutting costs, are having serious consequences in the inner cities. They threaten not only the standard of care available to the people of the inner city but also the health of the "safety-net providers" who offer those services.

In *Mama Might Be Better Off Dead*, Abraham[20] puts a real human face on an inner city family dealing with the multiple layers of the health bureaucracy. Abraham spent 3 years with a poor inner city family documenting the family's encounters with chronic illness and the chaos of the current health care system. Additional problems have been created by severe cutbacks in aid to refugees and by changes in federal welfare law, which have been implemented differently from state to state. Unless new ways can be found to help the residents of the inner cities enter the economic mainstream, their problems may grow worse.

A 29-year epidemiologic study conducted by Lynch and associates[21] from the University of Michigan School of Public Health stated in its conclusion, "sustained economic hardship leads to poorer physical, psychological, and cognitive functioning."[21] This may seem obvious to members of the communities and to health care providers working in the inner city. However, the Michigan study is able to draw a direct and clear connection between poverty and the increased incidence of illness (and not the reverse).

THE CHILDREN, THE FUTURE

A further disturbing trend in the United States is the effect of poverty on children. Studies provide persuasive data to show an increase in the rate of young children up to 5 years of age living in low-income families, up from 44% in 2005 to 48% in 2010.[22] The National Center for Children in Poverty notes evidence that due to the outdated formula for determining the official federal poverty level, families need approximately twice the poverty-level income to meet essential needs.[23] That figure rises to approximately 2.5 times the poverty level in high-cost urban settings.[23] Poor children lack health insurance at twice the rate of nonpoor children and suffer from generally worse health outcomes.[24]

- In 2010, the number of children younger than 6 years of age living in poverty (below the poverty line) was 5.9 million (25%),[22] of whom 3 million were 3 or younger.[25]
- Forty-eight percent (11.4 million) of all U.S. children younger than 6 are in low-income (poor and near-poor) families.[22]
- African American (70%), American Indian (69%), and Hispanic (66%) children younger than 6 are more likely than their white (35%) or Asian (30%) counterparts to be living in low-income families.[22]

Health professionals must wrestle with these issues and become involved with their solution.

There are a few rays of hope. Many immigrant communities seem to be successfully gaining a foothold in the mainstream economy by pooling their resources and cooperating with one another in establishing new enterprises. In some cities, past investments in the downtown commercial areas have created the prospect of employment opportunities for inner city residents. Whether these trends continue to grow will depend on the health of the economy and on the creativity and determination of those who care about the future of inner-city neighborhoods.

Ironically, the challenges of inner-city health care create unique opportunities for PAs to take on more responsibility and accomplish greater good than might be possible in less complex environments. Regardless of which practice setting PAs might choose, they will be asked to work at their full potential. Inner-city PAs will be allowed to enter into the most intimate and important decisions of families whose language they do not speak and whose cultural beliefs they must struggle to comprehend. They will have to learn to improvise treatment regimens for patients who have no health insurance, shelter, or decent food. They will need to learn everything there is to know about diseases that their colleagues in the suburbs may never see in their lifetime. They also will be called on to advocate for patients who are caught in red tape in ways that Orwell[26] himself could have never imagined.

The reward can be immense; it will never be dull, and at the end of many days, those who commit to this challenging setting will be able to truly believe that they have made a difference in the lives of their patients and in the community that will welcome them as members.

KEY POINTS

- According to the latest national census in 2010, 23% of the U.S. population was born outside the United States or was a first-generation American.[3]
- For a PA practicing in the inner city, cultural competence is critical knowledge. In Seattle, for example, more than 100 different languages are spoken in the homes of public school children.[1]
- The 2002 report *Unequal Treatment: Confronting Racial and Ethnic Disparities in Healthcare*,[4] published by The Institute of Medicine, presents numerous study citations that describe health care disparities. For example, asthma kills three times as many African Americans than it does white Americans; minority patients are less likely to be referred for some procedures; American Indians are twice as likely to have diabetes than are white Americans; and Asian Americans are twice as likely to have hepatitis B than are white Americans.
- Community health centers were created with four criteria. First, provide comprehensive primary and preventative care; second, provide care on a sliding-payment scale to make it affordable for all; third (maybe the most important), create a board of directors from the community members being served; and fourth, be a community institution that sparks community development. Unfortunately, this fourth element was never realized by a majority of the communities the clinics served.
- Forty-eight percent of young children (younger than age 6) are in low-income families. African American, American Indian, and Hispanic children are much more likely to be in low-income families.[22]
- A majority of hospital emergency department visits continue to be made by low-income or no-income members of our inner city communities.[14]
- PAs have historically provided the medical stability and continuity of care in community health centers. They do this for many reasons, including having been raised in the low-income communities they now serve.

References

1. English Language Learners (ELL) and International Programs. Seattle Public Schools. *http://www.seattleschools.org*. Accessed February 9, 2012.
2. Gibson C, Jung K. Historical census statistics on the foreign-born population of the United States: 1850–2000. U.S. Census Bureau. *http://www.census.gov/population/www/documentation/twps0081/twps0081.html*. Accessed February 9, 2012.
3. Current population survey data on the foreign-born population. U.S. Census Bureau. *http://www.census.gov/population/foreign/data/cps.html*. Accessed February 9, 2012.
4. Smedley BD, Stith AY, Nelson AR (eds). Unequal Treatment: Confronting Racial and Ethnic Disparities in Healthcare. Washington, DC: National Academies Press; 2002.
5. American Lung Association. State of Lung Disease in Diverse Communities 2010. *http://www.lung.org/finding-cures/our-research/solddc-index.html*. Accessed February 9, 2012.
6. Centers for Disease Control and Prevention. A comprehensive immunization strategy to eliminate transmission of hepatitis B virus infection in the United States. Recommendations of the advisory committee on immunization practices (ACIP) Part II: immunization of adults. MMWR 2006;55(RR-16):1–33.
7. American Diabetes Association. Diabetes Statistics. *http://www.diabetes.org/diabetes-basics/diabetes-statistics/*. Accessed February 9, 2012.
8. Centers for Disease Control and Prevention. 2007 National Health Interview Survey (NHIS) Data, Table 4–1. *http://www.cdc.gov/asthma/nhis/07/table4-1.htm*. Accessed February 9, 2012.

9. Mathews TJ, MacDorman MF. Infant mortality statistics from the 2007 period linked birth/infant death data set. Natl Vital Stat Rep 2011;59(6):1–30.
10. Massey DS. Segregation and separation: a biosocial model. DuBois Rev 2004;1:7–25.
11. Kaiser Commission on Medicaid and the Uninsured. The Uninsured: A Primer. Key Facts about Americans without Health Insurance; October 2011. Washington, DC: The Henry J. Kaiser Family Foundation, 2011. *http://www.kff.org/uninsured/7451.cfm*; Accessed February 9, 2012.
12. Murray CJ, Kulkarni SC, Michaud C, et al. Eight Americas: investigating mortality disparities across races, counties, and race-counties in the United States. PLoS Med [serial online] 2006;3(9):e260. *http://medicine.plosjournals.org*; Accessed February 9, 2012.
13. Frey WH. The new metro minority map: regional shifts in Hispanics, Asians and Blacks from Census 2010. Washington, DC: The Brookings Institution; August 2011, *http://www.brookings.edu/papers/2011/0831_census_race_frey.aspx*; Accessed January 9, 2012.
14. Ruger JP, Richter CJ, Spitznagel EL, Lewis LM. Analysis of costs, length of stay, and utilization of emergency department services by frequent users: implications for health policy. Acad Emerg Med 2004;11(12):1311–1317.
15. San Agustin M, Cohen P, Rubin D, et al. The Montefiore community children's project: a controlled study of cognitive and emotional problems of homeless mothers and children. J Urban Health 1999;76(1):39–50.
16. Andrulis DP. The Urban Health Penalty: New Dimensions and Directions in Inner-City Health Care. Philadelphia: American College of Physicians, 1997.
17. American College of Physicians. Inner city health care. Ann Intern Med 1997;126:485–490.
18. Greenberg M. American cities: good and bad news about public health. Bull NY Acad Med 1991;67:17–21.
19. House JS, Lepkowski JM, Williams DR, et al. Excess mortality among urban residents: how much, for whom, and why? Am J Public Health 2000;90(12):1898–1904.
20. Abraham LK. Mama Might Be Better Off Dead: The Failure of Health Care in Urban America. Chicago: University of Chicago Press, 1994.
21. Lynch JW, Kaplan GA, Shema SJ. Cumulative impact of sustained economic hardship on physical, cognitive, psychological, and social functioning. N Engl J Med 1997;337:1889–1895.
22. Addy S, Wight VR. Basic facts about low-income children, 2010. Children under age 6. National Center for Children in Poverty. New York: Columbia University Mailman School of Public Health, 2012. *http://nccp.org/publications/pub_1054.html*. Accessed February 16, 2012.
23. Cauthen NK, Fass S. Measuring income and poverty in the United States. National Center for Children in Poverty. New York: Columbia University Mailman School of Public Health; 2007. *http://nccp.org/publications/pub_707.html*; Accessed February 16, 2012.
24. Seith D, Isakson E. Who are America's poor children? Examining health disparities among children in the United States. National Center for Children in Poverty. New York: Columbia University Mailman School of Public Health; 2011. *http://nccp.org/publications/pub_1001.html*; Accessed February 16, 2012.
25. Addy S, Wight VR. Basic facts about low-income children, 2010. Children under age 3. National Center for Children in Poverty. New York: Columbia University Mailman School of Public Health; 2012. *http://nccp.org/publications/pub_1056.html*; Accessed February 16, 2012.
26. Orwell G. Nineteen Eighty-Four. London: Secker and Warburg, 1949.

The resources for this chapter can be found at www.expertconsult.com.

CHAPTER 48

Rural Health Care

Steven Meltzer

WHY YOU SHOULD READ THIS CHAPTER

The PA profession was envisioned and created, in part, to fulfill a growing gap in access to health care due to a shortage of primary care physicians. Using the field-tested skills of ex-military corpsmen as an "assistant to the primary care physician," it was felt that PAs could extend the practice reach of physicians to underserved communities and populations with less cost. Although changing demographics have shifted PAs to more urban practices and less primary care focus, there remains tremendous potential for the profession to help shape the health of rural communities and individuals and continue to fulfill the vision of its originators.

CHAPTER CONTENTS

WHAT IS RURAL? AND WHY DOES IT MATTER?

Our perspectives on the definition and culture of rural America today are very different from how we perceived rural in the mid-20th century or even in the current context of the 21st century.[1] For many, the word *rural* often paints a picture of "open farmlands, untouched forests, rolling hills, and a sparsely populated, rustic environment."[2] Although many rural people do live in such surroundings, other rural residents live in areas just adjacent to urban areas and their sense of being rural comes as much from their lifestyle as from the actual environment (Figure 48-1).

The U.S. population shift over the past century from rural to urban occurred steadily as a result of changing lifestyles, economics, and postdepression/postwar transitions. In 1910, the rural population accounted for 71.6% of the total population but by 1940 had dropped to 52.2%; 1950 was the first time the U.S. population had become predominantly urban with only 43.9% rural. Over the next 50 years, rural communities continued to erode and in 2000, the rural population was 19.7%.[3] The growth in urban populations was not primarily in the "core" inner cities; in fact, the majority of growth in urban areas from 1930 to the present was in the suburbs, increasing from 13.8% to 50% of the total urban population (80%).[3] Between 2000 and 2010, this trend has continued and the nonmetro population has dropped to 16.5%, with a significant decline in population in those areas with fewer than 2500 people.[4]

When considering rural America, caution should be used to not put everyone into the same basket; each rural community is distinct, and each U.S. region has distinct characteristics that help define its rurality.[1] For example, small towns in rural New England are different in character from the open plains and communities of Montana or Wyoming; these characteristics reflect the economic, ethnic, and social differences unique to each area.

So why does defining "rural" matter? ore than 40 federal programs use rural definitions to allocate facility and grant funding and support resources—for example, the National Health Service Corps, Rural Health Clinic and Federally Qualified Health Center designations, Critical Access Hospital designation, and Universal Services Telecommunications Grants. In addition, the physician assistant (PA) concept was envisioned at a time when there was a significant shortage of primary care physicians nationally, particularly in rural and suburban areas. Understanding the dynamics of rural health care, then, is important to understanding the evolution of the PA profession and future opportunities for PAs in rural practice settings.

CHARACTERISTICS OF RURAL POPULATIONS AND COMMUNITIES

Definitions of Rural

Federal and state policy makers are often required to define "rural" and "urban" in order to develop and apply policies appropriately. What seems like a simple task, however, can become complicated because agencies at both levels of government use differing methodologies to define those terms depending on the population targeted and the specific purpose of the program. There are at least three major federal agencies that define rural: the U.S. Census Bureau, the Office of Management and Budget (OMB), and the U.S. Department of Agriculture Economic Research Center (USDA/ERS).

The U.S. Census Bureau has defined *rural* as those areas of open country and settlements of less than 2500 population and uses the term *urbanized area* to define areas that include a central city and the surrounding densely settled territory that together have a population of 50,000 or more, as well as a population generally exceeding 1000 people per square mile. The OMB uses the terms *metropolitan* and *nonmetropolitan*, where a *metropolitan* county must have an urban population center of 50,000 or more people; and adjoining counties may be included in the metropolitan region according to specific criteria. Any area that does not meet these criteria is classified as *nonmetropolitan*. The OMB made a number of modifications to its definitions for specific programs, such as the 1977 Rural Health Clinics Act and Universal Service Provisions of the Telecommunications Act of 1996.[5]

The U.S. Department of Agriculture Economic Research Center (USDA/ERS), however, took a different approach and developed rural-urban continuum codes in the 1970s to distinguish between rural and urban areas. The *Rural-Urban Continuum Codes* have been refined each decade to form a classification scheme that helps distinguish metropolitan (metro) counties by the population size of their metro area and nonmetropolitan (nonmetro) counties by the degree of urbanization and adjacency to a metro area or areas. The metro and nonmetro categories have been subdivided into three metro and six nonmetro groupings, resulting in a nine-part county codification.[6]

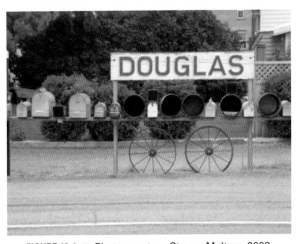

FIGURE 48-1 Photo courtesy Steven Meltzer, 2003.

To make things more interesting, in June 2003 the OMB released a revised definition of metropolitan (metro) and nonmetropolitan (nonmetro) areas. In this most recent update, nonmetro America comprises 2052 counties, contains 75% of the nation's land, and is home to 17.4% (49 million) of the U.S. population. The new version classifies 298 formerly nonmetro counties (10.3 million residents) as metro; 45 metro counties (3 million people) were reclassified as nonmetro. Thus, the new set of nonmetro counties contains a net of 7.3 million fewer residents than the former (1993) set based on the 1990 census.[6] The Bureau of the Census, also in 2003, released its revised definitions for urban area and urban centers that also expanded the number of geographic areas defined as urban.[6,7] An excellent overview of all the definitions and policy implications can be found at the Rural Policy Research Institute website: *http://www.rupri.org/Forms/RuralDefinitionsBrief.pdf.*

Frontier counties, a designation created for federal programs in 1990, were initially described as counties with very low population densities of no more than six people per square mile (compared with a national average of 73). The *frontier* designation was used inconsistently by the agencies that track rural populations and health, so a national consensus process was implemented by the Frontier Education Center and funded by the Federal Office of Rural Health in 1997. The purpose of the process was to develop a new definition recognizing that "frontier" described not only physically isolated areas but also those areas relatively isolated due to geography, weather, or other factors. The final report was published in April 1998 and provides a matrix, based on a maximum of 105 points, which can be used to determine the relative frontier status of any area. The determinants include population density per square mile, distance in miles to services/markets, and distance in time to services and markets.[8]

TABLE 48-1 **Selected Social and Economic Indicators 2010**

Indicator	Nonmetro	Metro
Unemployment (%)*	9.2	9.7
Annual per capita earnings*	$31,415	$41,244
Median household income*	$40,287	$51,244
Poverty rate—overall (%)*,†	17.8	14.8
By age‡:		
0–17	24.4	21.6
18–64	14.8	13.5
65 and older	10.3	8.7

* *http://www.ers.usda.gov/StateFacts/US.htm*

† U.S. Census Bureau, Current Population Reports, P60-239, Income, Poverty, and Health Insurance Coverage in the United States: 2010, U.S. Government Printing Office, Washington, D.C., 2011.

‡ *http://www.ers.usda.gov/Briefing/IncomePovertyWelfare/PovertyDemographics.htm*

RURAL DEMOGRAPHICS

Several features set rural communities apart, such as employment, income, poverty, and age, as noted in Tables 48-1 and 48-2.

In general, rural areas have higher rates of poverty, elderly, health disparities, low income, occupational injury, and unemployment.[7] Rural populations are less likely to have health insurance, retirement plans, and other benefits because the majority of employers have fewer than 50 employees and often are not able to provide those benefits at reasonable cost. Workers are often seasonally employed and may work in high-injury occupations, such as mining, timber, fishing, and farming. Non-metro populations typically have a lower education level than metro areas.

Although the prevailing impression of rural America is that it is primarily agricultural in nature, the percentage of population involved in traditional agricultural work (farming, forestry, and fishing) has declined from about 11% in the 1980s to 6.5% in the 1990s; in 2011 less than 2% of the population was directly involved in farming. Manufacturing (34.8%),

TABLE 48-2 **Metropolitan and Nonmetropolitan Population Trends**

Location	Population* 2000	Population* 2010	% Population 65 and Older 2009†	% Population Change 2010‡
U.S.	281,421,906	308,745,538	12.9	3.7
Nonmetro	48,841,966	51,043,753	16.9	2.3
Metro	232,579,949	257,701,785	12.6	4.1

* *http://www.ers.usda.gov/StateFacts/US.htm*

† *http://factfinder.census.gov/servlet/GCTTable?_bm=y&-state=gct&-ds_name=ACS_2009_1YR_G00_&-mt_name=ACS_2009_1YR_G00_GCT0103_US37&-CONTEXT=gct&-redoLog=true&-geo_id=&-format=US-37&-_lang=en*

‡ *http://www.ers.usda.gov/Briefing/IncomePovertyWelfare/PovertyDemographics.htm*

tourism and recreation services (16.7%), and destination retirement living (16.5%) now account for the bulk of employment in nonmetro areas of the country.[9-11]

Farm productivity has continued to increase due to changes in technology, equipment, and techniques, and therefore the transformation of farmland to other uses has been much slower than the decline in employment.[10] Farm households that do remain in agriculture are likely to also have nonfarm revenues from other sources in order to supplement income and maintain the farm.[10] In addition to these changes, farm lands are under increasing pressure from urban fringe expansion to be sold and developed for large housing tracts, recreation areas, manufacturing plants, and retirement villages.

Aging Populations

There are multiple challenges regarding the aging population in nonmetro areas stemming from factors such as out-migration of youth, aging in place of the existing population, increased migration of metro population to nonmetro areas, fewer health resources and access points, and declining number of rural health care services.[12]

The role of population aging on Medicare and access to health care will intensify, especially now that the large Baby Boomer generation began to turn 65 in 2010. Key issues that will effect change:

- Nonmetro areas will continue to have an increasing percent of elderly population.
- Compared with metro areas, nonmetro elderly generally have less income, lower educational attainment, and a higher dependence on Social Security income, creating demand for medical, social, and financial assistance.
- Continuing difficulty in accessing health care due to a reduced number of primary care and specialty providers and services.[12]
- One of the more recent trends that counteracts the previous information is the increasing number of metro aging populations that have moved, and continue to move, to nonmetro retirement communities typically adjacent to metro areas. This population group skews the data because they are often more affluent and mobile, have higher education levels, are more likely to be married rather than living alone, and typically have private insurance.[12,13]

Minority Population Trends

Compared with the 2000 U.S. Census, 2010 Census data show that racial and ethnic minorities increased from 18.3% of nonmetro residents to almost 20%, with Hispanics and Asians the fastest-growing minority groups.[13] American Indian numbers increased also, but this is believed to be due to the increased number of people reporting American Indian heritage on the census questionnaires. African Americans are the largest minority group in nonmetro areas (8.4%) compared with Hispanics (6.4%), American Indian (1.8%), Asian (1.0%), and Mixed Race (1.4%), a new category continued from the 2000 census.[13-15]

Although immigration brings new and diverse populations to nonmetro areas, which can revitalize small towns economically and demographically, those same increases create pressures in the local economic structure and raise concerns about increased demands for social services, education, and barriers to assimilation.[13] The Hispanic population had been primarily an urban-based group with roughly 90% of all Hispanics living in metro areas throughout the 1990s, but recent census data reflect a wider dispersion across the country and into more urbanized areas.[16] Although legal and illegal immigration generated the primary increase in Hispanic population before 9/11, the subsequent decrease in illegal immigration from Mexico due to multiple major Congressional Acts significantly reduced the flow of Hispanics into the United States. The Hispanic population had the greatest increase in population by 43% in the past decade due primarily to increased birth rates.[17]

One of the significant trends noted in the census is the geographic diversification over the past decade of Hispanic populations from metro areas primarily in the Southwest to metro and nonmetro areas across the nation, with more than half of all nonmetro Hispanics now living outside the Southwest.[15] As noted earlier, this trend has long-reaching effects for the social, cultural, economic, and political makeup of rural communities. As rural economies began to shift from farming to other agribusinesses, such as meat, poultry, and produce processing plants, there was a high demand for low-wage, skilled workers. Both documented and undocumented Hispanics are often employed in such industries, locked in due to low education levels (only 49% completed high school), less proficiency in English, and undocumented status.

This earlier influx of immigrants and the continuing shift from metro to nonmetro areas creates significant challenges for rural communities that for generations have had populations based in European cultures, often from the same regions or cities. These changes require a paradigm shift for communities in regard to accommodating language differences in schools and businesses, religious beliefs and the availability of churches, clothing and food purchases and social and health accessibility.

Rural America will continue to face many challenges with the continuing population shift to metropolitan areas and aging of the rural population, increasing presence of immigrant populations, changing economies, and lack of resources. Health policy makers will need to be creative in recognizing and meeting local and regional and national health care needs.

ACCESS TO HEALTH CARE

Two central concerns frame the issue of access to health care: being able to physically get to a source of care and the availability of services. Geography plays an important role in limiting access because rural residents must often travel longer distances and may have natural boundaries, such as mountains, rivers, and federal parks and forests that have no through roads. Distance is often compounded by weather conditions, which can make travel hazardous or limit air evacuation efforts; twisty two-lane roads; and lack of public transportation in rural areas (Figure 48-2).

Location and availability of health and social services create access issues as well. Health care providers are often found in county seats or similar population centers and often are not able to provide adequate outreach to less populated areas for financial, staffing, or other reasons. Those with special needs—such as people with physical or mental disabilities— who may need personal assistance to access care, are even more disadvantaged by these factors. In addition, federal and state programs set up to address these issues are often targeted toward children with special needs or the elderly. Unfortunately, many rural communities do not have the population to qualify for the special funding or to support the services.

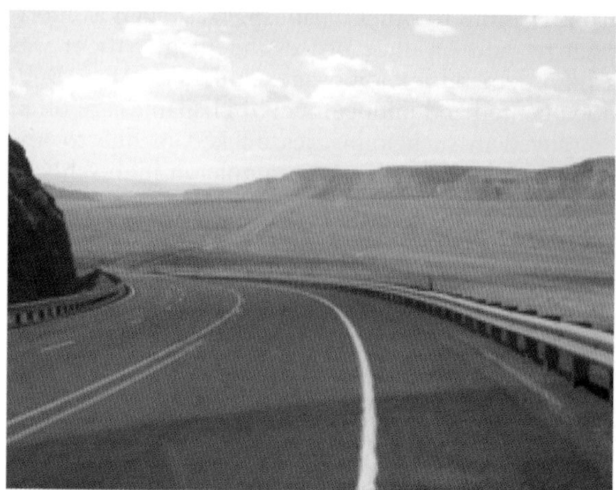

FIGURE 48-2 ■ Photo courtesy Steven Meltzer, 2003.

In looking at rural population data, it is frequently noted that many people do not have health care insurance, a significant barrier in accessing services. Rural populations tend on average to be older, poorer, and have lower levels of education—all of which can contribute to a lower health status and a higher need for health care. The 2010 Census shows there are 49.9 million people without health insurance in the United States—16.3% of the population; this is up from 46.6 million in 2006. Census 2010 shows that nationally, the metropolitan uninsured rate is 19% overall, while the nonmetro rate (communities under 2,500) is considerably higher at 23%. There are multiple reasons why there are fewer insured individuals: many small businesses cannot afford to pay full benefits for their workers; many rural jobs are seasonal and/or require only part-time work and therefore are not covered for benefits. Extended benefits to family members, dental coverage, and sick leave are also less often available to workers.[18]

Another critical aspect of access to health care is the availability of qualified health professionals. Recent data reflect that although slightly less than 20% of the population is rural, only 9% of physicians practice in those areas.[19,20] Comparatively, the 2009 and 2010 AAPA annual surveys[21,22] report that 15% of PAs work in nonmetro areas and 8.3% are employed in Community Health Centers, FQHCs, Critical Access Hospitals, and Indian Health Service Clinics, reflecting the continued important role nonphysician providers play in ensuring access to health care services in underserved areas. In addition to the general maldistribution of physicians, the imbalance of physicians by ethnicity as noted in the 17th COGME Report on Minorities in Medicine[23] also contributes to the overall lack of access:

- Whites and Asians are overrepresented in the U.S. physician population. Whites comprise 75.1% of the U.S. population and 73.8% of the physician population. Asians and Native Hawaiians and Other Pacific Islanders (NHOPIs) comprise 3.7% of the U.S. population and 14.9% of the physician population.
- Hispanics, Blacks, and AI/ANs are underrepresented in the U.S. physician population, comprising 12.5%, 12.3%, and 0.9% of the U.S. population and 5.1%, 4.4%, and 0.002% of the physician population, respectively.[23]

This becomes an important note when considering the growth of Hispanic and other nonwhite populations in nonmetro areas, as well as the need for greater numbers of culturally and linguistically appropriate health care providers and facilities.

According to multiple media reports and federal job sites, the growth of the PA profession continues to climb. Projections for the future indicate it will be one of the top jobs for the next decade or more, especially in rural and urban underserved areas. The challenge will be for the profession to capture potential applicants who increasingly match the new demographics of the nation and especially rural populations.

RURAL HEALTH CARE SYSTEMS: HOSPITALS, CLINICS, AND THE SAFETY NET

The health status of rural populations tends to be poorer than that of urban populations and is often compounded by higher levels of poverty, aging, and unemployment as noted earlier. Rural populations tend to have higher rates of chronic diseases, and health outcomes are dependent on factors such as adequate access to necessary and affordable health care services, distance and geography, and personal behaviors that contribute to poor health. Ethnic minorities, a growing population in rural communities as noted, have higher incidences of health disparities and lack of access to services, lack of health care insurance, and higher poverty rates. Almost 10% (9.8%) of children younger than age 18 were uninsured, as well as 20.8% of African Americans, 30.7% of Hispanics, and 11.7% of non-Hispanic Whites.[9,24]

The health care delivery system in rural America is trying to respond to many and varied problems. Although some of these also exist in urban underserved areas, many are unique to rural America. The rural health care system is often more loosely organized than its urban counterpart and much more thinly spread. Its component parts are similar, but many of the more familiar ones are missing or are present in only skeletal form. What appears in any given system varies with the degree of remoteness and the resources of the community. Mounting evidence of the relative decline in rural health care includes the closure and deteriorating financial condition of local hospitals and, more importantly, the difficulty of recruiting and retaining physicians, midlevel providers (PAs and nurse practitioners), nurses, and other health care personnel.

Over the past four decades, a wide range of health policies and programs have been developed and implemented to mitigate these issues and assist rural Americans in improving their personal and community health status. The overall effect has been to create a health care "safety net" that includes clinics, hospitals, free clinics, and public health services that improve access to care regardless of ability to pay.

HOSPITALS: TRANSITION FROM TRADITIONAL SERVICE TO LIMITED-SERVICE FACILITIES

As the demographics and economic basis of rural communities changed over the past four decades, rural hospitals faced significant challenges in maintaining services, staff, and providers. Several federal initiatives were created to assist these hospitals in finding a new way to not only survive but also continue to meet community needs in a more effective and efficient way (Figure 48-3).

Post World War II, as the nation's population began shifting to suburban and rural areas, Congress passed the Hill-Burton Act in 1946 that gave hospitals, nursing homes, and other health facilities grants and loans for construction and modernization. State plans were to be developed to encourage expansion of health care facilities so that all people in the state would have access to care. By applying for and accepting the grants, the facilities agreed to provide free or reduced-cost emergency and other services to persons unable to pay, they had to serve all persons residing in the facility's area, and later had to participate in the Medicare/Medicaid program. The Hill-Burton program stopped providing funds in 1997, but about 300 health care facilities nationwide are still obligated to provide free or reduced-cost care. Many of these facilities are still original buildings and struggle to find the capital resources to build new facilities or modernize.

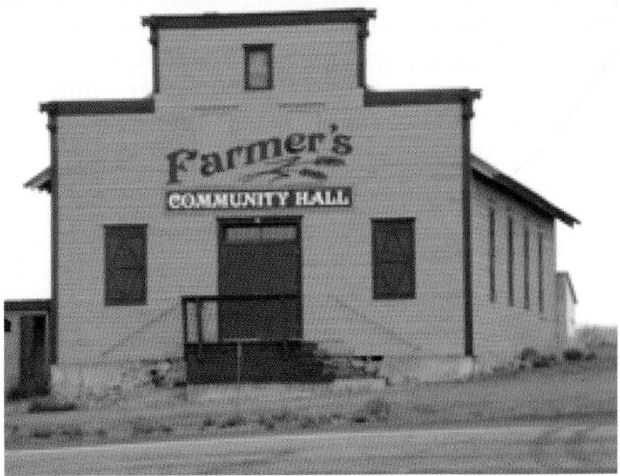

FIGURE 48-3 ■ Photo courtesy Steven Meltzer, 2003.

MAF Model

From 1974 to 1990, there were various alternative hospital models proposed and explored, many of which did not come to fruition. In the late 1970s and early 1980s, the federal government was exploring ways to reduce payments to hospitals for inpatient services in an attempt to salvage the system.[25] On the basis of academic research and tested in New Jersey, Congress established a prospective payment system centered around 600+ diagnostic-related groups (DRGs) that reimbursed hospitals a predetermined rate based on the patient's diagnosis, rather than whatever the hospital wanted to charge Medicare. This model was considered revolutionary at the time because it gave the government leverage to control hospitals costs for the first time. The result, however, was the closing of 193 hospitals—mostly small and rural facilities—between 1987 and 1991.[26]

To prevent further loss and ensure access to its remote and rural population, the Montana State Legislature, working in collaboration with the Montana Hospital Association in 1987, developed the concept, rules, and operating principles for a limited-service hospital that could provide emergent, limited inpatient and other health care services on a smaller scale than a fully licensed facility. The legislature submitted a grant proposal to the federal Health Care Financing Administration (HCFA) in 1990, and nine hospitals were initially selected to participate in the demonstration: three as actual participants as Medical Assistance Facility (MAF) sites and six as controls. One additional hospital was added the next year as a participant.

The MAF model in Montana was the first national demonstration program of the limited-service hospital concept. Implemented in 1990 after several years of development and political wrangling, the MAF concept was particularly well suited to Montana, given its relative size (the fourth largest state) and its sparse and aging population. Of Montana's 56 counties, 45 are currently considered frontier. Montana has lost significant numbers of the younger rural population to urban areas and as a result has increased the rural population median age. In addition, Montana residents have to contend with not only the state's size but also the most severe weather conditions in a winter that may last as long as half the year.

An important component of the MAF was the reliance on PAs or nurse practitioners as key providers and, in some situations, sole providers. Core elements of the program included:

- MAF facilities were limited to a 96-hour admission. Longer stays required discharging patients or transferring them to a full-service hospital.
- MAFs had to be located in a county with fewer than six residents per square mile, or the MAF could be located more than 35 miles from the nearest hospital.
- MAFs had to provide emergency services and basic laboratory services. More complex diagnostic services could be available by contract.
- There had to be a provider on call at all times who was able to respond within 1 hour to the MAF site.
- All MAFs were required to have formal agreements with hospitals, skilled nursing facilities, and home health agencies for services the MAF could not provide.
- Where there was a PA or nurse practitioner working as the sole provider at an MAF hospital, the rules required that a physician must review all admissions by telecommunication within 24 hours of admission and visit the facility every 30 days.[19]

In the ensuing 10 years, the MAF project was instrumental in creating new models of health care delivery in rural hospitals. Proponents of the MAF model pointed out that the rules imposed less service restriction and focused on saving a small hospital without the complex formal networking and restructuring of local health systems that were required by some other models. The importance of the MAF for the PA profession is that it created an opportunity to expand the role of PAs in hospital settings and solidified the utilization of midlevel practitioners (PA/NP) in helping to maintain access to health care services to underserved populations. Later programs would continue to mimic the MAF guidelines and include PAs as key providers in the safety net.

EACH/RPCH

About the same time as the MAF was getting under way, Congress passed the Omnibus Budget and Reconciliation Act of 1989 (OBRA), which established the Essential Access Community Hospital/Rural Primary Care Hospital (EACH/RPCH) program, a second model to allow rural and frontier communities to have a limited-service hospital. The program also relied on the use of PAs and nurse practitioners as core providers in the model. Key features of the program were the provision of a higher cost-based Medicare reimbursement rate for the RPCH facilities and recognition of the larger EACH hospitals as sole community providers, thus raising their Medicare reimbursement rates. Sole community provider rates are based more on historical costs than Medicare's prospective payment system normally allows.[27]

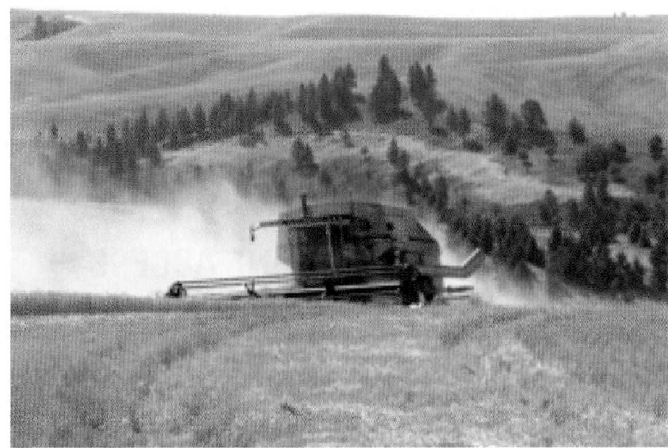

FIGURE 48-4 Morning Star Farms, Inc., Colfax, Washington. (Courtesy Willard and Heidi Morgan, 2006.)

Seven states were selected to start the program in early 1990: California, Colorado, Kansas, New York, North Carolina, South Dakota, and West Virginia. Much like the MAF model, the duration of admission was held to an average of 72 hours for all admissions on an annual basis. As the EACH/RPCH program demonstrated early success in helping rural communities build local networks of providers beyond the hospital-to-hospital link, researchers found that networking had generally been challenging for rural facilities. Some of the factors making it difficult to create a viable network included local politics, changes in personnel, variable interest at the larger referral hospital, community concerns related to historical rivalries or control, and a situation wherein the designated referral facility was not historically the facility with a previous strong relationship with the community[26,27] (Figure 48-4).

Critical Access Hospitals

Congress passed the Balanced Budget Act in 1997, which included provisions building on the successes of the MAF and EACH/RPCH models. The Medicare *Rural Hospital Flexibility Program* was established to continue to allow hospitals to refine the limited-service models, and in October 1999 all MAF and EACH/RPCH programs were grandfathered into the federally designated Critical Access Hospital (CAH) program. Its purpose was to improve rural health by addressing access and quality of care issues for rural citizens through partnerships between the federal government, state government, rural CAHs, acute care hospitals, emergency medical services (EMS), and rural communities.

The Flex Program consists of two separate but complementary components:

- A Medicare reimbursement program that provides reasonable cost reimbursement for Medicare-certified CAHs is administered by the Centers for Medicare & Medicaid Services; and
- A State grant program that supports the development of community-based rural organized systems of care in participating states is administered by the Health Resources and Services Administration through the Federal Office of Rural Health Policy.

To receive funds under the grant program, states must apply for the funds and engage in rural health planning through the development and maintenance of a State Rural Health Plan that:

- Designates and supports the conversions of CAHs
- Promotes emergency medical services (EMS) integration initiatives by linking local EMS with CAHs and their network partners
- Develops rural health networks to assist and support CAHs
- Develops and supports quality improvement initiatives
- Evaluates State programs within the framework of national program goals.[27]

State entities, typically State Offices of Rural Health, could apply for federal "Flex" grants to support development of CAHs and networks to meet the program objectives. As of 2011, there are a total of 1327 active CAHs overseen by the Federal Office of Rural Health Policy.

Modifications to the program have resulted from the enactment of the Balanced Budget Refinement Act (BBRA) of 1999, the Benefits Improvement and Protection Act (BIPA) of 2000, and the Medicare Prescription Drug Improvement and Modernization Act (MMA) of 2003. These changes have been incorporated into the information presented next.

Criteria for CAH Certification

"A rural hospital may be designated as a CAH if the following criteria are met:

- Owned by a public or nonprofit entity
- Located in a participating State Rural Hospital Flexibility state
- One or more of the following is true:
  - More than 35 miles from any other CAH or hospital
  - More than 15 miles from another hospital or CAH in mountainous terrain or in areas with only secondary roads
  - Designated a necessary provider under criteria published in the State CAH Plan

- Offers 24-hour emergency care
- Provides no more than 25 beds for acute care
- May operate distinct part units of up to 10 beds for psychiatric or rehabilitation services
- Keeps inpatients no more than an average of 96 hours except during inclement weather or other emergencies
- Meets staffing and other requirements established in General Acute Hospital or Primary Care Hospital licensing and the State Plan for CAHs
- Must have a formal agreement for participation as part of a rural health network. Rural health network defined as an organization of at least one CAH and one acute hospital"[29]

Over the past decade, as hospitals faced further implementation costs for new federal policies and regulations, rural and small hospitals again faced financial challenges. To offset those requirements and costs, more recent policy developments include the federal Office of Rural Health Policy's Small Rural Hospital Improvement (SHIP) Grant Program, which provides funding to small rural hospitals to help them do any or all of the following: (1) pay for costs related to the implementation of Prospective Payment Services (PPS); (2) comply with provisions of the Health Insurance Portability and Accountability Act (HIPAA); and (3) reduce medical errors and support quality improvement.

To be eligible for these grants, a hospital must be: (1) *small*—49 or fewer available beds; (2) *rural*—located outside a metropolitan statistical area (MSA) or located in a rural census tract of an MSA as defined by the Goldsmith Modification or the Rural Urban Commuting Areas; and (3) *a hospital*—which is a non-federal, short-term, general acute care facility. All designated CAHs were included as eligible, as well as hospitals with 50 or fewer beds located in an area designated by any State law or regulation as a rural area or as a rural hospital. Unlike other programs, there is no requirement for matching funds with this program.[30]

CAH—Physician Practice Mergers and Acquisitions

The combination of recruitment and retention difficulties for rural practices and downward spiralling reimbursement payments from public and private payers, and added expense of new federal requirements such as electronic medical records has encouraged the merging of physician practices with rural hospitals, many of which are CAH certified. As the overhead costs of owning and managing a practice continues to grow, physicians are more willing and interested in seeking relief through this mechanism. Additionally, such extended hospital linkages help capture market share by creating referral resources within the network. Federal health care reform requirements, such as creation of Accountable Care Organizations and Meaningful Use of Electronic Medical Records, have pushed providers to seek collaborations that allow for flexibility and efficient use of resources to maintain adequate levels of local services.

RURAL CLINICS: FRONTLINE ACCESS

Community/Migrant Health Centers

Access to health care for underserved populations such as migrant farm workers and their families was recognized as a problem as early as the 1960s. Congress passed the Migrant Health Act of 1962 (P.L. 87-692), which provided for development of dedicated health clinics to serve the needs of these workers and families. President Lyndon Johnson's "War on Poverty" in the mid-1960s was responsible for passage of the Economic Opportunity Act of 1964, which added to community health centers by creating neighborhood health centers in urban areas with high poverty populations. All these centers were transferred to the Public Health Service in the early 1970s and later authorized in 1975 under Section 330 of the Public Health Service Act (P.L. 94-63). The new Community Health Centers (CHCs) were established to provide quality care to a wide range of underserved populations in both rural and urban areas and encouraged collaborative partnerships between public and private providers.

Over the next two decades, new programs were added to the CHC program to include the Migrant Health Center program, Healthcare for the Homeless Centers, and the Public Housing Primary Care Program.[31] Later, the Omnibus Budget Reconciliation Acts of 1989, 1990, and 1993 created a new entity under Medicare and Medicaid known as the Federally Qualified Health Center (FQHC); the Social Security Act also expanded the definitions to add amendments describing FQHC Look-Alikes. These clinics received federal enhanced reimbursement but did not receive core federal grants under Section 330 for construction or operating costs.

Community Health Centers are characterized by five essential elements that differentiate them from other providers:

- They must be located in or serve a high-need community (i.e., "medically underserved areas" or "medically underserved populations")
- They must provide comprehensive primary care services and supportive services, such as translation and transportation services that promote access to health care.

- Their services must be available to all residents of their service areas, with fees adjusted according to patients' ability to pay.
- They must be governed by a community board with a majority of members being health center patients.
- They must meet other performance and accountability requirements regarding their administrative, clinical, and financial operations.

The Bush administration established the *President's Health Centers Initiative* in 2002, which was to increase the system by 1200 expanded or new access points, thereby pushing the number of patients served from approximately 15 million to 19.8 million.[32] There are now 1200 CHCs with more than 8000 clinical service units serving 20 million people. Under current ACA provisions, an additional $11 billion has been allocated for the period 2010-2015 to expand the number of centers ($9.5 billion) to eventually serve 40 million people or about double current capacity. There is also $1.5 billion set aside to upgrade current facilities. Additional funds are also included under Title VII training to create Teaching Health Center collaboratives to increase the actual time medical students and residents spend in CHCs, RHCs, and other similar sites as part of their training.[33-35]

CHCs often provide comprehensive health services including medical, dental, mental health, pharmacy, and social services. Although there are no specific requirements, the CHCs use all types of health care providers, including PAs and nurse practitioners. A 2004 study of CHC personnel shortages completed by Rosenblatt and colleagues[36] looked at the implications for the planned expansion under the President's Initiative and found that the CHCs were already understaffed and having difficulty recruiting and retaining providers.

The largest groups of physicians employed in CHCs are family physicians, internists, and pediatricians. Significantly, the study found that "in rural CHCs, 46% of the direct clinical providers of care are nonphysician clinicians (PA/NP/CNM) compared with 38.9% in urban CHCs." Obstetrician/gynecologists, psychiatrists, and dentists are the other main providers, although in much smaller numbers. Although there has been a slight incline in the past couple years, given the significant declining trend in family medicine residency matches since 1997 (a loss of almost 52%) and the relatively small number of graduates of the other specialties noted, the recruitment and retention challenges facing CHCs with further expansion will increase proportionately (Figure 48-5).

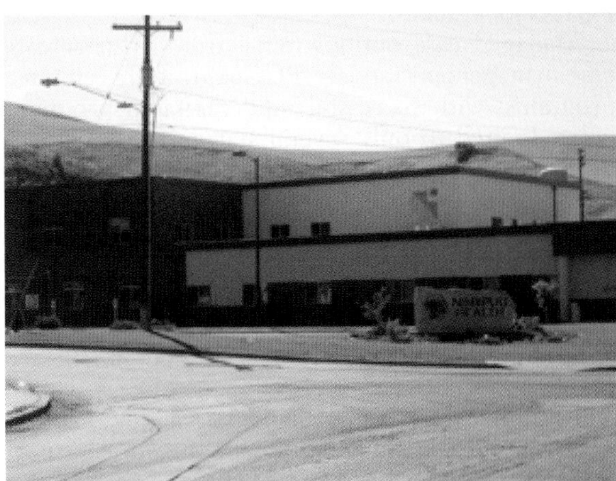

FIGURE 48-5 Photo courtesy Steven Meltzer, 2003.

Rural Health Clinics

The Rural Health Clinic Act of 1977 (P.L. 95-210) established CMS/Medicare recognized rural health clinics (RHCs) to help address the continuing shortages of health care access in rural areas. The purpose of the legislation was twofold: to increase access in rural, underserved communities and to encourage utilization of nonphysician providers such as PAs, nurse practitioners, and certified nurse midwives (PA/NP/CNM) in collaborative models to expand the reach of physicians in those communities.

The RHC program was the first federal initiative to mandate the utilization of a team approach to health care delivery. Each federally certified RHC must have:

- One or more physicians (does not have to be full time at the site)
- One or more PAs, NPs, or CNMs on-site and available to see patients 50% of the time the clinic is open for patients
- Written patient care policies developed by the physician, PA/NP/CNM, and one practitioner not employed at the clinic
- The ability to provide emergency services to stabilize patients with life-threatening or acute illness
- An accurate and confidential/secure record keeping system that is also in compliance with HIPAA regulations
- Diagnostic and treatment services commonly furnished in a physician's office including the following laboratory services: chemical examinations of urine, hemoglobin or hematocrit, blood sugar, examination of stool specimens for occult blood, pregnancy test, and primary culturing for transmittal to reference labs.

In addition, RHCs may have other services provided by arrangement to include:

- In-patient hospital care
- Specialized physician services
- Specialized diagnostic and laboratory services
- Interpreter for foreign language if indicated
- Interpreter for deaf and devices to assist communication with blind patients

Initially, the RHC qualification process under PL 95-210 was onerous and excessively cumbersome. Congress had expected several thousand clinics to apply, but by 1990, there were only about 600. In the late 1980s and early 1990s, Congress reviewed the program to see why there were so many fewer clinics than expected. This resulted in a number of changes that improved the certification process. By 1997, more than 3000 clinics were certified and there are were about 3800 clinics in 2011. The creation of the National Association of Rural Health Clinics has resulted in the availability of valuable technical assistance and networking support among clinics and clinicians. This association has also been effective in promoting rural health clinics at the state and community levels.[37]

New Models for Frontier Communities

Discussions about how to serve more remote communities and populations began in 1997 with establishment of the Rural Hospital Flexibility program. However, even the relaxed parameters of the CAH designation were not seen as reasonable for the outlying areas of Alaska, open spaces of Wyoming, or other remote areas of the country that did not have a hospital facility; there needed to be an expanded definition that would allow clinics to fill the gap in access to inpatient care. The Frontier Education Center (now the National Center for Frontier Communities), based in Arizona, helped spur the dialogue at state, regional, and national levels for more than a decade using the support of groups such as the National Rural Health Association.

As a result of these discussions, along with strong support from the Congressional representatives from Alaska, the Medicare Prescription Drug Improvement and Modernization Act of 2003 included provisions for testing a new model of clinics for more remote areas designated as the Frontier Extended Stay Clinic (FESC). There were two parts to the projected action: First, the Medicare Modernization Act of 2003 gave authority to the Centers for Medicare and Medicaid Services (CMS) at the Department of Health and Human Services (DHHS) to conduct a demonstration program to reimburse extended stay care received by Medicare beneficiaries. Second, the Consolidated Appropriations Acts of 2004, 2005, and 2006 included funding for the federal Office of Rural Health Policy (ORHP) "to examine the effectiveness and appropriateness of a new type of provider, the FESC, in providing health care services in certain remote locations." This became the Frontier Extended Stay Clinic (FESC) Cooperative Agreement Program.[38] Applicants for this Cooperative Agreement competed nationally, and the Southeast Alaska Regional Health Consortium (SEARHC), an Alaska Native corporation, was awarded the funding. The Alaska FESC Consortium is a partnership of providers in Alaska and Washington states, as well as evaluators from the University of Alaska, Anchorage, and the Sheps Center at the University of North Carolina, Chapel Hill.

A facility can be designated a *frontier extended stay clinic* if it (1) is located in a community where the closest short-term acute care hospital or critical access hospital is at least 75 miles away from the community or is inaccessible by public road and (2) is designed to address the needs of seriously or critically ill or injured patients who, due to adverse weather conditions or other reasons, cannot be transferred quickly to acute care referral centers, or patients who need monitoring and observation for a limited period of time.

FUNDING AND REIMBURSEMENT FOR RURAL HEALTH SERVICES

Finances for rural facilities are complex and underscored by periodic changes at the state and federal level. A more complete discussion can be found in Chapters 5 and 44. Important to recognize, however, are the various efforts to help stabilize rural hospitals and clinics including the enhanced payments from Medicare for Critical Access Hospitals, Rural Health Clinics, and Community Health Centers (including FQHC look-alikes).

Managed care options range from primary care case management models (PCCM) to fully capitated programs, with successful fully capitated programs being limited to only several states. The most significant barriers to implementation are absence of health plans willing to extend to rural areas and/or lack of providers; low population base; distance and time factors to get to primary care or hospital/specialty services; 24-hour coverage options; and protection of the safety-net providers via cost-based reimbursement. Felt-Lisk and colleagues[39]published a study in 1999 that challenged many of these issues. They found that if insurance networks took the extra time and effort to include as many health care providers as possible in an area, allowed for reasonable distance and travel times, and provided reasonable cost reimbursement to providers, then capitated programs could be fairly successful.

Alternatively, a study by Chan and colleagues,[40] published in 2006, researched geographic access issues for rural Medicare beneficiaries and found that covered patients living in small and isolated rural areas have less access to primary care providers but are restricted in seeking specialty services due to time and distance factors. In fact, most relied more on their generalist providers locally for care and not on urban areas for much of their care (≤30% of the time).

Rural Incentives for Providers

Several programs implemented over the years to create incentives for providers to stay in rural areas have been successful to some degree. These included a 10% Medicare bonus payment if the provider practiced in an HPSA and, more recently as a part of the MMA 2003, an additional 5% bonus if the provider was also in a Physician Shortage Area. Such incentives can become meaningful financially if the practice is busy and has significant Medicare patients. Under the new Affordable Care Act (ACA), physicians, hospitals, and Community Health Centers will receive varying amounts of financial support to maintain and increase services. For example, the 10% bonus payment to physicians will be extended to all physicians in rural areas meeting specific criteria, such as 60% of services being "primary care services" as defined by the ACA.[41]

RURAL HEALTH WORKFORCE ISSUES

Recruitment and retention of health care providers at every level and in every discipline for rural areas has remained a problem nationally even with the various programs and incentives described. Part of the problem is an absolute shortage of health professions available; the other factor is maldistribution toward urban/suburban communities.

Briefly, the shortages for medical practitioners for rural areas involve several factors:

- Applicant pools: multiple studies have shown that medical school applicants increasingly come from urban, higher-income areas and not from rural areas. Although the number of applicants waned for a short period several years ago, the applicant pool seems to be rising again but is not representative of the geographic areas that need physicians.
- Lengthy timelines for completion of training: The timeline for generalist physicians is a minimum of 11 years from start of an undergraduate program to the end of residency training; this increases with certain specialty programs, such as surgery, psychiatry, OB-GYN, and internal medicine subspecialties. As some disciplines move to the master's or doctorate level, such as the Doctor of Physical Therapy (DPT) and Doctor of Pharmacy (PharmD), additional time is required to graduate and enter the workforce.
- Institutional capacity: Classroom space and availability of qualified faculty have been major barriers to meeting the significant shortages of nurses, as an example of this issue. State higher-education budgets have not been a priority in many states, and resources are not available to support program expansion. The other factor is the inability of education programs to provide competitive salaries to attract personnel from the private sector. Nursing schools, in particular, have struggled to recruit and retain advanced nursing faculty because hospital and clinic salaries have increased significantly as a result of the nursing shortage nationally. For PA programs, the expansion of accredited programs in the past few years from 137 to 156 and the change to the master's degree has also created a gap of readily available academically prepared faculty.
- Program availability: Starting a new program or even expanding current programs is costly and has a long timeline due to approvals at the institutional and state levels. For example, there have only been two new allopathic medical schools started in the past 20 years. According to the COGME 16th report on Physician Workforce,[19] the number of medical students increased only 7% between 1981 and 2001, whereas the general population increased 23%, leading to a 13% decrease in physicians per capita. That gap is expected to increase between 2000 and 2020 as the population increases 18%, while medical schools increase the number of students by only 4%. On the other hand, the number of PA programs increased dramatically from three programs in 1967 to 65 in the 1970s and 1980s, to 156 in 2010 turning out about 5964 graduates each year.
- Changing discipline accreditation/graduation standards: As noted earlier, some disciplines have moved to more advanced degrees over the past decade. This has lengthened training time, changed the demographics of the applicant pool, and potentially influenced practice site decisions. Increased costs of education and graduate debt load push providers toward

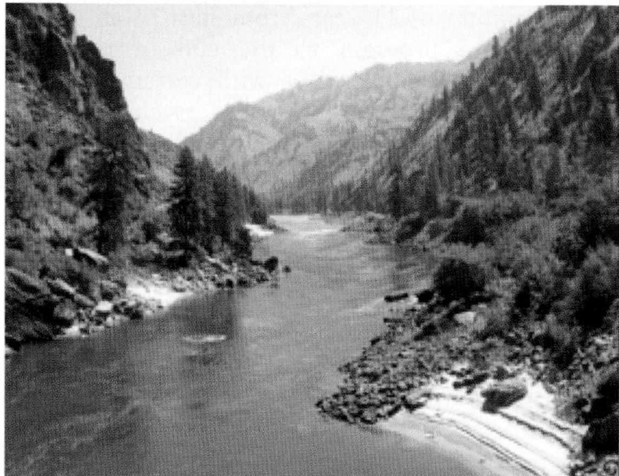

FIGURE 48-6 Photo courtesy Steven Meltzer, 2003.

higher-paying jobs in urban areas rather than rural practices (Figure 48-6).

- Recruitment costs and retention issues: With physician recruitment costs averaging $30,000 or more just for the search company fees, frequent turnover of providers creates a financial drain on facilities. If start-up salaries, travel, and relocation costs are included, a typical recruitment cost could be closer to $100,000. Most sources indicate that good recruitment tactics result in better retention with satisfied providers and family. With the number of positions opening for PAs in specialty and generalist practices, there is a growing similarity in competition and recruiting costs for PAs as well.

PHYSICIAN ASSISTANTS AND RURAL MEDICINE

Census data of the American Academy of Physician Assistants (AAPA) allows us to track PA involvement in rural health. The AAPA Annual survey reported that in 2010 that there were 83,466 individuals in practice.[22] The AAPA census notes that 31% are in primary care (as compared with 38% in 2006, 48.5% in 2003, 52.7% in 1997, and 37% in 1986). The primary care field breakdown includes family/general medicine (24.8%), general internal medicine/specialities (14.3%), general pediatrics (3.7%), and obstetrics/gynecology (2%). Other prevalent specialties for PAs include general surgery/surgical subspecialties (25.9%), emergency medicine (10.9%), the subspecialties of internal medicine (10.3%), and dermatology (3.5%).[42]

Currently, 15% of PAs describe themselves as working in nonmetro settings, a drop from 22.7% in 2003. A total of 16.1% work in communities of fewer than 20,000. About 1.7% work in communities of fewer than 2500. Geographic distribution across the nation is fairly even with the exception of South Central: 22.7% in the Northeast, 23.7% in the Southeast, 21% in North Central, 13.4% in South Central, and 19.1% in the Western states.[21]

Recruitment and retention issues are similar to physicians with multiple factors influencing rural practice. Factors such as the changing applicant pool with a significant increase in women applying and matriculating will have an increasing impact on practice profiles and lifestyles. A number of research studies have shown that women physicians and PAs tend to select urban practice settings to a greater extent than men. Another potential factor is the move by some institutions toward more advanced academic degrees, which may also affect rural deployment. A recent study of all PA graduates of the University of Washington MEDEX Physician Assistant program by Evans and colleagues[43] showed an almost inverse relationship between academic degrees awarded and rurality of employment, whereby graduates with higher degrees tend to practice to a greater extent in metro areas, a cause for concern for education programs targeting rural primary care.

Retention of rural PAs was examined by Larson and colleagues[44] who found that a high percentage of PAs who started practice in rural areas (41%) were likely to leave for urban practice during the first 4 years and that female PAs were slightly more likely to leave than men. This was mitigated by urban PAs transitioning to rural settings (10%), however, thereby keeping the number of rural PAs between 15% and 20%. Issues related to leaving included difficulties around prescriptive authority, reimbursement, and availability of insurance. Factors influencing retention of rural PAs were published by Muus and colleagues[45] and included good relationships with the supervising physician and a relative degree of autonomy, reasonable practice hours and responsibilities, and satisfaction with living in the community.

FEDERAL AND STATE POLICY IMPLICATIONS FOR RURAL HEALTH CARE

Over the past several decades there has always been a general lack of access to health care services in rural and frontier communities. Large-scale federal initiatives to deal with the problem consisted of provisions for medical research, construction of health centers, and money for medical education. Examples discussed earlier include the Hill-Burton Act of 1946, the Rural Health Clinic Act of 1977, implementation of Prospective Payment Systems and Diagnostic Related Group payment (PPS/DRG) in 1983, the Omnibus Budget Reconciliation Act of 1989, the Balanced Budget Act of 1997 and the Balanced Budget Revision Act of 1999, and more recently the Medicare Modernization Act of 2003—all of which defined or redefined funding or facility opportunities for health care systems. The recent passage of the Patient Protection and Affordable Care Act of 2010 (ACA) will be implemented over a 5-year period and has significant implications for rural health.[41] Specific federal initiatives have focused around the following areas:

- Personnel (Public Health Services Act Title VII (medicine/allied health) and VIII (nursing) funding for education, National Health Service Corps, 3R-Network)
- Reduction of inequities (the creation of designations for Health Professional Shortage Areas and Medically Underserved Areas, enhanced Medicare/Medicaid reimbursement for rural clinics and hospitals)
- Support for the actual delivery system (Rural Health Clinics, Community and Migrant Health Centers, Rural Hospital Flex Program, Frontier Extended Stay Clinic)
- Development of infrastructure to support the rural health care delivery system (Area Health Education Centers Program, Federal and State Offices of Rural Health, and State Primary Care Offices)

The *National Health Service Corps* (NHSC), established in 1970, was designed to provide health personnel to the areas of greatest need. Initially the NHSC was a program that linked scholarships with service obligations for "payback" in medically underserved communities. Although it was initially successful in placing new physicians—and later PAs, NPs, and certified nurse midwives (CNMs)—in needy clinics, the program was criticized when many providers moved on after their time was up. In response, the NHSC expanded its scope to include loan repayment and scholarship opportunities. This combination has given the NHSC more flexibility in responding to the needs of specific communities and individual providers. Over time, the NHSC has expanded the number of slots available to both PAs and NPs. The NHSC also supports the training of dentists and mental health providers. Lack of retention and the resulting disruption in continuity of care have been critical issues in continued congressional funding for the Corps. New funding under the ACA increases the NHSC substantially to expand both scholarship and loan repayment slots targeting FQHCs and RHCs and other underserved areas.

Parallel to the development of the NHSC, the federal government began investing directly in the training of primary care providers, including family medicine residencies and PA and nurse practitioner educational training programs through Title VII/VIII of the Public Health Service Act. Funding formulas for these programs provided incentives for the development and support of rural training opportunities. Many PA programs specifically received support for the recruitment of individuals from rural communities to be trained for rural practice. Federal funding for these critical programs has increased significantly under the ACA, which is promoting enhanced recruitment to the health professions, expanded primary care training for physicians, PAs, allied health fields, and nursing. Specific funding to increase the number of PA programs and students has already been initiated, and new programs targeting the transition of military and veteran PAs are being developed.

Federal designations—Health Professional Shortage Areas (HPSAs), Medically Underserved Areas (MUAs), and Medically Underserved Populations (MUPs)—are used to direct scarce public moneys to areas of greatest need. As noted, these criteria are critically important to rural communities since eligibility for over 40 programs—such as NHSC, Medicare bonus payments, Rural Health/FQHC Clinics, and Critical Access Hospitals—depend on these designations.

Although all three types of designation have been helpful in bringing more resources to rural America, they have also generated significant controversy. Some of the dissatisfaction has been with specific formulas—and cut-off points—in use at any given time. There has been a more general dissatisfaction with the cumbersome process involved in achieving these designations. The sad fact is that none of these designations gives a clear picture of the level of the "underservedness" that exists in this country. The granting of each of these designations involves a fairly high level of sophistication, the prior existence of an administrative infrastructure, and the availability of complex data sets. Thus, some of our most underserved areas have difficulty in meeting the administrative criteria for these designations even though they are clearly "eligible."

The creation of the *Federal Office of Rural Health Policy* (FORHP) was a significant juncture for rural communities. It was created by the Administration in 1987 and was tasked to promote better health care service in rural America. The FORHP was also charged with keeping the Department of Health and Human Services advised on matters affecting rural hospitals and health care, coordinating activities within the department that relate to rural health care, and maintaining a national information clearinghouse. Working with government at federal, state, and local levels, as well as with associations, foundations, providers, and community leaders, it seeks solutions to rural health care problems. The FORHP does the following:

- Helps shape rural health policy
- Works with state offices of rural health
- Promotes rural health research
- Funds innovative rural health programs
- Provides support to the National Advisory Committee on Rural Health and Human Services
- Acts as a voice for the concerns of rural hospitals, clinics, and other rural health care providers
- Acts as a liaison with national, state, and local rural health organizations
- Works with minority populations in rural areas
- Sponsors a national clearinghouse of rural health information
- Evaluates programs[38]

A significant outcome of the FOHRP was the development of a matching grant program for *State Offices of Rural Health*, which began in 1991, and has accomplished the creation of state offices in all 50 states. Each state office helps their local rural communities build health care delivery systems. Goals of the offices are to collect and disseminate information; provide technical assistance; help to coordinate rural health interests statewide; and support efforts to improve recruitment and retention of health professionals. Subsequently, the National Organization of State Offices of Rural Health was created as a representative body to provide states a voice in addressing legislative and policy issues at the national level.[46]

The AHEC *(Area Health Education Centers)* has a mission "to enhance access to quality health care, particularly primary and preventive care, by improving the supply and distribution of health care professionals through community/academic educational partnerships." The program was part of the Comprehensive Manpower Training Act of 1971, which Congress created to recruit, train, and retain a health professions workforce committed to underserved populations. The HETC (Health Education Training Centers) program was later created in 1989 to provide programs for specific populations with persistent, severe unmet health needs, particularly along the southern border of the United States. Together the AHEC and HETC programs help create a "town-gown" partnership between academic health centers and communities in addressing local community health needs. There are 56 AHEC programs with more than 235 centers operating in almost every state and the District of Columbia connecting more than 120 medical schools and 600 nursing and allied health schools collaborating with AHECs to improve health for underserved and underrepresented populations.[47]

REQUISITES FOR A RURAL PHYSICIAN ASSISTANT

Depending on the type of practice setting—solo in a satellite clinic or in a multiphysician clinic—PAs would benefit from having a broad range of skills beyond just their medical knowledge. Business knowledge and skills can be helpful in not only managing clinic operations if necessary but also tracking your own contributions and value to the practice. This is helpful in negotiating salary or benefit increases, expanding scope of practice, or even supporting a need for more advanced education for skills enhancement.

A number of published papers indicate that confidence is one of the primary factors that contributes to the success and retention of PAs in rural areas. Having confidence in your medical knowledge and skills provides the basis for a relatively high degree of autonomy, a significant factor in retention; this also enables PAs to engage the community through participation in outreach activities and social and community organizations. Factors that negatively affect retention include isolation (both from the precepting physicians/facilities and other professionals); frustration with lack of resources, such as equipment, no pharmacy in town, or adequate transportation for patients to travel for referred care; and lack of support for vacations or CME time off.

Studies have also shown that PAs who grew up in rural or similar communities are more satisfied with rural practice; this is also true for spouses. Gender also plays a role in that women are less likely to seek or remain in rural settings for a variety of reasons. With more marriages including two professionals, adequate job opportunities for the non-PA spouse is an important factor in long-term family satisfaction.[48-50]

Rural PAs certainly need to have a level of confidence in their knowledge and skills to manage routine and emergency situations, and they should have all their advanced skills certifications updated as appropriate (e.g., ACLS, PALS, ATLS). Familiarity with simple laboratory procedures, phlebotomy, taking routine radiographs, and enhanced computer skills can allow the PA to operate in a wider variety of settings comfortably, recognizing that often there are limited staff and ancillary services available locally.

Much of this may depend on the degree of remoteness and autonomy in the position, as well as the type of community population and practice. An important element of rural practice, which every PA needs to be mindful of, is the legal liability involved in autonomous decision-making and recognizing their own knowledge level, as well as knowing the limits of the physician-PA relationship.

CHALLENGES AND REWARDS OF RURAL PRACTICE

Some liken the challenge and/or the attraction of rural practice to being "a big frog in a little pond." There are many opportunities in a smaller community to influence the health and well-being of individuals, as well as the community as a whole, whether it is assisting with sports team coverage, participating in teaching health subjects in the schools at all levels, establishing chronic disease management programs, teaching EMS classes, or being asked to serve on various boards and committees. As a health care professional, PAs are often seen as having advanced knowledge and skills that can serve the community in many ways.

Why consider rural practice? Many see the lifestyle as personally attractive, including a safer environment in which to raise a family, often a more relaxed lifestyle (except for on-call time), and accessibility to superb recreational facilities. Care should be taken, however, to ensure that each member of the family has input into the decision to move to a rural community. Access to social and recreational amenities may be lacking or far enough away to limit frequent trips. Salaries and benefits may be somewhat lower than in urban practices, but market forces determine ranges as much as size of the practice. It is not unusual to hear of starting salaries in the $75,000 to $90,000 range even in small communities as an incentive to practitioners to relocate; other initial benefits may include assistance with housing and moving expenses.

Professionally, there is often the opportunity to have a wider scope of practice. Some of the professional rewards that one finds in a rural setting include the ability to use most, if not all, of one's training. The most common exceptions to this are obstetrical and surgical skills. Rural PAs usually have a much greater degree of independence (often regulatory as well as actual) than they would have in an urban setting, although this can be a two-edged sword because of the temptation to overstep limits. In rural practice, one can take pleasure in the fact that one can have a tremendous impact on the well-being of patients and can be involved in all aspects of their lives, from taking care of a newborn and reinforcing parenting skills to helping ease the pain of an elderly patient who is dying. Rural PAs also find that they truly are meeting a need, one that might well go unmet if they were not present. Medical needs in underserved rural and inner city areas are what PAs were originally created to meet. The PA profession has consistently shown that it can do an excellent job of meeting them.

CLINICAL APPLICATIONS

1. Current health care reform efforts focus on implementing Primary Care Medical Homes utilizing provider-based interdisciplinary teams of physicians, physician assistants, nurse practitioners, and others. Given the discussion and cited studies in regard to adequate access (RHC, CHC, CAH facilities), workforce shortages in primary care, and financial pressures caused by mandated technology implementation, how realistic is it to achieve this goal in rural communities?
2. Policy decisions, particularly at the federal level, often have unintended consequences for rural areas and health care. Issues such as health care reform, rigid immigration laws, decreased CMS reimbursement for physician services, decreased support for health professions education and training, and mandatory implementation of electronic medical records for Medicare reimbursement have all had significant effect on rural population access and health care system survival. Discuss possible options for rural community responses to these policy issues.
3. The PA profession was founded, in part, to meet the needs of rural and underserved communities and populations. As the profession shifts to more advanced degrees, what are the implications for PAs to continue to meet rural workforce needs? Likewise, most recent workforce studies show that a decreasing number of physicians will select rural communities to practice in; what initiatives might be helpful in encouraging PAs to meet that deficit?

KEY POINTS

Rural health involves a complex system that is determined in part by how we define "rural," the changing demographics of the population, state and federal programs that determine licensing, and certification and funding, as well as meeting geographic challenges in accessing care.

Rural communities and health care systems are always being challenged but have been resilient in meeting the health needs of their communities.

- Continued expansion of Community Health Centers, Rural Health Clinics, and specialty disciplines will provide new employment opportunities for PAs.
- Federal and state policies play a significant role in rural health care survival through development and support of new facility models, funding of health systems infrastructure, setting of reimbursement policies for public programs, funding public insurance programs, and establishing funds to pay for services.
- Rural health care practice, with all its pros and cons, can be rewarding personally and professionally.
- Self-actualization is the key to success in rural practice!

References

1. One Department Serving Rural America. HHS Rural Health Task Force Report to the Secretary, Section 1: Rural America in 2001: Challenges and Opportunities. *http://www.eric.ed.gov/PDFS/ED469138.pdf*; Accessed July 2002.
2. Blakely R. What is rural? And why does it matter? Rural New York Minute. Community and Rural Development Institute Number 1: Cornell University; *http://cals.cornell.edu/cals/devsoc/outreach/cardi/publications/loader.cfm?csModule=security/getfile&PageID=205428*; Accessed January 2007.
3. U.S. Census Bureau. Demographic Trends in the 20th Century. pp 9, 32–34, *http://www.census.gov/prod/2002pubs/censr-4.pdf*; Accessed November 2002.
4. Rural America at a Glance: 2011. *www.ers.usda.gov/Publications/EIB85/.* Accessed January 2012.
5. Ricketts T, Johnson-Webb K, Taylor P. Definitions of Rural: A Handbook for Health Policy Makers and Researchers. Federal Office of Rural Health Policy, HRSA/US DHHS June 1998:2–11.
6. Measuring Rurality. New Definitions in 2003. Economic Research Service/US Department of Agriculture, *http://www.ers.usda.gov/briefing/rurality/NewDefinitions*; Accessed August 21, 2003.
7. Measuring Rurality. Rural-Urban Continuum Codes. Economic Research Service/US Department of Agriculture, *http://www.ers.usda.gov/briefing/rurality/RuralUrbCon/*; Accessed April 28, 2004.
8. National Center for Frontier Communities. The Consensus Definition, *http://www.frontierus.org/documents/consensus.htm*; Accessed January 2012.
9. Jones CA, Parker TS, Ahern M, et al. Health Status and Health Care Access of Farm and Rural Populations. Economic Research Service/US Department of Agriculture, *http://www.ers.usda.gov/publications/eib57/*; Accessed August 2009.
10. Ricketts TC. Rural Health in the United States. New York: Oxford University Press, 1999, p. 3–19.
11. Rural Employment at a Glance. Economic Research Service/US Department of Agriculture, *http://www.ers.usda.gov/publications/EIB21*; Accessed December 2006.
12. Rural Population and Migration. Trend 6—Challenges from an Aging Population. Economic Research Service/US Department of Agriculture, *http://www.ers.usda.gov/Briefing/Population/Challenges.htm*; Accessed February 1, 2007.
13. Rural America at a Glance: 2006. *http://www.ers.usda.gov/publications/rdrr-91-1.pdf*; Accessed January 2008.
14. Kandel W. The Changing Face of Rural America: Growing Ethnic Diversity. Economic Research Service/US Department of Agriculture 2008, *http://www.usda.gov/oce/forum/2008_Speeches/PDFPPT/Kandel.pdf*; Accessed September 2012.
15. Rural Population and Migration. Trend 5—Diversity Increases in Nonmetro America. Economic Research Service/US Department of Agriculture, *http://www.ers.usda.gov/Briefing/Population/Diversity.htm*; Accessed February 1, 2007.
16. Rural Hispanics. Employment and Residential Trends. Amber Waves, Economic Research Service/US Department of Agriculture, *http://www.ers.usda.gov/AmberWaves/Scripts/print.asp?page=/June04/Features/RuralHispanic.htm*; Accessed June 2004.
17. Johnson K. Demographic Trends in Rural and Small Town America. Carsey Institute: Reports on Rural America 2006. University of New Hampshire, *http://www.carseyinstitute.unh.edu/publications/Report_Demographics.pdf*; Accessed September 2012.
18. Overview of the Uninsured in the United States. A Summary of the 2011 Current Population Survey. Office of the Assistant Secretary for Planning and Evaluation. Department of Health and Human Services, *http://aspe.hhs.gov/health/reports/2011/CPSHealthIns2011/ib.pdf*; Accessed September 2012.
19. Physician Workforce Policy Guidelines for the United States. 2000-2020. Council on Graduate Medical Education Sixteenth Report January 2005.
20. Recruitment and Retention of a Quality Health Workforce in Rural Areas. A Series of Policy Papers on The Rural Health Careers Pipeline, Number 1: Physicians. National Rural Health Association, *http://www.nrharural.org/pubs/index.htm*; Accessed November 2006.
21. 2009 AAPA Physician Assistant Census Report. American Academy of Physician Assistants. *http://www.aapa.org/uploadedFiles/content/Research/2009%20Census%20PUMF_Public%20View_Final.pdf*; Accessed September 2010.
22. 2010 AAPA Physician Assistant Census Report. American Academy of Physician Assistants, *http://www.aapa.org/uploadedFiles/content/Research/2010%20Census%20Report%20National%20_Final.pdf*; Accessed September 2012.
23. Minorities in Medicine. An Ethnic and Cultural Challenge for Physician Training. Council on Graduate Medical Education Seventeenth Report—An Update April 2005.

24. Income, Poverty and Health Insurance Coverage in the United States. 2010. U.S. Census Bureau/Department of Commerce, *http://www.census.gov/prod/2011pubs/p60-239.pdf*; Accessed September 2011.
25. Medical Assistance Facilities. A Demonstration Program to Provide Access to Health Care in Frontier Communities. U.S. DHHS/Office of the Inspector General, *http://oig.hhs.gov/oei/reports/oei-04-92-00731.pdf*; Accessed July 1993.
26. Mayes R. The origin, development and passage of Medicare's revolutionary prospective payment system. J Hist Med Allied Sci 2007 Jan;62(1):21–55.
27. HCFA Finalizes Rule to Improve Hospital, Emergency Treatment Access: Health Care Policy Report. Washington, DC: Bureau of National Affairs, May 31, 1993.
28. Wright G, Felt S, Wellever AL, et al. Limited Service Hospital Pioneers: Challenges and Successes of the Essential Access Community Hospital/Rural Primary Care Hospital (EACH/RPCH) Program and Medical Assistance Facility (MAF) Demonstration. Draft Final Report. Washington, DC: Mathematica Policy Research, March 28, 1995.
29. Critical Access Hospital fact Sheet. Medicare Learning Network. CMS/DHHS 2009, *https://www.cms.gov/MLNProducts/downloads/CritAccessHospfctsht.pdf*; Accessed September 2012.
30. Small Hospital Improvement Grant. Rural Assistance Center. US Department of Health and Human Services. *http://www.raconline.org/funding/details.php?funding_id=64*
31. Health Center History. Bureau of Primary Health Care/Health Resources Services Administration/DHHS. *www.bphc.hrsa.gov/about/history.htm http://bphc.hrsa.gov/about/index.html http://www.chcchronicles.org/main.cfm?actionId=globalShowStaticContent&screenKey=cmpHistory&s=chronicles&htmlKey=movementHistory*
32. President's Health centers Initiative. Bureau of Primary Health Care/Health Resources Services Administration/DHHS. *www.bphc.hrsa.gov/chc/pi.htm*.
33. America's Health Centers Fact Sheet. National Association of Community Health Centers, *http://www.nachc.org/client//America's%20Health%20Centers%20Fact%20Sheet%20August%202011.pdf*; Accessed August 2011.
34. Expanding Health Centers under Health Care Reform. Doubling Patient Capacity and Bringing Down Costs. National Association of Health Centers, *http://www.nachc.org/client/documents/HCR_New_Patients_Final.pdf*; Accessed June 2010.
35. Rieselbach RE, Crouse BJ, Frohna JG. Teaching primary care in community health centers: addressing the workforce crisis for the underserved. Ann Intern Med 2010;152:118–122.
36. Rosenblatt R, Andrilla CH, Curtin T, Hart LG. Shortages of medical personnel at community health centers. JAMA March 1, 2006;293:1042–1049.
37. Rural Health Clinic Fact Sheet. Medicare Learning Network, CMS/DHHS, *https://www.cms.gov/MLNProducts/downloads/RuralHlthClinfctsht.pdf*; Accessed October 2011.
38. Frontier Extended Stay Clinic (FESC) Cooperative Agreement Program. Office of Rural Health Policy/HRSA/DHHS, *http://ruralhealth.hrsa.gov/funding/fesc.htm* and *http://www.frontierus.org/index-current.htm*; Accessed September 2012.
39. Felt-Lisk S, Silberman P, Hoag S, Slifken R. Medicaid managed care in rural areas: a ten state follow-up study. Health Affairs, Vol 18, No. 2: 238–245.
40. Chan L, Hart LG, Goodman D. Geographic access to health care for rural Medicare beneficiaries. J Rural Health 2006;22:140–146.
41. Coburn AF, Lundblad JP, MacKinney AC, et al. The Patient Protection and Affordable Care Act of 2010: Impacts on Rural People, Places, and Providers: A First Look. RUPRI Health Panel, *http://www.rupri.org/Forms/Health_PPACAImpacts_Sept2010.pdf*; Accessed September 16, 2010.
42. PA Fact Sheet VITAL STATISTICS. American Academy of Physician Assistants 2010, *http://www.aapa.org/uploadedFiles/content/News_and_Publications/For_the_Media/VitalStats_Factsheet_Update_final.pdf*; Accessed September 2012.
43. Evans T, Wick K, Brock D, Academic degrees and clinical practice characteristics, et al. The University of Washington Physician Assistant program: 1969-2000. J Rural Health Summer 2006;Vol. 22(No. 3):212–219.
44. Larson EH, Hart LG, Goodwin MK, et al. Dimensions of retention: a national study of the locational histories of physician assistants. J Rural Health 1999;15:391.
45. Muus KJ, Geller JM, Williams JD, et al. Job satisfaction among rural physician assistants. J Rural Health 1998;14:100–108.
46. Federal Office of Rural Health Policy. *http://hrsa.gov/ruralhealth/about/index.html*; Accessed September, 2012
47. National AHEC Organization. *http://www.nationalahec.org*; Accessed September 2012.
48. Henry LR, Hooker RS. Retention of physician assistants in rural health clinics. J Rural Health 2007;23:207–214.
49. Daniels ZM, VanLeit BJ, Skipper BJ, et al. Factors in recruiting and retaining professionals for rural practice: National Rural Health Association Workforce Issues Series. J Rural Health 2007;Vol. 23:62–71.
50. Henry LR, Hooker RS, Yates KL. The role of physician assistants in rural health care: a systematic review of the literature. J Rural Health 2011;27:220–229.

The resources for this chapter can be found at www.expertconsult.com.

CHAPTER 49

INTERNATIONAL HEALTH CARE

David H. Kuhns

CHAPTER CONTENTS

The opportunity to work abroad in a clinical setting, whether updating the skills and knowledge of local providers for a couple of weeks or a longer-term commitment of months providing essential health care to displaced populations suffering from the ravages of war, will likely have long-term effects for the physician assistant (PA) who rises to such a challenge. For many PAs it is simply a heightened sense of adventure that makes such service appealing. For others it is the heartfelt sense of moral obligation to help wherever in world the needs are great and the resources scarce. Regardless of the motive, such service as a PA will likely be a life-altering event.

PAs have actively participated in the delivery of international health care since the inception of the PA profession. PAs work with many international organizations, both private and governmental. PAs have served, and continue to serve, with international relief organizations in Cambodia, Brazil, Tonga, Peru, Guatemala, Nicaragua, Sudan, Djibouti, and Somalia, to name but a few. Other PAs are employed by private multinational corporations, supporting the oil-drilling crews above the Arctic Circle in Siberia or providing primary care to expatriates and their families living in China and Saudi Arabia. Many more PAs serve with U.S. Armed Forces throughout the world in a variety of environments where they are often tasked to provide medical care to the indigent populations. Still other PAs work in other branches of the U.S. government as well. Some PAs serve as Peace Corps workers, while more experienced PAs serve as Peace Corps Medical Officers (PCMOs). As PCMOs, PAs provide the medical support for Peace Corps volunteers in a given country. Recent developments have brought the PA concept to the U.S. Foreign Service. Also of note is the fact that PAs are now being recruited for service with the Central Intelligence Agency and private firms for deployment overseas in "hardship" environments like Iraq and Afghanistan. In a much less volatile setting, American PAs have been working in the United Kingdom's National Health Service for the past 10 years. There they have served as both clinicians and role models for the recently qualified UK-trained PAs. PAs who want to practice internationally now have many more options than they did just a few years ago. Nonetheless, the overall number of PAs who work internationally remains relatively small.

The actual clinical roles and responsibilities of international PAs are as varied and diverse as the many countries and cultures in which they work. Thus, for the same reasons that it is difficult to describe the role of a "typical" PA practicing anywhere in the United States, it is equally difficult to identify the "typical" PA role in foreign countries.

PAs who choose to work in an international environment have many options. These options largely depend on the PAs themselves. First they must determine whether they will seek formal "paid" employment with financial compensation of salary and benefits or serve on a "volunteer" basis. PAs then need to identify the target population (expatriates or indigenous) they are interested in serving. Once they have decided where, how, and with whom they want to work, PAs can begin an often lengthy application process. Passports, visa application forms, references, security clearances and background checks, screening health examinations, necessary vaccines, language skills and other pertinent training, and formal interviews are just some of the many steps that are likely to be required.

Working for the U.S. government, either in the capacity of the military PA or with other governmental organizations (e.g., Foreign Service), usually entails providing care to a generally young and otherwise healthy expatriate staff. The "standards of care" are expected to be similar to treatment for the same problem in a typical medical facility in the United States. Diagnostic equipment and supplies, although perhaps rudimentary, are likely to be familiar to even the inexperienced provider. Advanced care may sometimes only be available by transporting the patient back to the continental United States by air ambulance.

At the other end of the health care spectrum is work in developing countries. Providing health care to indigenous populations through nongovernmental organizations (NGOs) can offer PAs a far greater challenge on many levels. Novice PAs (in terms of international experience) will likely face a rather unsettling experience when they come to realize that many of their preconceptions about what constitutes a "norm" in medical standards of care in the United States cannot, and for a variety of reasons *must not*, apply to the delivery of health care in a developing country. PAs may face medical conditions that they never imagined, disease states of which they know little or nothing, and an overwhelming lack of resources, such as hospitals without running water or an oxygen delivery system. Frequently they will find that the medical and diagnostic equipment, if and when available, is basic. Laboratory studies might be limited to determination of a hemoglobin value and microscopic examinations of urine and blood (for cell count and differential, as well as thick and thin prep slides for malaria) and stool for ova and parasites. Unless they are fluent in the local language, common tasks such as diagnostic studies and hands-on physical evaluations frequently will have to be done through local interpreters, thus increasing the time required for even a simple examination. The organizations listed in the box can provide additional information.

ORGANIZATIONS FOR INTERNATIONAL HEALTH CARE

American Academy of Physician Assistants
www.aapa.org/advocacy-and practice-resources/international

- Physician Assistants for Global Health
  www.pasforglobalhealth.org
  E-mail: pasforglobalhealth@gmail.com
- Fellowship of Christian Physician Assistants
  www.fcpa.net
  PO Box 2006
  Bristol, TN 337621
  E-mail: ContactFCPA@fcpa.net

The PA who chooses to work with an indigenous population will have to decide if he or she wants shorter terms (e.g., 3 to 6 months doing emergency relief where conditions are likely to be stressful). The generally safer alternative is to work in developmental projects for longer terms (e.g., 9 to 12 months). These developmental projects typically have more infrastructure and are therefore likely to be in more stable countries.

The PA serving indigenous populations will likely confront many other hurdles beyond simple language differences. There may be significant cultural, societal, and religious issues to address. Despite these factors, and perhaps because of them, the rewards of investing oneself in such a venture are often immeasurable.

PRACTICAL CONSIDERATIONS

General Issues

The experience of many internationally experienced PAs demonstrates the need for a well-conceived plan. PAs who hope to practice internationally would be well advised to research all aspects of such a commitment. This section addresses a number of major hurdles that PAs have encountered. Although the following list of topics is comprehensive, it is by no means complete.

The box presents a set of guidelines for PAs considering international work, which were adopted by the American Academy of Physician Assistants (AAPA) in 2001. All PAs working internationally need to adhere to these guidelines, as well as to the *Guidelines for Ethical Conduct for the Physician Assistant Profession*.

Licensure/Registration

There is no universal means by which PAs are permitted to work in a foreign country. In some cases whereby PAs are serving an expatriate patient population, official approval from foreign governments may be obtained through a series of clinical competency examinations. More often, PAs may be breaking new ground as they explore the ways by which they can perform the tasks and deliver the level of care for which they are trained. One such groundbreaker, Donald Prater, worked in Nanjing, China, for a U.S.-based company, providing health care to hundreds of expatriates and their families who live in that region. Even though he was not providing medical services to the local residents, Chinese authorities required that he take the Chinese medical examination (in English) so that he could see his expatriate patients on a fee-for-service basis.

More commonly, governmental approval is awarded to the agency with which the PA is working (e.g., American Refugee Committee). Thus, the PA is allowed to work under the umbrella of that organization. Consequently, that agency will typically require that credentials and letters of recommendation be submitted as the first step in going "to the field." Experience indicates that PAs, as fully licensed, certified, and registered providers in the United States, can usually practice their clinical skills to the full scope of their training. However, the actual scope of practice for the international PA can, and often does, vary widely.

Physician–Physician Assistant Relationship

The physician-PA relationship in international settings can be informal or tightly structured. The supervising physician can be in immediate proximity, working alongside the PA in a refugee camp, or in the capital city of the country while the PA is working in the field. Another possibility is that the supervising physician may be based in the United States but available by satellite communications or another electronic format, a model that many private multinational companies follow. It is important to remember that because there are no distinct or universal rules that govern international PA practice (except those constraints of the state wherein the PA is duly licensed or registered), practice standards for PAs in international settings unfortunately remain vague and ill defined.

Malpractice

Although the myriad aspects of U.S.-based medical practice differ from those of international practice, and malpractice is not usually an issue in international practice, PAs must always provide the same high level of care for which they have trained, regardless of where in the world they find themselves. PAs should check with their insurance carriers before departing because insurance carriers rarely provide coverage outside the United States.

PAs must never represent themselves as physicians, either at home or abroad. The problems that could occur as a result of such misrepresentation may be devastating for an individual PA and may even have long-reaching effects on the PA profession.

When the PA is working overseas, it remains his or her responsibility to account for absences from clinical practice at home. This may require that adequate documentation be provided for any extended absences, including formal verification from the international employer or the organization.

Continuing Education

Continuing medical education (CME), although not usually an issue for the other countries in which the PA may work, is nonetheless a requirement for maintaining licensure and certification. Maintaining certification by the National Commission on Certification of Physician Assistants (NCCPA) becomes an issue only if the PA is outside of the United States for a year or longer. From a practical perspective, Category 1 CME credits are best obtained either by "stockpiling" before leaving the United States, or web-based formats. Technologic developments can allow the globetrotting PA to access various Category 1 CME programs online from Internet cafes around the world.

Salaries

From those PAs who work for a small nongovernmental organization who may have to pay for all of their own travel and lodging expenses to the few lucky PAs who are fully employed by a multinational corporation that may compensate them generously, PAs working in the international arena will find that the range of salaries and benefits will be as varied as the types of positions that they may encounter.

QUALIFICATIONS

Medical Skills

The ability to work with limited or improvised resources is an essential skill. Of particular value is a reliance on a basic hands-on approach to medicine. To highlight this issue, Cameron McCauley, an experienced international PA, tells of a time during his PA training when he was learning to evaluate heart murmurs. Like most of his peers, he scoffed at the need for physical assessment skills when technology such as echocardiograms would confirm the diagnosis. Cameron was humbled many years later, when he found himself working in a remote village without any hope of accessing such technology. Instead, he used those basic physical diagnostic skills he had learned years before to determine that a young patient had a ventricular septal defect. The child was then referred to the distant capital city, where his diagnosis was confirmed and the defect was surgically corrected.

It is important to remember that there are usually few advanced resources available. The PA will seldom find advanced diagnostic options, such as ultrasound or computed tomography (CT), or even the basics of plain radiography. As an example of the paucity of resources that can be faced, when I worked in Kabul, Afghanistan, in 2003, there was only one working electrocardiogram (ECG) machine in the entire country. Often the nearest x-ray unit is hours away and can only be reached only by driving over rough roads, with the patient bouncing along in the back of a beat-up Land Rover.

Tropical Medicine

Patients in developing countries typically do not have the same causes of morbidity and mortality as those in the United States. Instead of cancers and cardiovascular diseases, patients in developing countries typically succumb to the ravages of infectious diseases. Even such relatively straightforward illnesses as gastroenteritis, acute respiratory infections such as pneumonia, and measles are the leading causes of death. Treatment is usually simple *if* the patient can access the proper medication in time. Clinicians can spend years learning to specialize in infectious tropical disease; however, there are several short courses in American universities that can provide excellent training over a couple of weeks to a few months.

Public Health and Epidemiology

Because infectious diseases are so commonplace, especially in developing countries, a strong emphasis must be placed on prevention of these problems. Therefore, it is essential that PAs, especially those working in medical infrastructure development and public health capacity building, develop an understanding of the basic principles of public health. Many accredited schools of public health are available in the United States, but only a relative few offer specialty training in international health.

Human Resource Management and Teaching Expertise

Frequently, PAs are sought not just as clinical providers, but as trainers and/or managers of local operations. In Jalalabad, Afghanistan, I served as the Project Medical Coordinator for New Hadda, an emergency refugee camp of more than 80,000 people who, in the mid-1990s, had fled the fighting in Kabul, the capital, but were then unable to escape to neighboring Pakistan. Health care provided in the camp was the responsibility of the international humanitarian aid agency, Doctors Without Borders, which provided primary care through a series of clinics staffed by Afghan doctors and nurses. As the project medical coordinator, I was responsible for the overall delivery of medical care in the camp clinics, some limited clinical practice, clinical teaching, as well as all aspects of public health in the camp. To accomplish this, I regularly collaborated with representatives from other local and international NGOs, the local Ministry of Health, the United Nations International Children's Emergency Fund (UNICEF), and the World Health Organization (WHO).

Language Skills

A second language (e.g., French, Spanish, Portuguese, Arabic, Persian) can open many doors and allow for an ease of communication with patients and professional counterparts. The alternative—total reliance on interpreters—can result in frustration for all parties involved. As a result, nuances in conversation during the medical history or examination process can be missed, and the interpreter can sometimes act as a screen, perhaps keeping details vague or even misleading the clinician.

OTHER CONSIDERATIONS

Stress

It is a fact that living in harsh environments is stressful. Accommodations are typically Spartan. Insects and vermin can plague your living space. The sound of gunfire can fill the air throughout the night. Adequate rest becomes a precious commodity. The days are often long and physically and sometime emotionally demanding. In addition, working and living with the same group of people, day in and day out, provides additional challenges. It is common for expatriates working in large refugee camp environments to work 7 days a week, 12 or more hours each day. Workers share a common feeling that there is so much work that needs to be done and so little time in which to do it. There must be some opportunity for rest and recuperation to avoid what many see as inevitable burnout. Therefore, many NGOs insist that workers take time away, to the extent that this can be done without affecting the operations of the project.

Medications and Standards of Treatment

Medications, if and when they are available, may not be familiar to the PA because they are sometimes antiquated by most Western standards. Usually, the latest multigenerational cephalosporins are unavailable, not just because of the cost but because resistance has not yet been a significant issue in the area. As a result, inexpensive but nonetheless effective drugs such as chloramphenicol or penicillin G are still used extensively.

Another common observation is that patients from the local population often expect that when they come to a clinic or a hospital, they will be treated and will *always* receive some sort of medication. A patient encounter in which the patient does not walk out with medications can be felt to be unsatisfactory from the patient's perspective, even though the PA may have otherwise given appropriate treatment and provided proper patient education. A visit without receiving medications can be viewed by the patient as substandard care.

Traditional Health Care

Maintaining an open mind is important when one is confronted with traditional and folk medicines. These methods, although usually unfamiliar to U.S.-born PAs, often play a significant role for patients. We must remember that after the PA and other international expatriate staff members leave, the responsibility for ongoing health care usually falls back onto the traditional health care worker.

In Afghanistan, I learned of the traditional "resuscitation" technique used by traditional birth attendants (TBAs) for stillborn infants. The TBA places the placenta on the face of the infant, with the thought that the placenta had provided life to the child in the womb and it should do similarly after birth. To attempt to change this misconception would involve much work and more than a simple message that the TBA "is wrong." It is essential that changes be introduced according to a well-conceived approach. Undermining a community's confidence in a local provider would have long-term ramifications.

An awareness of how a community relies on traditional healers is important if one is to understand what the community expects of the PA. Expatriates must realize that their presence, however long, is still seen as transient by the indigenous populations. It is therefore important to remember that, especially in emergency relief settings, when the expatriate leaves, there will be little left but footprints in the sand.

Personal Health and Safety

Although working in war-ravaged and developing countries represents its own challenge, typically the greatest risk to expatriates occurs while they are traveling by car or truck. Injuries from motor vehicle accidents remain the primary reason for expatriates with Doctors Without Borders to return from the field for medical reasons. Other common maladies range from the nuisance of common traveler's diarrhea to life-threatening cerebral malaria.

Land Mines

More than 60 countries are still littered with millions of land mines; these indiscriminate killers represent a significant threat not just to the local population but to expatriate relief workers as well. It is imperative that a mine-awareness training program be completed by expatriate PAs before they go to work in a land mine–infested country. PAs must always maintain a keen sense of safety when working in such an environment. Elizabeth Sheehan, a PA with vast international experience, tells of an incident when she was traveling through a heavily mined area of Cambodia. In front of her car, a cow was wandering down the dirt road. Suddenly, the cow exploded as it stepped onto a mine, showering Liz's car with cow parts.

Security

Expatriate PAs can sometimes find themselves in dangerous environments. Although they may be volunteers, the stipend of a few hundred dollars a month that they may receive is still significantly more than the average annual income for many locals. As a result, volunteer relief workers have been held hostage, and others have been threatened at gunpoint. There have been robberies, kidnappings, assaults, and even deaths among field workers of most major international relief organizations. Although the economic motivation for these acts seems clear, perhaps less obvious are the political overtones common in some developing countries. One such tragedy occurred on December 17, 1996, when six workers with the International Committee of the Red Cross in Chechnya were murdered as they slept. The reason for the attack was believed to be political. The murderers were never identified. In 2004, five medical relief workers from Doctors Without Borders were ambushed and killed in Afghanistan.

Reentry

Returning home from an overseas experience often proves difficult, and returning PAs should not count on a smooth transition. Family members, other loved ones, and co-workers can seldom understand fully what the returned PA may have seen or experienced. Common experiences have been identified among returning relief workers. An example of such an experience is the "supermarket event." Kate Herlihy, who spent 2 years working for the American Refugee Committee in a Cambodian refugee camp, speaks of the disdain and shock that she felt when she entered a supermarket at home. She was overwhelmed by the variety of pet food, after she had cared for starving people just a few days earlier.

More serious symptoms of posttraumatic stress disorder can also occur. Depression and even suicide have been reported in returned volunteers. It is therefore important to provide a mechanism for adequate debriefing on return and a means to follow up in a timely manner. Many international organizations offer psychological debriefings as part of ongoing support for their workers, paid and volunteer. It can be helpful to speak with a psychologist, psychiatrist, or other mental health expert if the PA has a difficult time with the reentry process.

Topics for Preparation

When a PA is considering taking the time to work overseas, it is important that he or she learn about all the possible aspects of such a commitment. The list below includes a selection of topics to be researched:

- What is the overall mission of the organization?
- What is the organizational approach to the problems—individual and curative, or more utilitarian public health focused, or perhaps a blend of both?
- What happens if you get to the field and you discover it is not what you had expected?
- What security parameters will be followed?
- Will the PA be self-sufficient, functioning outside the established health care system, or will he or she work alongside local counterparts in existing health support structures?
- Will there be a salary or a stipend for you as a volunteer?
- What will happen if you have a needlestick or some other HIV risk exposure?
- Who will pay the necessary expenses of your travel, room, and board?
- What provisions are made for your medical and/or psychological care both during and after a mission?
- Will you have time off while in the field? If so, what are the options for that time?
- What about repatriation to the United States in case of medical or family emergencies?
- What about life insurance?
- Will medical supplies and equipment be provided, or will you have to bring everything yourself?
- Is there a training or orientation program available, or will you be expected to go directly to the field?
- Is the situation stable enough for the PA to be accompanied by a spouse or other family member?
- How do you relax when you are under stress?
- How do you function in a team? How do you feel about living and working, day in and day out, in a cramped living space, surrounded by smokers?
- What about the job that you will be leaving behind? Is there any chance that the job, as well as any promises regarding the security of that job, will not be maintained? If not, what is your fall-back plan?

Case Study 49-1, written from my personal experience, illustrates the challenges and satisfactions of work in international health care.

CASE STUDY 49-1

For my first mission in 1994 with Doctors Without Borders, or *Médecins Sans Frontières (MSF)*, I had asked for a "stable" situation on which to cut my teeth. The reply from headquarters was that I had the opportunity to go to Somaliland (northwestern Somalia), where MSF had been working for almost a decade. The area was considered stable by MSF standards because it had been a couple of years since fighting had dominated the area. Somaliland was also hundreds of miles, and a separate and distinct country, from Somalia, where the situation around Mogadishu was much more volatile. Our project, based in the city of Burao, was to continue to strengthen the existing health structures, a 200-bed hospital and a series of 10 primary care clinics out in the "bush." This was to be accomplished through a collaborative effort with counterparts from the Somaliland Ministry of Public Health (MOPH).

As the Country Medical Coordinator, I was the leader of the small team of two other expatriates, a Dutch nurse and an English logistician, as well as about 40 local staff, consisting of doctors, nurses, and a variety of nonmedical support staff.

Due to improving health indicators, MSF was in the process of scaling back the team's overall operational involvement. As a result, my job was supposed to be primarily nonclinical. However, I was also told that I could probably integrate my clinical background into my daily work. Between regular meetings and negotiations with my counterpart, the hospital director, I would make ward rounds and discuss management of patients with the Somali doctors and nurses. Overall, it was proving a rather interesting departure from my experience in emergency medicine. My focus was no longer centered on a single patient at a time as it was when I was working in the emergency department back home; instead, I now looked at improving the access to and the overall quality of medical care for a whole city and the regions beyond.

My first couple of weeks in Burao were overwhelming. I tried to establish some sense of order in my life. I had just left a busy emergency department in a tertiary care center in Portland, Maine, and I was now working in a hospital that lacked such amenities as running water or even continuous electricity for 24 hours a day. Goats and sheep wandered about the grounds of the hospital compound, leaving behind a different sort of "land mine" to discover. I could literally walk through a pile of sheep dung and then step into the operating theater. There, the patient could be found situated on a table with a large ceiling fan turning directly overhead. On the wards, patients lay on the bare springs of decrepit beds. If patients were fortunate enough to have a mattress or bed linens, the patient's family had provided them. Hospital windows had no intact glass or screens. The ceilings of the wards were stained from rain that had leaked through the countless bullet and shrapnel holes in the roof. During the rainy season, I saw the staff madly shuffling children in cribs around the room in a futile effort to avoid the many leaks that plagued the entire hospital. I developed an overwhelming sense of seeing that there was so much work that needed to be done and so little time or money to do what was really needed. Eventually, that sense of frustration grew less when, on several occasions, community elders would approach me and thank me for the "help that MSF was providing to this impoverished and forgotten country."

I eventually shifted my focus from trying to reproduce what I knew to be a standard of health care and turned to a more pragmatic approach. It would not matter if we could provide drugs, supplies, and diagnostic equipment like x-ray machines, if they would then be lost to damage from the rains. We turned our focus to rehabilitating the infrastructure of the hospital—repairing the roof, replacing windows, and other simple efforts. Our efforts were starting to pay off. A sense of accomplishment was shared by the whole team. Unfortunately, our joy was short-lived. The political climate was changing acutely, and tensions were rising. The night air became quieter as people started to hoard their precious ammunition.

One particularly quiet night was suddenly disrupted by the sound of tanks rolling through the city streets. The next morning, the expatriate team was evacuated back to our base of operations in the adjacent country of Djibouti, a postage stamp–sized country located about 2 hours flying time to the west. There we could relax over a beer and contemplate our next actions. Our downtime was limited to a short few hours. A freak storm had struck the area, resulting in a tremendous flash flood that hit the city of Djiboutiville. Walls of water spilled out of the rugged mountain areas and dumped into the flood plains from which the city arises. Shanty towns in the city's periphery suffered the most, with thousands of homes destroyed. More than a hundred people were swept away by the rapidly rising waters, while hundreds of others escaped to safety when they were eventually plucked from roofs and treetops by helicopters sent by the local detachment of the French military. While the fetid waters also struck the MSF office and forced my colleagues to flee to the roof, I was out of danger.

The flood was only the first blow. Another killer was stalking the population and awaiting the chance to pounce. With the flood came the opportunity for that culprit—cholera. Cholera is endemic in the area. These simple bacteria thrive in the milieu of a hot, humid environment and in the poor sanitation found in such a developing country. Untreated, cholera can result in a 50% mortality rate. Like so many other infectious diseases, the highest mortality is among the elderly, children, and those with significant medical problems. Within a few hours of exposure, the body responds to the infection with gastrointestinal symptoms. Abdominal cramps, nausea, vomiting, and profound diarrhea, often described as "rice water" in appearance, are the classic presentation.

The city was trying to recover from the flooding, dealing with the displacement from the floods, and planning for the inevitable cholera outbreak. MSF responded by offering our assistance. Within the world of emergency medical relief, MSF is well known as an authority on managing cholera epidemics. With huge stores of prepackaged supplies available in European warehouses, MSF can respond to an emergency in a matter of days. The logistical support network is well organized and quite efficient, the product of many similar responses during the past decades. In just 3 days, two additional expatriate staff, an experienced nurse and a logistician, joined our team. The tents, intravenous fluids, chlorine for water treatment and disinfections, and the remainder of our cholera treatment center (CTC) supplies arrived the next day from Amsterdam. Our job was to establish a CTC near the hardest-hit area of the city. The residents were already poor, with limited resources. Many were Somalis who had fled the fighting in their homeland and settled in Djibouti, awaiting peace in their homeland. In Djibouti, they lived in shanties—simple wood frame structures covered with corrugated sheets of metal and plastic sheeting. Drinking water supplies throughout the city had been contaminated. Children already suffered from malnutrition and were subject to malabsorption diarrheas.

As a novice to the ravages of cholera, I soon found myself in the uncomfortable role of being the senior medical person in charge of the CTC. The good news was that the treatment for cholera was simple: Replace fluids at a greater rate than they are being lost. If patients could tolerate oral fluids, they received oral rehydration salts (ORS). If unable to keep that down, patients received nasogastric (NG) feedings of ORS. If patients were profoundly dehydrated, as so many were, intravenous (IV) replacement of fluids was the only option left. The local staff that made up the backbone of our CTC was, as a rule, excellent in assessing and treating patients. My job was to ensure that we treated patients according to the protocols of the World Health Organization (WHO). As the senior medical person on the scene, I was also the one to whom the staff turned if they were unable to place an NG tube or find an IV site.

I still recall treating a child about 2 years old, weighing only 6 or 7 kilograms (the result of chronic malnutrition). He was floppy and unresponsive, with poor skin turgor and sunken eyes, and in shock from the profound fluid loss of his vomiting and diarrhea. The child was held suspended by his feet, while I waited for his neck veins to distend. I placed an external jugular line and started the process of rehydrating the child. Accustomed as I was to working in a level I trauma center, I was initially taken aback by the WHO protocol for the aggressive IV rate of 30 mL/kg/hr that is recommended in volume replacement for cholera. My skepticism ended when I saw the tremendous volume of liquid stools that just poured out of these children. To hold a child, floppy and lethargic, in shock from this dramatic gastroenteritis was eye-opening. Suddenly it became clear why cholera claims so many victims around the world each year. The days in the CTC were long and demanding, but my reward was seeing the child who had been at death's door a few hours earlier, now bright-eyed and alert in the arms of his grateful mother.

We soon handed over the day-to-day supervision of the CTC to the Djiboutian Ministry of Health. Meanwhile, our team made preparations to return to Somaliland. We learned that tens of thousands of civilians had fled the fighting in the cities and had returned to their traditional home in the Somali "bush" country. Because this displaced population had no provisions for medical care, MSF volunteered to help. My team was soon traveling back into Burao. There, we planned for a series of assessment missions to determine the extent of the problem we were facing.

It was on such a mission on December 23, 1994, that I found myself in the settlement of Hor Fadda, normally just a stopover in the desert for bands of nomadic shepherds. The "village" was little more than hundreds of simple huts surrounding a muddy watering hole the size of a tennis court. Countless goats, sheep, camels, and humans muddied the water as they all sought to quench their thirst. Surrounding the water hole were thousands of people who had fled the fighting in the capital city of Hargeisa. These refugees, mostly women, elderly men, and children (the young men were back in the city as fighters), were living in makeshift shelters constructed of branches and covered with plastic sheeting, while the men slept outside on the ground, wrapped from head to toe, shroudlike, with thin wool blankets. The only permanent structure in the village was a small, mud-walled hut that we converted to a temporary clinic where we initially treated patients. We then set up a large canvas tent that we had brought with us. That night, the tent would serve as our shelter. The following day, the tent served as the base for a clinic that provided health care to the 15,000 people in the camp.

Later that evening, we shared a meal of boiled mutton and rice. I sat back, enjoyed a cup of chai, relished the warmth from the fire, and took the time to relax a bit and to reflect on the events of the day. It had been a very long day that started at dawn with a 6-hour trip in an elderly Land Rover, bouncing over dirt roads, at times feeling like I was in the midst of a National Geographic special. The one thing that kept me from enjoying much of the journey was that the Somali countryside had been littered with land mines, the result of many years of civil war. We were now traveling roads that normally we would have avoided because of that threat from land mines. However, now the stakes were different: Thousands of people were in need of assistance and, if we did not go, no one else was available. We traveled the well-worn roads and kept our fingers crossed. As we sat around the campfire, it was quiet—much quieter than I had yet experienced during my time on the horn of Africa. My thoughts turned to my loved ones, safe at home on the other side of the world. Christmas was less than a day away, and here I was, in the desert, half a world away, sitting around a campfire.

The silence was broken when Mohammed, one of the staff, asked me if I watched Western movies. I turned to see his toothy smile as he told me that the scene we were in was "just like in the movies." I chuckled and wondered what this man's image of America really was. I was surprised as he then described the typical cowboy scenario portrayed by John Wayne or Gary Cooper. He continued, "We could make a movie and call it 'Night in Hor Fadda,'" which caused us to laugh as we both continued to build the image upon the foundation that he had so accurately depicted.

It was during that evening that I realized how much I had experienced in a little over 2 weeks. I had been through the start of a civil war, a flash flood, a cholera outbreak, and a journey into the bush, where I had witnessed the devastating effects of war on civilians. Although physically and emotionally exhausted, I had survived. More important, at least to me, I felt good about what I had done. I started to lose some of my self-pity and instead started to feel that I was here for a purpose, and that I had, in some small way, made a difference. Even today, years later, on some clear nights as I look skyward, Mohammed's voice and handsome face echo in my mind. I smile when I see him.

CLINICAL APPLICATIONS

1. If you were interested in a position in international health care, how would you research the opportunities for PAs? How would you match your skills to the health care needs and practice settings of international communities?
2. If you secured an international position as a PA, how would you obtain information about the language, culture, politics, infrastructure, and health care system of the area? What else would you want to know before going to an international setting?

KEY POINTS

- Although sometimes dangerous, and usually clinically challenging, working as a PA in a developing country can also be demanding, both physically and emotionally. Nonetheless, it can be a rich and rewarding experience.
- Thoroughly researching the organization's mission statement and having a knowledge of the countries where they work will help you to better determine if you will be a fit in that organization.
- Personal preparation, including appropriate foreign language skills and supplemental training in tropical medicine, epidemiology, and disease control, will increase your marketability to international organizations.

The resources for this chapter can be found at the www.expertconsult.com.

CHAPTER 50

PATIENTS WITH DISABILITIES

Lisa K. Walker • Mary Vacala

CHAPTER CONTENTS

In July 2005 the U.S. Surgeon General issued a Call to Action to Improve the Health and Wellness of Persons with Disabilities. According to this Call to Action, an estimated 54 million people of all ages, races, ethnicities, socioeconomic status, and education levels in the United States (20% of the population) are living with at least one disability. These disabilities range from spinal cord injuries causing paralysis to patients who are born with hearing loss or cognitive disabilities. More than 3 million people 15 and older use a wheelchair. Another 10 million use a walking aid, such as a cane, crutches, or walker. Millions more live with hearing and/or visual losses that significantly impact activities of daily living.[1] Despite these overwhelming statistics and the fact that July 26, 2011, marked the 20th anniversary of the signing of the Americans with Disabilities Act (ADA),* the literature shows significant disparities continue to exist when comparing the health of people with disabilities with the general population. Access to acute and preventive health care services is lacking for these patients. Consequently, morbidity and mortality are high among the disabled patient population, according to the U.S. federal government's initiative Healthy People 2020. Some of the barriers that prevent people with disabilities from receiving appropriate health care include physical barriers, inadequate communication, and attitudinal and social policy barriers. Adequate access to care is not only a legal obligation but a necessity that could prevent catastrophic outcomes and prolong life. Clearly, we can, and must, improve our practice and do more to ensure equal access for patients with disabilities.

Disability can be defined many ways. The legal definition from the ADA is as follows:

> A disabled person is someone with a physical or mental impairment that substantially limits one or more major life activities (as well as someone with a history of such

*The ADA is a federal law that guarantees equal opportunity for people with disabilities in public accommodations, commercial facilities, employment, transportation, state and local government services and telecommunications.

an impairment or someone currently regarded as such). This includes people with obvious, visible disabilities, as well as the majority of people with disabilities who have hidden conditions such as arthritis, diabetes, or hearing impairment.

Information in this chapter is designed to enable students to identify and eliminate many of the barriers faced by patients with disabilities, thereby improving health outcomes for this population. Each section addresses appropriate terms and definitions when working with patients with disabilities. This is followed by a discussion of the appropriate approach, common challenges, and methods to avoid errors in diagnosis and treatment when providing care to patients with specific disabilities, including patients who are deaf and hard of hearing, patients with mobility disabilities, patients with visual impairments, and patients with intellectual and developmental disabilities. Although there is evidence that patients with severe mental illness experience disparities in access to care, a comprehensive discussion of the primary health care needs of patients with mental illness is beyond the scope of this chapter.[2]

Many people with disabilities are accustomed to having others evaluate and circumscribe their lives and opportunities. Stereotypic and stigmatizing views of living with disabilities erect barriers to comprehensive care, such as limiting discussions of mental health or sexuality, and overemphasizing isolated symptoms and diagnoses rather than overall health.

From Reis JP, Breslin ML, Iezzoni LI, Kirschner KL. It takes more than ramps to solve the crisis of healthcare for people with disabilities. *http://www.ric.org/pdf/RIC_whitepaperfinal82704.pdf.* Accessed December 8, 2011.

PROVIDING APPROPRIATE CARE FOR PATIENTS WHO ARE DEAF AND HARD OF HEARING

For the 28 million (1 in 10) Americans who are living with hearing loss, access to appropriate health care is limited primarily by the ability of the health care team to effectively communicate with the patient. A survey of people with varying degrees of hearing loss reveals that they often feel marginalized by their health care providers, that the "medical community holds a pathologic view of deaf people," and using inadequate modes of communication, such as lipreading, writing, or asking family members to interpret, is far too common.[3]

TABLE 50-1 Definitions of Hearing Loss Based on Audiometric Testing

Hearing	Measured Threshold in Decibels (dB)	Ability to Hear
Normal hearing	0-20	Soft whisper
Mild loss	20-40	Soft-spoken voice
Moderate loss	40-60	Normal speech
Severe loss	60-80	Loud-spoken voice
Profound loss*	>80	Shouting

Modified from McPhee SJ, Papadakis MA (eds). Lange's Current Medical Diagnosis and Treatment 2012, 51st ed. New York; McGraw-Hill, 2012.

*Other sources define profound hearing loss as greater than 90 dB, or the ability to hear a jet engine at 1000 feet.

Hearing loss can be defined in many ways. The medical definition of hearing loss is based on audiometric testing and measured in decibels[4] (Table 50-1). In general, a person with a severe hearing loss is unable to hear speech when a person is talking at a normal level and those with a profound hearing loss may only hear very loud sounds.[5] As with other types of physical disabilities, medical professionals view hearing loss as an illness that requires treatment. People with intact hearing tend to think of deafness as a terrible loss. However, many people with hearing loss, particularly those who call themselves Deaf (see following definitions), do not view themselves as ill or having suffered a tragic loss. Indeed, their deafness is as much a part of their identity as one's cultural or ethnic heritage. This distinction is critical in your approach to and appropriate care of patients with hearing loss.

Terms and Definitions

Prelingual deafness: Deafness occurring before the acquisition of spoken language, either congenital or before the age of 2 or 3.

Postlingual deafness: Deafness occurring after the acquisition of spoken language.

Presbycusis: Loss of hearing as part of the aging process. Estimates are as high as 80% of those older than age of 65 as having a hearing loss.

Deaf Culture: A culture is defined by a group of people who share similar beliefs, customs, and language. If American Sign Language is a deaf person's primary language, if he or she attended a school for the deaf, and if he or she seeks opportunities to socialize with other deaf people, then he or she most likely considers himself or herself part of the Deaf Culture. In this section of the text, you will see culturally deaf persons referred to as Deaf (capital "D") and persons who have a severe or profound hearing loss, but do not affiliate with the Deaf Community, as deaf (lower case "d"). This is important in terms of identifying the most appropriate method of communication and therefore ensuring accessible, quality health care for individual patients with hearing loss.

American Sign Language (ASL): A visual-gestural language used by the Deaf Community in the United States. ASL is a true language, as different from English as any other language. It has a distinct word order and grammatical structure. It is NOT a visual representation of English nor is it rudimentary gestures. Signed languages are not universal. As a matter of fact, British Sign Language is practically incomprehensible to Deaf people raised in the United States. There is more similarity between ASL and French Sign Language because the development of ASL was heavily influenced by a Deaf French man, Laurent Clerc, who came to the United States from France to teach deaf children in the late 1800s.

Interpreter: Someone who is fluent in two or more languages and renders messages from one spoken or signed language into another spoken or signed language.

It is important to note the use of the term *interpret* in contrast with the term *translate*, which means to render a message from one written language to another written language and is often incorrectly used when referring to interpreting. ASL interpreters have received special training. Some may have been raised in a Deaf family where ASL was their first language. They should have national or state certification, to ensure competency in the language, knowledge of the interpreting process, and adherence to a professional code of ethics. In some states, sign language interpreting is a licensed profession.

Best Practices

Always ask patients what their preferred mode of communication is: lip-reading and speaking, writing, or using an interpreter. Do not assume that all patients with hearing loss know sign language or are expert lip-readers.

When working with a patient who prefers lip-reading, speak in a normal tone of voice. Do not yell, exaggerate your lip movements, or speak excessively slowly. Maintain eye contact when speaking with your patient. Do not turn away or look down when speaking. Make sure the room is well lit and if at all possible, avoid back lighting, such as standing in front of a bright window. Remember that facial hair may interfere with accurate lip-reading. Do not wear a mask if a patient is relying on lip-reading for communication.

Even the best lip-readers can only understand approximately 30% to 40% of what is actually said on the lips.[6] The rest is educated guess work, gleaned from context and prior experiences. Therefore, it is important to have clear transitions from one topic to another. For example, if you are talking with a patient about his or her medication and then switch the topic suddenly to his or her upcoming surgery, most lip-readers will have difficulty following the conversation at that point. To ensure accuracy, always check for understanding. If something is not clear after one or two repetitions, try rephrasing the information or present it in writing. Do not say "Never mind" or "It's not important." This may be perceived as dismissive or condescending by the patient.

When working with a patient who prefers written communication, you will need to allow extra time for the encounter. Your communication with the patient should be written in short, simple phrases, but do not edit or eliminate information you would provide to any other patient. Avoid abbreviations and medical jargon. Do not assume a patient has fluency in written English. For many Deaf people who use ASL, English is their second language. Feel free to use brochures and patient education materials that are preprinted and readily available. Ask the patient to read any printed materials during the visit so that you can assess understanding. For lengthy visits requiring in-depth patient education (such as a patient newly diagnosed with diabetes), consider using Computer Assisted Real Time captioning (CART or C-Print). This service provides a transcriptionist who has special training and computer software that allows English text to be projected onto a screen as the speaker talks.

Health care facilities (public or private) are required to provide a sign language interpreter for Deaf patients who communicate in ASL. Interpreters can be scheduled through local medical centers or deaf service organizations, and some on-call availability is typical in major metropolitan areas. Interpreter requests should be made as soon as the need becomes known because there is a shortage of qualified interpreters in most communities. There are video relay services available at some locations, allowing immediate access to interpreters any time of the day or night. Not all Deaf people are comfortable with the video relay interpreters because trust plays a critical a role in potentially sensitive situations.

If you need to communicate with your deaf or hard-of-hearing patient by phone, you first need to assess his or her preferred mode of telecommunication. Many deaf people use text messaging or other computer-based communication such as e-mail. Some rely on a telecommunication device for the deaf (TDD or TTY). Your clinic or hospital should be equipped with a TDD, but if it is not, you can use a telephone relay service similar to the video relay mentioned earlier, by dialing 711 in most areas. There is no charge for this service. Some people with hearing loss have phone amplifiers and enough residual hearing to use the telephone directly. Never convey personal medical information through household members who can use the phone, unless you have written permission from the patient.

Challenges

Many health care providers do not know how to access the services of an interpreter. Be proactive. Know the resources in your community and how to locate qualified ASL interpreters.

Patients do not always get sick on our schedule, and they may not be able to tell you their preferred mode of communication; therefore, it is critical to have an on-call list of interpreters for urgent or emergent visits. A sign-language interpreter would have the skills to identify communication styles and recognize the communication needs of patients who are unable to do so. As always, if patients are able to communicate, ask first about their preferences before relying on a companion, family member, or interpreter to identify these needs.

Methods to Ensure Access

If 80% of our diagnoses come from the history, then how important is clear and accurate communication with the patient in our ability to provide appropriate care? Working effectively with interpreters is key to providing good care to patients who do not or cannot use spoken English as a primary means of communication. An interpreter should be someone who has fluency in both languages (the language of the patient and that of the health care worker) and training in the role and ethics of interpreting. Guidance from the federal Department of Health and Human Services Office of Civil Rights makes it clear that a family member or friend should not be relied on to provide objective interpretation. And, unless you are certain of a staff person's fluency and skill in functioning in the interpreter role, it is not advisable to use a staff member who happens to "know some signs" or "took some Spanish classes." Numerous examples (and lawsuits) exist regarding negative health outcomes as a result of using these well-intentioned but unqualified individuals to transmit medical information.

Interpreters have a distinct and limited role in medical settings. The ultimate goal is to allow the patient to function as autonomously and independently as anyone else in a similar situation (see Case Study 50-1). Interpreters are not advocates. They most likely do not know the medical or social history of the patient, nor would it be appropriate for them to share this information if they did know. Although they may periodically provide clarification, especially around cultural norms (this is called "cultural brokering"), it is not the role of an interpreter to explain things beyond what you have told the patient, check for understanding, or ensure appropriate follow-up. That is your job as the provider. The role of the interpreter is to afford individuals who do not share a common language the ability to effectively communicate with one another.

Working with sign language interpreters differs in some subtle ways from working with a spoken language interpreter. Although spoken language interpreters usually prefer to sit so that they can see both you and the patient, sign language interpreters need to sit beside and slightly behind the provider so that the patient can see the interpreter and provider at the same time. This positioning, particularly during history taking, will enhance rapport and improve clarity of communication.

Spoken language interpreters need to interpret consecutively (you speak, then pause and allow the interpreter to repeat what you have said, in the patient's language) because they cannot interpret while you are speaking. Sign language interpreting can, for the most part, be done simultaneously. The interpreter will sign as you are speaking, usually a phrase or two behind you. You should address the patient directly. Do not say, "tell him" or "ask her." Expect pauses in the conversation as the interpreter completes a phrase and receives the patient's response. The patient will respond in his or her native language, and the interpreter will voice the patient's response in the first person. When you hear the interpreter say, "I have a pain in my side," he or she is simply repeating what was said or signed by the patient.

Interpreters may need to periodically ask for clarification of terms or concepts. If this is the case, a professional interpreter will make the request by stating, "The interpreter needs clarification." This allows for distinction in role and clarity for the participants as to who is speaking at any given time.

At times, a hearing sign language interpreter will work in tandem with a Deaf interpreter: someone who is Deaf, a native user of ASL, trained as an interpreter, and familiar with many communication modalities used by a wide range of deaf people. Deaf interpreters are typically needed to communicate with Deaf patients who do not use standard ASL such as those from other countries using that country's sign language, or with Deaf people who have cognitive or physical barriers to using ASL and who rely on idiosyncratic or "home" signs.

Interpreter errors do occur. One study revealed a mean of 31 errors per encounter made by interpreters in medical settings.[7] As you should for any patient with whom you do not share a common language, check with your deaf patient frequently for understanding. As a supplement to your on-site communication through the interpreter or with your lip-reading patients, provide a written copy of critical material (such as medication dosage changes or follow-up instructions) whenever possible. Give complete information regarding new or changed medication orders because there will likely be no interpreter available at the pharmacy.

CASE STUDY 50-1

A Deaf woman was in the emergency department for acute pharyngitis. The sign language interpreter with her that day had worked with this patient before and, as a result, knew a great deal about her medical history, including the fact that she was on oral contraceptive pills (OCPs).

During the visit, as the provider was handing the patient her prescription, the provider asked if the patient was taking any medications. The patient said, "No."

The interpreter repeated and rephrased the question, asking the provider for clarification, making sure the patient understood the importance of the question. The patient persisted in her denial, and the interpreter faithfully interpreted her denial. The appointment ended, and the patient went on her way, a prescription for antibiotics in hand (which can decrease the efficacy of OCPs).

Should the interpreter have disclosed the patient's situation to the provider? Existing Codes of Ethics for medical interpreters support the actions of this interpreter.[8] If the patient and provider did not need an interpreter, the patient would have the right to withhold information. It is the patient's right to choose what information will be shared during the medical visit. This ethical tenet may be violated in situations where the patient's life or the safety of others is in jeopardy.

PROVIDING APPROPRIATE CARE FOR PATIENTS WITH MOBILITY DISABILITIES

As medical professionals, it is our duty to be aware of the challenges faced by millions of individuals with mobility disabilities in accessing proper medical care and to do everything we can to eliminate barriers. First and foremost, our role as physician assistants (PAs) is to improve the health of all patients so that they can live full, productive, and independent lives. However, according to *Healthy People 2020*, patients with severe difficulty walking receive fewer screening and preventive services than their counterparts without mobility disabilities. This lack of screening and prevention, along with inadequate accessibility to services, leads to unnecessary health disparities and poor outcomes (see Case Study 50-2).

Patients with mobility disabilities may rely on wheelchairs and other ambulatory aids as a primary means of mobilization while others may require no assistive devices at all. And although some individuals may only use a device temporarily, many need some form of ambulatory assistance on a permanent basis. Spinal cord injuries, stroke, cerebral palsy, amputations, and a variety of neuromuscular diseases (Huntington disease, muscular dystrophy, and multiple sclerosis, to name a few) are some of the more common reasons that individuals may rely on a wheelchair or ambulatory aid. As a health care provider, you should have a basic understanding of the special needs and complications associated with mobility disabilities.

Terms and Definitions

Spinal cord injury (SCI): Trauma causing damage to a segment of the spinal cord and nerve fibers. The location and degree of damage to the neurologic tissues determine the sensory, motor, and autonomic effect as a result of SCI. Of the 11,000 new cases of SCI per year in the United States, 82% of those injured are men, and the average age is 38 years.

Autonomic dysreflexia (AD): a potentially life-threatening increase in blood pressure, sweating, and other autonomic reflexes in reaction to some type of stimulus below the level of the lesion in a patient with a spinal cord injury. Autonomic dysreflexia occurs in 85% of the people with spinal cord injuries above T6. The elevated blood pressure can lead to renal failure, cardiopulmonary failure, and loss of consciousness, seizures, apnea, stroke, coma, and death.

Spina bifida: This neural tube defect results when the spinal cord, its surrounding nerves, and/or the spinal column develops abnormally during the first 28 days of gestation. It can affect the nervous, urinary, muscular, and skeletal systems, often causing bowel and bladder complications and paralysis below the spinal defect. It has been estimated that approximately 40% of the U.S. population may have spina bifida occulta, with little or no symptoms. The use of prenatal folic acid dietary supplementation has decreased the incidence of spina bifida and other neural tube defects.

Amputation: The surgical or traumatic loss of a limb or digits. There are approximately 1.9 million people living with limb loss in the United States. Each year, the majority of new amputations occur because of complications of the vascular system, especially from diabetes.

Phantom sensations and phantom pain: Sensations such as movement, touch, pressure, itching, posture, and heat and cold can still be felt, although the body part is no longer present. Patients with amputations often feel intense pain that comes from a missing limb, finger, or toe.

A comprehensive description of all conditions causing mobility disabilities, such as cerebral palsy, multiple sclerosis, muscular dystrophy, Huntington disease, and peripheral vascular disease, is beyond the scope of this chapter.

Best Practices

Patients with mobility disabilities should be treated with dignity in all aspects of the health care encounter. It is imperative that your interaction with the patient be respectful, appropriate, and reassuring. In addition to talking to your patient about his or her disability and inherent complications or conditions associated with it, you also need to address the same topics you address with every patient, such as immunizations, risk assessment, and sexual health. Studies show that patients with mobility disabilities suffer from increased morbidity and mortality when providers do not address *all* aspects of their health and well-being.[9]

When introduced to a person with a mobility disability, it is appropriate to offer to shake hands. People with limited hand use or those who wear an artificial limb can usually shake hands. Shaking hands with the left hand may be acceptable depending on the patient's cultural background. For those who cannot shake hands, touch them on the shoulder or arm to welcome them and acknowledge their presence.

It is important to respect the patient's personal space, including wheelchairs and other mobility aids. Avoid propelling the patient's wheelchair, unless asked. Sit across from the patient in a chair for eye-to-eye contact. Do not squat down in front of the patient or stand over them as you converse. This may be perceived as offensive and demeaning by the patient.

If the patient arrives with an assistant or companion, address the patient directly. Do not assume that patients with spasticity, paralysis, or speech difficulties also have an intellectual disability. Most patients with a mobility impairment have normal intelligence and can participate fully in their health care. Provide an opportunity for these patients to speak with you alone. Be aware that all patients with disabilities are at increased risk for abuse and neglect.

Your patients with disabilities are your best resources when it comes to accommodations and assistance they may or may not need. If there are concerns about barriers to performing a comprehensive examination, such as undressing, accessing the examination table, and positioning, ask your patients with movement disabilities for their recommendations to remove these potential barriers. It is important to remember that not all mobility disabilities are the same. Each individual may use mobility devices of different types, transfer in different ways, and have varying levels of physical ability. Working with the patients is the best way to ensure safe, efficient, and accessible health care for all individuals with mobility disabilities.

In order to ensure that the patient with a mobility disability receives equal medical care to that received by a person without a disability, ask the patient to disrobe and perform the examination on the examination table if this is required to provide comprehensive, appropriate care. Ask if assistance is necessary with transfers and dressing/undressing, and be aware that offering assistance with these tasks may require additional time or the assistance of another individual. Never leave the patient unattended unless he or she asks to be left alone. You should be alert to the potential for fainting due to a gravitational pooling of blood when transferring the patient. Seek out rehabilitation specialists in your community for training and assistance. Ask the patient which positions are most comfortable during the examination, and ask if assistance is necessary before giving it. Examination tables with varying height capabilities, back supports, and whole-leg rests are available.[10] If your employer does not have an accessible examination table, you may want to discuss its value with the providers in your practice. An accessible table will benefit more than just your patients who use wheelchairs. Many patients, including elders with arthritis and women in the last months of pregnancy, will appreciate a table that lowers and allows them to sit upright.

Ensure that the patient is positioned comfortably if he or she is going to be sitting or lying still for an extended period of time. Pillows or pads may have to be adjusted between legs and wedged against the patient to decrease discomfort and reduce the risk of developing pressure sores. Those patients with spasticity problems may need assistance holding still during procedures or examinations.

A complete examination should always include a sexual history. The sexual history is often neglected due to assumptions that people with limited mobility or paralysis cannot or do not have intimate relationships. These patients are still competent to maintain emotional and sexual relationships. The health care provider should perform the same inquiry for a patient with a mobility disability as he or she would for any other patient. It is also important to acknowledge the patient's needs, desires, anxieties, and questions pertaining to sexuality.

When examining a patient with a mobility disability, it is critical to perform a comprehensive visual inspection of the skin to assess for pressure sores and open wounds. Provide appropriate annual health promotion and disease prevention screenings, such as Pap smears, mammography, prostate and rectal examinations, and oral health examinations for all patients.

Challenges

Be cautious not to attribute all symptoms to an individual's primary disability. As with any patient, patients with disabilities can present with heart disease, gastroenteritis, and migraines—all unrelated to their particular disabling condition. Do not let a patient's disability keep you from developing a comprehensive differential diagnosis list when assessing a patient's problem. Although aging with a disability may be somewhat of an uncharted subject, the underlying cause for unusual symptoms should always be pursued.

Careful medical management and skilled supportive care are necessary to prevent complications in the patient with a mobility disability. Functional goals are defined as realistic expectations of activities that individuals with mobility disabilities eventually should be able to perform. It is important to continue with long-term physical therapy treatments to attempt to improve or maintain gross-motor skills and help prevent problems, such as muscle contractures and loss of strength.

Certain health issues must be followed closely to prevent complications in patients with mobility disabilities. Difficulties such as urinary tract infections, pressure sores, and autonomic dysreflexia could become life-threatening if not treated properly and promptly. Common serious challenges faced by these individuals include exaggerated reflexes, impaired cardiovascular function, loss of bladder and bowel control, loss of normal thermoregulation, lost or decreased breathing capacity; impaired cough reflexes, and muscle spasticity.

Autonomic dysreflexia (AD) is considered a medical emergency for the patient with a spinal cord injury. The patient may become frightened during an AD episode. You must remain calm and at the same time react quickly. It is critical to lower the patient's blood pressure as quickly as possible. This may be accomplished by raising the head of the examination table as high as possible. Sitting the patient straight up is best. Lower the legs, and remove any abdominal binders and compression hose. You must remove or correct any potential stimulus, such as a vaginal speculum. Methods to prevent AD include performing a bowel program and catheterizations on a regular schedule, checking and emptying indwelling catheter leg bags often, changing catheters every 4 weeks to prevent any clogging, checking for pressure sores regularly, and maintaining good toenail hygiene to prevent ingrown toenails because any of these may trigger an episode of AD. It is important to educate the patient and caregivers about AD and the possible associated complications.

Methods to Ensure Access

Patients with mobility disabilities may find it difficult to access health care services primarily because of problems with physical accommodations. From parking to being able to get onto an examination table, people with mobility disabilities are faced with many obstacles at medical facilities. Consequently, these patients are less likely to seek out and receive health services. As a health care provider, you can make a real difference in promoting the health of a population that is typically underserved. It is important to provide access to examination areas with wheelchair and other specialty orthopedic devices. Ask patients if they require assistance, and be respectful of their wishes.

Access to specialized medical services is often limited and could put the patient's health in jeopardy. The PA should make efforts to work closely with vocational rehabilitation, medical rehabilitation centers, and other agencies that could potentially influence the quality of the lives of patients with mobility disabilities.

When referring a patient for routine screening or specialty care, it is important to ensure there is accessible parking, including wheelchair van parking, which should include adequate space for a lift or ramp to deploy. Ensure that there is an accessible entrance to the facility and that it is clearly marked. Check to see if your local radiology service has an accessible mammogram machine and can accommodate patients in wheelchairs. When prescribing medication, ensure that the pharmacy can supply medication in easy-to-open containers that are accessible to individuals with hand disabilities. Office and medical staff should be educated to be respectful and to assume that a patient who is also a wheelchair user is potentially fully employed, competent, and knowledgeable about self-care.

For more information about providing accessible care to patients with limited mobility, the U.S. Department of Health and Human Services in collaboration with the Department of Justice has produced an excellent guide for clinics and hospitals. This guide, titled *Access to Medical Care for Individuals with Mobility Disabilities*, can be viewed at *http://www.ada.gov/medcare_ta.htm.*

CASE STUDY 50-2

A 49-year-old C5 quadriplegic female presented to the emergency department (ED) with a chief complaint of fever, chills, increased spasticity, hypertension, headache, and malaise. She had an ileal conduit and a colostomy bag. Her caregiver stated that she noticed an increased foul smell to her urine in the past several days. The ED staff decided to put her on an antibiotic and send her home. Three days later her symptoms progressively worsened.

The patient again reported to the ED with a fever and worsening symptoms. Urine cultures and blood cultures were ordered, and she was admitted for observation. The urine cultures grew out *Staphylococcus aureus* and *Clostridium difficile,* and the blood cultures showed methicillin-resistant *Staphylococcus aureus* (MRSA). The patient's health quickly deteriorated, and she had to be intubated for respiratory failure.

She recovered but continued to complain of severe leg spasms and headache. The patient's astute PA noticed a large abrasion and hematoma on the patient's lower leg and ordered a radiograph, which confirmed a healing nondisplaced fracture of the tibia. Once the fracture was stabilized, the hypertension, headaches, and spasms dissipated. In hindsight, it is thought that she was experiencing autonomic dysreflexia (AD) as a result of the fracture. If appropriate care had been provided immediately and a complete physical exam had been performed, this would have been observed and diagnosed earlier. The urinary tract infection (UTI) and subsequent septicemia do not justify the elimination of a complete physical exam.

CASE STUDY 50-3

For 18 years, a patient with quadriplegia urged his primary care clinic to obtain an adjustable examination table and for 18 years the clinic refused. He frequently underwent cursory examinations while seated in his wheelchair. It was not until he was hospitalized with an infected pressure ulcer and a successful ADA lawsuit was filed against the clinic that steps were taken to improve access for patients with mobility disabilities.[9] This story illustrates the need to look at our existing facilities and their accessibility BEFORE patients suffer from adverse outcomes.

PROVIDING APPROPRIATE CARE FOR PATIENTS WITH VISUAL IMPAIRMENTS

Approximately 10 million individuals who are blind or visually impaired live in the United States.[11] Approximately half of these individuals are elders, and although the vast majority of people living with visual loss lead active and productive lives, unemployment statistics range from 50% to 75% for visually impaired adults. For people with visual loss, the biggest obstacle to improved quality of life, including access to appropriate health care, is overcoming assumptions and stereotypes regarding their abilities and challenges.

Terms and Definitions

Visual impairment: Any vision problem that is severe enough to affect an individual's ability to carry out the activities of daily living. This may include people with low vision and those with no vision at all.

Legal blindness: A level of visual impairment that has been defined by law to determine eligibility for benefits. It refers to central visual acuity of 20/200 or less in the better eye with the best possible correction, as measured on the Snellen vision chart, or a visual field of 20 degrees or less.

Total or profound blindness: Absence of vision or the ability to determine only the existence, not the source, of light (also called *light perception*).

Braille: A tactile code system of raised dots in specific patterns, representing printed letters and words, which is used by some visually impaired individuals. If you have materials available in Braille, ask your patient if Braille is preferred before offering them.

Dog guide: Assistance dogs trained to lead people with visual impairments around obstacles. Not all people with visual impairments use canes or dog guides. The use of dog guides and canes for mobility depends on personal preference and the individual's travel skills. The presence or absence of a cane or dog guide does not indicate the level of assistance a person might require to navigate a hallway or hospital room. The best way to find out if assistance is needed is to ask.

Sighted-guide technique: A specific technique for providing mobility assistance to a person with a visual impairment. If a person with a visual impairment accepts your offer of guidance, this technique should always be used. First, stand one step ahead of the person you are guiding. Tap the back of your hand against his or her hand. The person will grasp your arm directly above the elbow. Relax and walk at a comfortable, normal pace, always staying one step ahead of the person you are guiding. Pause when there is a change in terrain, such as a curb or set of stairs. Verbal cues are not necessary but may be helpful. Never walk away from the person you are guiding without warning or explanation. To guide the person to a seat, place the hand of your guiding arm on the back of the seat and the person you are guiding will be able to find the seat.

Patients with visual impairment (VI) often receive less than optimal care because of assumptions made by health care providers.

I think it is really important that they know that most VI patients with diabetes can learn to measure insulin and monitor blood sugar and use a pump, so they don't just put them on the simplest routines and not the one that will give them the best management.

A diabetic patient with visual loss

From the IRIS Network: Association for Education and Rehabilitation of the Blind and Visually Impaired (website). *http://aerbvi.org/modules.php?name=Content&pa=showpage&pid=1.* Accessed May 17, 2007.

Best Practices

Most people with a visual impairment do not have hearing impairments or intellectual disabilities. Speak in a normal tone of voice and communicate directly with the patient.

Relax. It is okay to say things like "I see" or "it looks like." Sighted references used in everyday conversation will not be offensive to your patients with visual impairment.

Introduce yourself by name and function, and state the reason you are there. Every time you enter the room of a person with a visual impairment, state who you are, even if you only left the room for a brief time. Be sure others do the same. Stay in one place when addressing the patient. It is difficult to face someone who is moving constantly. Let the patient know when you move from one place to another and describe what you are doing (i.e., setting up for a procedure). It is disconcerting to hear drawers being opened and closed, instruments clanging, and wheels rolling across the floor when you do not know what is happening.

Most patients will not need assistance when changing, but do not forget to orient the patient to the room and the location of the gown. Be specific with directions, saying to your right, your left, or directly in front of you. Ask the patient if he or she needs assistance moving from chair to examination table. Guide patients using the sighted-guide technique described earlier, and make the patient aware if the step is pulled out before guiding him or her to the examination table. Always let the patient know when you are about to touch him or her for any reason, but particularly for the different components of the physical examination.

Residual sight is critical to patients with any degree of visual impairment. Routine eye examinations should be arranged. Changes in vision or new onset of eye symptoms may create tremendous anxiety and should be given your full concern and attention.

Challenges

There is a tremendous variety of residual sight in the visually impaired population. Some people can only see objects in the central field of vision (due to peripheral visual field deficits caused by glaucoma or retinitis pigmentosa), and others can only see at the periphery (as in macular degeneration). Some have only light perception, yet others can read a bold, 18-point font print with eyeglasses.

The patient's ability to use residual sight is greatly affected by lighting conditions and contrast. A patient may have difficulty navigating a dimly lit x-ray room or finding an examination table covered with white paper in a room painted white but has little or no trouble locating a dark blue chair on a white tile floor in the well-lit waiting room.

Methods to Ensure Access

Do not eliminate or abbreviate your history and physical examination. Include your usual patient education discussions, even if the health maintenance you are recommending requires sight. For example, if you want your patient to collect stool samples for guaiac testing, describe the process for collecting a specimen, let the patient handle the materials used, and confirm that the patient will be able to follow through with the collection. Your patients with disabilities often have the best suggestions for modifications and accommodations that will allow them to participate in self-care.

Ask your patients how they prefer to receive their patient education materials. Some may request material in Braille, some may prefer a particular font style, and yet others may prefer to record your instructions on a handheld tape recorder. It is helpful to have a preprinted sheet of paper with a variety of font styles and sizes (Times New Roman and Arial are typically preferred) in bold and normal print. This will allow your patients to choose the style they are best able to read. Transferring your patient education materials to a Word Document format will ensure accessibility for a majority of your patients with visual impairments.

CASE STUDY 50-4

An elderly woman with macular degeneration was brought to the emergency department (ED) after passing out in the grocery store. She was found to be severely anemic.

The patient had recently seen her primary care provider for symptoms of "diarrhea and fatigue." As a result of her syncopal episode and visit to the ED, a comprehensive history and thorough workup were pursued. Rectal bleeding was eventually revealed to be the source of her anemia.

It was not until this patient presented urgently to the ED that it became clear that what she had described as simple "diarrhea" was actually a much more serious symptom. It is important to be sensitive to these types of symptoms (those that rely on sight) in low-vision patients. Further investigation might be necessary in your visually impaired patients to avoid situations like the one described.

PROVIDING APPROPRIATE CARE FOR PATIENTS WITH INTELLECTUAL AND DEVELOPMENTAL DISABILITIES

In 2002 the U.S. Surgeon General issued the National Blueprint for Improving the Health of Persons with Mental Retardation (MR). Upon introduction of this Blueprint, the Surgeon General noted that, "Compared with other populations, adults, adolescents, and children with mental retardation experience poorer health and more difficulty in finding, getting to, and paying for appropriate health care." The Blueprint outlines a broad set of goals for improving the health of persons with intellectual and developmental disabilities, which includes improved training of health care providers. The Blueprint states, "The number one issue is lack of training to support healthy lifestyles for individuals with MR across the lifespan" and notes that didactic and clinical training of all health care providers is critical in meeting the goals of improved health.[12] According to the Declaration on Health Parity for Persons with Intellectual and Developmental Disabilities, "Health services for persons with intellectual and developmental disabilities often continue to be discriminatory, inappropriate, inefficient, uninformed, and insufficient" (see Case Study 50-5).[13]

Terms and Definitions

Mental retardation: Although this term has been around for decades, its pejorative use and negative connotation has led to a change in its acceptance and use by those in the field of intellectual and developmental disabilities. The best example of this is the recent name change of the American Association on Mental Retardation (AAMR), a 130-year-old association representing developmental disability professionals, clients, and their families nationwide. In November 2006, the AAMR announced its new name; the American Association on Intellectual and Developmental Disabilities.[14] With this in mind, throughout the remainder of this section, this population will be referred to as patients with intellectual and developmental disabilities.

Intellectual and developmental disability: A developmental disability is not a mental disorder. It is a disability that originates before the age of 18 and is characterized by limitations both in intellectual functioning and in adaptive behavior. Diagnosis is often based on an IQ test score of approximately 70 or below. An intellectual disability may be developmental or acquired. An acquired intellectual disability may be the result of a traumatic brain injury or stroke, for example. The functional abilities of the person with an intellectual or developmental disability can be positively affected by early intervention and individualized supports.

Autism spectrum disorders (ASDs): Previously called pervasive developmental disorders. A constellation of symptoms, which include a varying degree of impaired communication, difficulty with social interactions, and restricted, repetitive, and stereotyped patterns of behavior, are often seen. Although these disorders can be reliably detected by age 3 and, in some cases, as early as 18 months, it is estimated that only 50% are diagnosed before kindergarten. This has a profound impact on functioning because at least 2 years of early intervention has been shown to benefit long-term functional abilities in children with ASD. Many, but not all, people with ASD have some degree of intellectual disability, and one in four have a seizure disorder.[15]

Down syndrome: A chromosomal anomaly that occurs in 1 out of every 733 live births, which causes developmental delay and is associated with a number of physical conditions. In addition to intellectual disabilities, children with Down syndrome may have congenital heart defects, thyroid disease, and blood and nervous system disorders. Until the past few decades, the average age of survival for a person with Down syndrome was only 19 or 20. With recent advancements in clinical treatment, up to 80% of adults with Down syndrome reach age 55, and many live even longer. People with Down syndrome are at much greater risk for developing Alzheimer disease than the general population.[16]

Traumatic brain injury (TBI): A blow or jolt to the head, or a penetrating head injury that disrupts the function of the brain. Severity ranges from "mild" (brief change in mental status) to "severe," resulting in long-term problems with independent function. Recent data show that approximately 1.7 million people sustain a traumatic brain injury annually.[17] Depending on the severity of the injury, functional limitations may include memory problems, difficulty with problem solving, managing emotions, and vocational skills.

Best Practices

Because of the great variety in functional ability, it is critical that you know your patients with intellectual and developmental disabilities. Taking the time to assess their communication, level of understanding, and ability to follow through in self-care will greatly increase your ability to provide appropriate care for these patients across the life span.

Even if the patient arrives with a caregiver (often staff or family member), engage the patient in the history taking, examination, and patient education process as much as possible. Begin with the assumption that the patient can participate in his or her care. As is the case with all patients with disabilities, if you are unsure, ask. When needed, check with caregivers or review available documentation to ensure accuracy, but do not assume that staff members are familiar with any given patient's medical history.[18]

Many people with intellectual and developmental disabilities are literal, concrete thinkers. Therefore, keep your communication simple and straightforward, without being condescending or "talking down" to the patient. Avoid questions or instructions that require multitasking. If something requires several steps, ask the patient to complete one step before moving on to the next. Be thorough and inclusive. Discuss sexual health, and assess for smoking, as well as drug and alcohol use, when appropriate.

Perform a comprehensive physical examination when appropriate. Take the time to explain what you will be doing, and answer any questions before you begin the examination. Visuals can be helpful. Make sure you schedule adequate time for the more sensitive examinations like breast and pelvic. Because people with intellectual and developmental disabilities are vulnerable to sexual abuse, these examinations should be approached with great sensitivity, and any reaction that makes you concerned about abuse should be thoroughly explored. There are times when mild, conscious sedation may be necessary to accomplish an examination or procedure, but this should only be done if absolutely necessary to prevent pain and suffering on the part of the patient and not for the convenience of the providers or staff.

When discussing patient instructions or follow-up, give thorough explanations and always check for understanding. Simple written instructions should be provided. Ask the patient if he or she has any questions.

You should not hesitate to refer all patients for any recommended or required diagnostic screening. Routine health promotion and disease prevention should be provided to patients with intellectual and developmental disabilities, and as life expectancy continues to increase, more of these patients will be in need of screening examinations such as mammograms and colonoscopy. Good communication with your patient, caregivers, and other health care providers will ensure that these patients will be able to successfully participate in any necessary testing. When obtaining consent for testing or procedures, you need to ask about guardianship. Many patients with intellectual and developmental disabilities are their own guardians and can consent independently.[18]

Challenges

Assessing your patient's ability to participate in his or her own health care takes time and patience. You will need to work with your facility, supervising physicians, and support staff to ensure quality and continuity of care for your patients with intellectual and developmental disabilities. As much as possible, these patients should be given the opportunity to make choices and experience self-determination in areas that affect their health.

Preventive health screening and education regarding lifestyle modification should be undertaken with all patients, regardless of intellectual ability. You will need to get to know the auxiliary health services and providers in your area who are skilled in providing appropriate care for this population.

Methods to Ensure Access

A multidisciplinary approach and the enlistment of the assistance of experts in the field will ensure that your patients with intellectual and developmental disabilities get the best, most comprehensive care. Recommended by *Healthy People 2020*, a "medical home," defined as "a health professional who provides comprehensive, culturally sensitive, coordinated, continuous, family-centered, and accessible care," will ensure the provision of coordinated care across multiple providers and service systems, thereby improving access and outcomes.[19]

CASE STUDY 50-5

After several visits to his primary care provider for fever and rash, a 21-year-old man with a developmental disability was finally diagnosed with bacterial endocarditis. By the time he arrived at the hospital, he was suffering from bacteremia and shock. Before initiating any treatment, the providers responsible for his care in the hospital approached his parents and asked if "everything possible should be done." Horrified, they responded, "Of course!"

Before he fell ill, this young man was attending college classes, working part-time, and participating in an active social life through a local service organization. To insinuate that a patient with a developmental disability deserves anything less than comprehensive, aggressive treatment of a life-threatening illness is inexcusable and constitutes illegal discrimination.

CLINICAL APPLICATIONS

1. What experiences or encounters have you had with people with disabilities? How are people with disabilities portrayed in the media (movies, television)? How have these experiences and portrayals shaped your attitudes and opinions toward people with disabilities?
2. Seek out individuals with various disabilities and interview them regarding their challenges in obtaining appropriate, comprehensive health care services. Ask them about good and bad experiences they have had when interacting with health care professionals and the health care system.
3. As a community service project with your classmates, offer to speak to local groups that provide support and services for people with disabilities about the PA profession and general health topics such as diet and exercise or cancer screening.

KEY POINTS

1. Speak directly to the patient. If the patient has an assistant or companion in attendance, do not assume that the patient cannot answer his or her own questions. Listen attentively to your patients with disabilities to understand their background and individual functional needs. The patient is often your best source of information about his or her disability.
2. Avoid stereotyping your patients. Do not make assumptions about anything (cognitive function, relationships, sexual activity).
3. Become aware of the barriers to care that exist for your patients with disabilities and work to eliminate these barriers. Advanced access planning in the clinic can save time and improve quality of care. Check accessibility when referring patients to diagnostic testing and specialty clinics.

4. Treat every patient equally, providing the same services to patients with disabilities as you do to those without one. Do not take short cuts. Do not eliminate information or services you would provide to any other patient.
5. Focus on the patients' overall health and well-being, not just the disabling condition. Defining "health" as the absence of disability or chronic illness negatively affects people with disabilities. Most lead active, fulfilling lives that may include school, sports, work, community involvement, relationships, and parenting.

References

1. Center of Assistive Technology. Cornucopia of Disability Information: Disability Statistics (website), *http://codi.buffalo.edu/graph_based/demographics/.statistics.htm*; Accessed December 8, 2011.
2. Kennedy C, Salsberry P, Nickel J, et al. The burden of disease in those with serious mental and physical illness. J Am Psychiatr Nurse Assoc 2005;11(1):45–51.
3. Iezzoni LI, O'Day BL, Killeen M, Harker H. Communicating about health care: observations from persons who are deaf or hard of hearing. Ann Intern Med 2004;140(5):356–362.
4. McPhee SJ, Papadakis MA (eds). Lange's Current Medical Diagnosis and Treatment 2012. 51st ed. New York: McGraw-Hill, 2012.
5. Center for Disease Control. Hearing Loss in Children, Types of Hearing Loss (website), *http://www.cdc.gov/NCBDDD/hearingloss/types.html*; Accessed December 8, 2011.
6. Steinberg AG, Barnett S, Meador HE, et al. Health care system accessibility: experiences and perceptions of deaf people. J Gen Intern Med 2006;21(3):260–266.
7. Flores G, Laws MD, Mayo SJ, et al. Errors in medical interpretation and their potential clinical consequences in pediatric encounters. Pediatrics 2003;111(6 Pt 1):1495–1497.
8. The National Council on Interpreting in Health Care. A National Code of Ethics for Interpreters in Health Care (July 2004) and National Standards of Practice for Interpreters in Health Care (September 2005) (website), *www.ncihc.org*; Accessed December 8, 2011.
9. Reis JP, Breslin ML, Iezzoni LI, Kirschner KL. It takes more than ramps to solve the crisis of healthcare for people with disabilities; *http://www.ric.org/pdf/RIC_whitepaperfinal82704.pdf*; Accessed December 8, 2011.
10. Center for Disability Issues in the Health Professions, Western University of Health Sciences. The Importance of Accessible Examination Tables, Chairs and Weight Scales (website), *http://www.cdihp.org/products.html#tables*; Accessed December 8, 2011.
11. American Foundation for the Blind. Blindness Statistics (website), *http://www.afb.org/Section.asp?SectionID=15*; Accessed December 8, 2011.
12. National Library of Medicine. Closing the Gap: A National Blueprint for Improving the Health of Persons with Mental Retardation (website), *http://www.ncbi.nlm.nih.gov/books/NBK44346/*; Accessed December 8, 2011.
13. American Association on Mental Retardation. The Declaration on Health Parity for Persons with Intellectual and Developmental Disabilities (website), *http://www.aaidd.org/content_25.cfm*; Accessed December 8, 2011.
14. American Association on Mental Retardation. World's Oldest Organization on Intellectual Disability Has a Progressive New Name [November 2, 2006] (website), *http://www.aamr.org/content_1314.cfm*; Accessed December 8, 2011.
15. National Institute of Mental Health. Autism Spectrum Disorders (website), *http://www.nimh.nih.gov/health/topics/autism-spectrum-disorders-pervasive-developmental-disorders/index.shtml*; Accessed December 8, 2011.
16. National Down Syndrome Society. General Information (website), *http://www.ndss.org/index.php?option=com_content&view=article&id=172%3Athe-health-of-adults-with-down-syndrome&catid=60%3Aassociated-conditions&Itemid=88&limitstart=1*; Accessed December 8, 2011.
17. Faul M, Xu L, Wald MM, Coronado VG. Traumatic brain injury in the United States: emergency department visits, hospitalizations, and deaths. Atlanta (GA): Centers for Disease Control and Prevention, National Center for Injury Prevention and Control, 2010.
18. The staff and students of STRIVE U. Focus group conducted by author; December 19, 2006.
19. Krauss MW, Gulley S, Sciegaj M, Wells N. Access to specialty medical care for children with mental retardation, autism, and other special health care needs. Mental Retardation 2003;41(5):329–339.

The resources for this chapter can be found at the www.expertconsult.com.

CHAPTER 51

END-OF-LIFE ISSUES

Barbara Coombs Lee

You matter because you are you.... You matter to the last moment of your life, and we will do all we can, not only to help you die peacefully but also to live until you die.

—Dame Cicely Saunders

CHAPTER CONTENTS

This chapter is designed to serve as an introduction to some of the issues that may be encountered when working with terminally ill patients. It offers a broad perspective on topics commonly encountered as patients begin to prepare for the end of their lives.

Medical decisions are simple throughout most of one's life. When you are young, you get vaccinations. When you have an infection, you take an antibiotic. When you have a cold, you rest. But as multiple medical problems develop, the situation becomes more complex. With the advent of modern medicine, many patients now face treatment options that offer little or no benefit. The treatments may be painful, and they may be burdensome to both the patient and his or her caregiver. There comes a time when the patient or family must weigh the benefits of a treatment against the burdens because the goals of care shift as the patient's condition changes.

We live in a society that attempts to deny death. No one wants to admit he or she, too, will die someday. Although we know everything is impermanent, we want permanence; we expect permanence. Our natural tendency is to seek security. We do not like change. We do not like that our bodies change shape. We do not like that we age. We are afraid of wrinkles. And most notably, we are afraid of the unknown death brings.

TRUTH-TELLING

Medicine is a moral enterprise grounded in a covenant of trust. Historically, patients innately trusted their health care providers (HCPs) to act in their best interests and did as they were told. Once medicine began to move away from such a paternalistic approach, patients were faced with a new dilemma. Were HCPs divulging the full story, or just enough information to prompt the patient to act as the HCP desired? Medicine cannot be a public-service calling without the virtues of humility, honesty, intellectual integrity, compassion, and effacement of excessive self-interest.[1]

One of the central issues in end-of-life care is the controversy over what the terminally ill patient should be told about his diagnosis and prognosis. In the Hippocratic tradition, the standard of practice in many cultures has been to refrain from telling patients about their impending death. This approach has been used in Japan, Eastern Europe, and many Latin American countries.[2]

In 1961, a survey examined physicians' attitudes toward disclosing a cancer diagnosis to their patients. Eighty-eight percent of respondents usually followed a policy of *nondisclosure*. The same study, repeated in 1979, showed that 98% of physicians now usually followed a policy of *disclosure*.[3] During this period, paternalism gave way to patient self-determination. The HCP no longer had final say in the patient's care; rather, it was the patient himself or herself, now operating on principles of autonomy and informed consent. Improvements in cancer treatment options, improved survival rates, fear of malpractice suits, altered social attitudes about cancer, and the increased recognition of communication as an effective means of enhancing patients' understanding and compliance also aided this shift in disclosure practices.[4]

There may be times when cautious or limited disclosures are necessary. But to maintain trust, the whole truth should be divulged in a manner appropriate to the patient's circumstances. Information about a serious illness or impending death should be shared or offered to patients, even if they do not specifically request the information. Patients have legal and moral rights that must be respected. The question must no longer be, "Should we tell?" but rather, "How do we share this information with the patient?"[5]

HELPING PATIENTS MAKE INFORMED DECISIONS

Focus. End-of-life care should focus on the patient's life and current experience. Too often death is seen as a failure of treatment, not a natural event. This deprives patients of the opportunity to enter what Kübler-Ross calls "the final stage of growth." Too often physicians either withdraw from patients in the terminal stage of illness or encourage them to continue intensive therapies and not "give up."

Self-determination. Individuals vary in their tolerance for pain and suffering. Only patients can determine whether they are suffering, or are suffering too much. They should receive state-of-the-art comfort care accordingly. Providers should prescribe opioid analgesics generously for pain and breathlessness. Patients should control the dose and frequency of administration. Symptoms such as hiccups, nausea, diarrhea, itching, and fatigue can be oppressive and should not be disregarded.

Autonomy. Decisions about end-of-life care begin and end with the autonomous patient. The answer to the questions "who should decide?" is "the patient decides." Even very ill patients usually retain decisional capacity. Loved ones and providers should avoid inadvertently usurping decisions when communication becomes difficult. If a patient is no longer capable of decision making, their known wishes still dictate decisions.

Personal Beliefs. Patients should feel empowered to make decisions based on their own deeply held values and beliefs, without fear of moral condemnation or political interference. Law and policy should not place the provider's moral beliefs above the patient's or protect providers who withhold vital information about treatment options. Dying patients should not be subject to subtle or overt suggestions that their choices are wrong or immoral.

Informed Consent. Patients must have comprehensive, candid information in order to make valid decisions and give informed consent. Patients should receive encouragement to exercise a "BRAIN" process assessing the:

- Benefits,
- Risks,
- Alternatives, their own
- Insight into what these mean to them,
- And consequences of doing Nothing, before giving consent to procedures and treatment.

Four crucial questions often go unasked or incompletely answered when a patient consents to disease-specific treatment:

- What is the chance it will prolong my life?
- By how much?
- What are the side effects?
- What are the alternatives?

Providers should never withhold information about legal alternatives. This deprives the patient of crucial information to give informed consent.

Balance. Patients should feel empowered to make decisions on the basis of their own assessment and the balance between quantity and quality of life. Patients may reject treatment because of unacceptable side effects.

Saying "no" to burdensome treatment may mean saying "yes" to the joyful experience of life for as long as possible.

PLANNING FOR DEATH

In 2010 (the most current information available at this writing), 2,437,163 people died in the United States.[6] Death can occur unannounced at any given moment. Although most of us will live well into our 70s, 80s, and even 90s, finally succumbing to heart disease, cancer, or stroke,[7] not all of us share this fate. Karen Ann Quinlan was only 21 years old when she suffered cardiopulmonary arrest and fell into a persistent vegetative state. In *In the Matter of Quinlan*, the Supreme Court of New Jersey ruled that her family could remove her from a ventilator. This landmark ruling led to the requirement of ethics committees in medical institutions and to the creation of advance directives.[8] Nancy Cruzan was only 25 years old when she fell into a persistent vegetative state after being involved in a car accident. In its landmark decision, the Supreme Court of the United States paved the path for surrogate decision-making in the removal of artificial nutrition and hydration.[9] Terri Schiavo was 26 years old when her heart stopped. She, too, fell into a persistent vegetative state and, in 2005, became one of the more than 300,000 Americans withdrawn from artificial food and fluids.[10] The sagas of these three young women illustrate the importance of planning.

When thinking about the end of life, personal values about quality of life need to be considered. What makes living meaningful must be carefully weighed. Urge patients to talk with loved ones about their views and to choose someone to speak for them, should they become unable to speak for themselves.

A patient's right to refuse medical intervention has become well-established in medical practice. Patients and families of incompetent patients routinely choose to stop or not start ventilators, artificial nutrition and hydration, and antibiotics. Patients voluntarily stop eating and drinking (VSED). Do not resuscitate orders (DNRs) are being replaced with orders to Allow Natural Death (AND). Either one can prevent the distress that attempts at cardiopulmonary resuscitation (CPR) can bring. Others elect for palliative or terminal sedation.

The purpose of completing end-of-life documents is to make intentional decisions and express them in writing. Completed documents, discussed and shared with family and friends, lay the foundation for rational decision-making at the end of life.

EMERGING ISSUES

Sectarian Health Care Directives. Some religiously affiliated health care institutions may decline to honor expressed health care choices that conflict with their doctrine and beliefs. A sectarian health care directive[11] specifically indicates admission to such a facility does not imply consent to particular care mandated by its ethical, religious, or other policies. If the facility declines to follow the preferences in an advance directive, it outlines that the patient be transferred to a hospital, nursing home, or other institution that will agree to honor the instructions set forth in the directive.

Lesbian, Gay, Bisexual, Transgender (LGBT) Families. The LGBT community faces additional challenges at the end of life. Until recently, the partners of LGBT patients were routinely not allowed to participate in the medical treatment of their loved ones or even visit them in the hospital. Varying degrees of legal partnership and marital status still exist in the United States for same-sex couples, yet few in this community have advance directives or understand the potential need for a Hospital Visitation Authorization.[12] Lambda Legal (lambdalegal.org) has a comprehensive state-by-state listing of the nationwide status for same-sex couples.

ADVANCE DIRECTIVES

Every adult needs an advance directive for health care (AD). Regardless of age and health status, none of us knows when an event might leave us unable to speak for ourselves. If patients are not able to make or communicate decisions about medical treatment, a written record of their health care wishes is invaluable.

Advance directive is a generic term used for documents that traditionally include a living will and the appointment of a health care agent. These documents allow individuals to provide instructions relating to their future health care, such as when they want to receive medical treatment or when they want to stop or refuse life-sustaining medical treatments.

The living will portion of an AD allows the patient to specify which kinds of treatment and care are desired if he or she were unable to speak for himself or herself. The second part, often referred to as the *durable power of attorney for health care*, allows the appointment of someone to act on the patient's behalf in matters concerning his or her health care when the patient is unable to speak for himself or herself due to illness or incapacitation. Please note that the person appointed to speak on behalf of the patient may be called a *health care agent*, *proxy*, *surrogate*, or *representative*.

An AD allows patients to express their wishes about any aspect of their health care, including decisions regarding life-sustaining treatments. Remember, it can include treatments and procedures a patient *does or does not* want. Statements regarding organ and tissue donation may also be included. The instructions provided in this portion of the form serve as evidence of the patient's wishes.

The durable power of attorney portion of an AD allows the appointment of an agent to speak on behalf of the patient and communicate his or her wishes when the patient is not able to do so. Appointing an agent and making sure the agent is aware of and understands the wishes is one of the most important things that can be done. If the time comes for a decision to be made, the agent can participate in relevant discussions, weighing the pros and cons of treatment decisions on the basis of the patient's previously expressed wishes. The agent can act on behalf of a patient even when decision-making capacity is only temporarily affected. The degree of authority (how much or how little) the patient wants his agent to have can be defined in this document. Alternate agents can also be appointed, in case the primary agent is unwilling or unable to act. Additionally, the patient may name specific individuals who are NOT to participate in decision-making. If an agent is not appointed, the law in most states provides for other decision-makers by default, usually beginning with the spouse and adult children and ending with the patient's physician. When physicians tend to err on the side of prolonging life, their decisions may not be consistent with the patient's desires. In some cases, if the patient does not have an AD, a court may be required to appoint a guardian.

ADs ease the burden of family members. They help relieve the stress and doubt associated with having to make important health care decisions on behalf of someone you care about, but without clear instruction. By making wishes known in advance, patients can help guide their families and friends, who may otherwise struggle to decide the best course.

Advance directives are legally valid in every state. Each state and the District of Columbia have laws that permit individuals to sign documents stating their health care decisions when they cannot speak for themselves. The specifics of these laws vary, but the basic principle of listening to the patient's wishes is the same everywhere. The law gives great weight to any form of written directive. If the courts become involved, they usually attempt to follow the patient's stated values and preferences, especially if they are in written form. An AD may be the most concrete evidence of wishes possible. It is important to note that although it is legal to have an AD in every state, states vary in the degree to which they require adherence to the directive. Most states offer legal protection to HCPs for following, or deciding not to follow, the instructions contained in an AD.

An AD can be changed or cancelled at any time. This can be accomplished by notifying the agent and/or HCP, in writing, of the decision to do so. It is best to destroy all copies of the old AD and create a new one. Make sure to provide copies of the new form to the appropriate individuals. It is strongly recommended to review ADs every year and re-sign and re-date them to indicate that the document continues to reflect current wishes.

Physician Orders for Life-Sustaining Treatment

Another health care planning document is the Physician Orders for Life-Sustaining Treatment form, more commonly known as the POLST. It is also known as a MOLST (Medical Order for Life-Sustaining Treatment). The POLST is designed to help HCPs honor the end-of-life wishes of their patients. The form documents physician orders that adhere to the patient's wishes and treatment goals and are readily accessible to emergency medical personnel, assisted living facility staff, and other caregivers. They follow a patient from home, to emergency services, and to a hospital or other facility. Not all states have POLST programs in place.

Currently, New York, California, Oregon, Washington, West Virginia, Idaho, North Carolina, Tennessee, Utah, Colorado, Hawaii, and parts of Wisconsin have fully implemented programs. Fifteen other states and five metropolitan areas are developing POLST programs.[13]

Out-of-Hospital Do Not Resuscitate Orders

On average, only 5% to 10% of people who receive CPR survive.[14] Most states have some type of documentation that tells emergency medical services (EMS) personnel not to attempt resuscitation or perform heroic measures on a particular patient who has reached a point of medical futility. In states that do not have POLST programs, these documents can be called *out-of-hospital DNR orders, nonhospital DNRs, bedside DNR orders, EMS DNR orders, prehospital DNR orders*, or a *CPR advance directive*. Like the POLST, these documents are signed by the patient's HCP. Their intent is to prevent medical staff or EMS personnel from performing unwanted medical interventions on a seriously ill patient.

To avoid unwanted intubations or CPR during transport to or between medical facilities, patients must have appropriate state-specific forms that can be provided to those involved with their transport. Having a living will, health care power of attorney, and a DNR order in a hospital chart will *not* prevent this from occurring. The patient *must* have the appropriate POLST or out-of-hospital DNR orders to safeguard his or her wishes reliably.[15]

HOSPICE

In Latin, "hospice" means *host* and *guest* or *a place of shelter*. Hospice is a concept of care for the terminally ill patient that places an emphasis on life and living. Modern-day hospice began in 1967 in London when Dame Cecily Saunders founded St. Christopher's Hospice. The first U.S. hospice opened in Connecticut in 1974.

Hospice care is palliative care. To palliate means to "ease (symptoms) without curing the underlying disease; to moderate the intensity of."[16] Hospice provides aggressive pain and symptom management by using an interdisciplinary team comprising physicians; physician assistants (PAs); nurses; social workers; spiritual care providers; therapists (psychiatric, art, music, physical, occupational, and speech); and volunteers. The focus of hospice is comfort-oriented care when disease-specific therapy is no longer helpful and end-of-life decisions come to the fore. Living life as fully as possible is emphasized; entering hospice care does not mean all treatments must end. Hospice treatments aim to relieve the physical, emotional, and spiritual distress that often accompany a life-threatening illness. Hospice supports families while they care for their loved ones and provides grief support after the death occurs.

To qualify for hospice care, a patient must have a terminal illness. Although lung, breast, and prostate cancers are the three most common diagnoses,[17] a patient may have any diagnosis and be any age. Hospice patients must usually have a prognosis of 6 months or less. In recent years, there has been a movement within hospice to admit people with conditions that are often not deemed terminal and account for most noncancer diagnoses. These diagnoses may include unspecified debility of age (a chronic "disease" diagnosis with no single major illness), dementia, and heart and lung diseases. An HCP should refer patients to hospice when they have a prognosis measured in months versus years and once the goals of care have switched from cure to comfort. The question to ask is, "Would you be surprised if the patient died within the next year?" As long as the clinical criteria are met, a patient may usually be referred to hospice, regardless of his or her ability to pay. Having an AD or caregiver, being homebound, and ceasing treatment are not required to qualify for hospice care. Not all hospice programs require that a patient have a DNR order, but resuscitation attempts in the hospice setting are rare. Remember, hospice is not an end to treatment; rather, it is a shift to intensive palliative care that focuses on helping the patient to live life to the fullest. It is comfort-oriented care with end-of-life closure. In general, hospice care occurs wherever a person calls home and can be either community or institutionally based.

A more recent option now available in some states (Oregon 1994, Washington 2008, and Montana 2010) is legalized aid-in-dying. Although controversial in some forums, aid-in-dying provides a process for dignified dying that may be appropriate for individuals who are decisionally capable, terminally ill, suffering, and determined to stay in charge of their own end of life. In the previously mentioned states, this option is available through a strict and thoughtful medical process to allow a physician to prescribe medication in a life-ending dose. Patients who decide to ingest the medication must do so themselves.

Various other end-of-life options are supported in law and medicine to enable individuals to advance the time of death. Competent adults or their appointed health care agents may have the power to direct the commencement or discontinuation of any medical treatment in accordance with individual state law. Competent adults are permitted to refuse unwanted treatment regardless of the reason for their refusal or the nature of their illness; they need not be terminally ill. These same patients also have the legal right to stop life-sustaining medications or treatments, including voluntary stopping of eating and drinking. Although not for everyone, more people are learning about these voluntary end-of-life choices and discussing them with their families and health care providers.

HAVING THE CONVERSATION

One of the most productive ways to help patients as they approach the end of life is to encourage them to have a conversation with their loved ones about their preferences for treatment and end-of-life wishes. This conversation should include family members, friends, HCPs, and religious or spiritual leaders—anyone in the patient's life and involved with their care. In addition to promoting this conversation, you can enable it. Set a time for the patient to meet with his or her family and/or friends to discuss these issues. If possible, attend the meeting to help keep the conversation going and to help address any questions or concerns that may arise. Table 51-1 lists questions that may help patients as they begin to sort out these issues, whereas Table 51-2 provides questions patients may ask of you as they begin to come to terms with their own mortality.

Death is an uncomfortable topic. Many people believe that if they do not talk about it, it will not happen, especially to them. In reality, death must be discussed. Discussions are most useful if a plan is in place long before crucial decisions arise.

Although these conversations may seem awkward at first, they often bring families closer together. Talking about death is deeply personal; sharing beliefs and desires with those closest to you produces a more intimate relationship. It takes courage to have these conversations.

TABLE 51-1 **Representative Questions for Initiating the Discussion about End-of-Life Issues**

Domain	Representative Questions
Goals	Given the severity of your illness, what is most important for you to achieve? How do you think about balancing quality of life with length of life in terms of your treatment? What are your most important hopes? What are your biggest fears?
Values	What makes life most worth living for you? Would there be any circumstances under which you would find life not worth living? What do you consider your quality of life to be like now? Have you seen or been with someone who had a particularly good death or particularly difficult death?
Advance directives	If with future progression of your illness you are not able to speak for yourself, who would be best able to represent your views and values? (health care proxy) Have you given any thought to what kinds of treatment you would want (and not want) if you become unable to speak for yourself in the future? (living will)
Do-not-resuscitate order	If you were to die suddenly, that is, you stopped breathing or your heart stopped, we could try to revive you by using cardiopulmonary resuscitation (CPR). Are you familiar with CPR? Have you given thought as to whether you would want it? Given the severity of your illness, CPR would in all likelihood be ineffective. I would recommend that you choose not to have it, but that we continue all potentially effective treatments. What do you think?
Palliative care (pain and other symptoms)	Have you ever heard of hospice (palliative care)? What has been your experience with it? Tell me about your pain. Can you rate it on a 10-point scale? What is your breathing like when you feel at your best? How about when you are having trouble?
Palliative care ("unfinished business")	If you were to die sooner rather than later, what would be left undone? How is your family handling your illness? What are their reactions? Has religion been an important part of your life? Are there any spiritual issues you are concerned about at this point?

From Rando TA. Grief, Dying, and Death: Clinical Interventions for Caregivers. Champaign, IL: Research Press Publishers, 1984. Reprint courtesy Timothy E. Quill, MD.

TABLE 51-2 **Some Difficult Questions from Patients**

"Why me?"
"Why didn't you catch this earlier? Did you make a mistake?"
"How long do I have?
"What would you do in my shoes?"
"Should I try long-shot or experimental therapy?"
"Should I go to a 'medical Mecca' for treatment or a second opinion?"
"If my suffering gets really bad, will you help me die?"
"Will you work with me all the way through to my death, no matter what?"

From Rando TA. Grief, Dying, and Death: Clinical Interventions for Caregivers. Champaign, IL: Research Press Publishers, 1984. Reprint courtesy Timothy E. Quill, MD.

STAGES OF DYING

Death is a process, not an event. Every tissue of the body participates, each in its own way and at its own pace. The living-dying interval is the period of time between the normal processes of living and the point at which death occurs. There are three stages: acute crisis, chronic living-dying, and terminal.[18]

The physical changes that occur as death nears may happen over a few hours or several days. When the changes begin, the patient is considered to have begun actively dying.

As death approaches the patient may feel cool to the touch and skin color may change. The patient may sleep more. He or she may appear uncommunicative or unresponsive and may be difficult to arouse. Disorientation may occur. Incontinence of bowel and bladder occurs as muscles begin to relax. Congestion in the lungs and throat occur as fluid intake decreases, secretions thicken, and the patient becomes unable to cough. Restlessness, such as pulling at bedding or clothing, is common. Urine output decreases. The patient's regular breathing pattern may change. Periods of rapid breaths may alternate with periods of very slow, drawn-out breaths. The time between breaths can range from 5 seconds to 1 full minute.

Emotional, spiritual, and mental changes occur leading to death. The patient may withdraw as he or she begins to let go. He or she may want to be with only a very few people. The patient may talk about speaking with deceased relatives or friends. He or she may also claim to see things not visible to you. The following statements are commonly heard as a patient nears death:

- Where's the map?
- I'm getting ready to travel.
- I'm not alone.
- I see (name of deceased relative or friend).
- An angel is in the room.
- I'll be there soon.
- I know when I will die (day of week, time of day).

The patient is beginning to detach from life. Although you cannot hear or see what the patient does, it feels real to him or her, so it is best not to challenge or contradict the experience. Although this may be unnerving to you, it is not distressing to the patient and may be comforting.

Patients have strong feelings about the care they receive as they near the end of their lives. They worry how their decisions will affect their families, both emotionally and financially. Although they want to work with their HCPs to make the best treatment decisions, they often fear these same HCPs may stop caring for them when death is near. Dying patients desire emotional and spiritual care along with good medical care. Most want to die as peacefully as possible, free from pain, suffering, and prolonged dependence. Dying patients often want to forgive others, forgive themselves, say thank you, and say good-bye. They fear a loss of control, being in pain, and being rejected and isolated from family and friends.

STAGES OF GRIEF

Grief is the mental and/or physical pain experienced when the loss of a significant object, person, or part of the self is realized. This begins with the terminal diagnosis and includes a profound part of the loss of future dreams and goals (realization of all of the things that will not happen).

Because aging often leads to loss of independence, strength, health, and mobility, it commonly causes grief as well. This type of self-grief can result in depressive symptoms and profound sadness, but it is separate from clinical depression. Self-grief can be a normal, natural response to the changes and limitations older individuals experience.

In 1969, Elisabeth Kübler-Ross published a book detailing the grief process.[19] Her research identified five stages of grief: denial, anger, bargaining, depression, and acceptance. Hope can remain throughout all stages, even though what is hoped for is likely to change from hope for cure, for example, to hope for one last family gathering or hope for a peaceful death.

The grieving process is an individual process, unique to each person. There is no "right" or "wrong" way through the grieving process; there are just different ways. It is worth noting that not everyone experiences every stage of grief, and the stages may overlap, repeat, or appear in different order.

Grief is an intensely personal process and can be quite complicated. If the survivor sees the death as appropriate, it will moderate the grief. We often see unresolved, morbid, or exceptional grief reactions where the significance of the loss is unrecognized or discounted. Another form of grief is anticipatory grief, grief that allows for major emotional reaction before an expected loss. This does not replace the occurrence of postdeath grief. Disenfranchised grief is experienced when a loss is suffered that cannot or is not openly acknowledged, publicly mourned, or socially supported. Chronic sorrow is grieving a loss that cannot be fully resolved because there will be an ever-present sadness that will reoccur with its original pain at periodic intervals. Individual psychological and cultural differences can foster one form of grief over another. A broad range of literature is available on grief and the grieving process.

To quote Sherwin B. Nuland, "every life is different from any that has gone before it, and so is every death. The uniqueness of each of us extends even to the way we die."[20] The truth is that every last one of us will die. Some of us will die as our lives are just getting on track, whereas others will die of debilitating conditions many decades from now. Few of us will have the privilege of sitting with someone as they die. But for those of us who do, it will be a defining moment in our lives; it will be one that will leave deep impressions and ultimately guide us as we venture forth in the health care profession. Working with patients as they approach the end of their lives is not for everyone. But those who discover their niche in this area will find it to be a profoundly rewarding experience.

CLINICAL APPLICATIONS

1. An 88-year-old is hospitalized with advanced lung disease. His condition has deteriorated and he is unconscious, in the ICU on a ventilator. Medical staff agrees further treatment is probably futile, but the family disagrees on a course of action. There is no living will or durable power of attorney. What do you do?
2. A patient with early-stage lung cancer approaches you to discuss end-of-life options. What do you include in the discussion?
3. A male patient declines to follow your recommended course of treatment for stage 4 pancreatic cancer and instead opts to allow his disease to progress to a natural death. What recommendations would you make to him to allow for a comfortable death?

GLOSSARY

Advance directive: Encompasses both living wills and medical durable power of attorney.
Aid in dying: A practice specifically legalized in Oregon, Washington, and Montana, which allows mentally competent, terminally ill adults to request a prescription for life-ending medication from their physician. This medication must be self-administered.
Autonomy: The capacity of a rational individual to make an informed, uncoerced decision.
Hospice: An organization offering comfort care for the dying when medical treatment is no longer expected to cure the disease or prolong life. Hospice is provided wherever the person resides. The term may also apply to an insurance benefit that pays the costs of comfort care (usually at home) for patients with a prognosis of 6 months or less.
Informed consent: The communication process between a doctor and a patient that results in the patient having clear, unbiased information about treatment options in order to arrive at the best decision.
Living will: A term commonly substituted for advance directive, or for the portion of an advance directive containing specific instructions.
Out-of-hospital DNR: An order written by an HCP directing other providers in the out-of-hospital setting to withhold or withdraw specific life-sustaining treatments in the event of respiratory or cardiac arrest.
Palliative/total sedation: Also referred to as *terminal sedation.* The continuous administration of medication to relieve severe, intractable symptoms that cannot be controlled while keeping the patient conscious. An unconscious or semiconscious state is maintained until death occurs.
POLST: Physician Orders for Life-Sustaining Treatment. A medical order governing life-sustaining treatment that remains in effect across treatment settings and in the home.
Terminal, terminally: Describes an illness for which the medical expectation is death within the foreseeable future, usually 6 months.
VSED: Voluntary stopping eating and drinking.

KEY POINTS

- Patients act on principles of autonomy and informed consent. HCPs are almost always obligated to divulge the truth of the patient's diagnosis and prognosis to them.
- It is never too early to begin to plan and discuss treatment preferences at the end of life.
- Every adult needs an advance directive for health care and, where appropriate, a POLST or out-of-hospital DNR order.
- Conversations with family and friends help lay the foundation for rational end-of-life decision-making. These conversations can prove invaluable.
- Hospice provides aggressive palliative pain and symptom management to terminally ill patients, allowing them to live as fully as possible until they die.
- Dying is a process. It is a personal journey, unique to each of us.
- There are five stages of grief, but not everyone will experience every stage.
- Working with dying patients can be a profoundly rewarding experience.

References

1. Crawshaw R, Rogers DE, Pellegrino ED, et al. Patient-physician covenant (1995). In: Beauchamp TL, Walters L, (eds). Contemporary Issues in Bioethics. 5th ed. Belmont, CA: Wadsworth Publishing, 1999.
2. Beauchamp TL, Veatch RM. Ethical Issues in Death and Dying. 2nd ed. Upper Saddle River, NJ: Prentice Hall, 1996. p 64.
3. Beauchamp TL, Veatch RM. Ethical Issues in Death and Dying. 2nd ed. Upper Saddle River, NJ: Prentice Hall, 1996. p 69.
4. Beauchamp TL, Childress JF. Principles of Biomedical Ethics. 5th ed. New York: Oxford University Press, 2001, p. 285.
5. deBlois JC, Norris P, O'Rourke K. A Primer for Health Care Ethics: Essays for a Pluralistic Society. Washington, DC: Georgetown University Press, 1994, pp. 27–29.
6. CDC FastStats. Deaths and Mortality: Preliminary Data for 2010, *http://www.cdc.gov/nchs/fastats/deaths.htm*; Accessed September 12, 2012.
7. CDC National Center for Injury Prevention and Control. Leading Causes of Death Reports, 1999-2004, *http://www.cdc.gov/injury/wisqars/pdf/Death_by_Age_2007-a.pdf*; Accessed November 26, 2011.
8. Matter of Quinlan 70 N.J. 10; 355 A.2d 647; 1976 N.J.
9. Cruzan v. Director, Missouri Department of Health, 497 U.S. 261, 278, 110 S. Ct. 2841, 111 L. Ed. 2d 224 (1990).
10. Fritz M. How Simple Device Set Off a Fight over Elderly Care. Wall Street J Dec. 8, 2005:A1.
11. Compassion & Choices. My Directive Regarding Health Care Institutions Refusing to Honor My Health Care Choices, *http://community.compassionandchoices.org/document.doc?id=484*; Accessed November 26, 2011.

12. Human Rights Campaign. Hospital Visitation Authorization, *http://www.hrc.org/resources/entry/hospital-visitation-authorization*; Accessed November 26, 2011.
13. Center for Ethics in Health Care, Oregon Health & Science University. Physician Orders for Life-Sustaining Treatment Paradigm, *http://www.ohsu.edu/polst/*; Accessed November 26, 2011.
14. Mann D. Real CPR Isn't Everything It Seems to Be, *http://www.webmd.com/content/article/32/1728_79637.htm*; Accessed November 26, 2011.
15. Pennsylvania Department of Health. Out-Of-Hospital Do-Not-Resuscitate (DNR) Orders, *http://www.portal.health.state.pa.us/portal/server.pt/community/emergency_medical_services/14138/polst_-_out-of-hospital_dnr_orders/556979*; Accessed November 26, 2011.
16. Merriam-Webster OnLine Dictionary. *http://www.m-w.com/dictionary/palliate*; Accessed May 24, 2011.
17. National Hospice and Palliative Care Organization. Professional Resources: Hospice Statistics and Research, *http://www.nhpco.org/i4a/pages/Index.cfm?pageid=3274*; Accessed November 26, 2011.
18. Rando TA. Grief, Dying, and Death: Clinical Interventions for Caregivers. Champaign, IL: Research Press Publishers; 1984.
19. Kübler-Ross E. On Death and Dying. New York: MacMillan Publishing Company, 1969.
20. Nuland SB. How We Die: Reflections on Life's Final Chapter. New York: Alfred A. Knopf, 1994, p. 3.

The resources for this chapter can be found at www.expertconsult.com.

CHAPTER 52

MASS CASUALTY AND DISASTER MANAGEMENT

Martha Petersen • Linda G. Allison

CHAPTER CONTENTS

There are multiple definitions of disasters. A useful one is " … a nonroutine event that exceeds the capacity of the affected area to respond to it in such a way as to save lives; to preserve property; and to maintain the social, ecological, economic, and political stability of the affected region."[1] Inherent in this definition is to preserve and maintain health and health care. A mass casualty is defined similarly as an event that overwhelms available medical resources with injuries and deaths.

The impact of natural disasters is predicted to intensify due to several factors. The global population continues to increase, and larger numbers of those are becoming concentrated in urban or coastal areas, so greater numbers of people are vulnerable to a potential mass calamity and the aftermath. The trend in climate change affects weather and geological stability, raising the probability of certain natural disasters, making it more likely that such an event will exceed the coping capacity of the community or region.[2] According to the Center for Epidemiology on Disasters (CRED), during the period from 2000 to 2009, there were 385 disasters, an increase of 233 percent since 1980 to 1989 and an increase of 67 percent since 1990 to 1999.[3]

As a key member of the health care team, the physician assistant (PA) plays an essential role in disaster preparedness and management. That role may be in the office, hospital, community, and/or at the site of a disaster. Every geographical region is at risk for some type of disaster. Whether the "nonroutine event" is a hurricane, tornado, flood, earthquake, blizzard, fire, or something rarer, the need for preparedness is comparable. Advanced planning is the most valuable tool in assisting in a local or regional disaster. It is a natural urge to rush to the site immediately; however, this action can be detrimental. Effective relief in any disaster requires organization and communication among many different participants. A PA, no matter how well trained in a specialty, if not trained for mass casualty situations, may be more of a liability than a benefit. This chapter addresses the various responsibilities and possible limitations a PA may have in being prepared for a mass casualty situation or in managing the impact and aftermath of one.

PHYSICIAN ASSISTANTS AS EDUCATORS

The fundamental job of the majority of PAs in emergency preparedness is patient education. Although responding to a disaster in person may be perceived as dramatic or heroic, simple patient education may have a greater influence on reducing morbidity and mortality in any overwhelming event. A survey conducted by the Centers for Disease Control and Prevention (CDC) found that 48.7%, or almost half of all residents living in Florida, had no evacuation plans before the 2004 hurricane season, a year when there were four major storms requiring evacuations.[4] The Red Cross and the Federal Emergency Management Agency (FEMA) use the slogan "Get a Kit; Have a Plan; Be Informed."[5] This provides a basis for PAs to educate patients. All patients should have an updated emergency plan and kit. If people are informed and ready for a disaster, even one as simple as loss of electrical power, the negative effect on the individual and public can be decreased. Certain populations may be more at risk in a disaster situation, including families with small children, the elderly, and chronically ill and disabled people. It is especially important for these patients to have definitive emergency plans in place, and it is the clinician's job to ensure that they are aware, educated, and prepared.

When taking the social history, questions should be asked about risk behavior such as smoking, seat belt use, smoke detectors in the home, etc. PAs also need to ask about disaster planning. It is a simple step to ask a patient if he or she is prepared for a disaster as part of a routine history or as a question on an intake form. Posters and brochures can be placed in the waiting room, at the front desk, in hallways, or in examination rooms. Free downloadable forms for developing personal emergency kits and plans are available at the FEMA site, specifically at *http://www.ready.gov/research-publications*. The "Preparing and Getting Trained" section on the Red Cross website, *http://www.redcross.org/*, offers checklists, handouts, and posters in different languages, many designed for a particular type of disaster, allowing for customization for the type of disaster most common to an area. Under the Shop link on the Red Cross website, patients can purchase readymade kits. PAs, especially in primary care settings, should provide verbal and written education and resources for their patients.

In some emergency situations there is time for people to be warned and prepared. In these conditions, the public may have hours or days to organize and evacuate the area or relocate to a designated shelter. Other times, there is little or no warning and people must take shelter in their own homes (known as *shelter in place*): Either situation requires certain unique preparations that patients need to know. PAs should educate patients about both circumstances. Evacuation will necessitate knowledge about emergency routes, portable supplies, and possible long-term absence from the home. Shelter-in-place plans can include a larger supply of food and water. Basic provisions are the same in either scenario. PAs should encourage all their patients to have an emergency kit, a plan, and know how to get accurate information for a disaster (Table 52-1).

TABLE 52-1 **Resources for Clinicians, Patients, and Patient Education**

Agency	Website	Resources Offered
American Academy of Family Physicians	*http://www.aafp.org/online/en/home/clinical/disasterprep.html*	General disaster preparedness information, links, and resources (free downloads)
American Academy of Pediatrics	*http://www.aap.org/terrorism/index.html*	Patient information on preparation for all types of disasters (free downloads)
Centers for Disease Control and Prevention	*http://www.bt.cdc.gov/preparedness/*	Information and links on emergency planning
Department of Homeland Security and the Federal Emergency Management Agency	*http://www.dhs.gov/* *http://www.ready.gov/* *http://www.citizencorps.gov/*	• General emergency preparedness resources for families. • Ready.gov offers state and local information on and appropriate plans for types of emergencies most likely to occur in specific areas. • How to prepare and protect yourself, family and property in any type of disaster. • Brochures and checklists for families, businesses, and children. (free downloads)
Red Cross	*http://www.redcross.org/* *http://www.redcross.org/store/*	• Emergency plan brochure, education materials, and handouts (Under "Preparing and Getting Trained") • Prepared kits for purchase

Information available in various languages.
All sites active and accurate as of August 18, 2012.

GENERAL EMERGENCY PLAN AND KIT

Keep in mind the distinctive disasters most likely to your area: hurricanes, floods, tornados, blizzards, or wildfires and adapt your kit accordingly. Be sure to take into consideration the unique needs of your family: small children, pets, and handicapped or elderly people.

EMERGENCY PLAN

- Create an emergency contact list consisting of relatives or friends beyond your immediate area, and if possible identify one person as the primary contact. Be sure that all family members are familiar with this contact system. In an emergency it may be easier to call out of the area, or if not, once phone service can be used, one call can provide information to a designated family "clearinghouse."
- Post all emergency contact numbers both professional and personal, by the phone. If possible preprogram the numbers into the home and mobile phones.
- Select two meeting places—a church or school—one in the neighborhood and one farther away (in case no one can return to the immediate neighborhood) where the family can meet if it is impossible to get home.
- Keep family records and documents in a waterproof and fireproof box.

BASIC EMERGENCY KIT

- Water supply: 1 gallon of water per person per day for a minimum of 3 days.
- Canned or nonperishable food
- Blankets and bedding
- Radio (powered by batteries or solar or hand crank)
- Flashlight
- Extra batteries
- Cell phone and chargers (consider solar-powered chargers)
- First aid kit
- Medications
- Multipurpose tool
- Personal hygiene and sanitation objects
- Clothing
- Matches
- Plastic sheeting
- Duct tape
- Household bleach

Modified from CDC Emergency Preparedness and You. *http://www.bt.cdc.gov/preparedness*. Accessed November 26, 2011.

PHYSICIAN ASSISTANTS AS PROVIDERS

When a disaster happens, health care providers may feel the need to immediately go to the site and volunteer their services. This may be because an event happens within the community and PAs respond in the role of a medically trained professional that is part of the health care team. In any case where a health care professional responds by going to the site, he or she should identify himself or herself to the incident command personnel to ensure that services are provided where they are needed and not interfering with or endangering others. PAs must realize that the best assistance may not be medical but may be in some other aspect: digging latrines, passing out food or water, setting up temporary shelters, or transporting people. PAs must be flexible and willing to perform any activity that will be useful, whether they are trained as disaster responders or not.

If an emergency happens elsewhere, PAs need to be aware of several important aspects of disaster relief. It is important to recognize that any person showing up at a disaster site may encumber the process by adding to the demand for safety, shelter, water, or food. The best way to help may be to stay away and offer financial assistance through a reputable relief organization. If the PA is involved at the site at a non-local disaster, he or she may need to show proof of licensure and certification. The National Commission on the Certification of Physician Assistants (NCCPA) and many state medical boards give wallet-size replications of licensure and certification. PAs should carry these at all times. Although it may not always be practical to request and offer credentials in a disaster setting, for patient safety and for liability reasons it is valuable to have these credentials on hand if possible. Even with such documentation PAs must understand that despite a disaster situation, a given state may still require compliance with its own licensing standards.

In 2005, in reaction to the devastation of the hurricanes, governors of some states temporarily waived the requisite licensing process for PAs, whereas others simplified and streamlined the process.[6] States need to clarify the role of the supervising physician when a PA may be volunteering in another state without designated physician oversight. A volunteer PA at a disaster site may be practicing illegally. Practitioners must realize that the so-called Good Samaritan law does not guarantee liability protection in a disaster event.[6] The AAPA continues to work with states to amend laws that would allow PAs in a local or state emergency to "… render such care that they are able to provide without supervision … or with such supervision as is available."[7] Included in these changes is limited immunity from malpractice liability. Practicing PAs need to stay current on legislative issues affecting their scope of practice in all situations.

Advance preparation is the key to being effective in an emergency.

PHYSICIAN ASSISTANTS IN AFTERCARE

PAs need to be aware of federal and state surveillance and reporting requirements in order to protect patients and communities from epidemics following a disaster. Reporting requirements vary from state to state, so PAs should be familiar with the standards of the state where they practice, available from the individual state Department of Health office or website.

The best method of staying up to date with federal reporting is for clinicians to subscribe to the *Morbidity and Mortality Weekly Report (MMWR)* from the CDC. The *MMWR* is a summary of reported national and international incidents and is the best resource for a practicing PA to remain current on events that might threaten the health of patients and the community. This report can be received weekly via e-mail or in printed form. It is available at: *www.cdc.gov/mmwr*. Knowing that there is a surge in food poisonings; exposure to cleaning supplies, insecticides, or fungicides; or rabies in a nearby area can raise a clinician's level of suspicion, lead to a quicker diagnosis for their own patients, and help track outbreaks of any type.

Practicing PAs must remain informed about and use current evidence-based best practices as a means of preventing certain public health emergencies. For example, following the release of radioactive materials from a damaged nuclear reactor in Japan in 2011, many people in the United States asked for iodine to protect themselves but suffered iodine toxicity. The National Guideline Clearing House *(www.ngc.gov.)* guidelines on the judicious use of antibiotics help in controlling the increasing public health threat and impact of antibiotic resistant strains of bacteria. This emphasizes the PA's role as patient educator because many patients will continue to demand unnecessary prescriptions unless thoroughly informed about the personal and public health danger of inappropriate use of these medications.

LONG-TERM EFFECTS

When a community has been evacuated, people are often displaced into areas that are unfamiliar to them. Most people believe that loss of family and friends would be the most difficult part of displacement, but in actuality, it is the access to services that is most challenging. For example, where does one go to get money from a bank or automatic teller machine? Where does one go for groceries, post office, health care, and laundry facilities? Just surviving daily needs imposes stress on survivors of a disaster.

Once a community goes through a public health emergency (flood, hurricane, explosion, etc.) that threatens life, quality of life, and the sense of personal security, there are psychological effects to be expected. As health care providers, PAs need to anticipate and recognize both acute stress disorder (ASD) and post-traumatic stress disorder (PTSD). Given that the prevalence of PTSD is projected normally to be between 1% and 12% of the general population of the United States and as high as 18% in professional firefighters,[8] it is probable that patients will present with symptoms of ASD and/or PTSD after being involved in or witnessing a traumatic event. The clinical presentation of these conditions can vary extensively yet has common themes. An anxiety syndrome, ASD occurs within 4 weeks of the traumatic experience and is marked by a sense of dissociation or a sense of being "as if in a daze."[8]

Early intervention can usually prevent ASD progressing to PTSD. The diagnosis of PTSD is based on four categories of criteria, according to the *Diagnostic and Statistical Manual of Mental Health Disorders*, 4th ed. (DSM-IV) and is briefly summarized as follows:

1. The person has been exposed to a traumatic event.
2. The traumatic event is persistently re-experienced.
3. The person seeks to avoid trauma-related triggers and reports emotional "numbness."
4. The person experiences a sense of hyperarousal.

(See the DSM-IV for complete diagnostic criteria.)

The identification of PTSD depends on the symptoms occurring for more than 1 month and creating dysfunction in a personal, social, or occupational setting. The American Academy of Family Practice (AAFP, *www.aafp.org*) and the Department of Veterans Affairs *(www.ncptsd.va.gov)* offer practical information for primary care providers for screening, recognizing, and treating PTSD.

SPECIAL POPULATIONS

Children and the elderly are at higher risk for injury and illness during a disaster for several reasons. Cognitive impairment from dementia, limited mobility, impaired vision and hearing, and other chronic diseases can reduce an older person's ability to respond to an emergency in an appropriate or timely manner. Elderly with chronic diseases such as diabetes, asthma, or cardiovascular disease may have difficulty obtaining or using their medications. Likewise, children may not have the ability to recognize the appropriate actions or to move to safety. Both geriatric and pediatric populations may be more susceptible to infectious diseases. The American Academy of Pediatrics and the Agency for Healthcare Research and Quality (AHRQ) provide guidelines for disaster preparedness for children.[9-11] Although the Public Health Emergency Awareness Program (PHEP) is no longer funded, guidelines that were developed before June 2011 are archived through the AHRC website.[12]

PHYSICIAN ASSISTANTS IN POLICY

As clinicians, PAs are part of not only a health care team but also a policy-making team. Every practice, institution, and community needs to have a disaster action plan in place. This plan should be geared to emergencies that may be common to the region, but it must also include plans for unexpected situations such as epidemics, chemical or hazardous waste spills, explosions, terrorism, or an influx of evacuees. All health care systems are interconnected with each other, as well as with other community, regional, and state structures. Effective plans and policies must account for these multiple layers of people and organizations.[4] The interrelationships of the individual, family, workplace, community, state, federal and global aspects of emergency planning, response, and recovery must be taken into account in planning for a possible overwhelming event and casualties.

The foundation for a disaster response plan includes a flow chart that describes a list of incidents that are possible in the geographic area served, primary contacts, other responders and their roles, call trees, list of available resources, and communications options. The World Health Organization and the U.S. Environmental Protection Agency have developed multiple flow charts for responses to a large number of possible disasters, and they provide a starting place for a community or organization to develop plans specifically oriented to local potential disasters. An example of such a flow chart is available at: *http://www.epa.gov/oem/content/nrs/snapshot.htm.*

The World Health Organization provides a document with detailed flow charts for specific types of events and the related effects. Although directed toward emergency response in Africa, the flow charts are universally applicable for different disasters and are available at: *http://www.who.int/disasters/repo/5516.pdf*

POTENTIAL DISASTERS AND EFFECTS

Earthquakes; floods; droughts; landslides; volcanic eruptions; fires; hurricanes; tornadoes; snow storms; heat waves; violence/civil disturbance; power outage; disruption of water and/or food supplies; displacement and refugees; infectious disease epidemics

Flow charts for each available at: *http://www.who.int/disasters/repo/5516.pdf.* Accessed July 2, 2011.

Office

Every medical practice needs to have a policy for an event that could cause widespread illness, injury, or sudden disruption of electric, water, fire, police and emergency medical services. Will the clinicians report to the office or clinic, or to the local emergency department? If the local ER is nonfunctioning or overrun, are clinicians credentialed to report to other hospitals? Who on staff is trained to provide on-site disaster service? If the medical team and support staff of a practice has created a plan for an emergency they will be able to offer prompt and efficient assistance.

Hospitals and Clinics

The Joint Commission considers it critically important that hospitals are prepared to "screen, triage, and treat disaster survivors," which may include refugees from other areas where local health care has been overwhelmed by a disaster or by mass casualties.[4] FEMA created the Incident Command System (ICS) to provide for a common "language" for emergency preparation and response and focus on facilitating communication among local, regional, tribal, and national resources. It is a "standardized, on-scene, all-hazards incident management approach that:

- Allows for the integration of facilities, equipment, personnel, procedures, and communications operating within a common organizational structure.
- Enables a coordinated response among various jurisdictions and functional agencies, both public and private.
- Establishes common processes for planning and managing resources."[13]

Hospitals are required to have a Hospital Incident Command (HICS) plan in place that is coordinated with the community Incident Command System (ICS) which in turn is connected to the National Incident Management System (NMIS). Hospitals or health care systems that receive federal preparedness and response grants, contracts or cooperative agreements (e.g., Bioterrorism Hospital Preparedness Program, Department of Homeland Security grants) are required to be NIMS compliant. Any facility that routinely treats emergency medical and trauma patients should be NIMS compliant, as well as nursing homes, assisted living and long term living facilities and specialty hospitals. The essential elements of NIMS include planning, communications and resources. Information and training for ICS and NMIS is available on the Federal Emergency Management website: *http://www.fema.gov/prepared/train.shtm.* PAs with hospital privileges need to be aware of these systems and their expected individual role in the event of a catastrophe. They may serve on the committees that develop these policies. They may assist in training other members of the health care team. Hospitals and health care centers are required to run practice drills to ensure the ability to activate an efficient response.

Community

PAs can be involved in the development of the local emergency preparedness policies and plans. The first 72 hours in a disaster will mostly depend on the local resources, while state and federal assistance takes time to be mobilized. How will the community incident response system be activated? What buildings are safest to be designated as emergency shelters or triage areas? PAs can contribute medical expertise to the committees planning the local incident command system and emergency response (Table 52-2).

TABLE 52-2 **Disaster Management Organizations**

National Response Framework	NRF	Provides a general policy framework for disaster response
National Incident Management System	NIMS	Provides a policy framework for disaster response
Federal Emergency Management Agency	FEMA	Oversees property and infrastructures in disaster response
National Disaster Medical System	NDMS	Oversees the humanitarian and medical response
State and local organizations		Coordinates with federal and community response
Nongovernmental Organizations	NGO	Provide immediate local response and coordinate with local, state and national systems

PHYSICIAN ASSISTANT TRAINING FOR DISASTER RESPONSE

State, federal, and international organizations provide training and certification as a disaster relief responder. Any PA with an interest in disaster relief should investigate these opportunities. In most cases, this can ensure that the credentialing, licensing, and liability issues are covered and that the PA's skill and training can be used appropriately and safely. The National Disaster Life Support Foundation (NDLS) *(www.ndls.net)* in partnership with the American Medical Association (AMA) offers training in three levels of disaster response: Core, Basic, and Advanced Disaster Life Support (CDLS, BDLS, and ADLS, respectively). All PAs should consider certification in CDLS in addition to their cardiopulmonary resuscitation (CPR) and Advanced Cardiac Life Support (ACLS) training. As mentioned earlier, PAs must realize that the best assistance may not be medical but may be in some other aspect. They must be flexible and willing to perform any activity that will be useful, whether they are trained as disaster responders or not (Table 52-3).

Cases

The following examples of the major types of public health emergencies illustrate the extent to which an event can affect a population, the response and how the event impacted response capabilities, and general concepts related to the specific type of emergency.

Chemical Emergencies

CASE STUDY 52-1

On January 6, 2005, a freight train with three chlorine tankers and one sodium hydroxide tanker collided with a parked train in Graniteville, South Carolina. As a result of the collision, one of the chlorine tankers was damaged, releasing more than 11,000 gallons of chlorine gas, potentially exposing the 5453 residents to chlorine gas.

Chlorine gas is corrosive to the eye, skin, and respiratory tract, which can lead to chemical burns, pulmonary edema, and death, depending on the amount and duration of the exposure. More than 10% of the residents (529) sought medical attention; 511 were seen in emergency departments, with 69 of these being admitted to seven area hospitals. The remaining 18 were seen and treated at local physician offices.

TABLE 52-3 **Disaster Response Training Opportunities**

Agency	Website	Training
Centers for Disease Control and Prevention	*www.bt.cdc.gov/training*	Offers a variety of training opportunities
National Disaster Life Support Foundation	*http://www.bdls.com/*	Core, basic, and advanced disaster training classes and certification
Federal Emergency Management Agency	*http://www.fema.gov/about/training/emergency.shtm*	Emergency Management Training (for government and emergency personnel)
University of Northern California	*http://www.uncm.edu/departments/undergraduate/EHS.htm*	Online Associate of Science in Emergency Health and Safety degree
North Carolina Center for Public Health Preparedness	*http://cphp.sph.unc.edu/training/index.php*	Free brief online training in public health preparedness, surveillance, agents of bioterrorism, and emerging and reemerging disease agents
National Disaster Life Support Foundation	*http://www.ndlsf.org/common/content.asp?PAGE=345*	Multiple courses at various levels

This is a limited list with the goal of introducing PAs to a sample of training opportunities. Many other qualified agencies offer instruction in disaster relief preparation. All sites active and accurate as of November 11, 2012.

Impact

- The local health care system experienced a sudden increase in utilization, necessitating implementation of an existing disaster plan.
- Area businesses were closed due to the evacuation, leading to economic losses.
- Area schools were closed, with lost educational time.
- Cleanup of the spill required additional resources, both financial and manpower.
- Long-term health effects are not yet known, including physical and psychological effects on the 5453 residents.

Response

The initial response included a shelter-in-place for a 1-mile radius around the site, but this was changed to a mandatory evacuation for this same area approximately 14 hours after the initial event. A temporary repair of the damaged car was successful after 4 days. Federal responders from the Agency for Toxic Substances and Disease Registry (ATSDR), the U.S. Environmental Protection Agency, and the U.S. Coast Guard carried out air sampling in homes, schools, and factories within the 1-mile radius before allowing residents to move home.

Discussion

Chemical leaks and radiation leaks present a challenge for local EMS and law enforcement officials because communities may be required to evacuate and seek medical care about the same time. Health care systems can be overwhelmed by the numbers of persons affected but must also implement systems for decontamination of victims so that they pose no threat to the health care providers themselves.

A shelter-in-place response is used when leaving the area might take too long or would potentially expose people to more harm, or when going outside may be more dangerous than staying indoors. In this case, people should choose a room in the house that has the fewest windows, is most protected from outside air, and has a good water supply, such as a bathroom. This room should be at the highest possible place to avoid gases that are heavier than air and sink.

The CDC categorizes chemical toxins by the type of chemical or by the effect they have, including biotoxins, blistering agents/vesicants, caustics (acids), choking or pulmonary irritants, incapacitating agents, long-acting anticoagulants, metals, nerve agents, organic solvents, riot control agents (tear gas), toxic alcohols, and vomiting agents.

A radiation emergency is similar to a chemical emergency in that the effect will depend on the amount and duration of exposure to the radiation. Residents may be asked to shelter-in-place or evacuate, depending on the location and amount of radiation released. Decontamination is of primary importance for patients presenting to health care facilities so as not to contaminate these facilities or the health care workers.[14-16]

Mass Casualties

CASE STUDY 52-2

On April 19, 1995, a massive explosion destroyed nearly half of the nine-story Murrah Federal Building in downtown Oklahoma City. The explosion occurred just after 9:00 AM, after parents had dropped off children to the daycare center located in the building. There were 361 persons in the Murrah Federal Building at the time of the explosion; 319 (88%) were injured, and 163 died (19 of whom were children). The death rate was higher in the portion of the building that collapsed compared with the portion of the building that did not collapse. Injury rates in four adjacent buildings ranged from 38% to 100%, with three deaths occurring inside these buildings and one death occurring outside. A total of 759 persons were injured; of these, 168 people died, 83 were hospitalized, and 508 were treated as outpatients.

Impact

- This type of disaster, in which there are many survivors, puts a strain on existing emergency and health care resources. Many emergency departments are already working at maximum capacity on a regular basis, and there is little room for this type of additional demand on existing resources.
- The aftermath saw an increase in posttraumatic stress, especially children.
- Audiologic changes, respiratory problems, depression, anxiety, and posttraumatic stress syndrome affected a large proportion of those injured in the explosion 2 to 3 years after the event.

Response

The EMS response included immediately available local ambulances and staff; additional local ambulances staffed by recalled, off-duty personnel; and ambulances and personnel from surrounding communities. They transported 139 patients to area hospitals within the first hour, with a third of these in critical condition. Six transported patients died en route or at the hospital.

Nine hospitals put disaster plans into effect; two of these hospitals received bomb threats during the response. They dealt with security, hospital employees and volunteers, news media, victims, families and friends of victims, as well as countless concerned persons.

Volunteers flooded the scene with good intentions, but they created a logistical problem for the professionally trained rescue workers. Telephone lines and cell phones were overloaded with communications, but the emergency radio communications were only activated in three of the hospitals.

Discussion

The explosion destroyed the major supporting columns in front of the building, leading to a "pancaking" effect as the upper floors collapsed onto the lower ones. Of the 163 deaths at the Murrah Federal Building, 95% were due to blunt trauma related to the collapse. Additional injuries and one fatality occurred in the search and rescue effort.

This case illustrates the need for cooperation and collaboration of all community resources, including police, EMS, hospitals, and private practitioners. Training through drills improves performance and ability to successfully provide an appropriate response during a disaster.

The Commissioner of Health for the State of Oklahoma designated any injury or health-related condition related to the bombing a "reportable condition," including deaths, acute injuries directly related to the bombing, long-term health problems, and associated medical costs. There were 1259 survivors who were directly exposed to the bombing and four times as many nonfatal injuries as fatal injuries. As one would anticipate, those who sustained multiple injuries were more likely to die than those who did not. Injuries in survivors were generally related to flying glass and debris and falling ceilings, including soft tissue injuries, lacerations, fractures, sprains, and head injuries.

A follow-up study done 2 to 3 years after the bombing indicated that long-term survivors had an increased incidence of bombing-related medical conditions, including depression, anxiety, posttraumatic stress disorder, hearing problems, and respiratory problems. Primary care providers should be aware of these needs when caring for patients who have been exposed to and survived a mass casualty explosion.[17-20]

Natural Disasters and Severe Weather

CASE STUDY 52-3

During July 12-16, 1995, daily maximum high temperatures in Chicago ranged from 93° to 104° F; on July 13, the heat index peaked at 119° F. There were 485 heat-related deaths during July 11-27, with the peak of heat-related deaths occurring 2 days after the heat index peaked. There were no heat-related deaths from July 4 to 10. In 1988, a heat wave had resulted in 77 heat-related deaths.

Victims

Heat-related deaths were defined as those in which the core body temperature was greater than or equal to 105° F; the victim was found in an environment that indicated heat was a contributor to the death (such as being found a room without air conditioning, with windows closed, and a high room temperature); or there was no evidence of other cause of death in a victim who was found in a decomposed condition, and who had last been seen alive during the heat wave period. Of the 485 victims, 55% were male; 49% were black, 46% were white, and 5% were of other racial/ethnic groups. Victims ranged in age from 3 years to 103 years, with a median of 75 years and a mean of 72 years; 51% were 75 years or older.

Impact

- Most victims are elderly or disabled persons who live in non–air-conditioned houses or apartments.
- Other victims are younger but involved in heat-generating activities, such as sports.

Response

Chicago experienced two major heat waves in 1995 and 1999. In the first case, there were 485 heat-related deaths and 739 excess deaths. Following this, Chicago implemented an Extreme Weather Operations Plan to address the needs of those at most risk for heat-related death, including persons with an inability to care for themselves and advanced age. This plan increased the number of daily contacts for the elderly during periods of extreme heat. The heat wave in 1999 resulted in 103 heat-related deaths, a significant reduction over that which would have been expected.

Discussion

Exposure to extreme heat for long periods of time may lead to a number of heat-related illnesses, including heat exhaustion and heat stroke, and eventually death. The very young and the very old are more susceptible to heat-related illness, as are those with other chronic diseases, such as heart disease. Certain activities and medications may predispose a person to heat-related illness due to decreased ability to sweat (dehydration, many drugs) or increased heat production (physical activity). One of the most important factors in preventing heat illness or stroke is the availability of air conditioning.

A heat emergency response plan involves monitoring atmospheric and meteorologic conditions to determine when to implement strategies aimed at reducing heat injuries and deaths. A plan to check on elderly or disabled persons during a heat emergency will help to identify those persons at risk for injury so that preventive measures may be taken earlier. Sports activities should be curtailed. During a heat emergency, a community should use rolling energy blackouts during periods of high energy use to avoid complete loss of air conditioning in a single area, which would increase the risk of heat-related morbidity and mortality in that area. A community should provide support for low-income populations to allow for air-conditioning use during summer months. Fans themselves do not protect against heat injury when the ambient temperature exceeds 90°F, especially when the humidity exceeds 35%, but rather circulate hot air, which may actually increase heat stress.

Heat-related mortality is preventable. The time from onset of a major heat wave and the occurrence of heat-related deaths is long enough to implement a heat emergency response plan and to disseminate public health information to the community.[21,22]

CASE STUDY 52-4

Hurricane Katrina formed on August 23, 2005, and over the next week made landfall on both Florida and Louisiana, devastating much of the Gulf Coast from Florida to Louisiana, including Alabama and Mississippi, and the city of New Orleans. It started as a category 1 hurricane, strengthened to category 5, and was classified as a category 3 hurricane when it finally made landfall. The National Hurricane Center issued hurricane watches over 30 hours before and hurricane warnings over 19 hours before the first landfall in Florida.

Damage from the hurricane, storm surge, flooding, associated tornadoes, and wind extended from Florida up the eastern coast as far as New York, the Great Lakes region, and into Canada. More than 1800 persons died in the hurricane and resultant floods. More than 1.3 million persons were evacuated from New Orleans; more than 100,000 remained in the city, with 9000 initially housed in the Superdome. Most of those who did not evacuate had no available transportation. Outside of New Orleans, many other communities were also affected, with large numbers of people displaced by evacuations and loss of homes, contributing to the overall economic impact, health problems, and burden of suffering.

Impact

- More than 1800 people died in the United States.
- Initially more than 80% of the population of New Orleans was evacuated; approximately 26,000 remained in the city in shelters.
- Within 1 month, evacuees were scattered across the country, residing in every state; 240,000 households relocated to Houston and cities at least 250 miles away; 60,000 households relocated more than 750 miles away, including Chicago.
- More than 700,000 requested housing assistance from FEMA.
- The total economic impact in Mississippi and Louisiana alone exceeded $150 billion.

Response

When the National Hurricane Center issued watches and warnings, government officials issued evacuation orders. However, there was no transportation for those who had no way to evacuate, so shelters were set up in the Superdome and other areas in the city. Initially more than 9000 people were sheltered in the Superdome, but that number exceeded 30,000, with another 25,000 at the Convention Center as more people left their homes for higher ground and in preparation for evacuation by bus to Houston, Texas. During the first days after the storm, food and water supplies were used up and people waited for up to 4 days to be evacuated. Looting occurred, so National Guard troops were called in to restore order and provide food and water to victims. Conditions deteriorated over the first few weeks as local, state, and federal governmental agencies attempted to provide disaster relief and restore order.

A state-of-the-art mobile health care facility was set up in the parking lot of a supermarket. Health care workers encountered dehydration and infected wounds, as well as chronic illness in the first days; pregnant women were transported to hospitals that were equipped to manage them. There were a significant number of animal bites from domestic, wild, and marine animals. After the initial acute problems were taken care of, health care workers anticipated an increase in cholera, typhoid, and mosquito-borne illness such as malaria and West Nile virus; however, much of this did not occur. Surveillance by CDC for the month following hurricane Katrina revealed 7508 events; 4169 (55.6%) were illnesses, 2018 (26.9%) were injuries, and 1321 (17.5%) were nonacute health-related events (e.g., medication refills, wound checks, cast removals). Acute respiratory infections and noninfectious skin lesions accounted for a large proportion of the acute illnesses.

Discussion

Families who evacuated from their homes during and following hurricane Katrina face many of the same issues and concerns as refugees, including loss of access to their usual support system. Evacuees and refugees are faced with living in a community in which they do not know where basic services may be obtained, such as food (and available food may be unfamiliar), medical services, post office, and transportation. Chronically ill people may lose or run out of their medications and have difficulty replacing them. Family and friends may be hundreds of miles away or their status may be unknown. Evacuees and refugees may have no money or access to money, including cash or checkbook. If they are relocated to an unfamiliar city, it may be difficult for them to apply for or obtain financial assistance to even pay for food or shelter, and thus they are dependent on the government and charities for shelter and food.

Basic hygiene and sanitation are necessary to prevent the spread of infectious diseases, such as dysentery; crowded conditions contribute to the spread of respiratory illness. Dehydration can be a major problem for people in non–air-conditioned shelters during hot weather. A disaster kit that includes personal medications, drinking water, and other supplies can make a difference in how well a person fares during a major disaster.

As with any other mass casualty incident, communications and response by trained personnel are critical. Well-meaning volunteers can actually hinder rescue efforts without proper training and planning. The CDC has information on other natural disasters and severe weather-related events, including earthquakes, tsunamis, tornadoes, hurricanes, floods, volcanoes, wildfires, mudslides, winter weather, extreme heat, and power outages at *http://www.bt.cdc.gov/disasters/*, including information on preparation, what to do during and after a disaster, and other information for the public and health care providers.[23,24]

Infectious Disease Outbreaks

CASE STUDY 52-5

Between August 19 and September 26, 2006, at least 183 persons from 26 states had been infected with *Escherichia coli* O157:H7. Of these, at least 1 person died, 29 had hemolytic uremic syndrome, and more than half were hospitalized.

Impact and Response

News media began reporting these cases. Epidemiologists identified fresh spinach as the source of this infection, and on September 14, the U.S. Food and Drug Administration advised consumers to avoid eating any bagged fresh spinach and on September 16 extended this warning to any fresh spinach product. The farms producing the spinach suffered significant economic loss, along with vendors and grocery stores as the produce was pulled from market shelves and disposed of.

Discussion

Surveillance is a critical component of the public health response to any infectious disease outbreak. Identification of the source of an outbreak can help to reduce further cases. An outbreak may be confined to a single community or locale, such as the gastroenteritis cases on cruise ships caused by a virus, cases of salmonella in a community that originates from a single restaurant, or it may affect a geographically widespread area, as in the case of an *E. coli* outbreak.[25,26,27] In this age of rapid transportation, food supplies from one area can be distributed across the country, with any contaminant thus affecting a widely distributed population. Once a source has been identified, rapid response by the CDC and other public health agencies to educate the public and limit further exposure of consumers by removing the contaminated food from the market can reduce or prevent further cases.

Other infectious disease outbreaks that have occurred in recent years include mumps, measles, meningitis, multidrug-resistant tuberculosis in human immunodeficiency virus. Settings in which there is some crowding, such as prisons, dormitories, and military barracks, increase the chances that a single person with an infectious disease can expose others to that disease, leading to an increase in cases within that setting. In these cases, surveillance for an increased number of cases over the expected number helps to identify an outbreak so that a response can be initiated to reduce the further spread of the disease.[27,28]

SUMMARY

Mass casualty traumatic events and natural disasters such as severe weather, earthquakes, chemical spills, and infectious organisms can adversely affect the health and well-being of a population, leading to large numbers of deaths or high incidence of morbidity. In each of these emergencies, rapid response can minimize the adverse effects; communication systems are critical to coordinate the response of EMS, law enforcement, and local health care facilities. PAs play an important role in educating patients regarding preparedness; they may train to respond to emergencies through various training programs and agencies; they may participate in policy making at the local, state, and national levels.

CLINICAL APPLICATIONS

1. What are the most likely disasters in your area?
2. Based on the most likely disaster in your area:
   a. What would you advise your patients to have in their emergency kits and plans?
   b. What would be your role in such an emergency?
   c. What are the most likely reportable conditions that could occur?
3. How can patient education about preparedness be incorporated into your patient visits?
4. What would you do if a disaster occurred in a state near you?
5. How would your practice or hospital cope with an influx of disaster refugees?

KEY POINTS

- "Get a Kit; Have a Plan; Be Informed."
- PAs should educate patients on personal and family emergency preparedness.
- PAs need to know their role in the local Incident Command System.
- PAs can be trained in disaster response.

References

1. Pearce, Laurence Dominique Renee. An Integrated Approach for Community Hazard, Impact, Risk and Vulnerability Analysis: HIRV. Doctoral Dissertation: University of British Columbia, 2000.
2. James J, Subbarao I, Lanier W. Improving the Art and Science of Disaster Medicine and Public Health Preparedness. Mayo Clinic Proceedings May 2008;83:559–562.
3. Guha-Sapir D, Vos F, Below R, Ponserre S. Annual Disaster Statistical Review 2010: The Numbers and Trends. Brussels: CRED; 2011.
4. Beaton R, Bridges E, Salazar MK, et al. Ecological Model of Disaster Management. AAOHN J 2008;56(11):471–478.
5. Ready. *http://www.ready.gov*; Accessed November 26, 2011
6. The Physician Assistant in Disaster Response. Core Guidelines. Executive Summary. *http://www.aapa.org/uploadedFiles/content/Common/Files/15-ThePAinDisasterResponse.pdf*; Accessed December 4, 2011.
7. Physician Assistants and Medical Response to Disasters and Emergencies. Amending State Laws. Issue Brief. *http://www.aapa.org/uploadedFiles/content/The_PA_Profession/Federal_and_State_Affairs/Resource_Items/SL_PAs_MedicalResponse_v4-052611-UPDATED.pdf*; Accessed December 3, 2011.
8. Lange J, Lange C, Cabaltica R. Primary care treatment of post-traumatic stress disorder. Am Fam Physician 2000;62:1035–1040.
9. National Commission on Children and Disasters. *http://www.ahrq.gov/prep/nccdreport/*; Accessed July 16, 2011.
10. Children and Disasters. *http://www.aap.org/disasters/index.cfm*; Accessed November 26, 2011.
11. CDC's Disaster Planning Goal. Protect Vulnerable Older Adults. *http://www.cdc.gov/aging/pdf/disaster_planning_goal.pdf*; Accessed November 26, 2011.
12. Carolina Geriatric Education Center Disaster Preparedness Workgroup. Disaster and Emergency Preparedness. *http://www.med.unc.edu/aging/cgec/documents/Workgroups/DP%20OV.pdf*; Accessed July 16, 2011.
13. Incident Command Center. *http://www.fema.gov/emergency/nims/IncidentCommandSystem.shtm*; Accessed November 26, 2011.
14. CDC website. *http://www.cdc.gov/mmwr/preview/mmwrhtml/mm5403a2.htm*.
15. CDC website. *http://www.bt.cdc.gov/chemical/*; Accessed November 26, 2011.
16. CDC website. *http://www.bt.cdc.gov/radiation/*; Accessed November 26, 2011.
17. Shariat S, Mallonee S, Stidham S. Oklahoma City Bombing Injuries. *http://www.ok.gov/health/documents/OKC_Bombing.pdf*; Accessed December 3, 2011.
18. Mallonee S, Shariat S, Stennies G, et al. Physical injuries and fatalities resulting from the Oklahoma City bombing. JAMA 1996;276(5):382–387.
19. Shariat S, Mallonee S, Kruger E, et al. A prospective study of long-term health outcomes among Oklahoma City bombing survivors. J Okla State Med Assoc 1999;92(4):178–186.
20. Maningas PA, Robison M, Mallonee S. The EMS response to the Oklahoma City bombing. Prehospital Disaster Med 1997;12(2):80–85.
21. Centers for Disease Control and Prevention (CDC). Heat-related mortality—Chicago, July 1995. MMWR Morb Mortal Wkly Rep 1995;44:577–579.
22. *http://www.cdc.gov/mmwr/preview/mmwrhtml/00038443.htm*; Accessed November 26, 2011.
23. U.S. Department of Health and Human Services. Natural disasters. *http://www.phe.gov/emergency/naturaldisasters/Pages/default.aspx*; Accessed December 30, 2011.
24. Surveillance for Illness and Injury after Hurricane Katrina—New Orleans, September 8-25, 2005. MMWR 2005;54(40):1018–1021.
25. Outbreak of Gastrointestinal Illness Aboard Cruise Ship *MS Mercury*. San Diego: California; March 2006, *http://www.cdc.gov/nceh/vsp/surv/outbreak/2006/mercuryreport.pdf*. Accessed September18, 2012.
26. State-specific prevalence of obesity among adults—United States, 2007. MMWR Morbidity and Mortality Weekly Report 2008;57(28):11. *http://www.cdc.gov/mmwr/PDF/wk/mm5728.pdf*, Accessed September 18, 2012.
27. Ongoing Multistate Outbreak of *Escherichia coli* serotype O157:H7. Infections Associated with Consumption of Fresh Spinach—United States, September 2006. *http://www.cdc.gov/mmwr/preview/mmwrhtml/mm55d926a1.htm*; Accessed September 18, 2012.
28. Mumps epidemic—Iowa 2006. MMWR 2006;55(13):366–368. *http://www.cdc.gov/mmwr/preview/mmwrhtml/mm5513a3.htm*. Accessed September 12, 2012.

CHAPTER 53

Physician Assistants and Supervision

William C. Kohlhepp • Anthony Brenneman • Stephane VanderMeulen

CHAPTER CONTENTS

One of the defining features of the physician assistant (PA) profession is the relationship between PAs and physicians. When physicians created the PA profession, they envisioned PAs practicing medicine with physician delegation and supervision. Throughout the profession's more than 40-year history, PAs have consistently embraced the concept of the physician-directed team. In its Scope of Practice Issue Brief, the American Academy of Physician Assistants (AAPA) states: "This is unique; no other health profession sees itself as entirely complementary to the care provided by physicians."[1] The reason PAs believe that the physician-PA team relationship is fundamental is that the framework of practice is designed to ensure the delivery of high-quality health care.

The key features of this unique relationship were recognized by the PEW Health Professions Commission in its 1998 report on the PA profession when it pointed to frequent consultation, referral, and review of PA practice by the supervising physician. The report concluded, "The characteristics of this relationship are also considered to be the elements of professional relationships in any well-designed health system."[2]

The dimensions of the clinical relationship between PAs and physicians are multifaceted and variable given the setting (solo practice vs. hospital, group vs. solo practice, rural vs. urban, teaching hospital vs. nursing home); the practice (family practice vs. specialty, subspecialty vs. Internal Medicine, hospitalist vs. emergency medicine); and employer (solo practitioner vs. health maintenance organization, free clinic vs. boutique clinic, preferred provider organization vs. Medicaid). Each of these settings provides its own unique sets of challenges and opportunities. When practitioners, health care systems, and employers are aware of the unique state rules and regulations governing PAs and communication is open on both sides (employer/employee, partner/supervisor, etc.), then the physician-PA relationship can flourish, leading to high levels of satisfaction, high-quality health care, and excellent patient outcomes. In addition to the clinical relationship that exists between PAs and physicians, it is important to realize that their association also exists on other levels, particularly the employment relationship and their relationship as colleagues. Successful team practice depends on all those involved having a clear understanding of what their responsibilities will include. This has been further refined in an AAPA issue brief, "Supervision of Physician Assistants: Access and Excellence in Patient Care," as well as in AAPA's "Model State Legislation for Physician Assistants." For the physician, it is an understanding that he or she is to maintain an active license to practice medicine, accept responsibility for the care delivered by the PA, and maintain a delegation agreement with the PA to be supervised that is fluid and should be modified as changes occur. For the PA, it is working within areas delegated by the physician, establishing and maintaining clear lines of accountability, and "maintaining the reciprocal responsibilities of providing supervision and seeking consultation when needed."[3,4] Physician-PA team practice can most effectively operate if each team member appropriately allocates his or her time and talents. "Ideally, physicians are not involved in care best provided by PAs and, similarly, PAs do not undertake tasks best provided by physicians."[3]

HISTORICAL PERSPECTIVE

The physician-PA relationship has evolved since the inception of the PA profession. The team-based model of care that exists today differs from the original concept envisioned by Eugene Stead, M.D., of Duke University, who is generally credited with founding the PA profession. In an early monograph describing his vision for the PA's role, Dr. Stead intended for PAs to be trained in laboratories and clinics to perform an array of procedures, diagnostic tests, and medical therapies. Noting that the physician would direct the activities and would be legally responsible for all acts of the PA, it was thought that PAs would provide medical care in clinics, hospital settings, patient homes, and in outlying communities. Dr. Stead also discussed administrative duties for which PAs would be responsible, including the organization of "medical care units," managing all aspects and elements of patient care, ranging from technicians and nursing staff to housekeeping and custodial personnel.[5] Although PAs would be trained to recognize certain medical conditions such as heart failure and shock, Stead posed that PAs would not be involved in the clinical diagnosis, decision-making, and treatment of medical problems.[5]

The scope of PA practice has evolved since Stead's early vision to include a global approach to medical care, spanning all aspects of patient management. The concept of physician supervision, however, has remained integral to the PA profession. Though he may not have anticipated these changes, Stead made this prescient prediction of the value of PAs to physician practice: "They will be capable of extending the arms and the brains of the physician so that he can care for more people."[6] This statement remains true today.

SHARED KNOWLEDGE BASE

The relationship between physicians and PAs begins at the training level. PA training is modeled after medical school curriculum; thus, PAs and physicians possess a shared knowledge base.[7] Shared educational elements include foundational knowledge of the basic sciences and medicine, patient interviewing and interpersonal communication skills, physical examination skills, and critical problem-solving.

The foundation of the physician-PA relationship is established during PA education, which is based on the medical model. Many PA programs are located within medical schools, academic health centers, and military medical facilities or are associated with hospitals. It is common for PA students to share classes, faculty, and clinical training sites with medical students. Some programs housed within medical schools have fully integrated the PA curriculum into the medical school's curriculum. Having both been trained in the medical model, physicians and PAs develop a similarity in medical reasoning that eventually leads them to use a consistent approach to patient care in the clinical workplace; "PAs think like doctors."[7-10]

Training side by side builds camaraderie and allows PAs and physicians to understand one another's competence, knowledge, and skill levels. This leads to mutual trust and respect and creates the foundation of the physician-PA relationship.

DEPENDENT PRACTICE VERSUS INTERDEPENDENT PRACTICE

As the profession has matured and health care needs have evolved, so too has the way in which physicians and PAs have formulated practice styles and plans. What once was clearly a dependent practice, relying on one sole practitioner to supervise a single physician assistant, thereby limiting scope of practice, has evolved to an interdependent practice, where the PA and physician rely on each other to provide high-quality health care to a wide range of patients in all settings.

The interdependent practice of physicians and PAs over time has shown itself to be a cost-effective, dynamic, and medically sound approach to health care.[10] This interdependent practice assures the patient of a high-level, quality health care experience, in the style of the supervising physician, while helping to maintain continuity in the system. The physician benefits by being in the best position to determine that care is provided at the standard the physician seeks to provide, as well as being freed up to see the most complex and critical problems.[11] As Kimball and Rothwell have noted, regardless of the structure of their practice, if a PA determines that a patient's condition is beyond their expertise, the PA will expedite referral to the supervising physician or another specialist.[12] The Institute of Medicine in its landmark report *Crossing the Quality Chasm* discussed the importance of "communication among members of a team, using all the expertise and knowledge of team members and, where appropriate, sensibly extending roles to meet patient needs." This approach clearly reflects the physician-PA team and all its attributes.[13] This reflects all the interdependent and interconnected roles that the PA-physician team strives to achieve. Through this interdependent role, there is assurance that the PA will receive the appropriate back-up when needed. This interdependence reassures the patient that his or her care is continuous, monitored, and of high quality. It also reassures the physician that care will be provided at the physician standard of care.

COMMUNICATION, COORDINATION, AND CONTINUITY OF CARE

Communication is vital to a successful interdependent practice. It also requires advanced interpersonal skills and the ability to coordinate care between multiple providers and systems. Interdependent practice can improve patient care, outcomes, and satisfaction for patients and providers. Interpersonal skills, which include all the hallmarks of professionalism (see Chapter 34), form the foundation of a developing working relationship with the supervising physician and lead toward fully developed and integrated/interdependent practice.

Without clear lines of communication, the system quickly falls apart, leading to mistakes, misunderstandings, and at its worst, harm to the patient. Initially, it is important to develop lines of communication that will benefit the physician, PA, and patient. This can be done through the development of practice plans, physician delegation of workloads as defined, and regular meetings to discuss current working arrangements. This fluid and ever-evolving approach allows for expansion of duties, reassignment of resources, and clearer defined working roles and relationships leading to expanded patient services.

In the joint policy statement from the American Academy of Family Physicians (AAFP) and AAPA, the associations recognize the need for a shared commitment to achieving positive working relationships. This occurs by first understanding each member's roles and then maintaining and enhancing the relationship by effective communication.[14] This is nowhere more obvious than when the physician and PA are located at different sites. Particularly in this situation the use of technology becomes extremely helpful to support and facilitate communication and the practice of medicine.[14] With the movement toward electronic medical records, communication and delegation of practice will expand with easier access to patient records, as well as improvement in the continuity of care within the practice and throughout the health care system.

Continuity of care has been defined as the "process by which the patient and the physician are cooperatively involved in ongoing health care management toward the goal of high-quality, cost-effective medical care."[15] The AAFP in its joint policy statement says that this continuity is facilitated by the physician-led team.[14]

With its focus on communication, coordination of medical care, and the provision of that care in a continuous model, the physician-PA relationship benefits the patient and helps expand health care and its limited resources. These same characteristics are hallmarks of an evolving model of care—the patient-centered medical home. Through interdependent practice, PAs can help to ensure comprehensive care, providing continuity and coordination of care, while working with their physician colleagues and other health care members.

DELEGATED SCOPE OF PRACTICE

As medical practice has evolved over the years, tremendous change has occurred in the specific tasks to be accomplished by medical professionals, including PAs. Despite such a changing scope of practice, the PA profession has been unwavering in its commitment to a delegated scope of practice. The delegation of responsibilities by the supervising physician determines the PA's scope of practice.[10] Although scope of practice is a key section of the law and regulations in each state, generally the state delegates to supervising physicians the authority to determine the scope of practice for PAs.[16] This approach was reaffirmed recently by the Federation of State Medical Boards (FSMB), which stated: "Supervising physicians should be legally responsible for the delegation of medical tasks, the performance and the acts of omissions of the physician assistant."[17] Scope of practice may also be further limited by policies established by hospitals and other health care facilities.

Because the role of the PA in a practice is highly individualized, physicians and PAs who are working together are in the best position to define the PA's scope of practice. They can evaluate the many factors that go into that PA's role, including the type of practice, setting, acuity of the patients, physician's needs and preferences, and PA's training and experience.[12]

Evaluating the knowledge, skills, and abilities of the PA is a key step in scope of practice delegation. While supervising the PA, the physician can observe the PA's performance and can make sure the PA possesses the requisite clinical knowledge and accomplishes tasks and procedures in a highly competent manner. This was reaffirmed in the policy statement jointly written by the AAFP and the AAPA, which stated: "The physician evaluates the PA's competency and performance, and together they develop a team approach based on both the PA's and physician's clinical skills and patient needs."[14] In its monograph on the physician-PA relationship written with the AAPA, the American College of Physicians (ACP) stated: "The physician has the ability to observe the PA's competency and performance and plan for PA utilization based on the PA's abilities, the physician's delegatory style, and the needs of the patients seen in the practice."[18]

Another important consideration is the performance of tasks by the PA that may not be within the scope of practice of the supervising physician. In recent years, a number of states have adopted the language suggested by the AAPA in its Model Legislation: "A physician assistant may perform a task not within the scope of practice of the supervising physician as long as the supervising physician has adequate training, oversight skills, and supervisory and referral arrangements to ensure competent provision of the service by the PA."[4]

It must also be recognized that the scope of practice of the PA is not static but evolves over time. Supervising physicians play a key role in the development of PAs by mentoring them in the clinical setting. This effort, combined with that learned from formal continuing medical education programs, allows PAs to gain the advanced or specialized knowledge needed for their scope of practice to grow and change and to keep up with advances in the medical profession.[1]

Although the attention is often focused on its legal aspects, scope of practice is also a key expression of the physician-PA relationship. How much and what is delegated in the scope of practice is a measure of the level of trust and confidence placed in the PA by the supervising physician.[10] Scope of practice decisions also affect the effectiveness of the physician-PA team. The AAFP-AAPA joint policy statement notes: "The most effective physician-PA team practices provide optimal patient care by designing practice models where the skills and abilities of each team member are used most efficiently."[14]

Scope of practice is also central to optimal patient care. PAs believe that patients are best served when the physician-PA team treats patients in a consistent practice style and the socialization of PAs facilitates their adoption of the individual practice patterns of supervising physicians.[10] It is most important when discussing scope of practice to realize that patients seen by the PA are evaluated and cared for with a level of skill and competency similar to the manner in which a physician would treat a similarly situated patient.[1]

AUTONOMOUS MEDICAL DECISION-MAKING

Autonomous decision-making has always been an issue for clinical providers other than physicians. In strict definition, autonomy is having the right or power to self-govern or to carry on without outside control.[19] Although this strictly defines autonomy, it fails to recognize the unique team-based approach that the physician and PA maintain. In this model, autonomy is delegated by the supervising physician, allowing the PA to practice medicine as trained, able to make health care decisions within the scope of practice delegated by the physician, without need for input on these decisions unless the PA determines that the patient will be best served by physician input.

In the AAFP-AAPA joint policy statement, they use the concept of "delegated autonomy" and compare the relationship of the physician-PA practice to that of attending and resident physicians. They outline the key components of this delegated autonomy that should include clear lines of accountability, as well as reciprocal responsibilities of seeking and providing supervision and consultation.[14]

Chumbler and colleagues[20] defined autonomy of practice for PAs as "the extent to which PAs can determine independently the range of tasks they will perform." The authors further defined the concept of autonomy of practice as having two components: clinical decision-making and prescriptive authority. What was noted was that as the profession has matured, so too has the level of autonomy within delegated roles of the PA. As White and Davis[10] noted, there has been a trend toward more physician-determined scope of practice, as delegated activities have increased, instead of trying to list in state and federal law all activities performed by a PA. This allows for the original premise of the physician-PA team–based practice to function as originally designed with "delegated autonomy" determined by the physician's comfort and the PA's demonstrated competence.[10] This trend may be due to physicians being trained alongside of PAs, understanding the PA role better, and/or the expansion of state and federal laws, as well as the movement of PAs into areas of medicine outside of the traditional primary care scope of training. It is anticipated that these roles will continue to evolve over time as practice plans and laws evolve and the profession continues to mature. This has been noted and born out in monograph statements from the AAPA,[3] AAFP,[14] and ACP,[18] as well as in works by White and Davis[10] and Chumbler, Weier, and Geller.[20]

AGENCY RELATIONSHIP

The AAPA's Model Legislation points to another key descriptor for the legal relationship between the supervising physician and the PA, noting: "Physician assistants shall be considered the agents of their supervising physicians in the performance of all practice-related activities."[4] Agency is a fundamental legal concept that is relevant to those situations when the PA acts on behalf of the supervising physician. Agency has been described as the "fiduciary relation which manifests from the consent by one person to another that the other shall act on his behalf and subject to his control, and consent by the other so to act."[21]

Three factors must be present for an agency relationship to exist between two parties, such as between the supervising physician and the PA. The supervising physician consents to the relationship, the supervising physician accrues some degree of benefits from the acts of the PA, and the supervising physician has some degree of control of, or right to control, the PA.[22] The "assent, benefit, and control test" can be applied even in those situations where assent can be implied in the absence of express consent by the supervising physician (such as when the supervising physician is hired by the hospital or practice and supervising the PA is one of the assigned duties).[21]

Another parallel legal concept applicable to the supervising physician-PA relationship is that of the master-servant relationship or *respondeat superior* (translated from Latin as "let the master speak"). "If the principal (i.e., supervising physician) has the necessary control of or right to control the physical conduct of the agent (i.e., PA), then our principal is called master, and the agent who is subject to such control is called the servant."[21]

Because they have no independent authority to act but rather gain the basis for action from the physician's authority, PAs must be considered as "agents of the physicians rather than independent practitioners."[23] The question of to whom the liability runs is central to agency analysis. Thus, once an agency relationship is established, both the physician and PA are liable for the acts of the PA.

Establishing the responsibility of the supervising physician for the actions of the PA was a key factor in recognizing that the PA possessed the authority to establish valid patient care orders in the hospital setting. In a key article on the topic, Bissonette recounted several key attorney general opinions that pointed to the agency relationship in regards to patient orders. "The Attorney General in Maryland concluded, 'it must be presumed that a properly credentialed and supervised PA issues orders with the authority delegated to him/her by a licensed physician.' The Michigan Attorney General noted that physician delegation to the PA confers authority to the agent (PA) to do things that otherwise the physician would have to do."[24] A key court decision also relied on this concept to establish PA authority for order writing. The Supreme Court of the State of Washington held that it was the intent of the legislature to establish PAs as agents of their supervising physicians, so every order given by a PA is considered as coming from the supervising physician.[16, 23]

SUPERVISION

Physician supervision is a fundamental principle that guides the model of team-based patient care and PA practice. The American Academy of Physician Assistants defines supervision as "overseeing the activities of and accepting responsibility for the medical services rendered by the PA."[4] The ultimate goal of supervision is to ensure the health, welfare, and safety of the patient. According to AAPA's Guidelines for State Regulations of PAs, "the guiding principles of supervision must be that it (1) protects the public health and safety and (2) preserves the PA's access to physician consultation when indicated."[25]

To underline the importance of the supervisory concept, a statement regarding supervision is included in the AAPA Policy Manual. The PA profession considers it to be so essential to PA practice that supervision is included in the definition of PAs.[3] It states: "Physician assistants are health professionals licensed, or in case of those employed by the federal government, credentialed, to practice medicine with physician supervision. Within the physician-PA relationship, physician assistants exercise autonomy in medical decision making and provide a broad range of diagnostic and therapeutic services."[26]

A central theme of the supervisory relationship between physicians and PAs is the recognition that the physician is the most comprehensively trained member of the team and therefore holds terminal responsibility for ensuring that all members of the team adhere to accepted standards of care. He or she assumes legal liability and professional responsibility for all medical actions of the PA.

Although the physician is ultimately responsible for the acts of the PA, the responsibility to ensure that PAs practice in accordance within ethical, legal, and medical standards is shared and reciprocal. It is the responsibility of the PA to seek advice and consultation when indicated. PAs are often credited with the strength of "knowing their limits" and understanding when physician input should be solicited. It is incumbent on physician-PA teams to clearly delineate the role and tasks for which the PA is authorized to perform. These are the key factors in "delegated autonomy."

The synergic nature of this compact is beneficial for physicians, PAs, and patients. It allows physicians to expand the capacity of their practice, assured that patients will be cared for in accordance with their own style and preferences. It frees the physician to focus on patients with more complex medical problems. For PAs, this arrangement ensures that a constant resource exists to provide guidance and input when difficult or complicated medical problems arise. The physician is always available to assume care of the patient, if necessary. Patients can be assured that the style of practice and standard of care they receive is comparable, whether they are being cared for by the physician or the PA, and that physician involvement in their care is available at all times.[11]

PAs are authorized to practice medicine in all 50 states, the District of Columbia, and the majority of U.S. territories. All state laws mandate physician supervision as a part of PA practice; however, the definition and degree of supervision vary widely. Ideally, a minimum level of standardization would exist across all states and jurisdictions, but owing to the dramatic differences in state regulations and medical practice acts, inequities are inevitable. AAPA has drafted model legislation language in order to assist state constituent chapters and legislative committees to revise and update state laws.

"It is the obligation of each team of physician(s) and physician assistant(s) to ensure that the physician assistant's scope of practice is identified; that delegation of medical tasks is appropriate to the physician assistant's level of competence; that the relationship of, and access to, the supervising physician is defined; and that a process for evaluation of the physician assistant's performance is established."[4]

Types of Supervision

Supervision can be divided into three general categories: prospective, concurrent, and retrospective. Although perhaps not using these terms, each state's supervision laws contain elements of one or more category.

Prospective Supervision

Prospective supervision refers to agreements, both formal and informal, made between the physician and PA at the time of employment that delineate the duties and responsibilities of both parties. These agreements are based on the anticipated scope of PA practice and assume the likely or expected scenarios and patient population that will be managed by the PA. Formal agreements are required in many states; however, in all situations an informal discussion about both parties' expectations should occur early in the PA's employment.

Many states require written agreements, known as *delegation agreements* or *practice agreements*. In general, these guidelines delineate the type of patient visits and procedures the PA is authorized by the physician to perform. The duties should generally fall within the physician's own scope of practice and be appropriate to the PA's level of training and competence. The agreement provides for a clear understanding by all parties about what the physician's supervisory role and the delegated duties of the PA will entail. Some states require formal approval of the agreement by the state medical board or licensing agency. The agreements are signed by all parties, and regular maintenance and updating are required. States usually require that formal agreements be kept on file at the state licensing agency, the practice, and/or any remote sites in which the PA practices. Ideally, the practice agreement should be specific enough to eliminate any ambiguity about each party's responsibilities but flexible enough to allow the physician and PA to design a plan that maximizes the effectiveness of the team and allows both members to practice to the fullest extent of their qualifications.

AAPA has developed model legislation on which many states' supervisory laws and regulations are based. The model language addresses the need for written agreements between physicians and PAs.

"A physician wishing to supervise a physician assistant must maintain a written delegation agreement with the physician assistant. The delegation agreement must state that the physician will exercise supervision over the physician assistant in accordance with this act and any rules adopted by the board and will retain professional and legal responsibility for the care rendered by the physician assistant. The delegation agreement must be signed by the physician and the physician assistant and updated annually. The delegation agreement must be kept on file at the practice site and made available to the board upon request."[4]

Another form of prospective supervision involves protocols. The term *protocol* can be confusing because it is sometimes used to refer to delegation or practice agreements. True protocols are detailed clinical protocols that prescribe specific clinical courses of action in the treatment of disease. Some states require the use of protocols to guide PA practice. The use of protocols to guide PA practice is unwarranted and is discouraged by the AAPA.[27] Protocols by their nature are rigid and rapidly outdated. Extensive clinical protocols neither enhance the clinical judgment exercised by PAs nor improve the diagnosis and treatment of disease. Requirement of protocols may actually hinder care because it decreases the ability to use clinical judgment and individualize treatment for a specific patient.[27] The use of protocols is too prescriptive and does not allow for the dynamic, patient-specific clinical decision-making that is often necessary in today's challenging and constantly changing health care environment.

Concurrent Supervision

Concurrent supervision is a term that describes the oversight and availability of the physician, which occurs on an ongoing, daily basis. Medicare's description of the three levels of physician supervision for diagnostic tests provides a reasonable framework for considering the availability of the supervising physician to the PA envisioned.[28]

General supervision means that the physician must be available to the PA at all times. This does not necessarily suggest that he or she must be physically present but should be available by either electronic or telephonic means. All states require general supervision, but wide variability exists regarding the geographic or time limits and the means by which the physician is available. For example, one state may require that the physician stay within 10 miles of the practice site, whereas another might require that the physician be able to reach the clinic within 15 minutes. Some states require telephone contact, whereas others may allow text messaging or e-mail contact.

Direct supervision means that the physician must be physically present in the building. Requirements for direct supervision also vary widely. Some states require the physician to be present at all times, and others require direct oversight for either a percentage of the time that the PA practices or a specific amount of time, such as one day per week. Direct supervision requirements may differ if the PA practices at a geographically remote or satellite clinic rather than the "home" clinic and can vary depending on the PA's level of experience, skill, or competence. Occasionally, a limited probationary period of more strict oversight is required.

Personal supervision is the most restrictive form of concurrent supervision, requiring the physician to be present in the room while the PA provides care. Because of the delegatory nature of the physician-PA team, this type of supervision is rarely necessary or required. Occasionally, new graduates are required to be personally supervised for a finite period of time upon hiring. Some states require physician presence in the room when PAs perform surgical or other procedures and during major surgical procedures.

Retrospective Supervision

Retrospective supervision is the process of evaluating the performance, clinical activities, and the quality of care provided by the PA. The evaluation may take place either in person, electronically or telephonically. It involves the periodic review of patient charts, prescriptions, and orders written by the PA and often includes case discussions. The timing, frequency, and magnitude of review are dictated by the state. This can include all charts, a percentage of charts, a representative sample, or certain predetermined types of patient visits. Some states require physicians to cosign charts, orders, and prescriptions, and others require that the physician sees the patient periodically (e.g., every third visit). Retrospective supervision is an integral part of the physician-PA relationship because it provides a mechanism for feedback, quality assurance, and a guarantee that standards of care are being met.

FLEXIBILITY IN SUPERVISION

Although the PA profession's commitment to working in team practice with physician supervision is unwavering, there is an increasing recognition that the manner in which supervision occurs needs to keep up with the changing practice of medicine. Today health care delivery requires a level of efficiency and effectiveness not seen previously. When considering these changes, the AAFP in its statement on the physician-PA team noted: "The most effective teams are defined by physicians at the practice level to maximize the skills of the providers and meet patient needs."[14] In its monograph, ACP expanded on that theme, stating: "Flexibility in federal and state regulation [is encouraged] so that each medical practice determines appropriate clinical roles within the medical team, physician-to-PA ratios, and supervision processes, enabling each clinician to work to the fullest extent of his or her license and expertise."[18]

It is thus not surprising that the AAPA in its Issue Brief entitled *Six Key Elements of a Modern Physician Assistant Practice* focuses four of those six elements on achieving adaptability in supervision, as well as specific change in two key areas: removing restriction on the ratios of PAs to supervising physicians and ending blanket requirements for chart cosignature.[29] There is no argument that state laws should require supervision and define it. When states use an approach that allows for customization of the health care team, the physician(s)-PA(s) teams can match supervision to the specific needs of the practice.[3]

As far back as the late 1990s, the American Medical Association's Council on Medical Services pointed to the adverse impact on patient care that occurs when ratios are implemented. The Council said: "Supervising physicians are the most knowledgeable of their own supervisory abilities and practice style, as well as the training and experience of [PAs] in their practice. . . . Specified ratios of supervisory physicians to [PAs] might restrict appropriate provision of care and could reduce access to care."[30] In its *Six Key Elements*, the AAPA states: "The appropriate number of PAs that one physician may supervise should depend on several factors that are unique to each individual situation, including: the training and experience of the PA(s) being supervised, the nature of the practice, the complexity of the patient population and the physician's supervisory approach."[29]

Although preserving supervision and oversight is critical, requiring supervising physicians to cosign every PA-written order or chart removes the doctors' discretion to exercise supervision in the way that works best for their practices. Such cosignature requirements can place unnecessary burden on the supervising physician, which makes less efficient the care delivered by the team. Thus, physician cosignature should only be required when it is deemed to be necessary by the supervising physician, the PA, or the facility. The AAPA believes that establishing supervision requirements like ratios and cosignature "should be based on the experience of the PA, the complexity of the patient populations, and additional methods of oversight that are already taking place in the practice."[30]

Earlier, arguments were outlined for relying on the supervising physician to determine scope of practice at the practice level. AAPA's *Six Key Elements* reinforce this practice, stating: "The supervising physician is in the best position to evaluate the PA's abilities and to delegate procedures and services that are both appropriate to the PA and the nature of the practice. Supervising physician and PA jointly establish a written agreement outlining the PA's scope of practice."[29]

As the nation moves to provide services to the millions of uninsured Americans, the health care system will need to rely more heavily on primary care clinicians, such as PAs. One model for reforming primary care can be seen in the patient-centered medical home. Such a model depends on primary care providers who function with great skill and at high levels of efficiency to ensure the needed continuity, comprehensiveness, and coordination of care. In its monograph, the AAFP argued that PAs are well-suited to the patient-centered medical home.[14] Adaptability of supervision requirements will allow PAs to be successful at delivering needed patient care within that model.

The FSMB agrees that customization of the physician-PA relationship is key to the ability of the team to meet changing needs. The FSMB states in the document *Essentials of the Modern Medical and Osteopathic Practice Act:* "A physician assistant should be permitted to provide those medical services delegated to them by the supervising physician that are within their training and experience, form a usual component of the supervising physician's scope of practice, and are provided pursuant to the supervising physician's instruction."[17]

PRACTICE OWNERSHIP

The patient-centered medical home is but one of many changes in health care delivery that have occurred since the founding of the PA profession. Initially it was assumed that the supervising physician-PA model would involve a designated PA working beside a single physician in a primary care setting. As the use of PAs as members of the health care team has expanded over the past 40-plus years, the model for PA utilization has changed. Today many PAs work for hospitals, group practices, or other business entities. Often, supervising physicians have separate business relationships with the employers of PAs, rather than serving themselves as direct employers of PAs.

In an effort to meet patient needs in certain situations, PAs have assumed full or part ownership or become shareholders of a professional corporation. A key requirement to become a shareholder in a professional corporation is for one to be licensed or otherwise legally authorized to provide the services the corporation offers. Thus, when physicians are not willing or able to step forward to maintain the professional corporations under which the practice is established, the PA can step in because he or she possesses that legal authorization. PA involvement in the business of practice ownership has occurred through outright PA ownership of practices through purchase, establishing corporations to own practices, and creating practice arrangements.[31] Even Medicare policies and most state laws now recognize that employment and supervision are separate and unrelated aspects of medical practice. In April 2002, the Medicare program adopted rules that allow PAs to have an ownership interest in an approved Medicare corporation that is eligible to bill the Medicare program.[32]

Regardless of the ownership or shareholder relationships that involved PAs, PAs remain fully committed to having the physician serve as the clinical leader of the physician-PA team with that physician retaining professional authority over medical decisions made by PAs.[31]

SUMMARY

Although PA practice has evolved over time, the tenet of PAs practicing with physician supervision remains steady. This interdependent practice assures the patient of a high-level, quality health care experience, in the style of the supervising physician, while helping to maintain continuity in the system. Variables affecting this relationship include type of practice, practice setting, individual state laws, clearly delineated roles, and expectations. Many of these variables are easily dealt with through maintaining open lines of communication, good interpersonal skills, and ability to coordinate care between multiple providers and systems.

An ideal physician-PA relationship uses team-based concepts in order to maximize the efficiency and effectiveness of the team as a whole, with the ultimate goal of excellent patient outcomes. The role of PAs within the team should optimize the use of their training and skills and allow for appropriate autonomy to practice medicine to the highest extent of their abilities. Future legislation should preserve the physician-PA relationship while providing for the flexibility to create a team to provide excellence in promoting patient health and providing patient care on the basis of the needs of the population and the environment in which they practice.

CLINICAL APPLICATIONS

1. Interview a physician-PA team and ask them individually how they see the concept of supervision and how it has evolved over their time together.
2. Consider what you might do when your supervising physician believes you should manage your patient differently than you had planned. What recourse do you have?
3. Discuss in a small group how you might handle the situation in which your physician does not provide you with enough supervision. With too much supervision?

KEY POINTS

- PAs consistently embrace the concept of the physician-directed team and believe it is fundamental to high-quality patient care.
- Having both been trained in the medical model, PAs and physicians share a similarity of medical reasoning.
- Scope of practice for the PA is best determined by the supervising physician who evaluates both the PA's clinical skills and patient needs.
- PAs exercise "delegated autonomy" making medical decisions within the physician-delegated scope of practice.
- PAs act as the "agents" of the supervising physician, allowing them to act on behalf of the physician, particularly when generating orders for the delivery of care to hospitalized patients.
- Physician supervision ensures high-quality patient care by the PA and involves a framework that includes prospective, concurrent, and retrospective elements.
- The manner in which physician supervision is provided for PAs needs to keep up with the changing practice of medicine.

References

1. American Academy of Physician Assistants. PA Scope of Practice (website), *http://www.aapa.org/uploadedFiles/content/Common/Files/PI_PA_Scope_Practice_v4-052611-UPDATED.pdf*; Accessed February 12, 2012.
2. The PEW Health Care Commission. Charting a Course for the Twenty-First Century: Physician Assistants and Managed Care. San Francisco: University of California San Francisco Center for the Health Professions, 1998.
3. American Academy of Physician Assistants. Supervision of Physician Assistants: Access and Excellence in Patient Care (website), *http://www.aapa.org/uploadedFiles/content/Common/Files/SL_Supervision_PAs_v1-052611-UPDATED.pdf*; Accessed February 12, 2012.
4. American Academy of Physician Assistants. Model State Legislation for Physician Assistants (website), *http://www.aapa.org/uploadedFiles/content/The_PA_Profession/Federal_and_State_Affairs/Resource_Items/model%20law%209-09.pdf*; Accessed February 12, 2012.
5. Stead E. Physician Assistant History Center. Exhibits: Development of PA Program at Duke University Medical Center; 1964, July, *http://www.pahx.org/pdf/Item145.pdf*; Accessed February 12, 2012.
6. Stead E. Physician Assistant History Center. Exhibits: Development of PA Program at Duke University Medical Center; 1964, September, *http://www.pahx.org/pdf/Item143.pdf*; Accessed February 12, 2012.
7. American Academy of Physician Assistants. Physician-PA Team (website), *http://www.aapa.org/uploadedFiles/content/Common/Files/PI_PhysicianPATeam_v5%20-%20052711%20UPDATED.pdf*; Accessed October 28, 2011.
8. White GL, Egerton CP, Myers R, Holbert RD. Physician assistants and Mississippi. J Miss State Med Assoc 1994;35(12):353–357.
9. White GL. Physicians, PAs, and the facts. J Miss State Med Assoc 1997;38(12):460.
10. White GL, Davis AM. Physician assistants as partners in physician-directed care. South Med J 1999;92(10):956–960.
11. Kohlhepp W. Contemporary concepts of physician supervision. JAAPA 2003;16:48–51.
12. Kimball BA, Rothwell WS. Physician assistant practice in Minnesota providing care as part of a physician-directed team. Minn Med 2008;91(5):45–48.
13. Committee on Quality of Health Care in America, Institute of Medicine. Crossing the Quality Chasm: A New Health System for the 21st Century. Washington, DC: National Academies Press, 2001.
14. Rathfon E, Jones G. Family Physicians and Physician Assistants: Team-Based Family edicine. A Joint Policy Statement of the American Academy of Family Physicians and American Academy of Physician Assistants, February 2011.
15. American Academy of Family Physicians. (2010) Continuity of Care, Definition of, AAFP Policies, *http://www.aafp.org/online/en/home/policy/policies/c/continuityofcaredefinition.html*; Accessed February 12, 2012.
16. Younger PA. Physician Assistant Legal Handbook. Burlington, MA: Jones & Bartlett Learning, 1997.
17. Federation of State Medical Boards. Essentials of a Modern Medical and Osteopathic Practice Act (website), *http://www.fsmb.org/pdf/GRPOL_essentials.pdf*; Accessed February 12, 2012.
18. American College of Physicians. Internists and Physician Assistants: Team-Based Primary Care (website), *http://www.acponline.org/advocacy/where_we_stand/policy/internists_asst.pdf*; Accessed February 12, 2012.
19. Merriam-Webster Dictionary. *http://www.merriam-webster.com/dictionary/autonomous*; Accessed July 18, 2011.
20. Chumbler NR, Weier AW, Geller JM. Practice Autonomy Among Primary Care Physician Assistants: The Predictive Abilities of Selected Practice Attributes. J Allied Health 2001;30(1):2–10.
21. Wyse RC. A framework of analysis for the law of agency. Montana Law Rev 1979;40:31–58.
22. Harbert KR. Inpatient systems. In: Ballweg R, Sullivan EM, Brown D, Vetrosky D (eds). Physician Assistant: A Guide to Clinical Practice. 4th ed. Philadelphia: Saunders Elsevier, 2008.
23. Delman JL. The use and misuse of physician extenders. J Legal Med 2003;24:249–280.
24. Bissonette DJ. The derivation of authority for medical order writing by PAs. JAAPA 1991;4:358–361.
25. American Academy of Physician Assistants. Guidelines for State Regulation of Physician Assistants (website), *http://www.aapa.org/uploadedFiles/content/Common/Files/05-GuideforStateRegs.pdf*; Accessed February 12, 2012.
26. American Academy of Physician Assistants. AAPA 2011-2012 Policy Manual (website), *http://www.aapa.org/uploadedFiles/content/About_AAPA/PM-11-12-Final.pdf*; Accessed February 12, 2012.
27. American Academy of Physician Assistants. Physician Assistants and Protocols (website), *http://www.aapa.org/uploadedFiles/content/Common/Files/SL_PAsProtocols_123010_v2%20-%20052711%20UPDATED.pdf*; Accessed February 12, 2012.
28. Highmark Medicare Services. Medicare Reference Manual: Chapter 28—Physician Supervision of Diagnostic Tests (website), *https://www.highmarkmedicareservices.com/refman/chapter-28.html*; Accessed December 12, 2011.
29. American Academy of Physician Assistants. Six Key Elements of Modern Physician Assistant Practice (website), *http://www.aapa.org/uploadedFiles/content/Common/Files/SL_KeyElements_v3.pdf*; Accessed February 12, 2012.
30. American Academy of Physician Assistants. Ratio of Physician Assistants to Supervising Physicians (website), *http://www.aapa.org/uploadedFiles/content/Common/Files/SL_RatioPAsSupPhys_v7%20-%20052711%20UPDATED.pdf*; Accessed February 12, 2012.
31. American Academy of Physician Assistants. Physician Assistants and Practice Ownership (website), *http://www.aapa.org/uploadedFiles/content/Common/Files/SL_PractOwn_Mill_Rd_March2011.pdf*; Accessed February 12, 2012.
32. Powe ML. Financing and reimbursement. In: Ballweg R, Sullivan EM, Brown D, Vetrosky D (eds). Physician Assistant: A Guide to Clinical Practice. 4th ed. Philadelphia: Saunders Elsevier, 2008.

The resources for this chapter can be found at www.expertconsult.com.

APPENDIX

COMPETENCIES FOR THE PHYSICIAN ASSISTANT PROFESSION

PREAMBLE

In 2003, the National Commission on Certification of Physicians Assistants (NCCPA) initiated an effort to define PA competencies in response to similar efforts being conducted within other health care professions and growing demand for accountability and assessment in clinical practice. The following year, representatives from three other national PA organizations, each bringing a unique perspective and valuable insights, joined NCCPA in that effort. Those organizations were the Accreditation Review Commission for Education of the Physician Assistant (ARC-PA), the body that accredits PA educational programs; the Association of Physician Assistant Programs (APAP), the membership association for PA educators and program directors; and the American Academy of Physician Assistants (AAPA), the only national membership association representing all PAs.

The resultant document, *Competencies for the Physician Assistant Profession*, is a foundation from which each of those four organizations, other PA organizations, and individual PAs themselves can chart a course for advancing the competencies of the PA profession.

INTRODUCTION

The purpose of this document is to communicate to the PA profession and the public a set of competencies that all PAs regardless of specialty or setting are expected to acquire and maintain throughout their careers. This document serves as a map for the individual PA, the physician-PA team, and organizations that are committed to promoting the development and maintenance of these professional competencies among PAs.

The clinical role of PAs includes primary and specialty care in medical and surgical practice settings. Professional competencies* for PAs include the effective and appropriate application of medical knowledge, interpersonal and communication skills, patient care, professionalism, practice-based learning and improvement, systems-based practice, as well as an unwavering commitment to continual learning, professional growth, and the physician-PA team, for the benefit of patients and the larger community being served. These competencies are demonstrated within the scope of practice, whether medical or surgical, for each individual PA because that scope is defined by the supervising physician and appropriate to the practice setting.

The PA profession defines the specific knowledge, skills, and attitudes required and provides educational experiences as needed in order for PAs to acquire and demonstrate these competencies.

MEDICAL KNOWLEDGE

Medical knowledge includes an understanding of pathophysiology, patient presentation, differential diagnosis, patient management, surgical principles, health promotion, and disease prevention. PAs must demonstrate core knowledge about established and evolving biomedical and clinical sciences and the application of this knowledge to patient care in their area of practice. In addition, PAs are expected to demonstrate an investigatory and analytic thinking approach to clinical situations. PAs are expected to:

- Understand etiologies, risk factors, underlying pathologic process, and epidemiology for medical conditions

*In 1999, the Accreditation Council for Graduate Medical Education (ACGME) endorsed a list of general competencies for medical residents. NCCPA's Eligibility Committee, with substantial input from representatives of AAPA, APAP, and ARC-PA, has modified the ACGME's list for PA practice, drawing from several other resources, including the work of Drs. Epstein and Hundert; research conducted by AAPA's EVP/CEO, Dr. Steve Crane; and NCCPA's own examination content blueprint.

- Identify signs and symptoms of medical conditions
- Select and interpret appropriate diagnostic or laboratory studies
- Manage general medical and surgical conditions to include understanding the indications, contraindications, side effects, interactions, and adverse reactions of pharmacologic agents and other relevant treatment modalities
- Identify the appropriate site of care for presenting conditions, including identifying emergent cases and those requiring referral or admission
- Identify appropriate interventions for prevention of conditions
- Identify the appropriate methods to detect conditions in an asymptomatic individual
- Differentiate between the normal and the abnormal in anatomic, physiologic, laboratory findings, and other diagnostic data
- Appropriately use history and physical findings and diagnostic studies to formulate a differential diagnosis
- Provide appropriate care to patients with chronic conditions

INTERPERSONAL AND COMMUNICATION SKILLS

Interpersonal and communication skills encompass verbal, nonverbal, and written exchange of information. PAs must demonstrate interpersonal and communication skills that result in effective information exchange with patients, their patients' families, physicians, professional associates, and the health care system. PAs are expected to:

- Create and sustain a therapeutic and ethically sound relationship with patients
- Use effective listening, nonverbal, explanatory, questioning, and writing skills to elicit and provide information
- Appropriately adapt communication style and messages to the context of the individual patient interaction
- Work effectively with physicians and other health care professionals as a member or leader of a health care team or other professional group
- Apply an understanding of human behavior
- Demonstrate emotional resilience and stability, adaptability, flexibility, and tolerance of ambiguity and anxiety
- Accurately and adequately document and record information regarding the care process for medical, legal, quality, and financial purposes

PATIENT CARE

Patient care includes age-appropriate assessment, evaluation, and management. PAs must demonstrate patient-centered care that is effective, timely, efficient, and equitable for the treatment of health problems and the promotion of wellness. PAs are expected to:

- Work effectively with physicians and other health care professionals to provide patient-centered care
- Demonstrate caring and respectful behaviors when interacting with patients and their families
- Gather essential and accurate information about their patients
- Make informed decisions about diagnostic and therapeutic interventions on the basis of patient information and preferences, up-to-date scientific evidence, and clinical judgment
- Develop and carry out patient management plans
- Counsel and educate patients and their families
- Competently perform medical and surgical procedures considered essential in the area of practice
- Provide health care services and education aimed at preventing health problems or maintaining health

PROFESSIONALISM

Professionalism is the expression of positive values and ideals as care is delivered. Foremost, it involves prioritizing the interests of those being served above one's own. PAs must know their professional and personal limitations. Professionalism also requires that PAs practice without impairment from substance abuse, cognitive deficiency, or mental illness. PAs must demonstrate a high level of responsibility, ethical practice, sensitivity to a diverse patient population, and adherence to legal and regulatory requirements. PAs are expected to demonstrate:

- Understanding of legal and regulatory requirements, as well as the appropriate role of the PA
- Professional relationships with physician supervisors and other health care providers
- Respect, compassion, and integrity
- Responsiveness to the needs of patients and society
- Accountability to patients, society, and the profession
- Commitment to excellence and ongoing professional development

- Commitment to ethical principles pertaining to provision or withholding of clinical care, confidentiality of patient information, informed consent, and business practices
- Sensitivity and responsiveness to patients' culture, age, gender, and disabilities
- Self-reflection, critical curiosity, and initiative

PRACTICE-BASED LEARNING AND IMPROVEMENT

Practice-based learning and improvement includes the processes through which clinicians engage in critical analysis of their own practice experience, medical literature, and other information resources for the purpose of self-improvement. PAs must be able to assess, evaluate, and improve their patient care practices. PAs are expected to:

- Analyze practice experience and perform practice-based improvement activities using a systematic methodology in concert with other members of the health care delivery team
- Locate, appraise, and integrate evidence from scientific studies related to their patients' health problems
- Obtain and apply information about their own population of patients and the larger population from which their patients are drawn
- Apply knowledge of study designs and statistical methods to the appraisal of clinical studies and other information on diagnostic and therapeutic effectiveness
- Apply information technology to manage information, access on-line medical information, and support their own education
- Facilitate the learning of students and/or other health care professionals
- Recognize and appropriately address gender, cultural, cognitive, emotional, and other biases; gaps in medical knowledge; and physical limitations in themselves and others

SYSTEMS-BASED PRACTICE

Systems-based practice encompasses the societal, organizational, and economic environments in which health care is delivered. PAs must demonstrate an awareness of and responsiveness to the larger system of health care to provide patient care that is of optimal value. PAs should work to improve the larger health care system of which their practices are a part. PAs are expected to:

- Use information technology to support patient care decisions and patient education
- Effectively interact with different types of medical practice and delivery systems
- Understand the funding sources and payment systems that provide coverage for patient care
- Practice cost-effective health care and resource allocation that does not compromise quality of care
- Advocate for quality patient care and assist patients in dealing with system complexities
- Partner with supervising physicians, health care managers, and other health care providers to assess, coordinate, and improve the delivery of health care and patient outcomes
- Accept responsibility for promoting a safe environment for patient care and recognizing and correcting systems-based factors that negatively impact patient care
- Apply medical information and clinical data systems to provide more effective, efficient patient care
- Use the systems responsible for the appropriate payment of services

INDEX

Page numbers followed by *f* refer to figures; *t*, tables; *b*, boxes.

B

C

D

E

I

J

K

N

Q

R

S

T